Federal C
Drug Enf
U.S. Department of Justice
Schedules

SCHEDULE I: No accepted medical use in the United States and a high abuse potential. Examples include heroin, marijuana, LSD, peyote, mescaline, psilocybin, and methaqualone.

SCHEDULE II: High abuse potential with severe dependence liability, but currently accepted medical use. Examples include opium, morphine, codeine, fentanyl, hydromorphone, methadone, meperidine, oxycodone, oxymorphone, cocaine, amphetamine, methamphetamine, phenmetrazine, methylphenidate, phencyclidine, amobarbital, pentobarbital, and secobarbital.

SCHEDULE III: Lesser abuse potential with moderate dependence liability, but currently accepted medical use. Examples include compounds containing limited quantities of certain opiates and other sedative-hypnotic drugs. Examples include codeine and hydrocodone with aspirin or acetaminophen, barbiturates, glutethimide, methyprylon, nalorphine, benzphetamine, chlorphentermine, clortermine, phendimetrazine, and paregoric; suppository dosage form containing amobarbital, secobarbital, or pentobarbital. Anabolic steroids are also included here.

SCHEDULE IV: Low abuse potential. Examples include barbital, phenobarbital, mephobarbital, chloral hydrate, ethchlorvynol, ethinamate, meprobamate, paraldehyde, methohexital, fenfluramine, diethylpropion, phentermine, chlordiazepoxide, diazepam, oxazepam, clorazepate, flurazepam, clonazepam, prazepam, lorazepam, alprazolam, halazepam, temazepam, triazolam, propoxyphene, pentazocine, zaleplon, and zolpidem.

SCHEDULE V: Low abuse potential. These products contain limited quantities of certain opiate drugs generally for antitussive or antidiarrheal purposes. The over-the-counter cough medicines with codeine are classified schedule V.

FDA Pregnancy Categories

A: Adequate studies in pregnant women have not demonstrated a risk to the fetus in the first trimester of pregnancy, and there is no evidence of risk in later trimesters.

B: Animal studies have not demonstrated a risk to the fetus, but there are no adequate studies in pregnant women; **OR** animal studies have shown an adverse effect, but adequate studies in pregnant women have not demonstrated a risk to the fetus during the first trimester of pregnancy, and there is no evidence of risk in later trimesters.

C: Animal studies have shown an adverse effect on the fetus, but there are no adequate studies in humans; **OR** there are no animal reproduction studies and no adequate studies in humans.

D: There is evidence of human fetal risk, but the potential benefits from the use of the drug in pregnant women may be acceptable despite its potential risks.

X: Studies in animals or humans demonstrate fetal abnormalities or adverse reaction; reports indicate evidence of fetal risk. The risk of use in a pregnant woman clearly outweighs any possible benefit.

Mosby's

2007 Medical Drug Reference

Allan J. Ellsworth, Pharm.D., PA-C

Professor of Pharmacy and Family Medicine
University of Washington Schools of Pharmacy and Medicine
Seattle, Washington

Lynn M. Oliver, M.D.

Associate Professor of Family Medicine
University of Washington School of Medicine
Seattle, Washington

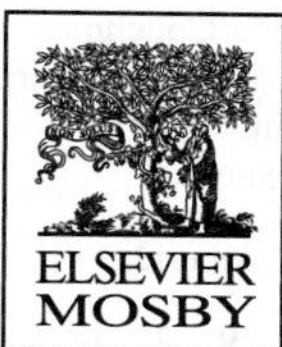

ELSEVIER
MOSBY

1600 John F. Kennedy Blvd.
Suite 1800
Philadelphia, PA 19103-2899

MOSBY'S 2007 MEDICAL DRUG REFERENCE ISBN 978-0-323-02223-1

NOTICE

Knowledge and best practice in this field are constantly changing. As new research and experience broaden our knowledge, changes in practice, treatment, and drug therapy may become necessary or appropriate. Readers are advised to check the most current information provided (i) on procedures featured or (ii) by the manufacturer of each product to be administered, to verify the recommended dose or formula, the method and duration of administration, and contraindications. It is the responsibility of the practitioner, relying on their own experience and knowledge of the patient, to make diagnoses, to determine dosages and the best treatment for each individual patient, and to take all appropriate safety precautions. To the fullest extent of the law, neither the Publisher nor the Editors assumes any liability for any injury and/or damage to persons or property arising out of or related to any use of the material contained in this book.

Some material was previously published.

ISBN: 978-0-323-02223-1

Senior Acquisitions Editor: Rolla Couchman
Publishing Services Manager: Melissa Lastarria
Senior Designer: Julia Dummitt
Multimedia Producer: Joseph Selby

Printed in the United States of America.

Last digit is the print number: 9 8 7 6 5 4 3 2 1

Instructions for Use

Mosby's Medical Drug Reference was conceived in the primary care environment in response to the demands of physicians and other healthcare providers who require an up-to-date, authoritative, comprehensive, portable drug prescribing reference for use at the point of care. This compact, easily accessible manual has been created in part from the renowned and objective drug database, *Mosby's Drug Consult,* which is updated continuously to provide timely drug information for accurate and efficient prescribing. As a standard reference, *Mosby's Drug Consult* is indispensable in its print and PDA formats; for those situations when the demands of patient care require a more portable drug prescribing guide, we proudly present *Mosby's 2007 Medical Drug Reference.*

Mosby's 2007 Medical Drug Reference is organized into several highly functional parts. The body of the book is an alphabetical listing, by generic name, of over 850 drugs in common clinical use, representing over 2800 products. An appendix of the book contains tables of comparative drug data and other information useful for choosing drug therapy. The comprehensive index provides rapid reference by listing all generic and trade names; index searches are further aided by the colored index paper. The inside front and back covers contain formulas for calculating drug dosages and useful conversion information. The comprehensive Therapeutic Index allows prescribers to locate drugs appropriate for a broad range of clinical indications.

Drug monographs in *Mosby's 2007 Medical Drug Reference* are organized uniformly as follows (when there is no information in a category applicable to a given drug, the category is deleted entirely):

Drug Name (generic)
Pronunciation (phonetic)
Trade Names
Chemical Class
Therapeutic Class
Clinical Pharmacology (including information about the mechanism of action and pharmacokinetics of the drug)
Indications and Dosages
Available Forms

Unlabelled Uses
Contraindications (if the only contraindication is hypersensitivity, this category has been deleted; hypersensitivity to the drug is always a contraindication)
Pregnancy and Lactation (see p. ix)
Side Effects (listed by frequency; anaphylaxis and hypersensitivity reactions are potentially possible for all drugs and have not been included routinely)
Serious Reactions Interactions, if applicable. The clinical significance of each drug interaction is derived from data presented in Hansten PD, Horn JR: Drug interactions analysis and management. Interactions are classified by potential severity as: ▲—Avoid combination, risk always outweighs benefit; ❷—Usually avoid combination, use combination only under special circumstances; or ▣—Minimize risk, take action as necessary to reduce risk of adverse outcome as a result of drug interaction. Interactions of lesser significance, either because they are minor or poorly documented, are not included. If no drug interactions are known, or if the interactions are of minimal risk, this category has been deleted.
Special Considerations (if applicable) such as patient education or monitoring.

Every possible effort has been made to ensure the accuracy and currency of the information contained within *Mosby's 2007 Medical Drug Reference*. However, drug information is constantly changing and is subject to interpretation. The authors, editors, or publishers cannot be responsible for information that has either changed or been erroneously published or for the consequences of such errors. Decisions regarding drug therapy for a specific patient must be based on the independent judgment of the clinician.

Allan J. Ellsworth
Lynn M. Oliver

ACKNOWLEDGMENTS

We are grateful for the support, stimulus, and suggestions of our colleagues in the Departments of Family Medicine, Medicine, and Pharmacy, University of Washington, Seattle, Washington. As usual, we also thank our families and friends for their continued support, patience, love, and understanding for time spent on *Mosby's 2007 Medical Drug Reference*.

Abbreviations

ABG arterial blood gas
ac before meals
ACE angiotensin-converting enzyme
ACTH adrenocorticotropic hormone
AD right ear
ADH antidiuretic hormone
aer aerosol
AIDS acquired immunodeficiency syndrome
ALT alanine aminotransferase, serum
ANA antinuclear antibody
aPTT activated partial thromboplastin time
ARB angiotensin receptor blocker
AS left ear
AST aspartate aminotransferase, serum
AT II angiotensin II
AU each ear
AUC area under curve
AV atrioventricular
bid twice a day
BP blood pressure
BUN blood urea nitrogen
c-AMP cyclic adenosine monophosphate
cap capsule
°C degrees Celsius (centigrade)
Ca calcium
CAD coronary artery disease
cath catheterize
cc cubic centimeter
CBC complete blood count
chew tab tablet, chewable
CHF congestive heart failure
Cl chloride
cm centimeter
CMV cytomegalovirus
CNS central nervous system
CO_2 carbon dioxide
COPD chronic obstructive pulmonary disease
CPAP continuous positive airway pressure
CPK creatine phosphokinase
CrCl creatinine clearance
cre cream
CRP c-reactive protein
Creat creatinine
CSF cerebrospinal fluid
CV cardiovascular
CVA cerebrovascular accident
CVP central venous pressure
CXR chest x-ray
D5W 5% dextrose in water
DIC disseminated intravascular coagulation
dL deciliter
D_LCO diffusing capacity of carbon monoxide
DMARDs disease-modifying antirheumatic drugs
DNA deoxyribonucleic acid
DUB dysfunctional uterine bleeding
ECG electrocardiogram
EDTA ethylenediaminetetraacetic acid
EEG electroencephalogram
EENT eye, ear, nose, throat
elix elixir
ESR erythrocyte sedimentation rate
ET via endotracheal tube
EXT REL extended release
°F degrees Fahrenheit
FEV_1 forced expiratory volume in 1 second
FSH follicle stimulating hormone
g gram
G6PD glucose-6-phosphate dehydrogenase
GGTP gamma glutamyl transpeptidase
GI gastrointestinal
gtt drop
GU genitourinary
H_2 histamine$_2$
Hct hematocrit

HCG human chorionic gonadotropin
HEME hematologic
Hgb hemoglobin
5-HIAA 5-hydroxyindoleacetic acid
HIV human immunodeficiency virus
H_2O water
HMG CoA 3-hydroxy-3-methylglutaryl coenzyme A
HPA hypothalamic-pituitary-adrenal
hr hour
hs at bedtime
HSV herpes simplex virus
IgG immunoglobulin G
IL-1 interleukin-1
IM intramuscular
in inch
INF infusion
INH inhalation
inj injection
INR international normalized ratio
IO intraosseous
IPPB intermittent positive pressure breathing
IU international units
IV intravenous
K potassium
kg kilogram
L liter
LA long acting
lb pound
LDH lactate dehydrogenase
LDL low density lipoprotein
LFTs liver function tests
LH luteinizing hormone
liq liquid
LMP last menstrual period
loz lozenge
lyphl lyophilized
m meter
m^2 square meter
MAOI monoamine oxidase inhibitor
mcg microgram
MDI metered dose inhaler
mEq milliequivalent
mg milligram
Mg magnesium
MI myocardial infarction
min minute
ml (mL) milliliter
mm millimeter
mmol millimole
mo month
MS musculoskeletal
Na sodium
neb nebulizer
NPO nothing by mouth
NS normal saline
NSAID nonsteroidal antiinflammatory drug
O_2 oxygen
OD right eye
oint ointment
OS left eye
OTC over the counter
OU each eye
oz ounce
$PaCO_2$ arterial partial pressure of carbon dioxide
PaO_2 arterial partial pressure of oxygen
pc after meals
PCWP pulmonary capillary wedge pressure
P_i inorganic phosphorus
po by mouth
PO_4 phosphate
pr per rectum
prn as needed
PT prothrombin time
PTH parathyroid hormone
PTT partial thromboplastin time
PVC premature ventricular contraction
q every
qAM every morning
qday every day
qh every hour
qid four times a day
qod every other day
qPM every night
q2h every 2 hours
q3h every 3 hours
q4h every 4 hours
q6h every 6 hours
q8h every 8 hours
q12h every 12 hours
RAIU radioactive iodine uptake
RBC red blood cell count
RESP respiratory
RNA ribonucleic acid
sc subcutaneous
sl sublingual
sol solution
SO_4 sulfate
ss one half
SSRI selective serotonin reuptake inhibitor
supp suppository

sus rel sustained release
susp suspension
sust sustained
syr syrup
T_3 triiodothyronine
T_4 thyroxine
tab tablet
TCA tricyclic antidepressant
tid three times a day
tinc tincture
top topical
trans transdermal
TSH thyroid stimulating hormone
TT thrombin time
U unit
UA urinalysis
URI upper respiratory infection
UTI urinary tract infection
UV ultraviolet
vag vaginal
VMA vanillylmandelic acid
vol volume
VS vital signs
WBC white blood cell count
wk week
-XL, -XR extended release preparations
yr year

Contents

abacavir sulfate

(a-ba-ka'-vir sul'-fate)

Rx: Ziagen

Combinations

Rx: with lamivudine (Epzicom); with zidovudine and lamivudine (Trizivir)

Chemical Class: Nucleoside analog

Therapeutic Class: Antiretroviral

CLINICAL PHARMACOLOGY

Mechanism of Action: An antiretroviral that inhibits the activity of HIV-1 reverse transcriptase by competing with the natural substrate deoxyguanosine-5'-triphosphate (dGTP) and by its incorporation into viral DNA. ***Therapeutic Effect:*** Inhibits viral DNA growth.

Pharmacokinetics

Rapidly and extensively absorbed after PO administration. Protein binding: 50%. Widely distributed, including to cerebrospinal fluid (CSF) and erythrocytes. Metabolized in the liver to inactive metabolites. Primarily excreted in urine. Unknown if removed by hemodialysis. ***Half-life:*** 1.5 hr.

INDICATIONS AND DOSAGES

HIV infection (in combination with other antiretrovirals)

PO

Adults. 300 mg twice a day or 600 mg once daily.

Children (3 mo-16 yr). 8 mg/kg twice a day. Maximum: 300 mg twice a day.

Dosage in hepatic impairment

Mild impairment: 200 mg twice a day.

Moderate to severe impairment: Not recommended.

AVAILABLE FORMS

- *Tablets:* 300 mg.
- *Oral Solution:* 20 mg/ml.

CONTRAINDICATIONS: Moderate or severe hepatic impairment

PREGNANCY AND LACTATION: Pregnancy category C; breast-feeding not recommended due to drug secretion and potential for HIV transmission

SIDE EFFECTS

Adult

Frequent

Nausea (47%), nausea with vomiting (16%), diarrhea (12%), decreased appetite (11%)

Occasional

Insomnia (7%)

Children

Frequent

Nausea with vomiting (39%), fever (19%), headache, diarrhea (16%), rash (11%)

Occasional

Decreased appetite (9%)

SERIOUS REACTIONS

- A hypersensitivity reaction may be life-threatening. Signs and symptoms include fever, rash, fatigue, intractable nausea and vomiting, severe diarrhea, abdominal pain, cough, pharyngitis, and dyspnea.
- Life-threatening hypotension may occur.
- Lactic acidosis and severe hepatomegaly may occur.

INTERACTIONS

Drugs

3 *Alcohol:* May increase abacavir blood concentration and half-life

3 *Amprenavir:* Mild increase in amprenavir plasma level with co-administration

3 *St. John's wort:* May decrease abacavir blood concentration and effect

SPECIAL CONSIDERATIONS

PATIENT/FAMILY EDUCATION

- May administer without regard for food
- If you miss a dose: take the missed dose as soon as you remember, then go back to your normal dosing schedule; skip the missed dose if it is time for your next dose; do not take 2 doses at the same time
- Do not take any other medication, including OTC drugs, without consulting the physician
- Abacavir is not a cure for HIV infection, nor does it reduce the risk of transmitting HIV to others

MONITORING PARAMETERS

- CBC, metabolic panel, CD4 lymphocyte count, HIV RNA level
- Pattern of daily bowel activity and stool consistency
- Weight

---

abciximab

(ab-siks'-ih-mab)

Rx: ReoPro

Chemical Class: Glycoprotein (GP) IIb/IIIa inhibitor

Therapeutic Class: Antiplatelet agent

CLINICAL PHARMACOLOGY

Mechanism of Action: A glycoprotein IIb/IIIa receptor inhibitor that rapidly inhibits platelet aggregation by preventing the binding of fibrinogen to GP IIb/IIIa receptor sites on platelets. ***Therapeutic Effect:*** Prevents closure of treated coronary arteries. Prevents acute cardiac ischemic complications.

Pharmacokinetics

Rapidly cleared from plasma. Initial-phase ***half-life*** is less than 10 min; second-phase ***half-life*** is 30 min. Platelet function generally returns within 48 hr.

INDICATIONS AND DOSAGES

Percutaneous coronary intervention (PCI)

IV Bolus

Adults. 0.25 mg/kg 10-60 min before angioplasty or atherectomy, then 12-hr IV infusion of 0.125 mcg/kg/min. Maximum: 10 mcg/min.

PCI (unstable angina)

IV Bolus

Adults. 0.25 mg/kg, followed by 18- to 24-hr infusion of 10 mcg/min, ending 1 hr after procedure.

AVAILABLE FORMS

- *Injection:* 2 mg/ml (5-ml vial).

CONTRAINDICATIONS: Active internal bleeding, arteriovenous malformation or aneurysm, cerebrovascular accident (CVA) with residual neurologic defect, history of CVA (within the past 2 years) or oral anticoagulant use within the past 7 days unless PT is less than 1.2 × control, history of vasculitis, hypersensitivity to murine proteins, intracranial neoplasm, prior IV dextran use before or during percutaneous transluminal coronary angioplasty (PTCA), recent surgery or trauma (within the past 6 weeks), recent (within the past 6 weeks or less) GI or GU bleeding, thrombocytopenia (less than 100,000 cells/mcl), and severe uncontrolled hypertension

PREGNANCY AND LACTATION: Pregnancy category C; excretion into breast milk unknown; use caution in nursing mothers

SIDE EFFECTS

Frequent

Nausea (16%), hypotension (12%)

Occasional (9%)

Vomiting

Rare (3%)

Bradycardia, confusion, dizziness, pain, peripheral edema, urinary tract infection

SERIOUS REACTIONS

• Major bleeding complications may occur. If complications occur, stop the infusion immediately.

• Hypersensitivity reaction may occur.

• Atrial fibrillation or flutter, pulmonary edema, and complete AV block occur occasionally.

INTERACTIONS

Drugs

3 *Antithrombotics (aspirin, heparin, warfarin, ticlopidine, clopidogrel):* Increased risk of bleeding

SPECIAL CONSIDERATIONS

• Fab fragment of the chimeric human-murine monoclonal antibody 7E3

• Intended to be used with aspirin and heparin

• Discontinue if bleeding occurs that is not controlled by compression

• Discontinue if PTCA fails

• Eptifibitide, tirofiban, and abciximab can all decrease the incidence of cardiac events associated with acute coronary syndromes; direct comparisons are needed to establish which, if any, is superior; for angioplasty, until more data become available, abciximab appears to be the drug of choice

PATIENT/FAMILY EDUCATION

• Use an electric razor and soft toothbrush to prevent bleeding

• Report signs of bleeding, including black or red stool, coffee-ground emesis, red or dark urine, or red-speckled mucus from cough

MONITORING PARAMETERS

• Baseline platelet count, prothrombin time, aPTT; during INF closely monitor platelet count and aPTT (heparin therapy)

• Stop abciximab and heparin infusion if serious bleeding uncontrolled by pressure occurs

• Assess skin for ecchymosis and petechiae; also, assess for GI, GU, and retroperitoneal bleeding and for bleeding at all puncture sites

• Assess for signs and symptoms of hemorrhage, including a decrease in blood pressure, increase in pulse rate, abdominal or back pain, and severe headache

• Assess urine for hematuria

acamprosate calcium

(ah-camp′-ro-sate kal′-see-um)

Rx: Campral

Chemical Class: Amino acid derivative

Therapeutic Class: Alcohol deterrent

CLINICAL PHARMACOLOGY

Mechanism of Action: An alcohol abuse deterrent that appears to interact with glutamate and gamma-aminobutyric acid neurotransmitter systems centrally, restoring their balance. ***Therapeutic Effect:*** Reduces alcohol dependence.

Pharmacokinetics

Slowly absorbed from the GI tract. Steady-state plasma concentrations are reached within 5 days. Does not undergo metabolism. Excreted in urine. ***Half-life:*** 20-33 hr.

INDICATIONS AND DOSAGES

Maintenance of alcohol abstinence in alcohol-dependent patients who are abstinent at initiation of treatment

PO

Adults, Elderly: Two tablets 3 times a day.

Dosage in renal impairment

For patients with creatinine clearance of 30-49 ml/min, dosage is decreased to one tablet 3 times a day.

AVAILABLE FORMS

• *Tablets:* 333 mg.

CONTRAINDICATIONS: Severe renal impairment (creatinine clearance of 30 ml/min or less)

PREGNANCY AND LACTATION: Pregnancy category C; teratogenicity has been demonstrated in animals; excreted in the milk of lactating rats, excretion into human milk is unknown; use caution in nursing mothers

SIDE EFFECTS

Frequent (17%)

Diarrhea

Occasional (6%-4%)

Insomnia, asthenia, fatigue, anxiety, flatulence, nausea, depression, pruritus

Rare (3%-1%)

Dizziness, anorexia, paresthesia, diaphoresis, dry mouth

SERIOUS REACTIONS

- Acute renal failure has been reported.

INTERACTIONS

Drugs

▲ *Antidepressants:* May cause weight gain or loss

3 *Naltrexone:* May increase acamprosate blood concentration

SPECIAL CONSIDERATIONS

- Does not cause disulfiram-like reaction with ingestion of alcohol
- Higher doses appear to be more effective for maintaining abstinence
- The optimal time to initiate therapy has not been identified

PATIENT/FAMILY EDUCATION

- Use caution operating hazardous machinery, including automobiles, until there is reasonable certainty that acamprosate will not affect ability to engage in such activities
- Continue use even in the event of a relapse and discuss any renewed drinking with prescriber
- To be used as part of a treatment program that includes psychosocial support

MONITORING PARAMETERS

- Maintenance of alcohol abstinence
- Pattern of daily bowel activity and stool consistency

acarbose

(ay'-car-bose)

Rx: Precose

Chemical Class: α-amylase inhibitor; α-glucosidase inhibitor

Therapeutic Class: Antidiabetic; hypoglycemic

CLINICAL PHARMACOLOGY

Mechanism of Action: An alpha glucosidase inhibitor that delays glucose absorption and digestion of carbohydrates, resulting in a smaller rise in blood glucose concentration after meals. ***Therapeutic Effect:*** Lowers postprandial hyperglycemia.

Pharmacokinetics

Low absorption within the GI tract. Extensive metabolism in the intestinal wall. Degraded in the intestine by bacterial and digestive enzymes. Excreted in feces and urine. ***Half-life:*** 2 hr.

INDICATIONS AND DOSAGES

Diabetes mellitus

PO

Adults, Elderly. Initially, 25 mg 3 times a day with first bite of each main meal. May increase at 4- to 8-wk intervals. Maximum: For patients weighing more than 60 kg, 100 mg 3 times a day; for patients weighing 60 kg or less, 50 mg 3 times a day.

AVAILABLE FORMS

- *Tablets:* 25 mg, 50 mg, 100 mg.

CONTRAINDICATIONS: Chronic intestinal diseases associated with marked disorders of digestion or absorption, cirrhosis, colonic ulceration, conditions that may deteriorate as a result of increased gas formation in the intestine, diabetic ketoacidosis, hypersensitivity to acarbose, inflammatory bowel disease, partial intestinal obstruction or predisposition to intestinal obstruction, significant renal dysfunction (serum creatinine level greater than 2 mg/dl)

PREGNANCY AND LACTATION: Pregnancy category B; excreted into breast milk in rats; no human data available

SIDE EFFECTS

Side effects diminish in frequency and intensity over time.

Frequent

Transient GI disturbances: flatulence (77%), diarrhea (33%), abdominal pain (21%)

SERIOUS REACTIONS

• None known.

INTERACTIONS

Drugs

3 *β-blockers:* May increase the risk of hypoglycemia, hyperglycemia, or hypertension

3 *Charcoal, digestive enzyme preparations:* Reduced effects of acarbose

3 *Cholestyramine:* Enhanced side effects of acarbose

3 *Fluoroquinolones:* May cause changes in blood glucose and increase the risk of hypoglycemia or hyperglycemia

3 *Neomycin:* Enhanced reduction of postprandial blood glucose and exacerbation of adverse effects

3 *Metformin:* Decreased metformin peak serum and AUC concentrations

3 *Sulfonylureas:* May increase the risk of hypoglycemia

3 *Warfarin:* May increase the risk of bleeding

SPECIAL CONSIDERATIONS

• Does not cause hypoglycemia
• Reduces HbAlc 0.5-1%
• Blood glucose; HbAlc 3-6 mo
• Consider ALT/AST during first yr

PATIENT/FAMILY EDUCATION

• Take glucose rather than complex carbohydrates to abort hypoglycemic episodes
• Decrease adverse GI effects by reducing dietary starch content
• Do not skip or delay meals
• Avoid alcohol
• Consult the physician when glucose demands are altered (such as with fever, heavy physical activity, infection, stress, trauma)
• Exercise, good personal hygiene (including foot care), not smoking, and weight control are essential parts of therapy

MONITORING PARAMETERS

• Food intake and blood glucose, glycosylated hemoglobin, and AST(SGOT) levels
• Assess for signs and symptoms of hypoglycemia (anxiety, cool wet skin, diplopia, dizziness, headache, hunger, numbness in mouth, tachycardia, tremors) or hyperglycemia (deep rapid breathing, dim vision, fatigue, nausea, polydipsia, polyphagia, polyuria, vomiting)
• Be alert to conditions that alter glucose requirements, including fever, increased activity or stress, or a surgical procedure

acebutolol hydrochloride

(a-se-byoo′-toe-lole hye-droe-klor′-ide)

Rx: Sectral

Chemical Class: β_1-adrenergic blocker, cardioselective

Therapeutic Class: Antianginal; antihypertensive

CLINICAL PHARMACOLOGY

Mechanism of Action: A beta_1-adrenergic blocker that competitively blocks beta_1-adrenergic receptors in cardiac tissue. Reduces the rate of spontaneous firing of the sinus pacemaker and delays AV conduction. ***Therapeutic Effect:*** Slows heart rate, decreases cardiac output, decreases BP, and exhibits antiarrhythmic activity.

Pharmacokinetics

Route	*Onset*	*Peak*	*Duration*
PO (hypotensive)	1-1.5 hr	2-8 hr	24 hr
PO (antiarrhythmic)	1 hr	4-6 hr	10 hr

Well absorbed from the GI tract. Protein binding: 26%. Undergoes extensive first-pass liver metabolism to active metabolite. Eliminated via bile, secreted into GI tract via intestine, and excreted in urine. Removed by hemodialysis. ***Half-life:*** 3-4 hr; metabolite, 8-13 hr.

INDICATIONS AND DOSAGES

Mild to moderate hypertension

PO

Adults. Initially, 400 mg/day in 12 divided doses. Range: Up to 1,200 mg/day in 2 divided doses. Maintenance: 400-800 mg/day.

Ventricular arrhythmias

PO

Adults. Initially, 200 mg q12h. Increase gradually to 600-1,200 mg/day in 2 divided doses.

Elderly. Initially, 200-400 mg/day. Maximum: 800 mg/day.

Dosage in renal impairment

Dosage is modified based on creatinine clearance.

Creatinine Clearance	*% of Usual Dosage*
less than 50 ml/min	50
less than 25 ml/min	25

AVAILABLE FORMS

- *Capsules:* 200 mg, 400 mg.

UNLABELED USES: Treatment of anxiety, chronic angina pectoris, hypertrophic cardiomyopathy, MI, pheochromocytoma, syndrome of mitral valve prolapse, thyrotoxicosis, tremors

CONTRAINDICATIONS: Cardiogenic shock, heart block greater than first degree, overt heart failure, severe bradycardia

PREGNANCY AND LACTATION: Pregnancy category B (D if used in second or third trimester); frequently used in the third trimester for treatment of hypertension; long-term use associated with intrauterine growth retardation; excreted into breast milk

SIDE EFFECTS

Frequent

Hypotension manifested as dizziness, nausea, diaphoresis, headache, cold extremities, fatigue, constipation, or diarrhea

Occasional

Insomnia, urinary frequency, impotence or decreased libido

Rare

Rash, arthralgia, myalgia, confusion (especially in the elderly), altered taste

SERIOUS REACTIONS

- Overdose may produce profound bradycardia and hypotension.
- Abrupt withdrawal may result in diaphoresis, palpitations, headache, and tremors.
- Acebutolol administration may precipitate CHF or MI in patients with heart disease; thyroid storm in those with thyrotoxicosis; or peripheral ischemia in those with existing peripheral vascular disease.
- Hypoglycemia may occur in patients with previously controlled diabetes.
- Signs of thrombocytopenia, such as unusual bleeding or bruising, occur rarely.

INTERACTIONS

Drugs

3 *α_1-adrenergic blockers:* Potential enhanced first dose response (marked initial drop in blood pressure, particularly on standing [especially prazosin])

3 *Amiodarone:* Bradycardia/ventricular dysrhythmia

3 *Anesthetics, local:* Enhanced sympathomimetic effects, hypertension due to unopposed α-receptor stimulation

3 *Antacids:* May reduce β-blocker absorption

3 *Antidiabetics:* Delayed recovery from hypoglycemia, hyperglycemia, attenuated tachycardia during hypoglycemia, hypertension during hypoglycemia

3 *Catecholamine-depleting drugs (e.g., reserpine):* Increased risk of bradycardia and syncope

3 *Clonidine:* Rebound hypertension; discontinue β-blocker prior to clonidine withdrawal

3 *Digoxin:* Additive prolongation of atrioventricular (AV) conduction time

3 *Dihydropyridine calcium channel blockers:* Severe hypotension or impaired cardiac performance; most prevalent with impaired left ventricular function, cardiac arrhythmias, or aortic stenosis

3 *Dipyridamole:* Bradycardia

3 *Disopyramide:* Additive decreases in cardiac output

3 *Diuretics:* Increases hypotensive effect of acebutolol

3 *Epinephrine:* Enhanced pressor response resulting in hypertension

3 *Neostigmine:* Bradycardia

3 *Neuroleptics:* Increased serum levels of both resulting in accentuated pharmacologic response to both drugs

3 *NSAIDs:* Reduced hypotensive effects

3 *Phenylephrine:* Acute hypertensive episodes

3 *Sympathomimetics, xanthines:* Mutually inhibit effects

3 *Tacrine:* Additive bradycardia

2 *Theophylline:* Antagonist pharmacodynamics

SPECIAL CONSIDERATIONS

- Fewer CNS and bronchospastic effects than other β-blockers

MONITORING PARAMETERS

- Heart rate, blood pressure
- EKG for arrhythmias
- Stool frequency and consistency, urine output
- Signs and symptoms of CHF

PATIENT/FAMILY EDUCATION

- Do not discontinue abruptly; may require taper; rapid withdrawal may produce rebound hypertension or angina
- Report excessive fatigue, headache, prolonged dizziness, shortness of breath, or weight gain
- Do not use nasal decongestants or OTC cold preparations (stimulants) without physician approval
- Restrict salt and alcohol intake

acetaminophen

(ah-seet'-ah-min-oh-fen)

OTC: Acephen, Apacet, Arthritis Pain Formula, Aspirin Free Pain Relief, Feverall, Genapap, Liquiprin, Neopap, Panadol, Tapanol Tempra, Tylenol

Combinations

Rx: with butalbital (Phrenilin); with butalbital and caffeine (Fioricet, Esgic, Isocet); with butalbital, caffeine and codeine (Amaphen, Fioricet w/codeine); with codeine (Tylenol, Phenaphen No. 2,3,4); with dichloralphenazone and isometheptene (Midrin, Midchlor); with hydrocodone (Vicodin, Lorcet, Lortab); with oxycodone (Percocet, Roxicet, Tylox); with pentazocine (Talacen); with propoxyphene (Wygesic, Darvocet-N)

OTC: with pamabrom + pyrilamine (Midol PMS, Pamprin); with antihistamine and decongestant (Actifed Plus, Drixoral Cold & Flu, Benadryl Sinus, Sine-Off, Sinarest); with decongestant, antihistamine, dextromethorphan (Nyquil)

Chemical Class: Para-aminophenol derivative

Therapeutic Class: Antipyretic; nonnarcotic analgesic

CLINICAL PHARMACOLOGY

Mechanism of Action: A central analgesic whose exact mechanism is unknown, but appears to inhibit prostaglandin synthesis in the central nervous system (CNS) and, to a lesser extent, block pain impulses through peripheral action. Acetaminophen acts centrally on hypothalamic heat-regulating center, producing peripheral vasodilation (heat loss, skin erythema, sweating). ***Therapeutic Effect:*** Results in antipyresis. Produces analgesic effect. Results in antipyresis.

Pharmacokinetics

Route	Onset	Peak	Duration
PO	15-30 mins	1-1.5 hrs	4-6 hrs

Rapidly, completely absorbed from gastrointestinal (GI) tract; rectal absorption variable. Protein binding: 20%-50%. Widely distributed to most body tissues. Metabolized in liver; excreted in urine. Removed by hemodialysis. ***Half-life:*** 1-4 hrs (half-life is increased in those with liver disease, elderly, neonates; decreased in children).

INDICATIONS AND DOSAGES

Analgesia and antipyresis

PO

Adults, Elderly. 325-650 mg q4-6h or 1 g 3-4 times/day. Maximum: 4 g/day.

Children. 10-15 mg/kg/dose q4-6h as needed. Maximum: 5 doses/24 hrs.

Neonates. 10-15 mg/kg/dose q6-8h as needed.

Rectal

Adults. 650 mg q4-6h. Maximum: 6 doses/24 hrs.

Children. 10-20 mg/kg/dose q4-6h as needed.

Neonates. 10-15 mg/kg/dose q6-8h as needed.

Dosage in renal impairment

Creatinine Clearance	Frequency
10-50 ml/min	q6h
less than 10 ml/min	q8h

AVAILABLE FORMS
• *Caplet (Genapap, Tylenol):* 500 mg.
• *Caplet, extended release (Mapap, Tylenol Arthritis Pain):* 650 mg.
• *Capsule (Mapap):* 500 mg.
• *Elixir:* 160 mg/5 ml.
• *Liquid, oral (Tylenol Extra Strength):* 500 mg/15 ml.
• *Solution, oral drops (Genapap Infant):* 80 mg/0.8 ml.
• *Suppository, rectal (Feverall):* 80 mg, *(Acephen, Feverall):* 120 mg, 325 mg, 650 mg.
• *Tablet (Genapap, Mapap, Tylenol):* 325 mg, 500 mg.
• *Tablet, chewable (Genapap, Mapap, Tylenol):* 80 mg.

CONTRAINDICATIONS: Active alcoholism, liver disease, or viral hepatitis, all of which increase the risk of hepatotoxicity

PREGNANCY AND LACTATION: Pregnancy category B; low concentrations in breast milk (1%-2% of maternal dose); compatible with breast-feeding

SIDE EFFECTS

Rare

Hypersensitivity reaction

SERIOUS REACTIONS
• Acetaminophen toxicity is the primary serious reaction.
• Early signs and symptoms of acetaminophen toxicity include anorexia, nausea, diaphoresis, and generalized weakness within the first 12 to 24 hrs.
• Later signs of acetaminophen toxicity include vomiting, right upper quadrant tenderness, and elevated liver function tests within 48 to 72 hrs after ingestion.
• The antidote to acetaminophen toxicity is acetylcysteine.

INTERACTIONS

Drugs

3 *Anticoagulants:* Enhanced hypoprothrombinemic response

3 *Anticonvulsants, Barbiturates, Rifabutin, Rifampin:* Enhanced hepatoxic potential in overdose

3 *Cholestyramine/Colestipol:* Reduced acetaminophen levels and response

3 *Ethanol:* Increased hepatoxicity in chronic, excessive alcohol ingestion

3 *Hepatotoxic medications (e.g., phenytoin), liver enzyme inducers (e.g., cimetidine):* Increases risk of hepatotoxicity with prolonged high dose or single toxic dose

3 *Isoniazid:* Increased acetaminophen levels & hepatotoxicity

Labs
• *False decrease:* Amylase
• *False increase:* Urine 5-HIAA
• *Interference:* Cannot assay ticarillin levels

SPECIAL CONSIDERATIONS

PATIENT/FAMILY EDUCATION
• Many OTC drugs contain acetaminophen; additive dosage may exceed 4 g/day maximum and increase risk of hepatotoxicity
• Consult with the physician before using acetaminophen in children under 2 years of age; oral use for more than 5 days in children, more than 10 days in adults, or fever lasting more than 3 days

acetaminophen; dichloralphenazone; isometheptene mucate

(ah-seet'-ah-min-oh-fen; dye-klor-al-fen'-a-zone; i-so-meh-thep'-tene)

Rx: I.D.A., Midrin, Migratine, Migrin-A

Chemical Class: Sympathomimetic amine

Therapeutic Class: Vasoconstrictor (in combination with analgesic and sedative)

CLINICAL PHARMACOLOGY

Mechanism of Action: Acetaminophen: A central analgesic whose exact mechanism is unknown, but appears to inhibit prostaglandin synthesis in the central nervous system (CNS) and, to a lesser extent, block pain impulses through peripheral action. Acetaminophen acts centrally on hypothalamic heat-regulating center, producing peripheral vasodilation (heat loss, skin erythema, sweating). Isometheptene: An indirect-acting sympathomimetic agent with vasoconstricting activity whose exact mechanism is unknown, but appears to constrict cerebral blood vessels and reduce pulsation in cerebral arteries that may be responsible for the pain of migraine headaches. Dichloralphenazone: A complex of chloral hydrate and antipyrine that acts as a mild sedative and relaxant. ***Therapeutic Effect:*** Relieves migraine headaches.

Pharmacokinetics

Rapidly, completely absorbed from gastrointestinal (GI) tract; rectal absorption variable. Widely distributed to most body tissues. Acetaminophen is metabolized in liver; excreted in urine. Dichloralphenazone is hydrolyzed to active compounds chloral hydrate and antipyrine. Chloral hydrate is metabolized in the liver and erythrocytes to the active metabolite trichloroethanol, which may be further metabolized to inactive metabolite. It is also metabolized in the liver and kidneys to inactive metabolites. The pharmacokinetics of isometheptene is not reported. Removed by hemodialysis. ***Half-life:*** Acetaminophen: 1-4 hrs (half-life is increased in those with liver disease, elderly, neonates; decreased in children).

INDICATIONS AND DOSAGES

Migraine headache

PO

Adults, Elderly. Initially, 2 capsules, followed by 1 capsule every hour until relief is obtained. Maximum: 5 capsules/12 hrs.

Tension headache

PO

Adults, Elderly. 1-2 capsules q4h. Maximum: 8 capsules/24 hrs.

AVAILABLE FORMS

- *Capsules:* Acetaminophen 325 mg, isometheptene mucate 65 mg, dichloralphenazone 100 mg (I.D.A., Midrin, Migrin-A).

CONTRAINDICATIONS: Glaucoma, hypersensitivity to acetaminophen, isometheptene, dichloralphenazone, or any component of the formulation, hepatic disease, hypertension, organic heart disease, MAO inhibitor therapy, severe renal disease

PREGNANCY AND LACTATION: Pregnancy category B; excretion into breast milk unknown

Controlled substance: Schedule IV

SIDE EFFECTS

Occasional

Transient dizziness

Rare

Hypersensitivity reaction

SERIOUS REACTIONS

- Acetaminophen toxicity is the primary serious reaction.
- Early signs and symptoms of acetaminophen toxicity include anorexia, nausea, diaphoresis, and generalized weakness within the first 12 to 24 hrs.
- Later signs of acetaminophen toxicity include vomiting, right upper quadrant tenderness, and elevated liver function tests within 48 to 72 hrs after ingestion.
- The antidote to acetaminophen toxicity is acetylcysteine.

INTERACTIONS

Drugs

⚠ *Bromocriptine:* Potential for hypertension and ventricular tachycardia

Labs

- *False positive:* Urine amphetamine

---

acetazolamide

(a-seat-a-zole′-a-mide)

Rx: Dazamide, Diamox, Diamox Sequels

Chemical Class: Carbonic anhydrase inhibitor; sulfonamide derivative

Therapeutic Class: Anticonvulsant; antiglaucoma agent; diuretic

---

CLINICAL PHARMACOLOGY

Mechanism of Action: A carbonic anhydrase inhibitor that reduces formation of hydrogen and bicarbonate ions from carbon dioxide and water by inhibiting, in proximal renal tubule, the enzyme carbonic anhydrase, thereby promoting renal excretion of sodium, potassium, bicarbonate, water. Ocular: Reduces rate of aqueous humor formation, lowers intraocular pressure. ***Therapeutic Effect:*** Produces anticonvulsant activity.

Pharmacokinetics

Rapidly absorbed. Protein binding: 95%. Widely distributed throughout body tissues including erythrocytes, kidneys, and blood brain barrier. Not metabolized. Excreted unchanged in urine. Removed by hemodialysis. ***Half-life:*** 2.4-5.8 hrs.

INDICATIONS AND DOSAGES

Glaucoma

PO

Adults. 250 mg 1-4 times/day. Extended-Release: 500 mg 1-2 times/day usually given in morning and evening.

Secondary glaucoma, preop treatment of acute congestive glaucoma

PO/IV

Adults. 250 mg q4h, 250 mg q12h; or 500 mg, then 125-250 mg q4h.

PO

Children. 10-15 mg/kg/day in divided doses.

IV

Children. 5-10 mg/kg q6h.

Edema

IV

Adults. 25-375 mg once daily.

Children. 5 mg/kg or 150 mg/m^2 once daily.

Epilepsy

Oral

Adults, Children. 375-1000 mg/day in 1-4 divided doses.

Acute mountain sickness

PO

Adults. 500-1,000 mg/day in divided doses. If possible, begin 24-48 hrs before ascent; continue at least 48 hrs at high altitude.

Usual elderly dosage

PO

Initially, 250 mg 2 times/day; use lowest effective dose.

Dosage in renal impairment

Creatinine Clearance	Dosage Interval
10-50 ml/min	q12h
less than 10 ml/min	avoid use

AVAILABLE FORMS

- *Capsules, sustained release:* 500 mg (Diamox Sequels).
- *Powder for reconstitution:* 500 mg.
- *Tablets:* 125 mg, 250 mg (Diamox).

UNLABELED USES: Urine alkalinization, respiratory stimulant in COPD

CONTRAINDICATIONS: Severe renal disease, adrenal insufficiency, hypochloremic acidosis, hypersensitivity to acetazolamide, to any component of the formulation, or to sulfonamides

PREGNANCY AND LACTATION: Pregnancy category C; premature delivery and congenital anomalies in humans; teratogenic (defects of the limbs) in mice, rats, hamsters, and rabbits; not recommended for nursing mothers

SIDE EFFECTS

Frequent

Unusually tired/weak, diarrhea, increased urination/frequency, decreased appetite/weight, altered taste (metallic), nausea, vomiting, numbness in extremities, lips, mouth

Occasional

Depression, drowsiness

Rare

Headache, photosensitivity, confusion, tinnitus, severe muscle weakness, loss of taste

SERIOUS REACTIONS

- Long-term therapy may result in acidotic state.
- Nephrotoxicity/hepatotoxicity occurs occasionally, manifested as dark urine/stools, pain in lower back, jaundice, dysuria, crystalluria, renal colic/calculi.
- Bone marrow depression may be manifested as aplastic anemia, thrombocytopenia, thrombocytopenic purpura, leukopenia, agranulocytosis, hemolytic anemia.

INTERACTIONS

Drugs

③ *Cyclosporine:* Increased trough cyclosporine levels with potential for neurotoxicity and nephropathy

③ *Flecainide, quinidine:* Alkalinization of urine increases quinidine serum levels

③ *Methenamine compounds:* Alkalinization of urine decreases antibacterial effects

③ *Phenytoin:* Increased risk of osteomalacia

③ *Primidone:* Decreased primidone levels

② *Salicylates:* Increased serum levels of acetazolamide—CNS toxicity

Labs

- *False increase:* 17 hydroxysteroid

SPECIAL CONSIDERATIONS

PATIENT/FAMILY EDUCATION

- Carbonated beverages taste flat
- If GI symptoms occur, take with food

MONITORING PARAMETERS

- Serum electrolytes, creatinine

acetic acid

(a-cee'-tik as'-id)

Rx: Acetasol, Acidic Vaginal Jelly, Acid Jelly, Aci-Jel, Borofair, Fem pH, Relagard, Vasotate, Vosol

Combinations

Rx: with hydrocortisone (Vo-Sol HC Otic, AA HC Otic, Acetasol HC) with oxyquinolone (Aci-Jel)

Chemical Class: Organic acid

Therapeutic Class: Antibacterial; antifungal

CLINICAL PHARMACOLOGY

Mechanism of Action: The mechanism by which acetic acid exerts its antibacterial and antifungal actions is unknown. ***Therapeutic Effect:*** Antibacterial and antifungal.

Pharmacokinetics

Unknown.

INDICATIONS AND DOSAGES

Superficial infections of the external auditory canal

Topical

Adults, Elderly, Children. Carefully remove all cerumen and debris to allow acetic acid to contact infected surfaces directly. To promote continuous contact, insert a wick saturated with acetic acid into the ear canal; the wick may also be saturated after insertion. Instruct the patient to keep the wick in for at least 24 hours and to keep it moist by adding 3-5 drops of acetic acid every 4-6 hours. The wick may be removed after 24 hours but the patient should continue to instill 5 drops of acetic acid 3 or 4 times daily thereafter, for as long as indicated. Dosing should be tapered gradually after apparent response to avoid relapse.

AVAILABLE FORMS

- *Solution (irrigation):* 0.25%
- *Solution (otic):* 2%
- *Gel (vaginal):* 0.92%
- *Solution (compounding):* 36%

CONTRAINDICATIONS: Hypersensitivity to acetic acid or any of the ingredients. Perforated tympanic membrane is frequently considered a contraindication to the use of any medication in the external ear canal.

PREGNANCY AND LACTATION: Pregnancy category C when combined with oxyquinoline

SIDE EFFECTS

Occasional

Stinging or burning

Rare

Local irritation, superinfection

SERIOUS REACTIONS

- Super infection with prolonged use

Alert: Discontinue promptly if sensitization or irritation occurs.

SPECIAL CONSIDERATIONS

PATIENT/FAMILY EDUCATION

- Carefully remove all cerumen and debris to allow acetic acid to contact infected surfaces directly. To promote continuous contact, insert a wick saturated with acetic acid into the ear canal; the wick may also be saturated after insertion. Keep the wick in for at least 24 hours and keep it moist by adding 3-5 drops of acetic acid every 4-6 hours. The wick may be removed after 24 hours but the patient should continue to instill 5 drops of acetic acid 3 or 4 times daily thereafter, for as long as indicated.

acetylcysteine

(a-se-teel-sis′-tay-een)

Rx: Acetadote, Mucomyst

Chemical Class: Amino acid, L-cysteine

Therapeutic Class: Antidote, acetaminophen; mucolytic

CLINICAL PHARMACOLOGY

Mechanism of Action: An intratracheal respiratory inhalant that splits the linkage of mucoproteins, reducing the viscosity of pulmonary secretions. ***Therapeutic Effect:*** Facilitates the removal of pulmonary secretions by coughing, postural drainage, mechanical means. Protects against acetaminophen overdose–induced hepatotoxicity.

Pharmacokinetics

Protein binding: 83% (injection). Rapidly and extensively metabolized in liver. Deacetylated by the liver to cysteine and subsequently metabolized. Excreted in urine. ***Half-life:*** 5.6 hr (injection).

INDICATIONS AND DOSAGES

Adjunctive treatment of viscid mucus secretions from chronic bronchopulmonary disease and for pulmonary complications of cystic fibrosis

Nebulization

Alert: Bronchodilators should be given 15 minutes before acetylcysteine.

Adults, Elderly, Children. 3-5 ml (20% solution) 3-4 times a day or 6-10 ml (10% solution) 3-4 times a day. Range: 1-10 ml (20% solution) q2-6h or 2-20 ml (10% solution) q2-6h.

Infants. 1-2 ml (20%) or 2-4 ml (10%) 3-4 times a day.

Treatment of viscid mucus secretions in patients with a tracheostomy

Intratracheal

Adults, Children. 1-2 ml of 10% or 20% solution instilled into tracheostomy q1-4h.

Acetaminophen overdose

PO (Oral solution 5%)

Adults, Elderly, Children. Loading dose of 140 mg/kg, followed in 4 hr by maintenance dose of 70 mg/kg q4h for 17 additional doses (unless acetaminophen assay reveals nontoxic level). Repeat dose if emesis occurs within 1 hour of administration. Continue until all doses are given, even if acetaminophen plasma level drops below toxic range.

IV

Adults, Elderly, Children. 150 mg/kg infused over 15 minutes, then 50 mg/kg infused over 4 hours, then 100 mg/kg infused over 16 hours. See administration and handling.

Prevention of renal damage from dyes used during certain diagnostic tests

PO (Oral solution 5%)

Adults, Elderly. 600 mg twice a day for 4 doses starting the day before the procedure.

AVAILABLE FORMS

- *Injection (Acedote):* 20% (200 mg/ml).
- *Inhalation Solution (Mucomyst):* 10% (100 mg/ml), 20% (200 mg/ml).

UNLABELED USES: Prevention of renal damage from dyes given during certain diagnostic tests (such as CT scans)

CONTRAINDICATIONS: None known.

PREGNANCY AND LACTATION: Pregnancy category B

SIDE EFFECTS
Frequent
Inhalation: Stickiness on face, transient unpleasant odor
Occasional
Inhalation: Increased bronchial secretions, throat irritation, nausea, vomiting, rhinorrhea
Rare
Inhalation: Rash
Oral: Facial edema, bronchospasm, wheezing

SERIOUS REACTIONS
• Large doses may produce severe nausea and vomiting.

INTERACTIONS
• Avoid contact with iron, copper, rubber

SPECIAL CONSIDERATIONS
• Disagreeable odor may be noted
• Solution in opened bottle may change color; of no significance

PATIENT/FAMILY EDUCATION
• Drink plenty of fluids

MONITORING PARAMETERS
• Respiratory rate, depth, and rhythm before treatment
• Check color, consistency, and amount of sputum

---

acitretin
(a-si-tre′-tin)
Rx: Soriatane
Chemical Class: Retinoid analog
Therapeutic Class: Antipsoriatic

CLINICAL PHARMACOLOGY
Mechanism of Action: A second-generation retinoid that adjusts factors influencing epidermal proliferation, RNA/DNA synthesis, controls glycoprotein, and governs immune response. ***Therapeutic Effect:*** Regulates keratinocyte growth and differentiation.
Pharmacokinetics
Well absorbed from the gastrointestinal (GI) tract. Food increases rate of absorption. Protein binding: greater than 99%. Metabolized in liver. Excreted in bile and urine. Not removed by hemodialysis. ***Half-life:*** 49 hrs.

INDICATIONS AND DOSAGES
Psoriasis
PO
Adults, Elderly. 25-50 mg/day as a single dose with main meal. May increase to 75 mg/day if necessary and dose tolerated. Maintenance: 25-50 mg/day after the initial response is noted. Continue until lesions have resolved.

AVAILABLE FORMS
• *Capsules:* 10 mg, 25 mg (Soriatane).

UNLABELED USES: Treatment of Darier's disease, palmoplantar pustulosis, lichen planus; children with lameliar ichthyosis, nonbullous and bullous ichthyosiform erythroderma, Sjogren-Larsson syndrome

CONTRAINDICATIONS: Pregnancy or those who intend to become pregnant within 3 years following discontinuation of therapy, severely impaired liver or kidney function, chronic abnormal elevated lipid levels, concomitant use of methotrexate or tetracyclines, ingestion of alcohol (in females of reproductive potential), hypersensitivity to acitretin, etretinate or other retinoids, sensitivity to parabenz (used as preservative in gelatin capsule)

PREGNANCY AND LACTATION: Pregnancy category X; breast milk excretion unknown

SIDE EFFECTS

Frequent

Lip inflammation, alopecia, skin peeling, shakiness, dry eyes, rash, hyperesthesia, paresthesia, sticky skin, dry mouth, epistaxis, dryness/thickening of conjunctiva

Occasional

Eye irritation, brow and lash loss, sweating, chills, sensation of cold, flushing, edema, blurred vision, diarrhea, nausea, thirst

SERIOUS REACTIONS

- Benign intracranial hypertension (pseudotumor cerebri) occurs rarely.

INTERACTIONS

Drugs

❷ *Methotrexate:* Increased potential for hepatotoxicity

❷ *Ethanol:* Drastically increases the $t_{1/2}$ of acitretin metabolite, etretinate

❷ *Progestin only contraceptives:* Decreased contraceptive effects

SPECIAL CONSIDERATIONS

PATIENT/FAMILY EDUCATION

- Avoid progestin only contraceptives
- Avoid exposure to sun and sunlamps

MONITORING PARAMETERS

- Transaminase levels monthly for first 6 mo then every 3 mo
- Lipid levels monthly for first 4 mo then every 2-3 mo
- Yearly radiographs to monitor for drug-induced vertebral abnormalities
- In children, measure PO_4, Ca levels in blood and urine and vitamin D and PTH levels every 6 mo

acyclovir

(ay-sye′-kloe-veer)

Rx: Zovirax, Zovirax Topical

Chemical Class: Acyclic purine nucleoside analog

Therapeutic Class: Antiviral

CLINICAL PHARMACOLOGY

Mechanism of Action: A synthetic nucleoside that converts to acyclovir triphosphate, becoming part of the DNA chain. ***Therapeutic Effect:*** Interferes with DNA synthesis and viral replication. Virustatic.

Pharmacokinetics

Poorly absorbed from the GI tract; minimal absorption following topical application. Protein binding: 9%-36%. Widely distributed. Partially metabolized in liver. Excreted primarily in urine. Removed by hemodialysis. ***Half-life:*** 2.5 hr (increased in impaired renal function).

INDICATIONS AND DOSAGES

Genital herpes (initial episode)

IV

Adults, Elderly, Children 12 yr and older. 5 mg/kg q8h for 5 days.

PO

Adults, Elderly, Children 12 yr and older. 200 mg q4h 5 times a day

Genital herpes (recurrent)

PO (Less than 6 episodes per year)

Adults, Elderly, Children 12 yr and older. 200 mg q4h 5 times a day for 5 days

PO (6 episodes or more per year:)

Adults, Elderly, Children 12 yr and older. 400 mg 2 times a day or 200 mg 3-5 times a day for up to 12 months.

Herpes simplex mucocutaneous

IV

Adults, Elderly, Children 12 yr and older. 5 mg/kg/dose q8h for 7 days

Children younger than 12 yr. 10 mg/kg q8h for 7 days.

Herpes simplex neonatal
IV
Children younger than 4 mo. 10 mg/kg q8h for 10 days.
Herpes simplex encephalitis
IV
Adults, Elderly, Children 12 yr and older. 10 mg/kg q8h for 10 days
Children 3 mos - younger than 12 yr. 20 mg/kg q8h for 10 days.
Herpes zoster (caused by varicella)
IV
Adults, Elderly, Children 12 yr and older. 10 mg/kg q8h for 7 days.
Children younger than 12 yr. 20 mg/kg q8h for 7 days.
Herpes zoster (shingles)
PO
Adults, Elderly, Children 12 yr and older. 800 mg q4h 5 times a day for 7-10 days.
Topical
Adults, Elderly. Apply to affected area 3-6 times a day for 7 days
Varicella (chickenpox)
PO
Adults, Elderly, Children older than 12 yr or children 2-12 yr, weighing 40 kg or more. 800 mg 4 times a day for 5 days.
Children 2-12 yr, weighing less than 40 kg. 20 mg/kg 4 times a day for 5 days. Maximum: 800 mg/dose
Children younger than 2 yr. 80 mg/kg/day.
Dosage in renal impairment
Dosage and frequency are modified based on severity of infection and degree of renal impairment.
PO, Normal dose 200 mg q4h: Creatinine clearance greater than 10 ml/min: Give usual dose and at normal interval, 200 mg q4h. *Creatinine clearance 10 ml/min and less:* 200 mg q12h.
PO, Normal dose 400 mg q12h: Creatinine clearance greater than 10 ml/min: Give usual dose and at normal interval, 400 mg q12h. *Creatinine clearance 10 ml/min and less:* 200 mg q12h.
PO, Normal dose 800 mg q4h: Creatinine clearance greater than 25 ml/min: Give usual dose and at normal interval, 800 mg q4h. *Creatinine clearance 10-25 ml/min:* 800 mg q8h. *Creatinine clearance less than 10 ml/min:* 800 mg q12h.
IV

Creatinine Clearance	*Dosage Percent*	*Dosage Interval*
greater than 50 ml/min	100	8 hr
25-50 ml/min	100	12 hr
10-24 ml/min	100	24 hr
less than 10 ml/min	50	24 hr

AVAILABLE FORMS
- *Capsules:* 200 mg.
- *Tablets:* 400 mg, 800 mg.
- *Injection Solution:* 50 mg/ml.
- *Oral Suspension:* 200 mg/5 ml.
- *Powder for Injection:* 500 mg, 1,000 mg.
- *Ointment:* 5%.

UNLABELED USES: *Oral, parenteral:* Prophylaxis of herpes simplex and herpes zoster infections, infectious mononucleosis.
Topical: Treatment adjunct for herpes zoster infections.
CONTRAINDICATIONS: Use in neonates when acyclovir is reconstituted with bacteriostatic water containing benzyl alcohol.
PREGNANCY AND LACTATION: Pregnancy category B; excreted into breast milk; compatible with breast-feeding
SIDE EFFECTS
Frequent
Parenteral (9%-7%): Phlebitis or inflammation at IV site, nausea, vomiting
Topical (28%): Burning, stinging

Occasional
Oral (12%-6%): Malaise, nausea
Parenteral (3%): Pruritus, rash, urticaria
Topical (4%): Pruritus
Rare
Oral (3%-1%): Vomiting, rash, diarrhea, headache
Parenteral (2%-1%): Confusion, hallucinations, seizures, tremors
Topical (less than 1%): Rash

SERIOUS REACTIONS

• Rapid parenteral administration, excessively high doses, or fluid and electrolyte imbalance may produce renal failure exhibited by such signs and symptoms as abdominal pain, decreased urination, decreased appetite, increased thirst, nausea, and vomiting.
• Toxicity has not been reported with oral or topical use.

INTERACTIONS

Drugs

3 *Nephrotoxic medications (such as aminoglycosides):* Increases the risk of nephrotoxicity

SPECIAL CONSIDERATIONS

• In recurrent herpes genitalis and herpes labialis in non-immunocompromised patients, no evidence of clinical benefit from topical acyclovir

PATIENT/FAMILY EDUCATION

• Drink adequate fluids during therapy
• Do not touch lesions to prevent spreading the infection to new sites
• Space doses evenly around the clock and continue taking acyclovir for the full course of treatment
• Use a finger cot or rubber glove when applying the ointment
• Avoid sexual intercourse while lesions are visible to prevent infecting the partner

adalimumab

(a-dal-aye′-mu-mab)
Rx: Humira
Chemical Class: Monoclonal antibody
Therapeutic Class: Disease-modifying antirheumatic drug (DMARD); immunomodulatory agent

CLINICAL PHARMACOLOGY

Mechanism of Action: A monoclonal antibody that binds specifically to tumor necrosis factor (TNF) alpha, blocking its interaction with cell surface TNF receptors. ***Therapeutic Effect:*** Reduces inflammation, tenderness, and swelling of joints; slows or prevents progressive destruction of joints in rheumatoid arthritis.

Pharmacokinetics

Half-life: 10-20 days.

INDICATIONS AND DOSAGES

Rheumatoid arthritis, psoriatic arthritis

Subcutaneous
Adults, Elderly. 40 mg every other week. Dose may be increased to 40 mg/wk in those not taking methotrexate.

AVAILABLE FORMS

• *Injection:* 40 mg/0.8 ml in prefilled syringes.

CONTRAINDICATIONS: Active infections

PREGNANCY AND LACTATION: Pregnancy category B; breast milk excretion unknown

SIDE EFFECTS

Frequent (20%)
Injection site, erythema, pruritus, pain, and swelling
Occasional (12%-9%)
Headache, rash, sinusitis, nausea

Rare (7%-5%)
Abdominal or back pain, hypertension

SERIOUS REACTIONS

• Rare reactions include hypersensitivity reactions, malignancies, respiratory tract infections, bronchitis, UTIs, and more serious infections (such as pneumonia, tuberculosis, cellulitus, pyelonephritis, and septic arthritis).

INTERACTIONS

Drugs

3 *Methotrexate:* Reduced apparent clearance after single and multiple dosing by 29% and 44%, respectively

SPECIAL CONSIDERATIONS

• Evaluate for latent tuberculosis infection with a tuberculin skin test before initiation of therapy
• Adalimumab does not contain preservatives—unused portions of drug should be discarded

PATIENT/FAMILY EDUCATION

• Injection sites should be rotated and injections should never be given into areas where the skin is tender, bruised, red, or hard
• Intended for use under the guidance and supervision of clinician; patients may self-inject if appropriate and with medical follow-up, after proper training in injection technique, including proper syringe and needle disposal
• Injection site reactions generally occur in the first month of treatment and decrease with continued therapy
• Avoid receiving live vaccines during adalimumab treatment

MONITORING PARAMETERS

• *Therapeutic:* Rheumatoid arthritis signs and symptoms (joint stiffness, pain, swollen/tender joints), mobility, quality of life, radiographs of affected joints, ESR, CRP
• *Toxicity:* Temperature, blood pressure periodically, signs and symptoms of respiratory infection, including tuberculosis, hypersensitivity, anti-adalimumab antibodies (ELISA) at least once during therapy, anti-dsDNA antibody determinations in patients presenting with lupus-like symptoms (*e.g.,* tiredness, rash, bone pain), CBC, routine blood chemistry periodically during long-term therapy

---

adapalene

(a-dap′-a-leen)
Rx: Differin
Chemical Class: Naphthoic acid derivative (retinoid-like)
Therapeutic Class: Antiacne agent

CLINICAL PHARMACOLOGY

Mechanism of Action: Binds to retinoic acid receptors in cell nuclei modulating cell differentiation, keratinization. Possesses anti-inflammatory properties. ***Therapeutic Effect:*** Normalizes differentiation of follicular epithelial cells.

Pharmacokinetics

Absorption through the skin is low. Trace amount found in plasma following topical application. Excreted primarily by biliary route.

INDICATIONS AND DOSAGES

Acne vulgaris

Topical

Adults, elderly, children > 12 years. Apply to affected area once daily at bedtime after washing.

AVAILABLE FORMS

• *Gel:* 0.1%
• *Cream:* 0.1%
• *Pledget (solution):* 0.1%

CONTRAINDICATIONS: Hypersensitivity to adapalene, vitamin A or any one of its components.

PREGNANCY AND LACTATION: Pregnancy category C; excretion in breast milk unknown

SIDE EFFECTS

Frequent

Erythema, scaling, dryness, pruritis, burning (likely to occur first 2-4 weeks, lessens with continued use)

Occasional

Skin irritation, stinging, sunburn, acne flares, erythema, photosensitivity, pruritis, xerosis

SERIOUS REACTIONS

• Concurrent use of other potential irritating topical products (soaps, cleansers, aftershave, cosmetics may produce severe topical irritation).

SPECIAL CONSIDERATIONS

• Avoid excessive exposure to sunlight
• Do not apply to lips or mucous membranes, or to cut, abraded, or sunburned skin
• May aggravate acne early in course of therapy
• Therapeutic results noticed in 8-12 wks
• Avoid contact with eyes

MONITORING PARAMETERS

• Skin for irritation

adefovir dipivoxil

(a-def'-o-veer)

Rx: Hepsera

Chemical Class: Nucleotide analog

Therapeutic Class: Antiviral

CLINICAL PHARMACOLOGY

Mechanism of Action: An antiviral that inhibits the enzyme DNA polymerase, causing DNA chain termination after its incorporation into viral DNA. ***Therapeutic Effect:*** Prevents cell replication of viral DNA.

Pharmacokinetics

Binds to proteins after PO administration. Protein binding: less than 4%. Excreted in urine. ***Half-life:*** 7 hr (increased in impaired renal function).

INDICATIONS AND DOSAGES

Chronic hepatitis B in patients with normal renal function

PO

Adults, Elderly. 10 mg once a day.

Chronic hepatitis B in patients with impaired renal function

Adults, Elderly with creatinine clearance 20-49 ml/min. 10 mg q48h.

Adults, Elderly with creatinine clearance 10-19 ml/min. 10 mg q72h.

Adults, Elderly on hemodialysis. 10 mg every 7 days following dialysis.

AVAILABLE FORMS

• *Tablets:* 10 mg.

CONTRAINDICATIONS: None known.

PREGNANCY AND LACTATION: Pregnancy category C; breast milk excretion unknown but breastfeeding not recommended

SIDE EFFECTS

Frequent (13%)

Asthenia

Occasional (9%-4%)

Headache, abdominal pain, nausea, flatulence

Rare (3%)

Diarrhea, dyspepsia

SERIOUS REACTIONS

• Nephrotoxicity (characterized by increased serum creatinine and decreased serum phosphorus levels) is a treatment-limiting toxicity of adefovir therapy.
• Lactic acidosis and severe hepatomegaly occur rarely, particularly in female patients.

INTERACTIONS

Drugs

3 *Ibuprofen:* Ibuprofen increases adefovir exposure by 23%

SPECIAL CONSIDERATIONS

- Offer HIV testing before treatment
- Effective in patients with HBV resistant to lamivudine
- Histologic improvement seen in 60% of treated patients, but long-term effect unknown

PATIENT/FAMILY EDUCATION

- Avoid behavior that may cause exposure to HIV
- Comply with follow-up laboratory testing; tests will help monitor kidney and liver function and hepatitis B virus levels
- Immediately notify the physician if unusual muscle pain, abdominal pain with nausea and vomiting, a cold feeling in arms and legs, and dizziness occurs; these signs and symptoms may signal the onset of lactic acidosis
- Continue to take adefovir as prescribed because a very serious form of hepatitis may develop if the drug is stopped
- Notify the physician of yellow skin color or whites of the eyes or other unusual signs or symptoms; it may indicate serious liver problems
- Use reliable methods of contraception during therapy

MONITORING PARAMETERS

- ALT, AST, bilirubin, HBV DNA level, INR, renal function
- Intake and output
- Closely monitor for serious reactions, especially in patients taking other drugs that are excreted by the kidneys or are known to affect renal function

adenosine

(ah-den'-oh-seen)

Rx: Adenocard, Adenojec, Adenoscan, My-O-Den

Chemical Class: Endogenous nucleoside

Therapeutic Class: Antiarrhythmic

CLINICAL PHARMACOLOGY

Mechanism of Action: A cardiac agent that slows impulse formation in the SA node and conduction time through the AV node. Adenosine also acts as a diagnostic aid in myocardial perfusion imaging or stress echocardiography. ***Therapeutic Effect:*** Depresses left ventricular function and restores normal sinus rhythm.

Pharmacokinetics

Rapidly cleared from the circulation via cellular uptake, primarily by erythrocytes and vascular endothelial cells. Extensively distributed and rapidly metabolized either via phosphorylation to adenosine monophosphate by adenosine kinase, or via deamination to inosine by adenosine deaminase in the cytosol. ***Half-life:*** 10 sec.

INDICATIONS AND DOSAGES

Paroxysmal supraventricular tachycardia (PSVT)

Rapid IV bolus

Adults, Elderly, Children weighing 50 kg and more. Initially, 6 mg given over 1-2 sec. If first dose does not convert within 1-2 min, give 12 mg; may repeat 12-mg dose in 1-2 min if no response has occurred

Children weighing less than 50 kg. Initially, 0.1 mg/kg (maximum: 6 mg). If ineffective, may give 0.2 mg/kg (maximum: 12 mg).

Diagnostic testing
IV infusion
Adults. 140 mcg/kg/min for 6 min.
AVAILABLE FORMS
• *Injection (Adenocard):* 3 mg/ml in 2 ml, 4 ml syringes.
• *Injection (Adenoscan):* 3 mg/ml in 20 ml, 30 ml vials.
CONTRAINDICATIONS: Atrial fibrillation or flutter, second- or third-degree AV block or sick sinus syndrome (with functioning pacemaker), ventricular tachycardia
PREGNANCY AND LACTATION: Pregnancy category C; fetal effects unlikely
SIDE EFFECTS
Frequent (18%-12%)
Facial flushing, dyspnea
Occasional (7%-2%)
Headache, nausea, light-headedness, chest pressure
Rare (less than or equal to 1%)
Numbness or tingling in arms; dizziness; diaphoresis; hypotension; palpitations; chest, jaw, or neck pain
SERIOUS REACTIONS
• May produce short-lasting heart block.
INTERACTIONS
Drugs
3 *β-blockers:* Bradycardia
3 *Dipyridamole:* Increased serum adenosine levels, potentiates pharmacologic effects of adenosine
3 *Nicotine:* Greater hemodynamic response to adenosine (hypotension, chest pain)
3 *Theophylline/caffeine:* Inhibits hemodynamic effects of adenosine
SPECIAL CONSIDERATIONS
PATIENT/FAMILY EDUCATION
• Report unusual signs and symptoms, including chest pain, chest pounding or palpitations, or difficulty breathing or shortness of breath
• Facial flushing, headache, and nausea may occur but these symptoms will resolve
MONITORING PARAMETERS
• Heart rate and rhythm, blood pressure, intake and output, electrolyte levels

albendazole
(al-ben'-da-zole)
Rx: Albenza
Chemical Class: Benzimidazole derivative
Therapeutic Class: Antihelmintic

CLINICAL PHARMACOLOGY
Mechanism of Action: A benzimidazole carbamate anthelmintic that degrades parasite cytoplasmic microtubules, irreversibly blocks cholinesterase secretion, glucose uptake in helminth and larvae (depletes glycogen, decreases ATP production, depletes energy). Vermicidal.
Therapeutic Effect: Immobilizes and kills worms.
Pharmacokinetics
Poorly and variable absorbed gastrointestinal (GI) tract. Widely distributed, cyst fluid and including cerebrospinal fluid (CSF). Protein binding: 70%. Extensively metabolized in liver. Primarily excreted in urine and bile. Not removed by hemodialysis. ***Half-life:*** 8-12 hrs.
INDICATIONS AND DOSAGES
Neurocysticercosis
PO
Adults, Elderly more than 60 kg. 400 mg 2 times/day. Continue for 28 days, rest 14 days, repeat cycle 3 times.
Adults, Elderly less than 60 kg. 15 mg/kg/day. Continue for 28 days, rest 14 days, repeat cycle 3 times.

Cystic hydatid
PO
Adults, Elderly more than 60 kg. 400 mg 2 times/day. Continue for 8-30 days.
Adults, Elderly less than 60 kg. 15 mg/kg/day. Continue for 8-30 days.

AVAILABLE FORMS
• *Tablets:* 200 mg (Albenza).

UNLABELED USES: Angiostrongyliasis, cysticerosis, gnathostomiasis, liver flukes, trichuriasis

CONTRAINDICATIONS: Hypersensitivity to albendazole or any component of the formulation, pregnancy

PREGNANCY AND LACTATION: Pregnancy category C; excreted in breast milk

SIDE EFFECTS
Frequent
Neurocysticerosis: Nausea, vomiting, headache
Hydatid: Abnormal liver function tests, abdominal pain, nausea, vomiting
Occasional
Neurocysticerosis: Increased intracranial pressure, meningeal signs
Hydatid: Headache, dizziness, alopecia, fever

SERIOUS REACTIONS
• Pancytopenia occurs rarely.
• In presence of cysticerosis, drug may produce retinal damage in presence of retinal lesions.

INTERACTIONS
Drugs
3 *Dexamethasone:* 56% increase in serum level of albendazole
3 *Praziquantel:* 50% increase in serum level of albendazole

SPECIAL CONSIDERATIONS
• For appropriate infections, retest stool 3 wk after treatment to detect residual ova
• Patients treated for neurocysticerosis should receive steroid and anticonvulsant therapy

PATIENT/FAMILY EDUCATION
• Avoid becoming pregnant during treatment or within 1 month following completion of treatment
• Notify the physician if fever, chills, sore throat, or unusual bleeding occurs

MONITORING PARAMETERS
• CBC and liver function

albuterol
(al-byoo′-ter-ole)
Rx: Accuneb, Proventil, Proventil-HFA, Proventil Repetabs, Ventolin, Ventolin HFA, Ventolin Rotacaps, Volmax, Vospire
Combinations
Rx: with ipratropium (Combivent)
Chemical Class: Sympathomimetic amine; β_2-adrenergic agonist
Therapeutic Class: Antiasthmatic; bronchodilator

CLINICAL PHARMACOLOGY
Mechanism of Action: A sympathomimetic that stimulates beta$_2$-adrenergic receptors in the lungs, resulting in relaxation of bronchial smooth muscle. ***Therapeutic Effect:*** Relieves bronchospasm and reduces airway resistance.
Pharmacokinetics

Route	Onset	Peak	Duration
PO	15-30 min	2-3 hr	4-6 hr
PO (extended-release)	30 min	2-4 hr	12 hr
Inhalation	5-15 min	0.5-2 hr	2-5 hr

Rapidly, well absorbed from the GI tract; gradually absorbed from the bronchi after inhalation. Metabolized in the liver. Primarily excreted in urine. ***Half-life:*** 2.7-5 hr (PO); 3.8 hr (inhalation).

INDICATIONS AND DOSAGES

Acute bronchospasm

Inhalation

Adults, Elderly, Children older than 12 yr. 4-8 puffs q20min up to 4 hours, then q1-4h as needed.

Children 12 yr and younger. 4-8 puffs q20min for 3 doses, then q1-4h as needed.

Nebulization

Adults, Elderly, Children older than 12 yr. 2.5-5 mg q20min for 3 doses, then 2.5-10 mg q1-4h or 10-15 mg/hr continuously.

Children 12 yr and younger. 0.15 mg/kg q20min for 3 doses (minimum: 2.5 mg), then 0.15-0.3 mg/kg q1-4h as needed.

Bronchospasm

PO

Adults, Children older than 12 yr. 2-4 mg 3-4 times a day. Maximum: 8 mg 4 times a day.

Elderly. 2 mg 3-4 times a day. Maximum: 8 mg 4 times a day.

Children 6-12 yr. 2 mg 3-4 times a day. Maximum: 24 mg/day.

Children 2-5 yr. 0.1-0.2 mg/kg/dose 3 times a day. Maximum: 12 mg/day.

PO (Extended-Release)

Adults, Children older than 12 yr. 4-8 mg q12h.

Nebulization

Adults, Elderly, Children older than 12 yr. 2.5 mg 3-4 times a day over 5-15 mins.

Children 12 yr and younger. 0.05 mg/kg q4-6h. Minimum: 1.25 mg/dose. Maximum: 2.5 mg/dose.

Chronic bronchospasm

Inhalation

Adults, Elderly, Children 4 yr and older. 1-2 puffs q4-6h. Maximum: 12 puffs per day.

Exercise-induced bronchospasm

Inhalation

Adults, Elderly, Children older than 12 yr. 2 puffs 15-30 mins before exercise.

Children 12 yr and younger. 1-2 puffs 5 mins before exercise.

AVAILABLE FORMS

- *Syrup:* 2 mg/5 ml.
- *Tablets (Proventil, Ventolin):* 2 mg, 4 mg.
- *Tablets (Extended-Release):* 4 mg (Proventil Repetabs, Volmax, VoSpire ER), 8 mg (Volmax, VoSpire ER).
- *Inhalation Aerosol (Proventil, Ventolin):* 90 mcg/spray.
- *Inhalation Solution (AccuNeb):* 0.75 mg/3 ml (0.63 mg/3 ml albuterol), 1.5 mg/3 ml (1.25 mg/3 ml albuterol).
- *Inhalation Solution:* 0.083% (Proventil), 0.5% (Proventil, Ventolin).

CONTRAINDICATIONS: History of hypersensitivity to sympathomimetics

PREGNANCY AND LACTATION: Pregnancy category C; excretion into breast milk unknown

SIDE EFFECTS

Frequent

Headache (27%); nausea (15%); restlessness, nervousness, tremors (20%); dizziness (less than 7%); throat dryness and irritation, pharyngitis (less than 6%); BP changes, including hypertension (5%-3%); heartburn, transient wheezing (less than 5%)

Occasional (3%-2%)

Insomnia, asthenia, altered taste

Inhalation: Dry, irritated mouth or throat; cough; bronchial irritation

Rare

Somnolence, diarrhea, dry mouth, flushing, diaphoresis, anorexia

SERIOUS REACTIONS

• Excessive sympathomimetic stimulation may produce palpitations, extrasystole, tachycardia, chest pain, a slight increase in BP followed by a substantial decrease, chills, diaphoresis, and blanching of skin.

• Too-frequent or excessive use may lead to decreased bronchodilating effectiveness and severe, paradoxical bronchoconstriction.

INTERACTIONS

Drugs

3 *β-blockers:* Decreased action of albuterol, cardioselective β-blockers preferable if concurrent use necessary

3 *Furosemide:* Potential for additive hypokalemia

3 *MAOIs:* Action of albuterol on the vascular system may be potentiated, caution if administered concomitantly or within 2 weeks of discontinuation of MAOIs

3 *Tricyclic antidepressants:* Action of albuterol on the vascular system may be potentiated, caution if administered concomitantly or within 2 weeks of discontinuation of tricyclics

SPECIAL CONSIDERATIONS

• Inhalation technique critical

• Consider spacer devices

• Rinse mouth immediately after inhalation

• Avoid excessive use of caffeine

MONITORING PARAMETERS

• 12-lead EKG, ABG determinations, pulse rate, respirations, serum potassium levels

PATIENT/FAMILY EDUCATION

• See clinician if using ≥4 inhalations/day on regular basis or >1 canister (200 inhalations) in 8 wks

alclometasone dipropionate

(al-kloe-met′-a-sone di-pro′-pee-on-ate)

Rx: Aclovate

Chemical Class: Corticosteroid, synthetic

Therapeutic Class: Corticosteroid, topical

CLINICAL PHARMACOLOGY

Mechanism of Action: Topical corticosteroids exhibit anti-inflammatory, antipruritic, and vasoconstrictive properties. Clinically, these actions correspond to decreased edema, erythema, pruritus, plaque formation and scaling of the affected skin.

Pharmacokinetics

Approximately 3% is absorbed during an 8-hr period. Metabolized in the liver. Excreted in the urine.

INDICATIONS AND DOSAGES

Atopic dermatitis, contact dermatitis, dermatitis, discoid lupus erythematosus, eczema, exfoliative dermatitis, granuloma annulare, lichen planus, lichen simplex, polymorphous light eruption, pruritis, psoriasis, Rhus dermatitis, seborrheic dermatitis, xerosis

Topical

Adults, adolescents, children 1 year and older. Apply a thin film to the affected area 2-3 times a day.

AVAILABLE FORMS

• *Cream:* (Aclovate)

• *Ointment:* (Aclovate)

CONTRAINDICATIONS: Hypersensitivity to alclometasone, other corticosteroids, or any of its components.

PREGNANCY AND LACTATION: Pregnancy category C; unknown whether topical application could result in sufficient systemic absorption to produce detectable amounts in breast milk (systemic corticosteroids are secreted into breast milk in quantities not likely to have detrimental effects on infant)

SIDE EFFECTS

Frequent

Burning, erythema, maculopapular rash, pruritis, skin irritation, xerosis

Occasional

Acneiform rash, contact dermatitis, folliculitis, glycosuria, growth inhibition, headache, hyperglycemia, infection, miliaria, papilledema, skin atrophy, skin hypopigmentation, skin ulcer, striae, telangiectasia

Rare

Adrenalcortical insufficiency, increased intracranial pressure, pseudotumor cerebri, impaired wound healing, Cushing's syndrome, HPA suppression, skin ulcers, tolerance, withdrawal, visual impairment, ocular hypertension, cataracts

SPECIAL CONSIDERATIONS

PATIENT/FAMILY EDUCATION

- Apply sparingly only to affected area
- Avoid contact with the eyes
- Do not put bandages or dressings over treated area unless directed by clinician
- Discontinue drug, notify clinician if local irritation or fever develops
- Do not use on weeping, denuded, or infected areas

alefacept

(a-la-fa'-cept)

Rx: Amevive

Chemical Class: Dimeric fusion protein

Therapeutic Class: Antipsoriatic; immunomodulatory agent

CLINICAL PHARMACOLOGY

Mechanism of Action: An immunologic agent that interferes with the activation of T-lymphocytes by binding to the lymphocyte antigen, thus reducing the number of circulating T-lymphocytes. ***Therapeutic Effect:*** Prevents T cells from becoming overactive, which may help reduce symptoms of chronic plaque psoriasis.

Pharmacokinetics

Half-life: 270 hr.

INDICATIONS AND DOSAGES

Plaque psoriasis

IV

Adults, Elderly. 7.5 mg once weekly for 12 wk.

IM

Adults, Elderly. 15 mg once weekly for 12 wk.

AVAILABLE FORMS

- *Powder for Injection:* 7.5 mg for IV administration, 15 mg for IM administration.

CONTRAINDICATIONS: History of systemic malignancy, concurrent use of immunosuppressive agents or phototherapy

PREGNANCY AND LACTATION: Pregnancy category B; effect on pregnancy and fetal development unknown (Biogen Pregnancy Registry available: 1-866-263-8483)

SIDE EFFECTS

Frequent (16%)

Injection site pain and inflammation (with IM administration)

Occasional (5%)
Chills
Rare (2% or less)
Pharyngitis, dizziness, cough, nausea, myalgia

SERIOUS REACTIONS

- Rare reactions include hypersensitivity reactions, lymphopenia, malignancies, and serious infections requiring hospitalization (such as abscess, pneumonia, and postoperative wound infection).
- Coronary artery disease and MI occur in less than 1% of patients.

INTERACTIONS

Drugs

3 *Immunosuppressive agents (steroids, chemotherapy, radiation):* potential excessive immunosuppression

3 *Phototherapy; photochemotherapy (light or laser):* potential excessive immunosuppression

3 *Vaccines, live or live-attenuated:* potential risk of disease

SPECIAL CONSIDERATIONS

PATIENT/FAMILY EDUCATION

- Inform patients of the need for monitoring of lymphocyte counts during therapy; increased risk of infection or a malignancy
- Avoid contact with infected individuals and situations that might place him or her at risk for infection

MONITORING PARAMETERS

- *Efficacy:* Psoriasis Area and Severity Index (PASI)—extent of area affected and severity of erythema, scaling, and thickness of plaques
- *Toxicity:* CD4+ lymphocyte counts weekly during 12-week course; withhold therapy if counts below 250 cells/μl

alendronate sodium

(a-len-droe′-nate soe′-dee-um)
Rx: Fosamax
Chemical Class: Pyrophosphate analog
Therapeutic Class: Antiosteoporotic; bisphosphonate; bone resorption inhibitor

CLINICAL PHARMACOLOGY

Mechanism of Action: A bisphosphonate that inhibits normal and abnormal bone resorption, without retarding mineralization. ***Therapeutic Effect:*** Leads to significantly increased bone mineral density; reverses the progression of osteoporosis.

Pharmacokinetics

Poorly absorbed after oral administration. Protein binding: 78%. After oral administration, rapidly taken into bone, with uptake greatest at sites of active bone turnover. Excreted in urine. ***Terminal half-life:*** Greater than 10 yr (reflects release from skeleton as bone is resorbed).

INDICATIONS AND DOSAGES

Osteoporosis (in men)
PO
Adults, Elderly. 10 mg once a day in the morning or 70 mg weekly.

Glucocorticoid-induced osteoporosis
PO
Adults, Elderly. 5 mg once a day in the morning.
Post-menopausal women not receiving estrogen. 10 mg once a day in the morning.

Post-menopausal osteoporosis
PO (treatment)
Adults, Elderly. 10 mg once a day in the morning or 70 mg weekly.
PO (prevention)
Adults, Elderly. 5 mg once a day in the morning or 35 mg weekly.

Paget's disease
PO
Adults, Elderly. 40 mg once a day in the morning for 6 mo.

AVAILABLE FORMS
- *Tablets:* 5 mg, 10 mg, 35 mg, 40 mg, 70 mg.
- *Oral Solution:* 70 mg/75 ml.

UNLABELED USES: Treatment of breast cancer

CONTRAINDICATIONS: GI disease, including dysphagia, frequent heartburn, gastrointestinal reflux disease, hiatal hernia, and ulcers; inability to stand or sit upright for at least 30 minutes; renal impairment; sensitivity to alendronate

PREGNANCY AND LACTATION: Pregnancy category C; contraindicated in nursing mothers

SIDE EFFECTS
Frequent (8%-7%)
Back pain, abdominal pain
Occasional (3%-2%)
Nausea, abdominal distention, constipation, diarrhea, flatulence
Rare (less than 2%)
Rash, severe bone, joint, muscle pain

SERIOUS REACTIONS
- Overdose causes hypocalcemia, hypophosphatemia, and significant GI disturbances.
- Esophageal irritation occurs if alendronate is not given with 6-8 ounces of plain water or if the patient lies down within 30 minutes of drug administration.

INTERACTIONS
Drugs
3 *Antacids:* Calcium, magnesium, and aluminum bind alendronate and reduce absorption
3 *Aspirin:* Increased risk of upper GI adverse effects
3 *Food (including coffee and orange juice):* Decreases bioavailability of alendronate by 40%-60%
3 *IV ranitidine:* May double the bioavailability of alendronate

SPECIAL CONSIDERATIONS
PATIENT/FAMILY EDUCATION
- Patients should receive supplemental calcium and vitamin D if dietary intake is inadequate
- Administer 30 min before the first food/beverage/medication of the day with 6-8 oz plain water; avoid lying down for at least 30 min
- Weekly administration may be an advantage
- Some experts recommend cessation of therapy after 5 yrs due to theoretical concerns of poor quality bone formation with prolonged therapy
- Consider beginning weight-bearing exercises and modifying behavioral factors, such as reducing alcohol consumption and stopping cigarette smoking

MONITORING PARAMETERS
- Serum electrolytes, including serum alkaline phosphatase and serum calcium levels

alfuzosin hydrochloride
(ale-fyoo-zoe′-sin)
Rx: Uroxatral
Chemical Class: Quinazoline
Therapeutic Class: α_1-adrenergic blocker

CLINICAL PHARMACOLOGY
Mechanism of Action: An alpha$_1$ antagonist that targets receptors around bladder neck and prostate capsule. ***Therapeutic Effect:*** Relaxes smooth muscle and improves urinary flow and symptoms of prostatic hyperplasia.

Pharmacokinetics

Rapidly absorbed and widely distributed. Protein binding: 90%. Extensively metabolized in the liver. Primarily excreted in urine. ***Half-life:*** 3-9 hr.

INDICATIONS AND DOSAGES

Benign prostatic hyperplasia

PO

Adults. 10 mg once a day, approximately 30 min after same meal each day.

AVAILABLE FORMS

• *Tablets (Extended-Release):* 10 mg.

CONTRAINDICATIONS: Hepatic disease, concomitant use of ketoconazole, itraconazole, ritonavir

PREGNANCY AND LACTATION: Pregnancy category B, but not indicated for use in women

SIDE EFFECTS

Frequent (7%-6%)

Dizziness, headache, malaise

Occasional (4%)

Dry mouth

Rare (3%-2%)

Nausea, dyspepsia (such as heartburn, and epigastric discomfort), diarrhea, orthostatic hypotension, tachycardia, drowsiness

SERIOUS REACTIONS

• Ischemia-related chest pain may occur rarely.

• Priapism has been reported.

INTERACTIONS

Drugs

3 *Atenolol:* Atenolol increases peak plasma alfuzosin level by 25%; alfuzosin increases plasma atenolol levels by 25%

3 *Cimetidine:* Cimetidine increases peak plasma alfuzosin level by 20%

❷ *Diltiazem:* Diltiazem increases peak plasma alfuzosin level by 50%; alfuzosin increases plasma diltiazem level by 50%

⚠ *Itraconazole:* Itraconazole markedly increases plasma alfuzosin level

⚠ *Ketoconazole:* Ketoconazole markedly increases plasma alfuzosin level

3 *Other alpha blockers, such as doxazosin, prazosin, tamsulosin, and terazosin:* May increase the alpha-blockade effects of both drugs

⚠ *Ritonavir:* Ritonavir markedly increases plasma alfuzosin level

SPECIAL CONSIDERATIONS

• In clinical trials, peak flow rates increase from a baseline of 10 ml/sec to 12 ml/sec; American Urological Association (AUA) scores decreased by 4-7 points from a baseline of 18

PATIENT/FAMILY EDUCATION

• Take immediately after the same meal each day

• Hypotension or postural hypotension may occur with first doses

• Avoid performing tasks that require mental alertness or motor skills until response to the drug has been established

• Notify the physician if headache occurs

• Do not chew or crush extended-release tablets

MONITORING PARAMETERS

• Liver function

allopurinol

(al-oh-pure'-i-nole)

Rx: Aloprim, Zyloprim

Chemical Class: Hypoxanthine isomer; xanthine oxidase inhibitor

Therapeutic Class: Antigout agent

CLINICAL PHARMACOLOGY

Mechanism of Action: A xanthine oxidase inhibitor that decreases uric acid production by inhibiting xanthine oxidase, an enzyme. ***Therapeutic Effect:*** Reduces uric acid concentrations in both serum and urine.

Pharmacokinetics

Route	*Onset*	*Peak*	*Duration*
PO/IV	2-3 days	1-3 wk	1-2 wk

Well absorbed from the GI tract. Widely distributed. Metabolized in the liver to active metabolite. Excreted primarily in urine. Removed by hemodialysis. ***Half-life:*** 1-3 hr; metabolite, 12-30 hr.

INDICATIONS AND DOSAGES

Chronic gouty arthritis

PO

Adults, Children older than 10 yr. Initially, 100 mg/day; may increase by 100 mg/day at weekly intervals. Maximum: 800 mg/day. Maintenance: 100-200 mg 2-3 times a day or 300 mg/day.

To prevent uric acid nephropathy during chemotherapy

PO

Adults: Initially, 600-800 mg/day starting 2-3 days before initiation of chemotherapy or radiation therapy.

Children 6-10 yr. 100 mg 3 times a day or 300 mg once a day.

Children less than 6 yr. 50 mg 3 times a day.

IV

Adults. 200-400 mg/m^2/day beginning 24-48 hr before initiation of chemotherapy.

Children. 200 mg/m^2/day. Maximum: 600 mg/day.

Alert: Maintenance dosage is based on serum uric acid levels. Discontinue following the period of tumor regression.

Prevention of uric acid calculi

PO

Adults. 100-200 mg 1-4 times a day or 300 mg once a day.

Recurrent calcium oxalate calculi

PO

Adults. 200-300 mg/day

Elderly. Initially, 100 mg/day, gradually increased until optimal uric acid level is reached.

Dosage in renal impairment

Dosage is modified based on creatinine clearance.

Creatinine Clearance	*Dosage Adjustment*
10-20 ml/min	200 mg/day
3-9 ml/min	100 mg/day
Less than 3 ml/min	100 mg at extended intervals

AVAILABLE FORMS

• *Tablets (Zyloprim):* 100 mg, 300 mg.

• *Powder for Injection (Aloprim):* 500 mg.

UNLABELED USES: In mouthwash following fluorouracil therapy to prevent stomatitis

CONTRAINDICATIONS: Asymptomatic hyperuricemia

PREGNANCY AND LACTATION: Pregnancy category C; allopurinol and oxypurinol have been found in the milk of a mother who was receiving allopurinol

SIDE EFFECTS

Occasional

Oral: Somnolence, unusual hair loss

IV: Rash, nausea, vomiting
Rare
Diarrhea, headache

SERIOUS REACTIONS

- Pruritic maculopapular rash possibly accompanied by malaise, fever, chills, joint pain, nausea, and vomiting should be considered a toxic reaction.
- Severe hypersensitivity may follow appearance of rash.
- Bone marrow depression, hepatic toxicity, peripheral neuritis, and acute renal failure occur rarely.

INTERACTIONS

Drugs

❷ *Angiotensin-converting enzyme inhibitors:* Predisposed to hypersensitivity reactions including Stevens-Johnson syndrome, skin eruptions, fever, and arthralgias

❸ *Antacids:* Aluminum hydroxide inhibits the response to allopurinol

❷ *Azathioprine:* Increased toxicity of azathioprine; requires dose adjustment

❸ *Cyclophosphamide:* May increase cyclophosphamide toxicity

❸ *Cyclosporine/tacrolimus:* Increased toxicity of immunosuppressive drug

❷ *Mercaptopurine:* Increased effect of mercaptopurine with increased risk of toxicity

❸ *Oral anticoagulants:* Enhanced hypoprothrombinemic response

❸ *Theophylline:* Large doses may increase serum theophylline levels

❸ *Thiazide diuretics:* Decreases the effects of allopurinol

SPECIAL CONSIDERATIONS

- Increased acute attacks of gout during early stages of allopurinol administration—cover with colchicine
- Maintenance doses of colchicine (0.6 mg qd-bid) should be given prophylactically along with starting with low doses of allopurinol
- To reduce risk of flare, begin with 100 mg qd and increase by 100 mg qwk until serum uric acid ≤6mg/dL
- Parenteral formulation available as orphan drug and in Canada

PATIENT/FAMILY EDUCATION

- It may take 1 week or longer of administration of the drug for it to reach full therapeutic effect
- Drink 10 to 12 eight-ounce glasses of fluid daily while taking medication
- Avoid tasks that require mental alertness or motor skills until response to the drug is established

MONITORING PARAMETERS

- Serum uric acid; can usually be achieved in 1-3 wks

---

almotriptan malate

(al-moh-trip′-tan mal′-ate)

Rx: Axert

Chemical Class: Serotonin derivative

Therapeutic Class: Antimigraine agent

CLINICAL PHARMACOLOGY

Mechanism of Action: A serotonin receptor agonist that binds selectively to vascular receptors, producing a vasoconstrictive effect on cranial blood vessels. ***Therapeutic Effect:*** Produces relief of migraine headache.

Pharmacokinetics

Well absorbed after PO administration. Metabolized by the liver, excreted in urine. ***Half-life:*** 3-4 hr.

INDICATIONS AND DOSAGES

Migraine headache

PO

Adults, Elderly. Initially, 6.25-12.5 mg as a single dose. If headache improves but then returns, dose may be repeated after 2 hr. Maximum: 2 doses/24 hr.

Dosage in renal impairment
For adult and elderly patients, recommended initial dose is 6.25 mg and maximum daily dose is 12.5 mg.

AVAILABLE FORMS

• *Tablets:* 6.5 mg, 12.5 mg.

CONTRAINDICATIONS: Arrhythmias associated with conduction disorders, hemiplegic or basilar migraine, ischemic heart disease (including angina pectoris, history of MI, silent ischemia, and Prinzmetal's angina), uncontrolled hypertension, use within 24 hours of ergotamine-containing preparation or another serotonin receptor antagonist, use within 14 days of MAOIs, Wolff-Parkinson-White syndrome

PREGNANCY AND LACTATION: Pregnancy category C; excretion in human breast milk unknown (but excreted into milk in lactating rats); use caution in nursing mothers

SIDE EFFECTS

Frequent
Nausea, dry mouth, paresthesia, flushing

Occasional
Changes in temperature sensation, asthenia, dizziness

SERIOUS REACTIONS

• Excessive dosage may produce tremor, red extremities, reduced respirations, cyanosis, seizures, and chest pain.

• Serious arrhythmias occur rarely, particularly in patients with hypertension or diabetes, obese patients, smokers, and those with a strong family history of coronary artery disease.

INTERACTIONS

Drugs

▲ *Egotomine-containing drugs:* Increased vasoconstriction

▲ *Other 5-HT$_1$-agonists:* Increased vasoconstriction

3 *MAO inhibitors:* Decreased almotriptan clearance

3 *Ketoconazole, itraconazole, ritonavir, erythromycin:* Increased plasma concentrations of almotriptan

2 *Sibutramine:* Theoretical increase in the risk of serotonin syndrome

SPECIAL CONSIDERATIONS

• Safety of treating, on average, more than 4 headaches in a 30-day period has not been established

• Controlled trials have not adequately established the effectiveness of a second dose if the initial dose is ineffective

• Superiority over other triptan migraine headache agents has not been demonstrated

PATIENT/FAMILY EDUCATION

• Use only to treat migraine headache, not for prevention

• Take a single dose of almotriptan as soon migraine symptoms appear

• Lie down in a quiet, dark room for additional benefit after taking this drug

• Avoid tasks that require mental alertness or motor skills until response to the drug has been established

• Notify the physician immediately if palpitations, pain or tightness in the chest or throat, or pain or weakness in the extremities occurs

MONITORING PARAMETERS

• Evaluate for relief of migraines and associated symptoms, including nausea and vomiting, photophobia, and phonophobia (sound sensitivity)

alprazolam

(al-pray'-zoe-lam)

Rx: Xanax, Niravam, Xanax XR

Chemical Class: Benzodiazepine

Therapeutic Class: Anxiolytic

DEA Class: Schedule IV

CLINICAL PHARMACOLOGY

Mechanism of Action: A benzodiazepine that enhances the action of the inhibitory neurotransmitter gamma-aminobutyric acid in the brain. ***Therapeutic Effect:*** Produces anxiolytic effect from its CNS depressant action.

Pharmacokinetics

Well absorbed from GI tract. Protein binding: 80%. Metabolized in the liver. Primarily excreted in urine. Minimal removal by hemodialysis. ***Half-life:*** 11-16 hr.

INDICATIONS AND DOSAGES

Anxiety disorders

PO (Immediate-Release)

Adults. Initially, 0.25-0.5 mg 3 times a day. May titrate q3-4 days. Maximum: 4 mg/day in divided doses.

Elderly, Debilitated patients, Patients with hepatic disease or low serum albumin. Initially, 0.25 mg 2-3 times a day. Gradually increase to optimum therapeutic response.

PO (Orally Disintegrating)

Adults. 0.25-0.5 mg 3 times a day. Maximum: 4 mg/day in divided doses.

Anxiety with depression

PO

Adults. 2.5-3 mg/day in divided doses.

Panic disorder

PO (Immediate-Release)

Adults. Initially, 0.5 mg 3 times a day. May increase at 3- to 4-day intervals. Range: 5-6 mg/day. Maximum: 10 mg/day.

Elderly. Initially, 0.125-0.25 mg twice a day. May increase in 0.125-mg increments until desired effect attained.

PO (Extended-Release)

Alert: To switch from immediate-release to extended-release form, give total daily dose (immediate-release) as a single daily dose of extended-release form.

Adults. Initially, 0.5-1 mg once a day. May titrate at 3- to 4-day intervals. Range: 3-6 mg/day. Maximum: 10 mg/day.

Elderly. Initially, 0.5 mg once daily.

PO (Orally Disintegrating)

Adults. Initially, 0.5 mg 3 times a day. May increase at 3- to 4-day intervals. Range: 5-6 mg/day. Maximum: 10 mg/day.

Premenstrual syndrome

PO

Adults. 0.25 mg 3 times a day.

AVAILABLE FORMS

- *Oral Solution (Alprazolam Intensol):* 1 mg/ml.
- *Tablets (Xanax):* 0.25 mg, 0.5 mg, 1 mg, 2 mg.
- *Tablets (Extended-Release [Xanax XR]):* 0.5 mg, 1 mg, 2 mg, 3 mg.
- *Tablets (Orally Disintegrating [Niravam]):* 0.25 mg, 0.5 mg, 1 mg, 2 mg.

UNLABELED USES: Management of premenstrual syndrome symptoms (mood disturbances, insomnia, and cramps), irritable bowel syndrome, treatment of agoraphobia, post-traumatic stress disorder, tremors, ethanol withdrawal, anxiety in children

CONTRAINDICATIONS: Acute alcohol intoxication with depressed vital signs, acute angle-closure glaucoma, concurrent use of itraconazole or ketoconazole, myasthenia gravis, severe COPD

PREGNANCY AND LACTATION: Pregnancy category D; children born of a mother receiving benzodiazepines may be at risk for withdrawal symptoms; neonatal flaccidity and respiratory problems have been reported; chronic administration of diazepam to nursing mothers has been reported to cause infants to become lethargic and lose weight

Controlled Substance: Schedule IV

SIDE EFFECTS

Frequent

Ataxia; lightheadedness; transient, mild somnolence; slurred speech (particularly in elderly or debilitated patients)

Occasional

Confusion, depression, blurred vision, constipation, diarrhea, dry mouth, headache, nausea

Rare

Behavioral problems such as anger, impaired memory; paradoxical reactions such as insomnia, nervousness, or irritability

SERIOUS REACTIONS

- Abrupt or too-rapid withdrawal may result in pronounced restlessness, irritability, insomnia, hand tremors, abdominal and muscle cramps, diaphoresis, vomiting, and seizures.
- Overdose results in somnolence, confusion, diminished reflexes, and coma.
- Blood dyscrasias have been reported rarely.

INTERACTIONS

Drugs

3 *Cimetidine:* Cimetidine inhibits metabolism, increases plasma levels

3 *Digoxin:* Inconsistently raises digoxin levels

3 *Erythromycin, clarithromycin, troleandomycin:* Possible increased sedation

3 *Ethanol:* Enhanced adverse psychomotor effects; difficulty performing tasks that require alertness

3 *Fluoxetine, fluvoxamine, ketoconazole, itraconazole, nefazadone (see contraindications):* Increases alprazolam plasma concentrations; increases in psychomotor impairment

3 *Grapefruit juice:* Increased alprazolam levels due to inhibition of presystemic (intestinal) enzyme CYP34A

3 *Phenytoin, carbamazepine:* Decreased benzodiazepine effect

3 *Kava kava, valerian:* Increases CNS depressant effect of alprazolam

SPECIAL CONSIDERATIONS

PATIENT/FAMILY EDUCATION

- Not for "everyday" stress or longer than 3 mo; avoid driving, activities that require alertness
- Caution when medication discontinued abruptly after long-term (>4 wks) use—may precipitate withdrawal syndrome
- Avoid tasks that require mental alertness or motor skills until response to the drug is established
- Smoking reduces alprazolam's effectiveness

alprostadil (prostaglandin E_1, PGE_1)

(al-pros'-ta-dil)

Rx: Caverject, Edex, Muse, Prostin VR Pediatric

Chemical Class: Prostaglandin E_1

Therapeutic Class: Anti-impotence agent; patent ductus arteriosus

CLINICAL PHARMACOLOGY

Mechanism of Action: A prostaglandin that directly affects vascular and ductus arteriosus smooth muscle and relaxes trabecular smooth muscle. ***Therapeutic Effect:*** Causes vasodilation; dilates cavernosal arteries, allowing blood flow to and entrapment in the lacunar spaces of the penis.

Pharmacokinetics

Absorption occurs from the urethral lining when inserted as a urethral suppository. Protein binding: 81%-99% (injection). Rapidly metabolized. Excreted in urine and lung. ***Half-life:*** 5-10 min (injection).

INDICATIONS AND DOSAGES

Maintain patency of ductus arteriosus

IV infusion

Neonates. Initially, 0.05-0.1 mcg/kg/min. Maintenance: 0.01-0.4 mcg/kg/min. Maximum: 0.4 mcg/kg/min.

Impotence

Pellet, Intracavernosal

Adults. Dosage is individualized.

AVAILABLE FORMS

- *Injection (Prostin VR Pediatric):* 500 mcg/ml.
- *Powder for Injection (Caverject, Edex):* 10 mcg, 20 mcg, 40 mcg.
- *Urethral Pellet (Muse):* 125 mcg, 250 mcg, 500 mcg, 1000 mcg.

UNLABELED USES: Treatment of atherosclerosis, gangrene, pain due to severe peripheral arterial occlusive disease, treatment of pulmonary hypertension in infants and children

CONTRAINDICATIONS: Conditions predisposing to anatomic deformation of penis, hyaline membrane disease, penile implants, priapism, respiratory distress syndrome

PREGNANCY AND LACTATION: Pregnancy category C

SIDE EFFECTS

Frequent

Intracavernosal (4%-1%): Penile pain (37%), prolonged erection, hypertension, localized pain, penile fibrosis, injection site hematoma or ecchymosis, headache, respiratory infection, flu-like symptoms

Intraurethral (3%): Penile pain (36%), urethral pain or burning, testicular pain, urethral bleeding, headache, dizziness, respiratory infection, flu-like symptoms

Systemic (greater than 1%): Fever, flushing, bradycardia, hypotension, tachycardia, diarrhea

Occasional

Intracavernosal (less than 1%): Hypotension, pelvic pain, back pain, dizziness, cough, nasal congestion

Intraurethral (less than 3%): Fainting, sinusitis, back and pelvic pain

Systemic (less than 1%): Anxiety, lethargy, myalgia, arrhythmias, respiratory depression, anemia, bleeding, hematuria

SERIOUS REACTIONS

Alert: Apnea is experienced by about 10%-12% of neonates with congenital heart defects.

- Overdose is manifested as apnea, flushing of the face and arms, and bradycardia.

• Cardiac arrest and sepsis occur rarely.
• Seizures, apnea, sepsis, and thrombocytopenia occur rarely.

INTERACTIONS

Drugs

3 *Anticoagulants:* Increases the risk of bleeding
3 *Sympathomimetics:* Decreases the effect of alprostadil
3 *Vasodilators:* Increases risk of hypotension

SPECIAL CONSIDERATIONS

• For intracavernosal use administer first dose under medical supervision. Use ½-inch 27-30-gauge needle along dorso-lateral aspect of proximal third of penis. Alternate sides.
• Urinate prior to intraurethral use to disperse pellet
• Use lowest dose allowing satisfactory erection lasting ≥1 h

MONITORING PARAMETERS

• Infant ABGs, arterial pH, arterial pressure, continuous ECG

alteplase, recombinant

(al-teep'-lase)
Rx: Activase, Cathflo Activase
Chemical Class: Tissue plasminogen activator (tPA)
Therapeutic Class: Thrombolytic

CLINICAL PHARMACOLOGY

Mechanism of Action: A tissue plasminogen activator that acts as a thrombolytic by binding to the fibrin in a thrombus and converting entrapped plasminogen to plasmin. This process initiates fibrinolysis. ***Therapeutic Effect:*** Degrades fibrin clots, fibrinogen, and other plasma proteins.

Pharmacokinetics

Rapidly metabolized in the liver. Primarily excreted in urine. ***Half-life:*** 35 min.

INDICATIONS AND DOSAGES

Acute MI

IV Infusion

Adults weighing greater than 67 kg. 100 mg over 90 min, starting with 15-mg bolus over 1-2 min, then 50 mg over 30 min, then 35 mg over 60 min. Or a 3-hour infusion, giving 60 mg over first hr (6-10 mg as bolus over 1-2 min), 20 mg over second hr, and 20 mg over third hr.

Adults weighing 67 kg or less: 100 mg over 90 min, starting with 15-mg bolus, then 0.75 mg/kg over 30 min (maximum: 50 mg), then 0.5 mg/kg over 60 min (maximum: 35 mg). Or 3-hour infusion of 1.25 mg/kg giving 60% of dose over first hr (6%-10% as 1- to 2-min bolus), 20% over second hr, and 20% over third hr.

Acute pulmonary emboli

IV Infusion

Adults. 100 mg over 2 hr. Institute or reinstitute heparin near end or immediately after infusion when aPTT or thrombin time (TT) returns to twice normal or less.

Acute ischemic stroke

IV Infusion

Adults. 0.9 mg/kg over 60 min (load with 0.09 mg/kg [10% of 0.9 mg/kg dose] as IV bolus over 1 min).

Alert: Dose should be given within the first 3 hours of the onset of symptoms.

Central venous catheter clearance

IV

Adults, Elderly. 2 mg; may repeat after 2 hr.

AVAILABLE FORMS

• *Powder for Injection:* 2 mg (Cathflo Activase), 50 mg (Activase), 100 mg (Activase).

UNLABELED USES: Acute peripheral occlusive disease, basilar artery occlusion, cerebral infarction, deep vein thrombosis, femoropopliteal artery occlusion, mesenteric or subclavian vein occlusion, pleural effusion (parapneumonic)

CONTRAINDICATIONS: Active internal bleeding, AV malformation or aneurysm, bleeding diathesis, intracranial neoplasm, intracranial or intraspinal surgery or trauma, recent (within past 2 months) cerebrovascular accident, severe uncontrolled hypertension

PREGNANCY AND LACTATION: Pregnancy category C; unknown if excreted in breast milk

SIDE EFFECTS

Frequent

Superficial bleeding at puncture sites, decreased BP

Occasional

Allergic reaction, such as rash or wheezing; bruising

SERIOUS REACTIONS

- Severe internal hemorrhage may occur.
- Lysis of coronary thrombi may produce atrial or ventricular arrhythmias or stroke.

INTERACTIONS

Drugs

3 *Heparin, oral anticoagulants, drugs that alter platelet function (i.e., aspirin, dipyridamole, abciximab, eptifibitide, tirofiban):* May increase the risk of bleeding

Labs

- *Decrease:* Fibrinogen (mitigated by collecting blood in presence of aprotinin)

SPECIAL CONSIDERATIONS

- Heparin (in doses sufficient to prolong the aPTT to 1.5-2 times control value) is usually administered in conjunction with thrombolytic therapy; aspirin may also be administered to inhibit platelet aggregation during and/or following post-thrombolytic therapy
- Compress arterial puncture sites at least 30 min

MONITORING PARAMETERS

- Prior to initiation of therapy: coagulation tests, hematocrit, platelet count
- Blood pressure

aluminum chloride hexahydrate

(a-loo′-mi-num klor′-ide hexa-hye′-drate)

Rx: Drysol, Xerac AC

OTC: powder, solution

Chemical Class: Trivalent cation

Therapeutic Class: Antihidrotic

CLINICAL PHARMACOLOGY

Mechanism of Action: Aluminum salts cause an obstruction of the distal sweat gland. This obstruction causes metal ions to precipitate with mucopolysaccharides, damaging epithelial cells along the lumen of the duct, and forming a plug to block sweat output. ***Therapeutic Effect:*** Results in decreased secretion of the sweat glands.

Pharmacokinetics

Not known.

INDICATIONS AND DOSAGES

Antiperspirant

Topical

Adults, Elderly, Children 12 yrs and older. Apply to each underarm once a day, at bedtime.

Hyperhidrosis

Topical

Adults, Elderly, Children 12 yrs and older. Apply to affected areas once a day, at bedtime.

AVAILABLE FORMS

• *Topical Solution:* 6.25% (Xerac AC), 20% (Drysol).

CONTRAINDICATIONS: Hypersensitivity to aluminum chloride or any one of its components.

PREGNANCY AND LACTATION: Pregnancy category C

SIDE EFFECTS

Frequent

Itching, burning, tingling sensation

Occasional

Rash

SERIOUS REACTIONS

• Hypersensitivity reaction, such as rash, may occur.

SPECIAL CONSIDERATIONS

PATIENT/FAMILY EDUCATION

• Do not apply to broken or irritated skin

• For maximum effect, cover treated area with saran wrap held in place by snug-fitting shirt, mitten or sock (never hold saran wrap in place with tape)

• Avoid contact with eyes

• May be harmful to cotton fibers or certain metals

• Do not apply other deodorants or antiperspirants while using this drug

aluminum salts

Combinations

OTC: Aluminum acetate and acetic acid (Otic Domeboro); aluminum hydroxide and magnesium carbonate (Gaviscon Extra Strength, Gaviscon Liquid); aluminum hydroxide and magnesium trisillicate (Gaviscon); aluminum hydroxide, magnesium hydroxide, and simethicone (Maalox Fast Release Liquid, Maalox Max, Mylanta Extra Strength Liquid, Mylanta Liquid); aluminum sulfate and calcium acetate (Bluboro, Domeboro, Pedi-Boro)

Chemical Class: Trivalent cation

Therapeutic Class: Antacid; phosphate adsorbent

CLINICAL PHARMACOLOGY

Mechanism of Action: An antacid that reduces gastric acid by binding with phosphate in the intestine, and then is excreted as aluminum carbonate in feces. Aluminum carbonate may increase the absorption of calcium due to decreased serum phosphate levels. The drug also has astringent and adsorbent properties.

Therapeutic Effect: Neutralizes or increases gastric pH; reduces phosphates in urine, preventing formation of phosphate urinary stones; reduces serum phosphate levels; decreases fluidity of stools.

Pharmacokinetics

Varies in each formulation.

INDICATIONS AND DOSAGES

Aluminum hydroxide

Peptic ulcer disease: PO: *Adults, Elderly, Children.* 5-15 ml as above.

15-45 ml q3-6h or 1 and 3 hr after meals and at bedtime.

Antacid: PO: *Adults, Elderly.* 30 ml 1 and 3 hr after meals and at bedtime.

Gastrointestinal (GI) bleeding prevention: PO: *Adults, Elderly.* 30-60 ml/hr. *Children.* 5-15 ml q1-2h.

Hyperphosphatemia: PO: *Adults, Elderly.* 500-1800 mg 1 and 3 hr after meals and at bedtime. *Children.* 50-150 mg/kg/24 hr q4-6h.

Aluminum acetate & acetic acid

Superficial infections of the external auditory canal: Otic: *Adults, Elderly.* Instill 4-6 drops in ear(s) q2-3h.

Aluminum hydroxide & magnesium carbonate

Antacid: PO: *Adults, Elderly.* 15-30 ml 4 times/day of the liquid; chew 2-4 tablets 4 times/day.

Aluminum hydroxide & magnesium hydroxide

Antacid: PO: *Adults, Elderly.* 5-10 ml 4-6 times/day.

Aluminum hydroxide & magnesium trisillicate

Antacid: PO: *Adults, Elderly.* Chew 2-4 tablets 4 times/day or as directed.

Aluminum hydroxide, magnesium hydroxide, and simethicone

Antacid (with flatulence): PO: *Adults, Elderly.* 10-20 ml or 2-4 tablets 4-6 times/day.

Aluminum sulfate & calcium acetate

Inflammatory skin conditions with weeping that occurs in dermatitis: Topical: *Adults, Elderly.* Soak affected area in solution 2-4 times/day for 15-30 min or apply wet dressing soaked in solution 2-4 times/day for 30-min treatment periods. Domeboro: Saturate dressing and apply to affected area and saturate every 15-30 min; or soak for 15-30 min 3 times/day.

AVAILABLE FORMS

Aluminum hydroxide

- *Capsules:* 400 mg (Alu-Cap), 500 mg (Dialume).
- *Liquid:* 600 mg/5 mg (ALternagel).
- *Suspension:* 320 mg/5 ml (Amphojel), 450 mg/5 ml, 675 mg/5 ml.
- *Tablets:* 300 mg (Amphojel), 500 mg (Alu-Tab), 600 mg (Amphojel).

Aluminum acetate & acetic acid

- *Otic solution:* 2% acetic acid and aluminum acetate (Otic Domeboro).

Aluminum hydroxide and magnesium carbonate

- *Liquid:* 31.7 mg aluminum hydroxide and 119.3 mg magnesium carbonate/5 ml (Gaviscon Liquid), 84.6 mg aluminum hydroxide and 79.1 mg magnesium carbonate/5 ml (Gaviscon Extra Strength).
- *Tablets, chewable:* 160 mg aluminum hydroxide and 1.5 mg magnesium carbonate (Gaviscon Extra Strength Relief).

Aluminum hydroxide & magnesium hydroxide

- *Suspension:* 225 mg aluminum hydroxide and 200 mg magnesium hydroxide/5 ml (Maalox).
- *Suspension:* 600 mg aluminum hydroxide and 300 mg magnesium hydroxide/5 ml (Maalox TC).

Aluminum hydroxide & magnesium trisillicate

- *Tablets, chewable:* 80 mg aluminum hydroxide and 20 mg magnesium hydroxide (Gaviscon).

Aluminum hydroxide, magnesium hydroxide, & simethicone

- *Liquid:* 200 mg aluminum hydroxide, 200 mg magnesium hydroxide, and 20 mg simethicone/5 ml (Mylanta), 400 mg aluminum hydroxide, 400 mg magnesium hydroxide, and 40 mg simethicone/5 ml (Maalox Max), 500 mg aluminum hydroxide, 450 mg magnesium hydroxide, and 20 mg simethicone/5 ml (Maalox Fast Release), 400 mg aluminum hydroxide, 400 mg magnesium hydroxide, and 40 mg simethicone/5 ml (Mylanta Extra Strength).

Aluminum sulfate & calcium acetate

• *Powder, for topical solution:* packets (Bluboro, Domeboro, Pedi-Boro).

• *Tablets, effervescent, for topical solution:* effervescent tablets (Domeboro).

CONTRAINDICATIONS: Children age 6 yrs or younger, intestinal obstruction, hypersensitivity to aluminum or any component of the formulation

PREGNANCY AND LACTATION: Pregnancy category C

SIDE EFFECTS

Frequent

PO: Chalky taste, mild constipation, stomach cramps

Topical: Burning, itching

Occasional

PO: Nausea, vomiting, speckling or whitish discoloration of stools

Otic: Burning or stinging in ear

Topical: New or continued redness, skin dryness

Rare

Otic: Skin rash, redness, swelling or pain in ear

SERIOUS REACTIONS

• Prolonged constipation may result in intestinal obstruction.

• Excessive or chronic use may produce hypophosphatemia manifested as anorexia, malaise, muscle weakness or bone pain and resulting in osteomalacia and osteoporosis.

• Prolonged use may produce urinary calculi.

INTERACTIONS

Drugs

3 *Allopurinol, atenolol, ketoconazole, itraconazole (not fluconazole):* Aluminum hydroxide inhibits GI absorption

3 *Cefpodoxime, cefuroxime:* Reduced antibiotic bioavailability and serum concentration

3 *Cyclosporine:* Reduced cyclosporine blood concentrations possible

3 *Glipizide, glyburide:* Enhanced absorption of hypoglycemic agent

3 *Iron:* Reduced GI absorption of iron; separate doses by 1-2 hr

3 *Isoniazid:* Some antacids reduce plasma concentration of isoniazid

3 *Penicillamine:* Reduced penicillamine bioavailability

3 *Quinolones:* Reduced serum concentration of antibiotics

3 *Salicylates:* Decreased serum salicylate concentrations

3 *Sodium polystyrene sulfonate resin:* Combined use may result in systemic alkalosis

3 *Tetracycline:* Reduced serum concentration and efficacy of tetracycline

3 *Vitamin C:* Increases aluminum absorption

SPECIAL CONSIDERATIONS

PATIENT/FAMILY EDUCATION

• Thoroughly chew chewable tablets before swallowing, follow with a glass of water

• May impair absorption of many drugs; do not take other drugs within 1-4 hr of aluminum hydroxide administration

• Stools may appear white or speckled

• Maintain adequate fluid intake

MONITORING PARAMETERS

• Consider monitoring for hypophosphatemia

• Daily bowel activity and stool consistency

amantadine hydrochloride

(a-man'-ta-deen hye-droe-klor'-ide)

Rx: Symmetrel

Chemical Class: Adamantane derivative; tricyclic amine

Therapeutic Class: Anti-Parkinson's agent; antiviral

CLINICAL PHARMACOLOGY

Mechanism of Action: A dopaminergic agonist that blocks the uncoating of influenza A virus, preventing penetration into the host and inhibiting M2 protein in the assembly of progeny virions. Amantadine also blocks the reuptake of dopamine into presynaptic neurons and causes direct stimulation of postsynaptic receptors. ***Therapeutic Effect:*** Antiviral and antiparkinsonian activity.

Pharmacokinetics

Rapidly and completely absorbed from the GI tract. Protein binding: 67%. Widely distributed. Primarily excreted in urine. Minimally removed by hemodialysis. ***Half-life:*** 11-15 hr (increased in the elderly, decreased in impaired renal function).

INDICATIONS AND DOSAGES

Treatment of Influenza A

PO

Adults, Children 13 yr and older. 100 mg twice a day. Initiate within 24-48 hr after onset of symptoms; discontinue as soon as possible based on clinical response.

Elderly. 100 mg once a day.

Children 10-12 yr, weighing 40 kg and more. 100 mg twice a day

Children 10 yr and older, weighing less than 40 kg. 5 mg/kg/day. Maximum: 150 mg/day.

Children 1-9 yr. 5 mg/kg/day. Maximum: 150 mg/day.

Prevention of Influenza A

PO

Adults, Children 13 yr and older. 100 mg twice a day

Parkinson's disease, extrapyramidal symptoms

PO

Adults, Elderly. 100 mg twice a day. May increase up to 400 mg/day in divided doses.

Dosage in renal impairment

Dose and frequency are modified based on creatinine clearance.

Creatinine Clearance	Dosage
30-50 ml/min	200 mg first day; 100 mg/day thereafter
15-29 ml/min	200 mg first day; 100 mg on alternate days
less than 15 ml/min	200 mg every 7 days

AVAILABLE FORMS

- *Capsules:* 100 mg.
- *Syrup:* 50 mg/5 ml.
- *Tablets:* 100 mg.

UNLABELED USES: Treatment of ADHD, fatigue associated with multiple sclerosis

CONTRAINDICATIONS: None known.

PREGNANCY AND LACTATION: Pregnancy category C; excreted in human milk; exercise caution when administering to nursing mothers because of potential for urinary retention, vomiting, and skin rash

SIDE EFFECTS

Frequent (10%-5%)

Nausea, dizziness, poor concentration, insomnia, nervousness

Occasional (5%-1%)

Orthostatic hypotension, anorexia, headache, livedo reticularis (reddish blue, netlike blotching of skin), blurred vision, urine retention, dry mouth or nose

Rare

Vomiting, depression, irritation or swelling of eyes, rash

SERIOUS REACTIONS

• CHF, leukopenia, and neutropenia occur rarely.

• Hyperexcitability, seizures, and ventricular arrhythmias may occur.

INTERACTIONS

Drugs

3 *Anticholinergics:* Increased anticholinergic effects

3 *Antihistamines:* Increased anticholinergic effects

3 *Benztropine:* Potentiation of amantadine's CNS side effects

3 *Hydrochlorothiazide:* Increased risk of amantadine toxicity

3 *Phenothiazines:* Increased anticholinergic effects

3 *Triamterene:* Increased amantadine toxicity

3 *Tricyclic antidepressants:* Increased anticholinergic effects

3 *Trihexyphenidyl:* Potentiation of amantadine's CNS side effects

SPECIAL CONSIDERATIONS

PATIENT/FAMILY EDUCATION

• Administer at least 4 hr before bedtime to prevent insomnia

• Take with meals for better absorption and to decrease GI symptoms

• Arise slowly from a reclining position; avoid hazardous activities if dizziness or blurred vision occurs

• Do not discontinue abruptly in Parkinson's disease

MONITORING PARAMETERS

• Renal function

• Intake and output

• Clinical reversal of symptoms

ambenonium chloride

(am-be-noe'-nee-um klor'-ide)

Rx: Mytelase

Chemical Class: Cholinesterase inhibitor; quaternary ammonium compound

Therapeutic Class: Cholinergic

CLINICAL PHARMACOLOGY

Mechanism of Action: A cholinesterase inhibitor that enhances and prolongs cholinergic function by increasing the concentration of acetylcholine through inhibition of the hydrolysis of acetylcholine. ***Therapeutic Effect:*** Increases muscle strength in myasthenia gravis.

Pharmacokinetics

Poorly absorbed after PO administration.

INDICATIONS AND DOSAGES

Myasthenia gravis

PO

Adults. 5-25 mg 3 or 4 times a day. If well tolerated, after 1 or 2 days, may increase to 50-75 mg 3 times a day. Range: 5-200 mg/day in divided doses.

AVAILABLE FORMS

• *Tablets:* 10 mg (Mytelase).

CONTRAINDICATIONS: Not recommended in patients receiving routine administration of atropine or other belladonna derivatives. Not recommended in patients receiving mecamylamine.

PREGNANCY AND LACTATION: Pregnancy category C; would not be expected to cross placenta or be excreted into breast milk because it is ionized at physiologic pH; although apparently safe for the fetus, may cause transient muscle weakness in the newborn

SIDE EFFECTS

Frequent

Abdominal pain, diarrhea, increased salivation, miosis, sweating, and vomiting

Occasional

Anxiety, blurred vision, and urinary urgency

Rare

Trembling, difficulty moving or controlling movement of the tongue, neck, or arms

SERIOUS REACTIONS

- Overdosage may result in cholinergic crisis, characterized by severe nausea, vomiting, diarrhea, increased salivation, diaphoresis, bradycardia, hypotension, flushed skin, stomach pain, respiratory depression, seizures, and paralysis of muscles.
- Increasing muscle weakness of myasthenia gravis may occur. Antidote: 0.5-1 mg IV atropine sulfate with other supportive treatment.

INTERACTIONS

Drugs

- *Atropine:* Suppresses the symptoms of ambenonium overdose

3 *Tacrine:* Increased cholinergic effects

SPECIAL CONSIDERATIONS

PATIENT/FAMILY EDUCATION

- Notify clinician of nausea, vomiting, diarrhea, sweating, increased salivation, irregular heartbeat, muscle weakness, severe abdominal pain, or difficulty in breathing
- Administer on an empty stomach

MONITORING PARAMETERS

- Narrow margin between first appearance of side effects and serious toxicity
- Symptoms of increasing muscle weakness may be due to cholinergic crisis (overdosage) or myasthenic crisis (increased disease severity); if crisis is myasthenia, patient will improve after 1-2 mg edrophonium; if cholinergic, withdraw ambenonium and administer atropine

amcinonide

(am-sin'-oh-nide)

Rx: Cylocort

Chemical Class: Corticosteroid, synthetic

Therapeutic Class: Corticosteroid, topical

CLINICAL PHARMACOLOGY

Mechanism of Action: Topical corticosteroids have anti-inflammatory, antipruritic, and vasoconstrictive properties. The exact mechanism of the anti-inflammatory process is unclear. ***Therapeutic Effect:*** Reduces or prevents tissue response to inflammatory process.

Pharmacokinetics

Well absorbed systemically. Large variation in absorption among sites: forearm 1%; scalp 4%, forehead 7%, scrotum 36%. Greatest penetration occurs at groin, axillae, and face. Protein binding in varying degrees. Metabolized in liver. Primarily excreted in urine.

INDICATIONS AND DOSAGES

Dermatoses

Topical

Adults, Elderly. Apply sparingly 2-3 times/day.

AVAILABLE FORMS

- *Lotion:* 0.1% (Cylocort).
- *Cream:* 0.1% (Cylocort).
- *Ointment:* 0.1% (Cylocort).

CONTRAINDICATIONS: History of hypersensitivity to amcinonide or other corticosteroids.

PREGNANCY AND LACTATION: Pregnancy category C; unknown whether topical application could result in sufficient systemic absorption to produce detectable amounts in breast milk (systemic corticosteroids are secreted into breast milk in quantities unlikely to have detrimental effects on breast-feeding infant)

SIDE EFFECTS

Frequent

Itching, redness, irritation, burning

Occasional

Dryness, folliculitis, hypertrichosis, acneiform eruptions, hypopigmentation, perioral dermatitis

Rare

Allergic contact dermatitis, maceration of the skin, secondary infection, skin atrophy

Systemic: Absorption more likely with occlusive dressings or extensive application in young children.

SERIOUS REACTIONS

- The serious reactions of long-term therapy and the addition of occlusive dressings are reversible hypothalamic-pituitary-adrenal (HPA) axis suppression, manifestations of Cushing's syndrome, hyperglycemia, and glucosuria.
- Abruptly withdrawing the drug after long-term therapy may require supplemental systemic corticosteroids.

SPECIAL CONSIDERATIONS

PATIENT/FAMILY EDUCATION

- Apply sparingly only to affected area
- Avoid contact with eyes
- Do not put bandages or dressings over treated area unless directed by clinician
- Do not use on weeping, denuded, or infected areas

MONITORING PARAMETERS

- Blood glucose levels, blood pressure, electrolytes

amikacin sulfate

(am-i-kay'-sin sul'-fate)

Rx: Amikin

Chemical Class: Aminoglycoside

Therapeutic Class: Antibiotic

CLINICAL PHARMACOLOGY

Mechanism of Action: An aminoglycoside antibiotic that irreversibly binds to protein on bacterial ribosomes. ***Therapeutic Effect:*** Interferes with protein synthesis of susceptible microorganisms.

Pharmacokinetics

Rapid, complete absorption after IM administration. Protein binding: 0%-10%. Widely distributed (does not cross the blood-brain barrier, low concentrations in CSF). Excreted unchanged in urine. Removed by hemodialysis. ***Half-life:*** 2-4 hr (increased in impaired renal function and neonates; decreased in cystic fibrosis and burn or febrile patients).

INDICATIONS AND DOSAGES

UTIs

IV, IM

Adults, Elderly. 250 mg q12h.

Moderate to severe infections

IV, IM

Adults, Elderly. 15 mg/kg/day in divided doses q8-12h. Maximum 1.5 g/day.

Children, Infants. 15-22.5 mg/kg/day in divided doses q8h.

Neonates. 7.5-10 mg/kg/dose q8-24h.

Dosage in renal impairment

Dosage and frequency are modified based on the degree of renal impairment and serum drug concentration. After a loading dose of 5-7.5 mg/kg, the maintenance dose and frequency are based on serum creatinine levels and creatinine clearance.

AVAILABLE FORMS

• *Injection:* 50 mg/ml (Amikin Pediatric), 62.5 mg/ml (Amikin), 250 mg/ml (Amikin).

CONTRAINDICATIONS: Hypersensitivity to amikacin, or other aminoglycosides (cross-sensitivity), or their components.

PREGNANCY AND LACTATION: Pregnancy category C; although fetal ototoxicity has occurred after *in utero* exposure to other aminoglycosides, 8th cranial nerve toxicity has not been reported with amikacin; excreted into breast milk in low concentrations; poor oral bioavailability reduces potential for ototoxicity for the infant

SIDE EFFECTS

Frequent

IM: Pain, induration

IV: Phlebitis, thrombophlebitis

Occasional

Hypersensitivity reactions (rash, fever, urticaria, pruritus)

Rare

Neuromuscular blockade (difficulty breathing, drowsiness, weakness)

SERIOUS REACTIONS

• Serious reactions may include nephrotoxicity (as evidenced by increased thirst, decreased appetite, nausea, vomiting, increased BUN and serum creatinine levels, and decreased creatinine clearance); neurotoxicity (manifested as muscle twitching, visual disturbances, seizures, and tingling); and ototoxicity (as evidenced by tinnitus, dizziness, and loss of hearing).

INTERACTIONS

Drugs

3 *Amphotericin B:* Synergistic nephrotoxicity

2 *Atracurium:* Amikacin potentiates respiratory depression by atracurium

3 *Carbenicillin:* Potential for inactivation of amikacin in patients with renal failure

3 *Carboplatin, Cisplatin:* Additive nephrotoxicity or ototoxicity

3 *Cephalosporins:* Increased potential for nephrotoxicity in patients with preexisting renal disease

3 *Cyclosporine:* Additive nephrotoxicity

2 *Ethacrynic acid:* Additive ototoxicity

3 *Indomethacin:* Reduced renal clearance of amikacin in premature infants

3 *Methoxyflurane:* Additive nephrotoxicity

3 *Neuromuscular blocking agents:* Amikacin potentiates respiratory depression by neuromuscular blocking agents

3 *NSAIDs:* May reduce renal clearance of amikacin

3 *Other aminoglycosides:* Increases the risk of nephrotoxicity or ototoxicity

3 *Pencillins (extended spectrum):* Potential for inactivation of amikacin in patients with renal failure

3 *Piperacillin:* Potential for inactivation of amikacin in patients with renal failure

2 *Succinylcholine:* Amikacin potentiates respiratory depression by succinylcholine

3 *Ticarcillin:* Potential for inactivation of amikacin in patients with renal failure

3 *Vancomycin:* Additive nephrotoxicity or ototoxicity

2 *Vecuronium:* Amikacin potentiates respiratory depression by vecuronium

Labs

• *False increase:* Urine amino acids

• *False decrease:* Bilirubin, cholesterol, serum creatine kinase, serum glucose, LDH, BUN

- *False positive:* Urine oligosaccharides
- *Interference:* Serum tobramycin, kanamycin

SPECIAL CONSIDERATIONS

MONITORING PARAMETERS

- Urine output, serum creatinine
- Serum peak, drawn 30-60 min after IV INF or 60 min after IM inj; trough level drawn just before next dose; adjust dosage per levels (usual therapeutic plasma levels; peak 20-35 mg/L, trough ≤10 mg/L)
- Skin for rash

---

amiloride hydrochloride

(a-mill'-oh-ride hye-droe-klor'-ide)

Rx: Midamor

Combinations

Rx: with hydrochlorothiazide (Moduretic)

Chemical Class: Pyrazine

Therapeutic Class: Antihypertensive; diuretic, potassium-sparing

---

CLINICAL PHARMACOLOGY

Mechanism of Action: A guanidine derivative that acts as a potassium-sparing diuretic, antihypertensive, and antihypokalemic by directly interfering with sodium reabsorption in the distal tubule. ***Therapeutic Effect:*** Increases sodium and water excretion and decreases potassium excretion.

Pharmacokinetics

Route	*Onset*	*Peak*	*Duration*
PO	2 hrs	6-10 hrs	24 hrs

Incompletely absorbed from the GI tract. Protein binding: Minimal. Primarily excreted in urine; partially eliminated in feces. ***Half-life:*** 6-9 hr.

INDICATIONS AND DOSAGES

To counteract potassium loss induced by other diuretics

PO

Adults, Children weighing more than 20 kg. 5-10 mg/day up to 20 mg.

Elderly. Initially, 5 mg/day or every other day.

Children weighing 6-20 kg. 0.625 mg/kg/day. Maximum: 10 mg/day.

Dosage in renal impairment

Creatinine Clearance	*Dosage*
10-50 ml/min	50% of normal
less than 10 ml/min	avoid use

AVAILABLE FORMS

- *Tablets:* 5 mg.

UNLABELED USES: Treatment of edema associated with CHF, liver cirrhosis, and nephrotic syndrome; treatment of hypertension, reduces lithium-induced polyuria, slows pulmonary function reduction in cystic fibrosis

CONTRAINDICATIONS: Acute or chronic renal insufficiency, anuria, diabetic nephropathy, patients on other potassium-sparing diuretics, serum potassium greater than 5.5 mEq/L

PREGNANCY AND LACTATION: Pregnancy category B; (D if used in pregnancy-induced hypertension); therapy for preexisting hypertension can be continued throughout pregnancy with minimal risk; initiating for simple edema not recommended; few unequivocal indications for diuretic therapy in pregnancy except for pulmonary edema or congestive heart failure; excretion into breast milk unknown; use caution in nursing mothers

SIDE EFFECTS

Frequent (8%-3%)

Headache, nausea, diarrhea, vomiting, decreased appetite

Occasional (3%-1%)
Dizziness, constipation, abdominal pain, weakness, fatigue, cough, impotence
Rare (less than 1%)
Tremors, vertigo, confusion, nervousness, insomnia, thirst, dry mouth, heartburn, shortness of breath, increased urination, hypotension, rash

SERIOUS REACTIONS

- Severe hyperkalemia may produce irritability, anxiety, a feeling of heaviness in the legs, paresthesia of hands, face, and lips, hypotension, bradycardia, tented T waves, widening of QRS, and ST depression.

INTERACTIONS

Drugs

3 *ACE inhibitors:* Hyperkalemia in predisposed patients
3 *Angiotensin II receptor antagonists:* Increased risk of hyperkalemia
3 *Anticoagulants:* Decreases the effect of anticoagulants
3 *Lithium:* Decreases lithium clearance and increases the risk of amiloride toxicity
3 *NSAIDs:* Decreases antihypertensive effect
2 *Potassium preparations:* Hyperkalemia in predisposed patients
3 *Quinidine:* Increased ventricular arrhythmias

SPECIAL CONSIDERATIONS

PATIENT/FAMILY EDUCATION

- Notify clinician of muscle weakness, fatigue, flaccid paralysis
- Take with food or milk for GI symptoms
- Take early in day to prevent nocturia
- Avoid large quantities of potassium-rich foods: oranges, bananas, salt substitutes

MONITORING PARAMETERS

- Electrolytes

aminocaproic acid

(a-mee-noe-ka-proe'-ik as'-id)
Rx: Amicar
Chemical Class: Monoaminocarboxylic acid, synthetic
Therapeutic Class: Hemostatic

CLINICAL PHARMACOLOGY

Mechanism of Action: A systemic hemostatic that acts as an antifibrinolytic and antihemorrhagic by inhibiting the activation of plasminogen activator substances. ***Therapeutic Effect:*** Prevents formation of fibrin clots.

Pharmacokinetics

Rapidly absorbed following PO administration. Does not appear to bind to plasma protein. Excreted rapidly in urine, mostly unchanged. ***Half-life:*** 2 hr.

INDICATIONS AND DOSAGES

Acute bleeding

PO, IV Infusion
Adults, Elderly. 4-5 g over first hr; then 1-1.25 g/hr. Continue for 8 hr or until bleeding is controlled. Maximum: 30 g/24 hr.
Children. 3 g/m^2 over first hr; then 1 g/m^2/hr. Maximum: 18 g/m^2/24 hr.

Dosage in renal impairment

Decrease dose to 25% of normal.

AVAILABLE FORMS

- *Syrup:* 250 mg/ml.
- *Tablets:* 500 mg.
- *Injection:* 250 mg/ml.

UNLABELED USES: Control of bleeding in thrombocytopenia, control of oral bleeding in congenital and acquired coagulation disorders, prevention of recurrence of subarachnoid hemorrhage, prevention of hemorrhage in hemophiliacs following dental surgery, treatment of traumatic hyphema

CONTRAINDICATIONS: Evidence of active intravascular clotting process, disseminated intravascular coagulation without concurrent heparin therapy, hematuria of upper urinary tract origin (unless benefit outweighs risk); newborns (parenteral form).

PREGNANCY AND LACTATION: Pregnancy category C; excretion in milk unknown; use caution in nursing mothers

SIDE EFFECTS

Occasional

Nausea, diarrhea, cramps, decreased urination, decreased BP, dizziness, headache, muscle fatigue and weakness, myopathy, bloodshot eyes

SERIOUS REACTIONS

- Too-rapid IV administration produces tinnitus, rash, arrhythmias, unusual fatigue, and weakness.
- Rarely, a grand mal seizure occurs, generally preceded by weakness, dizziness, and headache.

INTERACTIONS

Drugs

❷ *Anti-inhibitor coagulant complex, tretinoin:* Increases the risk of thrombosis

Labs

- *False increase:* Urine amino acids

SPECIAL CONSIDERATIONS

PATIENT/FAMILY EDUCATION

- Report any signs of bleeding or myopathy
- Change position slowly to decrease orthostatic hypotension
- No need to adjust INR in warfarin anticoagulated patients with topical hemostatic mouthwash use

MONITORING PARAMETERS

- Do **not** administer without a definite diagnosis and laboratory findings indicative of hyperfibrinolysis
- Blood studies including coagulation factors, platelets, fibrinolysin; CPK, urinalysis
- Blood pressure, heart rate

aminophylline/theophylline

(am-in-off'-i-lin)

Rx: (aminophylline) Phyllocontin

Rx: (theophylline) Elixophyllin, Quibron-T, Quibron-T/SR, Slo-Bid Gyrocaps, Theo-24, Theodur, Theolair, Theolair-SR, Theodur, Thoechron, T-Phyl, Uniphyl

Chemical Class: Ethylenediamine derivative

Therapeutic Class: COPD agent; antiasthmatic; bronchodilator

CLINICAL PHARMACOLOGY

Mechanism of Action: A xanthine derivative that acts as a bronchodilator by directly relaxing smooth muscle of the bronchial airways and pulmonary blood vessels. ***Therapeutic Effect:*** Relieves bronchospasm and increases vital capacity.

Pharmacokinetics

Rapidly and well absorbed. Protein binding: Moderate (to albumin). Extensively metabolized in liver. Partially excreted in urine. ***Half-life:*** 6-12 hr (varies).

INDICATIONS AND DOSAGES

Asthma

IV

Adults. Initially, 5 mg/kg bolus over 20-30 min (to provide serum theophylline of 5-15 mg/ml), then 0.4 mg/kg/hr continuous infusion.

Elderly. 5 mg/kg bolus, then 0.2 mg/kg/hr continuous infusion.

Children 9-6 yr. Initially, 5 mg/kg bolus, then 0.7 mg/kg/hr.

Children 1-8 yr. Initially, 5 mg/kg bolus, then 0.8 mg/kg/hr.

PO

Adults. Initially, 5 mg/kg (use ideal body weight), then 300-600 mg/day in 3-4 divided doses.

Elderly. Initially, 5 mg/kg, then 2 mg/kg q8h.

PO (Controlled-Release 12-Hour Formulations)

Adults, Children weighing 45 kg and more. Initially, 300 mg/day in 2 divided doses. May increase in 3 days to 400 mg/day in 2 divided doses. May increase in 3 days to 600 mg/day in 2 divided doses.

Children weighing less than 45 kg. Initially, 12-24 mg/kg/day in divided doses (maximum: 300 mg). May increase in 3 days to 16 mg/kg/day (maximum: 400 mg). May increase in 3 days to 20 mg/kg/day (maximum: 600 mg).

PO (Extended-Release 24-Hour Formulations)

Adults, Children weighing 45 kg and more. Initially, 300-400 mg/day. May increase in 3 days to 400-600 mg/day. May then titrate according to blood level.

Children weighing less than 45 kg. Initially, 12-24 mg/kg/day (maximum: 300 mg). May increase in 3 days to 16 mg/kg/day (maximum: 400 mg). May increase in 3 days to 20 mg/kg/day (maximum: 600 mg).

AVAILABLE FORMS

- *Capsules (Extended-Release [Theo-24]):* 100 mg, 200 mg, 300 mg, 400 mg.
- *Elixir (Elixophyllin):* 80 mg/15 ml.
- *Oral Solution:* 80 mg/15 ml.
- *Tablets (Controlled-Release [Theochron]):* 100 mg (Theochron), 200 mg (Theochron, T-Phyl), 300 mg (Quibron-T/SR, Theochron, Theolair-SR), 400 mg (Uniphyl), 500 mg (Theolair-SR), 600 mg (Uniphyl).
- *Infusion (theophylline):* 0.8 mg/ml, 1.6 mg/ml, 2 mg/ml, 3.2 mg/ml, 4 mg/ml.
- *Injection (aminophylline):* 25 mg/ml.

UNLABELED USES: Treatment of apnea in neonates

CONTRAINDICATIONS: History of hypersensitivity to caffeine or xanthine

PREGNANCY AND LACTATION: Pregnancy category C; pharmacokinetics of theophylline may be altered during pregnancy; monitor serum concentrations carefully; excreted into breast milk; may cause irritability in the nursing infant, otherwise compatible with breastfeeding

SIDE EFFECTS

Frequent

Altered smell (during IV administration), restlessness, tachycardia, tremor

Occasional

Heartburn, vomiting, headache, mild diuresis, insomnia, nausea

SERIOUS REACTIONS

- Too-rapid IV administration may produce marked hypotension with accompanying faintness, lightheadedness, palpitations, tachycardia, hyperventilation, nausea, vomiting, angina-like pain, seizures, ventricular fibrillation, and cardiac standstill.

INTERACTIONS

Drugs

3 *Adenosine:* Decreased hemodynamic effects of adenosine

3 *Allopurinol, Amiodarone, Cimetidine, Ciprofloxacin, Disulfiram, Erythromycin, Interferon alfa, Isoniazid, Methimazole, Metoprolol, Norfloxacin, Pefloxacin, Pentoxifylline, Propafenone, Propylthiouracil, Radioactive iodine, Tacrine,*

Thiabendazole, Ticlopidine, Verapamil: Increased theophylline concentrations

3 *Aminoglutethamide, Barbiturates, Carbamazepine, Moricizine, Phenytoin, Rifampin, Ritonavir, Thyroid hormone:* Reduced theophylline concentrations; decreased serum phenytoin levels

3 *β-blockers:* Reduced bronchodilating response to theophylline

❷ *Enoxacin, Fluvoxamine, Mexiletine, Propranolol, Troleandomycin:* Markedly increased theophylline concentrations

3 *Imipenem:* Some patients on theophylline have developed seizures following addition of imipenem

3 *Lithium:* Reduced lithium concentrations

3 *Smoking:* Increased aminophylline dosing requirements

SPECIAL CONSIDERATIONS

PATIENT/FAMILY EDUCATION

- Avoid large amounts of caffeine-containing products
- If GI upset occurs, take with 8 oz water
- Notify clinician if nausea, vomiting, insomnia, jitteriness, headache, rash, palpitations occur

MONITORING PARAMETERS

- Serum theophylline concentrations every 6-12 mo or with status changes (therapeutic level is 10-20 mcg/ml); toxicity may occur with small increase above 20 mcg/ml, especially in the elderly
- Serious side effects (ventricular dysrhythmias, seizures, death) may occur without preceding signs of less serious toxicity (nausea, restlessness)
- Arterial blood gases (ABGs)

aminosalicylic acid

(a-mee-noe-sal-i-si-lik as-id)

Rx: Paser

Chemical Class: Salicylate derivative

Therapeutic Class: Antituberculosis agent

CLINICAL PHARMACOLOGY

Mechanism of Action: An antitubercular agent active against *M. tuberculosis*. Thought to exhibit competitive antagonism of folic acid synthesis. ***Therapeutic Effect:*** Bacteriostatic activity in susceptible microorganisms.

Pharmacokinetics

Readily absorbed from the gastrointestinal (GI) tract. Protein binding: 50-60%. Widely distributed (including cerebrospinal fluid [CSF]). Metabolized in liver. Primarily excreted in urine. Removed by hemodialysis. ***Half-life:*** 1.1-1.62 hrs.

INDICATIONS AND DOSAGES

Tuberculosis

PO

Adults, Elderly. 4 g in divided doses 3 times/day.

Children. 150 mg/kg/day in divided doses 3 times/day. Maximum: 12 g/day.

AVAILABLE FORMS

- *Packet granules:* 4 g/packet granules (Paser).
- *Tablets, enteric-coated:* 7.7 grains (Paser).
- *Tablets, sustained-release:* 500 mg (Paser).

UNLABELED USES: Crohn's disease, hyperlipidemia, ulcerative colitis

CONTRAINDICATIONS: End-stage renal disease, hypersensitivity to aminosalicylic acid products

PREGNANCY AND LACTATION: Pregnancy category C; excreted into breast milk; use caution in nursing mothers

SIDE EFFECTS

Occasional

Abdominal pain, diarrhea, nausea, vomiting

Rare

Hypersensitivity reactions, hepatotoxicity, thrombocytopenia

SERIOUS REACTIONS

• Liver toxicity and hepatitis, blood dyscrasias occur rarely.

• Agranulocytosis, methemoglobinemia, thrombocytopenia have been reported.

INTERACTIONS

Drugs

❷ *Vitamin B_{12}:* Vitamin B_{12} absorption reduced by 55%; Vitamin B_{12} maintenance should be considered for therapy of more than 1 month

❸ *Digoxin:* Reduced digoxin levels

Labs

• Aminosalicylic acid has been reported to interfere technically with the serum determinations of albumin by dye-binding, SGOT by the azoene dye method and with qualitative urine test for ketones, bilirubin, urobilinogen, or porphobilinogen

SPECIAL CONSIDERATIONS

• If recognized promptly drug-induced hepatitis resolves quickly; 21% mortality if the reaction is unrecognized

• Desensitization has been accomplished with 10 mg aminosalicylic acid given as a single dose; double the dose q2 days until total of 1 gram then follow the regular schedule of administration; if a mild temperature rise or skin reaction develops, drop back one level or hold the progression for one cycle; reactions are rare after a total dosage of 1.5 g

PATIENT/FAMILY EDUCATION

• Sprinkle granules on applesauce or yogurt or add to acidic juice such as orange, tomato, grape, apple, grapefruit, or cranberry; swirl well, granules sink

• Protect from moisture, light, and extremes of temperature; do not use if packets are swollen or if granules turn dark brown or purple

• Notify clinician if fever, sore throat, unusual bleeding, bruising, or skin rashes occur

• The skeleton of the granules may be seen in the stool

• Avoid crowds or those with known infection

MONITORING PARAMETERS

• Monitor carefully in first 3 mo of therapy for signs of intolerance/drug-induced hepatitis (rash, fever, jaundice, hepatomegaly)

• Liver function

amiodarone hydrochloride

(a-mee'-oh-da-rone hye-droe-klor'-ide)

Rx: Cordarone, Cordarone IV, Pacerone

Chemical Class: Iodinated benzofuran derivative

Therapeutic Class: Antiarrhythmic, class III

CLINICAL PHARMACOLOGY

Mechanism of Action: A cardiac agent that prolongs duration of myocardial cell action potential and refractory period by acting directly on all cardiac tissue. Decreases AV and sinus node function. ***Therapeutic Effect:*** Suppresses arrhythmias.

Pharmacokinetics

Route	*Onset*	*Peak*	*Duration*
PO	3 days-3 wk	1 wk-5 mo	7-50 days after discontinuation

Slowly, variably absorbed from GI tract. Protein binding: 96%. Extensively metabolized in the liver to active metabolite. Excreted via bile; not removed by hemodialysis. ***Half-life:*** 26-107 days; metabolite, 61 days.

INDICATIONS AND DOSAGES

Life-threatening recurrent ventricular fibrillation or hemodynamically unstable ventricular tachycardia

PO

Adults, Elderly. Initially, 800-1600 mg/day in 2-4 divided doses for 1-3 wk. After arrhythmia is controlled or side effects occur, reduce to 600-800 mg/day for about 4 wk. Maintenance: 200-600 mg/day

Children. Initially, 10-20 mg/kg/day for 4-14 days, then 5 mg/kg/day for several wk. Maintenance: 2.5 mg/kg/day or lowest effective maintenance dose for 5 of 7 days/wk.

IV Infusion

Adults. Initially, 1050 mg over 24 hr; 150 mg over 10 min, then 360 mg over 6 hr; then 540 mg over 18 hr. May continue at 0.5 mg/min for up to 2-3 wk regardless of age or renal or left ventricular function.

AVAILABLE FORMS

- *Tablets:* 100 mg (Pacerone), 200 mg (Cordarone, Pacerone), 400 mg (Pacerone).
- *Injection (Cordarone IV):* 50 mg/ml.

UNLABELED USES: Control of hemodynamically stable ventricular tachycardia, control of rapid ventricular rate due to accessory pathway conduction in pre-excited atrial arrhythmias, conversion of atrial fibrillation to normal sinus rhythm, in cardiac arrest with persistent ventricular tachycardia or ventricular fibrillation, paroxysmal supraventricular tachycardia, polymorphic ventricular tachycardia or wide complex tachycardia of uncertain origin, prevention of post-operative atrial fibrillation

CONTRAINDICATIONS: Bradycardia-induced syncope (except in the presence of a pacemaker), second- and third-degree AV block, severe hepatic disease, severe sinus-node dysfunction

PREGNANCY AND LACTATION: Pregnancy category D; due to a very long $t_{1/2}$, amiodarone should be discontinued several months prior to conception to avoid early gestational exposure, reserve for refractory dysrhythmias; newborns exposed to amiodarone should have TFTs; excreted into breast milk; contains high proportions of iodine; breast-feeding not recommended

SIDE EFFECTS

Expected

Corneal microdeposits are noted in almost all patients treated for more than 6 months (can lead to blurry vision).

Frequent (greater than 3%)

Parenteral: Hypotension, nausea, fever, bradycardia.

Oral: Constipation, headache, decreased appetite, nausea, vomiting, paresthesias, photosensitivity, muscular incoordination.

Occasional (less than 3%)

Oral: Bitter or metallic taste; decreased libido; dizziness; facial flushing; blue-gray coloring of skin (face, arms, and neck); blurred vision; bradycardia; asymptomatic corneal deposits.

Rare (less than 1%)
Oral: Rash, vision loss, blindness.

SERIOUS REACTIONS

• Serious, potentially fatal pulmonary toxicity (alveolitis, pulmonary fibrosis, pneumonitis, acute respiratory distress syndrome) may begin with progressive dyspnea and cough with crackles, decreased breath sounds, pleurisy, CHF or hepatotoxicity.

• Amiodarone may worsen existing arrhythmias or produce new arrhythmias (called proarrhythmias).

INTERACTIONS

Drugs

3 *Aprinidine:* Increased aprinidine concentrations

3 *β-adrenergic blockers:* Bradycardia, cardiac arrest, or ventricular arrhythmia shortly after initiation of β-adrenergic blockers that undergo extensive hepatic metabolism (propranolol, sotalol, metoprolol)

3 *Calcium channel blockers:* Cardiotoxicity with bradycardia and decreased cardiac output with diltiazem and, potentially, verapamil

3 *Cholestyramine, Colestipol:* Decreased amiodarone plasma concentrations

3 *Cimetidine:* Increased amiodarone plasma concentrations (other H_2 blockers likely have no effect)

3 *Cyclosporine, Tacrolimus:* Increased cyclosporine, tacrolimus concentrations

3 *Digitalis glycosides:* Accumulation of digoxin

3 *Fentanyl:* In combination with amiodarone may cause hypotension, bradycardia, and decreased cardiac output

3 *Flecainide, Ecainide:* Increased flecainide, ecainide serum concentrations

3 *Methotrexate:* Impaired methotrexate metabolism with >2 weeks oral amiodarone administration

3 *Oral anticoagulants:* Enhanced hypoprothrombinemic response to warfarin (prothrombin time increased 100%), reduce warfarin dose ⅓-½

3 *Phenytoin:* Increased serum phenytoin concentrations, decreased amiodarone concentrations

3 *Procainamide:* Increased procainamide concentrations

3 *Protease inhibitors (Indinavir):* Inceased amiodarone plasma concentrations

3 *Quinidine:* Increased quinidine plasma concentrations, reduce quinidine dose by ⅓

3 *Rifampin:* Decreased amiodarone plasma concentrations

3 *St. John's Wort (Hypericum perforatum):* Potential for decreased amiodarone plasma concentrations

3 *Theophylline:* Increased theophylline levels

3 *Volatile anesthetic agents:* Increased sensitivity to myocardial depressant and conduction effects of halogenated inhalational anesthetics

Labs

• *Increase:* Serum T4 and serum reverse T3

• *Decrease:* Serum T3

SPECIAL CONSIDERATIONS

• Should be administered only by clinicians experienced in treatment of life-threatening dysrhythmias who are thoroughly familiar with the risks and benefits of amiodarone therapy

• IV amiodarone contains the preservative benzyl alcohol, which has been associated with fatal gasping syndrome in neonates

PATIENT/FAMILY EDUCATION

• Take with food and/or divide doses if GI intolerance occurs; do not take oral form with grapefruit juice

• Use sunscreen or stay out of sun to prevent burns

• Report side effects immediately
• Skin discoloration is usually reversible

MONITORING PARAMETERS
• Chest x-ray, ophth referral, and PFTs (baseline and q3 mo)
• Electrolytes
• LFTs
• ECG; QT interval prolongation of 10%-15% suggests therapeutic effect
• TFTs
• CNS symptoms

---

amitriptyline hydrochloride

(a-mee-trip'-ti-leen hye-droe-klor'-ide)

Rx: Elavil

Combinations

Rx: with chlordiazepoxide (Limbitrol); with perphenazine (Triavil)

Chemical Class: Dibenzocycloheptene derivative; tertiary amine

Therapeutic Class: Antidepressant, tricyclic; antineurolgic; anxiolytic

---

CLINICAL PHARMACOLOGY

Mechanism of Action: A tricyclic antidepressant that blocks the reuptake of neurotransmitters, including norepinephrine and serotonin, at presynaptic membranes, thus increasing their availability at postsynaptic receptor sites. Also has strong anticholinergic activity. ***Therapeutic Effect:*** Relieves depression.

Pharmacokinetics

Rapidly and well absorbed from the GI tract. Protein binding: 90%. Undergoes first-pass metabolism in the liver. Primarily excreted in urine. Minimal removal by hemodialysis. ***Half-life:*** 10-26 hr.

INDICATIONS AND DOSAGES

Depression

PO

Adults. 25-100 mg/day as a single dose at bedtime or in divided doses. May gradually increase up to 300 mg/day. Titrate to lowest effective dosage.

Elderly. Initially, 10-25 mg at bedtime. May increase by 10-25 mg at weekly intervals. Range: 25-150 mg/day.

Children 6-12 yr. 1-5 mg/kg/day in 2 divided doses.

IM

Adults. 20-30 mg 4 times a day.

Pain management

PO

Adults, Elderly. 25-100 mg at bedtime.

AVAILABLE FORMS

• *Tablets (Elavil):* 10 mg, 25 mg, 50 mg, 75 mg, 100 mg, 150 mg.
• *Injection (Elavil):* 10 mg/ml.

UNLABELED USES: Relief of neuropathic pain, such as that experienced by patients with diabetic neuropathy or postherpetic neuralgia; treatment of anxiety, bulimia nervosa, migraine, nocturnal enuresis, panic disorder, peptic ulcer

CONTRAINDICATIONS: Acute recovery period after MI, use within 14 days of MAOIs

PREGNANCY AND LACTATION: Pregnancy category C; excreted into breast milk; effect on nursing infant unknown but may be of concern

SIDE EFFECTS

Frequent

Dizziness, somnolence, dry mouth, orthostatic hypotension, headache, increased appetite, weight gain, nausea, unusual fatigue, unpleasant taste

Occasional

Blurred vision, confusion, constipation, hallucinations, delayed micturition, eye pain, arrhythmias, fine muscle tremors, parkinsonian syndrome, anxiety, diarrhea, diaphoresis, heartburn, insomnia

Rare

Hypersensitivity, alopecia, tinnitus, breast enlargement, photosensitivity

SERIOUS REACTIONS

- Overdose may produce confusion, seizures, severe somnolence, arrhythmias, fever, hallucinations, agitation, dyspnea, vomiting, and unusual fatigue or weakness.
- Abrupt discontinuation after prolonged therapy may produce headache, malaise, nausea, vomiting, and vivid dreams.
- Blood dyscrasias and cholestatic jaundice occur rarely.

INTERACTIONS

Drugs

3 *Altretamine:* Orthostatic hypotension

3 *Amphetamines:* Theoretical increase in effect of amphetamines, clinical evidence lacking

3 *Anticholinergics:* Excessive anticholinergic effects

3 *Antithyroid agents:* Increases the risk of agranulocytosis

3 *Barbiturates:* Reduced serum concentrations of cyclic antidepressants

2 *Bethanidine:* Reduced antihypertensive effect of bethanidine

3 *Carbamazepine:* Reduced antidepressant serum concentrations

3 *Cimetidine (other H_2 blockers less likely to have effect):* Inhibition of TCA metabolism

2 *Clonidine:* Reduced antihypertensive response to clonidine; enhanced hypertensive response with abrupt clonidine withdrawal

2 *Epinephrine, norepinephrine:* Enhanced pressor response

3 *Ethanol:* Additive impairment of motor skills; abstinent alcoholics may eliminate cyclic antidepressants more rapidly than non-alcoholics

3 *Fluoxetine, paroxetine:* Marked increases in cyclic antidepressant plasma concentrations

3 *Guanabenz, guanfacine, debrisoquin:* Inhibition of antihypertensive effect

2 *Guanethidine, guanadrel:* Inhibited antihypertensive response to guanethidine

3 *Hypoglycemics:* Enhanced hypoglemic effects

3 *Isoproterenol:* Increased cardiac arrhythmias

3 *Lithium:* Increased risk of neurotoxicity

2 *MAOIs:* Excessive sympathetic response, mania, or hyperpyrexia possible

2 *Moclobemide:* Potential association with fatal or non-fatal serotonin syndrome

3 *Neuroleptics:* Increased therapeutic and toxic effects of both drugs

2 *Norepinephrine:* Markedly enhanced pressor response to norepinephrine

2 *Phenothiazines:* Increases sedative and anticholinergic effects of amitriptyline

3 *Phenylephrine:* Enhanced pressor response

3 *Propoxyphene:* Enhanced effect of cyclic antidepressants

3 *Quinidine:* Increased cyclic antidepressant serum concentrations

3 *Rifampin:* Possible decreased TCA levels

3 *Ritonavir, indinavir:* Increased TCA levels

2 *Sympathomimetics:* Increases cardiac effects

Labs

• *False increase:* Carbamazepine levels

SPECIAL CONSIDERATIONS

PATIENT/FAMILY EDUCATION

• Therapeutic effects may take 2-3 wk

• Use caution in driving or other activities requiring alertness

• Avoid rising quickly from sitting to standing, especially elderly

• Avoid alcohol ingestion, other CNS depressants

• Do not discontinue abruptly after long-term use

• Wear sunscreen or large hat to prevent photosensitivity

• Increase fluids, bulk in diet if constipation occurs

• Gum, hard sugarless candy, or frequent sips of water for dry mouth

MONITORING PARAMETERS

• Mental status: mood, sensorium, affect, suicidal tendencies

• Determination of amitriptyline plasma concentrations is not routinely recommended but may be useful in identifying toxicity, drug interactions, or noncompliance (adjustments in dosage should be made according to clinical response not plasma concentrations)

• Therapeutic plasma levels 125-250 mcg/L (including active metabolites)

• Blood pressure, pulse

amlexanox

(am-lex'-an-ox)

Rx: Aphthasol

Chemical Class: Benzopyranobipyridine carboxylic acid derivative

Therapeutic Class: Antiinflammatory

CLINICAL PHARMACOLOGY

Mechanism of Action: A mouth agent that has anti-allergic and anti-inflammatory properties. Appears to inhibit formation and/or release of inflammatory mediators (e.g., histamine) from mast cells, neutrophils, mononuclear cells. ***Therapeutic Effect:*** Alleviates signs and symptoms of aphthous ulcers.

Pharmacokinetics

After topical application, most systemic absorption occurs from the gastrointestinal (GI) tract. Metabolized to inactive metabolite. Excreted in urine. ***Half-life:*** 3.5 hrs.

INDICATIONS AND DOSAGES

Aphthous ulcers

Topical

Adults, Elderly. Administer ¼ inch directly to ulcers 4 times/day (after meals and at bedtime) following oral hygiene.

AVAILABLE FORMS

• *Paste:* 5% (Apthasol).

CONTRAINDICATIONS: Hypersensitivity to amlexanox or any component of the formulation

PREGNANCY AND LACTATION: Pregnancy category B

SIDE EFFECTS

Rare

Stinging, burning at administration site, transient pain, rash

SERIOUS REACTIONS

• Ingestion of a full tube would result in nausea, vomiting, and diarrhea.

SPECIAL CONSIDERATIONS

PATIENT/FAMILY EDUCATION

- Discontinue if rash develops
- Apply after oral hygiene

MONITORING PARAMETERS

- Therapeutic response to therapy

amlodipine besylate

(am-loe'-di-peen be'-si-late)

Rx: Norvasc

Combinations

Rx: with atorvastatin (Caduet); with benazepril (Lotrel)

Chemical Class: Dihydropyridine

Therapeutic Class: Antianginal; antihypertensive; calcium channel blocker

CLINICAL PHARMACOLOGY

Mechanism of Action: A calcium channel blocker that inhibits calcium movement across cardiac and vascular smooth-muscle cell membranes. ***Therapeutic Effect:*** Relieves angina by dilating coronary arteries, peripheral arteries, and arterioles. Decreases total peripheral vascular resistance and BP by vasodilation.

Pharmacokinetics

Route	Onset	Peak	Duration
PO	0.5-1 hr	6-12 hr	24 hr

Slowly absorbed from the GI tract. Protein binding: 93%. Undergoes first-pass metabolism in the liver. Excreted primarily in urine. Not removed by hemodialysis. ***Half-life:*** 30-50 hr (increased in the elderly and those with liver cirrhosis).

INDICATIONS AND DOSAGES

Hypertension

PO

Adults. Initially, 5 mg/day as a single dose. Maximum: 10 mg/day.

Small-Frame, Fragile, Elderly. Initially, 2.5 mg/day as a single dose.

Children 6-17 yr. 2.5-5 mg/day.

Angina (chronic stable or vasospastic)

PO

Adults. 5-10 mg/day as a single dose.

Elderly, Patients with hepatic insufficiency. 5 mg/day as a single dose.

Dosage in renal impairment

Adults, Elderly. (Hypertension) 2.5 mg/day. (Angina) 5 mg/day.

AVAILABLE FORMS

- *Tablets:* 2.5 mg, 5 mg, 10 mg.

CONTRAINDICATIONS: Severe hypotension

PREGNANCY AND LACTATION: Pregnancy category C; unknown if excreted into milk; use caution in nursing mothers

SIDE EFFECTS

Frequent (greater than 5%)

Peripheral edema, headache, flushing

Occasional (less than 5%)

Dizziness, palpitations, nausea, unusual fatigue or weakness (asthenia)

Rare (less than 1%)

Chest pain, bradycardia, orthostatic hypotension

SERIOUS REACTIONS

- Overdose may produce excessive peripheral vasodilation and marked hypotension with reflex tachycardia.

INTERACTIONS

Drugs

3 *Barbiturates:* Reduced plasma concentrations of amlodipine

3 *Diltiazem:* Reduced clearance of amlodipine

3 *Erythromycin:* Reduced clearance of amlodipine

3 *Fentanyl:* Severe hypotension or increased fluid volume requirements

3 *Grapefruit juice:* Reduced clearance of amlodipine

3 *H_2 blockers:* Increased plasma concentration of amlodipine possible

3 *Proton pump inhibitors:* Increased plasma concentration of amlodipine possible

3 *Quinidine:* Increased plasma concentration of amlodipine; reduced plasma quinidine level

3 *Rifampin:* Reduced plasma concentration of amlodipine

3 *Vincristine:* Reduced vincristine clearance

SPECIAL CONSIDERATIONS

PATIENT/FAMILY EDUCATION

- Notify clinician of irregular heart beat, shortness of breath, swelling of feet and hands, pronounced dizziness, hypotension
- Do not abruptly discontinue amlodipine; compliance with therapy is essential to control hypertension
- Avoid tasks that require alertness and motor skills until response to the drug has been established
- Avoid drinking grapefruit juice while taking this drug

MONITORING PARAMETERS

- Blood pressure—if the patient's systolic BP is less than 90 mm Hg, withhold the medication and notify the physician
- Assess skin for flushing and peripheral edema, especially behind the medial malleolus and the sacral area

ammonium lactate

(ah-moe'-nee-um lack'-tate)

Rx: Amlactin, Lac-Hydrin, Lac-Hydrin Five, LAClotion

Chemical Class: α-hydroxy acid

Therapeutic Class: Emollient

CLINICAL PHARMACOLOGY

Mechanism of Action: Lactic acid is an alpha-hydroxy acid that influences hydration, decreases corneocyte cohesion, reduces excessive epidermal keratinization in hyperkeratotic conditions, and induces synthesis of mucopolysaccharides and collagen in photodamaged skin. The exact mechanism is not known.

Therapeutic Effect: Increases hydration of the skin.

Pharmacokinetics

Not known.

INDICATIONS AND DOSAGES

Treatment of ichthyosis vulgaris and xerosis

PO

Adults, Elderly. Apply sparingly and rub into area thoroughly q12h.

AVAILABLE FORMS

- *Cream:* 12% (Amlactin).
- *Lotion:* 5% (Lac-Hydrin Five), 12% (Amlactin, Lac-Hydrin, LAClotion).

CONTRAINDICATIONS: Hypersensitivity to ammonium lactate

PREGNANCY AND LACTATION: Pregnancy category C; unknown if excreted in breast milk; lactic acid is a normal constituent of blood and tissues

SIDE EFFECTS

Occasional (15%-2%)

Burning, stinging, rash, dry skin

INTERACTIONS

Drugs

3 *Calcipotriene:* Decreases the effects of calcipotriene

SPECIAL CONSIDERATIONS
- Side effects greater in fair-skinned individuals, if applied to abraded or inflamed areas, and in ichthyosis (where incidence of burning, stinging, and erythema is 10%)

PATIENT/FAMILY EDUCATION
- For external use only
- Avoid exposure to sunlight

amobarbital sodium

(am-oh-bar'-bi-tal soe'-dee-um)

Rx: Amytal sodium

Combinations

Rx: with secobarbital (Tuinal)

Chemical Class: Barbituric acid derivative

Therapeutic Class: Sedative/hypnotic

DEA Class: Schedule II

CLINICAL PHARMACOLOGY

Mechanism of Action: A barbiturate that depresses the sensory cortex, decreases motor activity, and alters cerebellar function. ***Therapeutic Effect:*** Produces drowsiness, sedation, and hypnosis.

Pharmacokinetics

Readily absorbed from the gastrointestinal (GI) tract and distributed. Protein binding: 60%. Metabolized in liver primarily by the hepatic microsomal enzyme system. Primarily excreted in urine. ***Half-life:*** 16-40 hrs.

INDICATIONS AND DOSAGES

Hypnotic

IM/IV

Adults, Children older than 6 yrs. 65-200 mg at bedtime.

IM: Administer deeply into a large muscle. Do not use more than 5 ml at any single site (may cause tissue damage). Maximum: 500 mg.

IV: Use only when IM administration is not feasible. Administer by slow IV injection. Maximum: 50 mg/min in adults.

Children younger than 6 yrs. 2-3 mg/kg/dose.

Preanesthetic

IM/IV

Adults, Children older than 6 yrs. 65-500 mg at bedtime.

Sedative

IV

Adults. 30-50 mg given 2 or 3 times/day.

AVAILABLE FORMS
- *Powder for injection:* 500 mg (Amytal sodium).

UNLABELED USES: Anticonvulsant

CONTRAINDICATIONS: History of manifest or latent porphyria, marked liver dysfunction, marked respiratory disease in which dyspnea or obstruction is evident, and hypersensitivity to amobarbital products

PREGNANCY AND LACTATION: Pregnancy category D; small amount excreted in breast milk; use caution in nursing mothers

Controlled substance: Schedule II

SIDE EFFECTS

Frequent

Somnolence, headache, confusion, dizziness

Occasional

Nausea, vomiting, visual abnormalities, such as spots before eyes, difficulty focusing, blurred vision, dry mouth or pharynx, tongue irritation, water retention, increased sweating, constipation, or diarrhea

SERIOUS REACTIONS
- Overdosage results in severe respiratory depression, skeletal muscle flaccidity, bronchospasm, cardiovascular disturbances, such as congestive heart failure (CHF), hypo-

tension or hypertension, arrhythmias, cold and clammy skin, cyanosis, and coma.

• Tolerance may occur with repeated use.

INTERACTIONS

Drugs

3 *Acetaminophen:* Enhanced hepatotoxic potential of acetaminophen overdoses

3 *Antidepressants:* Reduced serum concentration of cyclic antidepressants

3 *β-adrenergic blockers:* Reduced serum concentrations of β-blockers that are extensively metabolized

3 *Calcium channel blockers:* Reduced serum concentrations of verapamil and dihydropyridines

3 *Chloramphenicol:* Increased barbiturate concentrations; reduced serum chloramphenicol concentrations

3 *Corticosteroids:* Reduced serum concentrations of corticosteroids; may impair therapeutic effect

3 *Cyclosporine:* Reduced serum concentration of cyclosporine

3 *Digitoxin:* Reduced serum concentration of digitoxin

3 *Disopyramide:* Reduced serum concentrations of disopyramide

3 *Doxycycline:* Reduced serum doxycycline concentrations

3 *Estrogen:* Reduced serum concentration of estrogen

3 *Ethanol:* Excessive CNS depression

3 *Griseofulvin:* Reduced griseofulvin absorption

3 *Methoxyflurane:* Enhanced nephrotoxic effect

3 *MAOIs:* Prolonged effect of barbiturates

3 *Narcotic analgesics:* Increased toxicity of meperidine; reduced effect of methadone; additive CNS depression

3 *Neuroleptics:* Reduced effect of either drug

2 *Oral anticoagulants:* Decreased hypoprothrombinemic response to oral anticoagulants

3 *Oral contraceptives:* Reduced efficacy of oral contraceptives

3 *Phenytoin:* Unpredictable effect on serum phenytoin levels

3 *Propafenone:* Reduced serum concentration of propafenone

3 *Quinidine:* Reduced quinidine plasma concentrations

3 *Tacrolimus:* Reduced serum concentration of tacrolimus

3 *Theophylline:* Reduced serum theophylline concentrations

3 *Tranylcypromine:* Prolongs the effect of amobarbital

3 *Valproic acid:* Increased serum concentration of amobarbital

2 *Warfarin:* See oral anticoagulants

SPECIAL CONSIDERATIONS

PATIENT/FAMILY EDUCATION

• Indicated only for short-term treatment of insomnia; probably ineffective after 2 wk; physical dependency may result when used for extended time (45-90 days depending on dose)

• Avoid driving or other activities requiring alertness

• Avoid alcohol ingestion or CNS depressants

• Do not discontinue medication abruptly after long-term use

MONITORING PARAMETERS

• Serum folate, vitamin D (if on long-term therapy)

• PT in patients receiving anticoagulants

• Blood pressure, pulse

A

amoxapine

(a-mox'-a-peen)

Rx: Ascendin

Chemical Class: Dibenzocycloheptene derivative; secondary amine

Therapeutic Class: Antidepressant, tricyclic

CLINICAL PHARMACOLOGY

Mechanism of Action: A tricyclic antidepressant that blocks the reuptake of neurotransmitters, such as norepinephrine and serotonin, at central nervous system (CNS) presynaptic membranes, increasing their availability at postsynaptic receptor sites. The metabolite 7-OH-amoxapine has significant dopamine receptor blocking activity similar to haloperidol. ***Therapeutic Effect:*** Produces antidepressant effects.

Pharmacokinetics

Rapidly, well absorbed from the gastrointestinal (GI) tract. Protein binding: 90%. Metabolized in liver. Excreted in urine and feces. ***Half-life:*** 8 hrs.

INDICATIONS AND DOSAGES

Depression

PO

Adults. 25 mg 2-3 times/day. May increase to 100 mg 2-3 times/day.

Adolescents. Initially, 25-50 mg/day as single or divided doses. May increase to 100 mg/day.

Elderly. Initially, 25 mg at bedtime. May increase by 25 mg/day q3-7 days. Maximum: 400 mg/day (outpatient), 600 mg/day (inpatient).

AVAILABLE FORMS

- *Tablets:* 25 mg, 50 mg, 100 mg, 150 mg (Ascendin).

UNLABELED USES: Panic disorder

CONTRAINDICATIONS: Acute recovery period following myocardial infarction (MI), within 14 days of MAOI ingestion, hypersensitivity to dibenzoxazepine compounds

PREGNANCY AND LACTATION: Pregnancy category C; excreted into breast milk; effect on nursing infant unknown but may be of concern

SIDE EFFECTS

Frequent

Drowsiness, fatigue, xerostomia, constipation, weight gain

Occasional

Nausea, dizziness, headache, confusion, nervousness, restlessness, insomnia, edema, tremor, blurred vision, aggressiveness, muscle weakness

Rare

Paradoxical reactions (agitation, restlessness, nightmares, insomnia, extrapyramidal symptoms, particularly fine hand tremor), laryngitis, seizures

SERIOUS REACTIONS

- High dosage may produce cardiovascular effects, including severe postural hypotension, dizziness, tachycardia, palpitations, arrhythmias, and seizures. High dosage may also result in altered temperature regulation, such as hyperpyrexia or hypothermia.
- Abrupt withdrawal from prolonged therapy may produce headache, malaise, nausea, vomiting, and vivid dreams.

INTERACTIONS

Drugs

3 *Antithyroid agents:* Increases risk of agranulocytosis

3 *Barbiturates:* Reduced serum concentrations of cyclic antidepressants

2 *Bethanidine:* Reduced antihypertensive effect of bethanidine

3 *Carbamazepine:* Reduced serum concentrations of cyclic antidepressants
3 *Cimetidine:* Increased serum concentrations of cyclic antidepressants
3 *Clonidine:* Reduced antihypertensive effect of clonidine; enhanced hypertensive response with abrupt clonidine withdrawal
3 *Debrisoquin:* Reduced antihypertensive effect of debrisoquin
3 *Dilitiazem:* Increased serum concentrations of cyclic antidepressants
❷ *Epinephrine:* Markedly enhanced pressor response to IV epinephrine
3 *Estrogens:* Increases risk of amoxapine toxicity
3 *Ethanol:* Additive impairment of motor skills; abstinent alcoholics may eliminate cyclic antidepressants more rapidly than non-alcoholics
3 *Fluoroquinolones:* Increases cardiac effects
3 *Fluoxetine:* Marked increases in serum concentrations of cyclic antidepressants
3 *Fluvoxamine:* Marked increases in serum concentrations of cyclic antidepressants
3 *Guanabenz, guanadrel, guanethidine, guanfacine:* Reduced antihypertensive effect
3 *Lithium:* Increased risk of neurotoxicity
❷ *Moclobemide:* Potential association with fatal or non-fatal serotonin syndrome
⚠ *MAOIs:* Excessive sympathetic response, mania, or hyperpyrexia possible
3 *Neuroleptics:* Increased therapeutic and toxic effects of both drugs
❷ *Norepinephrine:* Markedly enhanced pressor response to IV norepinephrine
3 *Paroxetine:* Marked increases in serum concentrations of cyclic antidepressants
3 *Propoxyphene:* Increased serum concentrations of cyclic antidepressants
3 *Quinidine:* Increased serum concentrations of cyclic antidepressants
3 *Rifampin:* Reduced serum concentrations of cyclic antidepressants
3 *Ritonavir:* Marked increases in serum concentrations of cyclic antidepressants
3 *Sulfonylureas:* Cyclic antidepressants may increase hypoglycemic effect

SPECIAL CONSIDERATIONS

PATIENT/FAMILY EDUCATION

- Therapeutic effects may take 2-3 wk
- Use caution in driving or other activities requiring alertness
- Avoid rising quickly from sitting to standing, especially elderly
- Avoid alcohol ingestion, other CNS depressants
- Do not discontinue abruptly after long-term use
- Wear sunscreen or large hat to prevent photosensitivity
- Increase fluids, bulk in diet if constipation occurs
- Use gum, hard sugarless candy, or frequent sips of water for dry mouth
- Potential for tardive dyskinesia

MONITORING PARAMETERS

- Blood pressure, pulse

A

amoxicillin

(a-mox-i-sil′-in)

Rx: Amoxicot, Amoxil, Amoxil Pediatric Drops, Biomox, DisperMox, Moxilin, Polymox, Trimox, Wymox

Chemical Class: Penicillin derivative, aminopenicillin

Therapeutic Class: Antibiotic

CLINICAL PHARMACOLOGY

Mechanism of Action: A penicillin that inhibits bacterial cell wall synthesis. ***Therapeutic Effect:*** Bactericidal in susceptible microorganisms.

Pharmacokinetics

Well absorbed from the GI tract. Protein binding: 20%. Partially metabolized in the liver. Primarily excreted in urine. Removed by hemodialysis. ***Half-life:*** 1-1.3 hr (increased in impaired renal function).

INDICATIONS AND DOSAGES

Susceptible infections

PO

Adults, Elderly. 250-500 mg q8h or 500-875 mg q12h.

Children older than 3 mo. 25-50 mg/kg/day in 3 divided doses.

Children 3 mo and younger. 30 mg/kg/day in 2 divided doses.

Lower respiratory tract infection

PO

Adults, Elderly. 500 mg q8h or 875 mg q12h.

H. pylori infection

PO

Adults, Elderly. 1 g twice a day in combination with clarithromycin and lansoprazole for 14 days.

Otitis media

PO

Children. 80-90 mg/kg/day in 2 or 3 divided doses.

Gonorrhea

PO

Adults, Elderly. 3 g as a single dose.

Endocarditis prophylaxis

PO

Adults, Elderly. 2 g 1 hr before procedure.

Children. 50 mg/kg 1 hr before procedure. Maximum: 2 g.

Dosage in renal impairment

Dosage interval is modified based on creatinine clearance.

Creatinine clearance 10-30 ml/min. Usual dose q12h.

Creatinine clearance less than 10 ml/min. Usual dose q24h.

AVAILABLE FORMS

- *Capsules:* 250 mg (Amoxil, Biomox, Trimox, Wymox), 500 mg (Amoxil, Biomox, Trimox).
- *Powder for Reconstitution:* 50 mg/ml (Amoxil Pediatric Drops, Trimox), 125 mg/5 ml (Amoxil, Trimox), 200 mg/ml (Amoxil), 250 mg/ml (Amoxil, Biomox, Trimox), 400 mg/ml (Amoxil).
- *Tablets (Amoxil):* 500 mg, 875 mg.
- *Tablets (Chewable [Amoxil]):* 125 mg, 200 mg, 250 mg, 400 mg.
- *Tablets for Oral Suspension (DisperMox):* 200 mg, 400 mg.

UNLABELED USES: Treatment of Lyme disease and typhoid fever

CONTRAINDICATIONS: Hypersensitivity to any penicillin, infectious mononucleosis

PREGNANCY AND LACTATION: Pregnancy category B; excreted into breast milk in low concentrations; no adverse effects have been observed, but potential exists for modification of bowel flora and allergy/sensitization in nursing infant

SIDE EFFECTS

Frequent

GI disturbances (mild diarrhea, nausea, or vomiting), headache, oral or vaginal candidiasis

Occasional
Generalized rash, urticaria
SERIOUS REACTIONS
• Antibiotic-associated colitis and other superinfections may result from altered bacterial balance.
• Severe hypersensitivity reactions, including anaphylaxis and acute interstitial nephritis, occur rarely.
INTERACTIONS
Drugs
3 *Allopurinol:* Increased incidence of rash
3 *Atenolol:* Reduced serum concentration of atenolol
3 *Chloramphenicol:* Inhibited antibacterial activity of amoxicillin; administer amoxicillin 3 hours before chloramphenicol
3 *Macrolide antibiotics:* Inhibited antibacterial activity of amoxicillin; administer amoxicillin 3 hours before macrolides
3 *Methotrexate:* Increased serum methotrexate concentrations
3 *Oral contraceptives:* Occasional impairment of oral contraceptive efficacy; consider use of supplementary contraception during cycles in which amoxicillin is used
3 *Probenecid:* Increased amoxicillin blood concentration and risk of toxicity
3 *Tetracyclines:* Inhibited antibacterial activity of amoxicillin; administer amoxicillin 3 hours before tetracycline
SPECIAL CONSIDERATIONS
PATIENT/FAMILY EDUCATION
• May administer on a full or empty stomach
• Administer at even intervals
• Shake oral suspensions well before administering; discard after 14 days
• High rates of rash in patients on allopurinol, with mononucleosis, lymphocytic leukemia
• Chew or crush the chewable tablets before swallowing

amoxicillin/clavulanate potassium

(a-mox-i-sill'-in clav-u-lan'-ate)
Rx: Augmentin, Augmentin ES 600, Augmentin XR
Chemical Class: Penicillin derivative, aminopenicillin; β-lactamase inhibitor (clavulanate)
Therapeutic Class: Antibiotic

CLINICAL PHARMACOLOGY
Mechanism of Action: Amoxicillin inhibits bacterial cell wall synthesis, while clavulanate inhibits bacterial beta-lactamase. ***Therapeutic Effect:*** Amoxicillin is bactericidal in susceptible microorganisms. Clavulanate protects amoxicillin from enzymatic degradation.
Pharmacokinetics
Well absorbed from the GI tract. Protein binding: 20%. Partially metabolized in the liver. Primarily excreted in urine. Removed by hemodialysis. ***Half-life:*** 1-1.3 hr (increased in impaired renal function).
INDICATIONS AND DOSAGES
Mild to moderate infections
PO
Adults, Elderly. 500 mg q12h or 250 mg q8h.
Severe infections, respiratory tract infections
PO
Adults, Elderly. 875 mg q12h or 500 mg q8h.
Community-acquired pneumonia, sinusitis
PO
Adults, Elderly. 2 g (extended-release tablets) q12h for 7-10 days.

Sinusitis
PO
Adults, Elderly. 2 g (extended-release tablets) q12h for 7-10 days.
Children weighing 40 kg and less. 25-45 mg/kg/day (200 or 400 mg/5 ml powder or 200 or 400 mg chewable tablets) in 2 divided doses or 20-40 mg/kg/day (125 or 250 mg/5 ml powder or 125 or 250 mg chewable tablets) in 3 divided doses.
Otitis media
PO
Children. 90 mg/kg/day (600 mg/5 ml suspension) in divided doses q12h for 10 days.
Usual neonate dosage
PO
Neonates, Children younger than 3 mos. 30 mg/kg/day (125 mg/5 ml suspension) in divided doses q12h.
Dosage in renal impairment
Dosage and frequency are modified based on creatinine clearance.
Creatinine clearance 10-30 ml/min. 250-500 mg q12h.
Creatinine clearance less than 10 ml/min. 250-500 mg q24h.

AVAILABLE FORMS
- *Powder for Oral Suspension (Augmentin):* 125 mg-31.25 mg/5 ml, 200 mg-28.5 mg/5 ml, 250 mg-62.5 mg/5 ml, 400 mg-57 mg/5 ml, 600 mg-42.9 mg/5 ml.
- *Tablets (Augmentin):* 250 mg-125 mg, 500 mg-125 mg, 875 mg-125 mg.
- *Tablets (Extended-Release [Augmentin XR]):* 1000 mg-62.5 mg.
- *Tablets (Chewable [Augmentin]):* 125 mg-31.25 mg, 200 mg-28.5 mg, 250 mg-62.5 mg, 400 mg-57 mg.

UNLABELED USES: Treatment of bronchitis and chancroid

CONTRAINDICATIONS: Hypersensitivity to any penicillins, infectious mononucleosis

PREGNANCY AND LACTATION: Pregnancy category B; excreted into breast milk in low concentrations; no adverse effects have been observed

SIDE EFFECTS
Frequent
GI disturbances (mild diarrhea, nausea, vomiting), headache, oral or vaginal candidiasis
Occasional
Generalized rash, urticaria

SERIOUS REACTIONS
- Antibiotic-associated colitis and other superinfections may result from altered bacterial balance.
- Severe hypersensitivity reactions, including anaphylaxis and acute interstitial nephritis occur rarely.

INTERACTIONS
Drugs
3 *Allopurinol:* Increased incidence of rash
3 *Atenolol:* Reduced serum concentration of atenolol
3 *Chloramphenicol:* Inhibited antibacterial activity of amoxicillin; administer amoxicillin 3 hours before chloramphenicol
3 *Macrolide antibiotics:* Inhibited antibacterial activity of amoxicillin; administer amoxicillin 3 hours before macrolides
3 *Methotrexate:* Increased serum methotrexate concentrations
3 *Oral contraceptives:* Occasional impairment of oral contraceptive efficacy; consider use of supplementary contraception during cycles in which amoxicillin is used
3 *Probenecid:* Increased amoxicillin blood concentration and risk of toxicity
3 *Tetracyclines:* Inhibited antibacterial activity of amoxicillin; administer amoxicillin 3 hours before tetracycline

SPECIAL CONSIDERATIONS

- Augmentin XR indicated for treatment of community acquired pneumonia or bacterial sinusitis due to β-lactamase-producing strains with reduced penicillin susceptibility
- Augmentin ES indicated for otitis media (AOM) in pediatric patients with antibiotic treatment for AOM in previous 3 mos and either ≤age 2 or attending daycare

PATIENT/FAMILY EDUCATION

- Administer with food to decrease GI side effects and enhance absorption
- Administer at even intervals
- Shake oral suspensions well before administering; discard after 14 days; must be refrigerated

---

amphetamine sulfate

(am-fet'-ah-meen sul'-fate)

Combinations

Rx: with dextroamphetamine: (Adderall, Adderall XR)

Chemical Class: β-phenylisopropylamine (racemic)

Therapeutic Class: Central nervous system stimulant

DEA Class: Schedule II

CLINICAL PHARMACOLOGY

Mechanism of Action: A sympathomimetic amine that produces central nervous system (CNS) and respiratory stimulation, mydriasis, bronchodilation, a pressor response, and contraction of the urinary sphincter. Directly effects alpha and beta receptor sites in peripheral system. Enhances release of norepinephrine by blocking reuptake, inhibiting monoamine oxidase. ***Therapeutic Effect:*** Increases motor activity, mental alertness; decreases drowsiness, fatigue.

Pharmacokinetics

Well absorbed from the gastrointestinal (GI) tract. Protein binding: 20%. Widely distributed (including CSF). Metabolized in liver. Excreted in urine. Unknown if removed by hemodialysis. ***Half-life:*** 7-31 hrs.

INDICATIONS AND DOSAGES

Attention-deficit hyperactivity disorder (ADHD)

PO

Adults. 5-20 mg 1-3 times/day.

Adults, Children older than 12 yrs. Initially, 5 mg twice a day. Increase by 10 mg at weekly intervals until therapeutic response achieved.

Children 6-12 yrs. Initially, 2.5 mg twice a day. Increase by 5 mg/day at weekly intervals until therapeutic response achieved.

Children 3-6 yrs. Initially, 2.5 mg twice a day. Increase by 2.5 mg/day at weekly intervals until therapeutic response achieved.

Narcolepsy

PO

Adults. 5-20 mg 1-3 times/day.

Adults, Children older than 12 yrs. Initially, 5 mg twice a day. Increase by 10 mg at weekly intervals until therapeutic response achieved.

Children 6-12 yrs. Initially, 2.5 mg twice a day. Increase by 5 mg/day at weekly intervals until therapeutic response achieved.

AVAILABLE FORMS

- *Tablets:* 5 mg, 10 mg.

UNLABELED USES: Depression, obsessive-compulsive disorder

CONTRAINDICATIONS: Advanced arteriosclerosis, agitated states, glaucoma, history of drug abuse, history of hypersensitivity to sympathomimetic amines, hyperthyroidism, moderate to severe hypertension, symptomatic cardiovascular disease, within 14 days following discontinuation of an MAOI

PREGNANCY AND LACTATION: Pregnancy category C; use of amphetamine for medical indications not a significant risk to the fetus for congenital anomalies, mild withdrawal symptoms may be observed in the newborn; illicit maternal use presents significant risks to the fetus and newborn, including intrauterine growth retardation, premature delivery, and the potential for increased maternal, fetal, and neonatal morbidity; concentrated in breast milk; contraindicated during breastfeeding

Controlled substance: Schedule II

SIDE EFFECTS

Frequent

Irregular pulse, increased motor activity, talkativeness, nervousness, mild euphoria, insomnia

Occasional

Headache, chills, dry mouth, gastrointestinal (GI) distress, worsening depression in patients who are clinically depressed, tachycardia, palpitations, chest pain

SERIOUS REACTIONS

- Overdose may produce skin pallor or flushing, arrhythmias, and psychosis.
- Abrupt withdrawal following prolonged administration of high dosage may produce lethargy (may last for weeks).
- Prolonged administration to children with ADHD may produce a temporary suppression of normal weight and height patterns.

INTERACTIONS

Drugs

3 *Antacids:* May inhibit amphetamine excretion

3 *β-blockers:* Increased risk of bradycardia

3 *Ethosuximide:* Intestinal absorption of ethosuximide may be delayed

3 *Furazolidone:* Hypertensive reactions

3 *Guanadrel:* Inhibits antihypertensive response to guanadrel

3 *Guanethidine:* Inhibits antihypertensive response to guanethidine

3 *Lithium:* May inhibit effects of amphetamines

⚠ *MAOIs:* Severe hypertensive reactions possible

3 *Methenamine:* Urinary excretion of amphetamine is increased by acidifying agents

❷ *Norepinephrine:* Adrenergic effect of norepinephrine enhanced

3 *Phenobarbital:* Intestinal absorption of phenobarbital may be delayed; synergistic anticonvulsant effect possible

3 *Phenytoin:* Intestinal absorption of phenytoin may be delayed; synergistic anticonvulsant effect possible

⚠ *Propoxyphene:* In cases of propoxyphene overdosage, amphetamine CNS stimulation is potentiated, fatal convulsions can occur

❷ *Selegiline:* Severe hypertensive reactions possible

3 *Sodium bicarbonate:* May inhibit amphetamine excretion

❷ *Tricyclic antidepressants:* May enhance activity of tricyclics; increased amphetamine levels in the brain; CV effects potentiated

Labs

- *False positive:* Urine amino acids
- May interfere with urinary steroid determinations

SPECIAL CONSIDERATIONS

PATIENT/FAMILY EDUCATION

- Take early in the day
- Do not discontinue abruptly
- Avoid hazardous activities until stabilized on medication
- Sip tepid water and sugarless gum to relieve dry mouth

MONITORING PARAMETERS

- Heart rate, pulse
- Weight

amphotericin B / amphotericin B cholesteryl / amphotericin B lipid complex / liposomal amphotericin B

(am-foe-ter'-i-sin bee)

Rx: Abelcet (ABLC); AmBisome, Amphotec, Fungizone (IV and topical)

Chemical Class: Amphoteric polyene lipid complex (ABLC)

Therapeutic Class: Antifungal

CLINICAL PHARMACOLOGY

Mechanism of Action: The amphotericin B group is antifungal and antiprotozoal and generally fungistatic but may become fungicidal with high dosages or very susceptible microorganisms. This drug binds to sterols in the fungal cell membrane. ***Therapeutic Effect:*** Increases fungal cell-membrane permeability, allowing loss of potassium, and other cellular components.

Pharmacokinetics

Protein binding: 90%. Widely distributed. Metabolic fate unknown. Cleared by nonrenal pathways. Minimal removal by hemodialysis. Amphotec and Abelcet are not dialyzable. ***Half-life:*** 24 hrs (half-life increased in neonates, children). Amphotec ***Half-life:*** 26-28 hrs. Abelcet ***Half-life:*** 7.2 days. AmBisome ***Half-life:*** 100-153 hrs.

INDICATIONS AND DOSAGES

Invasive fungal infections unresponsive or intolerant to Fungizone (Abelcet)

IV Infusion

Adults, Children. 5 mg/kg at rate of 2.5 mg/kg/hr.

Empiric treatment for fungal infection in patients with febrile neutropenia; for aspergillus, candida, or cryptococcus infections unresponsive to Fungizone; or for patients with renal impairment or toxicity from Fungizone (AmBisome)

IV Infusion

Adults, Children. 3-5 mg/kg over 1 hr.

Invasive aspergillus in patients with renal impairment, renal toxicity, or treatment failure with Fungizone (Amphotec)

IV Infusion

Adults, Children. 3-4 mg/kg over 2-4 hrs.

Cutaneous and mucocutaneous infections caused by Candida albicans, such as paronychia, oral thrush, perlèche, diaper rash, and intertriginous candidiasis (Topical)

Adults, Elderly, Children. Apply liberally to the affected area and rub in 2-4 times/day.

Cryptococcosis; blastomycosis; systemic candidiasis; disseminated forms of moniliasis, coccidioidomycosis, and histoplasmosis; zygomycosis; sporotrichosis; and aspergillosis (Fungizone)

IV Infusion

Adults, Elderly. Dosage based on pt tolerance, severity of infection. Initially, 1-mg test dose is given over 20-30 min. If test dose is tolerated, 5-mg dose may be given the same day. Subsequently, increases of 5 mg/dose are made q12-24h until desired daily dose is reached. Alternatively, if test dose is tolerated, a dose of 0.25 mg/kg is given same day; increased to 0.5 mg/kg the second day. Dose increased until desired daily dose reached. Total daily dose: 1 mg/kg/day up to 1.5 mg/kg every other day. Do not exceed maximum total daily dose of 1.5 mg/kg.

Children. Test dose: 0.1 mg/kg/dose (maximum 1 mg) infused over 20-60 min. If tolerated, then initial dose: 0.4 mg/kg same day; Dose may be increased in 0.25 mg/kg increments. Maintenance dose: 0.25-1 mg/kg/day.

AVAILABLE FORMS

- *Injection:* 50 mg, 50 mg (Fungizone), 100 mg (Amphotec), 50 mg (AmBisone).
- *Suspension for Injection:* 5 mg/ml (Amphotericin B lipid complex, Abelcet).
- *Cream, Lotion, Ointment:* 3% (Fungizone).

CONTRAINDICATIONS: Hypersensitivity to amphotericin B, sulfite

PREGNANCY AND LACTATION: Pregnancy category B; excretion in human milk unknown; due to the potential toxicity, consider discontinuing nursing

SIDE EFFECTS

Frequent (greater than 10%)

Abelcet: Chills, fever, increased serum creatinine, multiple organ failure

AmBisome: Hypokalemia, hypomagnesemia, hyperglycemia, hypocalcemia, edema, abdominal pain, back pain, chills, chest pain, hypotension, diarrhea, nausea, vomiting, headache, fever, rigors, insomnia, dyspnea, epistaxis, increased liver/renal function test results

Amphotec: Chills, fever, hypotension, tachycardia, increased creatinine, hypokalemia, bilirubinemia

Fungizone: Fever, chills, headache, anemia, hypokalemia, hypomagnesemia, anorexia, malaise, generalized pain, nephrotoxicity

Topical: Local irritation, dry skin

Rare

Topical: Skin rash

SERIOUS REACTIONS

- Cardiovascular toxicity as evidenced by hypotension and ventricular fibrillation and anaphylaxis occur rarely.
- Vision and hearing alterations, seizures, liver failure, coagulation defects, multiple organ failure, and sepsis may be noted.

INTERACTIONS

Drugs

3 *Aminoglycosides:* Synergistic nephrotoxicity

3 *Cyclosporine:* Increased nephrotoxicity of both drugs

3 *Digoxin:* Digitalis toxicity may be enhanced by amphotericin B–induced hypokalemia

3 *Neuromuscular blocking agents:* Prolonged muscle relaxation due to hypokalemia

3 *Steroids:* May cause hypokalemia

Labs

- *Increase:* Serum bilirubin, serum conjugated bilirubin, serum cholesterol
- *Decrease:* Serum unconjugated bilirubin

SPECIAL CONSIDERATIONS

PATIENT/FAMILY EDUCATION

- Long-term therapy may be needed to clear infection (2 wk-3 mo depending on type of infection)
- Fever reaction may decrease with continued therapy
- Muscle weakness may occur from drug-related loss of potassium

MONITORING PARAMETERS

- BUN, serum creatinine; if BUN exceeds 40 mg/dl or serum creatinine exceeds 3 mg/dl, discontinue the drug or reduce dosage until renal function improves
- Regular monitoring of CBC, K, Na, Mg, LFTs

- Total dosage
- Blood pressure, pulse, respirations, and temperature every 15 minutes, then every 30 minutes for the first 4 hours of the infusion to assess for adverse reactions. Adverse reactions include abdominal pain, anorexia, chills, fever, nausea, vomiting, and tremors. If adverse reactions occur, slow the infusion rate and give prescribed drugs to provide symptomatic relief. For patients with a severe reaction and those without orders for symptomatic relief, stop the infusion and notify the physician.

ampicillin

(am-pi-sill'-in)

Rx: Amficot, Omnipen, Omnipen-N, Polycillin, Polycillin-N, Principen, Totacillin, Totacillin-N

Combinations

Rx: with probenecid (Polycillin PRB, Probampicin)

Chemical Class: Penicillin derivative, aminopenicillin

Therapeutic Class: Antibiotic

CLINICAL PHARMACOLOGY

Mechanism of Action: A penicillin that inhibits cell wall synthesis in susceptible microorganisms. ***Therapeutic Effect:*** Produces bactericidal effect.

Pharmacokinetics

Moderately absorbed from the gastrointestinal (GI) tract. Protein binding: 28%. Widely distributed. Partially metabolized in liver. Primarily excreted in urine. Removed by hemodialysis. ***Half-life:*** 1-1.9 hrs (half-life increased in impaired renal function).

INDICATIONS AND DOSAGES

Respiratory tract, skin/skin-structure infections

PO

Adults, Elderly, Children weighing more than 20 kg. 250-500 mg q6h.

Children weighing less than 20 kg. 50 mg/kg/day in divided doses q6h.

IM/IV

Adults, Elderly, Children weighing more than 40 kg. 250-500 mg q6h.

Children weighing less than 40 kg. 25-50 mg/kg/day in divided doses q6-8h. Bacterial meningitis, septicemia.

IM/IV

Adults, Elderly. 2 g q4h or 3 g q6h.

Children. 100-200 mg/kg/day in divided doses q4h. Gonococcal infections.

PO

Adults. 3.5 g one time with 1 g probenecid. Perioperative prophylaxis

IM/IV

Adults, Elderly. 2 g 30 min before procedure. May repeat in 8 hrs.

Children. 50 mg/kg using same dosage regimen. Usual neonate dosage.

IM/IV

Neonates 7-28 days old. 75 mg/kg/day in divided doses q8h up to 200 mg/kg/day in divided doses q6h.

Neonates 0-7 days old. 50 mg/kg/day in divided doses q12h up to 150 mg/kg/day in divided doses q8h.

AVAILABLE FORMS

- *Capsules:* 250 mg (Amficot), 500 mg (Omnipen, Principen, Totacillin).
- *Powder for PO Suspension:* 100/ml (Polycillin), 125 mg/5 ml (Omnipen, Polycillin, Principen, Totacillin), 250 mg/5 ml (Omnipen,

Polycillin, Principen, Totacillin), 500 mg/5 ml (Polycillin).

• *Powder for Injection:* 125 mg (Omnipen-N, Polycillin-N), 250 mg (Omnipen-N, Polycillin-N, Totacillin-N), 500 mg (Omnipen-N, Polycillin-N, Totacillin-N), 1 g (Omnipen-N, Polycillin-N, Totacillin-N), 2 g (Omnipen-N, Polycillin-N, Totacillin-N), 10 g (Omnipen-N, Polycillin-N).

CONTRAINDICATIONS: Hypersensitivity to any penicillin, infectious mononucleosis

PREGNANCY AND LACTATION: Pregnancy category B; excreted into breast milk in low concentrations; no adverse effects have been observed

SIDE EFFECTS

Frequent

Pain at IM injection site, GI disturbances, including mild diarrhea, nausea, or vomiting, oral or vaginal candidiasis

Occasional

Generalized rash, urticaria, phlebitis, thrombophlebitis with IV administration, headache

Rare

Dizziness, seizures, especially with IV therapy

SERIOUS REACTIONS

• Altered bacterial balance may result in potentially fatal superinfections and antibiotic-associated colitis as evidenced by abdominal cramps, watery or severe diarrhea, and fever.

• Severe hypersensitivity reactions, including anaphylaxis and acute interstitial nephritis, occur rarely.

INTERACTIONS

Drugs

3 *Allopurinol:* Increased incidence of rash

3 *Atenolol:* Reduced serum concentration of atenolol

3 *Chloramphenicol:* Inhibited antibacterial activity of ampicillin; administer ampicillin 3 hr before chloramphenicol

3 *Macrolide antibiotics:* Inhibited antibacterial activity of ampicillin; administer amoxicillin 3 hr before macrolides

3 *Methotrexate:* Increased serum methotrexate concentrations

3 *Oral contraceptives:* Occasional impairment of oral contraceptive efficacy; consider use of supplemental contraception during cycles in which ampicillin is used

3 *Probenecid:* Increased amoxicillin blood concentration and risk of toxicity

3 *Tetracyclines:* Inhibited antibacterial activity of ampicillin; administer ampicillin 3 hr before tetracycline

Labs

• *False positive:* Urine amino acids

• *Increase:* Urine glucose (Clinitest method), plasma phenyldanine (dried blood spot method), CSF protein (Ektachem method), serum protein (Biuret method), serum theophylline (3M Diagnostics TheoFast method), serum uric acid

• *Decrease:* Serum cholesterol (CHOD-iodide method only), serum folate (bioassay method only), urine glucose (Clinistix and Diastix methods)

SPECIAL CONSIDERATIONS

PATIENT/FAMILY EDUCATION

• Administer on an empty stomach

• Administer at even intervals

• Shake oral suspensions well before administering, discard after 14 days

• High rates of rash in patients on allopurinol, with mononucleosis, lymphatic leukemia

• Amoxicillin is better oral choice given greater ease of dosing and lower incidence of diarrhea

ampicillin/sulbactam sodium

(am'-pi-sill-in/sul-bac'-tam)

Rx: Unasyn

Chemical Class: Penicillin derivative, aminopenicillin; penicillinate (sulbactam)

Therapeutic Class: Antibiotic

CLINICAL PHARMACOLOGY

Mechanism of Action: Ampicillin inhibits bacterial cell wall synthesis, while sulbactam inhibits bacterial beta-lactamase. ***Therapeutic Effect:*** Ampicillin is bactericidal in susceptible microorganisms. Sulbactam protects ampicillin from enzymatic degradation.

Pharmacokinetics

Protein binding: 28%-38%. Widely distributed. Partially metabolized in the liver. Primarily excreted in urine. Removed by hemodialysis. ***Half-life:*** 1 hr (increased in impaired renal function).

INDICATIONS AND DOSAGES

Skin and skin-structure, intra-abdominal, and gynecologic infections

IV, IM

Adults, Elderly. 1.5 g (1 g ampicillin/500 mg sulbactam) to 3 g (2 g ampicillin/1 g sulbactam) q6h.

Skin and skin-structure infections

IV

Children 12 yr and younger. 150-400 mg/kg/day in divided doses q6h.

Dosage in renal impairment

Dosage and frequency are modified based on creatinine clearance and the severity of the infection.

Creatinine Clearance	*Dosage*
greater than 30 ml/min	0.5-3 g q6-8h
15-29 ml/min	1.5-3 g q12h
5-14 ml/min	1.5-3 g q24h
less than 5 ml/min	Not recommended

AVAILABLE FORMS

• *Powder for Injection:* 1.5 g (ampicillin 1 g/sulbactam 500 g), 3 g (ampicillin 2 g/sulbactam 1 g).

CONTRAINDICATIONS: Hypersensitivity to any penicillin or sulbactam, infectious mononucleosis

PREGNANCY AND LACTATION: Pregnancy category B; animal studies at doses 10× the human dose reveal no evidence of harm; low concentrations excreted in breast milk

SIDE EFFECTS

Frequent

Diarrhea and rash (most common), urticaria, pain at IM injection site, thrombophlebitis with IV administration, oral or vaginal candidiasis

Occasional

Nausea, vomiting, headache, malaise, urine retention

SERIOUS REACTIONS

• Severe hypersensitivity reactions, including anaphylaxis, acute interstitial nephritis, and blood dyscrasias may occur.

• Antibiotic-associated colitis and other superinfections may result from altered bacterial balance.

• Overdose may produce seizures.

INTERACTIONS

Drugs

3 *Allopurinol:* Increased incidence of rash

3 *Chloramphenicol:* Inhibited antibacterial activity of ampicillin/sulbactam; administer ampicillin/sulbactam 3 hr before chloramphenicol

3 *Macrolide antibiotics:* Inhibited antibacterial activity of ampicillin/

sulbactam; administer ampicillin/sulbactam 3 hr before macrolides

3 *Methotrexate:* Increased serum methotrexate concentrations

3 *Oral contraceptives:* Occasional impairment of oral contraceptive efficacy; consider use of supplemental contraception during cycles in which ampicillin/sulbactam is used

3 *Probenecid:* Increased amoxicillin blood concentration and risk of toxicity

3 *Tetracyclines:* Inhibited antibacterial activity of ampicillin/sulbactam; administer ampicillin/sulbactam 3 hr before tetracyclines

Labs

- *False positive:* Urine amino acids
- *Increase:* Urine glucose (Clinitest method), plasma phenyldanine (dried blood spot method), CSF protein (Ektachem method), serum protein (biuret method), serum theophylline (3M Diagnostics TheoFast method), serum uric acid, serum creatinine
- *Decrease:* Serum cholesterol (CHOD-iodide method only), serum folate (bioassay method only)

SPECIAL CONSIDERATIONS

- Do not reconstitute or administer with aminoglycosides (ampicillin inactivates aminoglycosides, may be administered separately)
- Safety and efficacy established for pediatric skin and soft tissue infections only

PATIENT/FAMILY EDUCATION

- Administer at even intervals

amprenavir

(am-pren′-a-veer)

Rx: Agenerase

Chemical Class: Protease inhibitor, HIV

Therapeutic Class: Antiretroviral

CLINICAL PHARMACOLOGY

Mechanism of Action: An antiretroviral that inhibits HIV-1 protease by binding to the enzyme's active site, thus preventing processing of viral precursors and resulting in the formation of immature, noninfectious viral particles. ***Therapeutic Effect:*** Impairs HIV replication and proliferation.

Pharmacokinetics

Rapidly absorbed after PO administration. Protein binding: 90%. Metabolized in the liver. Primarily excreted in feces. ***Half-life:*** 7.1-10.6 hr.

INDICATIONS AND DOSAGES

HIV-1 infection (in combination with other antiretrovirals)

PO

Adults, Children 17 yr and older, Children 13-16 yr weighing 50 kg and more. 1200 mg twice a day.

Children 4-12 yr, Children 13-16 yr weighing less than 50 kg. 20 mg/kg twice a day or 15 mg/kg 3 times a day. Maximum: 2400 mg/day.

Oral solution

Adults, Children 17 yr and older, Children 13-16 yr weighing 50 kg and more. 1400 mg twice a day.

Children 4-12 yr, Children 13-16 yr weighing less than 50 kg. 22.5 mg/kg/day (1.5 ml/kg) oral solution twice a day or 17 mg/kg/day (1.1 ml/kg) 3 times a day. Maximum: 2800 mg/day.

Dosage in hepatic impairment

Dosage and frequency are modified based on the Child-Pugh score.

Child-Pugh Score	*Capsules*	*Oral Solution*
5-8	450 mg bid	513 mg bid
9-12	300 mg bid	342 mg bid

AVAILABLE FORMS

- *Capsules:* 50 mg.
- *Oral Solution:* 15 mg/ml.

CONTRAINDICATIONS: None known.

PREGNANCY AND LACTATION: Pregnancy category C; excreted in breast milk of animals

SIDE EFFECTS

Frequent

Diarrhea or loose stools (56%), nausea (38%), oral paresthesia (30%), rash (25%), vomiting (20%)

Occasional

Peripheral paresthesia (12%), depression (4%)

SERIOUS REACTIONS

- Severe hypersensitivity reactions or Stevens-Johnson syndrome as evidenced by blisters, peeling of the skin, loosening of skin and mucous membranes, and fever may occur.

INTERACTIONS

Drugs

3 *Abacavir:* Mild increase in amprenavir plasma level when given with abacavir

3 *Antacids:* May decrease amprenavir absorption

▲ *Astemizole:* Increased plasma levels of astemizole

3 *Barbiturates:* Increased clearance of amprenavir; reduced clearance of barbiturates

❷ *Carbamazepine:* Increased clearance of amprenavir; reduced clearance of carbamazepine

▲ *Cisapride:* Increased plasma levels of cisapride

3 *Delavirdine:* Chronic dosing of delavirdine increases amprenavir concentrations, while chronic amprenavir administration decreases delavirdine plasma concentrations

▲ *Ergot alkaloids:* Increased plasma levels of ergot alkaloids

3 *Erythromycin:* Reduced clearance of amprenavir; amprenavir reduces clearance of erythromycin

3 *High-fat meals:* May decrease amprenavir absorption

3 *Ketoconazole:* Increases both drugs' plasma concentrations

▲ *Lovastatin:* Amprenavir reduces clearance of lovastatin

▲ *Midazolam:* Increased plasma levels of midazolam and prolonged effect

3 *Nevirapine:* Reduces plasma amprenavir levels

3 *Oral contraceptives:* Amprenavir may reduce efficacy

3 *Phenytoin:* Increased clearance of amprenavir; reduced clearance of phenytoin

❷ *Rifabutin:* Increased clearance of amprenavir; reduced clearance of rifabutin

▲ *Rifampin:* Increased clearance of amprenavir

3 *Ritonavir:* Decreased clearance of amprenavir

3 *Saquinavir:* Decreased clearance of saquinavir; reduce dose of Fortovase (saquinavir soft gel capsule) to 800 mg tid

3 *Sildenafil:* Decreased clearance of sildenafil

▲ *Simvastatin:* Amprenavir reduces clearance of simvastatin

3 *St. John's Wort:* May decrease amprenavir blood concentration

▲ *Terfenadine:* Increased plasma levels of terfenadine

▲ *Triazolam:* Increased plasma levels of triazolam and prolonged effect

SPECIAL CONSIDERATIONS

PATIENT/FAMILY EDUCATION

- May take with or without food, but do not take with a high-fat meal
- Do not take supplemental vitamin E; capsule and liquid forms have vitamin E in them
- Amprenavir is not a cure for HIV infection, nor does it reduce the risk of transmitting HIV to others

MONITORING PARAMETERS

- CBC, metabolic panel, hepatic function panel, CD4 lymphocyte count, HIV RNA level
- Skin for rash
- Pattern of daily bowel activity and stool consistency

---

amyl nitrite

(am'-il nye'-trate)

Rx: Amyl nitrite

Chemical Class: Nitrate, organic

Therapeutic Class: Antianginal; antidote, cyanide; vasodilator

---

CLINICAL PHARMACOLOGY

Mechanism of Action: A nitrite vasodilator that relaxes smooth muscles. Reduces afterload and improves vascular supply to the myocardium. ***Therapeutic Effect:*** Dilates coronary arteries, improves blood flow to ischemic areas within myocardium. Following inhalation, systemic vasodilation occurs.

Pharmacokinetics

The vapors are absorbed rapidly through the pulmonary alveoli and metabolized rapidly. Partially excreted in the urine.

INDICATIONS AND DOSAGES

Acute relief of angina pectoris

Nasal inhalation

Adults, Elderly. Place crushed capsule to nostrils for 0.18-0.3 ml inhalation of vapors. Repeat at 5-10 min intervals. No more than 3 doses in 15-30 min period.

AVAILABLE FORMS

- *Solution:* 0.3 ml (Amyl nitrite).

UNLABELED USES: Cyanide toxicity

CONTRAINDICATIONS: Closed-angle glaucoma, severe anemia, head injury, postural hypotension, pregnancy, hypersensitivity to nitrates

PREGNANCY AND LACTATION: Pregnancy category C; markedly reduces systemic blood pressure and blood flow on maternal side of the placenta

SIDE EFFECTS

Frequent

Headache (may be severe) occurs mostly in early therapy, diminishes rapidly in intensity, usually disappears during continued treatment; transient flushing of face and neck; dizziness (especially if patient is standing immobile or is in a warm environment); weakness; postural hypotension

Occasional

Nausea, rash, vomiting

Rare

Involuntary passage of urine and feces, restlessness, weakness

SERIOUS REACTIONS

- Large doses may produce hemolytic anemia or methemoglobinemia.
- Severe postural hypotension manifested by fainting, pulselessness, cold or clammy skin, and profuse sweating may occur.
- Tolerance may occur with repeated, prolonged therapy.
- High dose tends to produce severe headache.

INTERACTIONS

Drugs

3 *Alcohol:* Exaggerated hypotension and cardiac collapse

■3 *Calcium channel blockers:* Exaggerated symptomatic orthostatic hypotension
■3 *Dihydroergotamine:* Increases the bioavailability of dihydroergotamine with resultant increase in mean standing systolic blood pressure; functional antagonism, decreasing effects
■3 *Sildenafil:* Excessive hypotensive effects

Labs

- False decrease in cholesterol via Zlatkis-Zak color reaction

SPECIAL CONSIDERATIONS

- Volatile nitrites abused for sexual stimulation; transient dizziness, weakness, or other signs of cerebral hypoperfusion may develop following inhalation

PATIENT/FAMILY EDUCATION

- Drug should be inhaled while the patient is seated or lying down
- Taking after drinking alcohol may worsen side effects
- Alert to probable headache, dizziness, or flushing side effects
- Amyl nitrite is very flammable
- Tolerance may develop with repeated use

MONITORING PARAMETERS

- Blood pressure, pulse
- Onset, type, location, intensity, and duration of anginal pain

anagrelide

(an-ag′-gre-lide)

Rx: Agrylin

Chemical Class: Quinazoline derivative

Therapeutic Class: Antiplatelet agent

CLINICAL PHARMACOLOGY

Mechanism of Action: A hematologic agent that reduces platelet production and prevents platelet shape changes caused by platelet aggregating agents. ***Therapeutic Effect:*** Inhibits platelet aggregation.

Pharmacokinetics

After oral administration, plasma concentration peak within 1 hr. Extensively metabolized. Primarily excreted in urine. ***Half-life:*** About 3 days.

INDICATIONS AND DOSAGES

Thrombocythemia

PO

Adults, Elderly. Initially, 0.5 mg 4 times a day or 1 mg twice a day. Adjust to lowest effective dosage, increasing by up to 0.5 mg/day or less in any 1 wk. Maximum: 10 mg/day or 2.5 mg/dose.

Children. Initially, 0.5 mg/day. Range: 0.5 mg 1-4 times a day.

AVAILABLE FORMS

- *Capsules:* 0.5 mg, 1 mg.

CONTRAINDICATIONS: Severe hepatic impairment

PREGNANCY AND LACTATION: Pregnancy category C; not recommended in women who are or may become pregnant; excretion into breast milk unknown

SIDE EFFECTS

Frequent (5% or more)

Headache, palpitations, diarrhea, abdominal pain, nausea, flatulence, bloating, asthenia, pain, dizziness

Occasional (less than 5%)

Tachycardia, chest pain, vomiting, paresthesia, peripheral edema, anorexia, dyspepsia, rash

Rare

Confusion, insomnia

SERIOUS REACTIONS

- Angina, heart failure, and arrhythmias occur rarely.

SPECIAL CONSIDERATIONS

PATIENT/FAMILY EDUCATION

- Platelet count should respond within 7 to 14 days of beginning therapy

• Anagrelide is not for pregnant women; they should use contraceptives while taking the drug

MONITORING PARAMETERS

• Platelet count q2 days during first wk, then weekly thereafter until maintenance dose reached

• BUN and serum creatinine levels and hepatic enzyme test

• Assess the patient with suspected heart disease for tachycardia, palpitations, and signs and symptoms of CHF, such as dyspnea

• Assess skin for bruises or petechiae, and inspect catheter and needle insertion sites for bleeding; also assess for signs and symptoms of GI bleeding

anakinra

(an-a-kin′-ra)

Rx: Kineret

Chemical Class: Recombinant interleukin receptor antagonist (IL-1Ra)

Therapeutic Class: Disease-modifying antirheumatic drug (DMARD); immunomodulatory agent

CLINICAL PHARMACOLOGY

Mechanism of Action: An interleukin-1 (IL-1) receptor antagonist that blocks the binding of IL-1, a protein that is a major mediator of joint disease and is present in excess amounts in patients with rheumatoid arthritis. ***Therapeutic Effect:*** Inhibits the inflammatory response.

Pharmacokinetics

No accumulation of anakinra in tissues or organs was observed after daily subcutaneous doses. Excreted in urine. ***Half-life:*** 4-6 hr.

INDICATIONS AND DOSAGES

Rheumatoid arthritis

Subcutaneous

Adults, Elderly. 100 mg/day, given at same time each day.

AVAILABLE FORMS

• *Solution:* 100-mg syringe.

CONTRAINDICATIONS: Known hypersensitivity to *Escherichia coli*–derived proteins, serious infection

PREGNANCY AND LACTATION: Pregnancy category B; excretion into breast milk unknown; use caution in nursing mothers

SIDE EFFECTS

Occasional

Injection site ecchymosis, erythema, and inflammation

Rare

Headache, nausea, diarrhea, abdominal pain

SERIOUS REACTIONS

• Infections, including upper respiratory tract infection, sinusitis, flulike symptoms, and cellulitis, have been noted.

• Neutropenia may occur, particularly when anakinra is used in combination with tumor necrosis factor–blocking agents.

INTERACTIONS

Drugs

❷ *Etanercept:* increased rate of serious infections, neutropenia

❸ *Live-virus vaccines:* May cause the vaccines to be ineffective

SPECIAL CONSIDERATIONS

• Currently recommended for management of rheumatoid arthritis after failure of other DMARD agents

PATIENT/FAMILY EDUCATION

• Signs and symptoms of allergic reactions, injection site reactions, and infections and advised of appropriate actions

• Proper disposal of needles, syringes

MONITORING PARAMETERS

- Patient reported outcomes (disability index, patient global assessment), physician assessments (tender/painful/swollen joints, physician's global assessment), objective measures (ESR, CRP); neutrophil counts baseline, q3mo, then quarterly qyr

anastrozole

(an-as'-troe-zole)

Rx: Arimidex

Chemical Class: Benzyltriazole derivative

Therapeutic Class: Antineoplastic

CLINICAL PHARMACOLOGY

Mechanism of Action: Decreases the circulating estrogen level by inhibiting aromatase, the enzyme that catalyzes the final step in estrogen production. ***Therapeutic Effect:*** Inhibits the growth of breast cancers that are stimulated by estrogens.

Pharmacokinetics

Well absorbed into systemic circulation (absorption not affected by food). Protein binding: 40%. Extensively metabolized in the liver. Eliminated by biliary system and, to a lesser extent, kidneys. ***Mean half-life:*** 50 hr in postmenopausal women. Steady-state plasma levels reached in about 7 days.

INDICATIONS AND DOSAGES

Breast cancer

PO

Adults, Elderly. 1 mg once a day.

AVAILABLE FORMS

- *Tablets:* 1 mg.

CONTRAINDICATIONS: None known.

PREGNANCY AND LACTATION: Pregnancy category D; excretion into breast milk unknown

SIDE EFFECTS

Frequent (16%-8%)

Asthenia, nausea, headache, hot flashes, back pain, vomiting, cough, diarrhea

Occasional (6%-4%)

Constipation, abdominal pain, anorexia, bone pain, pharyngitis, dizziness, rash, dry mouth, peripheral edema, pelvic pain, depression, chest pain, paresthesia

Rare (2%-1%)

Weight gain, diaphoresis

SERIOUS REACTIONS

- Thrombophlebitis, anemia, leukopenia, and vaginal hemorrhage occur rarely.

SPECIAL CONSIDERATIONS

- No difference between doses of 1-10 mg qd
- Objective response in 10% of patients
- Usually ineffective in estrogen receptor negative patients and those unresponsive to prior tamoxifen

PATIENT/FAMILY EDUCATION

- Notify the physician if asthenia, hot flashes, and nausea become unmanageable

MONITORING PARAMETERS

- Body weight, edema
- Thromboembolic events
- CBC, blood chemistry, LFTs, serum lipids

anthralin

(an′-thra-lin)

Rx: A-Fil, Anthra-Derm, Drithocreme, Dritho-Scalp, Micanol, Psoriatec

OTC: (capsules, tablets, chewable tablets, syrup, elixir, cream, spray)

Chemical Class: Anthratriol derivative

Therapeutic Class: Antipsoriatic; keratolytic

CLINICAL PHARMACOLOGY

Mechanism of Action: A topical agent that binds DNA, inhibiting synthesis of nucleic protein, and reduces mitotic activity. ***Therapeutic Effect:*** Results in damage to DNA sugar and enhances membrane lipid peroxidation, which may play a critical role in the antipsoriatic action.

Pharmacokinetics

Poorly absorbed systemically, but excellent epidermal absorption. Auto-oxidized to inactive metabolites—danthrone and dianthrone. Rapid urinary excretion, so significant levels do not accumulate in the blood or other tissues. ***Half-life:*** 6 hrs.

INDICATIONS AND DOSAGES

Psoriasis

Topical

Adults, Elderly. Apply in a thin layer to affected areas q12h or q24h.

AVAILABLE FORMS

- *Cream:* 0.1% (Drithocreme), 0.25% (Drithocreme, Dritho-Scalp), 0.5 % (Drithocreme, Dritho-Scalp), 1% (Anthra-Derm).
- *Ointment:* 0.1% (Anthra-Derm), 0.25% (Anthra-Derm), 0.5 % (Anthra-Derm), 1% (Micanol, Psoriatec).

UNLABELED USES: Inflammatory linear verrucous epidermal nevus

CONTRAINDICATIONS: Acute psoriasis where inflammation is present, erythroderma, hypersensitivity to anthralin

PREGNANCY AND LACTATION: Pregnancy category C; excretion into human milk unknown; because of the potential for tumorigenicity shown in animal studies, use with caution in nursing mothers

SIDE EFFECTS

Frequent

Irritation

Rare

Neutrophilia, proteinuria, staining of the skin

SERIOUS REACTIONS

- Patients with renal disease should have routine urine tests for albuminuria.
- Hypersensitivity reaction, such as burning, erythema, and dermatitis, may occur.

SPECIAL CONSIDERATIONS

PATIENT/FAMILY EDUCATION

- Use plastic gloves for application and wear a plastic cap over treated scalp at bedtime to avoid staining
- Apply a protective film of petrolatum to areas surrounding plaque
- May stain fabrics
- Notify the physician if severe irritation or edema occurs

aprepitant

(ap-re′-pi-tant)

Rx: Emend, Emend 3-Day

Chemical Class: Triazolone derivative

Therapeutic Class: Antiemetic

CLINICAL PHARMACOLOGY

Mechanism of Action: A selective human substance P and neurokinin-1 (NK_1) receptor antagonist that inhibits chemotherapy-induced nausea and vomiting centrally in the chemoreceptor trigger zone. ***Therapeutic Effect:*** Prevents the acute and delayed phases of chemotherapy-induced emesis, including vomiting caused by high-dose cisplatin.

Pharmacokinetics

Crosses the blood-brain barrier. Extensively metabolized in the liver. Eliminated primarily by liver metabolism (not excreted renally). ***Half-life:*** 9-13 hr.

INDICATIONS AND DOSAGES

Prevention of chemotherapy-induced nausea and vomiting

PO

Adults, Elderly. 125 mg 1 hr before chemotherapy on day 1 and 80 mg once a day in the morning on days 2 and 3.

AVAILABLE FORMS

- *Capsules (Emend):* 80 mg, 125 mg.
- *Kit (Emend 3-Day):* 125 mg-80 mg.

CONTRAINDICATIONS: Breastfeeding, concurrent use of astemizole, cisapride, pimozide, or terfenadine

PREGNANCY AND LACTATION: Pregnancy category B; excretion into breast milk unknown, use caution in nursing mothers

SIDE EFFECTS

Frequent (17%-10%)

Fatigue, nausea, hiccups, diarrhea, constipation, anorexia

Occasional (8%-4%)

Headache, vomiting, dizziness, dehydration, heartburn

Rare (3% or less)

Abdominal pain, epigastric discomfort, gastritis, tinnitus, insomnia

SERIOUS REACTIONS

- Neutropenia and mucous membrane disorders occur rarely.

INTERACTIONS

Drugs

▲ *Pimozide, terfenadine, astemizole, cisapride:* Increased risk of fatal cardiac dysrhythmia through CYP 3A4 inhibition

3 *Antineoplastics (docetaxel, paclitaxel, etoposide, irinotecan, ifosfamide, imatinib, vinorelbine, vinblastine, vincristine):* Increased concentrations of these drugs through CYP 3A4 inhibition

3 *Benzodiazepines (midazolam, alprazolam, triazolam):* Increased concentrations of these drugs through CYP 3A4 inhibition

3 *Warfarin:* Increased hypoprothrombinemic response to warfarin

3 *Oral contraceptives:* Reduced contraceptive effectiveness

3 *Dexamethasone:* Oral dexamethasone doses should be reduced by approximately 50% when coadministered with aprepitant to achieve exposures of dexamethasone similar to those obtained when it is given without aprepitant

3 *Methylprednisolone:* IV methylprednisolone doses should be reduced by approximately 25%, and oral methylprednisolone doses should be reduced by approximately 50% when coadministered with aprepitant to achieve exposures of methylprednisolone similar to those obtained when it is given without aprepitant

3 *Tolbutamide:* Reduced effect of this drug

3 *CYP 3A4 inhibitors (ketoconazole, itraconazole, nefazodone, troleandomycin, clarithromycin, ritonavir, nelfinavir, diltiazem, paroxetine):* Increased plasma concentrations of aprepitant

3 *CYP 3A4 inducers (rifampin, carbamazepine, phenytoin):* Reduced plasma concentrations of aprepitant

SPECIAL CONSIDERATIONS

• Augments the antiemetic activity of the 5-HT_3-receptor antagonist ondansetron and the corticosteroid dexamethasone and inhibits both the acute and delayed phases of cisplatin-induced emesis

PATIENT/FAMILY EDUCATION

• Nausea and vomiting should be relieved shortly after drug administration

• Notify the physician if headache or persistent vomiting occurs

MONITORING PARAMETERS

• Assess pattern of daily bowel activity and stool consistency; also auscultate bowel sounds for peristalsis and record time of evacuation

---

argatroban

(ar-gat'-tro-ban)

Rx: Acova

Chemical Class: L-arginine derivative; thrombin inhibitor

Therapeutic Class: Anticoagulant; direct thrombin inhibitor

CLINICAL PHARMACOLOGY

Mechanism of Action: A direct thrombin inhibitor that reversibly binds to thrombin-active sites. Inhibits thrombin-catalyzed or thrombin-induced reactions, including fibrin formation, activation of coagulant factors V, VIII, and XIII; also inhibits protein C formation; and platelet aggregation. ***Therapeutic Effect:*** Produces anticoagulation.

Pharmacokinetics

Following IV administration, distributed primarily in extracellular fluid. Protein binding: 54%. Metabolized in the liver. Primarily excreted in the feces, presumably through biliary secretion. ***Half-life:*** 39-51 min.

INDICATIONS AND DOSAGES

To prevent and treat heparin-induced thrombocytopenia

IV Infusion

Adults, Elderly. Initially, 2 mcg/kg/min administered as a continuous infusion. After initial infusion, dose may be adjusted until steady state aPTT is 1.5-3 times initial baseline value, not to exceed 100 sec.

Percutaneous coronary intervention

IV Infusion

Adults, Elderly. Initially, 25 mcg/kg/min and administer bolus of 350 mcg/kg over 3-5 min. ACT (activated clotting time) checked in 5-10 min following bolus. If ACT is less than 300 sec, give additional bolus 150 mcg/kg, increase infusion to 30 mcg/kg/min. If ACT is greater than 450 sec, decrease infusion to 15 mcg/kg/min. Once ACT of 300-450 sec achieved, proceed with procedure.

Dosage in hepatic impairment

Adults, Elderly. Initially, 0.5 mcg/kg/min.

AVAILABLE FORMS

• *Injection:* 100 mg/ml.

UNLABELED USES: Cerebral thrombosis, MI

CONTRAINDICATIONS: Overt major bleeding

PREGNANCY AND LACTATION: Pregnancy category B; excretion into human milk unknown; use caution in nursing mothers

SIDE EFFECTS

Frequent (8%-3%)

Dyspnea, hypotension, fever, diarrhea, nausea, pain, vomiting, infection, cough

SERIOUS REACTIONS

• Ventricular tachycardia and atrial fibrillation occur occasionally.

• Major bleeding and sepsis occur rarely.

INTERACTIONS

Drugs

3 *Antiplatelet agents:* Increased bleeding risk

3 *Ginkgo biloba:* Increased risk of bleeding

3 *Heparin:* Allow heparin's effect on the aPTT to decrease prior to initiation of argatroban; co-administration is unlikely since heparin is contraindicated in patients with HIT

3 *Warfarin:* Increased prolongation of prothrombin time and INR (see SPECIAL CONSIDERATIONS)

Labs

• *Increased:* aPTT, PT, INR, activated clotting time, thrombin time

SPECIAL CONSIDERATIONS

• Discontinue all parenteral anticoagulants prior to administration

• Recognize the potential for combined effects on INR with co-administration of argatroban and warfarin; an INR should be measured daily while argatroban and warfarin are co-administered; in general, with doses of argatroban up to 2 mcg/kg/min, argatroban can be discontinued when the INR is >4 on combined therapy; after argatroban is discontinued, repeat the INR measurement in 4-6 hr; resume the argatroban infusion if the repeat INR is below the desired therapeutic range; repeat this procedure daily until the desired therapeutic range on warfarin alone is reached; for argatroban doses greater than 2 mcg/kg/min, temporarily reduce the dose of argatroban to a dose of 2 mcg/kg/min; repeat the INR on argatroban and warfarin 4-6 hr after reduction of the argatroban dose and follow the process outlined above for administering argatroban at doses up to 2 mcg/kg/min

PATIENT/FAMILY EDUCATION

• Use an electric razor and soft toothbrush to prevent bleeding

• Report black or red stool, coffee-ground vomitus, red or dark urine, or blood-tinged mucus from cough

MONITORING PARAMETERS

• aPTT, hemoglobin, hematocrit, platelet count

• Monitor for any complaints of abdominal or back pain, a decrease in blood pressure, increase in pulse rate, and severe headache, which indicates hemorrhage

---

aripiprazole

(ay-ri-pip'-ray-zole)

Rx: Abilify

Chemical Class: Quinolinone derivative

Therapeutic Class: Antipsychotic

CLINICAL PHARMACOLOGY

Mechanism of Action: An antipsychotic agent that provides partial agonist activity at dopamine and serotonin (5-HT_{1A}) receptors and antagonist activity at serotonin (5-HT_{2A}) receptors. ***Therapeutic Effect:*** Diminishes schizophrenic behavior.

Pharmacokinetics

Well absorbed through the GI tract. Protein binding: 99% (primarily albumin). Reaches steady levels in 2 wk. Metabolized in the liver. Eliminated primarily in feces and, to a lesser extent, in urine. Not removed by hemodialysis. ***Half-life:*** 75 hr.

INDICATIONS AND DOSAGES

Schizophrenia

PO

Adults, Elderly. Initially, 10-15 mg once a day. May increase up to 30 mg/day.

Bipolar disorder
PO
Adults, Elderly. 30 mg once a day. May decrease to 15 mg/day based on patient tolerance.

AVAILABLE FORMS

- *Tablets:* 5 mg, 10 mg, 15 mg, 20 mg, 30 mg.
- *Oral solution:* 1 mg/ml.

UNLABELED USES: Schizoaffective disorder

CONTRAINDICATIONS: None known.

PREGNANCY AND LACTATION: Pregnancy category C; excreted in milk of rats during lactation; no human information

SIDE EFFECTS

Frequent (11%-5%)
Weight gain, headache, insomnia, vomiting

Occasional (4%-3%)
Light-headedness, nausea, akathisia, somnolence

Rare (2% or less)
Blurred vision, constipation, asthenia or loss of energy and strength, anxiety, fever, rash, cough, rhinitis, orthostatic hypotension

SERIOUS REACTIONS

- Extrapyramidal symptoms and neuroleptic malignant syndrome occur rarely.
- Prolonged QT interval occurs rarely.

INTERACTIONS

Drugs

[3] *Alcohol:* Additive CNS depression and psychomotor depression

[3] *α-blockers (doxazocin, prazocin, terazocin):* Potential for enhanced blood pressure lowering effect

❷ *Amiodarone:* Hepatic metabolism inhibition; consider decreasing aripiprazole dose

❷ *Azole antifungals (fluconazole, itraconazole, ketoconazole, miconazole, variconazole):* Increased aripiprazole and metabolite concentrations via CYP3A4 inhibition; reduce dose of aripiprazole

[3] *Bosentan:* Hepatic metabolism induced; consider doubling aripirazole dose

❷ *Carbamazepine, oxcarbazepine:* Reductions in aripiprazole and metabolite concentrations via CYP3A4 induction; double dose of aripiprazole

[3] *Centrally acting agents (i.e., opiates, antidepressants, antihistamines, sedative/hypnotics):* Additive CNS depression and psychomotor depression

[3] *Cimetidine:* Hepatic metabolism inhibition; consider reducing aripiprazole dose or use alternate H_2 receptor blocker

[3] *Cyclosporine:* Hepatic metabolism inhibition; consider reducing aripiprazole dose

[3] *Danazole:* Hepatic metabolism inhibition; consider reducing aripiprazole dose

[3] *Delavirdine:* Hepatic metabolism inhibition; consider reducing aripiprazole dose

[3] *Dexamethasone:* Hepatic metabolism induced; consider doubling aripirazole dose

[3] *Diltiazem:* Hepatic metabolism inhibition; consider reducing aripiprazole dose

[3] *Droperidol:* Increased risk of extrapyrimidal reactions, CNS depression, QT prolongation with similar drug (ziprasidone)

❷ *Efavirenz:* Hepatic metabolism induced; consider doubling aripiprazole dose

❷ *Estrogen:* Hepatic metabolism inhibition; consider reducing aripiprazole dose

[3] *Grapefruit juice:* Increased aripiprazole and metabolite concentrations via CYP3A4 inhibition

❷ *Griseofulvin:* Hepatic metabolism induced; consider doubling aripiprazole dose
❷ *Isoniazid:* Hepatic metabolism induced; consider doubling aripiprazole dose
❸ *Macrolide antibiotics (erythromycin, clairithromycin):* Increased aripiprazole and metabolite concentrations via CYP3A4 inhibition
❷ *Protease inhibitors (indinivir, saquinivir, ritonavir, nelfinavir, amprenivir, lopinavir):* Hepatic metabolism inhibition; consider reducing aripiprazole dosage
❷ *Quinidine:* Increased aripiprazole and metabolite concentrations via CYP2D6 inhibition; reduce dose of aripiprazole by approximately 50%
❷ *SSRIs (fluoxetine, fluvoxamine, paroxetine):* Increased aripiprazole and metabolite concentrations via CYP2D6 inhibition; reduce dose of aripiprazole by approximately 50%

SPECIAL CONSIDERATIONS

• Reports of efficacy in acutely relapsed schizophrenia and schizoaffective disorder, and has an improved tolerability profile compared to haloperidol

PATIENT/FAMILY EDUCATION

• Understanding of potential interference with cognitive and motor performance, potential for drug interactions, and risk factors for neuroleptic malignant syndrome (overheating, dehydration)
• Avoid alcohol
• Avoid tasks that require mental alertness or motor skills until response the drug has been established

MONITORING PARAMETERS

• Improvement of both positive and negative schizophrenic symptoms; periodic BP and heart rate; abnormal movement monitoring; weight

ascorbic acid (vitamin C)

(a-skor'-bic)

Rx: Ascor L 500, Cenolate, CEE-500, Mega-C/A Plus
OTC: Ascorbicap, Cecon, Cevi-Bid, Ce-Vi-Sol, C-Crystals, Cebid Timecelles, Dull-C, Flavorcee, N'ice Vitamin C Drops
Chemical Class: Vitamin, water soluble
Therapeutic Class: Acidifier, urinary; vitamin

CLINICAL PHARMACOLOGY

Mechanism of Action: Assists in collagen formation and tissue repair and is involved in oxidation reduction reactions and other metabolic reactions. ***Therapeutic Effect:*** Involved in carbohydrate use and metabolism, as well as synthesis of carnitine, lipids, and proteins. Preserves blood vessel integrity.

Pharmacokinetics

Readily absorbed from the GI tract. Protein binding: 25%. Metabolized in the liver. Excreted in urine. Removed by hemodialysis.

INDICATIONS AND DOSAGES

Dietary supplement

PO

Adults, Elderly. 50-200 mg/day.
Children. 35-100 mg/day.

Acidification of urine

PO

Adults, Elderly. 4-12 g/day in 3-4 divided doses.
Children. 500 mg q6-8h.

Scurvy

PO

Adults, Elderly. 100-250 mg 1-2 times a day.
Children. 100-300 mg/day in divided doses.

Prevention and reduction of severity of colds
PO
Adults, Elderly. 1-3 g/day in divided doses.

AVAILABLE FORMS

- *Capsules (Controlled-Release):* 500 mg.
- *Liquid:* 500 mg/5 ml.
- *Oral Solution:* 500 mg/5 ml.
- *Tablets:* 100 mg, 250 mg, 500 mg, 1 g.
- *Tablets (Chewable):* 100 mg, 250 mg, 500 mg.
- *Tablets (Controlled-Release):* 500 mg, 1 g, 1500 mg.
- *Injection:* 222 mg/ml (Mega-C/A Plus, Vitamin C), 250 mg/ml (Cenolate), 500 mg/ml (Ascor L 500, Cee-500, Cenolate, Vitamin C).

UNLABELED USES: Chronic iron toxicity, control of idiopathic methemoglobinemia, macular degeneration, prevention of common cold, urine acidifier

CONTRAINDICATIONS: None known.

PREGNANCY AND LACTATION: Pregnancy category A if doses do not exceed the RDA, otherwise pregnancy category C; excreted into breast milk via a saturable process; the RDA during lactation is 90-100 mg; maternal supplementation up to the RDA is needed only in those women with poor nutritional status

SIDE EFFECTS

Rare

Abdominal cramps, nausea, vomiting, diarrhea, increased urination with doses exceeding 1 g

Parenteral: Flushing, headache, dizziness, sleepiness or insomnia, soreness at injection site.

SERIOUS REACTIONS

- Ascorbic acid may acidify urine, leading to crystalluria.
- Large doses of IV ascorbic acid may lead to deep vein thrombosis.
- Abrupt discontinuation after prolonged use of large doses may produce rebound ascorbic acid deficiency.

INTERACTIONS

Drugs

3 *Antacids:* Vitamin C increases the amount of aluminum absorbed from aluminum-containing antacids

3 *Deferoxamine:* Increased risk of iron toxicity

Labs

- *False negative:* Amine-dependent stool occult blood, urine bilirubin, blood, leukocyte determinations
- *False positive:* Urine glucose
- *Decrease:* Urine amphetamine, serum AST (Ames Seralyzer method), urine barbiturate (Abbott TDx method), serum bicarbonate (Kodak Ektachem 700 method), serum bilirubin (Jendrassik method), serum cholesterol (Olympus, Abbott TDx, CHOD-PAP methods), serum CK (Kodak Ektachem Systems), serum creatinine (Merck, Wako, Boehringer Mannheim methods), urine glucose (glucose oxidase methods), serum HDL-cholesterol (Kodak Ektachem Systems), urine oxalate (oxalate decarboxylase methods), urine porphobilinogen, serum triglycerides (GPO-PAP, Boehringer Mannheim methods), serum urea nitrogen (Ames Seralyzer), serum uric acid (Ames Seralyzer), urine uric acid (Kodak Ektachem Systems)
- *Increase:* Serum amylase (only at toxic ascorbic acid levels), serum AST (SMA 12/60 method), serum bilirubin (SMA 12/60 method), serum glucose (SMA 12/60 and O-toluidine methods), serum HbAlc (electrophoretic method), urine β-hydroxybutyrate, urine 17-hydroxy corticosteroids, urine iodide, urine 17-ketosteroids, urine oxalate (chromatographic methods), serum

phosphate (Boehringer-Mannheim method), CSF and urine protein (Kodak Ektachem Systems), serum uric acid (Klein and phosphotungstate methods)

SPECIAL CONSIDERATIONS

PATIENT/FAMILY EDUCATION

- Reduce ascorbic acid dosage gradually because abrupt discontinuation may produce rebound deficiency

---

aspirin/acetylsalicylic acid/ASA

(as'-pir-in)

Rx: Entaprin, YSP Aspirin, Zero-Order Release, ZORprin

OTC: Ascriptin, Aspergum, Bayer, Bayer Children's Aspirin, Ecotrin, Ecotrin Maximum Strength, 8-Hour Bayer Extended Release, Empirin, Maximum Bayer, Norwich

Combinations

Rx: with butalbital (Fiorinal); with codeine (Empirin); with dihydrocodeine and caffeine (Synalgos DC); with dipyridamole (Aggrenox); with oxycodone (Percodan); with propoxyphene (Darvon)

OTC: with antacids (Ascriptin, Bufferin, Magnaprin)

Chemical Class: Salicylate derivative

Therapeutic Class: Antiinflammatory; antiplatelet agent; antipyretic; nonnarcotic analgesic

---

CLINICAL PHARMACOLOGY

Mechanism of Action: A nonsteroidal salicylate that inhibits prostaglandin synthesis, acts on the hypothalamus heat-regulating center, and interferes with the production of thromboxane A, a substance that stimulates platelet aggregation. ***Therapeutic Effect:*** Reduces inflammatory response and intensity of pain; decreases fever; inhibits platelet aggregation.

Pharmacokinetics

Route	*Onset*	*Peak*	*Duration*
PO	1 hr	2-4 hr	4-6 hr

Rapidly and completely absorbed from GI tract; enteric-coated absorption delayed; rectal absorption delayed and incomplete. Protein binding: High. Widely distributed. Rapidly hydrolyzed to salicylate. ***Half-life:*** 15-20 min (aspirin); 2-3 hr (salicylate at low dose); more than 20 hr (salicylate at high dose).

INDICATIONS AND DOSAGES

Analgesia, fever

PO, Rectal

Adults, Elderly. 325-1000 mg q4-6h

Children. 10-15 mg/kg/dose q4-6h. Maximum: 4 g/day.

Anti-inflammatory

PO

Adults, Elderly. Initially, 2.4-3.6 g/day in divided doses; then 3.6-5.4 g/day.

Children. Initially, 60-90 mg/kg/day in divided doses; then 80-100 mg/kg/day.

Platelet aggregation inhibitor

PO

Adults, Elderly. 80-325 mg/day.

Kawasaki disease

PO

Children. 80-100 mg/kg/day in divided doses.

AVAILABLE FORMS

- *Tablets:* 162 mg (Halfprin), 325 mg (Bayer), 500 mg (Bayer).
- *Tablets (Chewable [Bayer, St. Joseph]):* 81 mg.

• *Tablets (Enteric-Coated [Bayer, Ecotrin, St. Joseph]):* 81 mg, 325 mg, 500 mg, 650 mg.
• *Caplets (Bayer):* 81 mg, 325 mg, 500 mg.
• *Gelcaps (Bayer):* 325 mg, 500 mg.
• *Suppositories:* 60 mg, 120 mg, 125 mg, 200 mg, 325 mg, 600 mg, 650 mg.

UNLABELED USES: Acute ischemic stroke, complications of pregnancy (prophylaxis), MI (prophylaxis), prevention of thromboembolism, rheumatic fever, treatment of Kawasaki disease

CONTRAINDICATIONS: Allergy to tartrazine dye, bleeding disorders, chickenpox or flu in children and teenagers, GI bleeding or ulceration, hepatic impairment, history of hypersensitivity to aspirin or NSAIDs

PREGNANCY AND LACTATION: Pregnancy category C (category D if full doses used in third trimester); use in pregnancy should generally be avoided; in pregnancies at risk for the development of pregnancy-induced hypertension and preeclampsia, and in fetuses with intrauterine growth retardation, low-dose aspirin (40-150 mg/day) may be beneficial; excreted into breast milk in low concentrations

SIDE EFFECTS

Occasional

GI distress (including abdominal distention, cramping, heartburn, and mild nausea); allergic reaction (including bronchospasm, pruritus, and urticaria)

SERIOUS REACTIONS

• High doses of aspirin may produce GI bleeding and gastric mucosal lesions.
• Dehydrated, febrile children may experience aspirin toxicity quickly. Reye's syndrome may occur in children with the chickenpox or the flu.
• Low-grade toxicity characterized is by tinnitus, generalized pruritus (possibly severe), headache, dizziness, flushing, tachycardia, hyperventilation, diaphoresis, and thirst.
• Market toxicity is characterized by hyperthermia, restlessness, seizures, abnormal breathing patterns, respiratory failure, and coma.

INTERACTIONS

Drugs

3 *ACE inhibitors:* Reduced antihypertensive effect

2 *Acetazolamide:* Increased concentrations of acetazolamide, possibly leading to CNS toxicity

3 *Antacids:* Decreased serum salicylate concentrations; high dose salicylates only

3 *Corticosteroids:* Increased incidence and/or severity of GI ulceration; enhanced salicylate excretion

3 *Diltiazem:* Enhanced antiplatelet effect of aspirin

3 *Ethanol:* Enhanced aspirin-induced GI mucosal damage and aspirin-induced prolongation of bleeding time

3 *Griseofulvin:* Reduced serum salicylate level

3 *Intrauterine contraceptive device:* May reduce contraceptive effectiveness

2 *Methotrexate:* Increased serum methotrexate concentrations and enhanced methotrexate toxicity

3 *NSAIDs:* Increased risk of adverse GI effects

2 *Oral anticoagulants:* Increased risk of bleeding by inhibiting platelet function and possibly by producing gastric erosions

3 *Probenecid:* Salicylates inhibit the uricosuric activity of probenecid

3 *Sulfinpyrazone:* Salicylates inhibit the uricosuric activity of sulfinpyrazone

3 *Sulfonylureas:* Enhanced hypoglycemic response to sulfonylureas

❷ *Warfarin:* Enhanced hypoprothrombinemic effect of warfarin
❸ *Valproic acid:* Increased risk of bleeding
❸ *Vancomycin:* Increased risk of ototoxicity
❸ *Zafirlukast:* Increased plasma concentrations of zafirlukast

Labs

• *Increase:* Serum acetaminophen (Glynn-Kendal method), urine acetoacetate (Gerhardt ferric chloride procedure), urine glucose (Ames Clinitest method), serum HbAlc (chromatographic and electrophoretic, but not colorimetric methods), urine hippuric acid, urine homogentisic acid, urine homovanillic acid, urine ketones (Gerhardt's test), urine phenyl ketones, CSF and urine protein (Folm-Ciocalteu method), serum and urine uric acid (non-specific methods only)
• *Decrease:* Serum albumin, urine glucose (glucose oxidase methods), total serum phenytoin (but not free serum phenytoin)

SPECIAL CONSIDERATIONS

• 81 mg qd may be as effective as higher doses in primary and secondary MI prevention

PATIENT/FAMILY EDUCATION

• Administer with food
• Do not exceed recommended doses
• Read label on other OTC drugs, many contain aspirin
• Therapeutic response may take 2 wk (arthritis)
• Avoid alcohol ingestion, GI bleeding may occur
• Not to be given to children with flu-like symptoms or chickenpox; Reye's syndrome may develop
• Do not crush or chew enteric-coated or extended-release tablets
• Report ringing in ears or resistant abdominal pain

MONITORING PARAMETERS

• AST, ALT, bilirubin, creatinine, CBC, hematocrit if patient is on long-term therapy
• Urine pH for signs of sudden acidification

atazanavir sulfate

(at-a-za-na'-veer sul'-fate)

Rx: Reyataz

Chemical Class: Protease inhibitor, HIV

Therapeutic Class: Antiretroviral

CLINICAL PHARMACOLOGY

Mechanism of Action: An antiviral that acts as an HIV-1 protease inhibitor, selectively preventing the processing of viral precursors found in cells infected with HIV-1. ***Therapeutic Effect:*** Prevents the formation of mature HIV cells.

Pharmacokinetics

Rapidly absorbed after PO administration. Protein binding: 86%. Extensively metabolized in the liver. Excreted primarily in urine and, to a lesser extent, in feces. ***Half-life:*** 5-8 hr.

INDICATIONS AND DOSAGES

HIV-1 infection

PO

Adults, Elderly (antiretroviral-naive). 400 mg (2 capsules) once a day with food.

Adults, Elderly (antiretroviral-experienced). 300 mg and ritonavir (Norvir) 100 mg once a day.

HIV-1 infection (concurrent therapy with efavirenz)

PO

Adults, Elderly. 300 mg atazanavir, 100 mg ritonavir, and 600 mg efavirenz as a single daily dose with food.

HIV-1 infection (concurrent therapy with didanosine)
PO
Adults, Elderly. Give atazanavir with food 2 hrs before or 1 hr after didanosine.
HIV-1 infection (concurrent therapy with tenofovir)
PO
Adults, Elderly. 300 mg atazanavir and 100 mg ritonavir and 300 mg tenofovir given as a single daily dose with food.
HIV-1 infection in patients with mild to moderate hepatic impairment
PO
Alert: Avoid use in patients with severe hepatic impairment.
Adults, Elderly. 300 mg once a day with food.

AVAILABLE FORMS
- *Capsules:* 100 mg, 150 mg, 200 mg.

CONTRAINDICATIONS: Concurrent use with ergot derivatives, midazolam, pimozide, or triazolam; severe hepatic insufficiency

PREGNANCY AND LACTATION: Pregnancy category B; breast milk excretion unknown (breast-feeding not advised for HIV-infected women)

SIDE EFFECTS
Frequent (16%-14%)
Nausea, headache
Occasional (9%-4%)
Rash, vomiting, depression, diarrhea, abdominal pain, fever
Rare (3% or less)
Dizziness, insomnia, cough, fatigue, back pain

SERIOUS REACTIONS
- A severe hypersensitivity reaction (marked by angioedema and chest pain) and jaundice may occur.

INTERACTIONS
- **(competitively inhibits CYP1A2, CYP2C9 systems)**

Drugs
❷ *Amiodarone:* Increased plasma levels of amiodarone
3 *Antacids:* Antacids reduce absorption of atazanavir, take atazanavir 2 hr before or 1 hr after antacids
⚠ *Astemizole:* Increased plasma levels of astemizole
❷ *Atorvastatin:* Atazanavir reduces clearance of atorvastatin
3 *Barbiturates:* Increased clearance of atazanavir; reduced clearance of barbiturates
⚠ *Bepridil:* Increased plasma levels of bepridil
3 *Calcium channel blockers:* Atazanavir reduces clearance of calcium channel blockers
3 *Carbamazepine:* Increased clearance of atazanavir; reduced clearance of carbamazepine
⚠ *Cisapride:* Increased plasma levels of cisapride
❷ *Clarithromycin:* Atazanavir reduces clearance of clarithromycin; reduce clarithromycin dose by 50%
3 *Cyclosporine:* Atazanavir reduces clearance of cyclosporine, monitor plasma levels
3 *Desipramine:* Atazanavir increases AUC of desipramine, monitor plasma levels
❷ *Didanosine (buffered formulation):* Didanosine, buffered formulation (but not didanosine EC) reduces absorption of atazanavir, take atazanavir 2 hr before or 1 hr after didanosine, buffered formulation
❷ *Diltiazem:* Atazanavir reduces diltiazem clearance, reduce diltiazem dose by 50%
❷ *Efavirenz:* Efavirenz increases atazanavir clearance, give atazanavir 300 mg qday with ritonavir 100 mg qday, when coadministered with efavirenz; no change in efavirenz dose

▲ *Ergot alkaloids:* Increased plasma levels of ergot alkaloids
❷ *Flecainide:* Increased plasma levels of flecainide
3 *High-fat meals:* May decrease atazanavir absorption
❷ *H2 receptor antagonists:* H2 receptor antagonists reduce absorption of atazanavir, separate dosing by 12 hrs
▲ *Indinavir:* Potential for additive hyperbilirubinemia
▲ *Irinotecan:* Atazanavir increases plasma levels of irinotecan
❷ *Lidocaine:* Increased plasma levels of lidocaine
▲ *Lovastatin:* Atazanavir markedly reduces clearance of lovastatin
▲ *Midazolam:* Increased plasma levels of midazolam and prolonged effect
❷ *Oral contraceptives:* Atazanavir increases ethinyl estradiol and norethindrone plasma levels
3 *Phenytoin:* Increased clearance of atazanavir; reduced clearance of phenytoin
▲ *Pimozide:* Increased plasma levels of pimozide
▲ *Proton pump inhibitors:* Marked reduction of atazanavir absorption and lower plasma levels
❷ *Quinidine:* Increased plasma levels of quinidine
❷ *Rifabutin:* Increased clearance of atazanavir; reduced clearance of rifabutin; reduce rifabutin dose to 150 mg qod
▲ *Rifampin:* Increased clearance of atazanavir
▲ *Rifapentine:* Increased clearance of atazanavir
❷ *Ritonavir:* Ritonavir decreases clearance of atazanavir, reduce atazanavir does to 300 mg qday
❷ *Saquinavir:* Decreased clearance of saquinavir, dose adjustment may be needed but optimal dose not established
❷ *Sildenafil:* Atazanavir markedly reduces clearance of sildenafil, reduce sildenafil dose to 25 mg q48h
3 *Sirolimus:* Atazanavir reduces clearance of sirolimus, monitor plasma levels
▲ *St. John's wort:* St. John's wort reduces plasma levels of atazanavir
3 *Tacrolimus:* Atazanavir reduces clearance of tacrolimus, monitor plasma levels
▲ *Terfenadine:* Increased plasma levels of terfenadine
▲ *Triazolam:* Increased plasma levels of triazolam and prolonged effect
❷ *Vardenafil:* Atazanavir reduces clearance of vardenafil, reduce vardenafil dose to 2.5 mg q24h
❷ *Warfarin:* Atazanavir increases warfarin effect

SPECIAL CONSIDERATIONS

- Reduced susceptibility to atazanavir is conferred by the following mutations of the HIV protease gene: N88S, I50L, I84V, A71V, and M46I
- In patients with no prior antiretroviral therapy, a randomized trial found atazanavir equivalent to efavirenz when both were part of a 3-drug combination including zidovudine and lamivudine; another trial found atazanavir equivalent to nelfinavir when both were part of a 3-drug combination including lamivudine and stavudine
- In patients with prior antiretroviral therapy, a randomized trial found that viral suppression rates for atazanavir were lower than with lopinavir/ritonavir (HIV RNA <400 copies/ml after 24 weeks of therapy: 54% vs 75%; HIV RNA <50 copies/ml after 24 weeks of therapy: 34% vs 50%; CD4 count change after 24 weeks of therapy: +101 cells/mm^3 vs 121 cells/mm^3

• Always check updated treatment guidelines before initiating or changing antiretroviral therapy (http://AIDSinfo.nih.gov)

PATIENT/FAMILY EDUCATION

• Antacids or buffered medications; reduce absorption of atazanavir; take atazanavir 2 hrs before or 1 hr after antacids or buffered medications

• Any medications that reduce stomach acid also reduce absorption of atazanavir; consult prescriber before using

• Take with food; eating small, frequent meals may offset the drug's side effects of nausea and vomiting

• Atazanavir is not a cure for HIV infection, nor does it reduce the risk of transmitting HIV to others

MONITORING PARAMETERS

• CBC, ALT, AST, bilirubin, HIV RNA, CD4 count

• Pattern of daily bowel activity and stool consistency

• Skin for rash

• Monitor for onset of depression

• Determine if the patient experiences headache

atenolol

(a-ten′-oh-lol)

Rx: Tenormin

Combinations

Rx: with chlorthalidone (Tenoretic)

Chemical Class: β_1-adrenergic blocker, cardioselective

Therapeutic Class: Antianginal; antihypertensive

CLINICAL PHARMACOLOGY

Mechanism of Action: A beta$_1$-adrenergic blocker that acts as an antianginal, antiarrhythmic, and antihypertensive agent by blocking beta$_1$-adrenergic receptors in cardiac tissue. ***Therapeutic Effect:*** Slows sinus node heart rate, decreasing cardiac output and BP. Decreases myocardial oxygen demand.

Pharmacokinetics

Route	Onset	Peak	Duration
PO	1 hr	2-4 hr	24 hr

Incompletely absorbed from the GI tract. Protein binding: 6%-16%. Minimal liver metabolism. Primarily excreted unchanged in urine. Removed by hemodialysis. ***Half-life:*** 6-7 hr (increased in impaired renal function).

INDICATIONS AND DOSAGES

Hypertension

PO

Adults. Initially, 25-50 mg once a day. May increase dose up to 100 mg once a day.

Elderly. Usual initial dose, 25 mg a day.

Children. Initially, 0.8-1 mg/kg/dose given once a day. Range: 0.8-1.5 mg/kg/day. **Maximum:** 2 mg/kg/day or 100 mg/day.

Angina pectoris

PO

Adults. Initially, 50 mg once a day. May increase dose up to 200 mg once a day.

Elderly. Usual initial dose, 25 mg a day.

Acute MI

IV

Adults. Give 5 mg over 5 min; may repeat in 10 min. In those who tolerate full 10-mg IV dose, begin 50-mg tablets 10 min after last IV dose followed by another 50-mg oral dose 12 hr later. Thereafter, give 100 mg once a day or 50 mg twice a day for 6-9 days. Or, for those who do not tolerate full IV dose, give 50 mg orally twice a day or 100 mg once a day for at least 7 days.

Dosage in renal impairment

Dosage interval is modified based on creatinine clearance.

Creatinine Clearance	Dosage Interval
15-35 ml/min	50 mg a day
less than 15 ml/min	50 mg every other day

AVAILABLE FORMS

- *Tablets:* 25 mg, 50 mg, 100 mg.
- *Injection:* 5 mg/10 ml.

UNLABELED USES: Acute alcohol withdrawal; arrhythmia (especially supraventricular and ventricular tachycardia); improved survival in diabetics with heart disease, mild to moderately severe CHF (adjunct); prevention of migraine, thyrotoxicosis, tremors; treatment of hypertrophic cardiomyopathy, pheochromocytoma, and syndrome of mitral valve prolapse

CONTRAINDICATIONS: Cardiogenic shock, overt heart failure, second- or third-degree heart block, severe bradycardia

PREGNANCY AND LACTATION: Pregnancy category D; frequently used in the third trimester for treatment of hypertension (many studies of efficacy and safety of atenolol in pregnancy-induced hypertension); long-term use has been associated with intrauterine growth retardation; excreted into breast milk; observe for signs of β-blockade

SIDE EFFECTS

Atenolol is generally well tolerated, with mild and transient side effects.

Frequent

Hypotension manifested as cold extremities, constipation or diarrhea, diaphoresis, dizziness, fatigue, headache, and nausea

Occasional

Insomnia, flatulence, urinary frequency, impotence or decreased libido, depression

Rare

Rash, arthralgia, myalgia, confusion (especially in the elderly), altered taste

SERIOUS REACTIONS

- Overdose may produce profound bradycardia and hypotension.
- Abrupt atenolol withdrawal may result in diaphoresis, palpitations, headache, and tremors.
- Atenolol administration may precipitate CHF or MI in patients with cardiac disease; thyroid storm in those with thyrotoxicosis; and peripheral ischemia in those with existing peripheral vascular disease.
- Hypoglycemia may occur in patients with previously controlled diabetes.
- Thrombocytopenia, manifested as unusual bruising or bleeding, occurs rarely.

INTERACTIONS

Drugs

3 *Adenosine:* Bradycardia aggravated

3 *α_1-adrenergic blockers:* Potential enhanced first dose response (marked initial drop in blood pressure, particularly on standing [especially prazosin])

3 *Amoxicillin, Ampicillin:* Reduced atenolol bioavailability

3 *Antacids:* Reduced atenolol absorption

3 *Antidiabetics, insulin:* Delayed recovery from hypoglycemia, hyperglycemia; attenuated tachycardia during hypoglycemia; hypertension during hypoglycemia

3 *Calcium channel blockers:* Enhanced effects of both drugs, particularly AV node conduction slowing; reduced atenolol clearance

3 *Clonidine:* Exacerbation of rebound hypertension upon discontinuation of clonidine

3 *Cimetidine:* Increased atenolol blood concentration

3 *Digoxin:* Additive prolongation of atrioventricular (AV) conduction time
3 *Dipyridamole:* Bradycardia aggravated
3 *Disopyramide:* Additive decreases in cardiac output
3 *Diuretics:* Increased hypotensive effect of atenolol
3 *Lidocaine:* Increased serum lidocaine concentrations possible
3 *Neostigmine:* Increased bradycardia
3 *NSAIDs:* Reduced antihypertensive effects of atenolol
3 *Physostigmine:* Increased bradycardia
3 *Sympathomimetics:* Mutually inhibit effects
3 *Tacrine:* Increased bradycardia
2 *Theophylline:* Antagonistic pharmacodynamic effects

SPECIAL CONSIDERATIONS

- Properties of low lipid solubility and competitive cardioselectivity yield less CNS and bronchospastic adverse effects than propranolol

PATIENT/FAMILY EDUCATION

- Do not discontinue abruptly, may precipitate angina
- Report bradycardia, dizziness, confusion, depression, fever, shortness of breath, swelling of the extremities
- Take pulse at home, notify clinician if <50 beats/min
- Avoid hazardous activities if dizziness, drowsiness, lightheadedness are present
- May mask the symptoms of hypoglycemia, except for sweating, in diabetic patients
- Restrict alcohol and salt intake

MONITORING PARAMETERS

- Blood pressure, heart rate
- Pattern of daily bowel activity and stool consistency
- Intake and output
- Weight

atomoxetine hydrochloride

(at′-oh-mox-e-teen hye-droe-klor′-ide)

Rx: Strattera

Chemical Class: Propylamine derivative

Therapeutic Class: Selective norepinephrine transporter inhibitor

CLINICAL PHARMACOLOGY

Mechanism of Action: A norepinephrine reuptake inhibitor that enhances noradrenergic function by selective inhibition of the presynaptic norepinephrine transporter. ***Therapeutic Effect:*** Improves symptoms of attention-deficit hyperactivity disorder (ADHD).

Pharmacokinetics

Rapidly absorbed after PO administration. Protein binding: 98% (primarily to albumin). Eliminated primarily in urine and, to a lesser extent, in feces. Not removed by hemodialysis. ***Half-life:*** 4-5 hr in general population, 22 hr in 7% of Caucasians and 2% of African-Americans; (increased in moderate to severe hepatic insufficiency).

INDICATIONS AND DOSAGES

ADHD

PO

Adults, Children weighing 70 kg and more. 40 mg once a day. May increase after at least 3 days to 80 mg as a single daily dose or in divided doses. Maximum: 100 mg.

Children weighing less than 70 kg. Initially, 0.5 mg/kg/day. May increase after at least 3 days to 1.2 mg/kg/day. Maximum: 1.4 mg/kg/day or 100 mg.

Dosage in hepatic impairment

Expect to administer 50% of normal atomoxetine dosage to patients with moderate hepatic impairment and 25% of normal dosage to those with severe hepatic impairment.

AVAILABLE FORMS

• *Capsules:* 10 mg, 18 mg, 25 mg, 40 mg, 60 mg, 80 mg, 100 mg.

UNLABELED USES: Treatment of depression

CONTRAINDICATIONS: Angle-closure glaucoma, use within 14 days of MAOIs

PREGNANCY AND LACTATION: Pregnancy category C; excretion into breast milk unknown; use caution in nursing mothers

SIDE EFFECTS

Frequent

Headache, dyspepsia, nausea, vomiting, fatigue, decreased appetite, dizziness, altered mood

Occasional

Tachycardia, hypertension, weight loss, delayed growth in children, irritability

Rare

Insomnia, sexual dysfunction in adults, fever

SERIOUS REACTIONS

• Urine retention or urinary hesitance may occur.

• In overdose, gastric emptying and repeated use of activated charcoal may prevent systemic absorption.

• Severe hepatic injury occurs rarely.

INTERACTIONS

Drugs

❷ *MAOIs:* Hypertensive crisis

❸ *Albuterol, other β-agonists:* Potentiated effects on the cardiovascular system

❸ *CYP2D6 inhibitors (fluoxetine, paroxetine, quinidine):* Increased levels of atomoxetine

SPECIAL CONSIDERATIONS

• Promoted as a "milder" but equally efficacious agent; inadequate comparisons available—should not be considered over conventional therapy

PATIENT/FAMILY EDUCATION

• Take the last daily dose of atomoxetine early in the evening to avoid insomnia

• Avoid tasks that require mental alertness and motor skills until response to the drug has been established

• Notify the physician if fever, irritability, palpitations, or vomiting occurs

MONITORING PARAMETERS

• Pretreatment blood samples for PCR-CYP2D6 genotyping (poor-metabolizer alleles) in selected patients (e.g., those with a history of super sensitivity/marked clinical response to other medications)

• History: Improvement of ADHD symptoms such as inattentiveness, hyperactivity, anxiety, impaired academic/social functioning; interviewing via ADHD Rating Scale-IV (parent version); routine blood chemistry periodically during prolonged administration; BP, pulse rate, body weight periodically during prolonged administration; signs and symptoms of toxicity

atorvastatin

(a-tore'-va-sta-tin)

Rx: Lipitor

Combinations

Rx: with amlodipine (Caduet)

Chemical Class: Substituted hexahydronaphthalene

Therapeutic Class: HMG-CoA reductase inhibitor; antilipemic

CLINICAL PHARMACOLOGY

Mechanism of Action: An antihyperlipidemic that inhibits hydroxamethylglutaryl-CoA (HMG-CoA) reductase, the enzyme that catalyzes the early step in cholesterol synthesis. ***Therapeutic Effect:*** Decreases LDL and VLDL cholesterol, and plasma triglyceride levels; increases HDL cholesterol concentration.

Pharmacokinetics

Poorly absorbed from the GI tract. Protein binding: greater than 98%. Metabolized in the liver. Minimally eliminated in urine. Plasma levels are markedly increased in chronic alcoholic hepatic disease, but are unaffected by renal disease. ***Half-life:*** 14 hr.

INDICATIONS AND DOSAGES

Prevention of cardiovascular disease (CVD)

PO

Adults, Elderly. 10 mg once daily.

Hyperlipidemias

PO

Adults, Elderly. Initially, 10-20 mg/day (40 mg in patients requiring greater than 45% reduction in LDL-C). Range: 10-80 mg/day.

Heterozygous hypercholesterolemia

PO

Children 10-17 yr. Initially, 10 mg/day. Maximum: 20 mg/day.

AVAILABLE FORMS

• *Tablets:* 10 mg, 20 mg, 40 mg, 80 mg.

UNLABELED USES: Secondary prevention of ischemia in patients with CHF

CONTRAINDICATIONS: Active hepatic disease, lactation, pregnancy, unexplained elevated liver function test results

PREGNANCY AND LACTATION: Pregnancy category X; not recommended for nursing mothers

SIDE EFFECTS

Atorvastatin is generally well tolerated. Side effects are usually mild and transient.

Frequent (16%)

Headache

Occasional (5%-2%)

Myalgia, rash or pruritus, allergy

Rare (2%-1%)

Flatulence, dyspepsia

SERIOUS REACTIONS

• Cataracts may develop, and photosensitivity may occur.

INTERACTIONS

Drugs

3 *Antacids:* Decreases atorvastatin activity

3 *Azole antifungals (fluconazole, itraconazole, ketoconazole, miconazole):* Increased atorvastatin levels; increased risk of rhabdomyolysis

3 *Bile acid sequestrants (cholestyramine, colestipol):* 25% reduction in atorvastatin plasma levels if coadministered

3 *Clarithromycin:* Increases atorvastatin plasma concentrations

3 *Cyclosporine:* Concomitant administration increases risk of severe myopathy or rhabdomyolysis

3 *Digoxin:* Elevation of digoxin level (approximately 20%)

■3 *Erythromycin:* Increased atorvastatin concentrations (approximately 40%); increased risk of rhabdomyolysis
■3 *Fibric acid:* Increased risk of severe myopathy, especially with high statin doses
■3 *Gemfibrozil:* Increased risk of rhabdomyolysis
■3 *Nefazodone:* Increased atorvastatin levels; increased risk of rhabdomyolyisis
■3 *Nelfinavir:* Increases atorvastatin concentrations
■3 *Niacin:* Concomitant administration increases risk of severe myopathy or rhabdomyolysis
■3 *Oral contraceptives:* Co-administration increases AUC for norethindrone and ethinyl estradiol by approximately 30% and 20%, respectively
■3 *Warfarin:* May increase atorvastatin blood concentration, producing severe muscle inflammation, pain, and weakness

SPECIAL CONSIDERATIONS

- Base statin selection on lipid-lowering prowess, cost, and availability
- Potency and ability to lower serum triglycerides is unique among the HMG-CoA reductase inhibitors. However, no outcome data available

PATIENT/FAMILY EDUCATION

- Report symptoms of myalgia, muscle tenderness, or weakness
- Take daily doses in the evening for increased effect
- Follow prescribed diet
- Periodic laboratory tests are an essential part of therapy
- Do not take other medications without physician approval

MONITORING PARAMETERS

- Cholesterol (max therapeutic response 4-6 wk)
- LFTs (AST, ALT) at baseline and at 12 wk of therapy: if no change, no further monitoring necessary (discontinue if elevations persist at >3 × upper limit of normal)
- CPK in patients complaining of diffuse myalgia, muscle tenderness, or weakness
- Assess skin for rash

atovaquone

(a-toe'-va-kwone)
Rx: Mepron
Combinations
Rx: with proguanil (Malarone)
Chemical Class: Hydroxynapthoquinone derivative
Therapeutic Class: Antiprotozoal

CLINICAL PHARMACOLOGY

Mechanism of Action: A systemic anti-infective that inhibits the mitochondrial electron-transport system at the cytochrome bc1 complex (Complex III), which interrupts nucleic acid and adenosine triphosphate synthesis. ***Therapeutic Effect:*** Antiprotozoal and antipneumocystic activity.

Pharmacokinetics

Absorption increased with a high-fat meal. Protein binding: greater than 99%. Metabolized in liver. Primarily excreted in feces. ***Half-life:*** 2-3 days.

INDICATIONS AND DOSAGES

Pneumocystis carinii pneumonia (PCP)

PO

Adults, Children older than 12 yr. 750 mg twice a day with food for 21 days.

Children 12 yr and younger. 40 mg/kg/day in 2 divided doses. Maximum: 1500 mg/day.

Prevention of PCP
PO
Adults. 1500 mg once a day with food.
Children 4-24 mo. 45 mg/kg/day as single dose. Maximum: 1500 mg/day.
Children 1-3 mo and older than 24 mo. 30 mg/kg/day as single dose. Maximum: 1500 mg/day.

AVAILABLE FORMS
- *Oral Suspension:* 750 mg/5 ml.

CONTRAINDICATIONS: Development or history of potentially life-threatening allergic reaction to the drug

PREGNANCY AND LACTATION: Pregnancy category C; human breast milk studies not available; in rats, concentrations in milk 30% of maternal serum

SIDE EFFECTS
Frequent (greater than 10%)
Rash, nausea, diarrhea, headache, vomiting, fever, insomnia, cough
Occasional (less than 10%)
Abdominal discomfort, thrush, asthenia, anemia, neutropenia

SERIOUS REACTIONS
- None known.

INTERACTIONS
Drugs
3 *Rifampin:* May decrease atovaquone blood concentration and increase rifampin blood concentration

SPECIAL CONSIDERATIONS
- Plasma concentrations have been shown to correlate with the likelihood of successful treatment and survival

PATIENT/FAMILY EDUCATION
- Take for the full course of treatment
- Do not take any other medications without first notifying the physician
- Notify the physician if diarrhea, rash, or other new symptoms occur

MONITORING PARAMETERS
- Pattern of daily bowel activity and stool consistency
- Skin for rash
- Hgb levels, intake and output, and renal function test results
- Monitor elderly patients closely because of age-related cardiac, hepatic, and renal impairment

atropine sulfate
(a'-troe-peen sul'-fate)
Rx: Atropine Care, Atropen Autoinjector, Atropisol, Atrosulf-1, Isopto Atropine, Ocu-Tropine, Sal-Tropine
Chemical Class: Belladonna alkaloid
Therapeutic Class: Antiasthmatic; anticholinergic; antispasmodic; bronchodilator; gastrointestinal; mydriatic; ophthalmic anticholinergic

CLINICAL PHARMACOLOGY
Mechanism of Action: An acetylcholine antagonist that inhibits the action of acetylcholine by competing with acetylcholine for common binding sites on muscarinic receptors, which are located on exocrine glands, cardiac and smooth-muscle ganglia, and intramural neurons. This action blocks all muscarinic effects. ***Therapeutic Effect:*** Decreases GI motility and secretory activity, and GU muscle tone (ureter, bladder); produces ophthalmic cycloplegia, and mydriasis.
Pharmacokinetics
AtroPen auto injector: Rapidly and well absorbed after IM administration. Much of the drug is destroyed by enzymatic hydrolysis, particularly in the liver. Partially excreted unchanged in urine.

INDICATIONS AND DOSAGES

Asystole, slow pulseless electrical activity

IV

Adults, Elderly. 1 mg; may repeat q3-5min up to total dose of 0.04 mg/kg.

Pre-anesthetic

IV, IM, Subcutaneous

Adults, Elderly. 0.4-0.6 mg 30-60 min pre-op.

Children weighing 5 kg and more. 0.01-0.02 mg/kg/dose to maximum of 0.4 mg/dose.

Children weighing less than 5 kg. 0.02 mg/kg/dose 30-60 min pre-op.

Bradycardia

IV

Adults, Elderly. 0.5-1 mg q5min not to exceed 2 mg or 0.04 mg/kg.

Children. 0.02 mg/kg with a minimum of 0.1 mg to a maximum of 0.5 mg in children and 1 mg in adolescents. May repeat in 5 min. Maximum total dose: 1 mg in children, 2 mg in adolescents.

Cycloplegic refraction, postoperative mydriasis, uveitis

Ophthalmic Solution

Adults, Elderly. Instill 1 drop of 1% or 2% solution in affected eye(s) up to 4 times a day.

Ophthalmic Ointment

Adults, Elderly. Apply ointment several hours prior to examination when used for refraction.

Poisoning by susceptible organophosphorous nerve agents having cholinesterase activity, organophosphorous or carbamate insecticides

IM

Adults, Children weighing more than 90 kg. AtroPen 2 mg (green).

Children weighing 40-90 kg. AtroPen 1 mg (dark red).

Children weighing 15-39 kg. AtroPen 0.5 mg (blue).

Infants weighing less than 15 kg. AtroPen 0.25 mg (yellow).

AVAILABLE FORMS

- *Injection:* 0.05 mg/ml, 0.1 mg/ml, 0.4 mg/0.5 ml, 0.4 mg/ml, 0.5 mg/ml, 1 mg/ml.
- *IM Injection (AtroPen):* 0.25 mg, 0.5 mg, 1 mg, 2 mg.
- *Ophthalmic ointment:* 0.5%, 1%.
- *Ophthalmic solution:* 0.5% (Isopto Atropine), 1% (Atropisol, Isopto Atropine), 2% (Atropisol).

UNLABELED USES: Malignant glaucoma

CONTRAINDICATIONS: Bladder neck obstruction due to prostatic hypertrophy, cardiospasm, intestinal atony, myasthenia gravis in those not treated with neostigmine, narrow-angle glaucoma, obstructive disease of the GI tract, paralytic ileus, severe ulcerative colitis, tachycardia secondary to cardiac insufficiency or thyrotoxicosis, toxic megacolon, unstable cardiovascular status in acute hemorrhage

PREGNANCY AND LACTATION: Pregnancy category C; passage into breast milk still controversial; neonates particularly sensitive to anticholinergic agents; compatible with breast-feeding

SIDE EFFECTS

Frequent

Dry mouth, nose, and throat that may be severe; decreased sweating, constipation, irritation at subcutaneous or IM injection site

Occasional

Swallowing difficulty, blurred vision, bloated feeling, impotence, urinary hesitancy

Ophthalmic: Mydriasis, blurred vision, photophobia, decreased visual acuity, tearing, dry eyes or dry conjunctiva, eye irritation, crusting of eyelid

Rare
Allergic reaction, including rash and urticaria; mental confusion or excitement, particularly in children; fatigue

SERIOUS REACTIONS

- Overdosage may produce tachycardia, palpitations, hot, dry or flushed skin, absence of bowel sounds, increased respiratory rate, nausea, vomiting, confusion, somnolence, slurred speech, dizziness and CNS stimulation.
- Overdosage may also produce psychosis as evidenced by agitation, restlessness, rambling speech, visual hallucinations, paranoid behavior, and delusions, followed by depression.
- Increased intraocular pressure occurs rarely with the use of the ophthalmic form.

INTERACTIONS

Drugs

3 *Amantadine:* Enhanced anticholinergic effect of atropine; enhanced CNS effect of amantadine
3 *Antacids, antidiarrheals:* Decreased effects of atropine
3 *Anticholinergics:* Increased effects of atropine
3 *Ketoconazole:* Decreased absorption of ketoconazole
3 *Neuroleptics:* Reduced neuroleptic effect
3 *Potassium chloride:* Increased severity of GI lesions (wax matrix)
3 *Rimantadine:* Enhanced anticholinergic effect of atropine; enhanced CNS effect of rimantadine
3 *Tacrine:* May reduce anticholinergic effect of atropine; atropine may reduce CNS effect of tacrine

SPECIAL CONSIDERATIONS

PATIENT/FAMILY EDUCATION

- Warm, dry, flushing feeling may occur upon administration

MONITORING PARAMETERS

- Blood pressure, heart rate, temperature
- Skin turgor and mucous membranes to evaluate hydration status
- Bowel sounds for presence of peristalsis
- Intake and output

atropine sulfate; diphenoxylate hydrochloride

(a'-troe-peen sul'-fate; dye-fen-ox'-i-late hye-droe-klor'-ide)
Rx: Lomocot, Lomotil, Lonox, Vi-Atro
Chemical Class: Meperidine analog
Therapeutic Class: Antidiarrheal
DEA Class: Schedule V

CLINICAL PHARMACOLOGY

Mechanism of Action: A meperidine derivative that acts locally and centrally on gastric mucosa. ***Therapeutic Effect:*** Reduces intestinal motility.

Pharmacokinetics

Well absorbed from the GI tract. Metabolized in the liver to active metabolite. Primarily eliminated in feces. ***Half-life:*** 2.5 hr; metabolite, 12-24 hr.

INDICATIONS AND DOSAGES

Diarrhea

PO

Adults, Elderly. Initially, 15-20 mg/day in 3-4 divided doses; then 5-15 mg/day in 2-3 divided doses.
Children 9-12 yr. 2 mg 5 times a day.
Children 6-8 yr. 2 mg 4 times a day.
Children 2-5 yr. 2 mg 3 times a day.

AVAILABLE FORMS

- *Tablets (Lomotil, Lonox):* 2.5 mg diphenoxylate/0.025 mg atropine.
- *Liquid (Lomotil):* 2.5 mg/5 ml.

CONTRAINDICATIONS: Children younger than 2 years, dehydration, jaundice, narrow-angle glaucoma, severe hepatic disease

PREGNANCY AND LACTATION: Pregnancy category C; excreted in breast milk

SIDE EFFECTS

Frequent

Somnolence, light-headedness, dizziness, nausea

Occasional

Headache, dry mouth

Rare

Flushing, tachycardia, urine retention, constipation, paradoxical reaction (marked by restlessness and agitation), blurred vision

SERIOUS REACTIONS

- Dehydration may predispose to diphenoxylate toxicity.
- Paralytic ileus and toxic megacolon (marked by constipation, decreased appetite, and stomach pain with nausea or vomiting) occur rarely.
- Severe anticholinergic reaction, manifested by severe lethargy, hypotonic reflexes, and hyperthermia, may result in severe respiratory depression and coma.

INTERACTIONS

Drugs

3 *Anticholinergics:* Increased effects of atropine

3 *Ethanol, CNS depressants:* Increased effects of diphenoxylate and atropine

2 *MAOIs:* Possible hypertensive crisis

3 *Barbiturates, tranquilizers, narcotics, alcohol:* Potentiation of effects

SPECIAL CONSIDERATIONS

- Equally effective as codeine or loperamide

PATIENT/FAMILY EDUCATION

- Prolonged use not recommended
- Drowsiness or dizziness may occur; use caution when driving or operating dangerous machinery
- Avoid alcohol

MONITORING PARAMETERS

- Bowel sounds and bowel activity

auranofin/aurothioglucose

(au-rane'-oh-fin/aur-oh-thye-oh-gloo'-kose)

Rx: Ridaura, Solganal

Chemical Class: Gold compound

Therapeutic Class: Disease-modifying antirheumatic drug (DMARD)

CLINICAL PHARMACOLOGY

Mechanism of Action: Gold compounds that alter cellular mechanisms, collagen biosynthesis, enzyme systems, and immune responses. ***Therapeutic Effect:*** Suppress synovitis in the active stage of rheumatoid arthritis.

Pharmacokinetics

Auranofin (29% gold): Moderately absorbed from the GI tract. Protein binding: 60%. Rapidly metabolized. Primarily excreted in urine. ***Half-life:*** 21-31 days. Aurothioglucose (50% gold): Slowly and erratically absorbed after IM administration. Protein binding: 95%-99%. Primarily excreted in urine. ***Half-life:*** 3-27 days (increased with increased number of doses).

INDICATIONS AND DOSAGES

Rheumatoid arthritis

PO

Adults, Elderly. 6 mg/day as a single or 2 divided doses. If there is no response in 6 mo, may increase to 9 mg/day in 3 divided doses. If response is still inadequate, discontinue.

Children. 0.1 mg/kg/day as a single or 2 divided doses. Maintenance: 0.15 mg/kg/day. Maximum: 0.2 mg/kg/day.

IM

Adults, Elderly. Initially, 10 mg, followed by 25 mg for 2 doses, then 50 mg weekly until total dose of 0.8-1 g has been given. If patient has improved and shows no signs of toxicity, may give 50 mg q3-4wk for many months.

Children. 0.25 mg/kg; may increase by 0.25 mg/kg each week. Maintenance: 0.75-1 mg/kg/dose. Maximum: 25 mg/dose for 20 doses, then repeated q2-4wk.

AVAILABLE FORMS

- *Capsules (Ridaura):* 3 mg.
- *Injection (Solganal):* 50-mg/ml suspension.

UNLABELED USES: Treatment of pemphigus, psoriatic arthritis

CONTRAINDICATIONS: Bone marrow aplasia, history of gold-induced pathologies (including blood dyscrasias, exfoliative dermatitis, necrotizing enterocolitis, and pulmonary fibrosis), severe blood dyscrasias

PREGNANCY AND LACTATION: Pregnancy category C; nursing not recommended; gold appears in breast milk

SIDE EFFECTS

Frequent

Auranofin: Diarrhea (50%), pruritic rash (26%), abdominal pain (14%), stomatitis (13%), nausea (10%)

Aurothioglucose: Rash (39%), stomatitis (19%), diarrhea (13%).

Occasional

Aurothioglucose: Nausea, vomiting, anorexia, abdominal cramps

SERIOUS REACTIONS

- Signs and symptoms of gold toxicity, the primary serious reaction, include decreased Hgb level, decreased granulocyte count (less than 150,000/mm^3), proteinuria, hematuria, stomatitis, blood dyscrasias (anemia, leukopenia [WBC count less than 4000/mm^3], thrombocytopenia, and eosinophilia), glomerulonephritis, nephrotic syndrome, and cholestatic jaundice.

SPECIAL CONSIDERATIONS

- Pruritus is a warning sign for development of cutaneous reactions
- Metallic taste may be a warning sign of stomatitis development

MONITORING PARAMETERS

- CBC, platelet count, urinalysis, renal function, and LFTs before treatment
- CBC, platelet count, urinalysis every month during therapy
- Gold toxicity

---

aurothioglucose/gold sodium thiomalate

Rx: Solganal; Myochrysine

Chemical Class: Heavy metal, active gold compound (50%)

Therapeutic Class: Disease-modifying antirheumatic drug (DMARD)

CLINICAL PHARMACOLOGY

Mechanism of Action: Aurothioglucose: A gold compound that alters cellular mechanisms, collagen biosynthesis, enzyme systems, and immune responses. ***Therapeutic Effect:*** Suppresses synovitis of the active stage of rheumatoid arthritis.

Gold sodium thiomalate: A gold compound whose mechanism of action is unknown. May decrease prostaglandin synthesis or alter cellular mechanisms by inhibiting sulfhydryl systems. ***Therapeutic Effect:*** Decreases synovial inflammation, retards cartilage and bone destruction, suppresses or prevents but does not cure, arthritis, synovitis.

Pharmacokinetics
Aurothioglucose (50% gold): Slow, erratic absorption after IM administration. Protein binding: 95%-99%. Primarily excreted in urine. ***Half-life:*** 3-27 days (half-life increased with increased number of doses).
Gold sodium thiomalate: Well absorbed. Protein binding: 95%. Widely distributed. Metabolized in liver. Excreted in urine and feces. Not removed by hemodialysis. ***Half-life:*** 5 days.

INDICATIONS AND DOSAGES
Rheumatoid arthritis (Aurothioglucose)
IM
Adults, Elderly. Initially, 10 mg, then 25 mg for 2 doses, then 50 mg weekly thereafter until total dose of 0.8-1 g given. If patient is improved and there are no signs of toxicity, may give 50 mg at 3- to 4-wk intervals for many months.
Children. 0.25 mg/kg, may increase by 0.25 mg/kg each week. Maintenance: 0.75-1 mg/kg/dose. Maximum: 25-mg dose for total of 20 doses, then q2-4wks.
Rheumatoid arthritis (Gold sodium thiomalate)
IM
Adults, Elderly. Initially, 10 mg, then 25 mg for second dose. Follow with 25-50 mg/wk until improvement noted or total of 1 g administered. Maintenance: 25-50 mg q2wks for 2-20 wks; if stable, may increase to q3-4wk intervals.
Children. Initially, 10 mg, then 1 mg/kg/wk. Maximum single dose: 50 mg. Maintenance: 1 mg/kg/dose at 2- to 4-wk intervals.
Dosage in renal impairment

Creatinine Clearance	***Dosage***
50-80 ml/min	50% of usual dosage
less than 50 ml/min	not recommended

AVAILABLE FORMS
Aurothioglucose
• *Injection:* 50 mg/ml suspension (Solganal).
Gold sodium thiomalate
• *Injection:* 50 mg/ml (Myochrysine).

UNLABELED USES: Treatment of pemphigus, psoriatic arthritis

CONTRAINDICATIONS:
Aurothioglucose
Bone marrow aplasia, history of gold-induced pathologies, including blood dyscrasias, exfoliative dermatitis, necrotizing enterocolitis, and pulmonary fibrosis, serious adverse effects with previous gold therapy, severe blood dyscrasias
Gold sodium thiomalate
Colitis, concurrent use of antimalarials, immunosuppressive agents, penicillamine, or phenylbutazone, congestive heart failure (CHF), exfoliative dermatitis, history of blood dyscrasias, severe liver or renal impairment, systemic lupus erythematosus

PREGNANCY AND LACTATION: Pregnancy category C; gold has been demonstrated in breast milk and in the serum and red blood cells of a nursing infant; the slow excretion and persistence of gold in the mother, even after discontinuing therapy, must also be considered

SIDE EFFECTS
Frequent
Aurothioglucose: Rash, stomatitis, diarrhea
Gold sodium thiomalate: Pruritic dermatitis, stomatitis, marked by erythema, redness, shallow ulcers of oral mucous membranes, sore throat, and difficulty swallowing, diarrhea or loose stools, abdominal pain, nausea
Occasional
Aurothioglucose: Nausea, vomiting, anorexia, abdominal cramps

Gold sodium thiomalate: Vomiting, anorexia, flatulence, dyspepsia, conjunctivitis, photosensitivity
Rare
Gold sodium thiomalate: Constipation, urticaria, rash
SERIOUS REACTIONS
- Gold toxicity is the primary serious reaction. Signs and symptoms of gold toxicity include decreased hemoglobin, leukopenia (WBC count less than 4000/mm^3), reduced granulocyte counts (less than 150,000/mm^3), proteinuria, hematuria, stomatitis (sores, ulcers and white spots in the mouth and throat), blood dyscrasias (anemia, leukopenia, thrombocytopenia and eosinophilia), glomerulonephritis, nephritic syndrome, and cholestatic jaundice.

INTERACTIONS
Drugs
3 *Penicillamine:* May increase the risk of hematologic or renal adverse effects of aurothioglucose
SPECIAL CONSIDERATIONS
- Administer in gluteal muscle with patient recumbent for 10 min after injection
- Pruritus is a warning sign for development of cutaneous reactions
- Metallic taste may be a warning sign of stomatitis development

PATIENT/FAMILY EDUCATION
- Avoid exposure to sunlight because it may cause a gray to blue pigment to appear on the skin
- Maintain diligent oral hygiene to prevent stomatitis

MONITORING PARAMETERS
- CBC, platelet count, urinalysis, renal function, and LFTs before treatment
- CBC, platelet count, urinalysis every month during therapy
- Gold toxicity

azathioprine
(ay-za-thye'-oh-preen)
Rx: Azasan, Azathioprine Sodium, Imuran
Chemical Class: 6-mercaptopurine derivative; purine analog
Therapeutic Class: Immunosuppressant

CLINICAL PHARMACOLOGY
Mechanism of Action: An immunologic agent that antagonizes purine metabolism and inhibits DNA, protein, and RNA synthesis. ***Therapeutic Effect:*** Suppresses cell-mediated hypersensitivities; alters antibody production and immune response in transplant recipients; reduces the severity of arthritis symptoms.
Pharmacokinetics
Well absorbed from the GI tract following PO administration. Protein binding: 30%. Metabolized in liver. Excreted in urine. ***Half-life:*** 5 hr.
INDICATIONS AND DOSAGES
Adjunct in prevention of renal allograft rejection
PO, IV
Adults, Elderly, Children. 2-5 mg/kg/day on day of transplant, then 1-3 mg/kg/day as maintenance dose.
Rheumatoid arthritis
PO
Adults. Initially, 1 mg/kg/day as a single dose or in 2 divided doses. May increase by 0.5 mg/kg/day after 6-8 wk at 4-wk intervals up to maximum of 2.5 mg/kg/day. Maintenance: Lowest effective dosage. May decrease dose by 0.5 mg/kg or 25 mg/day q4wk (while other therapies, such as rest, physiotherapy, and salicylates, are maintained).
Elderly. Initially, 1 mg/kg/day (50-100 mg); may increase by 25 mg/day until response or toxicity.

Dosage in renal impairment

Dosage is modified based on creatinine clearance.

Creatinine Clearance	Dose
10-50 ml/min	75% of usual dose
less than 10 ml/min	50% of usual dose

AVAILABLE FORMS

• *Tablets:* 25 mg (Azasan), 50 mg (Azasan, Imuran), 75 mg (Azasan), 100 mg (Azasan).

• *Injection (Imuran):* 100-mg vial.

UNLABELED USES: Treatment of biliary cirrhosis, chronic active hepatitis, glomerulonephritis, inflammatory bowel disease, inflammatory myopathy, multiple sclerosis, myasthenia gravis, nephrotic syndrome, pemphigoid, pemphigus, polymyositis, systemic lupus erythematosus

CONTRAINDICATIONS: Pregnant patients with rheumatoid arthritis

PREGNANCY AND LACTATION: Pregnancy category D

SIDE EFFECTS

Frequent

Nausea, vomiting, anorexia (particularly during early treatment and with large doses)

Occasional

Rash

Rare

Severe nausea and vomiting with diarrhea, abdominal pain, hypersensitivity reaction

SERIOUS REACTIONS

• Azathioprine use increases the risk of developing neoplasia (new abnormal-growth tumors).

• Significant leukopenia and thrombocytopenia may occur, particularly in those undergoing kidney transplant rejection.

• Hepatotoxicity occurs rarely.

INTERACTIONS

Drugs

❷ *Allopurinol:* Allopurinol may increase toxicity of azathioprine; dosage adjustment is necessary

❷ *Bone marrow depressants:* Increased myelosuppression

❷ *Liver-virus vaccines:* Potentiates virus replication, increases the vaccine's side effects, and decreases the antibody response to the vaccine

❷ *Other immunosuppressants:* Increased risk of infection or neoplasms

❸ *Warfarin:* Reduced warfarin effect

SPECIAL CONSIDERATIONS

• Severe leukopenia and/or thrombocytopenia may occur, as well as macrocytic anemia and bone marrow depression; fungal, viral, bacterial, and protozoal infections may be fatal; may increase the patient's risk of neoplasia via mutagenic and carcinogenic properties (skin cancer and reticulum cell or lymphomatous tumors); temporary depression in spermatogenesis

PATIENT/FAMILY EDUCATION

• The drug's therapeutic response may take up to 12 wks to appear

• Notify the physician if abdominal pain, fever, mouth sores, sore throat, or unusual bleeding occurs

• Women of childbearing age should avoid pregnancy during treatment

MONITORING PARAMETERS

• Hgb, WBC, monthly

• D/C if leukocytes are $<3000/mm^3$

• Therapeutic response may take 3-4 mo in rheumatoid arthritis

• CBC (especially platelet count) and serum hepatic enzyme levels weekly during the first month of therapy, twice monthly during the second and third months of treatment, and monthly thereafter

azelaic acid

(ay-zeh-lay'-ic as'-id)

Rx: Azelex, Finevin

Chemical Class: Dicarboxylic acid

Therapeutic Class: Antiacne agent

CLINICAL PHARMACOLOGY

Mechanism of Action: A hypopigmentation agent that possesses antimicrobial action by inhibiting cellular protein synthesis in aerobic and anaerobic microorganisms. ***Therapeutic Effect:*** Improves acne vulgaris, normalizing keratin process.

Pharmacokinetics

Minimal absorption after topical administration. Metabolized in liver. Excreted in urine as unchanged drug. ***Half-life:*** 12 hrs.

INDICATIONS AND DOSAGES

Antiacne, hypopigmentation

Topical

Adults, Adolescents. Apply topically to affected area 2 times/day (morning and evening).

AVAILABLE FORMS

• *Cream:* 20% (Azelex, Finevin).

CONTRAINDICATIONS: Hypersensitivity to azelaic acid or any component of the formulation

PREGNANCY AND LACTATION: Pregnancy category B

SIDE EFFECTS

Occasional

Pruritus, stinging, burning, tingling

Rare

Erythema, dryness, rash, peeling, irritation, contact dermatitis

SERIOUS REACTIONS

• None reported.

SPECIAL CONSIDERATIONS

• Wash hands after application; avoid contact with mucous membranes; if drug gets into eyes, wash with large quantities of water

• If skin irritation occurs, decrease frequency of application or temporarily discontinue treatment

• Azelaic acid is a naturally occurring substance found in the human diet

MONITORING PARAMETERS

• Skin for erythema and dryness

azelastine

(a-zel'-as-teen)

Rx: Astelin (nasal), Optivar (ophthalmic)

Chemical Class: Phthalazinone derivative

Therapeutic Class: Antihistamine

CLINICAL PHARMACOLOGY

Mechanism of Action: An antihistamine that competes with histamine for histamine receptor sites on cells in the blood vessels, GI tract, and respiratory tract. ***Therapeutic Effect:*** Relieves symptoms associated with seasonal allergic rhinitis such as increased mucus production and sneezing and symptoms associated with allergic conjunctivitis, such as redness, itching, and excessive tearing.

Pharmacokinetics

Route	*Onset*	*Peak*	*Duration*
Nasal spray	0.5-1 hr	2-3 hr	12 hr
Ophthalmic	N/A	3 min	8 hr

Well absorbed through nasal mucosa. Primarily excreted in feces. ***Half-life:*** 22 hr.

INDICATIONS AND DOSAGES
Allergic rhinitis
Nasal
Adults, Elderly, Children 12 yr and older. 2 sprays in each nostril twice a day.
Children 5-11 yr. 1 spray in each nostril twice a day.
Allergic conjunctivitis
Ophthalmic
Adults, Elderly, Children 3 yr or older. 1 drop into affected eye twice a day.

AVAILABLE FORMS
- *Nasal Spray (Astelin):* 137 mcg/spray.
- *Ophthalmic Solution (Optivar):* 0.05%.

CONTRAINDICATIONS: Breast-feeding women; history of hypersensitivity to antihistamines; neonates or premature infants; third trimester of pregnancy

PREGNANCY AND LACTATION: Pregnancy category C; excretion into breast milk unknown

SIDE EFFECTS
Frequent (20%-15%)
Headache, bitter taste
Rare
Nasal burning, paroxysmal sneezing, somnolence
Ophthalmic: Transient eye burning or stinging, bitter taste, headache

SERIOUS REACTIONS
- Epistaxis occurs rarely.

INTERACTIONS
3 *Alcohol, other CNS depressants:* May increase CNS depression
3 *Cimetidine:* May increase azelastine blood concentration

SPECIAL CONSIDERATIONS
- Low sedating antihistamine nasal spray with first-dose activity; note: onset of action not as fast as decongestant nasal sprays, but appropriate for prn use

PATIENT/FAMILY EDUCATION
- Advise caution with use concomitant with activities that require concentration or while operating machinery; may cause drowsiness
- Preservative in ophth sol, benzlkonium chloride, may be absorbed by soft contact lenses, wait at least 10 min after instilling ophth sol before inserting soft contacts
- Clear nasal passages before using azelastine
- Prime the pump with 4 sprays or until a fine mist appears before using the nasal spray the first time. After the first use and if the pump has not been used for 3 or more days, prime the pump with 2 sprays or until a fine mist appears
- Wipe the applicator tip with a clean, damp tissue and replace the cap immediately after use
- Avoid spraying the nasal drug into the eyes
- Avoid drinking alcoholic beverages during azelastine therapy

MONITORING PARAMETERS
- Therapeutic response to medication

azithromycin
(ay-zi-thro-mye'-sin)
Rx: Zithromax, Zithromax TRI-PAK, Zithromax Z-PAK, Zmax
Chemical Class: Macrolide derivative
Therapeutic Class: Antibiotic

CLINICAL PHARMACOLOGY
Mechanism of Action: A macrolide antibiotic that binds to ribosomal receptor sites of susceptible organisms, inhibiting RNA-dependent protein synthesis. ***Therapeutic Effect:*** Bacteriostatic or bactericidal, depending on the drug dosage.

Pharmacokinetics
Rapidly absorbed from the GI tract. Protein binding: 7%-50%. Widely distributed. Eliminated primarily unchanged by biliary excretion. ***Half-life:*** 68 hr.

INDICATIONS AND DOSAGES
Acute exacerbations of chronic obstructive pulmonary disease (COPD)
PO
Adults, Elderly, Children 16 yr and older. 500 mg/day for 3 days or 500 mg on day 1, then 250 mg/day on days 2-5.
Acute bacterial sinusitis
PO (Zmax)
Adults, Elderly. 2 g as a single dose.
PO
Adults, Elderly. 500 mg/day for 3 days.
Children 6 mo and older. 10 mg/kg for 3 days. Maximum: 500 mg/day.
Cervicitis
PO
Adults, Elderly. 1-2 g as single dose.
Chancroid
PO
Adults, Elderly: 1 g as single dose.
Mycobacterium avium complex (MAC) prevention
PO
Adults, Elderly. 1200 mg once weekly.
Children. 20 mg/kg once weekly. Maximum: 1200 mg/dose.
MAC treatment
PO
Adults, Elderly. 600 mg/day with ethambutol 15 mg/kg/day.
Children. 5-20 mg/kg/day for 1 mo or longer.
Otitis media
PO
Children 6 mo and older. 30 mg/kg as single dose or 10 mg/kg/day for 3 days or 10 mg/kg on day 1 then 5 mg/kg on days 2-5.
Pharyngitis, tonsillitis
PO
Adults, Elderly, Children 16 yr and older. 500 mg on day 1, then 250 mg on days 2-5.
Children 2-15 yr. 12 mg/kg daily for 5 days.
Pneumonia, community acquired
PO (Zmax)
Adults, Elderly. 2 g as a single dose.
PO
Adults, Elderly, Children 16 yr and older. 500 mg on day 1, then 250 mg on days 2-5 or 500 mg/day IV for 2 days, then 500 mg/day PO to complete course of therapy.
Children 6 mo-15 yr. 10 mg/kg on day 1, then 5 mg/kg on days 2-5.
Skin/skin-structure infections
PO
Adults, Elderly, Children 16 yr and older. 500 mg on day 1, then 250 mg on days 2-5.
Pelvic inflammatory disease (PID)
IV
Adults, Elderly. 500 mg/day for at least 2 days, then 250 mg/day to complete a 7-day course of therapy.

AVAILABLE FORMS
- *Oral Suspension (Zithromax):* 100 mg/5 ml, 200 mg/5 ml.
- *Oral Suspension (Extended-Release [Zmax]):* 1 g single-dose packet, 2 g single-dose packet.
- *Tablets:* 250 mg, 500 mg, 600 mg (Zithromax). Tri-Pak: 3×500 mg (Zithromax TRI-PAK). Z-Pak: 6×250 mg (Zithromax Z-PAK).
- *Powder for Injection (Zithromax):* 500 mg.
- *Powder for Reconstitution (Zithromax):* 1 g.

UNLABELED USES: Chlamydial infections, gonococcal pharyngitis, uncomplicated gonococcal infections of the cervix, urethra, and rectum

CONTRAINDICATIONS: Hypersensitivity to other macrolide antibiotics

PREGNANCY AND LACTATION: Pregnancy category B; excretion into breast milk unknown

SIDE EFFECTS

Occasional

Nausea, vomiting, diarrhea, abdominal pain

Rare

Headache, dizziness, allergic reaction

SERIOUS REACTIONS

• Antibiotic-associated colitis and other superinfections may result from altered bacterial balance.

• Acute interstitial nephritis and hepatotoxicity occur rarely.

INTERACTIONS

Drugs

3 *Aluminum- or magnesium-containing antacids:* May decrease azithromycin blood concentration

3 *Carbamazepine, cyclosporine, theophylline, warfarin:* May increase the serum concentrations of these drugs

3 *Penicillins:* Azithromycin may inhibit antibacterial activity of penicillins

Labs

• *Increase:* Serum 17 Hydroxycorticosteroids, 17 ketosteroids

• *Decrease:* Serum folate (bioassay only)

SPECIAL CONSIDERATIONS

• Otitis media: single dose and 3d therapy similar efficacy but fewer side effects than amoxicillin/clavulanate × 10d

• Group A strep pharyngitis; 12 mg/kg/d × 5d shown to have superior cure rate to PCN × 10d but no data on rheumatic fever prophylaxis

PATIENT/FAMILY EDUCATION

• Tablet may be taken without regard to food. Suspension and capsule should be taken on an empty stomach

• Space doses evenly around the clock and continue taking azithromycin for the full course of treatment

• If the patient must take an antacid containing aluminum or magnesium, take the drug 1 hr before or 2 hrs after the antacid

MONITORING PARAMETERS

• Evaluate the patient for signs and symptoms of superinfection, including genital or anal pruritus, sore mouth or tongue, and moderate to severe diarrhea

• Pattern of daily bowel activity and stool consistency

• Liver function

• Assess the patient for signs and symptoms of hepatotoxicity, such as abdominal pain, fever, GI disturbances, and malaise

---

aztreonam

(az'-tree-oh-nam)

Rx: Azactam

Chemical Class: Monobactam

Therapeutic Class: Antibiotic

CLINICAL PHARMACOLOGY

Mechanism of Action: A monobactam antibiotic that inhibits bacterial cell wall synthesis. ***Therapeutic Effect:*** Bactericidal.

Pharmacokinetics

Completely absorbed after IM administration. Protein binding: 56%-60%. Partially metabolized by hydrolysis. Primarily excreted unchanged in urine. Removed by hemodialysis. ***Half-life:*** 1.4-2.2 hr (increased in impaired renal or hepatic function).

INDICATIONS AND DOSAGES

UTIs

IV, IM

Adults, Elderly. 500 mg-1 g q8-12h.

Moderate to severe systemic infections
IV, IM
Adults, Elderly. 1-2 g q8-12h.
Severe or life-threatening infections
IV
Adults, Elderly. 2 g q6-8h.
Cystic fibrosis
IV
Children. 50 mg/kg/dose q6-8h up to 200 mg/kg/day. Maximum: 8g/d.
Mild to severe infections in children
IV
Children. 30 mg/kg q6-8h. Maximum: 120 mg/kg/day.
Neonates. 60-120 mg/kg/day q6-12h.
Dosage in renal impairment
Dosage and frequency are modified based on creatinine clearance and the severity of the infection:

Creatinine Clearance	Dosage
10-30 ml/min	1-2 g initially, then ½ usual dose at usual intervals
less than 10 ml/min	1-2 g initially, then ¼ usual dose at usual intervals

AVAILABLE FORMS
• *Injection Powder for Reconstitution:* 500 mg, 1 g, 2 g.
UNLABELED USES: Treatment of bone and joint infections
CONTRAINDICATIONS: None known
PREGNANCY AND LACTATION: Pregnancy category B; excreted in breast milk in concentrations <1% of maternal serum concentrations
SIDE EFFECTS
Occasional (less than 3%)
Discomfort and swelling at IM injection site, nausea, vomiting, diarrhea, rash
Rare (less than 1%)
Phlebitis or thrombophlebitis at IV injection site, abdominal cramps, headache, hypotension
SERIOUS REACTIONS
• Antibiotic-associated colitis and other superinfections may result from altered bacterial balance.
• Severe hypersensitivity reactions, including anaphylaxis, occur rarely.
INTERACTIONS
Drugs
3 *Aminoglycosides:* Potential increased nephrotoxicity, ototoxicity
3 *Cephalosporins, imipenem:* Antagonism secondary to antibiotic-induced high levels of β-lactamase
SPECIAL CONSIDERATIONS
• Minimal cross-reactivity between aztreonam and penicillins and cephalosporins; aztreonam and aminoglycosides have been shown to be synergistic *in vitro* against most strains of *P. aeruginosa,* many strains of *Enterobacteriaceae,* and other gram-negative aerobic bacilli
MONITORING PARAMETERS
• Daily bowel activity and stool consistency
• Signs and symptoms of superinfections, including anal or genital pruritus, black hairy tongue, vomiting, diarrhea, fever, sore throat, and ulceration or changes of oral mucosa

bacitracin

(bass-i-tray′-sin)

Rx: Ak-Tracin, Baci-IM, Baci-Rx, Ocu-Tracin, Ziba-Rx

Combinations

Rx: with neomycin, polymixin, and hydrocortisone (Cortisporin)

OTC: with neomycin and polymixin (Neosporin); with polymixin (Polysporin)

Chemical Class: Bacillus subtilis derivative

Therapeutic Class: Antibacterial; ophthalmic antibiotic

CLINICAL PHARMACOLOGY

Mechanism of Action: An antibiotic that interferes with plasma membrane permeability and inhibits bacterial cell wall synthesis in susceptible bacteria. ***Therapeutic Effect:*** Bacteriostatic.

Pharmacokinetics

Not significantly absorbed following topical or ophthalmic administration.

INDICATIONS AND DOSAGES

Superficial ocular infections

Ophthalmic

Adults. ½-inch ribbon in conjunctival sac q3-4h.

Skin abrasions, superficial skin infections

Topical

Adults, Children. Apply to affected area 1-5 times a day.

Surgical treatment and prophylaxis

Irrigation

Adults, Elderly. 50,000-150,000 units, as needed.

Pneumonia and empyema caused by staphylococci

IM

Infants weighing 2500 g and less. 900 units/kg/24 hrs in 2 or 3 divided doses.

Infants weighing more than 2500 g. 1000 units/kg/24 hrs in 2 or 3 divided doses.

AVAILABLE FORMS

- *Powder for Irrigation:* 50,000 units.
- *Powder for Injection (Baci-IM):* 50,000 units.
- *Ophthalmic Ointment (AK-Tracin):* 500 units/g.
- *Topical Ointment (Ocu-Tracin):* 500 units/g.

CONTRAINDICATIONS: None known

PREGNANCY AND LACTATION: Pregnancy category C

SIDE EFFECTS

Rare

Ophthalmic: Burning, itching, redness, swelling, pain

IM injection: Nausea, vomiting, pain at injection site, rash, azotemia, rising blood levels without any increase in dosage

Topical: Hypersensitivity reaction (allergic contact dermatitis, burning, inflammation, pruritus)

SERIOUS REACTIONS

Alert: Bacitracin used intramuscularly may cause renal failure due to tubular and glomerular necrosis. Its use should be restricted to infants with staphylococci pneumonia and empyema.

- Severe hypersensitivity reactions, including apnea and hypotension, occur rarely.

SPECIAL CONSIDERATIONS

- Administer IM in deep muscle mass; rotate injection site; do *not* give IV/SC

PATIENT/FAMILY EDUCATION

- Administer at even intervals
- Report burning, itching, increased irritation, or rash

MONITORING PARAMETERS

- Using the topical ointment, be alert for signs and symptoms of hypersensitivity, such as burning, inflammation, and pruritus

baclofen

(bak'-loe-fen)

Rx: Lioresal, Lioresal Intrathecal

Chemical Class: GABA chlorophenyl derivative

Therapeutic Class: Skeletal muscle relaxant

CLINICAL PHARMACOLOGY

Mechanism of Action: A direct-acting skeletal muscle relaxant that inhibits transmission of reflexes at the spinal cord level. ***Therapeutic Effect:*** Relieves muscle spasticity.

Pharmacokinetics

Well absorbed from the GI tract. Protein binding: 30%. Partially metabolized in the liver. Primarily excreted in urine. ***Half-life:*** 2.5-4 hr; intrathecal: 1.5 hr.

INDICATIONS AND DOSAGES

Spasticity

PO

Adults. Initially, 5 mg 3 times a day. May increase by 15 mg/day at 3-day intervals. Range: 40-80 mg/day. Maximum: 80 mg/day.

Elderly. Initially, 5 mg 2-3 times a day. May gradually increase dosage.

Children. Initially, 10-15 mg/day in divided doses q8h. May increase by 5-15 mg/day at 3-day intervals. Maximum: 40 mg/day (children 2-7 yr); 60 mg/day (children 8 yr and older).

Usual intrathecal dosage

Intrathecal

Adults, Elderly, Children older than 12 yr. 300-800 mcg/day.

Children 12 yr and younger. 100-300 mcg/day.

AVAILABLE FORMS

• *Tablets:* 10 mg, 20 mg.

• *Intrathecal Injection:* 50 mcg/ml, 500 mcg/ml, 2000 mcg/ml.

UNLABELED USES: Treatment of bladder spasms, cerebral palsy, intractable hiccups or pain, Huntington's chorea, trigeminal neuralgia

CONTRAINDICATIONS: Skeletal muscle spasm due to cerebral palsy, Parkinson's disease, rheumatic disorders, CVA, cough, intractable hiccups, neuropathic pain

PREGNANCY AND LACTATION: Pregnancy category C; present in breast milk, 0.1% of mother's dose; compatible with breast-feeding

SIDE EFFECTS

Frequent (greater than 10%)

Transient somnolence, asthenia, dizziness, light-headedness, nausea, vomiting

Occasional (10%-2%)

Headache, paresthesia, constipation, anorexia, hypotension, confusion, nasal congestion

Rare (less than 1%)

Paradoxical CNS excitement or restlessness, slurred speech, tremor, dry mouth, diarrhea, nocturia, impotence

SERIOUS REACTIONS

• Abrupt discontinuation of baclofen may produce hallucinations and seizures.

• Overdose results in blurred vision, seizures, myosis, mydriasis, severe muscle weakness, strabismus, respiratory depression, and vomiting.

INTERACTIONS

Drugs

3 *Alcohol, CNS depressants:* Increases CNS depression

SPECIAL CONSIDERATIONS

• Abrupt discontinuation may lead to hallucinations, spasticity, tachycardia; drug should be tapered off over 1-2 wk

PATIENT/FAMILY EDUCATION

- Do not abruptly discontinue after long-term therapy
- Avoid hazardous activities if dizziness, drowsiness, lightheadedness are present
- Avoid alcohol and CNS depressants during therapy

MONITORING PARAMETERS

- CBC, liver and renal function

balsalazide disodium

(bal-sal'-a-zide dye-soe'-dee-um)

Rx: Colazal

Chemical Class: 5-amino derivative of salicylic acid

Therapeutic Class: Gastrointestinal antiinflammatory

CLINICAL PHARMACOLOGY

Mechanism of Action: A 5-aminosalicylic acid derivative that changes intestinal microflora, altering prostaglandin production and inhibiting function of natural killer cells, mast cells, neutrophils, and macrophages. ***Therapeutic Effect:*** Diminishes inflammatory effect in colon.

Pharmacokinetics

Low and variable absorption following PO administration. Protein binding: greater than 99%. Extensively metabolized in colon. Minimal elimination in urine and feces. ***Half-life:*** Unknown.

INDICATIONS AND DOSAGES

Ulcerative colitis

PO

Adults, Elderly. Three 750-mg capsules 3 times a day for 8 wk.

AVAILABLE FORMS

- *Capsules:* 750 mg.

CONTRAINDICATIONS: Hypersensitivity to salicylates

PREGNANCY AND LACTATION: Pregnancy category B; excretion into breast milk unknown; mesalamine has produced adverse effects in a nursing infant and should be used with caution during breastfeeding; observe nursing infant closely for changes in stool consistency

SIDE EFFECTS

Frequent (8%-6%)

Headache, abdominal pain, nausea, diarrhea

Occasional (4%-2%)

Vomiting, arthralgia, rhinitis, insomnia, fatigue, flatulence, coughing, dyspepsia

SERIOUS REACTIONS

- Liver toxicity occurs rarely.

INTERACTIONS

Drugs

3 *Orally administered antibiotics:* Theoretical interference with the release of mesalamine in the colon

SPECIAL CONSIDERATIONS

- The recommended dose of 6.75 g/day provides approximately 2.4 g of free mesalamine to the colon

PATIENT/FAMILY EDUCATION

- Take as directed
- Do not chew or open balsalazide capsules
- Notify the physician if abdominal pain, severe headache or chest pain, or unresolved diarrhea occurs

MONITORING PARAMETERS

- Liver function test
- Pattern of daily bowel activity and stool consistency

becaplermin

(be-kap'-ler-min)

Rx: Regranex

Chemical Class: Recombinant human platelet-derived growth factor (rhPDGF-BB)

Therapeutic Class: Diabetic neuropathic ulcer agent

CLINICAL PHARMACOLOGY

Mechanism of Action: A platelet-derived growth factor that heals open wounds. ***Therapeutic Effect:*** Stimulates body to grow new tissue.

Pharmacokinetics

None reported.

INDICATIONS AND DOSAGES

Ulcers

Topical

Adults, Elderly. Apply once daily (spread evenly; cover with saline-moistened gauze dressing). After 12 hrs, rinse ulcer, re-cover with saline gauze.

AVAILABLE FORMS

- *Gel:* 0.01% (Regranex).

CONTRAINDICATIONS: Neoplasms at site of application, hypersensitivity to becaplermin or any component of the formulation

PREGNANCY AND LACTATION: Pregnancy category C; excretion into breast milk is unknown but would be expected to be low given the systemic bioavailability of the drug

SIDE EFFECTS

Occasional

Local rash near ulcer

SERIOUS REACTIONS

- None reported.

SPECIAL CONSIDERATIONS

PATIENT/FAMILY EDUCATION

- Refrigerate
- Wash hands before applying

MONITORING PARAMETERS

- If the ulcer does not decrease in size by approximately 30% after 10 wk of treatment or complete healing has not occurred in 20 wk, continued treatment should be reassessed
- Dose requires recalculation weekly or bi-weekly, depending on rate of change in the width and length of ulcer

beclomethasone dipropionate

(be-kloe-meth'-a-sone)

Rx: Beconase AQ, Beconase, Beclovent, Qvar, Vancenase, Vancenase AQ, Vancenase AQ DS, Vanceril, Vanceril DS

Chemical Class: Glucocorticoid, synthetic

Therapeutic Class: Corticosteroid, antiinflammatory

CLINICAL PHARMACOLOGY

Mechanism of Action: An adrenocorticosteroid that prevents or controls inflammation by controlling the rate of protein synthesis; decreasing migration of polymorphonuclear leukocytes and fibroblasts; and reversing capillary permeability. ***Therapeutic Effect:*** Inhalation: Inhibits bronchoconstriction, produces smooth muscle relaxation, decreases mucus secretion. Intranasal: Decreases response to seasonal and perennial rhinitis.

Pharmacokinetics

Rapidly absorbed from pulmonary, nasal, and GI tissue. Undergoes extensive first-pass metabolism in the liver. Protein binding: 87%. Primarily eliminated in feces. ***Half-life:*** 15 hr.

INDICATIONS AND DOSAGES

Long-term control of bronchial asthma, reduces need for oral corticosteriod therapy for asthma

Oral Inhalation

Adults, Elderly, Children 12 yr and older. 40-160 mcg twice a day. Maximum: 320 mcg twice a day.

Rhinitis, prevention of recurrence of nasal polyps

Nasal Inhalation

Adults, Elderly, Children 12 yr and older. 1 spray in each nostril 2-4 times a day or 2 sprays twice a day. Maintenance: 1 spray 3 times a day.

Children 6-12 yr. 1 spray 3 times a day.

AVAILABLE FORMS

• *Oral Inhalation (QVAR):* 40 mcg per inhalation, 80 mcg/inhalation.

• *Nasal spray (Beconase AQ):* 42 mcg/inhalation.

UNLABELED USES: Prevention of seasonal rhinitis (nasal form)

CONTRAINDICATIONS: Hypersensitivity to beclomethasone, acute exacerbation of asthma, status asthmaticus

PREGNANCY AND LACTATION: Pregnancy category C; breast milk excretion unknown; other corticosteroids excreted in low concentrations with systemic administration; compatible with breast-feeding

SIDE EFFECTS

Frequent

Inhalation (14%-4%): Throat irritation, dry mouth, hoarseness, cough

Intranasal: Nasal burning, mucosal dryness

Occasional

Inhalation (3%-2%): Localized fungal infection (thrush)

Intranasal: Nasal-crusting epistaxis, sore throat, ulceration of nasal mucosa

Rare

Inhalation: Transient bronchospasm, esophageal candidiasis

Intranasal: Nasal and pharyngeal candidiasis, eye pain

SERIOUS REACTIONS

• An acute hypersensitivity reaction, as evidenced by urticaria, angioedema, and severe bronchospasm, occurs rarely.

• A transfer from systemic to local steroid therapy may unmask previously suppressed bronchial asthma condition.

SPECIAL CONSIDERATIONS

PATIENT/FAMILY EDUCATION

• Rinse mouth with water following INH to decrease possibility of fungal infections, dysphonia

• Review proper MDI administration technique regularly

• Systemic corticosteroid effects from inhaled and nasal steroids inadequate to prevent adrenal insufficiency in patients withdrawn from corticosteroids abruptly

• Response to nasal steroids seen in 3 days-2 wk; discontinue if no improvement in 3 wk

• For prophylactic use, no role in acute treatment of asthma/allergy

• Taper dosage gradually; do not change dosage schedule or stop taking the drug abruptly

MONITORING PARAMETERS

• Relief of symptoms, such as wheezing, congestion, and dyspnea

belladonna alkaloids

(bell-a-don-a al-kuh-loydz)

Rx: Antispas, Antispasmodic, Barbidonna, Barophen, Bellalphen, Bellatal, Chardonna-2, Donnapine, D-Tal, Haponal, Spacol, Spasmolin, Spasquid

Combinations

Rx: with butalbital (Butibel); with ergotamine and phenobarbital (Bellergal-S, Phenerbel-S); with phenobarbital (Donnatal, Donnatal Extentabs)

Chemical Class: Belladonna alkaloid

Therapeutic Class: Anticholinergic; antispasmodic; gastrointestinal

CLINICAL PHARMACOLOGY

Mechanism of Action: Competitive inhibitors of the muscarinic actions of acetylcholine, acting at receptors located in exocrine glands, smooth and cardiac muscle, and intramural neurons. Composed of 3 main constituents: atropine, scopolamine and hyoscyamine. Scopolamine exerts greater effects on the CNS, eye, and secretory glands than the constituents atropine and hyoscyamine. Atropine exerts more activity on the heart, intestine, and bronchial muscle and exhibits a more prolonged duration of action compared to scopolamine. Hyoscyamine exerts similar actions to atropine but has more potent central and peripheral nervous system effects. ***Therapeutic Effect:*** Peripheral anticholinergic and antispasmodic action, mild sedation.

Pharmacokinetics

None known.

INDICATIONS AND DOSAGES

Irritable bowel syndrome, acute enterocolitis

PO

Adults: 1-2 tablets or capsules 3-4 times daily or 1-2 teaspoonfuls of elixir 3-4 times daily according to conditions and severity of symptoms.

Children: Dosage varies depending on body weight and may be dosed every 4 or 6 hours.

AVAILABLE FORMS

- *Tablet:* 40 mg phenobarbital, 0.6 mg ergotamine tartrate, 0.2 mg levorotatory alkaloids of belladonna (Bellergal, Bellergal-S, Bellergal-R, Spasmolin, Bellalphen, Antispas, Spacol, Chardonna-2, Barbidonna)
- *Tablet, extended release:* 0.0582 mg-48.6 mg-0.0195 mg (Donnatal Extendtabs)
- *Elixir:* 0.0194 mg-0.1037 mg-16.2 mg-0.0065 mg/5 ml (Barophen, Donnapine, Antispasmodic, Spacol, Donnatal, D-Tal, Spasquid)

CONTRAINDICATIONS: Glaucoma, obstructive uropathy, obstructive disease of gastrointestinal tract, paralytic ileus, intestinal atony of the elderly or debilitated patient, unstable cardiovascular status in acute hemorrhage, severe ulcerative colitis especially if complicated by toxic megacolon, myasthenia gravis, hiatal hernia associated with reflux esophagitis, hypersensitivity to any component of the formulation, acute intermittent porphyria

PREGNANCY AND LACTATION: Pregnancy category C; excretion into breast milk is controversial; neonates may be particularly sensitive to anticholinergic agents; use caution in nursing mothers

SIDE EFFECTS

Frequent

Dry mouth, urinary retention, pupillary dilation, constipation, confusion, redness of the skin, flushing, dry skin, allergic contact dermatitis, headache, excitement, agitation, dizziness, lightheadedness, drowsiness, unsteadiness, confusion, slurred speech, sedation, hyperreflexia, convulsions, vertigo, coma, mydriasis, photophobia, blurred vision, dilation of pupils

Rare

Hallucinations, acute psychosis, Stevens-Johnson syndrome, photosensitivity

SERIOUS REACTIONS

• Signs and symptoms of overdose include headache, nausea, vomiting, blurred vision, dilated pupils, hot and dry skin, dizziness, dryness of the mouth, difficulty in swallowing, and CNS stimulation.

• Treatment should consist of gastric lavage, emetics, and activated charcoal. If indicated, parenteral cholinergic agents such as physostigmine or bethanechol chloride should be added.

INTERACTIONS

Drugs

3 *Amantadine:* Enhanced anticholinergic effect; enhanced CNS effect of amantadine

3 *Neuroleptics:* Reduced neuroleptic effect

3 *Rimantadine:* Enhanced anticholinergic effect; enhanced CNS effect of rimantadine

3 *Tacrine:* May reduce anticholinergic effect of atropine; belladonna may reduce CNS effect of tacrine

SPECIAL CONSIDERATIONS

• Product contains hyoscyamine, atropine, and scopolamine

PATIENT/FAMILY EDUCATION

• Avoid hot environments, heat stroke may occur

• Use sunglasses when outside to prevent photophobia

• Change positions slowly to avoid lightheadedness

• Avoid alcohol, CNS depressants, and tasks that require mental alertness

• Constipation, difficulty urinating, decreased sweating, drowsiness, dry mouth, increased heart rate, headache, orthostatic hypotension may occur

belladonna and opium

(bell-a-don'-a)

Rx: B&O Supprettes 15-A, B&O Supprettes 16-A

Chemical Class: Belladonna alkaloid; opiate

Therapeutic Class: Antispasmodic; narcotic analgesic

DEA Class: Schedule II

CLINICAL PHARMACOLOGY

Mechanism of Action: Anticholinergic alkaloids that inhibit the action of acetylcholine at post-ganglionic (muscarinic) receptor sites. Morphine (10% of opium) depresses cerebral cortex, hypothalamus, and medullary centers. ***Therapeutic Effect:*** Decreases digestive secretions, increases GI muscle tone, reduces GI force, alters pain perception and emotional response to pain.

Pharmacokinetics

Onset of action occurs within 30 min. Absorption is dependent on body hydration. Metabolized in liver to form glucuronide metabolites.

INDICATIONS AND DOSAGES

Analgesic, antispasmodic

Rectal

Adults, Elderly. 1 suppository 1-2 times/day. Maximum: 4 doses/day.

AVAILABLE FORMS

• *Suppository:* 16.2 mg belladonna extract/30 mg opium (B&O Supprettes 15-A), 16.2 mg belladonna extract/60 mg opium (B&O Supprettes 16-A).

UNLABELED USES: Glaucoma, severe renal or hepatic disease, bronchial asthma, respiratory depression, convulsive disorders, acute alcoholism, premature labor, hypersensitivity to belladonna or opium or its components

CONTRAINDICATIONS: None known

PREGNANCY AND LACTATION: Pregnancy category C; excretion of belladonna into breast milk is controversial; neonates may be particularly sensitive to anticholinergic agents, therefore use caution in nursing mothers

Controlled Substance: Schedule II

SIDE EFFECTS

Frequent

Dry mouth, nose, skin, and throat, decreased sweating, constipation, irritation at site of administration, drowsiness, urinary retention, dizziness

Occasional

Blurred vision, decreased flow of breast milk, bloated feeling, drowsiness, headache, intolerance to light, nervousness, flushing

Rare

Dizziness, faintness, pruritis, urticaria

SERIOUS REACTIONS

• Respiratory depression, increased intraocular pain, loss of memory, orthostatic hypotension, tachycardia, and ventricular fibrillation rarely occur.

• Tolerance to the drug's analgesic effect and physical dependence may occur with repeated use.

INTERACTIONS

Drugs

3 *Amantadine:* Enhanced anticholinergic effect; enhanced CNS effect of amantadine

3 *Anticholinergics:* Increased effects of belladonna and opium

3 *Ethanol, CNS depressants:* Increased CNS or respiratory depression

3 *Neuroleptics:* Reduced neuroleptic effect

3 *Phenothiazines:* Decreased antipsychotic effects of these drugs

3 *Rimantadine:* Enhanced anticholinergic effect; enhanced CNS effect of rimantadine

3 *Tacrine:* May reduce anticholinergic effect; belladonna may reduce CNS effect of tacrine

SPECIAL CONSIDERATIONS

PATIENT/FAMILY EDUCATION

• Moisten finger and suppository with water before inserting

• May cause drowsiness, dry mouth, and blurred vision

• Store at room temperature; DO NOT refrigerate

MONITORING PARAMETERS

• Bowel activity

---

benazepril hydrochloride

(ben-ay'-ze-pril hye-droe-klor'-ide)

Rx: Lotensin

Combinations

Rx: with hydrochlorothiazide (Lotensin HCT)

Rx: with amlodipine (Lotrel)

Chemical Class: Angiotensin-converting enzyme (ACE) inhibitor, nonsulfhydryl

Therapeutic Class: Antihypertensive

CLINICAL PHARMACOLOGY

Mechanism of Action: An angiotensin-converting enzyme (ACE)

inhibitor that decreases the rate of conversion of angiotensin I to angiotensin II, a potent vasoconstrictor. Reduces peripheral arterial resistance. ***Therapeutic Effect:*** Lowers BP.

Pharmacokinetics

Route	*Onset*	*Peak*	*Duration*
PO	1 hr	2-4 hr	24 hr

Partially absorbed from the GI tract. Protein binding: 97%. Metabolized in the liver to active metabolite. Primarily excreted in urine. Minimal removal by hemodialysis. ***Half-life:*** 35 min; metabolite 10-11 hr.

INDICATIONS AND DOSAGES

Hypertension (monotherapy)

PO

Adults. Initially, 10 mg/day. Maintenance: 20-40 mg/day as single dose or in 2 divided doses. Maximum: 80 mg/day.

Elderly. Initially, 5-10 mg/day. Range: 20-40 mg/day.

Hypertension (combination therapy)

PO

Adults. Discontinue diuretic 2-3 days prior to initiating benazepril, then dose as noted above. If unable to discontinue diuretic, begin benazepril at 5 mg/day.

Usual pediatric dosage

PO

Children 6 yr and older. Initially, 0.2 mg/kg/day. Range: 0.1-0.6 mg/kg/day. Maximum: 40 mg/day.

Dosage in renal impairment

For adult patients with creatinine clearance less than 30 ml/min, initially, 5 mg/day titrated up to maximum of 40 mg/day.

AVAILABLE FORMS

- *Tablets:* 5 mg, 10 mg, 20 mg, 40 mg.

UNLABELED USES: Treatment of CHF

CONTRAINDICATIONS: History of angioedema from previous treatment with ACE inhibitors, pregnancy

PREGNANCY AND LACTATION: Pregnancy category C (first trimester), category D (second and third trimesters); ACE inhibitors can cause fetal and neonatal morbidity and death when administered to pregnant women; detectable in breast milk in trace amounts, a newborn would receive <0.1% of the mg/kg maternal dose; effect on nursing infant has not been determined

SIDE EFFECTS

Frequent (6%-3%)

Cough, headache, dizziness

Occasional (2%)

Fatigue, somnolence or drowsiness, nausea

Rare (less than 1%)

Rash, fever, myalgia, diarrhea, loss of taste

SERIOUS REACTIONS

- Excessive hypotension ("first-dose syncope") may occur in patients with CHF and in those who are severely salt or volume depleted.
- Angioedema (swelling of the face and lips) and hyperkalemia occur rarely.
- Agranulocytosis and neutropenia may be noted in those with collagen vascular disease, including scleroderma and systemic lupus erythematosus, and impaired renal function.
- Nephrotic syndrome may be noted in patients with history of renal disease.

INTERACTIONS

Drugs

3 *Alcohol:* May increase the effects of benazepril

2 *Allopurinol:* Combination may predispose to hypersensitivity reactions

3 *α-adrenergic blockers:* Exaggerated first-dose hypotensive response when added to benazepril
3 *Aspirin:* May reduce hemodynamic effects of benazepril; less likely at doses under 236 mg; less likely with nonacetylated salicylates
3 *Azathioprine:* Increased myelosuppression
3 *COX-2 inhibitors:* May reduce hemodynamic effects of benazepril
3 *Cyclosporine:* Combination may cause renal insufficiency
3 *Insulin:* Benazepril may enhance insulin sensitivity
3 *Iron:* Benazepril may increase chance of systemic reaction to IV iron
3 *Lithium:* Reduced lithium clearance
3 *Loop diuretics:* Initiation of benazepril may cause hypotension and renal insufficiency in patients taking loop diuretics
3 *NSAIDs:* May reduce hemodynamic effects of benazepril
3 *Potassium-sparing diuretics:* Increased risk of hyperkalemia
3 *Trimethoprim:* Additive risk of hyperkalemia, especially in patient predisposed to renal insufficiency

Labs

- ACE inhibition can account for approximately 0.5 mEq/L rise in serum potassium

SPECIAL CONSIDERATIONS

PATIENT/FAMILY EDUCATION

- Caution with salt substitutes containing potassium chloride
- Rise slowly to sitting/standing position to minimize orthostatic hypotension
- Dizziness, fainting, lightheadedness may occur during first few days of therapy
- May cause altered taste perception or cough; persistent dry cough usually does not subside unless medication is stopped
- Full therapeutic effect of benazepril may take 2 to 4 wks to appear
- Noncompliance with drug therapy or skipping drug doses may produce severe, rebound hypertension

MONITORING PARAMETERS

- BUN, creatinine, potassium within 2 wk after initiation of therapy (increased levels may indicate acute renal failure)
- Blood pressure, CBC, urine protein levels

bentoquatam

(ben′-toe-kwa-tam)

Rx: Ivy Block

Chemical Class: Organoclay compound

Therapeutic Class: Rhus dermatitis protectant

CLINICAL PHARMACOLOGY

Mechanism of Action: An organoclay substance that absorbs and binds to urushiol, the active principle in poison oak, ivy, and sumac. ***Therapeutic Effect:*** Blocks urushiol skin contact and absorption.

Pharmacokinetics

None reported.

INDICATIONS AND DOSAGES

Contact dermatitis prophylaxis caused by poison oak, ivy, or sumac

Topical

Adults, Elderly, Children 6 yrs and older. Apply thin film over skin at least 15 mins before potential exposure. Re-apply q4h or sooner if needed.

AVAILABLE FORMS

- *Lotion:* 5% (Ivy Block).

CONTRAINDICATIONS: Hypersensitivity to bentoquatam or any of its components such as methylparabens

PREGNANCY AND LACTATION: Pregnancy category NR

SIDE EFFECTS

Occasional

Erythema

SERIOUS REACTIONS

• None reported.

SPECIAL CONSIDERATIONS

PATIENT/FAMILY EDUCATION

• To be used prior to exposure only
• Avoid using near eyes
• Re-apply every 4 hrs as needed

MONITORING PARAMETERS

• Therapeutic response

benzocaine

(ben'-zoe-kane)

OTC: Americaine Anesthetic Lubricant, Americaine Otic, Anbesol, Anbesol Baby Gel, Anbesol Maximum Strength, Babee Teething, Benzodent, Cepacol, Cetacaine, Chiggerex, Chiggertox, Cylex, Dermoplast, Detaine, Foille, Foille Medicated First Aid, Foille Plus, HDA Toothache, Hurricane, Lanacane, Mycinettes, Omedia, Orabase-B, Orajel, Orajel Baby, Orajel Baby Nighttime, Orajel Maximum Strength, Orasol, Otricaine, Otocain, Retre-Gel, Solarcaine, Trocaine, Zilactin, Zilactin Baby

Combinations

Rx: with antipyrine (Allergen, Auralgan, Auroto); with benzethonium chloride (Americaine, Otocain); with phenylephrine (Tympagesic)

Chemical Class: Benzoic acid derivative

Therapeutic Class: Anesthetic, local

CLINICAL PHARMACOLOGY

Mechanism of Action: A local anesthetic that blocks nerve conduction in the autonomic, sensory, and motor nerve fibers. Competes with calcium ions for membrane binding. Reduces permeability of resting nerves to potassium and sodium ions. ***Therapeutic Effect:*** Produces local analgesic effect.

Pharmacokinetics

Poorly absorbed by topical administration. Well absorbed from mucous membranes and traumatized skin. Metabolized in liver and by hydrolysis with cholinesterase. Minimal excretion in urine.

INDICATIONS AND DOSAGES

Canker sores

Topical

Adults, Elderly, Children older than 2 yrs. Apply gel, liquid, or ointment to affected area. Maximum: 4 times/day.

Denture irritation

Topical

Adults, Elderly. Apply thin layer of gel to affected area up to 4 times/day or until pain is relieved.

General lubrication

Topical

Adults, Elderly, Children older than 2 yrs. Apply gel to exterior of tube or instrument prior to use.

Otitis externa, otitis media

Otic

Adults, Elderly, Children older than 1 yr. Instill 4-5 drops into external ear canal of affected ears. Repeat q1-2h as needed.

Pain and itching associated with sunburn, insect bites, minor cuts, scrapes, minor burns, minor skin irritations

Topical

Adults, Elderly, Children older than 2 yrs. Apply to affected area 3-4 times/day.

Pharyngitis

PO

Adults, Elderly. 1 lozenge q2h. Maximum 8 lozenges/day.

Toothache/teething pain

Topical

Adults, Elderly, Children older than 2 yrs. Apply gel, liquid, or ointment to affected areas. Maximum: 4 times/day.

Anesthesia

Topical

Adults, Elderly. Apply aerosol, gel, ointment, liquid q4-12h as needed.

AVAILABLE FORMS

- *Cream:* 5%, 20% (Lanacane).
- *Lozenge:* 10 mg (Cepacol, Trocaine), 15 mg (Cyclex, Mycinettes).
- *Oral Aerosol:* 14% (Cetacaine), 20% (Hurricane).
- *Oral Gel:* 6.3% (Anbesol), 6.5% (HDA Toothache), 7.5% (Anbesol Baby, Detaine, Orajel Baby), 10% (Orajel, Orajel Baby Nighttime, Zilactin-B, Zilactin Baby), 20% (Anbesol Maximum Strength, Hurricane).
- *Oral Liquid:* 6.3% (Anbesol), 7.5% (Orajel Baby), 10% (Orajel), 20% (Anbesol Maximum Strength, Hurricane).
- *Oral Lotion:* 2.5% (Babee Teething).
- *Oral Ointment:* 20% (Benzadent).
- *Otic Solution:* 20% (Americane Otic, Omedia, Otricaine, Otocain).
- *Paste:* 20% (Orabase-B).
- *Topical Aerosol:* 5%, (Foille, Foille Plus), 20% (Dermoplast, Solarcaine).
- *Topical Gel:* 5% (Retre-Gel), 20% (Americaine Anesthetic Lubricant).
- *Topical Liquid:* 2% (Chiggertox).
- *Topical Ointment:* 2% (Chiggerex), 5% (Foille Medicated First Aid).

UNLABELED USES: Obesity, spasticity

CONTRAINDICATIONS: Hypersensitivity to benzocaine or ester-type local anesthetics, perforated tympanic membrane or ear discharge (otic preparations)

PREGNANCY AND LACTATION: Pregnancy category C; excretion in breast milk unknown; use caution in nursing mothers

SIDE EFFECTS

Occasional

Burning, stinging, angioedema, contact dermatitis, taste disorders

SERIOUS REACTIONS

- Methemoglobinermia occurs rarely in infants and young children.

SPECIAL CONSIDERATIONS

PATIENT/FAMILY EDUCATION

- Protect the solution from light and heat, do not use if it is brown or contains a precipitate
- Discard this product 6 mo after dropper is first placed in the drug solution
- Avoid contact with eyes
- Clean hands with soap and water before using benzocaine
- Do not eat for 1 hr after oral application

---

benzonatate

(ben-zoe'-na-tate)

Rx: Tessalon, Tessalon Perles

Chemical Class: Tetracaine derivative

Therapeutic Class: Antitussive

CLINICAL PHARMACOLOGY

Mechanism of Action: A non-narcotic antitussive that anesthetizes stretch receptors in respiratory passages, lungs, and pleura. ***Therapeutic Effect:*** Reduces cough production.

Pharmacokinetics

Onset	*Duration*
15-20 min	Up to 8 hr

INDICATIONS AND DOSAGES

Antitussive

PO

Adults, Elderly, Children older than 10 yr. 100 mg 3 times a day or q4h up to 600 mg/day.

AVAILABLE FORMS

- *Capsules (Tessalon):* 100 mg, 200 mg.

CONTRAINDICATIONS: None known

PREGNANCY AND LACTATION: Pregnancy category C; excretion into breast milk unknown; use with caution in nursing mothers

SIDE EFFECTS

Occasional

Mild somnolence, mild dizziness, constipation, GI upset, skin eruptions, nasal congestion

SERIOUS REACTIONS

- A paradoxical reaction, including restlessness, insomnia, euphoria, nervousness, and tremor, has been noted.

INTERACTIONS

Drugs

3 *CNS depressants:* Increase effects of benzonatate

SPECIAL CONSIDERATIONS

PATIENT/FAMILY EDUCATION

- Avoid driving, other hazardous activities until stabilized on this medication
- Do not chew or break capsules, will anesthetize mouth

MONITORING PARAMETERS

- Clinical improvement, onset of cough relief

benzoyl peroxide

(ben'-zoe-il per-ox'-side)

Rx: Benzac, Benzac AC, Benzac AC Wash, Benzac W, Benzac W Wash, Benzagel, Benzagel Wash, Benzashave, Brevoxyl, Brevoxyl Cleansing, Brevoxyl Wash, Clearplex, Clinac BPO, Del Aqua, Desquam-E, Desquam-X, Exact Acne Medication, Fostex 10% BPO, Loroxide, Neutrogena Acne Mask, Neutrogena On The Spot Acne Treatment, Oxy 10 Balanced Medicated Face Wash, Oxy 10 Balance Spot Treatment, Palmer's Skin Success Acne, PanOxyl, PanOxyl-AQ, PanOxyl Aqua Gel, PanOxylBar, Triaz, Triaz Cleanser, Zapzyt

Chemical Class: Benzoic acid derivative

Therapeutic Class: Antiacne agent

CLINICAL PHARMACOLOGY

Mechanism of Action: A keratolytic agent that releases free-radical oxygen, which oxidizes bacterial proteins in the sebaceous follicles, decreasing the number of anaerobic bacteria and decreasing irritating-type free fatty acids. ***Therapeutic Effect:*** Bactericidal action against *Propionbacterium acnes* and *Staphlococcus epidermidis*.

Pharmacokinetics

Minimal absorption through skin. Gel is more penetrating than cream. Metabolized to benzoic acid in skin. Excreted in urine as benzoate.

INDICATIONS AND DOSAGES

Acne

Topical

Adults. Apply 2.5%-10% concentration 1-2 times/day.

AVAILABLE FORMS

- *Cream, topical:* 2.5% (Neutrogena On The Spot Acne Treatment), 5% (Benzashave, Exact Acne Medication, Neutrogena Acne Mask), 10% (Benzashave).
- *Gel, topical:* 2.5% (Benzac, Benzac AC, Benzac W, Desquam-E), 4% (Brevoxyl), 5% (Benzac, Benzac AC, Benzac W, Benzagel, Clearplex, Desquam-E, Desquam-X, Oxy 10 Balance Spot Treatment, PanOxyl, PanOxyl AQ, Seba-Gel), 6% (Triaz, Triaz Cleanser), 7% (Clinac BPO), 8% (Brevoxyl), 10% (Benzac, Benzac AC, Benzac W, Benzagel, Benzagel Wash, Clearplex, Desquam-E, Desquam-X, Fostex, Oxy 10 Balance Spot Treatment, PanOxyl, PanOxyl AQ, PanOxyl Aqua Gel, Seba-Gel, Triaz, Triaz Cleanser, Zapzyt).
- *Liquid, topical:* 2.5% (Benzac AC Wash), 5% (Benzac AC Wash, Benzac W Wash, Del-Aqua, Desquam-X), 10% (Benzac AC Wash, Benzac W Wash, Del-Aqua, Oxy-10 Balance Medicated Face Wash).
- *Lotion, topical:* 4% (Brevoxyl Cleansing, Brevoxyl Wash), 5.5% (Loroxide), 8% (Brevoxyl Cleansing, Brevoxyl Wash), 10% (Fostex, Palmer's Skin Success Acne).
- *Soap bar, topical:* 5% (PanOxyl Bar), 10% (Desquam-X, Fostex, PanOxyl Bar).

UNLABELED USES: Dermal ulcers, seborrheic dermatitis, surgical wounds, tinea pedis, tinea versicolor

CONTRAINDICATIONS: Hypersensitivity to benzoyl peroxide or any component of the formulation

PREGNANCY AND LACTATION: Pregnancy category C; excretion into milk unknown

SIDE EFFECTS

Occasional

Irritation, dryness, burning, peeling, stinging, contact dermatitis, bleaching of hair

SERIOUS REACTIONS

- Hypersensitivity reactions have been reported with benzoyl peroxide use.

INTERACTIONS

Drugs

3 *Tretinoin:* Excess skin irritation

SPECIAL CONSIDERATIONS

PATIENT/FAMILY EDUCATION

- Keep away from eyes, mouth, inside of nose and other mucous membranes
- May cause transitory feeling of warmth or slight stinging
- Expect dryness and peeling, discontinue use if rash or irritation develops. Use lower concentration in fair-skinned individuals
- Water-based cosmetics may be used over drug; do not counter-treat dryness with emollients

MONITORING PARAMETERS

- Skin for irritation

---

benztropine mesylate

(benz'-troe-peen mes'-sil-ate)

Rx: Cogentin

Chemical Class: Tertiary amine

Therapeutic Class: Anti-Parkinson's agent; anticholinergic

CLINICAL PHARMACOLOGY

Mechanism of Action: An antiparkinson agent that selectively blocks central cholinergic receptors, helping to balance cholinergic and dopaminergic activity. ***Therapeutic Effect:*** Reduces the incidence and severity of akinesia, rigidity, and tremor.

Pharmacokinetics

Well absorbed following oral and IM administration. Oral onset of action: 1-2 hr, IM onset of action: minutes. The pharmacologic effects may not be apparent until 2-3 days after initiation of therapy and may persist for up to 24 hr after discontinuation of the drug. ***Half-life:*** Extended.

INDICATIONS AND DOSAGES

Parkinsonism

PO

Adults. 0.5-6 mg/day as a single dose or in 2 divided doses. Titrate by 0.5 mg at 5-6 day intervals.

Elderly. Initially, 0.5 mg once or twice a day. Titrate by 0.5 mg at 5-6 day intervals. Maximum: 4 mg/day.

Drug-induced extrapyramidal symptoms

PO, IM

Adults. 1-4 mg once or twice a day.

Children older than 3 yr. 0.02-0.05 mg/kg/dose once or twice a day.

Acute dystonic reactions

IV, IM

Adults. Initially, 1-2 mg; then 1-2 mg PO twice a day to prevent recurrence.

AVAILABLE FORMS

- *Tablets:* 0.5 mg, 1 mg, 2 mg.
- *Injection:* 1 mg/ml.

CONTRAINDICATIONS: Angle-closure glaucoma, benign prostatic hyperplasia, children younger than 3 years, GI obstruction, intestinal atony, megacolon, myasthenia gravis, paralytic ileus, severe ulcerative colitis

PREGNANCY AND LACTATION: Pregnancy category C; an inhibitory effect on lactation may occur; infants may be particularly sensitive to anticholinergic effects

B

SIDE EFFECTS

Frequent

Somnolence, dry mouth, blurred vision, constipation, decreased sweating or urination, GI upset, photosensitivity

Occasional

Headache, memory loss, muscle cramps, anxiety, peripheral paresthesia, orthostatic hypotension, abdominal cramps

Rare

Rash, confusion, eye pain

SERIOUS REACTIONS

• Overdose may produce severe anticholinergic effects, such as unsteadiness, somnolence, tachycardia, dyspnea, skin flushing, and severe dryness of the mouth, nose, or throat.

• Severe paradoxical reactions, marked by hallucinations, tremor, seizures, and toxic psychosis, may occur.

INTERACTIONS

Drugs

3 *Alcohol, other CNS depressants:* Increases sedation

3 *Anticholinergics:* Excess anticholinergic side effects

3 *Amantadine:* Potentiates CNS side effects of amantadine

3 *Neuroleptics:* Inhibition of therapeutic response to neuroleptics; excessive anticholinergic effects

3 *Tacrine:* Reduced therapeutic effects of both drugs

3 *Tricyclic antidepressants:* Causes excessive anticholinergic effects

SPECIAL CONSIDERATIONS

PATIENT/FAMILY EDUCATION

• Do not discontinue abruptly

• Administer with or after meals to prevent GI upset

• Drug may increase susceptibility to heat stroke

• Dizziness, drowsiness, and dry mouth are expected responses to the drug

• Avoid tasks that require mental alertness or motor skills until response to the drug has been established

MONITORING PARAMETERS

• Relief of symptoms, such as an improvement of masklike facial expression, muscular rigidity, shuffling gait, and resting tremors of the hands and head

benzylpenicilloyl-polylysine

(ben'-zil-pen-i-sil'-oyl-pol-i-lie'-seen)

Rx: Pre-Pen

Chemical Class: Penicillin derivative

Therapeutic Class: Penicillin allergy skin test

CLINICAL PHARMACOLOGY

Mechanism of Action: A diagnostic agent that invokes immunoglobulin E, which produces type I accelerated urticarial reactions to penicillins. ***Therapeutic Effect:*** A positive reaction will suggest penicillin sensitivity.

Pharmacokinetics

Not known.

INDICATIONS AND DOSAGES

Penicillin sensitivity

Intradermal

Adults, Children. Use a tuberculin syringe with a 26-30 gauge, short bevel needle. A dose of 0.01-0.02 ml is injected intradermally. A control of 0.9% sodium chloride should be injected about 1½ inches from the test site. Skin response usually occurs within 5-15 min.

Scratch test

Adults, Children. Use a 20-gauge needle to make 3-5 mm nonbleeding scratch of the epidermis. Apply a small drop of solution to scratch and rub gently with applicator or toothpick. A positive reaction consists of a pale wheal surrounding the scratch site, develops within 10 minutes, and ranges from 5-15 mm in diameter.

AVAILABLE FORMS

• *Solution:* 0.25 ml (Pre-Pen).

CONTRAINDICATIONS: Systemic or marked local reaction to its previous administration or hypersensitivity to penicillin

PREGNANCY AND LACTATION: Pregnancy category C

SIDE EFFECTS

Frequent

Skin rash

Occasional

Nausea

SERIOUS REACTIONS

• None significant.

SPECIAL CONSIDERATIONS

• Does not identify those patients who react to a minor antigenic determinant (i.e., anaphylaxis); does not reliably predict the occurrence of late reactions; patients with a negative skin test may still have allergic reactions to therapeutic penicillin

• (−) Negative response: No increase in size of original bleb and/or no greater reaction than the control site

• (±) Ambiguous response: Wheal being only slightly larger than initial injection bleb, with or without accompanying erythematous flare and larger than the control site

• (+) Positive response: Itching and marked increase in size of original bleb. Wheal may exceed 20 mm in diameter and exhibit pseudopods

PATIENT/FAMILY EDUCATION

• Contact the physician if pain or discomfort is severe or continues for more than 5 hrs

bepridil hydrochloride

(be'-pri-dil hye-droe-klor'-ide)

Rx: Vascor

Chemical Class: Diarylaminopropylamine ether

Therapeutic Class: Antianginal; calcium channel blocker

CLINICAL PHARMACOLOGY

Mechanism of Action: A calcium channel blocker that inhibits calcium ion entry across cell membranes of cardiac and vascular smooth muscle; decreases heart rate, myocardial contractility, slows SA and AV conduction. ***Therapeutic Effect:*** Dilates coronary arteries, peripheral arteries/arterioles.

Pharmacokinetics

Rapidly, completely absorbed from GI tract. Undergoes first-pass metabolism in liver to active metabolite. Primarily excreted in urine. Not removed by hemodialysis. ***Half-life:*** less than 24 hrs.

INDICATIONS AND DOSAGES

Chronic stable angina

PO

Adults, Elderly: Initially, 200 mg/day; after 10 days, dosage may be adjusted. Maintenance: 200-400 mg/day.

AVAILABLE FORMS

• *Tablets:* 200 mg, 300 mg (Vascor).

CONTRAINDICATIONS: Sick sinus syndrome/second- or third-degree AV block (except in presence of pacemaker), severe hypotension (<90 mm Hg, systolic), history of serious ventricular arrhythmias, uncompensated cardiac insufficiency, congenital QT interval prolongation, use with other drugs prolonging QT interval

PREGNANCY AND LACTATION: Pregnancy category C; excreted in breast milk; use caution in nursing mothers

SIDE EFFECTS

Frequent

Dizziness, lightheadedness, nervousness, headache, asthenia (loss of strength), hand tremor, nausea, diarrhea

Occasional

Drowsiness, insomnia, tinnitus, abdominal discomfort, palpitations, dry mouth, shortness of breath, wheezing, anorexia, constipation

Rare

Peripheral edema, anxiety, flatulence, nasal congestion, paresthesia

SERIOUS REACTIONS

• CHF, second- and third-degree AV block occur rarely.

• Serious arrhythmias can be induced.

• Overdosage produces nausea, drowsiness, confusion, slurred speech, profound bradycardia.

INTERACTIONS

Drugs

3 *β-blockers:* Additive depressant effects on myocardial contractility or AV conduction

3 *Digitalis glycosides:* Reduced clearance; increased digitalis levels; potential toxicity

3 *Hypokalemia-producing agents:* Increased risk of arrhythmias

3 *Procainamide, quinidine:* Increased risk of QT interval prolongation

SPECIAL CONSIDERATIONS

PATIENT/FAMILY EDUCATION

• ECGs will be necessary during initiation of therapy and after dosage changes

• Notify provider immediately for irregular heartbeat, shortness of breath, pronounced dizziness, constipation, or hypotension

• May be taken with food or meals

• Rise slowly from lying to sitting position to avoid hypotensive effect

MONITORING PARAMETERS

• Blood pressure, pulse, respiration, ECG intervals (PR, QRS, QT) at initiation of therapy and again after dosage increases prologation of QT interval by >0.52 sec predisposes to proarrythmia

• Serum potassium (normalize before initiation)

---

betamethasone

(bay-ta-meth'-a-sone)

Rx: Abdeon, Alphatrex, Beta-Phos/AC, Betatrex, Beta-Val, Celestone, Celestone Phosphate, Celestone Soluspan, Diprolene, Luxiq, Maxivate

Combinations

Rx: with clotrimazole (Lotrisone)

Chemical Class: Glucocorticoid, synthetic

Therapeutic Class: Corticosteroid, systemic; corticosteroid, topical

CLINICAL PHARMACOLOGY

Mechanism of Action: An adrenocortical steroid that controls the rate of protein synthesis, depresses the migration of polymorphonuclear leukocytes and fibroblasts, reduces capillary permeability and prevents or controls inflammation. ***Therapeutic Effect:*** Decreases tissue response to inflammatory process.

Pharmacokinetics

Rapidly and almost completely absorbed following PO administration. After topical application, limited absorption systemically. Metabolized in liver. Excreted in urine. ***Half-life:*** 36-54 hr.

INDICATIONS AND DOSAGES

Anti-inflammation, immunosuppression, corticosteroid replacement therapy

PO

Adults, Elderly. 0.6-7.2 mg/day.

Children. 0.0175-0.25 mg/kg/day in 3-4 divided doses.

IM

Adults, Elderly. 0.5-9 mg/day in 2 divided doses.

Children. 0.0175-0.125 mg/kg/day in 3-4 divided doses.

Relief of inflamed and pruritic dermatoses

Topical

Adults, Elderly. 1-3 times a day. Foam: Apply twice a day.

AVAILABLE FORMS

- *Tablets (Celestone):* 0.6 mg.
- *Cream:* 0.05% (Alphatrex, Diprolene, Maxivate), 0.1% (Betatrex, Beta-Val).
- *Foam (Luxiq):* 0.12%.
- *Gel (Diprolene):* 0.05%.
- *Lotion:* 0.05% (Alphatrex, Diprolene, Maxivate), 0.1% (Betatrex, Beta-Val).
- *Ointment:* 0.05% (Alphatrex, Diprolene, Maxivate), 0.1% (Betatrex).
- *Syrup (Celestone):* 0.6 mg/5 ml.
- *Injection Solution (Abdeon, Celestone Phosphate):* 4 mg/ml.
- *Injection Suspension (Beta-Phos/AC, Celestone Soluspan):* 3 mg acetate/3 mg betamethasone sodium phosphate.

CONTRAINDICATIONS: Hypersensitivity to betamethasone, systemic fungal infections

PREGNANCY AND LACTATION: Pregnancy category C (D if used in first trimester); used in patients with premature labor at about 24-36 wk gestation to stimulate fetal lung maturation (see dosage); excreted in breast milk; could suppress infant's growth and interfere with endogenous corticosteroid production

SIDE EFFECTS

Frequent

Systemic: Increased appetite, abdominal distention, nervousness, insomnia, false sense of well-being

Topical: Burning, stinging, pruritus

Occasional

Systemic: Dizziness, facial flushing, diaphoresis, decreased or blurred vision, mood swings

Topical: Allergic contact dermatitis, purpura or blood-containing blisters, thinning of skin with easy bruising, telangiectases or raised dark red spots on skin

SERIOUS REACTIONS

- Overdose may cause systemic hypercorticism and adrenal suppression.

INTERACTIONS

Drugs

3 *Aminoglutethamide:* Enhanced elimination of corticosteroids; marked reduction in corticosteroid response; increased clearance of prednisone; doubling of dose may be necessary

3 *Amphotericin:* Increases the risk of hypokalemia

3 *Antidiabetics:* Increased blood glucose

3 *Barbiturates, carbamazepine:* Reduced serum concentrations of corticosteroids; increased clearance of prednisone

3 *Cholestyramine, colestipol:* Possible reduced absorption of corticosteroids

3 *Cyclosporine:* Possible increased concentration of both drugs, seizures

3 *Digoxin:* Increases digoxin toxicity secondary to hypokalemia

3 *Erythromycin, troleandomycin, clarithromycin, ketoconazole:* Possible enhanced steroid effect

3 *Estrogens, oral contraceptives:* Enhanced effects of corticosteroids
3 *Isoniazid:* Reduced plasma concentrations of isoniazid
3 *IUDs:* Inhibition of inflammation may decrease contraceptive effect
3 *Live-virus vaccines:* Decrease the patient's antibody response to vaccine, increase vaccine side effects, and potentiate virus replication
3 *NSAIDs:* Increased risk of GI ulceration
3 *Potassium supplements:* Decreases the effects of these drugs
3 *Rifampin:* Reduced therapeutic effect of corticosteroids; may reduce hepatic clearance of prednisone
3 *Salicylates:* Subtherapeutic salicylate concentrations possible

Labs

- *False negative:* Skin allergy tests

SPECIAL CONSIDERATIONS

- Recommend single daily doses in a.m.
- Signs of adrenal insufficiency include fatigue, anorexia, nausea, vomiting, diarrhea, weight loss, weakness, dizziness, and low blood sugar; drug-induced secondary adrenocorticoid insufficiency may be minimized by gradual systemic dosage reduction; relative insufficiency may exist for up to 1 yr after discontinuation of therapy; be prepared to supplement in situations of stress
- May mask infections
- Do not give live virus vaccines to patients on prolonged therapy
- Patients on chronic steroid therapy should wear medic alert bracelet
- Do not use topical products on weeping, denuded, or infected areas

PATIENT/FAMILY EDUCATIONs

- Take oral betamethasone in the morning with food or milk
- Do not abruptly discontinue drug

MONITORING PARAMETERS

- Serum K and glucose
- Growth of children on prolonged therapy
- Blood pressure
- Electrolytes

betaxolol hydrochloride

(bay-tax'-oh-lol hye-droe-klor'-ide)

Rx: Betoptic, Betoptic S, Kerlone

Chemical Class: β_1-adrenergic blocker, cardioselective

Therapeutic Class: Antianginal; antihypertensive

CLINICAL PHARMACOLOGY

Mechanism of Action: An antihypertensive and antiglaucoma agent that blocks beta$_1$-adrenergic receptors in cardiac tissue. Reduces aqueous humor production. ***Therapeutic Effect:*** Slows sinus heart rate, decreases BP, and reduces intraocular pressure (IOP).

Pharmacokinetics

Well absorbed from the GI tract. Minimal absorption after ophthalmic administration. Protein binding: 50%-60% (oral). Metabolized in liver. Primarily excreted in urine. Removed by hemodialysis. ***Half-life:*** 12-22 hr (half-life is increased in the elderly and patients with impaired renal function). Ophthalmic: Systemic absorption may occur.

INDICATIONS AND DOSAGES

Hypertension

PO

Adults. Initially, 5-10 mg/day. May increase to 20 mg/day after 7-14 days.

Elderly. Initially, 5 mg/day.

Chronic open-angle glaucoma and ocular hypertension
Ophthalmic (solution)
Adults, Elderly. 1 drop twice a day.
Ophthalmic (suspension)
Adults, Elderly. 1-2 drops twice a day.
Dosage in renal impairment
For adult and elderly patients who are on dialysis, initially give 5 mg/day; increase by 5 mg/day q2wk. Maximum: 20 mg/day.

AVAILABLE FORMS
- *Tablets (Kerlone):* 10 mg, 20 mg.
- *Ophthalmic Solution (Betoptic):* 0.5%.
- *Ophthalmic Suspension (Betoptic-S):* 0.25%.

UNLABELED USES: Treatment of angle-closure glaucoma during or after iridectomy, malignant glaucoma, secondary glaucoma; with miotics, to decrease IOP in acute and chronic angle-closure glaucoma

CONTRAINDICATIONS: Cardiogenic shock, overt cardiac failure, second- or third-degree heart block, sinus bradycardia

PREGNANCY AND LACTATION: Pregnancy category C (D if used in second or third trimester); excretion into breast milk unknown; use caution in nursing mothers

SIDE EFFECTS
Betaxolol is generally well tolerated, with mild and transient side effects.
Frequent
Systemic: Hypotension manifested as dizziness, nausea, diaphoresis, headache, fatigue, constipation or diarrhea, dyspnea
Ophthalmic: Eye irritation, visual disturbances
Occasional
Systemic: Insomnia, flatulence, urinary frequency, impotence or decreased libido
Ophthalmic: Increased light sensitivity, watering of eye
Rare
Systemic: Rash, arrhythmias, arthralgia, myalgia, confusion, altered taste, increased urination
Ophthalmic: Dry eye, conjunctivitis, eye pain

SERIOUS REACTIONS
- Overdose may produce profound bradycardia, hypotension, and bronchospasm.
- Abrupt withdrawal may result in diaphoresis, palpitations, headache, and tremors.
- Betaxolol administration may precipitate CHF or MI in patients with cardiac disease; thyroid storm in those with thyrotoxicosis; and peripheral ischemia in those with existing peripheral vascular disease.
- Hypoglycemia may occur in patients with previously controlled diabetes.
- Ophthalmic overdose may produce bradycardia, hypotension, bronchospasm, and acute cardiac failure.

INTERACTIONS
Drugs
3 *α_1-adrenergic blockers:* Potential enhanced first-dose response (marked initial drop in blood pressure, particularly on standing [especially prazosin])
3 *Amiodarone:* Bradycardia/ventricular dysrhythmia
3 *Anesthetics, local:* Enhanced sympathomimetic effects, hypertension due to unopposed α-receptor stimulation
3 *Antacids:* May reduce β-blocker absorption
3 *Antidiabetics, insulin:* Delayed recovery from hypoglycemia, hyperglycemia, attenuated tachycardia during hypoglycemia, hypertension during hypoglycemia

3 *Clonidine:* Rebound hypertension; discontinue β-blocker prior to clonidine withdrawal
3 *Cimetidine:* Increased betaxolol blood concentration
3 *Digoxin:* Additive prolongation of atrioventricular (AV) conduction time
3 *Dihydropyridine calcium channel blockers:* Severe hypotension or impaired cardiac performance; most prevalent with impaired left ventricular function, cardiac arrhythmias, or aortic stenosis
3 *Dipyridamole:* Bradycardia
3 *Disopyramide:* Additive decreases in cardiac output
3 *Diuretics:* Increased hypotensive effect of betaxolol
3 *Epinephrine:* Enhanced pressor response resulting in hypertension
3 *Neostigmine:* Bradycardia
3 *Neuroleptics:* Increased serum levels of both resulting in accentuated pharmacologic response to both drugs
3 *NSAIDs:* Reduced hypotensive effects
3 *Phenylephrine:* Acute hypertensive episodes
3 *Sympathomimetics:* Mutually inhibit effects
3 *Tacrine:* Additive bradycardia
2 *Theophylline:* Antagonist pharmacodynamics

SPECIAL CONSIDERATIONS

- Do not discontinue oral drug abruptly, may precipitate angina or MI
- Anaphylactic reactions may be more severe and not be as responsive to usual doses of epinephrine
- Transient stinging/discomfort is relatively common with ophthalmic preparations, notify clinician if severe
- Avoid hazardous activities if dizziness, drowsiness, lightheadedness are present
- May mask the symptoms of hypoglycemia, except for sweating, in diabetic patients

MONITORING PARAMETERS

- Blood pressure, pulse, intraocular pressure (ophth)
- Pattern of daily bowel activity and stool consistency
- Intake and output
- Weight

bethanechol chloride

(be-than'-e-kole klor'-ide)

Rx: Duvoid, Urecholine

Chemical Class: Choline ester

Therapeutic Class: Cholinergic stimulant

CLINICAL PHARMACOLOGY

Mechanism of Action: A cholinergic that acts directly at cholinergic receptors in the smooth muscle of the urinary bladder and GI tract. Increases detrusor muscle tone. ***Therapeutic Effect:*** May initiate micturition and bladder emptying. Improves gastric and intestinal motility.

Pharmacokinetics

Poorly absorbed following PO administration. Does not cross the blood-brain barrier. Metabolism, ***Half-life:*** Unknown.

INDICATIONS AND DOSAGES

Postoperative and postpartum urine retention, atony of bladder

PO

Adults, Elderly. 10-50 mg 3-4 times a day. Minimum effective dose determined by giving 5-10 mg initially, then repeating same amount at 1-hr intervals until desired response is achieved.

Children. 0.6 mg/kg/day in 3-4 divided doses.

Subcutaneous

Adults, Elderly. Initially, 2.5-5 mg. Minimum effective dose determined by giving 2.5 mg (0.5 ml), repeating same amount at 15- to 30-min intervals up to a maximum of 4 doses. Minimum dose repeated 3-4 times a day.

Children. 0.2 mg/kg/day in 3-4 divided doses.

AVAILABLE FORMS

- *Tablets:* 5 mg (Urecholine), 10 mg (Duvoid, Urecholine), 25 mg (Duvoid, Urecholine), 50 mg (Duvoid, Urecholine).
- *Subcutaneous solution:* 5 mg/ml (Urecholine).

UNLABELED USES: Treatment of congenital megacolon, gastroesophageal reflux, postoperative gastric atony

CONTRAINDICATIONS: Active or latent bronchial asthma, acute inflammatory GI tract conditions, anastomosis, bladder wall instability, cardiac or coronary artery disease, epilepsy, hypertension, hyperthyroidism, hypotension, mechanical GI or urinary tract obstruction or recent GI resection, parkinsonism, peptic ulcer, pronounced bradycardia, vasomotor instability

PREGNANCY AND LACTATION: Pregnancy category C; abdominal pain and diarrhea have been reported in a nursing infant exposed to bethanechol in milk; use caution in nursing mothers

SIDE EFFECTS

Occasional

Belching, changes in vision, blurred vision, diarrhea, frequent urinary urgency

Rare

Subcutaneous: Shortness of breath, chest tightness, bronchospasm

SERIOUS REACTIONS

- Overdosage produces CNS stimulation, including insomnia, nervousness, and orthostatic hypotension, and cholinergic stimulation, such as headache, increased salivation and diaphoresis, nausea, vomiting, flushed skin, abdominal pain, and seizures.

INTERACTIONS

Drugs

3 *β-blockers:* Additive bradycardia

3 *Cholinesterase inhibitors:* Increases the effects and risk of toxicity of bethanechol

3 *Procainamide, quinidine:* Decreases the effects of bethanechol

3 *Tacrine:* Increased cholinergic effects

SPECIAL CONSIDERATIONS

- Recommend taking on an empty stomach to avoid nausea and vomiting

PATIENT/FAMILY EDUCATION

- Notify the physician if patient experiences diarrhea, difficulty breathing, increased salivary secretions, irregular heartbeat, muscle weakness, nausea, severe abdominal pain, sweating, and vomiting

MONITORING PARAMETERS

- Fluid intake and output

biperiden hydrochloride

(bye-per′-i-den hye-droe-klor′-ide)

Rx: Akineton

Chemical Class: Tertiary amine

Therapeutic Class: Anti-Parkinson's agent; anticholinergic

CLINICAL PHARMACOLOGY

Mechanism of Action: A weak anticholinergic that exhibits competitive antagonism of acetylcholine at cholinergic receptors in the corpus striatum, which restores balance. ***Therapeutic Effect:*** Antiparkinson activity.

Pharmacokinetics
Well absorbed from gastrointestinal (GI) tract. Protein binding: 23%-33%. Widely distributed. ***Half-life:*** 18-24 hr.

INDICATIONS AND DOSAGES

Extrapyramidal symptoms
PO
Adults, Elderly. 2 mg 3-4 times/day. Dosage in renal impairment.

Parkinsonism
PO
Adults, Elderly. 2 mg 1-3 times/day.

AVAILABLE FORMS

• *Tablets:* 2 mg (Akineton HCl).

UNLABELED USES: Adjunct to methadone maintenance

CONTRAINDICATIONS: None known

PREGNANCY AND LACTATION: Pregnancy category C; breast milk excretion not known, nursing infants particularly sensitive to anticholinergic effects

SIDE EFFECTS

Frequent
Orthostatic hypotension, anorexia, headache, blurred vision, urinary retention, dry mouth or nose
Occasional
Insomnia, agitation, euphoria
Rare
Vomiting, depression, irritation or swelling of eyes, rash

SERIOUS REACTIONS

• Overdosage may vary from severe anticholinergic effects, such as unsteadiness, severe drowsiness, dryness of mouth, nose, or throat, tachycardia, shortness of breath, and skin flushing.
• Also produces severe paradoxical reaction, marked by hallucinations, tremor, seizures, and toxic psychosis.

INTERACTIONS

Drugs
3 *Amantadine:* Potentiates CNS side effect of amantadine
3 *Anticholinergics:* Increased anticholinergic effects
3 *Antihistamines, phenothiazines, tricyclic antidepressants:* Increased anticholinergic effects
3 *Neuroleptics:* Inhibition of therapeutic response to neuroleptics; excessive anticholinergic effects
3 *Tacrine:* Reduced therapeutic effects of both drugs

SPECIAL CONSIDERATIONS

• Give parenteral dose with patient recumbent to prevent postural hypotension

PATIENT/FAMILY EDUCATION

• May increase susceptibility to heatstroke
• Do not discontinue drug abruptly; taper off over 1 wk
• Avoid tasks that require mental alertness or motor skills until response to the drug is established
• Dizziness, drowsiness, and dry mouth are expected responses to the drug

MONITORING PARAMETERS

• Relief of symptoms such as an improvement of masklike facial expression, muscular rigidity, shuffling gait, and resting tremors of hands and head

bisacodyl

(bis-a-koe′-dill)
OTC: Alophen, Dulcolax, Fleet, Gentlax, Modane, Veracolate
Chemical Class: Diphenylmethane derivative
Therapeutic Class: Laxative, stimulant

CLINICAL PHARMACOLOGY

Mechanism of Action: A GI stimulant that has a direct effect on colonic smooth musculature by stimulating the intramural nerve plexi. ***Thera-***

peutic Effect: Promotes fluid and ion accumulation in the colon, increasing peristalsis and producing a laxative effect.

Pharmacokinetics

Route	Onset	Peak	Duration
PO	6-12 hr	N/A	N/A
Rectal	15-60 min	N/A	N/A

Minimal absorption following oral and rectal administration. Absorbed drug is excreted in urine; remainder is eliminated in feces.

INDICATIONS AND DOSAGES

Treatment of constipation

PO

Adults, Children older than 12 yr. 5-15 mg as needed. Maximum: 30 mg.

Children 3-12 yr. 5-10 mg or 0.3 mg/kg at bedtime or after breakfast.

Elderly. Initially, 5 mg/day.

Rectal, enema

Adults, Children 12 yr and older. One 1.25-oz bottle in a single daily dose.

Rectal, suppository

Adults, Children 12 yr and older. 10 mg to induce bowel movement.

Children 2-11 yr. 5-10 mg as a single dose.

Children younger than 2 yr. 5 mg.

Elderly. 5-10 mg/day.

AVAILABLE FORMS

- *Tablets (Enteric-Coated [Dulcolax, Fleet]):* 5 mg.
- *Rectal enema (Fleet):* 10 mg/1.25 oz.
- *Suppositories (Dulcolax, Fleet):* 10 mg.

CONTRAINDICATIONS: Abdominal pain, appendicitis, intestinal obstruction, nausea, undiagnosed rectal bleeding, vomiting

PREGNANCY AND LACTATION: Pregnancy category C; excreted in breast milk

SIDE EFFECTS

Frequent

Some degree of abdominal discomfort, nausea, mild cramps, faintness

Occasional

Rectal administration: burning of rectal mucosa, mild proctitis

SERIOUS REACTIONS

- Long-term use may result in laxative dependence, chronic constipation, and loss of normal bowel function.
- Prolonged use or overdose may result in electrolyte or metabolic disturbances (such as hypokalemia, hypocalcemia, and metabolic acidosis or alkalosis), as well as persistent diarrhea, vomiting, muscle weakness, malabsorption, and weight loss.

INTERACTIONS

Drugs

3 *Antacids, cimetidine, famotidine, ranitidine:* Rapid dissolution of bisacodyl, producing abdominal cramping and vomiting

3 *Oral medications:* Decreases transit time of concurrently administered oral medications, decreasing absorption of bisacodyl

Labs

- *False decrease:* glucose (Clinistix, Diastix); no effect with Tes-tape

SPECIAL CONSIDERATIONS

PATIENT/FAMILY EDUCATION

- Do not take within 1 hr of antacids or milk
- Increasing fluid intake, exercising, and eating a high-fiber diet will promote defecation
- Notify the physician if unrelieved constipation, dizziness, muscle cramps or pain, rectal bleeding, or weakness occurs

MONITORING PARAMETERS

- Fluid intake
- Pattern of daily bowel activity
- Electrolytes

bismuth subsalicylate

(bis′-muth sub-sal-ih′-sah-late)

OTC: Colo-Fresh, Devrom, Kaopectate, Pepto-Bismol, Pink Bismuth

Combinations

Rx: with metronidazole, tetracycline (Helidac)

Chemical Class: Salicylate derivative

Therapeutic Class: Antidiarrheal; antiulcer agent; gastrointestinal

CLINICAL PHARMACOLOGY

Mechanism of Action: An antinauseant and antiulcer agent that absorbs water and toxins in the large intestine and forms a protective coating in the intestinal mucosa. Also possesses antisecretory and antimicrobial effects. ***Therapeutic Effect:*** Prevents diarrhea. Helps treat *Helicobacter-pylori*-associated peptic ulcer disease.

Pharmacokinetics

Rapidly and completely absorbed following PO administration. Protein binding: greater than 90%. Primarily excreted in feces. Terminal ***half-life:*** 21-72 days.

INDICATIONS AND DOSAGES

Diarrhea, gastric distress

PO

Adults, Elderly. 2 tablets (30 ml) q30-60min. Maximum: 8 doses in 24 hr.

Children 9-12 yr. 1 tablet or 15 ml q30-60min. Maximum: 8 doses in 24 hr.

Children 6-8 yr. Two-thirds of a tablet or 10 ml q30-60min. Maximum: 8 doses in 24 hr.

Children 3-5 yr. One-third of a tablet or 5 ml q30-60min. Maximum: 8 doses in 24 hr.

H. pylori–associated duodenal ulcer, gastritis

PO

Adults, Elderly. 525 mg 4 times a day, with 500 mg amoxicillin and 500 mg metronidazole, 3 times a day after meals, for 7-14 days.

Chronic infant diarrhea

PO

Children 2-24 mo. 2.5 ml q4h.

AVAILABLE FORMS

- *Caplets (Devrom):* 200 mg.
- *Liquid (Kaopectate, Pepto-Bismol):* 262 mg/15 ml, 525 mg/15 ml.
- *Tablets (Colo-Fresh):* 324 mg.
- *Tablets (Chewable):* 200 mg (Devrom), 262 mg (Pepto-Bismol).

UNLABELED USES: Prevention of traveler's diarrhea

CONTRAINDICATIONS: Bleeding ulcers, gout, hemophilia, hemorrhagic states, renal impairment

PREGNANCY AND LACTATION: Pregnancy category C; salicylate excreted in breast milk

SIDE EFFECTS

Frequent

Grayish black stools

Rare

Constipation

SERIOUS REACTIONS

- Debilitated patients and infants may develop impaction.

INTERACTIONS

Drugs

3 *Anticoagulants, heparin, thrombolytics:* Increases risk of bleeding

3 *Aspirin, other salicylates:* Increases the risk of salicylate toxicity

3 *Oral antidiabetics, insulin:* Large dose may increase the effects of insulin and oral antidiabetics

2 *Tetracyclines:* Decreased absorption of tetracyclines

Labs

- *Color:* Blackens or discolors stool
- *Glucose (urine):* Interferes with Benedict's reaction

SPECIAL CONSIDERATIONS

PATIENT/FAMILY EDUCATION

- Chew or dissolve in mouth; do not swallow whole
- Shake suspension before using
- Stop use if symptoms do not improve within 2 days or become worse, or if diarrhea is accompanied by high fever or severe abdominal pain
- Avoid bismuth if taking aspirin or other salicylates because of the increased risk of toxicity
- Stool may appear black or gray

MONITORING PARAMETERS

- Bowel sounds and daily bowel activity

bisoprolol fumarate

(bis-oh′-proe-lol fyoo′-muh-rate)

Rx: Zebeta

Combinations

Rx: with hydrochlorothiazide: (Ziac)

Chemical Class: β_1-adrenergic blocker, cardioselective

Therapeutic Class: Antihypertensive

CLINICAL PHARMACOLOGY

Mechanism of Action: An antihypertensive that blocks beta$_1$-adrenergic receptors in cardiac tissue. ***Therapeutic Effect:*** Slows sinus heart rate and decreases BP.

Pharmacokinetics

Well absorbed from the GI tract. Protein binding: 26%-33%. Metabolized in the liver. Primarily excreted in urine. Not removed by hemodialysis. ***Half-life:*** 9-12 hr (increased in impaired renal function).

INDICATIONS AND DOSAGES

Hypertension

PO

Adults. Initially, 2.5-5 mg/day. May increase up to 20 mg/day.

Elderly. Initially, 2.5 mg/day. May increase by 2.5-5 mg/day. Maximum: 20 mg/day.

Dosage in hepatic impairment

For adults and elderly patients with cirrhosis or hepatitis whose creatinine clearance is less than 40 ml/minute, initially give 2.5 mg.

AVAILABLE FORMS

- *Tablets:* 5 mg, 10 mg.

UNLABELED USES: Angina pectoris, premature ventricular contractions, supraventricular arrhythmias

CONTRAINDICATIONS: Cardiogenic shock, marked sinus bradycardia, overt cardiac failure, second- or third-degree heart block

PREGNANCY AND LACTATION: Pregnancy category C; similar drug, atenolol, frequently used in the third trimester for treatment of hypertension (many studies of efficacy and safety of atenolol in pregnancy-induced hypertension); long-term use has been associated with intrauterine growth retardation; excreted into breast milk; observe for signs of β-blockade

SIDE EFFECTS

Frequent

Hypotension manifested as dizziness, nausea, diaphoresis, headache, cold extremities, fatigue, constipation or diarrhea

Occasional

Insomnia, flatulence, urinary frequency, impotence or decreased libido

Rare

Rash, arthralgia, myalgia, confusion (especially in the elderly), altered taste

SERIOUS REACTIONS

- Overdose may produce profound bradycardia and hypotension.
- Abrupt withdrawal may result in diaphoresis, palpitations, headache, and tremulousness.

• Bisoprolol administration may precipitate CHF and MI in patients with heart disease, thyroid storm in those with thyrotoxicosis, and peripheral ischemia in those with existing peripheral vascular disease.
• Hypoglycemia may occur in patients with previously controlled diabetes.
• Thrombocytopenia, including unusual bruising and bleeding, occurs rarely.

INTERACTIONS

Drugs

3 *Adenosine:* Additive bradycardia
3 *α_1-adrenergic blockers:* Potential enhanced first-dose response [marked initial drop in blood pressure, particularly on standing (especially prazosin)]
3 *Amiodarone:* Increased bradycardic effect of bisoprolol
3 *Antidiabetics:* Reduced response to hypoglycemia (sweating persists)
3 *Barbiturates:* Enhanced bisoprolol metabolism
3 *Cimetidine:* Plasma levels of β-blocker may be elevated
3 *Clonidine:* Rebound hypertension; discontinue beta blocker prior to clonidine withdrawal
3 *Cocaine:* Bisoprolol potentiates cocaine-induced coronary vasoconstriction
3 *Contrast media:* Increased risk for anaphylaxis
3 *Digoxin, digitoxin:* Potentiation of bradycardia; additive prolongation of atrioventricular (AV) conduction time
3 *Dipyridamole:* Additive bradycardia
3 *Disopyramide:* Additive decreases in cardiac output
3 *Diuretics:* May increase the hypotensive effect of bisoprolol
3 *Fluoxetine:* Fluoxetine inhibits CYPD26, partially responsible for bisoprolol metabolism; increased β-blocker effects
3 *Lidocaine:* β-blocker-induced reductions in cardiac output and hepatic blood flow may yield increased lidocaine concentrations
3 *Neostigmine:* Additive bradycardia
3 *Neuroleptics:* Decreased bisoprolol metabolism; decreased neuroleptic metabolism
3 *NSAIDs:* Reduced antihypertensive effect
3 *Physostigmine:* Additive bradycardia
3 *Rifampin:* Increases clearance by 51%, reduced β-blocker effects
3 *Sympathomimetics, xanthines:* May mutually inhibit effects
3 *Tacrine:* Additive bradycardia
❷ *Theophylline:* Bisoprolol reduces clearance of theophylline; antagonistic pharmacodynamics

SPECIAL CONSIDERATIONS

• Property of competitive cardioselectivity yields less bronchospastic adverse effects

PATIENT/FAMILY EDUCATION

• Do not abruptly discontinue bisoprolol; compliance with the therapy regimen is essential to control hypertension
• If dizziness occurs, sit or lie down immediately
• Avoid tasks that require mental alertness or motor skills until response to the drug has been established
• Do not use nasal decongestants and OTC cold preparations, especially those containing stimulants, without physician approval
• Limit alcohol and salt intake

MONITORING PARAMETERS

• Heart rate, blood pressure
• Pattern of daily bowel activity and stool consistency
• Assess for peripheral edema

bitolterol mesylate

(bye-tole′-ter-ol mes′-sil-ate)

Chemical Class: Sympathomimetic amine; β_2-adrenergic agonist

Therapeutic Class: Antiasthmatic; bronchodilator

CLINICAL PHARMACOLOGY

Mechanism of Action: An antiadrenergic, sympatholytic agent that stimulates beta$_2$-adrenergic receptors in lungs. ***Therapeutic Effect:*** Relaxes bronchial smooth muscle, relieves bronchospasm, reduces airway resistance.

Pharmacokinetics

Onset of action is rapid with duration of 4-8 hrs. Rapidly absorbed following aerosol administration. Primarily distributed to lungs. Metabolized in liver. Excreted in urine and feces. ***Half-life:*** 3 hrs.

INDICATIONS AND DOSAGES

Bronchospasm

Inhalation

Adults, Elderly, Children 12 yrs and older. Use 2 inhalations, separated by 1-3-min interval. A third inhalation may be required.

Prevention of bronchospasm

Inhalation

Adults, Elderly, Children 12 yrs and older. Use 2 inhalations q8h. Do not exceed 3 inhalations q6h, or 2 inhalations q4h.

AVAILABLE FORMS

- *Aerosol for oral inhalation:* 0.8% (Tornalate).
- *Solution for oral inhalation:* 0.2% (Tornalate).

UNLABELED USES: Chronic obstructive pulmonary disease

CONTRAINDICATIONS: History of hypersensitivity to sympathomimetics, bitolterol, or any of its components.

PREGNANCY AND LACTATION: Pregnancy category C; excretion into breast milk unknown

SIDE EFFECTS

Frequent

Tremor

Occasional

Cough, dry or irritated mouth/throat, headache, nausea, vomiting

Rare

Dizziness, vertigo, palpitations, insomnia

SERIOUS REACTIONS

- Although tolerance to the bronchodilating effect has not been observed, prolonged or too-frequent use may lead to tolerance.
- Severe paradoxical bronchoconstriction may occur with excessive use.

INTERACTIONS

Drugs

3 *Aminophylline:* Increased risk of cardiotoxicity

2 *β-blockers:* Decreased action of bitolterol, cardioselective β-blockers preferable if concurrent use necessary

3 *Digoxin:* Increased risk of arrhythmias

3 *Furosemide:* Potential for additive hypokalemia

3 *MAOIs, tricyclic antidepressants, sympathomimetic agents, inhaled anesthetics:* Increased risk of toxicity

SPECIAL CONSIDERATIONS

- No real clinical advantage over less expensive agents (e.g., albuterol, metaproterenol)

PATIENT/FAMILY EDUCATION

- Wash inhaler in warm water and dry qd
- If previously effective dosage regimen fails to provide usual relief, seek medical advice immediately

• Rinse mouth with water immediately after inhalation to prevent mouth/throat dryness
• May cause nervousness, restlessness, and insomnia; if these effects persist, notify the physician

MONITORING PARAMETERS

• Rate, depth, rhythm, type of respiration, and quality and rate of pulse

bivalirudin

(bye-va-leer′-u-din)

Rx: Angiomax

Chemical Class: Hirudin derivative; thrombin inhibitor
Therapeutic Class: Anticoagulant; direct thrombin inhibitor

CLINICAL PHARMACOLOGY

Mechanism of Action: An anticoagulant that specifically and reversibly inhibits thrombin by binding to its receptor sites. ***Therapeutic Effect:*** Decreases acute ischemic complications in patients with unstable angina pectoris.

Pharmacokinetics

Route	Onset	Peak	Duration
IV	Immediate	N/A	1 hr

Primarily eliminated by kidneys. Twenty-five percent removed by hemodialysis. ***Half-life:*** 25 min (increased in moderate to severe renal impairment).

INDICATIONS AND DOSAGES

Anticoagulant in patients with unstable angina who are undergoing percutaneous transluminal coronary angioplasty (PTCA) in conjunction with aspirin

IV

Adults, Elderly. 0.75 mg/kg as IV bolus followed by IV infusion at rate of 1.75 mg/ kg/hr for duration of procedure. After initial 4-hr infusion is completed, may give additional IV infusion at rate of 0.2 mg/kg/hr for 20 hr or less, if necessary.

Dosage in renal impairment

GFR	Dosage Reduced By
30-59 ml/min	20%
10-29 ml/min	60%
Dialysis	90%

AVAILABLE FORMS

• *Injection, Powder for Reconstitution:* 250 mg.

CONTRAINDICATIONS: Active major bleeding

PREGNANCY AND LACTATION: Pregnancy category B; because of possible adverse effects on the neonate and the potential for increased maternal bleeding, particularly during the third trimester, should be used during pregnancy only if clearly needed; excretion into breast milk unknown; use caution in nursing mothers

SIDE EFFECTS

Frequent (42%)
Back pain
Occasional (15%-12%)
Nausea, headache, hypotension, generalized pain
Rare (8%-4%)
Injection site pain, insomnia, hypertension, anxiety, vomiting, pelvic or abdominal pain, bradycardia, nervousness, dyspepsia, fever, urine retention

SERIOUS REACTIONS

• A hemorrhagic event occurs rarely and is characterized by a fall in BP or Hct.

INTERACTIONS

Drugs

3 *Ginkgo biloba:* Increased risk of bleeding

3 *Heparin, thrombolytics, warfarin:* Increased risk of major bleeding

SPECIAL CONSIDERATIONS

- Safety and effectiveness have not been established in patients with unstable angina who are not undergoing PTCA or in patients with other acute coronary syndromes
- In comparative studies of PTCA in unstable angina, incidence of major bleeding lower than heparin (4% vs 9%)
- Safety and efficacy with platelet inhibitors other than aspirin (e.g., glycoprotein IIb/IIIa inhibitors) not established

PATIENT/FAMILY EDUCATION

- The female patient should be aware that her menstrual flow may be heavier than usual
- Report blood in urine or stool
- Report discomfort or pain, especially chest pain, after treatment
- Remain on bed rest and keep the leg used during PTCA immobile, as ordered

MONITORING PARAMETERS

- In clinical trials, the dose of bivalirudin was not titrated according to the activated clotting time (ACT)
- aPTT, Hct, BUN, and serum creatinine levels, and stool or urine cultures for occult blood
- Blood pressure, pulse rate
- Assess for an increase in menstrual flow
- Assess urine for hematuria

bosentan

(boe-sen′-tan)
Rx: Tracleer
Chemical Class: Pyrimidine derivative
Therapeutic Class: Endothelin receptor antagonist

CLINICAL PHARMACOLOGY

Mechanism of Action: An endothelin receptor antagonist that blocks endothelin-1, the neurohormone that constricts pulmonary arteries. ***Therapeutic Effect:*** Improves exercise ability and slows clinical worsening of pulmonary arterial hypertension (PAH).

Pharmacokinetics

Highly bound to plasma proteins, mainly albumin. Metabolized in the liver. Eliminated by biliary excretion. ***Half-life:*** Approximately 5 hr.

INDICATIONS AND DOSAGES

PAH in those with World Health Organization Class III or IV symptoms

PO

Adults, Elderly. 62.5 mg twice a day for 4 wk; then increase to maintenance dosage of 125 mg twice a day. **Alert:** When discontinuing, reduce dosage to 62.5 mg twice a day for 3-7 days to avoid clinical deterioration.

Children weighing less than 40 kg. 62.5 mg twice a day.

Dosage based on transaminase elevations

Any elevation accompanied by symptoms of liver injury or serum bilirubin 2 or more times upper limit of normal, stop treatment.

AST/ALT greater than 3 or less than 6 times upper limit of normal, reduce dose or interrupt treatment.

AST/ALT greater than 5 or less than 9 times upper limit of normal, stop treatment.

AST/ALT greater than 8 times upper limit of normal, stop treatment.

AVAILABLE FORMS

• *Tablets:* 62.5 mg, 125 mg.

UNLABELED USES: CHF, pulmonary hypertension secondary to scleroderma

CONTRAINDICATIONS: Administration with cyclosporine or glyburide, pregnancy

PREGNANCY AND LACTATION: Pregnancy category X; expected to cause fetal harm if administered to pregnant women; excretion into human breast milk unknown

SIDE EFFECTS

Occasional

Headache, nasopharyngitis, flushing

Rare

Dyspepsia (heartburn, epigastric distress), fatigue, pruritus, hypotension

SERIOUS REACTIONS

• Abnormal hepatic function, lower extremity edema, and palpitations occur rarely.

INTERACTIONS

Drugs

3 *Hormonal contraceptives:* Induction of CYP3A4 by bosentan may increase metabolism of contraceptive with possible failure

⚠ *Cyclosporine A:* Increased bosentan trough concentrations of 3-30-fold and decreased cyclosporine A levels by 50% with concomitant administration

❷ *Glyburide:* Increased risk of liver enzyme elevations

3 *Ketoconazole:* Ketoconazole is a potent CYP3A4 inhibitor; concurrent administration increases bosentan levels 2-fold

3 *Simvastatin and other statins:* Concurrent administration decreased simvastatin and metabolites by 50%

3 *Warfarin:* Concurrent administration reduces both S-warfarin (CYP2C9 substrate) and R-warfarin (CYP3A4 substrate) by 29% and 38%, respectively, but without clinical changes in INR

SPECIAL CONSIDERATIONS

• Because of potential liver injury and in an effort to decrease the risk of fetal exposure, the drug may only be prescribed through the TRACLEER Access Program by calling 1-866-228-3546

PATIENT/FAMILY EDUCATION

• The female patient should be aware of the importance of pregnancy testing and the avoidance of pregnancy while taking bosentan

MONITORING PARAMETERS

• Blood pressure, blood chemistries to include transaminases, before therapy begins and monthly thereafter monthly pregnancy test, hemoglobin levels at 1 and 3 months

• Clinical symptoms of hepatic injury, including abdominal pain, fatigue, jaundice, nausea, and vomiting

bretylium tosylate

(bre-til'-ee-um)

Rx: Bretylium Tosylate-Dextrose

Chemical Class: Bromobenzyl quaternary ammonium compound

Therapeutic Class: Antiarrhythmic, class III

CLINICAL PHARMACOLOGY

Mechanism of Action: An antiarrhythmic that directly affects myocardial cell membranes. ***Therapeutic Effect:*** Contributes to suppression of ventricular tachycardia.

Pharmacokinetics

Absorption is not expected to be present in peripheral blood at recommended doses. Protein binding: 1-6%. Not metabolized. Excreted unchanged in urine. Removed by hemodialysis. ***Half-life:*** 6-13.5 hrs.

INDICATIONS AND DOSAGES

Ventricular arrhythmias, immediate, life threatening

IV

Adults, Elderly. 5 mg/kg undiluted by rapid IV injection. May increase to 10 mg/kg, repeat as needed. Maintenance: 5-10 mg/kg diluted over 8 mins or longer, q6h or IV infusion at 1-2 mg/min.

Children. 5 mg/kg, then 10 mg/kg at 15-30-min intervals. Maximum: 30 mg/kg total dose. Maintenance: 5-10 mg/kg q6h.

Ventricular arrhythmias, other

IM

Adults, Elderly. 5-10 mg/kg undiluted, may repeat at 1-2-hr intervals. Maintenance: 5-10 mg/kg q6-8h

IV

Adults, Elderly. 5-10 mg/kg diluted over 8 mins or longer, may repeat at 1-2-hr intervals. Maintenance: 5-10 mg/kg q6h or IV infusion at 1-2 mg/min.

Children. 5-10 mg/kg/dose diluted q6h.

AVAILABLE FORMS

• *Injection:* 50 mg/ml (Bretylium Tosylate-Dextrose).

• *Premix Solutions:* 500 mg/250 ml, 1000 mg/250 ml (Bretylium Tosylate-Dextrose).

UNLABELED USES: Treatment of cervical dystonia in patients who have developed resistance to botulinum toxin type A.

CONTRAINDICATIONS: Hypersensitivity to bretylium or any component of the formulation

PREGNANCY AND LACTATION: Pregnancy category C

SIDE EFFECTS

Frequent

Transitory hypertension followed by postural and supine hypotension in 50% of pts observed as dizziness, lightheadedness, faintness, vertigo

Occasional

Diarrhea, loose stools, nausea, vomiting

Rare

Angina, bradycardia

SERIOUS REACTIONS

• Respiratory depression from possible neuromuscular blockade.

INTERACTIONS

Drugs

3 *Catecholamines:* Enhanced pressor effects

2 *Class I antiarrhythmics, Class IA antiarrhythmics, other Class III antiarrhythmics:* Increases risk of cardiotoxicity

3 *Digoxin:* Digitalis toxicity may be aggravated by the initial norepinephrine release

SPECIAL CONSIDERATIONS

PATIENT/FAMILY EDUCATION

• Rise slowly from lying to sitting position and permit legs to dangle from bed for at least 5 mins before standing 1 hr after dose administration

MONITORING PARAMETERS

• ECG, electrolytes, BP

bromocriptine mesylate

(broe-moe-krip'-teen mes'-sil-ate)

Rx: Parlodel

Chemical Class: Ergot alkaloid derivative

Therapeutic Class: Anti-Parkinson's agent; dopaminergic; ovulation stimulant

CLINICAL PHARMACOLOGY

Mechanism of Action: A dopamine agonist that directly stimulates dopamine receptors in the corpus striatum and inhibits prolactin secretion. Also suppresses secretion of growth hormone. ***Therapeutic Effect:*** Improves symptoms of parkinsonism, suppresses galactorrhea, and reduces serum growth hormone concentrations in acromegaly.

Pharmacokinetics

Indication	*Onset*	*Peak*	*Duration*
Prolactin lowering	2 hr	8 hr	24 hr
Antiparkinson	0.5-1.5 hr	2 hr	N/A
Growth hormone suppressant	1-2 hr	4-8 wk	4-8 hr

Minimally absorbed from the GI tract. Protein binding: 90%-96%. Metabolized in the liver. Excreted in feces by biliary secretion. ***Half-life:*** 15 hr.

INDICATIONS AND DOSAGES

Hyperprolactinemia

PO

Adults, Elderly. Initially, 1.25-2.5 mg at bedtime. May increase by 2.5 mg q3-7days up to 5-7.5 mg/day in divided doses. Maintenance: 2.5 mg 2-3 times a day.

Pituitary prolactinomas

PO

Adults, Elderly. Initially, 1.25 mg 2-3 times a day. May gradually increase over several weeks to 10-20 mg/day in divided doses. Maintenance: 2.5-20 mg/day in divided doses.

Parkinsonism

PO

Adults, Elderly. Initially, 1.25 mg 1-2 times a day. May take single doses at bedtime. May increase by 2.5 mg/day at 14-28-day intervals. Maintenance: 2.5-40 mg/day in divided doses. Maximum: 100 mg/day.

Acromegaly

PO

Adults, Elderly. Initially, 1.25-2.5 mg at bedtime. May increase by 1.25-2.5 mg q3-7days up to 30 mg/day in divided doses. Maintenance: 10-30 mg/day in divided doses. Maximum: 100 mg/day.

AVAILABLE FORMS

• *Capsules:* 5 mg.
• *Tablets:* 2.5 mg.

UNLABELED USES: Treatment of cocaine addiction, hyperprolactinemia associated with pituitary adenomas, neuroleptic malignant syndrome

CONTRAINDICATIONS: Hypersensitivity to ergot alkaloids, peripheral vascular disease, pregnancy, severe ischemic heart disease, uncontrolled hypertension

PREGNANCY AND LACTATION: Pregnancy category C; since it prevents lactation, should not be administered to mothers who elect to breast-feed infants

SIDE EFFECTS

Frequent

Nausea (49%), headache (19%), dizziness (17%)

Occasional (7%-3%)
Fatigue, lightheadedness, vomiting, abdominal cramps, diarrhea, constipation, nasal congestion, somnolence, dry mouth
Rare
Muscle cramps, urinary hesitancy
SERIOUS REACTIONS
• Visual or auditory hallucinations have been noted in patients with Parkinson's disease.
• Long-term, high-dose therapy may produce continuing rhinorrhea, syncope, GI hemorrhage, peptic ulcer, and severe abdominal pain.
INTERACTIONS
Drugs
3 *Erythromycin:* Marked elevations in bromocriptine levels
3 *Estrogens, progestins:* Decreases the effects of bromocriptine
▲ *Isometheptene:* Case report of hypertension and ventricular tachycardia with combination
3 *Levodopa:* Increases the effects of bromocriptine
3 *Neuroleptics:* Neuroleptic drugs probably inhibit the ability of bromocriptine to lower serum prolactin concentrations in patients with pituitary adenomas; theoretically, bromocriptine should inhibit the antipsychotic effects of neuroleptic agents, but clinical evidence suggests that this may be uncommon
▲ *Phenylpropanolamine:* Increased risk of hypertension and seizures
SPECIAL CONSIDERATIONS
• Routine use for suppression of lactation not recommended
• Use measures to prevent orthostatic hypotension
PATIENT/FAMILY EDUCATION
• Change positions slowly and to dangle the legs momentarily before standing to avoid lightheadedness
• Avoid tasks that require mental alertness or motor skills until response to the drug has been established
MONITORING PARAMETERS
• Therapeutic response

brompheniramine maleate

(brome-fen-ir'-a-meen mal'-ee-ate)
Rx: BroveX, BroveX CT, Codimal A, Colhist, Dimetane, Dimetane Extentabs, Dimetapp, Lodrane 12 Hour, Nasahist B, ND Stat
Combinations
Rx: with phenylpropanolamine, codeine (Bromanate DC, Bromphen DC with Codeine, Dimetane-DC Cough, Myphetane DC Cough, Polyhistine CS); with pseudoephedrine, dextromethorphan (Bromadine-DM, Bromarest DX, Bromatane DX, Bromfed DM, Bromphen DX, Dimetane DX, Myphetane DX)
OTC: with phenylpropanolamine (Bromaline, Bromanate, Dimaphen, Dimetane Decongestant, Dimetapp, Vicks DayQuil Allergy); with pseudoephedrine (Bromfed, Drixoral)
Chemical Class: Alkylamine derivative
Therapeutic Class: Antihistamine

CLINICAL PHARMACOLOGY
Mechanism of Action: An alklamine that competes with histamine at histaminic receptor sites. Inhibits central acetylcholine. ***Thera-***

peutic Effect: Results in anticholinergic, antipruritic, antitussive, antiemetic effects. Produces antidyskinetic, sedative effect.

Pharmacokinetics

Rapidly absorbed after PO administration. Widely distributed. Metabolized in liver. Primarily excreted in urine. ***Half-life:*** 25 hrs.

INDICATIONS AND DOSAGES

Allergic rhinitis, anaphylaxis, urticarial transfusion reactions, urticaria

PO

Adults, Elderly, Children 12 yrs and older. 4 mg q4-6h or 8-12 mg extended/timed-release q12h.

Children younger than 12 yrs. 1-2 mg q4-6h.

Amelioration of allergic reactions to blood or plasma, anaphylaxis as an adjunct to epinephrine and other standard measures after the acute symptoms have been controlled, other uncomplicated allergic conditions of the immediate type when oral therapy is impossible or contraindicated

IM/IV/SC

Adults, Elderly, Children 12 yrs and older. 5-20 mg/day in 2 divided doses. Maximum: 40 mg/day.

Children younger than 12 yrs. 0.125 mg/kg/day or 3.75 mg/m2 in 3-4 divided doses.

AVAILABLE FORMS

- *Tablets:* 4 mg (Dimetane).
- *Tablets, chewable (extended-release):* 12 mg (BroveX CT).
- *Tablets (extended-release):* 6 mg (Lodrane 12 Hour).
- *Tablets (timed-release):* 8 mg, 12 mg (Dimetane Extentabs).
- *Elixir:* 2 mg/5 ml (Dimetapp). Oral Suspension: 12 mg/5 ml (BroveX).

CONTRAINDICATIONS: Concurrent MAOI therapy, focal CNS lesions, newborn or premature infants, hypersensitivity to brompheniramine or related drugs

PREGNANCY AND LACTATION: Pregnancy category B; an association between first trimester exposure and congenital defects has been found in humans; excreted into breast milk; compatible with breastfeeding

SIDE EFFECTS

Frequent

Drowsiness, dizziness, dry mouth, nose, or throat, urinary retention, thickening of bronchial secretions

Elderly: Sedation, dizziness, hypotension

Occasional

Epigastric distress, flushing, blurred vision, tinnitus, paresthesia, sweating, chills

SERIOUS REACTIONS

- Children may experience dominant paradoxical reactions, including restlessness, insomnia, euphoria, nervousness, and tremors.
- Overdosage in children may result in hallucinations, seizures, and death.
- Hypersensitivity reaction, such as eczema, pruritus, rash, cardiac disturbances, and photosensitivity, may occur.

INTERACTIONS

Drugs

3 *Anticholinergics:* Increases anticholinergic effects

3 *MAOIs:* Increases anticholinergic and CNS depressant effects

Labs

- *Aminoacids:* Urine, increase; on thin-layer chromatography
- *Amphetamine:* Urine, increase; false positives
- *False negative:* Skin allergy tests

SPECIAL CONSIDERATIONS

PATIENT/FAMILY EDUCATION

- Do not crush or chew sustained release forms
- Use hard candy, gum, frequent rinsing of mouth for dryness
- Avoid consuming alcohol during brompheniramine therapy
- Dizziness, drowsiness, and dry mouth are expected responses to the drug
- Avoid performing tasks that require mental alertness or motor skills until response to the drug is established

MONITORING PARAMETERS

- Blood pressure, especially in the elderly

budesonide

(byoo-des'-oh-nide)

Rx: Entocort EC, Pulmicort Respules, Pulmicort Turbuhaler, Rhinocort, Rhinocort Aqua

Chemical Class: Glucocorticoid, synthetic

Therapeutic Class: Antiasthmatic; corticosteroid, antiinflammatory

CLINICAL PHARMACOLOGY

Mechanism of Action: A glucocorticoid that inhibits the accumulation of inflammatory cells and decreases and prevents tissues from responding to the inflammatory process. ***Therapeutic Effect:*** Relieves symptoms of allergic rhinitis or Crohn's disease.

Pharmacokinetics

Minimally absorbed from nasal tissue; moderately absorbed from inhalation. Protein binding: 88%. Primarily metabolized in the liver. ***Half-life:*** 2-3 hr.

INDICATIONS AND DOSAGES

Rhinitis

Intranasal (Rhinocort Aqua)

Adults, Elderly, Children 6 yr and older. 1 spray in each nostril once a day. Maximum: 8 sprays/day for adults and children 12 yr and older; 4 sprays/day for children younger than 12 yr.

Bronchial asthma

Nebulization

Children 6 mo-8 yr. 0.25-1 mg/day titrated to lowest effective dosage.

Inhalation

Adults, Elderly, Children 6 yr and older. Initially, 200-400 mcg twice a day. Maximum: Adults: 800 mcg twice a day. Children: 400 mcg twice a day.

Crohn's disease

PO

Adults, Elderly. 9 mg once a day for up to 8 wk.

AVAILABLE FORMS

- *Capsules (Entocort EC):* 3 mg.
- *Powder for Oral Inhalation (Pulmicort Turbuhaler):* 200 mcg per inhalation.
- *Suspension for Oral Inhalation (Pulmicort Respules):* 0.25 mg/2 ml; 0.5 mg/2 mg.
- *Nasal Spray (Rhinocort Aqua):* 32 mcg/spray.

UNLABELED USES: Treatment of vasomotor rhinitis

CONTRAINDICATIONS: Hypersensitivity to any corticosteroid or its components, persistently positive sputum cultures for *Candida albicans,* primary treatment of status asthmaticus, systemic fungal infections, untreated localized infection involving nasal mucosa

PREGNANCY AND LACTATION: Pregnancy category B

SIDE EFFECTS

Frequent (greater than 3%)

Nasal: Mild nasopharyngeal irritation, burning, stinging, or dryness; headache; cough

Inhalation: Flu-like symptoms, headache, pharyngitis

Occasional (3%-1%)

Nasal: Dry mouth, dyspepsia, rebound congestion, rhinorrhea, loss of taste

Inhalation: Back pain, vomiting, altered taste, voice changes, abdominal pain, nausea, dyspepsia

SERIOUS REACTIONS

• An acute hypersensitivity reaction marked by urticaria, angioedema, and severe bronchospasm, occurs rarely.

INTERACTIONS

Drugs

3 *Ketoconazole:* Increases budesonide plasma concentrations; increased systemic steroid effects are likely to occur

SPECIAL CONSIDERATIONS

• May allow discontinuation of chronic systemic corticosteroids in many patients with asthma

• 3-7 days required for maximum benefit (nasal)

PATIENT/FAMILY EDUCATION

• To be used on regular basis, not for acute symptoms

• Use bronchodilators before oral inhaler (for patients using both)

• Nasal vehicle may cause rhinitis

• Notify the physician if nasal irritation occurs or if symptoms, such as sneezing, fail to improve

MONITORING PARAMETERS

• Monitor children for growth as well as for effects on the HPA axis during chronic therapy

• Monitor patients switched from chronic systemic corticosteroids to avoid acute adrenal insufficiency in response to stress

bumetanide

(byoo-met′-a-nide)

Rx: Bumex

Chemical Class: Sulfonamide derivative

Therapeutic Class: Diuretic, loop

CLINICAL PHARMACOLOGY

Mechanism of Action: A loop diuretic that enhances excretion of sodium, chloride, and to a lesser degree, potassium, by direct action at the ascending limb of the loop of Henle and in the proximal tubule. ***Therapeutic Effect:*** Produces diuresis.

Pharmacokinetics

Route	Onset	Peak	Duration
PO	30-60 min	60-120 min	4-6 hr
IV	Rapid	15-30 min	2-3 hr
IM	40 min	60-120 min	4-6 hr

Completely absorbed from the GI tract (absorption decreased in CHF and nephrotic syndrome). Protein binding: 94%-96%. Partially metabolized in the liver. Primarily excreted in urine. Not removed by hemodialysis. ***Half-life:*** 1-1.5 hr.

INDICATIONS AND DOSAGES

Edema

PO

Adults, Children older than 18 yr. 0.5-2 mg as a single dose in the morning. May repeat at q4-5hr.

Elderly. 0.5 mg/day, increased as needed.

IV, IM

Adults, Elderly. 0.5-2 mg/dose; may repeat in 2-3 hr. Or 0.5-1 mg/hr by continuous IV infusion.

Hypertension
PO
Adults, Elderly. Initially, 0.5 mg/day. Range: 1-4 mg/day. Maximum: 5 mg/day. Larger doses may be given 2-3 doses/day.

Usual pediatric dosage
PO, IV, IM
Children. 0.015-0.1 mg/kg/dose q6-24h. Maximum: 10 mg/day.

AVAILABLE FORMS
- *Tablets:* 0.5 mg, 1 mg, 2 mg.
- *Injection:* 0.25 mg/ml.

UNLABELED USES: Treatment of hypercalcemia, hypertension

CONTRAINDICATIONS: Anuria, hepatic coma, severe electrolyte depletion

PREGNANCY AND LACTATION: Pregnancy category C (D if used in pregnancy-induced hypertension); cardiovascular disorders such as pulmonary edema, severe hypertension, or CHF are probably the only valid indications for loop diuretics during pregnancy; excretion into breast milk unknown

SIDE EFFECTS
Expected
Increased urinary frequency and urine volume
Frequent
Orthostatic hypotension, dizziness
Occasional
Blurred vision, diarrhea, headache, anorexia, premature ejaculation, impotence, dyspepsia
Rare
Rash, urticaria, pruritus, asthenia, muscle cramps, nipple tenderness

SERIOUS REACTIONS
- Vigorous diuresis may lead to profound water and electrolyte depletion, resulting in hypokalemia, hyponatremia, dehydration, coma, and circulatory collapse.
- Ototoxicity—manifested as deafness, vertigo, or tinnitus—may occur, especially in patients with severe renal impairment and those taking other ototoxic drugs.
- Blood dyscrasias and acute hypotensive episodes have been reported.

INTERACTIONS
Drugs
3 *Aminoglycosides (gentamicin, kanamycin, neomycin, streptomycin):* Additive ototoxicity (ethacrynic acid > furosemide, torsemide, bumetanide)
3 *Amphotericin B, nephrotoxic and ototoxic medications:* Increase the risk of nephrotoxicity and ototoxicity
3 *Anticoagulants, heparin:* Decreases the effects of these drugs
3 *Angiotensin converting enzyme inhibitors:* Initiation of ACEI with intensive diuretic therapy may result in precipitous fall in blood pressure; ACEIs may induce renal insufficiency in the presence of diuretic-induced sodium depletion
3 *Barbiturates (phenobarbital):* Reduced diuretic response
3 *Bile acid-binding resins (cholestyramine, colestipol):* Resins markedly reduce the bioavailability and diuretic response of furosemide
3 *Carbenoxolone:* Severe hypokalemia from co-administration
3 *Cephalosporins (cephaloridine, cephalothin):* Enhanced nephrotoxicity with co-administration
❷ *Cisplatin:* Additive ototoxicity (ethacrynic acid > furosemide, torsemide, bumetanide)
3 *Clofibrate:* Enhanced effects of both drugs, especially in hypoalbuminemic patients
3 *Corticosteroids:* Concomitant loop diuretic and corticosteroid

therapy can result in excessive potassium loss

3 *Digitalis glycosides (digoxin, digitoxin):* Diuretic-induced hypokalemia may increase risk of digitalis toxicity

3 *Lithium:* Increases the risk of lithium toxicity

3 *Nonsteroidal antiinflammatory drugs (flurbiprofen, ibuprofen, indomethacin, naproxen, piroxicam, sulindac):* Reduced diuretic and antihypertensive effects

3 *Phenytoin:* Reduced diuretic response

3 *Serotonin-reuptake inhibitors (fluoxetine, paroxetine, sertraline):* Case reports of sudden death; enhanced hyponatremia proposed; causal relationships not established

3 *Terbutaline:* Additive hypokalemia

3 *Tubocurarine:* Prolonged neuromuscular blockade

Labs

- *Cortisol:* False increases
- *Glucose:* Falsely low urine tests with Clinistix and Diastix
- *Thyroxine:* Increased serum concentration
- *T_3 uptake:* Interference causes increased serum values

SPECIAL CONSIDERATIONS

- Cross-sensitivity with furosemide rare; may substitute bumetanide at a 1:40 ratio with furosemide in patients allergic to furosemide; may show cross-hypersensitivity to sulfonamides

PATIENT/FAMILY EDUCATION

- Take early in the day
- Rise slowly from a sitting or lying position

MONITORING PARAMETERS

- *Frequent:* electrolyte, calcium, glucose, uric acid, CO_2, BUN, creatinine during first months, then periodically
- *Consider:* CBC, LFTs
- Monitor for tinnitus, hearing loss (IV doses >120 mg; concomitant ototoxic drugs, renal disease)

B

bupivacaine hydrochloride

(byoo-piv'-a-caine hye-droe-klor'-ide)

Rx: Marcaine, Marcaine Spinal, Sensorcaine, Sensorcaine-MPF

Combinations

Rx: with epinephrine (Marcaine with Epinephrine, Sensorcaine with Epinephrine, Sensorcaine-MPF with Epinephrine)

Chemical Class: Amide derivative

Therapeutic Class: Anesthetic, local

CLINICAL PHARMACOLOGY

Mechanism of Action: An amide-type anesthetic that stabilizes neuronal membranes and prevents initiation and transmission of nerve impulses thereby effecting local anesthetic actions. ***Therapeutic Effect:*** Produces local analgesia.

Pharmacokinetics

Onset of action occurs within 4-10 minutes depending on route of administration. Duration is 1.5-8.5 hrs. Well absorbed. Protein binding: 95%. Metabolized in liver. Excreted in urine. ***Half life:*** 1.5-5.5 hrs (Adults), 8.1 hrs (Neonates).

INDICATIONS AND DOSAGES: Dose varies with procedure, depth of anesthesia, vascularity of tissues, duration of anesthesia, and condition of patient.

Analgesic, epidural (partial to moderate motor blockade)
IV
Adults, Elderly. 10-20 ml (25-50 mg) of a 0.25% solution. Repeat once q3h as needed.
Children weighing more than 10 kg. 1-2.5 mg/kg single dose as a 0.125% or 0.25% solution or 0.2-0.4 mg/kg/hr continuous infusion as a 0.1%, 0.125%, or 0.25% solution. Maximum: 0.4 mg/kg/hr.
Children weighing less than 10 kg. 1-1.25 mg/kg single dose as a 0.125% or 0.25% solution or 0.1-0.2 mg/kg/hr continuous infusion as a 0.1%, 0.125%, or 0.25% solution. Maximum: 0.2 mg/kg/hr.
Analgesic, epidural (moderate to complete motor blockade)
IV
Adults, Elderly. 10-20 ml (50-100 mg) as a 0.5% solution. Repeat once q3h as needed.
Children weighing more than 10 kg. 1-2.5 mg/kg single dose as a 0.125% or 0.25% solution or 0.2-0.4 mg/kg/hr continuous infusion as a 0.1%, 0.125%, or 0.25% solution. Maximum: 0.4 mg/kg/hr.
Children weighing less than 10 kg. 1-1.25 mg/kg single dose as a 0.125% or 0.25% solution or 0.1-0.2 mg/kg/hr continuous infusion as a 0.1%, 0.125%, or 0.25% solution. Maximum: 0.2 mg/kg/hr.
Analgesic, epidural (complete motor blockade)
IV
Adults. 10-20 ml (75-150 mg) as a 0.75% solution. Repeat once q3h as needed.
Children weighing more than 10 kg. 1-2.5 mg/kg single dose as a 0.125% or 0.25% solution or 0.2-0.4 mg/kg/hr continuous infusion as a 0.1%, 0.125%, or 0.25% solution. Maximum: 0.4 mg/kg/hr.
Children weighing less than 10 kg. 1-1.25 mg/kg single dose as a 0.125% or 0.25% solution or 0.1-0.2 mg/kg/hr continuous infusion as a 0.1%, 0.125%, or 0.25% solution. Maximum: 0.2 mg/kg/hr.
Analgesic, intrapleural
IV
Adults, Elderly. 10-30-ml bolus of 0.25%, 0.375%, or 0.5% q4-8h or 0.375% solution with epinephrine continuous infusion at 6 ml/hr after 20-ml loading dose.
Analgesic, caudal (moderate to complete blockade)
IV
Adults, Elderly. 15-30 ml of 0.5% solution (75-150 mg) or 0.25% solution (37.5-75 mg), repeated once every 3 hr as needed.
Children weighing more than 10 kg. 1-2.5 mg/kg single dose as a 0.125% or 0.25% solution or 0.2-0.4 mg/kg/hr continuous infusion as a 0.1%, 0.125%, or 0.25% solution. Maximum: 0.4 mg/kg/hr.
Children weighing less than 10 kg. 1-1.25 mg/kg single dose as a 0.125% or 0.25% solution or 0.1-0.2 mg/kg/hr continuous infusion as a 0.1%, 0.125%, or 0.25% solution. Maximum: 0.2 mg/kg/hr.
Analgesic, dental
IV
Adults, Elderly. 1.8-3.6 ml of 0.5% solution (9-18 mg) with epinephrine. A second dose of 9 mg may be administered. Maximum: 90 mg total dose.
Analgesic, peripheral nerve block (moderate to complete motor blockade)
IV
Adults, Elderly. 5-37.5 ml (25-175 mg) of 0.5% solution or 5-70 ml

(12.5-175 mg) of 0.25% solution. Repeat q3h as needed. Maximum: up to 400 mg/day.
Children 12 yrs and older. 0.3-2.5 mg/kg as a 0.25% or 0.5% solution. Maximum: 1 ml/kg of 0.25% solution or 0.5 ml/kg of 0.5% solution.
Analgesic, retrobulbar (complete motor blockade)
IV
Adults, Elderly. 2-4 ml (15-30 mg) of 0.75% solution.
Analgesic, sympathetic blockade
IV
Adults, Elderly. 20-50 ml (50-125 mg) of 0.25% (no epinephrine) solution. Repeat once q3h as needed.
Analgesic, hyperbaric spinal (obstetrical, normal vaginal delivery)
IV
Adults, Elderly. 0.8 ml (6 mg) bupivacaine in dextrose as 0.75% solution.
Analgesic, hyperbaric spinal (obstetrical, cesarean section)
IV
Adults, Elderly. 1-1.4 ml (7.5-10.5 mg) bupivacaine in dextrose as 0.75% solution.
Anesthesia, hyperbaric spinal (surgical, lower extremity and perineal procedures)
IV
Adults, Elderly. 1 ml (7.5 mg) bupivacaine in dextrose as 0.75% solution.
Children 12 yrs and older. 0.3-0.6 mg/kg bupivacaine in dextrose as a 0.75% solution.
Anesthesia, spinal (surgical, lower abdominal procedures)
IV
Adults, Elderly. 1.6 ml (12 mg) bupivacaine in dextrose as 0.75% solution.
Children 12 yrs and older. 0.3-0.6 mg/kg bupivacaine in dextrose as a 0.75% solution.
Anesthesia, spinal (surgical, hyperbaric, upper abdominal procedures)
IV
Adults, Elderly. 2 ml (15 mg) bupivacaine in dextrose administered in horizontal position.
Children 12 yrs and older. 0.3-0.6 mg/kg bupivacaine in dextrose as a 0.75% solution.
Analgesic, local infiltration
IV
Adults, Elderly. 0.25% solution. Maximum: 225 mg with epinephrine or 175 mg without epinephrine.
Children 12 yrs and older. 0.5-2.5 mg/kg as a 0.25% or 0.5% solution. Maximum: 1 ml/kg of 0.25% solution or 0.5 ml/kg of 0.5% solution.

AVAILABLE FORMS

- *Injection:* 0.25% (Marcaine, Sensorcaine-MPF, 0.5% (Marcaine, Sensorcaine-MPF, 0.75% (Marcaine, Marcaine Spinal, Sensorcaine-MPF).

CONTRAINDICATIONS: Local infection at the site of proposed lumbar puncture (spinal anesthesia), obstetrical paracervical block anesthesia, septicemia (spinal anesthesia), severe hemorrhage, severe hypotension or shock, arrhythmias such as complete heart block, which severely restrict cardiac output (spinal anesthesia), sulfite allergy (epinephrine containing solutions only), hypersensitivity to bupivacaine products or to other amide-type anesthetics

PREGNANCY AND LACTATION: Pregnancy category C; excretion into breast milk unknown; regional use may prolong labor and delivery

SIDE EFFECTS

Occasional
Hypotension, bradycardia, palpitations, respiratory depression, dizzi-

ness, headache, vomiting, nausea, restlessness, weakness, blurred vision, tinnitus, apnea

SERIOUS REACTIONS

• Arterial hypotension, bradycardia, ventricular arrhythmias, central nervous system (CNS) depression and excitation, convulsions, respiratory arrest, tinnitus have been reported.

• Solutions with epinephrine contain metabisulfite, a sulfite that may cause allergic-type reactions, including anaphylaxis.

INTERACTIONS

Drugs

3 *β-blockers:* Hypertensive reactions possible, especially with local anesthetics containing epinephrine; acute discontinuation of β-blockers before local anesthesia may increase the risk of side effects due to anesthetic

3 *MAOIs, tricyclic antidepressants:* May produce prolonged hypertension

SPECIAL CONSIDERATIONS

• Amide-type local anesthetic

PATIENT/FAMILY EDUCATION

• Do not chew gum or food while mouth is numb from injection

• Notify the physician immediately if rash or hives occurs

MONITORING PARAMETERS

• Blood pressure, pulse, respiration during treatment, ECG

• Fetal heart tones if drug is used during labor

buprenorphine

(byoo-pre-nor′-feen)

Rx: Buprenex, Subutex (sublingual)

Combinations

Rx: with naloxone (Suboxone)

Chemical Class: Opiate derivative; thebaine derivative

Therapeutic Class: Narcotic agonist-antagonist analgesic

DEA Class: Schedule V

CLINICAL PHARMACOLOGY

Mechanism of Action: An opioid agonist-antagonist that binds with opioid receptors in the CNS. ***Therapeutic Effect:*** Alters the perception of and emotional response to pain; blocks the effects of heroin and produces minimal opioid withdrawal symptoms.

Pharmacokinetics

Rapidly absorbed following IM administration. Protein binding: Very high. Metabolized in liver. Primarily excreted in feces; minimal excretion in urine. ***Half-life:*** 2 hr.

INDICATIONS AND DOSAGES

Analgesia

IV, IM

Adults, Children older than 12 yr. 0.3 mg q6-8h as needed. May repeat once in 30-60 min. Range: 0.15-0.6 mg q4-8h as needed.

Children 2-12 yr. 2-6 mcg/kg q4-6h as needed.

Elderly. 0.15 mg q6h as needed.

Opioid dependence

Sublingual

Adults, Elderly, Children older than 16 yr. Initially, 12-16 mg/day, beginning at least 4 hr after last use of heroin or short-acting opioid. Maintenance: 16 mg/day. Range: 4-24 mg/day. Patients should be switched to buprenorphine and naloxone combination, which is preferred for maintenance treatment.

AVAILABLE FORMS

• *Tablets (Sublingual [Subutex]):* 2 mg, 8 mg.

• *Tablets (Sublingual [Suboxone]):* 2 mg buprenorphine/0.5 mg naloxone, 8 mg buprenorphine/2 mg naloxone.

• *Injection (Buprenex):* 0.3 mg/ml.

CONTRAINDICATIONS: Hypersensitivity to buprenorphine; hypersensitivity to naloxone for those receiving the fixed combination product containing naloxone (Suboxone)

PREGNANCY AND LACTATION: Pregnancy category C; safe use in labor and delivery has not been established; excretion into breast milk unknown

Controlled Substance: Schedule V (opioid agonist), III (tablet)

SIDE EFFECTS

Frequent

Tablet: Headache, pain, insomnia, anxiety, depression, nausea, abdominal pain, constipation, back pain, weakness, rhinitis, withdrawal syndrome, infection, diaphoresis

Injection (more than 10%): Sedation

Occasional

Injection: Hypotension, respiratory depression, dizziness, headache, vomiting, nausea, vertigo

SERIOUS REACTIONS

• Overdose results in cold and clammy skin, weakness, confusion, severe respiratory depression, cyanosis, pinpoint pupils, and extreme somnolence progressing to seizures, stupor, and coma.

INTERACTIONS

Drugs

3 *CNS depressants, MAOIs:* May increase CNS or respiratory depression and hypotension

3 *Other opioid analgesics:* May decrease the effects of other opioid analgesics

SPECIAL CONSIDERATIONS

• Effective long-acting opioid agonist-antagonist; unconfirmed reported lower physical dependence; no significant advantages

• Use of SL tabs restricted to physicians licensed to treat opioid dependence

• In opioid dependence use Subutex during induction and Suboxone for unsupervised administration

PATIENT/FAMILY EDUCATION

• Do not swallow SL tablets

• Change positions slowly to avoid dizziness

• Avoid tasks requiring mental alertness or motor skills until response to the drug has been established

MONITORING PARAMETERS

• Respiration rate

• Blood pressure, pulse rate

bupropion hydrochloride

(byoo-proe′-pee-on hye-droe-klor′-ide)

Rx: Wellbutrin, Wellbutrin SR, Zyban

Chemical Class: Aminoketone derivative

Therapeutic Class: Antidepressant

CLINICAL PHARMACOLOGY

Mechanism of Action: An aminoketone that blocks the reuptake of neurotransmitters, including serotonin and norepinephrine at CNS presynaptic membranes, increasing their availability at postsynaptic receptor sites. Also reduces the firing rate of noradrenergic neurons. ***Therapeutic Effect:*** Relieves depression and nicotine withdrawal symptoms.

Pharmacokinetics
Rapidly absorbed from the GI tract. Protein binding: 84%. Crosses the blood-brain barrier. Undergoes extensive first-pass metabolism in the liver to active metabolite. Primarily excreted in urine. ***Half-life:*** 14 hr.

INDICATIONS AND DOSAGES

Depression
PO (Immediate-Release)
Adults. Initially, 100 mg twice a day. May increase to 100 mg 3 times a day no sooner than 3 days after beginning therapy. Maximum: 450 mg/day.
Elderly. 37.5 mg twice a day. May increase by 37.5 mg q3-4 days. Maintenance: Lowest effective dosage.
PO (Sustained-Release)
Adults. Initially, 150 mg/day as a single dose in the morning. May increase to 150 mg twice a day as early as day 4 after beginning therapy. Maximum: 400 mg/day.
Elderly. Initially, 50-100 mg/day. May increase by 50-100 mg/day q3-4 days. Maintenance: Lowest effective dosage.
PO (Extended-Release)
Adults. 150 mg once a day. May increase to 300 mg once a day. Maximum: 450 mg a day.

Smoking cessation
PO
Adults. Initially, 150 mg a day for 3 days; then 150 mg twice a day for 7-12 wk.

Dosage in liver impairment
Mild-moderate: use caution, reduce dosage
Severe: use extreme caution, maximum dose:
Wellbutrin: 75 mg/day
Wellbutrin SR: 100 mg/day or 150 mg every other day
Wellbutrin XL: 150 mg every other day
Zyban: 150 mg every other day

AVAILABLE FORMS
• *Tablets (Wellbutrin):* 75 mg, 100 mg.
• *Tablets (Extended-Release [Wellbutrin XL]):* 150 mg, 300 mg.
• *Tablets (Sustained-Release [Wellbutrin SR]):* 100 mg, 150 mg, 200 mg.
• *Tablets (Sustained-Release [Zyban SR, Zyban SR Refill]):* 150 mg.

UNLABELED USES: Treatment of attention deficit hyperactivity disorder in adults and children

CONTRAINDICATIONS: Current or prior diagnosis of anorexia nervosa or bulimia, seizure disorder, use within 14 days of MAOIs, concomitant use of other bupropion products

PREGNANCY AND LACTATION: Pregnancy category B; excretion into breast milk unknown

SIDE EFFECTS
Frequent (32%-18%)
Constipation, weight gain or loss, nausea, vomiting, anorexia, dry mouth, headache, diaphoresis, tremor, sedation, insomnia, dizziness, agitation
Occasional (10%-5%)
Diarrhea, akinesia, blurred vision, tachycardia, confusion, hostility, fatigue

SERIOUS REACTIONS
• The risk of seizures increases in patients taking more than 150 mg/dose of bupropion, in patients with a history of bulimia or seizure disorders, and in patients discontinuing drugs that may lower the seizure threshold.

INTERACTIONS

Drugs
3 *Alcohol, lithium, ritonavir, steroids, trazodone, tricyclic antidepressants:* Increases the risk of seizures

3 *Fosphenytoin, phenytoin, phenobarbital:* May decrease the effectiveness of bupropion

3 *Haloperidol:* May increase plasma levels of haloperidol

3 *Levodopa:* Increases the risk of adverse effects including nausea, vomiting, excitation, restlessness, and postural tremor

⚠ *MAOIs:* Increases the risk of neuroleptic malignant syndrome and acute bupropion toxicity

SPECIAL CONSIDERATIONS

- Equal efficacy as tricyclic antidepressants; advantages include minimal anticholinergic effects, lack of orthostatic hypotension, no cardiac conduction problems, absence of weight gain, no sedation
- Fewer sexual side effects than TCAs or SSRIs
- Prescribe in equally divided doses of 3 or 4 times daily to minimize risk of seizures

PATIENT/FAMILY EDUCATION

- Ability to perform tasks requiring judgment or motor and cognitive skills may be impaired
- Therapeutic effects may take 2-4 wk
- Do not discontinue medication quickly after long-term use
- Take sips of tepid water or chew sugarless gum to relieve dry mouth

MONITORING PARAMETERS

- Assess the patient's appearance, behavior, level of interest, mood, and sleep pattern to determine the drug's therapeutic effect

buspirone hydrochloride

(byoo-spye'-rone hye-droe-klor'-ide)

Rx: BuSpar, BuSpar Dividose

Chemical Class: Azaspirodecanedione

Therapeutic Class: Anxiolytic

CLINICAL PHARMACOLOGY

Mechanism of Action: Although its exact mechanism of action is unknown, this nonbarbiturate is thought to bind to serotonin and dopamine receptors in the CNS. The drug may also increase norepinephrine metabolism in the locus ceruleus. ***Therapeutic Effect:*** Produces anxiolytic effect.

Pharmacokinetics

Rapidly and completely absorbed from the GI tract. Protein binding: 95%. Undergoes extensive first-pass metabolism. Metabolized in the liver to active metabolite. Primarily excreted in urine. Not removed by hemodialysis. ***Half-life:*** 2-3 hr.

INDICATIONS AND DOSAGES

Short-term management (up to 4 weeks) of anxiety disorders

PO

Adults. 5 mg 2-3 times a day or 7.5 mg twice a day. May increase by 5 mg/day every 2-4 days. Maintenance: 15-30 mg/day in 2-3 divided doses. Maximum: 60 mg/day.

Elderly. Initially, 5 mg twice a day. May increase by 5 mg/day every 2-3 days. Maximum: 60 mg/day.

Children. Initially, 5 mg/day. May increase by 5 mg/day at weekly intervals. Maximum: 60 mg/day.

AVAILABLE FORMS

- *Tablets:* 5 mg (BuSpar), 7.5 mg, 10 mg (BuSpar), 15 mg (BuSpar, BuSpar Dividose), 30 mg (BuSpar Dividose).

UNLABELED USES: Augmenting medication for antidepressants; management of aggression in mental retardation and secondary mental disorders, major depression, panic attack; premenstrual syndrome (aches, pain, fatigue, irritability),

CONTRAINDICATIONS: Concurrent use of MAOIs, severe hepatic or renal impairment

PREGNANCY AND LACTATION: Pregnancy category B; excretion into breast milk unknown; use caution in nursing mothers

SIDE EFFECTS

Frequent (12%-6%)

Dizziness, somnolence, nausea, headache

Occasional (5%-2%)

Nervousness, fatigue, insomnia, dry mouth, lightheadedness, mood swings, blurred vision, poor concentration, diarrhea, paraesthesia

Rare

Muscle pain and stiffness, nightmares, chest pain, involuntary movements

SERIOUS REACTIONS

- Buspirone does not appear to cause drug tolerance, psychologic or physical dependence, or withdrawal syndrome.
- Overdose may produce severe nausea, vomiting, dizziness, drowsiness, abdominal distention, and excessive pupil contraction.

INTERACTIONS

Drugs

3 *Alcohol, other CNS depressants:* Potentiates effects of buspirone and may increase sedation

3 *Erythromycin:* Increases buspirone blood concentration and risk of toxicity

3 *Fluoxetine:* Reduced therapeutic response to both drugs

▲ *MAOIs:* Elevated blood pressure, do not give concomitantly

3 *Ginkgo biloba, St. John's wort:* May cause changes in mental status

3 *Haloperidol:* Increased serum concentration of haloperidol

3 *CYP3A4 inhibitors (diltiazem, verapamil, erythromycin, itraconazole, nefazodone, ketoconazole, ritonavir, grapefruit juice):* Plasma buspirone concentration increased, adverse events likely, may need to adjust dose

3 *CYP3A4 inducers (rifampin, dexamethasone, phenytoin, phenobarbital, carbamazepine):* Plasma buspirone concentration decreased, may need to adjust dose to maintain anxiolytic effect

SPECIAL CONSIDERATIONS

- Advantages include less sedation (preferable in elderly), less effect on psychomotor and psychologic function, minimal propensity to interact with ethanol and other CNS depressants
- Will not prevent benzodiazepine withdrawal

PATIENT/FAMILY EDUCATION

- Optimal results may take 3-4 wk of treatment, some improvement may be seen after 7-10 days
- Drowsiness usually disappears with continued therapy
- Change positions slowly—from recumbent to sitting before standing —to avoid dizziness
- Avoid tasks that require mental alertness and motor skills until response to buspirone has been established

MONITORING PARAMETERS

- Hepatic and renal function

butalbital compound

(byoo-tal'-bi-tal)

Combinations

Rx: Butalbital/acetaminophen/caffeine: Amaphen, Anolor-300, Anoquan, Arcet, Butacet, Dolmar, Endolor, Esgic, Esgic-Plus, Ezol, Femcet, Fioricet, Isocet, Medigesic, Pacaps, Pharmagesic, Repan, Tencet, Triad, Two-Dyne, Zebutal

Rx: Butalbital/acetaminophen/caffeine with codeine: Ezol III, Fioricet w/codeine

Rx: Butalbital/acetaminophen: Bancap, Phrenilin, Phrenilin Forte, Sedapap-10, Triaprin

Rx: Butalbital/aspirin: Axotal

Rx: Butalbital/aspirin/caffeine: Butalgen, Fiorinal, Fiorgen, Fiormor, Fortabs, Isobutal, Isobutyl, Isolin, Isollyl, Laniroif, Lanorinal, Marnal, Tecnal, Virbutal

Rx: Butalbital/aspirin/caffeine with codeine: Ascomp with Codeine No. 3, Butalbital Compound with Codeine, Butinal with Codeine No. 3, Fiorinal with Codeine No. 3, Idenal with Codeine, Isollyl with Codeine

Chemical Class: Barbituric acid derivative

Therapeutic Class: Nonnarcotic analgesic

CLINICAL PHARMACOLOGY

Mechanism of Action: A barbiturate that depresses the central nervous system. ***Therapeutic Effect:*** Pain relief and sedation.

Pharmacokinetics

Well absorbed from the gastrointestinal (GI) tract. Widely distributed to most tissues in the body. Protein binding: varies. Excreted in the urine as unchanged drug or metabolites. ***Half-life:*** 35 hrs (butalbital).

INDICATIONS AND DOSAGES

Relief of mild to moderate pain, tension headaches

PO

Adults, Elderly. 1-2 tablets/capsules q4h. Maximum: 6 tablets/capsules daily.

AVAILABLE FORMS

Butalbital/acetaminophen

- *Capsules:* 50 mg butalbital and 325 mg acetaminophen (Bancap, Triaprin).
- *Capsules:* 50 mg butalbital and 650 mg acetaminophen (Bucet, Conten, Phrenilin Forte, Tencon).
- *Tablets:* 50 mg butalbital and 325 mg acetaminophen (Phrenilin).
- *Tablets:* 50 mg butalbital and 650 mg acetaminophen (Sedapap).

Butalbital/caffeine/acetaminophen

- *Capsules:* 50 mg butalbital, 40 mg caffeine, and 325 mg acetaminophen (Amaphen, Anolor-300, Anoquan, Butacet, Dolmar, Endolor, Esgic, Ezol, Femcet, Medigesic, Pacaps, Repan, Tencet, Triad, Two-Dyne).
- *Tablets:* 50 mg butalbital, 40 mg caffeine, and 325 mg acetaminophen (Arcet, Dolmar, Esgic, Fioricet, Isocet, Pharmagesic, Repan), 50 mg butalbital, 40 mg caffeine, and 500 mg acetaminophen (Esgic-Plus, Zebutal).

Butalbital/caffeine/acetaminophen/codeine

- *Capsules:* 50 mg butalbital, 40 mg caffeine, 325 mg acetaminophen, and 30 mg codeine phosphate (Fioricet with Codeine)

Butalbital/aspirin
• *Tablets:* 50 mg butalbital and 650 mg aspirin (Axotal).
Butalbital/caffeine/aspirin
• *Capsules:* 50 mg butalbital, 40 mg caffeine, and 325 mg aspirin (Butalgen, Fiorinal, Isobutal, Isollyl, Laniroif, Lanorinal, Marnal), 50 mg butalbital, 40 mg caffeine, and 330 mg aspirin (Fiorinal, Tecnal).
• *Tablets:* 50 mg butalbital, 40 mg caffeine, and 325 mg aspirin (Butalgen, Fiorgen, Fiorinal, Fiormor, Fortabs, Isobutal, Isobutyl, Isolin, Isollyl, Laniroif, Lanorinal, Marnal, Virbutal), 50 mg butalbital, 40 mg caffeine, and 330 mg aspirin (Fiorinal, Tecnal).
Butalbital/caffeine/aspirin/codeine
• *Capsules:* 50 mg butalbital, 40 mg caffeine, 325 mg aspirin, 30 mg codeine phosphate (Ascomp with Codeine No. 3, Butalbital Compound with Codeine, Butinal with Codeine No. 3, Fiorinal with Codeine No. 3, Idenal with Codeine, Isollyl with Codeine).

CONTRAINDICATIONS: Hypersensitivity to butalbital or any component of the formulation, porphyria

PREGNANCY AND LACTATION: Pregnancy category C (category D if used for prolonged periods or in high doses at term); excretion into breast milk unknown (see also aspirin, acetaminophen, and caffeine)

SIDE EFFECTS

Frequent
Drowsiness, excitation, confusion, excitement, mental depression, lightheadedness, dizziness, stomach upset, nausea, sleep disturbances

Rare
Rapid/irregular heartbeat, rash, itching, swelling, severe dizziness, trouble breathing, toxic epidermal necrolysis

SERIOUS REACTIONS

• Symptoms of overdose may include vomiting, unusual drowsiness, lack of feeling alert, slow or shallow breathing, cold or clammy skin, loss of consciousness, dark urine, stomach pain, and extreme fatigue.

INTERACTIONS

Drugs

3 *Alcohol, other CNS depressants:* May enhance CNS depression

2 *Oral anticoagulants:* Barbiturates inhibit the hypoprothrombinemic response to oral anticoagulants; fatal bleeding episodes have occurred when barbiturates were discontinued in patients stabilized on an anticoagulant (see also aspirin, acetaminophen, and caffeine)

SPECIAL CONSIDERATIONS

PATIENT/FAMILY EDUCATION

• May cause psychologic and/or physical dependence
• May cause drowsiness, use caution driving or operating machinery
• Avoid alcohol and other CNS depressants

MONITORING PARAMETERS

• Liver and renal function

butenafine hydrochloride

(byoo-ten′-a-feen)

Rx: Mentax

OTC: Lotrimin Ultra

Chemical Class: Benzylamine derivative

Therapeutic Class: Antifungal

CLINICAL PHARMACOLOGY

Mechanism of Action: An antifungal agent that locks biosynthesis of ergosterol, essential for fungal cell

membrane. Fungicidal. ***Therapeutic Effect:*** Relieves athlete's foot.
Pharmacokinetics
Total amount absorbed into systemic circulation has not been determined. Metabolized in liver. Excreted in urine. ***Half-life:*** 35 hrs.
INDICATIONS AND DOSAGES
Tinea pedis, tinea corporis, tinea cruris, tinea versicolor
Topical
Adults, Elderly, Children 12 yrs and older. Apply to affected area and immediate surrounding skin daily for 4 wks.
AVAILABLE FORMS
- *Cream:* 1% (Mentax).

UNLABELED USES: Onychomycosis, seborrheic dermatitis
CONTRAINDICATIONS: Hypersensitivity to butenafine or any component of the formulation
PREGNANCY AND LACTATION: Pregnancy category B
SIDE EFFECTS
Occasional (2%)
Contact dermatitis, burning/stinging, worsening of the condition
Rare (less than 2%)
Erythema, irritation, pruritus
SERIOUS REACTIONS
- None known.

SPECIAL CONSIDERATIONS
- Good cutaneous absorption, prolonged skin retention, and fungicidal activity are potential advantages. Comparative trials with other agents necessary

PATIENT/FAMILY EDUCATION
- Wash hands after applying medication
- Avoid contact with eyes, nose, and mouth
- Use the medication for the full length of treatment, even if symptoms have improved

MONITORING PARAMETERS
- Skin for evidence of contact dermatitis or erythema

butoconazole nitrate
(byoo-toe-ko′-na-zole)
Rx: Gynazole-1
OTC: Mycelex-3 2%
Chemical Class: Imidazole derivative
Therapeutic Class: Antifungal

CLINICAL PHARMACOLOGY
Mechanism of Action: An antifungal similar to imidazole derivatives that inhibits the steroid synthesis, a vital component of fungal cell formation, thereby damaging the fungal cell membrane. ***Therapeutic Effect:*** Fungistatic.
Pharmacokinetics
Not known.
INDICATIONS AND DOSAGES
Treatment of candidiasis
Topical
Adults, Elderly. Insert 1 applicatorful intravaginally at bedtime for up to 3 or 6 days.
AVAILABLE FORMS
- *Cream:* 2% (Mycelex-3, OTC)
- *Cream:* 2% (Gynazole-1, prefilled applicator)

CONTRAINDICATIONS: Hypersensitivity to butoconazole or any of its components
PREGNANCY AND LACTATION: Pregnancy category C; excretion into breast milk unknown
SIDE EFFECTS
Occasional
Vaginal itching, burning, irritation
SERIOUS REACTIONS
- Soreness, swelling, pelvic pain or cramping rarely occurs.

SPECIAL CONSIDERATIONS
PATIENT/FAMILY EDUCATION
- Do not use if abdominal pain, fever, or foul-smelling discharge is present
- Do not use tampons while using butoconazole

butorphanol tartrate

(byoo-tor'-fa-nole tar'-trate)
Rx: Stadol, Stadol NS
Chemical Class: Morphinian congener; opiate derivative
Therapeutic Class: Narcotic agonist-antagonist analgesic
DEA Class: Schedule IV

CLINICAL PHARMACOLOGY

Mechanism of Action: An opioid that binds to opiate receptor sites in the CNS. Reduces intensity of pain stimuli incoming from sensory nerve endings. ***Therapeutic Effect:*** Alters pain perception and emotional response to pain.

Pharmacokinetics

Route	Onset	Peak	Duration
IM	10-30 min	30-60 min	3-4 hr
IV	less than 1 min	30 min	2-4 hr
Nasal	15 min	1-2 hr	4-5 hr

Rapidly absorbed after IM injection. Protein binding: 80%. Extensively metabolized in the liver. Primarily excreted in urine. ***Half-life:*** 2.5-4 hr.

INDICATIONS AND DOSAGES

Analgesia

IV

Adults. 0.5-2 mg q3-4h as needed.
Elderly. 1 mg q4-6h as needed.

IM

Adults. 1-4 mg q3-4h as needed.
Elderly. 1 mg q4-6h as needed.

Migraine

Nasal

Adults. 1 mg or 1 spray in one nostril. May repeat in 60-90 min. May repeat 2-dose sequence q3-4h as needed. Alternatively, 2 mg or 1 spray each nostril if patient remains recumbent, may repeat in 3-4 hrs.

AVAILABLE FORMS

- *Injection (Stadol):* 1 mg/ml, 2 mg/ml.
- *Nasal Spray (Stadol NS):* 10 mg/ml.

CONTRAINDICATIONS: CNS disease that affects respirations, hypersensitivity to the preservative benzethonium chloride, physical dependence on other opioid analgesics, preexisting respiratory depression, pulmonary disease

PREGNANCY AND LACTATION: Pregnancy category C, D if used for prolonged time, high dose at term
Controlled Substance: Schedule IV

SIDE EFFECTS

Frequent

Parenteral: Somnolence (43%), dizziness (19%)
Nasal: Nasal congestion (13%), insomnia (11%)

Occasional

Parenteral (3%-9%): Confusion, diaphoresis, clammy skin, lethargy, headache, nausea, vomiting, dry mouth
Nasal (3%-9%): Vasodilation, constipation, unpleasant taste, dyspnea, epistaxis, nasal irritation, upper respiratory tract infection, tinnitus

Rare

Parenteral: Hypotension, pruritus, blurred vision, sensation of heat, CNS stimulation, insomnia
Nasal: Hypertension, tremor, ear pain, paresthesia, depression, sinusitis

SERIOUS REACTIONS

- Abrupt withdrawal after prolonged use may produce symptoms of narcotic withdrawal, such as abdominal cramping, rhinorrhea, lacrimation, anxiety, increased temperature, and piloerection or goose bumps.
- Overdose results in severe respiratory depression, skeletal muscle flaccidity, cyanosis, and extreme somnolence progressing to seizures, stupor, and coma.

• Tolerance to analgesic effect and physical dependence may occur with chronic use.

INTERACTIONS

Drugs

• *Nasal vasoconstrictors:* Slower onset of action of butorphanol (nasal spray)

3 *CNS depressants:* May increase CNS or respiratory depression and hypotension

3 *Buprenorphine:* Effects may be decreased with buprenorphine

3 *MAOIs:* May produce a severe, fatal reaction unless dose is reduced by one-fourth

SPECIAL CONSIDERATIONS

• Chronic use can precipitate withdrawal symptoms of anxiety, agitation, mood changes, hallucinations, dysphoria, weakness, and diarrhea

• Although not classified as a controlled substance by the FDA, prolonged use can result in habituation and drug-seeking behavior

• 2 mg = 1 spray in each nostril

PATIENT/FAMILY EDUCATION

• Change positions slowly to avoid dizziness

• Avoid tasks that require mental alertness or motor skills until response to the drug is established

• Avoid alcohol or CNS depressants during butorphanol therapy

MONITORING PARAMETERS

• Blood pressure, heart rate, respirations

cabergoline

(ca-ber'-goe-leen)

Rx: Dostinex

Chemical Class: Ergoline derivative

Therapeutic Class: Anti-Parkinson's agent; dopaminergic

CLINICAL PHARMACOLOGY

Mechanism of Action: Agonist at dopamine D2 receptors suppressing prolactin secretion. ***Therapeutic Effects:*** Shrinks prolactinomas, restores gonadal function.

Pharmacokinetics

Cabergoline is administered orally and undergoes significant first-pass metabolism following systemic absorption. Extensively metabolized in the liver. Elimination is primarily in the feces. ***Half-life:*** 80 hrs.

INDICATIONS AND DOSAGES

Hyperprolactemia (idiopathic or primary pituitary adenomas)

PO

Adults, Elderly. 0.25 mg 2 times per wk, titrate by 0.25 mg/dose no more than every 4 wks up to 1 mg 2 times per wk.

PV

Adults. 0.5 mg 2 to 5 times per wk.

Parkinson's disease

PO

Adults. 0.5 mg/day and titrate to response. Mean effective dose is 3 mg/day and ranges from 0.5-6 mg/day.

Restless leg syndrome (RLS)

PO

Adults. 0.5 mg once daily at bedtime, slowly titrate up until symptoms resolve or drug-intolerance limits further adjustment. Mean effective dose is 2 mg/day and ranges from 1-4 mg/day.

AVAILABLE FORMS
- *Tablet:* 0.5 mg

UNLABELED USES: Parkinson's disease, restless leg syndrome (RLS)

CONTRAINDICATIONS: Hypersensitivity to cabergoline, ergot alkaloids, or any one of its components; uncontrolled hypertension

PREGNANCY AND LACTATION: Pregnancy category B; unknown if excreted in breast milk

SIDE EFFECTS

Frequent

Nausea, orthostatic hypotension, confusion, dyskinesia, hallucinations, peripheral edema

Occasional

Headache, vertigo, dizziness, dyspepsia, postural hypotension, constipation, asthenia, fatigue, abdominal pain, drowsiness

Rare

Vomiting, dry mouth, diarrhea, flatulence, anxiety, depression, dysmenorrhea, dyspepsia, mastalgia, paresthesias, vertigo, visual impairment, pleuropulmonary changes, pleural effusion, pulmonary fibrosis, heart failure, peptic ulcer

SERIOUS REACTIONS
- Overdosage may produce nasal congestion, syncope, or hallucinations.

INTERACTIONS

Drugs

3 *Antihypertensives:* May increase the hypotensive effect

SPECIAL CONSIDERATIONS

- More potent with longer half-life than bromocriptine or pergolide, allowing for less frequent dosing
- Initial treatment produces dramatic response; as disease progresses, response duration decreases

PATIENT/FAMILY EDUCATION
- To reduce the hypotensive effect, rise slowly from lying to sitting position and permit legs to dangle momentarily before rising

MONITORING PARAMETERS
- Monitor prolactin levels monthly until prolactin levels equalize

caffeine

(kaf'-feen)

Rx: Caffedrine, Dexitac Stay Alert Stimulant, Enerjets, Keep Alert, NoDoz, Pep-Back, Ultra Pep-Back, Quick Pep, Vivarin

Chemical Class: Xanthine derivative

Therapeutic Class: Analeptic; central nervous system stimulant

CLINICAL PHARMACOLOGY

Mechanism of Action: A methylxanthine and competitive inhibitor of phosphodiesterase that blocks antagonism of adenosine receptors. ***Therapeutic Effect:*** Stimulates respiratory center, increases minute ventilation, decreases threshold of or increases response to hypercapnia, increases skeletal muscle tone, decreases diaphragmatic fatigue, increases metabolic rate, and increases oxygen consumption.

Pharmacokinetics

Protein binding: 36%. Widely distributed through the tissues and CSF. Metabolized in liver. Excreted in urine. ***Half-life:*** 3-7 hrs.

INDICATIONS AND DOSAGES

Drowsiness, fatigue

Adults, Elderly. 200 mg no sooner than every 3-4 hrs, as needed.

AVAILABLE FORMS

• *Tablets:* 75 mg (Enerjets), 100 mg (Pep-Back), 150 mg (Quick Pep), 200 mg (Caffedrine Caplets, Dexitac Stay Alert Stimulant, Keep Alert, NoDoz, Ultra Pep-Back Vivarin)

CONTRAINDICATIONS: Hypersensitivity to caffeine, xanthines, or any other component of the formulation

PREGNANCY AND LACTATION: Pregnancy category C; amounts in breast milk after maternal ingestion of caffeinated beverages not clinically significant; accumulation can occur in heavy-using mothers

SIDE EFFECTS

Occasional

Agitation, insomnia, nervousness, restlessness, GI irritation

SERIOUS REACTIONS

• At high doses, caffeine can cause arrhythmias, palpitations, and tachycardia.

INTERACTIONS

Drugs

3 *β-adrenergic agents:* Enhanced β-adrenergic stimulating effects

3 *Cimetidine:* Impairs caffeine metabolism resulting in excessive CNS or cardiovascular effects

3 *Clozapine:* Caffeine inhibits CYP1A2, with elevations of clozapine levels

3 *Contraceptives, oral:* Impair caffeine metabolism resulting in excessive CNS or cardiovascular effects

3 *Disulfiram:* Impairs caffeine metabolism resulting in excessive CNS or cardiovascular effects

3 *Fluroquinolone antibiotics:* Increases caffeine concentrations and may enhance its side effects

3 *Fluconazole:* Increased caffeine concentrations

3 *Ketoconazole:* Increases effects of caffeine

3 *Mexiletine:* 30%-50% reduction in caffeine clearance; potentially increased risk of CNS or cardiovascular effects

3 *Phenobarbital:* Decreases the effects of caffeine

3 *Phenylpropanolamine:* Additive effects

3 *Phenytoin:* Induced hepatic metabolism of caffeine; decreased caffeine effects

3 *Pipemidic acid:* Produces a large increase in caffeine concentrations and may increase side effects

3 *Terbinafine:* Impairs caffeine metabolism resulting in excessive CNS or cardiovascular effects

3 *Theophylline:* Caffeine reduces theophylline clearance by 30%; may affect serum theophylline levels

Labs

• *False positive elevations:* Serum uric acid levels, urine levels of VMA, catecholamines, 5-hydroxyindoleacetic acid

SPECIAL CONSIDERATIONS

PATIENT/FAMILY EDUCATION

• Gradual taper if used long-term to prevent withdrawal syndrome, especially headache

• Most authorities believe caffeine and other analeptics should not be used in overdose with CNS depressants and recommend other supportive therapy

MONITORING PARAMETERS

• Blood pressure, heart rate

calcipotriene

(kal-si-poe-try′-een)

Rx: Dovonex

Chemical Class: Vitamin D analog

Therapeutic Class: Antipsoriatic

CLINICAL PHARMACOLOGY

Mechanism of Action: A synthetic vitamin D_3 analogue that regulates skin cell (keratinocyte) production and development. ***Therapeutic Effect:*** Prevents abnormal growth and production of psoriasis (abnormal keratinocyte growth).

Pharmacokinetics

Minimal absorption through intact skin. Metabolized in liver.

INDICATIONS AND DOSAGES

Psoriasis

Topical

Adults, Elderly, Children 12 yrs and older. Apply thin layer to affected skin twice daily (morning and evening); rub in gently and completely.

Scalp psoriasis

Topical Solution

Adults, Elderly, Children 12 yrs and older. Apply to lesions after combing hair.

AVAILABLE FORMS

- *Cream:* 0.005% (Dovonex).
- *Ointment:* 0.005% (Dovonex).
- *Topical Solution:* 0.005% (Dovonex).

CONTRAINDICATIONS: Hypercalcemia or evidence of vitamin D toxicity, use on face, hypersensitivity to calcipotriene or any component of the formulation

PREGNANCY AND LACTATION: Pregnancy category C

SIDE EFFECTS

Frequent

Burning, itching, skin irritation

Occasional

Erythema, dry skin, peeling, rash, worsening of psoriasis, dermatititis

Rare

Skin atrophy, hyperpigmentation, folliculitis

SERIOUS REACTIONS

- Potential for hypercalcemia may occur.

SPECIAL CONSIDERATIONS

PATIENT/FAMILY EDUCATION

- Avoid contact with eyes
- Wash hands after application
- Report any signs of local reaction

MONITORING PARAMETERS

- Serum calcium (if elevated discontinue therapy until normal calcium levels are restored); topical administration can yield systemic effects with excessive use
- Skin for irritation

calcitonin

(kal-si-toe′-nin)

Rx: Calcimar, Cibacalcin, Fortical, Miacalcin, Miacalcin Nasal

Chemical Class: Polypeptide hormone

Therapeutic Class: Antidote, hypercalcemia; antiosteoporotic

CLINICAL PHARMACOLOGY

Mechanism of Action: A synthetic hormone that decreases osteoclast activity in bones, decreases tubular reabsorption of sodium and calcium in the kidneys, and increases absorption of calcium in the GI tract. ***Therapeutic Effect:*** Regulates serum calcium concentrations.

Pharmacokinetics

Injection form rapidly metabolized (primarily in kidneys); primarily excreted in urine. Nasal form rapidly absorbed. ***Half-life:*** 70-90 min (injection); 43 min (nasal).

INDICATIONS AND DOSAGES

Skin testing before treatment in patients with suspected sensitivity to calcitonin-salmon

Intracutaneous

Adults, Elderly. Prepare a 10-international units/ml dilution; withdraw 0.05 ml from a 200-international units/ml vial in a tuberculin syringe; fill up to 1 ml with 0.9% NaCl. Take 0.1 ml and inject intracutaneously on inner aspect of forearm. Observe after 15 min; a positive response is the appearance of more than mild erythema or wheal.

Paget's disease

IM, Subcutaneous

Adults, Elderly. Initially, 100 international units/day. Maintenance: 50 international units/day or 50-100 international units every 1-3 days.

Intranasal

Adults, Elderly. 200-400 international units/day.

Osteoporosis imperfecta

IM, Subcutaneous

Adults. 2 international units/kg 3 times a week.

Postmenopausal osteoporosis

IM, Subcutaneous

Adults, Elderly. 100 international units/day with adequate calcium and vitamin D intake.

Intranasal

Adults, Elderly. 200 international units/day as a single spray, alternating nostrils daily.

Hypercalcemia

IM, Subcutaneous

Adults, Elderly. Initially, 4 international units/kg q12h; may increase to 8 international units/kg q12h if no response in 2 days; may further increase to 8 international units/kg q6h if no response in another 2 days.

AVAILABLE FORMS

- *Injection (Miacalcin):* 200 international units/ml (calcitonin-salmon), 500 mg (calcitonin-human).
- *Nasal Spray (Fortical, Miacalcin Nasal):* 200 international units/activation (calcitonin-salmon).

UNLABELED USES: Treatment of secondary osteoporosis due to drug therapy or hormone disturbance

CONTRAINDICATIONS: Hypersensitivity to gelatin desserts or salmon protein

PREGNANCY AND LACTATION: Pregnancy category C; inhibits lactation in animals

SIDE EFFECTS

Frequent

IM, Subcutaneous (10%): Nausea (may occur 30 min after injection, usually diminishes with continued therapy), inflammation at injection site

Nasal (12%-10%): Rhinitis, nasal irritation, redness, sores

Occasional

IM, Subcutaneous (5%-2%): Flushing of face or hands

Nasal (5%-3%): Back pain, arthralgia, epistaxis, headache

Rare

IM, Subcutaneous: Epigastric discomfort, dry mouth, diarrhea, flatulence

Nasal: Itching of earlobes, pedal edema, rash, diaphoresis

SERIOUS REACTIONS

- Patients with a protein allergy may develop a hypersensitivity reaction.

SPECIAL CONSIDERATIONS

PATIENT/FAMILY EDUCATION

- Before first dose, new bottle of nasal spray pump must be activated by holding upright and pumping nozzle 6 times until a faint spray is emitted
- Nausea usually decreases with continued therapy

• Notify the physician immediately of itching, rash, shortness of breath, or significant nasal irritation

calcitriol

(kal-si-trye′-ole)

Rx: Calcijex, Rocaltrol

Chemical Class: Vitamin D analog

Therapeutic Class: Antiosteoporotic; vitamin D analog

CLINICAL PHARMACOLOGY

Mechanism of Action: A fat-soluble vitamin that is essential for absorption, utilization of calcium phosphate, and normal calcification of bone. ***Therapeutic Effect:*** Stimulates calcium and phosphate absorption from small intestine, promotes secretion of calcium from bone to blood, promotes renal tubule phosphate resorption, acts on bone cells to stimulate skeletal growth and on parathyroid gland to suppress hormone synthesis and secretion.

Pharmacokinetics

Rapidly absorbed from small intestine. Extensive metabolism in kidneys. Primarily excreted in feces; minimal excretion in urine. ***Half-life:*** 5-8 hrs.

INDICATIONS AND DOSAGES

Renal failure

PO

Adults, Elderly. 0.25 mcg/day or every other day.

Children. 0.25-2 mcg/day with hemodialysis; 0.014-0.41 mcg/kg/day without hemodialysis.

IV

Adults, Elderly. 0.5 mcg/day (0.01 mcg/kg) 3 times/week. Dose range: 0.5-3 mcg (0.01-0.05 mcg/kg) 3 times/week.

Children. 0.01-0.05 mcg/kg 3 times/week with hemodialysis.

Hypoparathyroidism/pseudohypoparathyroidism

PO

Adults, Elderly. 0.5-2 mcg/day

Children 6 yrs and older. 0.5-2 mcg once daily.

Children 5-1 yr. 0.25-0.75 mcg once daily

Children less than 1 yr. 0.04-0.08 mcg/kg once daily.

Vitamin D-dependent rickets

PO

Adults, Elderly, Children. 1 mcg once daily.

Vitamin D-resistant rickets

PO

Adults, Elderly, Children. 0.015-0.02 mcg/kg once daily. Maintenance: 0.03-0.06 mcg/kg once daily. Maximum: 2 mcg once daily.

AVAILABLE FORMS

• *Capsule:* 0.25 mcg, 0.5 mcg (Rocaltrol).
• *Injection:* 1 mcg/ml, 2 mcg/ml (Calcijex).
• *Oral Solution:* 1 mcg/ml (Rocaltrol).

CONTRAINDICATIONS: Hypercalcemia, malabsorption syndrome, vitamin D toxicity, hypersensitivity to other vitamin D products or analogs

PREGNANCY AND LACTATION: Pregnancy category A; may be excreted in breast milk

SIDE EFFECTS

Occasional

Hypercalcemia, headache, irritability, constipation, metallic taste, nausea, polyuria

SERIOUS REACTIONS

• Early signs of overdosage are manifested as weakness, headache, somnolence, nausea, vomiting, dry mouth, constipation, muscle and bone pain, and metallic taste sensation.

• Later signs of overdosage are evidenced by polyuria, polydipsia, anorexia, weight loss, nocturia, photophobia, rhinorrhea, pruritus, disorientation, hallucinations, hyperthermia, hypertension, and cardiac arrhythmias.

INTERACTIONS

Drugs

3 *Cholestyramine:* May impair intestinal absorption of calcitriol

3 *Digitalis:* May precipitate cardiac arrhythmias

3 *Ketoconazole:* May cause reductions in calcitriol concentrations

3 *Magnesium:* May cause hypermagnesemia

3 *Phenytoin:* Reduces blood levels of calcitriol

3 *Phenobarbital:* Reduces blood levels of calcitriol

3 *Phosphate-binding agents:* Since calcitriol has an effect on phosphate transport in the intestine, kidneys, and bones, the dosage of phosphate-binding agents should be adjusted in accordance with the serum phosphate concentration

3 *Thiazide diuretics:* Increased risk of hypercalcemia

3 *Verapamil:* Hypercalcemia may inhibit the activity of verapamil

3 *Vitamin D:* Causes additive effects and hypercalcemia

SPECIAL CONSIDERATIONS

PATIENT/FAMILY EDUCATION

• Adequate dietary calcium is necessary for clinical response to vitamin D therapy

• Drink plenty of liquids

MONITORING PARAMETERS

• Blood Ca^{2+} and phosphate determinations must be made every week until stable, or more frequently if necessary

• Vitamin D levels also helpful, although less frequently

• Height and weight in children

• BUN

calcium salts

(kal'-see-um)

Rx: *Calcium acetate:* PhosLo

OTC: *Calcium carbonate:* Amitone, Cal-Carb Forte, Calci-Chew, Calci-Mix, Caltrate, Caltrate 600, Chooz, Dicarbosil, Florical, Maalox, Mallamint, Mylanta, Nephro-Calci, Os-Cal 500, Oysco 500, Oyst-Cal 500, Oyster Calcium, Quick Dissolve, Rolaids, Titralac, Tums, Tums Ex

OTC: *Calcium citrate:* Citracal, Citracal Prenatal Rx, Cal-Citrate

Rx: *Calcium glubionate:* Calcione, Calciquid

OTC: *Tricalcium phosphate:* Posture

Combinations

Rx: with cholecalciferol (Os-Cal-D)

OTC: with sodium fluoride (Caltrate, Florical)

Chemical Class: Divalent cation

Therapeutic Class: Antacid; antiosteoporotic; phosphate adsorbent (acetate)

CLINICAL PHARMACOLOGY

Mechanism of Action: An electrolyte that is essential for the function and integrity of the nervous, muscular, and skeletal systems. Calcium plays an important role in normal cardiac and renal function, respiration, blood coagulation, and cell membrane and capillary permeability. It helps regulate the release and storage of neurotransmitters and hormones, and it neutralizes or reduces gastric acid (increase pH). Calcium acetate combines with dietary phosphate to form insoluble calcium phosphate. ***Therapeutic Effect:*** Replaces calcium in deficiency states; controls hyperphosphatemia in end-stage renal disease.

Pharmacokinetics

Moderately absorbed from the small intestine (absorption depends on presence of vitamin D metabolites and patient's pH). Primarily eliminated in feces.

INDICATIONS AND DOSAGES

Hyperphosphatemia

PO (calcium acetate)

Adults, Elderly. 2 tablets 3 times a day with meals. May increase gradually to bring serum phosphate level to less than 6 mg/dl as long as hypercalcemia does not develop.

Hypocalcemia

PO (calcium carbonate)

Adults, Elderly. 1-2 g/day in 3-4 divided doses.

Children. 45-65 mg/kg/day in 3-4 divided doses.

PO (calcium glubionate)

Adults, Elderly. 6-18 g/day in 4-6 divided doses.

Children, Infants. 0.6-2 g/kg/day in 4 divided doses.

Neonates. 1.2 g/kg/day in 4-6 divided doses.

IV (calcium chloride)

Adults, Elderly. 0.5-1 g repeated q4-6h as needed.

Children. 2.5-5 mg/kg/dose q4-6h.

IV (calcium gluconate)

Adults, Elderly. 2-15 g/24 hr.

Children. 200-500 mg/kg/day.

Antacid

PO (calcium carbonate)

Adults, Elderly. 1-2 tabs (5-10 ml) q2h as needed.

Osteoporosis

PO (calcium carbonate)

Adults, Elderly. 1200 mg/day.

Cardiac arrest

IV (calcium chloride)

Adults, Elderly. 2-4 mg/kg. May repeat q10min.

Children. 20 mg/kg. May repeat in 10 min.

Hypocalcemia tetany

IV (calcium chloride)

Adults, Elderly. 1 g. May repeat in 6 hr.

Children. 10 mg/kg over 5-10 min. May repeat in 6-8 hr.

IV (calcium gluconate)

Adults, Elderly. 1-3 g until therapeutic response achieved.

Children. 100-200 mg/kg/dose q6-8h.

Supplement

PO (calcium citrate)

Adults, Elderly. 0.5-2 g 2-4 times a day.

AVAILABLE FORMS

Calcium acetate

- *Gelcap (Phoslo):* 667 mg (equivalent to 169 mg elemental calcium).
- *Tablet (Phoslo):* 667 mg (equivalent to 169 mg elemental calcium).

Calcium carbonate

- *Tablets:* Equivalent to 500 mg elemental calcium (Os-Cal 500), equivalent to 600 mg elemental calcium (Caltrate 600).
- *Tablets (chewable):* Equivalent to 200 mg elemental calcium (Tums), equivalent to 500 mg elemental calcium (Os-Cal 500), 600 mg (Maalox Quick Dissolve).

Calcium chloride

- *Injection:* 10% (100 mg/ml) equivalent to 27.2 mg elemental calcium per ml.

Calcium citrate

- *Tablets:* 125 mg (Citracal Prenatal Rx), 250 mg (equivalent to 53 mg elemental calcium) (Cal-Citrate), 950 mg (equivalent to 200 mg elemental calcium) (Citracal).

Calcium glubionate

- *Syrup:* 1.8 g/5 ml (equivalent to 115 mg of elemental calcium per 5 ml).

Calcium gluconate
• *Injection:* 10% (equivalent to 9 mg elemental calcium per ml).

UNLABELED USES: Treatment of hyperphosphatemia (calcium carbonate)

CONTRAINDICATIONS: Calcium renal calculi, digoxin toxicity, hypercalcemia, hypercalciuria, sarcoidosis, ventricular fibrillation
Calcium acetate: Decreased renal function, hypoparathyroidism

PREGNANCY AND LACTATION: Pregnancy category C; some oral supplemental calcium may be excreted in breast milk (chloride, gluconate, unknown); concentrations not sufficient to produce an adverse effect in neonates

SIDE EFFECTS
Frequent
PO: Chalky taste
Parenteral: Hypotension; flushing; feeling of warmth; nausea; vomiting; pain, rash, redness, or burning at injection site; diaphoresis
Occasional
PO: Mild constipation, fecal impaction, peripheral edema, metabolic alkalosis (muscle pain, restlessness, slow breathing, altered taste)
Calcium carbonate: Milk-alkali syndrome (headache, decreased appetite, nausea, vomiting, unusual tiredness)
Rare
Difficult or painful urination

SERIOUS REACTIONS
• Hypercalcemia is a serious adverse effect of calcium acetate use. Early signs include constipation, headache, dry mouth, increased thirst, irritability, decreased appetite, metallic taste, fatigue, weakness, and depression. Later signs include confusion, somnolence, hypertension, photosensitivity, arrhythmias, nausea, vomiting, and increased painful urination.

INTERACTIONS
Drugs
3 *Calcium channel blockers:* Calcium administration (especially parenteral) may inhibit calcium channel blocker activity
3 *Digoxin, digitoxin:* Elevated calcium concentrations associated with acute digitalis toxicity
3 *Doxycycline, tetracycline:* Cotherapy with a tetracycline and a divalent or trivalent cation can reduce the serum concentration and efficacy of tetracyclines
3 *Etidronate, gallium:* May antagonize the effects of these drugs
3 *Iron:* Some calcium antacids reduce the GI absorption of iron; inhibition of the hematologic response to iron has been reported
3 *Itraconazole, ketoconazole:* Antacids containing calcium may reduce antifungal concentrations
3 *Magnesium (parenteral), methanamine:* May decrease the effects of these drugs
3 *Quinidine:* Calcium antacids capable of increasing urine pH may increase serum quinidine concentrations
3 *Quinolones:* Reduced bioavailability of quinolone antibiotics
3 *Sodium polystyrene sulfonate resin:* Combined use with calcium-containing antacid may result in systemic alkalosis
3 *Thiazides:* Large doses of calcium with thiazides may lead to milk-alkali syndrome

Labs
• *False increase:* Chloride, green color, benzodiazepine (false positive)
• *False decrease:* Magnesium, oxylate, lipase

SPECIAL CONSIDERATIONS
• Percentage elemental calcium content of various calcium salts: calcium acetate (25%), calcium car-

bonate (40%), calcium chloride (27.2%), calcium citrate (21%), calcium glubionate (6.5%), calcium gluceptate (8.2%), calcium gluconate (9.3%), calcium lactate (13%), tricalcium phosphate, (39%)

PATIENT/FAMILY EDUCATION

- Take tablets with a full glass of water, 30 mins to 1 hr after meals
- Drink liquids before meals
- Take calcium within 2 hrs of consuming other oral drugs or fiber-containing foods
- Avoid consuming excessive amounts of alcohol, caffeine, and tobacco

MONITORING PARAMETERS

- Serum calcium or serum ionized calcium concentrations (ionized calcium concentrations are preferable to determine free and bound calcium, especially with concurrent low serum albumin)
- Alternatively, ionized calcium can be estimated using the following rule: Total serum calcium will fall by 0.8 mg/dL for each 1.0 g/dL decrease in serum albumin concentration
- Blood pressure, ECG, serum magnesium, phosphate, and potassium levels

candesartan cilexetil

(kan-de-sar'-tan)

Rx: Atacand

Chemical Class: Angiotensin II receptor antagonist

Therapeutic Class: Antihypertensive

CLINICAL PHARMACOLOGY

Mechanism of Action: An angiotensin II receptor, type AT_1, antagonist that blocks the vasoconstrictor and aldosterone-secreting effects of angiotensin II, inhibiting the binding of angiotensin II to the AT_1 receptors. ***Therapeutic Effect:*** Causes vasodilation, decreases peripheral resistance, and decreases BP.

Pharmacokinetics

Route	*Onset*	*Peak*	*Duration*
PO	2-3 hr	6-8 hr	Greater than 24 hr

Rapidly, completely absorbed. Protein binding: greater than 99%. Undergoes minor hepatic metabolism to inactive metabolite. Excreted unchanged in urine and in the feces through the biliary system. Not removed by hemodialysis. ***Half-life:*** 9 hr.

INDICATIONS AND DOSAGES

Hypertension alone or in combination with other antihypertensives

PO

Adults, Elderly, Patients with mildly impaired liver or renal function. Initially, 16 mg once a day in those who are not volume depleted. Can be given once or twice a day with total daily doses of 8-32 mg. Give lower dosage in those treated with diuretics or with severely impaired renal function.

Heart failure

PO

Adults, Elderly. Initially, 4 mg once daily. May double dose at approximately 2-wk intervals up to a target dose of 32 mg/day.

AVAILABLE FORMS

- *Tablets:* 4 mg, 8 mg, 16 mg, 32 mg.

CONTRAINDICATIONS: Hypersensitivity to candesartan

PREGNANCY AND LACTATION: Pregnancy category C (first trimester) and D (second and third trimester); use caution in nursing mothers

SIDE EFFECTS

Occasional (6%-3%)

Upper respiratory tract infection, dizziness, back and leg pain

Rare (2%-1%)
Pharyngitis, rhinitis, headache, fatigue, diarrhea, nausea, dry cough, peripheral edema

SERIOUS REACTIONS

• Overdosage may manifest as hypotension and tachycardia. Bradycardia occurs less often. Institute supportive measures.

INTERACTIONS

Drugs

3 *Cimetidine:* Increased levels of candesartan

3 *Fluconazole:* Decreased conversion to active metabolite (CYP2C9 inhibition), loss of antihypertensive effects

2 *Lithium:* Increased renal lithium reabsorption at the proximal tubular site due to the natriuresis associated with the inhibition of aldosterone secretion; increased risk of lithium toxicity

3 *Potassium-sparing diuretics, salt substitutes, potassium supplements:* Increased risk of hyperkalemia

3 *Phenobarbital:* Decreased levels of candesartan

3 *Rifampin:* Induced metabolism resulting in a decrease in the area under the concentration-time curve (AUC) and half-life and reduced efficacy of candesartan

SPECIAL CONSIDERATIONS

• Potentially as or more effective than angiotensin-converting enzyme inhibitors, without cough; no evidence for reduction in morbidity and mortality as first-line agents in hypertension yet; whether they provide the same cardiac and renal protection also still tentative; like ACE inhibitors, less effective in black patients

PATIENT/FAMILY EDUCATION

• Call your clinician immediately if the following side effects are noted: wheezing; lip, throat, or face swelling; hives or rash

• Female patients should be aware of the consequences of second- and third-trimester exposure to candesartan; the female patient should immediately notify the physician if she becomes pregnant

• Avoid tasks that require mental alertness or motor skills until response to the drug has been established

• Candesartan must be taken for the rest of the patient's life to control hypertension

• Avoid exercising outside during hot weather to avoid the risks of dehydration and hypotension

MONITORING PARAMETERS

• Baseline electrolytes, urinalysis, blood urea nitrogen, and creatinine with recheck at 2-4 wk after initiation (sooner in volume-depleted patients); monitor sitting BP; watch for symptomatic hypotension, particularly in volume-depleted patients

• Maintain hydration

capreomycin sulfate

(kap-ree-oh-mye′-sin sul′-fate)

Rx: Capastat

Chemical Class: Polypeptide antibiotic

Therapeutic Class: Antituberculosis agent

CLINICAL PHARMACOLOGY

Mechanism of Action: A cyclic polypeptide antimicrobial, but the mechanism of action is not well understood. ***Therapeutic Effect:*** Suppresses mycobacterial multiplication.

Pharmacokinetics

Not well absorbed from the gastrointestinal (GI) tract. Undergoes little metabolism. Primarily excreted unchanged in urine. ***Half-life:*** 4-6 hrs (half-life is increased with impaired renal function).

INDICATIONS AND DOSAGES

Tuberculosis

IM

Adults, Elderly, Children. 15-20 mg/kg/day for 60-120 days, followed by 1 g 2-3 times/wk. Maximum: 1 g/day.

AVAILABLE FORMS

• *Injection:* 100 mg/ml (Capastat sulfate).

UNLABELED USES: Treatment of atypical mycobacterial infections

CONTRAINDICATIONS: Concurrent use of other ototoxic or nephrotoxic drugs, hypersensitivity to capreomycin

PREGNANCY AND LACTATION: Pregnancy category C; breast milk excretion is unknown; however, problems in humans have not been documented (poorly absorbed from GI tract)

SIDE EFFECTS

Frequent

Ototoxicity, nephrotoxicity

Occasional

Eosinophilia

Rare

Rash, fever, urticaria, hypokalemia, thrombocytopenia, vertigo

SERIOUS REACTIONS

• Renal failure, ototoxicity, and thrombocytopenia can occur.

INTERACTIONS

Drugs

3 *Amphotericin B, cephalosporins, cyclosporine, methoxyflurane:* Additive nephrotoxicity risk

3 *Carboplatin:* Additive ototoxicity

❷ *Ethacrynic acid:* Additive ototoxicity

❷ *Neuromuscular blocking agents:* Potentiate the respiratory suppression produced by neuromuscular blocking agents

3 *Oral anticoagulants:* Enhanced hypoprothrombinemic response

3 *Other aminoglycosides:* May increase the risk of aminoglycoside toxicity

SPECIAL CONSIDERATIONS

• When used in renal insufficiency or preexisting auditory impairment, risks of additional 8th-nerve impairment or renal injury should be weighed against the benefits of therapy

PATIENT/FAMILY EDUCATION

• Notify the physician immediately of any auditory problems

MONITORING PARAMETERS

• Electrolytes, BUN, creatinine weekly

• Blood levels of drug

• Audiometric testing before, during, after treatment

capsaicin

(cap-say'-sin)

OTC: Zostrix, Zostrix HP

Chemical Class: Alkaloid derivative of solanaceae plant family

Therapeutic Class: Topical analgesic

CLINICAL PHARMACOLOGY

Mechanism of Action: A topical analgesic that depletes and prevents reaccumulation of the chemomediator of pain impulses (substance P) from peripheral sensory neurons to CNS.

Therapeutic Effect: Relieves pain.

Pharmacokinetics

None reported.

INDICATIONS AND DOSAGES
Treatment of neuralgia, osteoarthritis, rheumatoid arthritis
Topical
Adults, Elderly, Children older than 2 yrs. Apply directly to affected area 3-4 times/day. Continue for 14-28 days for optimal clinical response.
AVAILABLE FORMS
- *Cream:* 0.025%, 0.075% (Zostrix).

UNLABELED USES: Treatment of neurogenic pain
CONTRAINDICATIONS: Hypersensitivity to capsaicin or any component of the formulation
PREGNANCY AND LACTATION: Pregnancy category C
SIDE EFFECTS
Frequent
Burning, stinging, erythema at site of application
SERIOUS REACTIONS
- None known.

SPECIAL CONSIDERATIONS
- Pretreatment with topical lidocaine 5% ointment may relieve burning

PATIENT/FAMILY EDUCATION
- Wash hands following use
- Transient burning may occur upon application and usually disappears after 72 hrs

MONITORING PARAMETERS
- Therapeutic response to the medication

captopril
(cap′-toe-pril)
Rx: Capoten
Combinations
Rx: with hydrochlorothiazide (Capozide)
Chemical Class: Angiotensin-converting enzyme (ACE) inhibitor, nonsulfhydryl
Therapeutic Class: Antihypertensive

CLINICAL PHARMACOLOGY
Mechanism of Action: An angiotensin-converting enzyme (ACE) inhibitor that suppresses the renin-angiotensin-aldosterone system and prevents conversion of angiotensin I to angiotensin II, a potent vasoconstrictor; may also inhibit angiotensin II at local vascular and renal sites. Decreases plasma angiotensin II, increases plasma renin activity, and decreases aldosterone secretion. ***Therapeutic Effect:*** Reduces peripheral arterial resistance, pulmonary capillary wedge pressure; improves cardiac output and exercise tolerance.
Pharmacokinetics

Route	*Onset*	*Peak*	*Duration*
PO	0.25 hr	0.5-1.5 hr	Dose-related

Rapidly, well absorbed from the GI tract (absorption is decreased in the presence of food). Protein binding: 25%-30%. Metabolized in the liver. Primarily excreted in urine. Removed by hemodialysis. ***Half-life:*** less than 3 hr (increased in those with impaired renal function).
INDICATIONS AND DOSAGES
Hypertension
PO
Adults, Elderly. Initially, 12.5-25 mg 2-3 times a day. After 1-2 wk, may increase to 50 mg 2-3 times a

day. Diuretic may be added if no response in additional 1-2 wk. If taken in combination with diuretic, may increase to 100-150 mg 2-3 times a day after 1-2 wk. Maintenance: 25-150 mg 2-3 times a day. Maximum: 450 mg/day.

CHF

PO

Adults, Elderly. Initially, 6.25-25 mg 3 times a day. Increase to 50 mg 3 times a day. After at least 2 wk, may increase to 50-100 mg 3 times a day. Maximum: 450 mg/day.

Post-myocardial infarction, impaired liver function

PO

Adults, Elderly. 6.25 mg a day, then 12.5 mg 3 times a day. Increase to 25 mg 3 times a day over several days up to 50 mg 3 times a day over several weeks.

Diabetic nephropathy prevention of kidney failure

PO

Adults, Elderly. 25 mg 3 times a day.

Children. Initially 0.3-0.5 mg/kg/dose titrated up to a maximum of 6 mg/kg/day in 2-4 divided doses.

Neonates. Initially, 0.05-0.1 mg/kg/dose q8-24h titrated up to 0.5 mg/kg/dose given q6-24h.

Dosage in renal impairment

Creatinine clearance 10-50 ml/min. 75% of normal dosage.

Creatinine clearance less than 10 ml/min. 50% of normal dosage.

AVAILABLE FORMS

• *Tablets:* 12.5 mg, 25 mg, 50 mg, 100 mg.

UNLABELED USES: Diagnosis of anatomic renal artery stenosis, hypertensive crisis, rheumatoid arthritis

CONTRAINDICATIONS: History of angioedema from previous treatment with ACE inhibitors

PREGNANCY AND LACTATION: Pregnancy category C (first trimester) and D (second and third trimesters—fetal and neonatal hypotension, neonatal skull hypoplasia, anuria, reversible or irreversible renal failure, death, oligohydramnios); excreted into breast milk in small amounts; compatible with breast-feeding

SIDE EFFECTS

Frequent (7%-4%)

Rash

Occasional (4%-2%)

Pruritus, dysgeusia (altered taste)

Rare (less than 2%-0.5%)

Headache, cough, insomnia, dizziness, fatigue, paresthesia, malaise, nausea, diarrhea or constipation, dry mouth, tachycardia

SERIOUS REACTIONS

• Excessive hypotension ("first-dose syncope") may occur in patients with CHF and in those who are severely salt and volume depleted.

• Angioedema (swelling of face and lips) and hyperkalemia occur rarely.

• Agranulocytosis and neutropenia may be noted in those with collagen vascular disease, including scleroderma and systemic lupus erythematosus, and impaired renal function.

• Nephrotic syndrome may be noted in those with history of renal disease.

INTERACTIONS

Drugs

3 *Alcohol:* May increase effects of captopril

❷ *Allopurinol:* Increased risk of hypersensitivity reactions including Stevens-Johnson syndrome, skin eruptions, fever, and arthralgias

3 *α-blockers:* Possible exaggerated "first-dose" response

3 *Aspirin:* Reduced hemodynamic effects of captopril; less likely at doses <236 mg qd

3 *Azathioprine:* Increased risk of myelosuppression
3 *Cyclosporine:* Increased risk of nephrotoxicity
3 *Indomethacin:* Inhibits the antihypertensive response to ACE inhibition; other NSAIDs probably have similar effect
3 *Insulin:* ACE inhibitors enhance insulin sensitivity; hypoglycemia possible
3 *Iron:* Increased risk of systemic reaction (GI symptoms, hypotension) with parenteral iron
3 *Lithium:* Increased risk of lithium toxicity
3 *Loop diuretics:* Initiation of ACE inhibition therapy with concurrent intensive diuretic therapy may cause significant hypotension, renal insufficiency
3 *Mercaptopurine:* Increased risk of neutropenia
3 *Potassium, potassium-sparing diuretics:* ACE inhibition tends to increase potassium; increased risk of hyperkalemia in predisposed patients
3 *Trimethoprim:* Additive risk of hyperkalemia, especially in patient predisposed to renal insufficiency

Labs

- ACE inhibition can account for approximately 0.5mEq/L rise in serum potassium
- *Blood in urine:* Decreased reactivity with occult blood test
- *Fructosamine:* Captopril interferes with assay increasing serum fructosamine
- *Ketones in urine:* False positive dipsticks
- *False positive:* Urine acetone

SPECIAL CONSIDERATIONS

PATIENT/FAMILY EDUCATION

- Caution with salt substitutes containing potassium chloride
- Rise slowly to sitting/standing position to minimize orthostatic hypotension
- Dizziness, fainting, lightheadedness may occur during first few days of therapy
- May cause altered taste perception or cough; persistent dry cough usually does not subside unless medication is stopped; notify clinician if these symptoms persist
- Noncompliance with drug therapy or skipping captopril doses may cause severe, rebound hypertension

MONITORING PARAMETERS

- BUN, creatinine, potassium within 2 wk after initiation of therapy (increased levels may indicate acute renal failure)
- Urinalysis for proteinuria

carbamazepine

(kar-ba-maz'-e-peen)

Rx: Atretol, Carbatrol, Epitol, Tegretol, Tegretol-XR

Chemical Class: Iminostilbene derivative

Therapeutic Class: Anticonvulsant; antimanic; antineuralgic; antipsychotic

CLINICAL PHARMACOLOGY

Mechanism of Action: An iminostilbene derivative that decreases sodium and calcium ion influx into neuronal membranes, reducing post-tetanic potentiation at synapses. ***Therapeutic Effect:*** Reduces seizure activity.

Pharmacokinetics

Slowly and completely absorbed from the GI tract. Protein binding: 75%. Metabolized in the liver to active metabolite. Primarily excreted in urine. Not removed by hemodialysis. ***Half-life:*** 25-65 hr (decreased with chronic use).

INDICATIONS AND DOSAGES

Seizure control

PO

Adults, Children older than 12 yr. Initially, 200 mg twice a day. May increase dosage by 200 mg/day at weekly intervals. Range: 400-1200 mg/day in 2-4 divided doses. Maximum: 1.6-2.4 g/day.

Children 6-12 yr. Initially, 100 mg twice a day. May increase by 100 mg/day at weekly intervals. Range: 400-800 mg/day. Maximum: 1000 mg/day.

Children younger than 6 yr. Initially, 5 mg/kg/day. May increase at weekly intervals to 10 mg/kg/day up to 20 mg/kg/day. Maximum: 35 mg/kg/day.

Elderly. Initially, 100 mg 1-2 times a day. May increase by 100 mg/day at weekly intervals. Usual dose 400-1000 mg/day.

Trigeminal neuralgia, diabetic neuropathy

PO

Adults. Initially, 100 mg twice a day. May increase by 100 mg twice a day up to 400-800 mg/day. Maximum: 1200 mg/day.

Elderly. Initially, 100 mg 1-2 times a day. May increase by 100 mg/day at weekly intervals. Usual dose 400-1000 mg/day.

Bipolar disorder

PO (Equetro)

Adults, Elderly. Initially, 400 mg/day in 2 divided doses. May adjust dose in 200-mg increments. Maximum: 1600 mg/day in divided doses.

AVAILABLE FORMS

- *Capsules (Extended-Release):* 100 mg (Carbatrol, Equetro), 200 mg (Carbatrol, Equetro), 300 mg (Carbatrol, Equetro), 400 mg (Carbatrol).
- *Suspension (Tegretol):* 100 mg/5 ml.
- *Tablets (Epitol, Tegretol):* 200 mg.
- *Tablets (Chewable [Tegretol]):* 100 mg.
- *Tablets (Extended-Release [Tegretol XR]):* 100 mg, 200 mg, 400 mg.

UNLABELED USES: Treatment of alcohol withdrawal, diabetes insipidus, neurogenic pain, psychotic disorders

CONTRAINDICATIONS: Concomitant use of MAOIs, history of myelosuppression, hypersensitivity to tricyclic antidepressants

PREGNANCY AND LACTATION: Pregnancy category D; concentration in milk approximately 60% of maternal plasma concentration; compatible with breast-feeding

SIDE EFFECTS

Frequent

Drowsiness, dizziness, nausea, vomiting

Occasional

Visual abnormalities (spots before eyes, difficulty focusing, blurred vision), dry mouth or pharynx, tongue irritation, headache, fluid retention, diaphoresis, constipation or diarrhea, behavioral changes in children

SERIOUS REACTIONS

- Toxic reactions may include blood dyscrasias (such as aplastic anemia, agranulocytosis, thrombocytopenia, leukopenia, leukocytosis, and eosinophilia), cardiovascular disturbances (such as CHF, hypotension or hypertension, thrombophlebitis and arrhythmias), and dermatologic effects (such as rash, urticaria, pruritus, and photosensitivity).
- Abrupt withdrawal may precipitate status epilepticus.

INTERACTIONS

Drugs

3 *Acetaminophen:* Enhanced hepatotoxic potential; reduced acetaminophen response

3 *Antidepressants, tricyclic:* Carbamazepine reduces serum concentrations of imipramine and probably other cyclic antidepressants
3 *Benzodiazepines (alprazolam, diazepam, midazolam, triazolam):* Metabolized by CYP3A4; enzyme induced by carbamazepine; reduced benzo effect
❷ *Calcium channel blockers:* Verapamil and diltiazem reduce the metabolism of carbamazepine leading to increased carbamazepine toxicity when these CCBs are added to chronic carbamazepine therapy; enzyme induction by carbamazepine can reduce the bioavailability of CCBs that undergo extensive first-pass hepatic clearance, like felodipine (94% reduction)
3 *Cimetidine:* Transient (1 week) increases in carbamazepine levels
3 *Corticosteroids:* Carbamazepine reduces levels and therapeutic effect
3 *Cyclosporine:* Carbamazepine reduces cyclosporine blood levels
3 *Danazol:* Carbamazepine reduces doxycycline levels and antibiotic effects
3 *Erythromycin, clarithromycin:* Increased carbamazepine levels
3 *Ethinyl estradiol, Oral contraceptives:* Carbamazepine-induced metabolic induction may lead to menstrual irregularities and unplanned pregnancies
3 *Felbamate:* Reductions in carbamazepine levels and increases in 10,11-epoxide metabolite, along with decreased felbamate concentrations
3 *Fluoxetine, fluvoxamine:* Inhibits carbamazepine metabolism, increased levels and risk of toxicity
3 *Haloperidol:* May decrease serum haloperidol concentrations and inhibit the response haloperidol
3 *Isoniazid:* Increases carbamazepine levels with increased risk of toxicity
3 *Isotretinoin:* Reduced carbamazepine bioavailability
3 *Lamotrigine:* Increased carbamazepine metabolism and risk of toxicity; carbamazepine reduces lamotrigine levels
3 *Lithium:* Increased potential for neurotoxicity with normal lithium concentrations; reverses carbamazepine-induced leukopenia; additive antithyroidal effects
3 *Mebendazole:* Carbamazepine decreases mebendazole levels, significant only when large doses given
3 *Methadone:* Carbamazepine reduces levels and therapeutic effect
3 *Metronidazole:* Increases carbamazepine concentrations with toxicity
3 *Neuroleptics:* Reduced concentration of and therapeutic response to these agents when used with carbamazepine
3 *Omeprazole:* May increase carbamazepine concentrations
3 *Oral anticoagulants:* Decreased prothrombin time
3 *Phenytoin:* Concurrent use reduces serum concentrations of both
❷ *Propoxyphene:* Increases carbamazepine levels
3 *Theophylline:* Carbamazepine reduces levels and therapeutic effect
3 *Thyroid:* Carbamazepine reduces levels and therapeutic effect
3 *Valproic acid:* Valproic acid can increase, decrease, or have no effect on carbamazepine, monitor serum levels; carbamazepine decreases levels of valproic acid

Labs

- *Chloride, serum:* Falsely elevated at elevated carbamazepine concentrations

• *Thyroxine (T_4), free serum:* Falsely elevated by certain test methods
• *Tri-iodothyronine (T_3), free serum:* Falsely decreased by certain test methods
• *T_3 uptake:* Carbamazepine interference falsely increases assay
• *Uric acid, serum:* High carbamazepine levels falsely decrease uric acid

SPECIAL CONSIDERATIONS

PATIENT/FAMILY EDUCATION

• Caution about driving and other activities that require alertness, at least initially
• Drug may turn urine pink to brown
• Do not take oral suspension of carbamazepine simultaneously with other liquid medicines
• Do not abruptly discontinue carbamazepine after long-term use because this may precipitate seizures

MONITORING PARAMETERS

• CBC—aplastic anemia and agranulocytosis have been reported 5-8× greater than in the general public
• Liver function test
• Serum drug levels (therapeutic 4-12 mcg/ml) during initial treatment

carbamide peroxide

Rx: Auro Ear Drops, Debrox, E▪R▪O Ear, GlyOxide, Mollifene Ear Wax Removing, Murine Ear Drops, Orajel Perioseptic, Proxigel
OTC: (gel, solution)
Chemical Class: Urea compound and hydrogen peroxide
Therapeutic Class: Cerumenolytic; topical oral antiinflammatory

CLINICAL PHARMACOLOGY

Mechanism of Action: A cerumenolytic that releases oxygen on contact with moist mouth tissues to provide cleansing effects, reduce inflammation, relieve pain, and inhibit odor-forming bacteria. In the ear, oxygen is released and hydrogen peroxide is reduced to water, which enables the chemical reaction. ***Therapeutic Effect:*** Relieves inflammation of gums and lips. Emulsifies and disperses ear wax.

Pharmacokinetics

Not known.

INDICATIONS AND DOSAGES

Earwax removal

Topical, solution

Adults, Elderly, Children 12 yrs or older. Tilt head and administer 5-10 drops twice a day for up to 4 days.

Children 12 yrs or younger. Tilt head and administer 1-5 drops twice a day for up to 4 days.

Oral lesions

Topical, gel

Adults, Elderly, Children. Apply to affected area 4 times a day.

Topical, solution

Adults, Elderly, Children. Apply several drops undiluted on affected area 4 times a day after meals and at bedtime.

AVAILABLE FORMS

- *Gel, oral:* 10% (Proxigel).
- *Solution, oral:* 10% (Gly-Oxide), 15% (Orajel Perioseptic).
- *Solution, otic:* 6.5% (Auro Ear Drops, Debrox, E•R•O Ear, Mollifene Ear Wax Removing, Murine Ear Drops)

UNLABELED USES: Dental whitener

CONTRAINDICATIONS: Dizziness, ear discharge or drainage, ear injury, ear pain, irritation, or rash, hypersensitivity to carbamide peroxide or any one of its components

PREGNANCY AND LACTATION: Pregnancy category C

SIDE EFFECTS

Occasional

Oral: Gingival sensitivity

SERIOUS REACTIONS

- Opportunistic infections caused by organisms like *Candida albicans* is possible with prolonged use.

SPECIAL CONSIDERATIONS

PATIENT/FAMILY EDUCATION

- The tip of the applicator should not enter the ear canal

---

carbenicillin indanyl sodium

(kar-ben-ih-sill′-in)

Rx: Geocillin

Chemical Class: Penicillin derivative, extended-spectrum

Therapeutic Class: Antibiotic

CLINICAL PHARMACOLOGY

Mechanism of Action: A penicillin that inhibits cell wall synthesis in susceptible microorganisms. ***Therapeutic Effect:*** Produces bactericidal effect.

Pharmacokinetics

Moderately absorbed from the gastrointestinal (GI) tract. Protein binding: 50%. Widely distributed. Partially metabolized in liver. Primarily excreted in urine. Removed by hemodialysis. ***Half-life:*** 1-1.5 hrs (half-life increased in impaired renal function).

INDICATIONS AND DOSAGES

Prostatitis

PO

Adults, Elderly. 764 mg q6h.

Urinary tract infection

PO

Adults, Elderly. 382-764 mg q6h.

AVAILABLE FORMS

- *Tablet:* 382 mg (Geocillin).

UNLABELED USES: Perioperative prophylaxis

CONTRAINDICATIONS: Hypersensitivity to any penicillin

PREGNANCY AND LACTATION: Pregnancy category B

SIDE EFFECTS

Frequent

GI disturbances, including mild diarrhea, nausea, or vomiting, oral or vaginal candidiasis

Occasional

Generalized rash, urticaria, phlebitis, headache

Rare

Dizziness, seizures

SERIOUS REACTIONS

- Altered bacterial balance may result in potentially fatal superinfections and antibiotic-associated colitis as evidenced by abdominal cramps, watery or severe diarrhea, and fever.
- Severe hypersensitivity reactions, including seizures, occur rarely.

INTERACTIONS

Drugs

3 *Aminoglycosides:* Chemically inactivated by carbenicillin

3 *Gentamicin:* 25% increase in serum gentamicin concentration

3 *Methotrexate:* Increased methotrexate serum concentration

3 *Probenecid:* Increased carbenicillin concentrations

Labs

• *Albumin:* Decreased serum concentrations

• *Amino acids:* Increased urine concentrations

• *Bilirubin:* Increased serum bilirubin levels

• *Glucose:* False positive using Clinitest

• *Protein:* Increased serum levels

• *Triglycerides:* Increased serum levels

SPECIAL CONSIDERATIONS

NOTE: When high and rapid blood and urine levels of antibiotic are indicated, alternative parenteral therapy should be used

PATIENT/FAMILY EDUCATION

• Take the antibiotic for the full length of treatment and evenly space doses around the clock

• Take 1 hr before or 2 hrs after consuming food or beverages

• Notify the physician if diarrhea, rash, or other new symptoms occur

MONITORING PARAMETERS

• Intake and output, renal and hepatic function

carbidopa; levodopa

(kar-bi-doe'-pa; lee-voe-doe'-pa)

Rx: Atamet, Parcopa, Sinemet, Sinemet CR

Chemical Class: Catecholamine precursor

Therapeutic Class: Anti-Parkinson's agent; antidyskinetic

CLINICAL PHARMACOLOGY

Mechanism of Action: Levodopa is converted to dopamine in the basal ganglia thus increasing dopamine concentration in brain and inhibiting hyperactive cholinergic activity. Carbidopa prevents peripheral breakdown of levodopa, allowing more levodopa to be available for transport into the brain. ***Therapeutic Effect:*** Reduces tremor.

Pharmacokinetics

Carbidopa is rapidly and completely absorbed from the GI tract. Widely distributed. Excreted primarily in urine. Levodopa is converted to dopamine. Excreted primarily in urine. ***Half-life:*** 1-2 hr (carbidopa); 1-3 hr (levodopa).

INDICATIONS AND DOSAGES

Parkinsonism

PO

Adults. Initially, 25-100 mg 2-4 times a day. May increase up 200-2000 mg daily.

Elderly. Initially, 25-100 mg twice a day. May increase as necessary.

When converting a patient from Sinemet to Sinemet CR (50 mg/200 mg), dosage is based on the total daily dose of levodopa, as follows:

Sinemet	*Sinemet CR*
300-400 mg	1 tablet twice a day
500-600 mg	1.5 tablet twice a day or 1 tab 3 times a day
700-800 mg	4 tablets in 3 or more divided doses
900-1000 mg	5 tablets in 3 or more divided doses

Intervals between doses of Sinemet CR should be 4-8 hr while awake.

AVAILABLE FORMS

• *Tablets (Atamet, Sinemet):* 10 mg carbidopa/100 mg levodopa, 25 mg carbidopa/100 mg levodopa, 25 mg carbidopa/250 mg levodopa.

• *Tablets (Oral-Disintegrating [Parcopa]):* 10 mg carbidopa/100 mg levodopa, 25 mg carbidopa/100 mg levodopa, 25 mg carbidopa/250 mg levodopa.

• *Tablets (Extended-Release [Sinemet CR]):* 25 mg carbidopa/100 mg levodopa, 50 mg carbidopa/200 mg levodopa.

CONTRAINDICATIONS: Angle-closure glaucoma, use within 14 days of MAOIs, skin lesions (Sinemet CR), history of melanoma (Sinemet CR)

PREGNANCY AND LACTATION: Pregnancy category C; should not be given to nursing mothers

SIDE EFFECTS

Frequent (90%-10%)

Uncontrolled movements of face, tongue, arms, or upper body; nausea and vomiting (80%); anorexia (50%)

Occasional

Depression, anxiety, confusion, nervousness, urine retention, palpitations, dizziness, lightheadedness, decreased appetite, blurred vision, constipation, dry mouth, flushed skin, headache, insomnia, diarrhea, unusual fatigue, darkening of urine and sweat

Rare

Hypertension, ulcer, hemolytic anemia (marked by fatigue)

SERIOUS REACTIONS

- Patients on long-term therapy have a high incidence of involuntary choreiform, dystonic, and dyskinetic movements.
- Numerous mild to severe CNS and psychiatric disturbances may occur, including reduced attention span, anxiety, nightmares, daytime somnolence, euphoria, fatigue, paranoia, psychotic episodes, depression, and hallucinations.

INTERACTIONS

Drugs

3 *Antipsychotics (haloperidol, olanzapine, phenothiazines, quetiapine, risperdone, ziprasidone):* Inhibition of the antiparkinsonian effect of levodopa through dopamine receptor antagonism

3 *Benzodiazepines:* May exacerbate parkinsonism in patients receiving levodopa; inhibits antiparkinsonian effects of levodopa

3 *Buproprion:* Increased risk of adverse effects

3 *Food:* High-protein diets inhibit the efficacy of levodopa

3 *Iron (oral):* Reduces levodopa bioavailability by 50%

3 *Isoniazid:* May inhibit the clinical response to levodopa through dopamine receptor antagonism

3 *MAOIs:* May result in hypertensive response, do not use levodopa until MAOIs have been discontinued for 2 wk

3 *Methionine:* Inhibits the clinical response to levodopa

3 *Metoclopramide:* May inhibit the clinical response to levodopa through dopamine receptor antagonism, may increase the bioavailability of levodopa through delayed gastric emptying

3 *Phenytoin:* May inhibit the antiparkinsonian effect of levodopa

3 *Pyridoxine:* Inhibits the antiparkinsonian effect of levodopa; concurrent carbidopa negates the interaction

3 *Selegiline:* Increases levodopa-induced dyskinesias, nausea, orthostatic hypotension, confusion, and hallucinations

3 *Spiramycin:* Reduces the plasma concentration of levodopa, with reduction of antiparkinsonian efficacy

3 *Tacrine:* May inhibit the effect of levodopa in Parkinson's patients; dosage adjustments may be required

3 *Tricyclic antidepressants:* Increased risk of adverse effects, hypertension, and dyskinesias

Labs

- *Acid phosphatase:* Increased serum acid phosphatase
- *Amino acids:* Increased urine amino acids

• *Aspartate aminotransferase:* Increased serum aspartate aminotransferase
• *Bilirubin:* Decreased serum bilirubin at concentrations of 15 mg/dL (Kodak Ektachem systems 2083); increased bilirubin at concentrations above 80 mg/dL (methods of Jendrassik and Grof) and below 5 mg/dL (Kodak Ektachem systems 2083)
• *Bilirubin, conjugated:* Decreased serum levels by 0.3 mg/dL at therapeutic levels of levodopa; minimally increased serum levels at markedly elevated levodopa concentrations (i.e., >60 mg/dL)
• *Catecholamines:* Increased plasma catecholamines, reported as epinephrine and norepinephrine
• *Cholinesterase:* Increased serum cholinesterase activity
• *Sputum:* Brown discoloration reported
• *Creatinine:* Increased serum creatinine
• *Creatinine clearance:* Increased urinary creatinine clearance (Jaffe method)
• *Ferric chloride test:* False positive
• *Glucose:* Decreases serum glucose as measured by GODPERID method, Ames Seralyzer, and glucose oxidase method; increased serum glucose by alkaline ferricyanide procedure, Technicon SMA method, and glucokinase method of Scott; false negative urine glucose (inhibits glucose oxidase method)
• *Guaiacols Spot test:* False negative
• *Hydroxy-methoxymandelic acid:* Increased urinary levels
• *Lithium:* Positive bias on serum lithium levels measured with Kodak Ektachem systems 2083
• *Triglycerides:* Lowered triglyceride levels measured by GPOPAP method
• *Urea nitrogen:* Decreases BUN
• *Uric acid:* Lowers serum urate levels as measured by uricase PAP method

SPECIAL CONSIDERATIONS

• If previously on levodopa, discontinue for at least 12 hr before change to carbidopa-levodopa combination

PATIENT/FAMILY EDUCATION

• Limit protein taken with drug
• Arise slowly from a reclining position
• Wearing off effect may occur at end of dosing interval
• Saliva, urine, or sweat may turn dark color (red, brown, or black)
• Delayed onset up to 1 hr with controlled release formulation possible compared to immediate release formulation
• Avoid tasks that require mental alertness or motor skills until response to the drug has been established
• Avoid alcohol
• Notify the physician if difficulty urinating, irregular heartbeats, mental changes, severe nausea or vomiting, or uncontrolled movement of the hands, arms, legs, eyelids, face, mouth, or tongue occurs

MONITORING PARAMETERS

• Relief of symptoms, such as improvement of masklike facial expression, muscular rigidity, shuffling gait, and resting tremors of the hands and head

carboprost tromethamine

(kar'-boe-prost)

Rx: Hemabate

Chemical Class: Prostaglandin F_2-alpha analog

Therapeutic Class: Abortifacient; antihemorrhagic, uterine; uterine stimulant

CLINICAL PHARMACOLOGY

Mechanism of Action: A prostaglandin similar to prostaglandin F_2 alpha (dinoprost) that directly acts on myometrium and stimulates contraction in gravid uterus. ***Therapeutic Effect:*** Produces cervical dilation and softening.

Pharmacokinetics

None reported.

INDICATIONS AND DOSAGES

Abortion

IM

Adults. Initially, 100-250 mcg, may repeat at 1.5-3.5 hour intervals. May increase up to 500 mcg if uterine contractility inadequate. Maximum: 12 mg total dose or continuous administration for more than 2 days.

Postpartum hemorrhage

IM

Adults. Initially, 250 mcg, may repeat at 15-90 minute intervals. Maximum: 2 mg total dose.

AVAILABLE FORMS

- *Injection:* 250 mcg carboprost and 83 mcg tromethamine/ml (Hemabate).

UNLABELED USES: Treatment of incomplete abortion, benign hydatiform mole, induction of labor, ripening of cervix prior to abortion

CONTRAINDICATIONS: Acute pelvic inflammatory disease, active cardiac disease, pulmonary disease, renal disease, hepatic disease, pregnancy, hypersensitivity to carboprost or other prostaglandins

PREGNANCY AND LACTATION: Pregnancy category X; any dose that produces increased uterine tone could put the embryo or fetus at risk.

SIDE EFFECTS

Frequent

Nausea

Occasional

Facial flushing

Rare

Vomiting, diarrhea

SERIOUS REACTIONS

- Excessive dosing may cause uterine hypertonicity with spasm and tetanic contraction, leading to cervical laceration/perforation and uterine rupture and hemorrhage.

INTERACTIONS

Drugs

❷ *Oxytocic agents:* May augment the activity of other oxytocic agents; concomitant use is not recommended

SPECIAL CONSIDERATIONS

- Antiemetic, analgesic, and antidiarrheal medications should be considered concurrently to counter adverse GI effects
- In the treatment of uterine atony, IV oxytocin, uterine massage, and IM methylergonovine (unless contraindicated) should be used before carboprost

PATIENT/FAMILY EDUCATION

- Avoid smoking
- Notify the physician if fever, chills, foul-smelling/increased vaginal discharge, or uterine cramps/pain occurs

MONITORING PARAMETERS

- Vital signs
- Strength, duration, frequency of contractions

carisoprodol

(kar-i-so-pro′-dol)

Rx: Soma, Vanadom

Combinations

Rx: with aspirin (Soma Compound); with aspirin and codeine (Soma Compound with Codeine)

Chemical Class: Meprobamate congener

Therapeutic Class: Skeletal muscle relaxant

CLINICAL PHARMACOLOGY

Mechanism of Action: A centrally acting skeletal muscle relaxant whose exact mechanism is unknown. Effects may be due to its CNS depressant actions. ***Therapeutic Effect:*** Relieves muscle spasms and pain.

Pharmacokinetics

Metabolized in liver to meprobamate. Excreted in urine. ***Half-life:*** 8 hr.

INDICATIONS AND DOSAGES

Adjunct to rest, physical therapy, analgesics, and other measures for relief of discomfort from acute, painful musculoskeletal conditions

PO

Adults, Elderly. 350 mg 4 times a day. Use lower initial dose and increase gradually as needed and tolerated in patients with hepatic disease.

AVAILABLE FORMS

• *Tablets (Soma, Vanadom):* 350 mg.

CONTRAINDICATIONS: Acute intermittent porphyria, sensitivity to meprobamate, mebutamate, or tybamate

PREGNANCY AND LACTATION: Pregnancy category C; crosses placenta; excreted in breast milk (2-4× maternal plasma)

SIDE EFFECTS

Frequent (greater than 10%)

Somnolence

Occasional (10%-1%)

Tachycardia, facial flushing, dizziness, headache, lightheadedness, dermatitis, nausea, vomiting, abdominal cramps, dyspnea

SERIOUS REACTIONS

• Overdose may cause CNS and respiratory depression, shock, and coma.

INTERACTIONS

Drug

3 *Alcohol, other CNS depressants:* May increase CNS depression

SPECIAL CONSIDERATIONS

• Caution when used in addiction-prone individuals

• Abused on the street in conjunction with narcotics

PATIENT/FAMILY EDUCATION

• Abrupt cessation may precipitate mild withdrawal symptoms such as abdominal cramps, insomnia, chills, headache, and nausea

• The drug may cause dizziness or drowsiness

• Avoid alcohol and other CNS depressants during carisoprodol therapy

MONITORING PARAMETERS

• Relief of muscle spasm and pain

carteolol hydrochloride

(kar-tee'-oh-lole hye-droe-klor'-ide)

Rx: Cartrol, Ocupress

Chemical Class: β-adrenergic blocker, nonselective

Therapeutic Class: Antiglaucoma agent; antihypertensive

CLINICAL PHARMACOLOGY

Mechanism of Action: An antihypertensive that blocks $beta_1$-adrenergic receptor at normal doses and $beta_2$-adrenergic receptors at large doses. Predominantly blocks $beta_1$-adrenergic receptors in cardiac tissue. Reduces aqueous humor production. ***Therapeutic Effect:*** Slows sinus heart rate, decreases cardiac output, decreases blood pressure (BP), increases airway resistance, decreases intraocular pressure.

Pharmacokinetics

Well absorbed from the gastrointestinal (GI) tract. Protein binding: unknown. Minimally metabolized in liver. Primarily excreted unchanged in urine. Not removed by hemodialysis. ***Half-life:*** 6 hrs (increased in decreased renal function).

INDICATIONS AND DOSAGES

Hypertension

PO

Adults, Elderly. Initially, 2.5 mg/day as single dose either alone or in combination with diuretic. May increase gradually to 5-10 mg/day as a single dose. Maintenance: 2.5-5 mg/day.

Dosage in renal impairment

Creatinine Clearance	*Dosage Interval*
60 ml/min	24 hrs
20-60 ml/min	48 hrs
20 ml/min	72 hrs

Open-angle glaucoma, ocular hypertension

Ophthalmic

Adults, Elderly. 1 drop 2 times/day.

AVAILABLE FORMS

- *Ophthalmic solution:* 1% (Ocupress).
- *Tablets:* 2.5 mg, 5 mg (Cartrol).

UNLABELED USES: Combination with miotics decreases IOP in acute/chronic angle closure glaucoma, treatment of secondary glaucoma, malignant glaucoma, angle closure glaucoma during/after iridectomy

CONTRAINDICATIONS: Bronchial asthma, COPD, bronchospasm, overt cardiac failure, cardiogenic shock, heart block greater than first degree, persistently severe bradycardia

PREGNANCY AND LACTATION: Pregnancy category C; excreted in breast milk

SIDE EFFECTS

Frequent

Oral: Hypotension manifested as dizziness, nausea, diaphoresis, headache, cold extremities, fatigue, constipation/diarrhea

Ophthalmic: Redness of eye or inside of eyelids, decreased night vision

Occasional

Oral: Insomnia, flatulence, urinary frequency, impotence or decreased libido

Ophthalmic:

Blepharoconjunctivitis, edema, droopy eyelid, staining of cornea, blurred vision, brow ache, increased light sensitivity, burning, stinging

Rare

Rash, arthralgia, myalgia, confusion (especially elderly), taste disturbances

SERIOUS REACTIONS

• Abrupt withdrawal (particularly in those with coronary artery disease) may produce angina or precipitate MI.

• May precipitate thyroid crisis in those with thyrotoxicosis.

• Beta-blockers may mask signs and symptoms of acute hypoglycemia (tachycardia, BP changes) in diabetic patients.

INTERACTIONS

Drugs

3 *Adenosine:* Increased risk of bradycardic response

3 *Amiodarone:* Increased bradycardic effect of carteolol

3 *Antacids:* Decreased absorption of oral carteolol

3 *Antidiabetics:* Carteolol reduces response to hypoglycemia (sweating excepted)

3 *Antipyrine:* Many β-blockers increase serum concentrations of antipyrine; though antipyrine is not used therapeutically, this interaction has implications for other drugs whose metabolism is similarly inhibited

3 *Barbiturates, rifampin:* Enhanced carteolol metabolism

3 *Bupivacaine:* Potentiates cardiodepression and heart block

3 *Cimetidine, propafenone, propoxyphene, quinidine:* Decreased carteolol metabolism

3 *Cocaine:* β-Blockade increases angina-inducing potential of cocaine

3 *Contrast media:* Increased risk of anaphylaxis

3 *Digoxin, digitoxin:* Bradycardia potentiated

3 *Dipyridamole:* Bradycardia potentiated

3 *Epinephrine:* Enhanced pressor response resulting in hypertension and bradycardia

3 *Fluoxetine:* Fluoxetine may reduce hepatic metabolism; increased β-blocking activity

3 *Isoproterenol:* Reduced effectiveness of isoproterenol in the treatment of asthma

3 *Neuroleptics:* Decreased carteolol metabolism; decreased neuroleptic metabolism

3 *Nonsteroidal antiinflammatory drugs:* Reduced antihypertensive effect of carteolol

3 *Physostigmine:* Additive bradycardia

3 *Prazosin, terazosin:* Enhanced first-dose response to α-blockers

3 *Tacrine:* Additive bradycardia

3 *Theophylline:* Decreased metabolism of theophylline

SPECIAL CONSIDERATIONS

• Does not alter serum cholesterol or triglycerides

PATIENT/FAMILY EDUCATION

• Do not stop drug abruptly; taper over 2 wk

• Do not use OTC products containing α-adrenergic stimulants (nasal decongestants, cold remedies) unless directed by physician

• Restrict salt and alcohol intake

MONITORING PARAMETERS

• Blood pressure, heart rate

• Daily bowel activity and stool consistency

• Intake and output

carvedilol

(kar'-ve-dil-ol)

Rx: Coreg

Chemical Class: α-adrenergic blocker, peripheral; β-adrenergic blocker, nonselective

Therapeutic Class: Antihypertensive

CLINICAL PHARMACOLOGY

Mechanism of Action: An antihypertensive that possesses nonselective beta-blocking and alpha-adrenergic blocking activity. Causes vasodilation. ***Therapeutic Effect:*** Reduces cardiac output, exercise-induced tachycardia, and reflex orthostatic tachycardia; reduces peripheral vascular resistance.

Pharmacokinetics

Route	Onset	Peak	Duration
PO	30 min	1-2 hr	24 hr

Rapidly and extensively absorbed from the GI tract. Protein binding: 98%. Metabolized in the liver. Excreted primarily via bile into feces. Minimally removed by hemodialysis. ***Half-life:*** 7-10 hr. Food delays rate of absorption.

INDICATIONS AND DOSAGES

Hypertension

PO

Adults, Elderly. Initially, 6.25 mg twice a day. May double at 7- to 14-day intervals to highest tolerated dosage. Maximum: 50 mg/day.

CHF

PO

Adults, Elderly. Initially, 3.125 mg twice a day. May double at 2-wk intervals to highest tolerated dosage. Maximum: For patients weighing more than 85 kg, give 50 mg twice a day; for those weighing 85 kg or less, give 25 mg twice a day.

Left ventricular dysfunction

PO

Adults, Elderly. Initially, 3.125-6.25 mg twice a day. May increase at intervals of 3-10 days up to 25 mg twice a day.

AVAILABLE FORMS

- *Tablets:* 3.125 mg, 6.25 mg, 12.5 mg, 25 mg.

UNLABELED USES: Treatment of angina pectoris, idiopathic cardiomyopathy

CONTRAINDICATIONS: Bronchial asthma or related bronchospastic conditions, cardiogenic shock, pulmonary edema, second- or third-degree AV block, severe bradycardia

PREGNANCY AND LACTATION: Pregnancy category C (D if used in the second or third trimester)

SIDE EFFECTS

Carvedilol is generally well tolerated, with mild and transient side effects.

Frequent (6%-4%)

Fatigue, dizziness

Occasional (2%)

Diarrhea, bradycardia, rhinitis, back pain

Rare (less than 2%)

Orthostatic hypotension, somnolence, UTI, viral infection

SERIOUS REACTIONS

- Overdose may produce profound bradycardia, hypotension, bronchospasm, cardiac insufficiency, cardiogenic shock, and cardiac arrest.
- Abrupt withdrawal may result in diaphoresis, palpitations, headache, and tremors.
- Carvedilol administration may precipitate CHF and MI in patients with heart disease; thyroid storm in those with thyrotoxicosis; and peripheral ischemia in those with existing peripheral vascular disease.
- Hypoglycemia may occur in patients with previously controlled diabetes.

INTERACTIONS

Drugs

3 *α_1-adrenergic blockers:* Potential enhanced first-dose response (marked initial drop in blood pressure, particularly on standing)

3 *Amiodarone:* Symptomatic bradycardia and sinus arrest; AV node refractory period prolonged and sinus node automaticity decreased, especially patients with bradycardia, sick sinus syndrome, or partial AV block

3 *Benzodiazepines:* Increased benzodiazepine activity

3 *Catecholamine-depleting agents (reserpine, MAOIs):* Hypotension or bradycardia possible

3 *Cimetidine:* Via inhibition of hepatic metabolism, cimetidine increases β-blocker serum concentrations

3 *Clonidine:* Withdrawal of clonidine abruptly may exaggerate the hypertension due to unopposed alpha stimulation; safer than other β-blockers, however

3 *Cyclosporin:* Increased trough cyclosporin concentrations

3 *CYP2D6 inhibitors (quinidine, fluoxetine, paroxetine, propafenone):* Increased levels of carvedilol

3 *Digoxin:* Additive prolongation of AV conduction time

3 *Dihydropyridine calcium channel blockers:* Severe hypotension or impaired cardiac performance; most prevalent with impaired left ventricular function, cardiac arrhythmias, or aortic stenosis

3 *Diltiazem:* Potentiates β-adrenergic effects; hypotension, left ventricular failure, and AV conduction disturbances problematic in elderly, patients with left ventricular dysfunction, aortic stenosis, or with large doses of either drug

3 *Hypoglycemic agents:* Masked hypoglycemia, hyperglycemia

3 *Nonsteroidal antiinflammatory drugs:* Reduced antihypertensive effect

3 *Rifampin:* 70% decrease in carvedilol concentrations

3 *Verapamil:* Potentiates β-adrenergic effects; hypotension, left ventricular failure, and AV conduction disturbances problematic in elderly, patients with left ventricular dysfunction, aortic stenosis, or with large doses of either drug

SPECIAL CONSIDERATIONS

- Response less in African-Americans

PATIENT/FAMILY EDUCATION

- Do not discontinue abruptly; may require taper; rapid withdrawal may produce rebound hypertension or angina
- Careful monitoring essential when initiating therapy to detect and correct worsening symptoms of heart failure
- If heart rate drops below 55 beats per minute, reduce dosage
- Take with food
- Avoid driving, hazardous tasks during initiation of therapy
- Compliance is essential to control hypertension
- Avoid tasks that require mental alertness or motor skills until response to the drug has been established
- Do not take nasal decongestants and OTC cold preparations, especially those containing stimulants, without physician approval
- Avoid alcohol and salt intake

MONITORING PARAMETERS

- *Congestive heart failure:* Functional status, cough, dyspnea on exertion, paroxysmal nocturnal dyspnea, exercise tolerance, and ventricular function
- *Hypertension:* Blood pressure

cascara sagrada

(cass-care-ah sah-graud'-ah)

OTC: Aromatic Cascara Fluid extract, Cascara Sagrada, Cascara Aromatic

Chemical Class: Anthraquinone derivative

Therapeutic Class: Laxative, stimulant

CLINICAL PHARMACOLOGY

Mechanism of Action: A GI stimulant that has a direct effect on colonic smooth musculature, by stimulating intramural nerve plexi. ***Therapeutic Effect:*** Promotes fluid and ion accumulation in the colon, increasing peristalsis and promoting a laxative effect.

Pharmacokinetics

Poorly absorbed following PO administration. Metabolized in the intestinal wall. Excreted in urine and bile. ***Half-life:*** Unknown.

INDICATIONS AND DOSAGES

Treatment of constipation

PO

Adults, Elderly. 5 ml or 1-2 tablets at bedtime.

Children 2-11 yr. 2.5 ml, 1-3 ml as a single dose.

Infants. 1.25 ml, 0.5-2 ml as a single dose.

AVAILABLE FORMS

- *Liquid:* (18% alcohol) 1 g/ml.
- *Tablets:* 150 mg, 325 mg.

CONTRAINDICATIONS: Abdominal pain, appendicitis, intestinal obstruction, nausea, vomiting

PREGNANCY AND LACTATION: Pregnancy category C; excreted in breast milk

SIDE EFFECTS

Frequent

Pink-red, red-violet, red-brown, or yellow-brown discoloration of urine

Occasional

Some degree of abdominal discomfort, nausea, mild cramps, faintness

SERIOUS REACTIONS

- Long-term use may result in laxative dependence, chronic constipation, and loss of normal bowel function.
- Prolonged use or overdose may result in electrolyte or metabolic disturbances (such as hypokalemia, hypocalcemia, and metabolic acidosis or alkalosis), as well as persistent diarrhea, vomiting, muscle weakness, malabsorption, and weight loss.

INTERACTIONS

Drugs

3 *Oral medications:* May decrease transit time of concurrently administered oral medications, decreasing the absorption of cascara sagrada

Labs

- *Increase:* Color of urine (brown-acid; yellow-pink-alkaline); porphobilinogen; urobiligen

SPECIAL CONSIDERATIONS

- Stimulant laxatives are habit forming
- Long-term use may lead to colonic atony

PATIENT/FAMILY EDUCATION

- Urine may temporarily turn pink-red, red-violet, red-brown, or yellow-brown
- Take measures to promote defecation, such as increasing fluid intake, exercising, and eating a high-fiber diet
- Do not use cascara sagrada if abdominal pain, nausea, or vomiting lasting longer than 1 week occurs
- The liquid form contains alcohol

MONITORING PARAMETERS

- Bowel activity and stool consistency
- Electrolytes

castor oil

OTC: Emulsoil, Purge
Chemical Class: Fatty acid ester
Therapeutic Class: Laxative, stimulant

CLINICAL PHARMACOLOGY
Mechanism of Action: A laxative prepared from the bean of the castor plant, but the exact mechanism of action is unknown. Acts primarily in the small intestine. May be hydrolyzed to ricinoleic acid, which reduces net absorption of fluid and electrolytes and stimulates peristalsis. ***Therapeutic Effect:*** Increases peristalsis, promotes laxative effect.
Pharmacokinetics
Minimal absorption by the gastrointestinal (GI) tract. May be metabolized like other fatty acids.

INDICATIONS AND DOSAGES
Constipation
PO
Adults, Elderly, Children 12 yrs and older. 15-60 ml as a single dose.
Children 2-12 yrs. 5-15 ml as a single dose.
Children less than 2 yrs. 1-2 ml as a single dose. Maximum: 5 ml as a single dose.

AVAILABLE FORMS
- *Emulsion:* 36.4%/ml.
- *Oral liquid:* 95% (Emulsoil, Purge).

CONTRAINDICATIONS: Abdominal pain, appendicitis, intestinal obstruction, nausea, vomiting

PREGNANCY AND LACTATION: Pregnancy category X; excreted in breast milk

SIDE EFFECTS
Occasional
Some degree of abdominal discomfort, nausea, mild cramps, griping, faintness

SERIOUS REACTIONS
- Long-term use may result in laxative dependence, chronic constipation, and loss of normal bowel function.
- Chronic use or overdosage may result in electrolyte disturbances, such as hypokalemia, hypocalcemia, and metabolic acidosis or alkalosis, persistent diarrhea, malabsorption, and weight loss. Electrolyte disturbance may produce vomiting and muscle weakness.

SPECIAL CONSIDERATIONS
- Stimulant laxatives are habit forming
- Long-term use may lead to colonic atony

PATIENT/FAMILY EDUCATION
- Increasing fluid intake, exercising, and eating a high-fiber diet will promote defecation
- Do not take oral medications within 1 hr of taking castor oil

MONITORING PARAMETERS
- Daily bowel activity and stool consistency
- Electrolytes

cefaclor

(sef'-ah-klor)
Rx: Ceclor, Ceclor CD, Ceclor Pulvules
Chemical Class: Cephalosporin (2nd generation)
Therapeutic Class: Antibiotic

CLINICAL PHARMACOLOGY
Mechanism of Action: A second-generation cephalosporin that binds to bacterial cell membranes and inhibits cell wall synthesis. ***Therapeutic Effect:*** Bactericidal.
Pharmacokinetics
Well absorbed from the GI tract. Protein binding: 25%. Widely distributed. Primarily excreted un-

changed in urine. Moderately removed by hemodialysis. ***Half-life:*** 0.6-0.9 hr (increased in impaired renal function).

INDICATIONS AND DOSAGES

Bronchitis

PO (Extended-Release)

Adults, Elderly. 500 mg q12h for 7 days.

Lower respiratory tract infections

PO

Adults, Elderly. 250-500 mg q8h.

Otitis media

PO

Children. 20-40 mg/kg/day in 2-3 divided doses. Maximum: 1 g/day.

Pharyngitis, skin/skin structure infections, tonsillitis

PO (Extended-Release)

Adults, Elderly. 375 mg q12h.

PO (Regular-Release)

Adults, Elderly. 250-500 mg q8h.

Children. 20-40 mg/kg/day in 2-3 divided doses. Maximum: 1 g/day.

Urinary tract infections

PO

Adults, Elderly. 250-500 mg q8h.

Children. 20-40 mg/kg/day in 2-3 divided doses q8h. Maximum: 1 g/day

PO (Extended-Release)

Adults, Children older than 16 yr. 375-500 mg q12h.

Otitis media

PO

Children older than 1 mo. 40 mg/kg/day in divided doses q8h. Maximum: 1 g/day.

Dosage in renal impairment

Decreased dosage may be necessary in patients with creatinine clearance less than 40 ml/min.

AVAILABLE FORMS

• *Capsules (Ceclor Pulvules):* 250 mg, 500 mg.

• *Oral Suspension (Ceclor):* 125 mg/5 ml, 187 mg/5 ml, 250 mg/5 ml, 375 mg/5 ml.

• *Tablets (Extended-Release [Ceclor CD]):* 375 mg, 500 mg.

• *Tablets (Chewable [Raniclor]):* 125 mg, 187 mg, 250 mg, 375 mg.

CONTRAINDICATIONS: History of anaphylactic reaction to penicillins or hypersensitivity to cephalosporins

PREGNANCY AND LACTATION: Pregnancy category B; excreted in breast milk

SIDE EFFECTS

Frequent

Oral candidiasis, mild diarrhea, mild abdominal cramping, vaginal candidiasis

Occasional

Nausea, serum sickness–like reaction (marked by fever and joint pain; usually occurs after the second course of therapy and resolves after the drug is discontinued)

Rare

Allergic reaction (pruritus, rash, and urticaria)

SERIOUS REACTIONS

• Antibiotic-associated colitis and other superinfections may result from altered bacterial balance.

• Nephrotoxicity may occur, especially in patients with preexisting renal disease.

• Patients with a history of allergies, especially to penicillin, are at increased risk for developing a severe hypersensitivity reaction, marked by severe pruritus, angioedema, bronchospasm, and anaphylaxis.

INTERACTIONS

Drugs

3 *Aminoglycosides:* Additive nephrotoxicity

3 *Loop diuretics:* Increased nephrotoxicity

❷ *Warfarin:* Hypoprothrombinemic response enhanced

Labs

• *Creatinine:* Analytical increases and decreases depending on assay

SPECIAL CONSIDERATIONS

- Last-choice second generation cephalosporin given relative decreased activity against *S. pneumonia* and increased side effects

PATIENT/FAMILY EDUCATION

- Administer at even intervals
- Administer with food or milk if the drug causes GI upset
- Refrigerate oral suspension

MONITORING PARAMETERS

- Intake and output
- Renal function
- Daily bowel activity
- Signs and symptoms of superinfection

cefadroxil monohydrate

(sef-ah-drox'-il mon-oh-hye'-drate)

Rx: Duricef

Chemical Class: Cephalosporin (1st generation)

Therapeutic Class: Antibiotic

CLINICAL PHARMACOLOGY

Mechanism of Action: A first-generation cephalosporin that binds to bacterial cell membranes and inhibits its cell wall synthesis. ***Therapeutic Effect:*** Bactericidal.

Pharmacokinetics

Well absorbed from the GI tract. Protein binding: 15%-20%. Widely distributed. Primarily excreted unchanged in urine. Removed by hemodialysis. ***Half-life:*** 1.2-1.5 hr (increased in impaired renal function).

INDICATIONS AND DOSAGES

UTIs

PO

Adults, Elderly. 1-2 g/day as a single dose or in 2 divided doses.

Children. 30 mg/kg/day in 2 divided doses. Maximum: 2 g/day.

Skin and skin-structure infections, group A beta-hemolytic streptococcal pharyngitis, tonsillitis

PO

Adults, Elderly. 1-2 g in 2 divided doses.

Children. 30 mg/kg/day in 2 divided doses. Maximum: 2 g/day.

Impetigo

PO

Children. 30 mg/kg/day as a single or in 2 divided doses. Maximum: 2 g/day.

Dosage in renal impairment

After an initial 1-g dose, dosage and frequency are modified based on creatinine clearance and the severity of the infection.

Creatinine Clearance	*Dosage Interval*
25-50 ml/min	500 mg q12h
10-25 ml/min	500 mg q24h
0-10 ml/min	500 mg q36h

AVAILABLE FORMS

- *Capsules:* 500 mg.
- *Oral Suspension:* 125 mg/5 ml, 250 mg/5 ml, 500 mg/5 ml.
- *Tablets:* 1 g.

CONTRAINDICATIONS: History of anaphylactic reaction to penicillins or hypersensitivity to cephalosporins

PREGNANCY AND LACTATION: Pregnancy category B; low concentrations in milk

SIDE EFFECTS

Frequent

Oral candidiasis, mild diarrhea, mild abdominal cramping, vaginal candidiasis

Occasional

Nausea, unusual bruising or bleeding, serum sickness–like reaction (marked by fever and joint pain; usually occurs after the second course of therapy and resolves after the drug is discontinued)

Rare

Allergic reaction (rash, pruritus, urticaria), thrombophlebitis (pain, redness, swelling at injection site)

SERIOUS REACTIONS

• Antibiotic-associated colitis and other superinfections may result from altered bacterial balance.

• Nephrotoxicity may occur, especially in patients with preexisting renal disease.

• Patients with a history of allergies, especially to penicillin, are at increased risk for developing a severe hypersensitivity reaction, marked by severe pruritus, angioedema, bronchospasm, and anaphylaxis.

INTERACTIONS

Drugs

3 *Aminoglycosides:* Additive nephrotoxicity

3 *Loop diuretics:* Increased nephrotoxicity

SPECIAL CONSIDERATIONS

• No clinical advantage over less expensive cephalexin

PATIENT/FAMILY EDUCATION

• Administer at even intervals

• Administer with food or milk if the drug causes GI upset

• Refrigerate oral suspension

MONITORING PARAMETERS

• Intake and output

• Renal function

• Daily bowel activity

• Signs and symptoms of superinfection

cefamandole nafate

(sef-a-man′-dole na′-fate)

Rx: Mandol

Chemical Class: Cephalosporin (2nd generation)

Therapeutic Class: Antibiotic

CLINICAL PHARMACOLOGY

Mechanism of Action: A second-generation cephalosporin that binds to bacterial cell membranes. ***Therapeutic Effect:*** Inhibits synthesis of bacterial cell wall. Bactericidal.

Pharmacokinetics

Well absorbed from the gastrointestinal (GI) tract. Protein binding: 56%-78%. Widely distributed. Primarily excreted unchanged in urine and high concentrations in feces. Moderately removed by hemodialysis. ***Half-life:*** 0.5-1 hr (half-life is increased with impaired renal function).

INDICATIONS AND DOSAGES

Severe infections

IV/IM

Adults, Elderly. 500-1000 mg q4-8h. Maximum: 2 g q4h.

Children older than 1 mo. 50-150 mg/kg/day in divided doses q4-8h.

Creatinine Clearance	*Dose*
25-50 ml/min	1-2 g q8h
10-25 ml/min	1 g q8h
10 ml/min or less	1 g q12h

AVAILABLE FORMS

• *Injection:* 1 g, 2 g, 10 g (Mandol).

UNLABELED USES: None known.

CONTRAINDICATIONS: Hypersensitivity to cephalosporins, any component of the formulation, or other cephalosporins

PREGNANCY AND LACTATION: Pregnancy category B; low milk concentrations

SIDE EFFECTS

Frequent

Diarrhea, thrombophlebitis (pain, redness, swelling at injection site)

Occasional

Nausea, fever, vomiting

Rare

Allergic reaction as evidenced by pruritus, rash, and urticaria

SERIOUS REACTIONS

- Antibiotic-associated colitis manifested as severe abdominal pain and tenderness, fever, and watery and severe diarrhea, and other superinfections, may result from altered bacterial balance.
- Nephrotoxicity may occur, especially in patients with preexisting renal disease.
- Severe hypersensitivity reaction including severe pruritus, angioedema, bronchospasm, and anaphylaxis, particularly in patients with a history of allergies, especially to penicillin, may occur.

INTERACTIONS

Drugs

3 *Aminoglycosides:* Potential additive nephrotoxicity

3 *Ethanol:* Disulfiram-like reactions secondary to acetaldehyde accumulation

3 *Loop diuretics:* Increased nephrotoxicity

2 *Oral anticoagulants:* Additive hypoprothrombinemia

Labs

- *Creatinine:* Increases and decreases depending on assay
- *Erythromycin:* False positive
- *Metronidazole:* Interferes with assay

SPECIAL CONSIDERATIONS

PATIENT/FAMILY EDUCATION

- Administer at even intervals

MONITORING PARAMETERS

- Intake and output
- Renal function
- Daily bowel activity
- Signs and symptoms of superinfection

cefazolin sodium

(sef-a'-zoe-lin soe'-dee-um)

Rx: Ancef, Kefzol

Chemical Class: Cephalosporin (1st generation)

Therapeutic Class: Antibiotic

CLINICAL PHARMACOLOGY

Mechanism of Action: A first-generation cephalosporin that binds to bacterial cell membranes and inhibits its cell wall synthesis. ***Therapeutic Effect:*** Bactericidal.

Pharmacokinetics

Widely distributed. Protein binding: 85%. Primarily excreted unchanged in urine. Moderately removed by hemodialysis. ***Half-life:*** 1.4-1.8 hr (increased in impaired renal function).

INDICATIONS AND DOSAGES

Uncomplicated UTIs

IV, IM

Adults, Elderly. 1 g q12h.

Mild to moderate infections

IV, IM

Adults, Elderly. 250-500 mg q8-12h.

Severe infections

IV, IM

Adults, Elderly. 0.5-1 g q6-8h.

Life-threatening infections

IV, IM

Adults, Elderly. 1-1.5 g q6h. Maximum: 12 g/day.

Perioperative prophylaxis

IV, IM

Adults, Elderly. 1 g 30-60 min before surgery, 0.5-1 g during surgery, and q6-8h for up to 24 hrs postoperatively.

Usual pediatric dosage

Children. 50-100 mg/kg/day in divided doses q8h. Maximum: 6 g/day.

Neonates older than 7 days. 40-60 mg/kg/day in divided doses q8-12h.
Neonates 7 days and younger. 40 mg/kg/day in divided doses q12h.

Dosage in renal impairment

Dosing frequency is modified based on creatinine clearance.

Creatinine Clearance	*Dosage Interval*
10-30 ml/min	Usual dose q12h
less than 10 ml/min	Usual dose q24h

AVAILABLE FORMS

• *Powder for Injection (Ancef, Kefzol):* 500 mg, 1 g, 5 g, 10 g.
• *Ready-to-Hang Infusion (Ancef):* 500 mg/50 ml, 1 g/50 ml.

CONTRAINDICATIONS: History of anaphylactic reaction to penicillins or hypersensitivity to cephalosporins

PREGNANCY AND LACTATION: Pregnancy category B; low milk concentrations

SIDE EFFECTS

Frequent

Discomfort with IM administration, oral candidiasis, mild diarrhea, mild abdominal cramping, vaginal candidiasis

Occasional

Nausea, serum sickness–like reaction (marked by fever and joint pain; usually occurs after the second course of therapy and resolves after the drug is discontinued)

Rare

Allergic reaction (rash, pruritus, urticaria), thrombophlebitis (pain, redness, swelling at injection site)

SERIOUS REACTIONS

• Antibiotic-associated colitis and other superinfections may result from altered bacterial balance.
• Nephrotoxicity may occur, especially in patients with preexisting renal disease.
• Patients with a history of allergies, especially to penicillin, are at increased risk for developing a severe hypersensitivity reaction, marked by severe pruritus, angioedema, bronchospasm, and anaphylaxis.

INTERACTIONS

Drugs

3 *Aminoglycosides:* Additive nephrotoxicity
3 *Chloramphenicol:* Inhibits antibacterial activity of cefazolin
3 *Loop diuretics:* Increased nephrotoxicity
2 *Oral anticoagulants:* Additive hypoprothrombinemia

SPECIAL CONSIDERATIONS

PATIENT/FAMILY EDUCATION

• IM injections may cause discomfort

MONITORING PARAMETERS

• Intake and output
• Renal function
• Daily bowel activity
• Signs and symptoms of superinfection

cefdinir

(sef'-di-neer)

Rx: Omnicef

Chemical Class: Cephalosporin (3rd generation)
Therapeutic Class: Antibiotic

CLINICAL PHARMACOLOGY

Mechanism of Action: A third-generation cephalosporin that binds to bacterial cell membranes and inhibits cell wall synthesis. ***Therapeutic Effect:*** Bactericidal.

Pharmacokinetics

Moderately absorbed from the GI tract. Protein binding: 60%-70%. Widely distributed. Not appreciably metabolized. Primarily excreted unchanged in urine. Minimally removed by hemodialysis. ***Half-life:*** 1-2 hr (increased in impaired renal function).

INDICATIONS AND DOSAGES

Community-acquired pneumonia

PO

Adults, Elderly, Children 13 yrs and older. 300 mg q12h for 10 days.

Acute exacerbation of chronic bronchitis

PO

Adults, Elderly. 300 mg q12h for 5-10 days.

Acute maxillary sinusitis

PO

Adults, Elderly, Children 13 yrs and older. 300 mg q12h or 600 mg q24h for 10 days.

Children 6 mos-12 yrs. 7 mg/kg q12h or 14 mg/kg q24h for 10 days.

Pharyngitis or tonsillitis

PO

Adults, Elderly, Children 13 yrs and older. 300 mg q12h for 5-10 days or 600 mg q24h for 10 days.

Children 6 mos-12 yrs. 7 mg/kg q12h for 5-10 days or 14 mg/kg q24h for 10 days.

Uncomplicated skin or skin-structure infections

PO

Adults, Elderly, Children 13 yrs and older. 300 mg q12h for 10 days.

Children 6 mos-12 yrs. 7 mg/kg q12h for 10 days.

Acute bacterial otitis media

PO (Capsules)

Children 6 mos-12 yrs. 7 mg/kg q12h or 14 mg/kg q24h for 10 days.

Usual pediatric dosage for oral suspension

Children weighing 81-95 lb (37-43 kg). 12.5 ml (2.5 tsp) q12h or 25 ml (5 tsp) q24h.

Children weighing 61-80 lb (28-36 kg). 10 ml (2 tsp) q12h or 20 ml (4 tsp) q24h.

Children weighing 41-60 lb (19-27 kg). 7.5 ml (1 tsp) q12h or 15 ml (3 tsp) q24h.

Children weighing 20-40 lb (9-18 kg). 5 ml (1 tsp) q12h or 10 ml (2 tsp) q24h.

Infants weighing less than 20 lb (9 kg). 2.5 ml (½ tsp) q12h or 5 ml (1 tsp) q24h.

Dosage in renal impairment

For patients with creatinine clearance less than 30 ml/min, dosage is 300 mg/day as single daily dose. For hemodialysis patients, dosage is 300 mg or 7 mg/kg/dose every other day.

AVAILABLE FORMS

- *Capsules:* 300 mg.
- *Oral Suspension:* 125 mg/5 ml, 250 mg/5 ml.

CONTRAINDICATIONS: History of anaphylactic reaction to penicillins or hypersensitivity to cephalosporins

PREGNANCY AND LACTATION: Pregnancy category B; not detected in human milk after administration of single 600-mg dose

SIDE EFFECTS

Frequent

Oral candidiasis, mild diarrhea, mild abdominal cramping, vaginal candidiasis

Occasional

Nausea, serum sickness–like reaction (marked by fever and joint pain; usually occurs after the second course of therapy and resolves after the drug is discontinued)

Rare

Allergic reaction (rash, pruritus, urticaria)

SERIOUS REACTIONS

- Antibiotic-associated colitis and other superinfections may result from altered bacterial balance.
- Nephrotoxicity may occur, especially in patients with preexisting renal disease.

• Patients with a history of allergies, especially to penicillin, are at increased risk for developing a severe hypersensitivity reaction, marked by severe pruritus, angioedema, bronchospasm, and anaphylaxis.

INTERACTIONS

Drugs

3 *Aminoglycosides:* May increase the risk of nephrotoxicity

3 *Antacids, iron:* Interference with cefdinir absorption, take antibiotic 2 hr before or after (can be administered with iron-fortified infant formula)

3 *Probenecid:* Inhibits cefdinir excretion

3 *Live typhoid vaccine:* Interference with immune response to vaccine, give vaccine at least 24 hr after last dose

Labs

• *False positive:* Urine ketones using nitroprusside method, urine glucose using Clinitest, Benedict's or Fehling's solution, direct Coomb's test

SPECIAL CONSIDERATIONS

• May be taken without regard to food

• More active *in vitro* against *S. aureus* and *Enterococcus faecalis* than cefixime, but less active against some enterobacteraceae

PATIENT/FAMILY EDUCATION

• Space doses evenly around the clock and continue taking cefdinir for the full length of treatment

• Notify the physician of persistent diarrhea

• Take antacids 2 hrs before or after taking cefdinir

MONITORING PARAMETERS

• Assess pattern of daily bowel activity and stool consistency; although mild GI effects may be tolerable, severe symptoms may indicate the onset of antibiotic-associated colitis

• Be alert for signs and symptoms of superinfection, including abdominal pain or cramping, anal or genital pruritus or discharge, moderate to severe diarrhea, severe mouth or tongue soreness, and new or increased fever

• Monitor hematology reports

cefditoren pivoxil

(seff-di-tore′-en pi-vox′-il)

Rx: Spectracef

Chemical Class: Cephalosporin (3rd generation)

Therapeutic Class: Antibiotic

CLINICAL PHARMACOLOGY

Mechanism of Action: A third-generation cephalosporin that binds to bacterial cell membranes and inhibits cell wall synthesis. ***Therapeutic Effect:*** Bactericidal.

Pharmacokinetics

Moderately absorbed from the GI tract. Protein binding: 88%. Not metabolized. Excreted in the urine. Minimally removed by hemodialysis. ***Half-life:*** 1.6 hr (half-life increased with impaired renal function).

INDICATIONS AND DOSAGES

Pharyngitis, tonsillitis, skin infections

PO

Adults, Elderly, Children older than 12 yr. 200 mg twice a day for 10 days.

Acute exacerbation of chronic bronchitis

PO

Adults, Elderly, Children older than 12 yr. 400 mg twice a day for 10 days.

Community-acquired pneumonia

PO

Adults, Elderly, Children older than 12 yr. 400 mg 2 twice a day for 14 days.

Dosage in renal impairment

Dosage and frequency are modified based on creatinine clearance.

Creatinine Clearance	*Dosage*
50-80 ml/min	No adjustment necessary
30-49 ml/min	200 mg twice a day
less than 30 ml/min	200 mg once a day

AVAILABLE FORMS

• *Tablets:* 200 mg.

CONTRAINDICATIONS: Carnitine deficiency, inborn errors of metabolism, known allergy to cephalosporins, hypersensitivity to milk protein

PREGNANCY AND LACTATION: Pregnancy category B; excreted into breast milk

SIDE EFFECTS

Occasional (11%)

Diarrhea

Rare (4%-1%)

Nausea, headache, abdominal pain, vaginal candidiasis, dyspepsia, vomiting

SERIOUS REACTIONS

• Antibiotic-associated colitis and other superinfections may occur.

• Patients with a history of allergies, especially to penicillin, are at increased risk for developing a severe hypersensitivity reaction, marked by severe pruritus, angioedema, bronchospasm, and anaphylaxis.

INTERACTIONS

Drugs

3 *Antacids, H_2 blockers:* Reduced absorption of cefditoren

3 *Probenecid:* Decreased cefditoren excretion

Labs

• *False positive:* Urine glucose (Benedict's or Fehling's solution or Clinitest tablets)

• *False negative:* Urine, plasma glucose (glucose oxidase or hexokinase methods)

SPECIAL CONSIDERATIONS

• Older oral cephalosporins preferred; no more efficacious than second-generation oral cephalosporins, no advantage over penicillin in strep pharyngitis

• Not recommended for prolonged therapy as carnitine deficiency may result

PATIENT/FAMILY EDUCATION

• Take with meals

• Space doses evenly around the clock, do not skip doses, and continue taking cefditoren for the full course of treatment

MONITORING PARAMETERS

• Be alert for signs and symptoms of superinfection, including abdominal pain, moderate to severe diarrhea, severe anal or genital pruritus, and stomatitis

• Assess pattern of daily bowel activity and stool consistency; severe GI effects may indicate the onset of antibiotic-associated colitis

• Monitor for carnitine deficiency, as evidenced by confusion, fatigue, hypoglycemia, and muscle damage

cefepime hydrochloride

(sef'-e-pim)

Rx: Maxipime

Chemical Class: Cephalosporin (4th generation)

Therapeutic Class: Antibiotic

CLINICAL PHARMACOLOGY

Mechanism of Action: A fourth-generation cephalosporin that binds to bacterial cell membranes and inhibits cell wall synthesis. ***Therapeutic Effect:*** Bactericidal.

Pharmacokinetics

Well absorbed after IM administration. Protein binding: 20%. Widely distributed. Primarily excreted unchanged in urine. Removed by hemodialysis. ***Half-life:*** 2-2.3 hr (increased in impaired renal function, and in the elderly).

INDICATIONS AND DOSAGES

Pneumonia

IV

Adults, Elderly. 1-2 g q12h for 7-10 days.

Children 2 mo and older. 50 mg/kg q12h. Maximum: 2 g/dose.

Intraabdominal infections

IV

Adults, Elderly. 2 g q12h for 10 days.

Skin and skin structure infections

IV

Adults, Elderly. 2 g q12h for 10 days.

Children 2 mo and older. 50 mg/kg q12h. Maximum: 2 g/dose.

UTIs

IV

Adults, Elderly. 0.5-2 g q12h for 7-10 days.

Children 2 mo and older. 50 mg/kg q12h. Maximum: 2 g/dose.

Febrile neutropenia

IV

Adults, Elderly. 2 g q8h.

Children 2 mo and older. 50 mg/kg q8h. Maximum: 2 g/dose.

Dosage in renal impairment

Dosage and frequency are modified based on creatinine clearance and the severity of the infection.

Creatinine Clearance	Dose Range
30-60 ml/min	0.5 g q24h-2 g q12h
11-29 ml/min	0.5-2 g q24h
10 ml/min or less	0.25-1 g q24h

AVAILABLE FORMS

• *Powder for Injection:* 500 mg, 1 g, 2 g.

CONTRAINDICATIONS: History of anaphylactic reaction to penicillins or hypersensitivity to cephalosporins

PREGNANCY AND LACTATION: Pregnancy category B; excreted into breast milk in very low concentrations (0.5 mcg/ml)

SIDE EFFECTS

Frequent

Discomfort with IM administration, oral candidiasis, mild diarrhea, mild abdominal cramping, vaginal candidiasis

Occasional

Nausea, serum sickness–like reaction (marked by fever and joint pain; usually occurs after the second course of therapy and resolves after the drug is discontinued)

Rare

Allergic reaction (rash, pruritus, urticaria), thrombophlebitis (pain, redness, swelling at injection site)

SERIOUS REACTIONS

• Antibiotic-associated colitis manifested and other superinfections may result from altered bacterial balance.

• Nephrotoxicity may occur, especially in patients with preexisting renal disease.

• Patients with a history of allergies, especially to penicillin, are at increased risk for developing a severe hypersensitivity reaction, marked by severe pruritus, angioedema, bronchospasm, and anaphylaxis.

INTERACTIONS

Drugs

3 *Aminoglycosides:* Additive nephrotoxicity

3 *Loop diuretics:* Increased nephrotoxicity

2 *Oral anticoagulants:* Potential increase in hypoprothrombinemic response to oral anticoagulants

3 *Probenecid:* May increase cefepime blood concentration

Labs

• *False positive:* Positive direct Coomb's test, positive urine glucose test (copper reduction method, i.e., Clinitest)

SPECIAL CONSIDERATIONS

• Broad-spectrum, fourth-generation cephalosporin demonstrating a low potential for resistance due to lack of β-lactamase induction and low potential for selection of resistant mutant strains; as effective as ceftazidime and cefotaxime in comparative trials; twice daily dosing may add economic advantage

PATIENT/FAMILY EDUCATION

• IM injection may cause discomfort

MONITORING PARAMETERS

• Pattern of daily bowel activity and stool consistency; although mild GI effects may be tolerable, severe symptoms may indicate the onset of antibiotic-associated colitis
• Intake and output and renal function test results to assess for nephrotoxicity
• Evaluate the IM injection site for induration and tenderness
• Check mouth for white patches on the mucous membranes and tongue
• Be alert for signs and symptoms of superinfection, including abdominal pain or cramping, moderate to severe diarrhea, severe anal or genital pruritus or discharge, and severe mouth or tongue soreness

cefixime

(sef-ix'-zeem)

Rx: Suprax

Chemical Class: Cephalosporin (3rd generation)

Therapeutic Class: Antibiotic

CLINICAL PHARMACOLOGY

Mechanism of Action: A third-generation cephalosporin that binds to bacterial cell membranes and inhibits cell wall synthesis. ***Therapeutic Effect:*** Bactericidal.

Pharmacokinetics

Moderately absorbed from the GI tract. Protein binding: 65%-70%. Widely distributed. Primarily excreted unchanged in urine. Minimally removed by hemodialysis. ***Half-life:*** 3-4 hr (increased in renal impairment).

INDICATIONS AND DOSAGES

Otitis media, acute bronchitis, acute exacerbations of chronic bronchitis, pharyngitis, tonsillitis, and uncomplicated UTIs

PO

Adults, Elderly, Children weighing more than 50 kg. 400 mg/day as a single dose or in 2 divided doses.

Children 6 mo-12 yr weighing less than 50 kg. 8 mg/kg/day as a single dose or in 2 divided doses. Maximum: 400 mg.

Uncomplicated gonorrhea

PO

Adults. 400 mg as a single dose.

Dosage in renal impairment

Creatinine Clearance	*% of Usual Dose*
21-60 ml/min	75%
20 ml/min or less	50%

Dosage is modified based on creatinine clearance.

AVAILABLE FORMS

• *Oral Suspension:* 100 mg/5 ml.
• *Tablets:* 200 mg, 400 mg.

CONTRAINDICATIONS: History of anaphylactic reaction to penicillins, hypersensitivity to cephalosporins

PREGNANCY AND LACTATION: Pregnancy category B; excreted in breast milk

SIDE EFFECTS

Frequent

Oral candidiasis, mild diarrhea, mild abdominal cramping, vaginal candidiasis

Occasional

Nausea, serum sickness–like reaction (marked by arthralgia and fever;

usually occurs after second course of therapy and resolves after drug is discontinued)

Rare

Allergic reaction (rash, pruritus, urticaria)

SERIOUS REACTIONS

• Antibiotic-associated colitis and other superinfections may result from altered bacterial balance.

• Nephrotoxicity may occur, especially in patients with preexisting renal disease.

• Patients with a history of allergies, especially to penicillin, are at increased risk for developing a severe hypersensitivity reaction, marked by severe pruritus, angioedema, bronchospasm, and anaphylaxis.

INTERACTIONS

Drugs

3 *Aminoglycosides:* Additive nephrotoxicity

3 *Loop diuretics:* Increased nephrotoxicity

2 *Oral anticoagulants:* Enhanced hypoprothrombinemia

Labs

• *Cefotaxime:* Interferes with assay

• *Creatinine:* Increases or decreases depending on assay

SPECIAL CONSIDERATIONS

• No *S. aureus* coverage

PATIENT/FAMILY EDUCATION

• Administer at even intervals

• Administer with food or milk if the drug causes GI upset

MONITORING PARAMETERS

• Intake and output

• Renal function

• Daily bowel activity

• Signs and symptoms of superinfection

cefoperazone sodium

(sef-oh-per'-a-zone)

Rx: Cefobid

Chemical Class: Cephalosporin (3rd generation)

Therapeutic Class: Antibiotic

CLINICAL PHARMACOLOGY

Mechanism of Action: A third-generation cephalosporin that binds to bacterial cell membranes. ***Therapeutic Effect:*** Inhibits synthesis of bacterial cell wall. Bactericidal.

Pharmacokinetics

Widely distributed, including cerebrospinal fluid (CSF). Protein binding: 82%-93%. Metabolized and excreted in kidney and urine. Removed by hemodialysis. ***Half-life:*** 1.6-2.4 hrs (half-life is increased with impaired renal function).

INDICATIONS AND DOSAGES

Mild to moderate infections

IM/IV

Adults, Elderly. 2-4 g/day in 2 divided doses q12h.

Severe or life-threatening infections

IM/IV

Adults, Elderly. Total daily dose and/or frequency may be increased to 6-12 g/day divided into 2, 3, or 4 equal doses of 1.5-4 g per dose.

Dosage in renal and/or hepatic impairment

Do not exceed 4 g/day in those with liver disease and/or biliary obstruction. Modification of dose usually not necessary in those with renal impairment. Dose should not exceed 1-2 g/day in those with both hepatic and substantial renal impairment.

AVAILABLE FORMS

• *Injection, premixed frozen:* 1 g (Cefobid).

• *Powder for Injection:* 1 g, 2 g (Cefobid).

UNLABELED USES: Treatment of Lyme disease

CONTRAINDICATIONS: Anaphylactic reaction to penicillins, history of hypersensitivity to cephalosporins or any one of its components.

PREGNANCY AND LACTATION: Pregnancy category B; low concentrations excreted in human milk

SIDE EFFECTS

Frequent

Discomfort with IM administration, oral candidiasis, mild diarrhea, mild abdominal cramping, vaginal candidiasis

Occasional

Nausea, unusual bruising/bleeding, serum sickness reaction

Rare

Allergic reaction, rash, pruritus, urticaria, thrombophlebitis (pain, redness, swelling at injection site)

SERIOUS REACTIONS

- Antibiotic-associated colitis manifested as severe abdominal pain and tenderness, fever, and watery and severe diarrhea, and other superinfections may result from altered bacterial balance.
- Nephrotoxicity may occur, especially in patients with preexisting renal disease. Severe hypersensitivity reaction including severe pruritus, angioedema, bronchospasm, and anaphylaxis, particularly in patients with a history of allergies, especially to penicillins, may occur.

INTERACTIONS

Drugs

3 *Aminoglycosides:* Increased risk of nephrotoxicity

3 *Ethanol:* Disulfiram-like reactions

3 *Loop diuretics:* Increased nephrotoxicity

2 *Oral anticoagulants:* Via hypoprothrombinemia, may enhance anticoagulant effects

Labs

- *Creatinine:* Increased serum values

SPECIAL CONSIDERATIONS

- No dose adjustment necessary in renal failure when usual doses are administered

PATIENT/FAMILY EDUCATION

- Avoid alcohol during and for 3 days after use
- Discomfort may occur with IM injection

MONITORING PARAMETERS

- Intake and output
- Renal function
- Daily bowel activity
- Signs and symptoms of superinfection

---

cefotaxime sodium

(sef-oh-taks'-eem soe-dee-um)

Rx: Claforan

Chemical Class: Cephalosporin (3rd generation)

Therapeutic Class: Antibiotic

CLINICAL PHARMACOLOGY

Mechanism of Action: A third-generation cephalosporin that binds to bacterial cell membranes and inhibits its cell wall synthesis. ***Therapeutic Effect:*** Bactericidal.

Pharmacokinetics

Widely distributed, including to CSF. Protein binding: 30%-50%. Partially metabolized in the liver to active metabolite. Primarily excreted in urine. Moderately removed by hemodialysis. ***Half-life:*** 1 hr (increased in impaired renal function).

INDICATIONS AND DOSAGES

Uncomplicated infections

IV, IM

Adults, Elderly. 1 g q12h.

Mild to moderate infections
IV, IM
Adults, Elderly. 1-2 g q8h.
Severe infections
IV, IM
Adults, Elderly. 2 g q6-8h.
Life-threatening infections
IV, IM
Adults, Elderly. 2 g q4h.
Children: 2 g q4h. Maximum: 12 g/day.
Gonorrhea
IM
Adults. (Male): 1 g as a single dose. (Female): 0.5 g as a single dose.
Perioperative prophylaxis
IV, IM
Adults, Elderly. 1 g 30-90 min before surgery.
Cesarean section
IV
Adults. 1 g as soon as umbilical cord is clamped, then 1 g 6 and 12 hr after first dose.
Usual pediatric dosage
Children weighing 50 kg or more. 1-2 g q6-8h.
Children 1 mo-12 yr weighing less than 50 kg. 100-200 mg/kg/day in divided doses q6-8h.
Dosage in renal impairment
For patients with creatinine clearance less than 20 ml/min give half of dose at usual dosing intervals.

AVAILABLE FORMS
- *Powder for Injection:* 500 mg, 1 g, 2 g, 10 g.
- *Intravenous Solution:* 1 g/50 ml, 2 g/50 ml.

UNLABELED USES: Treatment of Lyme disease

CONTRAINDICATIONS: History of anaphylactic reaction to penicillins or hypersensitivity to cephalosporins

PREGNANCY AND LACTATION: Pregnancy category B; low milk concentrations

SIDE EFFECTS
Frequent
Discomfort with IM administration, oral candidiasis, mild diarrhea, mild abdominal cramping, vaginal candidiasis
Occasional
Nausea, serum sickness–like reaction (marked by fever and joint pain; usually occurs after the second course of therapy and resolves after the drug is discontinued)
Rare
Allergic reaction (rash, pruritus, urticaria), thrombophlebitis (pain, redness, swelling at injection site)

SERIOUS REACTIONS
- Antibiotic-associated colitis and other superinfections may result from altered bacterial balance.
- Nephrotoxicity may occur, especially in patients with preexisting renal disease.
- Patients with a history of allergies, especially to penicillin, are at increased risk for developing a severe hypersensitivity reaction, marked by severe pruritus, angioedema, bronchospasm, and anaphylaxis.

INTERACTIONS
Drugs
3 *Aminoglycosides:* Additive nephrotoxicity
3 *Chloramphenicol:* Inhibits antibacterial activity of cefotaxime
2 *Oral anticoagulants:* Hypoprothrombinemia
Labs
- *False serum increases:* Albumin, alkaline phosphatase, calcium ceftriaxone, cholesterol, creatine kinase, creatinine, glucose, iron, iron saturation, metronidazole, potassium, sodium, tetracycline, trimethoprim

• *False serum decreases:* Ammonia, amylase, chloride, γ-glutamyltransferase (GGT), lactate dehydrogenase, magnesium, phosphate, potassium, urea nitrogen, uric acid
• *False positive:* Clindamycin, colistin, erythromycin, polymyxin

SPECIAL CONSIDERATIONS

PATIENT/FAMILY EDUCATION
• IM injections may cause discomfort

MONITORING PARAMETERS
• Intake and output
• Renal function
• Daily bowel activity
• Signs and symptoms of superinfection

cefotetan disodium

(sef'-oh-tee-tan dye-soe'-dee-um)

Rx: Cefotan

Chemical Class: Cephamycin

Therapeutic Class: Antibiotic

CLINICAL PHARMACOLOGY

Mechanism of Action: A second-generation cephalosporin that binds to bacterial cell membranes and inhibits cell wall synthesis. ***Therapeutic Effect:*** Bactericidal.

Pharmacokinetics

Protein binding: 78%-91%. Primarily excreted unchanged in urine. Minimally removed by hemodialysis. ***Half-life:*** 3-4.6 hr (increased in impaired renal function).

INDICATIONS AND DOSAGES

UTIs

IV, IM

Adults, Elderly. 1-2 g in divided doses q12-24h.

Mild to moderate infections

IV, IM

Adults, Elderly. 1-2 g q12h.

Severe infections

IV, IM

Adults, Elderly. 2 g q12h.

Life-threatening infections

IV, IM

Adults, Elderly. 3 g q12h.

Perioperative prophylaxis

IV

Adults, Elderly. 1-2 g 30-60 min before surgery.

Cesarean section

IV

Adults. 1-2 g as soon as umbilical cord is clamped.

Usual pediatric dosage

Children. 40-80 mg/kg/day in divided doses q12h. Maximum: 6 g/day.

Dosage in renal impairment

Dosing frequency is modified based on creatinine clearance and the severity of the infection.

Creatinine Clearance	*Dosage Interval*
10-30 ml/min	Usual dose q24h
less than 10 ml/min	Usual dose q48h

AVAILABLE FORMS
• *Powder for Injection:* 1 g, 2 g, 10g.
• *Intravenous Solution:* 1 g/50 ml, 2 g/50 ml.

CONTRAINDICATIONS: History of anaphylactic reaction to penicillins or hypersensitivity to cephalosporins

PREGNANCY AND LACTATION: Pregnancy category B; small amounts excreted into breast milk

SIDE EFFECTS

Frequent

Discomfort with IM administration, oral candidiasis, mild diarrhea, mild abdominal cramping, vaginal candidiasis

Occasional

Nausea, unusual bleeding or bruising, serum sickness–like reaction (marked by fever and joint pain;

usually occurs after the second course of therapy and resolves after the drug is discontinued)

Rare

Allergic reaction (rash, pruritus, urticaria), thrombophlebitis (pain, redness, swelling at injection site)

SERIOUS REACTIONS

• Antibiotic-associated colitis and other superinfections may result from altered bacterial balance.

• Nephrotoxicity may occur, especially in patients with preexisting renal disease.

• Patients with a history of allergies, especially to penicillin, are at increased risk for developing a severe hypersensitivity reaction, marked by severe pruritus, angioedema, bronchospasm, and anaphylaxis.

INTERACTIONS

Drugs

3 *Aminoglycosides:* Additive nephrotoxicity

3 *Ethanol:* Disulfiram-like reaction

3 *Chloramphenicol:* Inhibits antibacterial activity of cefotetan

2 *Oral anticoagulants:* Additive hypoprothrombinemia; enhanced anticoagulant effects

SPECIAL CONSIDERATIONS

PATIENT/FAMILY EDUCATION

• Avoid alcohol during and for 3 days after use

• IM injections may cause discomfort

MONITORING PARAMETERS

• Intake and output

• Renal function

• Daily bowel activity

• Signs and symptoms of superinfection

cefoxitin sodium

(se-fox'-i-tin soe'-dee-um)

Rx: Mefoxin

Chemical Class: Cephamycin

Therapeutic Class: Antibiotic

C

CLINICAL PHARMACOLOGY

Mechanism of Action: A second-generation cephalosporin that binds to bacterial cell membranes and inhibits cell wall synthesis. ***Therapeutic Effect:*** Bactericidal.

Pharmacokinetics

Well distributed. Protein binding: 41%-75%. Primarily excreted in urine. Removed by hemodialysis. ***Half-life:*** 0.8-1 hr.

INDICATIONS AND DOSAGES

Mild to moderate infections

IV, IM

Adults, Elderly. 1-2 g q6-8h.

Severe infections

IV, IM

Adults, Elderly. 1 g q4h or 2 g q6-8h up to 2 g q4h.

Perioperative prophylaxis

IV, IM

Adults, Elderly. 2 g 30-60 min before surgery, then q6h for up to 24 hr after surgery.

Children older than 3 mo. 30-40 mg/kg 30-60 min before surgery, then q6h for up to 24 hr after surgery.

Cesarean section

IV

Adults. 2 g as soon as umbilical cord is clamped, then 2 g 4 and 8 hr after first dose, then q6h for up to 24 hr.

Usual pediatric dosage

Children older than 3 mo. 80-160 mg/kg/day in 4-6 divided doses. Maximum: 12 g/day.

Neonates. 90-100 mg/kg/day in divided doses q6-8h.

Dosage in renal impairment
After a loading dose of 1-2 g, dosage and frequency are modified based on creatinine clearance and the severity of the infection.

Creatinine Clearance	*Dosage*
30-50 ml/min	1-2 g q8-12h
10-29 ml/min	1-2 g q12-24h
5-9 ml/min	500 mg-1 g q12-24h
less than 5 ml/min	500 mg-1 g q24-48h

AVAILABLE FORMS
• *Powder for Injection:* 1 g, 2 g, 10 g.
• *Intravenous Solution:* 1 g/50 ml, 2 g/50 ml.

CONTRAINDICATIONS: History of anaphylactic reaction to penicillins or hypersensitivity to cephalosporins

PREGNANCY AND LACTATION: Pregnancy category B; low milk concentrations

SIDE EFFECTS
Frequent
Discomfort with IM administration, oral candidiasis, mild diarrhea, mild abdominal cramping, vaginal candidiasis
Occasional
Nausea, serum sickness–like reaction (marked by fever and joint pain; usually occurs after the second course of therapy and resolves after the drug is discontinued)
Rare
Allergic reaction (pruritus, rash, urticaria), thrombophlebitis (pain, redness, swelling at injection site)

SERIOUS REACTIONS
• Antibiotic-associated colitis and other superinfections may result from altered bacterial balance.
• Nephrotoxicity may occur, especially in patients with preexisting renal disease.
• Patients with a history of allergies, especially to penicillin, are at increased risk for developing a severe hypersensitivity reaction, marked by severe pruritus, angioedema, bronchospasm, and anaphylaxis.

INTERACTIONS
Drugs
3 *Aminoglycosides:* Additive nephrotoxicity
3 *Chloramphenicol:* Inhibits antibacterial activity of cefoxitin
❷ *Oral anticoagulants:* Additive hypoprothrombinemia, enhanced anticoagulant effects
Labs
• *False serum increases:* Creatinine (serum and urine), cefuroxime, gentamicin, metronidazole, potassium, tetracycline
• *False urine increases:* 17-hydroxycorticosteroids
• *False serum decreases:* Creatinine clearance
• *False positive:* Polymyxin

SPECIAL CONSIDERATIONS
PATIENT/FAMILY EDUCATION
• IM injections may cause discomfort

MONITORING PARAMETERS
• Intake and output
• Renal function
• Daily bowel activity
• Signs and symptoms of superinfection

cefpodoxime proxetil
(sef-pode-ox'-eem proks'-eh-till)
Rx: Vantin
Chemical Class: Cephalosporin (3rd generation)
Therapeutic Class: Antibiotic

CLINICAL PHARMACOLOGY
Mechanism of Action: A third-generation cephalosporin that binds to bacterial cell membranes and inhibits cell wall synthesis. ***Therapeutic Effect:*** Bactericidal.

Pharmacokinetics

Well absorbed from the GI tract (food increases absorption). Protein binding: 21%-40%. Widely distributed. Primarily excreted unchanged in urine. Partially removed by hemodialysis. ***Half-life:*** 2.3 hr (increased in impaired renal function and elderly patients).

INDICATIONS AND DOSAGES

Chronic bronchitis, pneumonia

PO

Adults, Elderly, Children older than 13 yrs. 200 mg q12h for 10-14 days.

Gonorrhea, rectal gonococcal infection (female patients only)

PO

Adults, Children older than 13 yrs. 200 mg as a single dose.

Skin and skin-structure infections

PO

Adults, Elderly, Children older than 13 yrs. 400 mg q12h for 7-14 days.

Pharyngitis, tonsillitis

PO

Adults, Elderly, Children older than 13 yrs. 100 mg q12h for 5-10 days.

Children 6 mos-13 yrs. 5 mg/kg q12h for 5-10 days. Maximum: 100 mg/dose.

Acute maxillary sinusitis

PO

Adults, Children older than 13 yrs. 200 mg twice a day for 10 days.

Children 2 mos-13 yrs. 5 mg/kg q12h for 10 days. Maximum: 200 mg/dose.

UTIs

PO

Adults, Elderly, Children older than 13 yrs. 100 mg q12h for 7 days.

Acute otitis media

PO

Children 6 mos-13 yrs. 5 mg/kg q12h for 5 days. Maximum: 400 mg/dose.

Dosage in renal impairment

For patients with creatinine clearance less than 30 ml/min, usual dose is given q24h. For patients on hemodialysis, usual dose is given 3 times/wk after dialysis.

AVAILABLE FORMS

- *Oral Suspension:* 50 mg/5 ml, 100 mg/5 ml.
- *Tablets:* 100 mg, 200 mg.

CONTRAINDICATIONS: History of anaphylactic reaction to penicillins or hypersensitivity to cephalosporins

PREGNANCY AND LACTATION: Pregnancy category B; excreted into breast milk; average 2% of serum levels at 4 hr following 200-mg dose

SIDE EFFECTS

Frequent

Oral candidiasis, mild diarrhea, mild abdominal cramping, vaginal candidiasis

Occasional

Nausea, serum sickness–like reaction (marked by fever and joint pain; usually occurs after the second course of therapy and resolves after the drug is discontinued)

Rare

Allergic reaction (pruritus, rash, urticaria)

SERIOUS REACTIONS

- Antibiotic-associated colitis and other superinfections may result from altered bacterial balance.
- Nephrotoxicity may occur, especially in patients with preexisting renal disease.
- Patients with a history of allergies, especially to penicillin, are at increased risk for developing a severe hypersensitivity reaction, marked by severe pruritus, angioedema, bronchospasm, and anaphylaxis.

INTERACTIONS

Drugs

3 *Aminoglycosides:* Additive nephrotoxicity

3 *Antacids:* Reduced bioavailability and serum cefpodoxime levels
3 *H_2-blockers (cimetidine, famotidine, nizatidine, ranitidine), proton pump inhibitors (lansoprazole, omeprazole):* Reduced bioavailability and serum cefpodoxime levels
3 *Loop diuretics:* Increased nephrotoxicity
3 *Probenecid:* May increase cefpodoxime blood concentration

SPECIAL CONSIDERATIONS

- Reserve use for otitis media to infections that fail to respond to less expensive agents (e.g., amoxicillin, co-trimoxazole)
- Suspension tastes very bitter

MONITORING PARAMETERS

- Pattern of daily bowel activity and stool consistency; mild GI effects may be tolerable, but severe symptoms may indicate the onset of antibiotic-associated colitis
- Intake and output and renal function test results to assess for nephrotoxicity
- Assess mouth for white patches on the mucous membranes and tongue
- Be alert for signs and symptoms of superinfection, including abdominal pain or cramping, moderate to severe diarrhea, severe anal or genital pruritus or discharge, and severe mouth or tongue soreness

cefprozil

(sef-pro'-zil)
Rx: Cefzil
Chemical Class: Cephalosporin (2nd generation)
Therapeutic Class: Antibiotic

CLINICAL PHARMACOLOGY

Mechanism of Action: A second-generation cephalosporin that binds to bacterial cell membranes and inhibits cell wall synthesis. ***Therapeutic Effect:*** Bactericidal.

Pharmacokinetics

Well absorbed from the GI tract. Protein binding: 36%-45%. Widely distributed. Primarily excreted unchanged in urine. Moderately removed by hemodialysis. ***Half-life:*** 1.3 hr (increased in impaired renal function).

INDICATIONS AND DOSAGES

Pharyngitis, tonsillitis

PO

Adults, Elderly. 500 mg q24h for 10 days.
Children 2-12 yr. 7.5 mg/kg q12h for 10 days. Maximum: 1 g/day.

Acute bacterial exacerbation of chronic bronchitis, secondary bacterial infection of acute bronchitis

PO

Adults, Elderly. 500 mg q12h for 10 days.

Skin and skin-structure infections

PO

Adults, Elderly, Children older than 12 yr. 250-500 mg q12h for 10 days.
Children 2-12 yr. 20 mg/kg q24h for 10 days. Maximum: 1 g/day.

Acute sinusitis

PO

Adults, Elderly. 250-500 mg q12h for 10 days.
Children 6 mo-12 yr. 7.5-15 mg/kg q12h for 10 days.

Otitis media

PO

Children 6 mo-12 yr. 15 mg/kg q12h for 10 days. Maximum: 1 g/day.

Dosage in renal impairment

Patients with creatinine clearance less than 30 ml/min receive 50% of usual dose at usual interval.

AVAILABLE FORMS

- *Oral Suspension:* 125 mg/5 ml, 250 mg/5 ml.
- *Tablets:* 250 mg, 500 mg.

CONTRAINDICATIONS: History of anaphylactic reaction to penicillins or hypersensitivity to cephalosporins

PREGNANCY AND LACTATION: Pregnancy category B; excreted into breast milk in low concentratons

SIDE EFFECTS

Frequent

Oral candidiasis, mild diarrhea, mild abdominal cramping, vaginal candidiasis

Occasional

Nausea, serum sickness–like reaction (marked by fever and joint pain; usually occurs after the second course of therapy and resolves after the drug is discontinued)

Rare

Allergic reaction (pruritus, rash, urticaria)

SERIOUS REACTIONS

- Antibiotic-associated colitis and other superinfections may result from altered bacterial balance.
- Nephrotoxicity may occur, especially in patients with preexisting renal disease.
- Patients with a history of allergies, especially to penicillin, are at increased risk for developing a severe hypersensitivity reaction, marked by severe pruritus, angioedema, bronchospasm, and anaphylaxis.

INTERACTIONS

Drugs

3 *Aminoglycosides:* Additive nephrotoxicity

3 *Loop diuretics:* Increased nephrotoxicity

3 *Probenecid:* Increases serum concentration of cefprozil

SPECIAL CONSIDERATIONS

- Reserve use for otitis media to infections that fail to respond to less expensive agents (e.g., amoxicillin, co-trimoxazole)
- Suspension contains phenylalanine 28 mg/5 ml

PATIENT/FAMILY EDUCATION

- Space drug doses evenly around the clock and continue cefprozil therapy for the full course of treatment
- Take with food if GI upset occurs

MONITORING PARAMETERS

- Pattern of daily bowel activity and stool consistency; mild GI effects may be tolerable, but severe symptoms may indicate the onset of antibiotic-associated colitis
- Intake and output and renal function test results to assess for nephrotoxicity
- Assess oral cavity for evidence of stomatitis
- Be alert for signs and symptoms of superinfection, including abdominal pain or cramping, moderate to severe diarrhea, severe anal or genital pruritus or discharge, and severe mouth or tongue soreness

ceftazidime

(sef′-tay-zi-deem)

Rx: Ceptaz, Fortaz, Tazicef, Tazidime

Chemical Class: Cephalosporin (3rd generation)

Therapeutic Class: Antibiotic

CLINICAL PHARMACOLOGY

Mechanism of Action: A third-generation cephalosporin that binds to bacterial cell membranes and inhibits cell wall synthesis. ***Therapeutic Effect:*** Bactericidal.

Pharmacokinetics

Widely distributed (including to cerebrospinal fluid [CSF]). Protein binding: 5%-17%. Primarily excreted unchanged in urine. Removed by hemodialysis. ***Half-life:*** 2 hr (increased in impaired renal function).

INDICATIONS AND DOSAGES

UTIs

IV, IM

Adults. 250-500 mg q8-12h.

Mild to moderate infections

IV, IM

Adults. 1 g q8-12h.

Uncomplicated pneumonia, skin and skin-structure infections

IV, IM

Adults. 0.5-1 g q8h.

Bone and joint infections

IV, IM

Adults. 2 g q12h.

Meningitis, serious gynecologic and intraabdominal infections

IV, IM

Adults. 2 g q8h.

Pseudomonal pulmonary infections in patients with cystic fibrosis

IV

Adults. 30-50 mg/kg q8h. Maximum: 6 g/day.

Usual elderly dosage

Elderly (normal renal function). 500 mg-1 g q12h.

Usual pediatric dosage

Children 1 mo-12 yr. 100-150 mg/kg/day in divided doses q8h. Maximum: 6 g/day.

Neonates 0-4 wk. 100-150 mg/kg/day in divided doses q8-12h.

Dosage in renal impairment

After an initial 1-g dose, dosage and frequency are modified based on creatinine clearance and the severity of the infection.

Creatinine Clearance	Dosage
31-50 ml/min	1 g q12h
16-30 ml/min	1 g q24h
6-15 ml/min	500 mg q24h
less than 5 ml/min	500 mg q48h

AVAILABLE FORMS

• *Powder for Injection (Fortaz, Tazicef, Tazidime):* 500 mg, 1 g, 2 g.

CONTRAINDICATIONS: History of anaphylactic reaction to penicillins or hypersensitivity to cephalosporins

PREGNANCY AND LACTATION: Pregnancy category B; excreted in human milk in low concentrations

SIDE EFFECTS

Frequent

Discomfort with IM administration, oral candidiasis, mild diarrhea, mild abdominal cramping, vaginal candidiasis

Occasional

Nausea, serum sickness–like reaction (marked by fever and joint pain; usually occurs after the second course of therapy and resolves after the drug is discontinued)

Rare

Allergic reaction (pruritus, rash, urticaria), thrombophlebitis (pain, redness, swelling at injection site)

SERIOUS REACTIONS

• Antibiotic-associated colitis and other superinfections may result from altered bacterial balance.

• Nephrotoxicity may occur, especially in patients with preexisting renal disease.

• Patients with a history of allergies, especially to penicillin, are at increased risk for developing a severe hypersensitivity reaction, marked by severe pruritus, angioedema, bronchospasm, and anaphylaxis.

INTERACTIONS

Drugs

3 *Aminoglycosides:* Additive nephrotoxicity

3 *Chloramphenicol:* Inhibition of the antibacterial activity of ceftazidime

3 *Loop diuretics:* Increased nephrotoxicity

SPECIAL CONSIDERATIONS

• Especially useful for infections due to *Pseudomonas aeruginosa* (with or without an aminoglycoside)

PATIENT/FAMILY EDUCATION
- IM injections may cause discomfort

MONITORING PARAMETERS
- Pattern of daily bowel activity and stool consistency; mild GI effects may be tolerable, but severe symptoms may indicate the onset of antibiotic-associated colitis
- Intake and output and renal function test results to assess for nephrotoxicity
- Evaluate the IV site for phlebitis, as evidenced by heat, pain, and red streaking over the vein
- Assess the IM injection site for induration and tenderness
- Assess mouth for white patches on the mucous membranes or tongue
- Be alert for signs and symptoms of superinfection, including abdominal pain or cramping, moderate to severe diarrhea, severe anal or genital pruritus or discharge, and severe mouth or tongue soreness

ceftibuten

(sef-tye'-byoo-ten)
Rx: Cedax
Chemical Class: Cephalosporin (3rd generation)
Therapeutic Class: Antibiotic

CLINICAL PHARMACOLOGY
Mechanism of Action: A third-generation cephalosporin that binds to bacterial cell membranes and inhibits cell wall synthesis. ***Therapeutic Effect:*** Bactericidal.

Pharmacokinetics
Rapidly absorbed from the gastrointestinal tract. Protein binding: 65%-77%. Excreted primarily in urine. ***Half-life:*** 2-3 hr.

INDICATIONS AND DOSAGES
Chronic bronchitis
PO
Adults, Elderly. 400 mg/day once a day for 10 days.
Pharyngitis, tonsillitis
PO
Adults, Elderly. 400 mg once a day for 10 days.
Children older than 6 mo. 9 mg/kg once a day for 10 days. Maximum: 400 mg/day.
Otitis media
PO
Children older than 6 mo. 9 mg/kg once a day for 10 days. Maximum: 400 mg/day.
Dosage in renal impairment
Dosage is modified based on creatinine clearance.

Creatinine Clearance	*Dosage*
50 ml/min and higher	400 mg or 9 mg/kg q24h
30-49 ml/min	200 mg or 4.5 mg/kg q24h
less than 30 ml/min	100 mg or 2.25 mg/kg q24h

AVAILABLE FORMS
- *Capsules:* 400 mg.
- *Oral Suspension:* 90 mg/5 ml.

CONTRAINDICATIONS: History of anaphylactic reaction to penicillins or hypersensitivity to cephalosporins

PREGNANCY AND LACTATION: Pregnancy category B; excreted into breast milk in negligible concentrations

SIDE EFFECTS
Frequent
Oral candidiasis, mild diarrhea (discharge, itching)
Occasional
Nausea, serum sickness–like reaction (marked by fever and joint pain; usually occurs after the second

course of therapy and resolves after the drug is discontinued)

Rare

Allergic reaction (rash, pruritus, urticaria)

SERIOUS REACTIONS

- Antibiotic-associated colitis and other superinfections may result from altered bacterial balance.
- Nephrotoxicity may occur, especially in patients with preexisting renal disease.
- Patients with a history of allergies, especially to penicillin, are at increased risk for developing a severe hypersensitivity reaction, marked by severe pruritus, angioedema, bronchospasm, and anaphylaxis.

INTERACTIONS

Drugs

3 *Aminoglycosides:* Additive nephrotoxicity

3 *Loop diuretics:* Increased nephrotoxicity

3 *Probenecid:* Increases serum ceftibuten level

SPECIAL CONSIDERATIONS

- Comparable to many other oral cephalosporins; may produce higher serum levels and better penetration, but unsubstantiated
- Clinical application as alternative in respiratory tract infections
- Recommend empty stomach administration for the suspension

PATIENT/FAMILY EDUCATION

- Space drug doses evenly around the clock and continue taking ceftibuten for the full course of treatment
- Take drug with food or milk if GI upset occurs

MONITORING PARAMETERS

- Pattern of daily bowel activity and stool consistency; mild GI effects may be tolerable, but severe symptoms may indicate the onset of antibiotic-associated colitis
- Intake and output and renal function test results to assess for nephrotoxicity
- Assess mouth for white patches on the mucous membranes and tongue
- Be alert for signs and symptoms of superinfection, including abdominal pain or cramping, moderate to severe diarrhea, severe anal or genital pruritus or discharge, and severe mouth or tongue soreness

ceftizoxime sodium

(sef-ti-zox'-eem)

Rx: Cefizox

Chemical Class: Cephalosporin (3rd generation)

Therapeutic Class: Antibiotic

CLINICAL PHARMACOLOGY

Mechanism of Action: A third-generation cephalosporin that binds to bacterial cell membranes and inhibits cell wall synthesis. ***Therapeutic Effect:*** Bactericidal.

Pharmacokinetics

Widely distributed (including to CSF). Protein binding: 30%. Primarily excreted unchanged in urine. Moderately removed by hemodialysis. ***Half-life:*** 1.7 hr (increased in impaired renal function).

INDICATIONS AND DOSAGES

Uncomplicated UTIs

IV, IM

Adults, Elderly. 500 mg q12h.

Mild, moderate, or severe infections of the biliary, respiratory, and GU tracts; skin, bone, and intraabdominal infections; meningitis; and septicemia

IV, IM

Adults, Elderly. 1-2 g q8-12h.

Life-threatening infections of the biliary, respiratory, and GU tracts; skin, bone, and intraabdominal infections; meningitis; and septicemia
IV
Adults, Elderly. 3-4 g q8h, up to 2 g q4h.
Pelvic inflammatory disease (PID)
IV
Adults. 2 g q4-8h.
Uncomplicated gonorrhea
IM
Adults. 1 g one time.
Usual pediatric dosage
Children older than 6 mo: 50 mg/kg q6-8h. Maximum: 12 g/day.
Dosage in renal impairment
After a loading dose of 0.5-1 g, dosage and frequency are modified based on creatinine clearance and the severity of the infection.

Creatinine Clearance	*Dosage*
50-79 ml/min	0.5 g-1.5 g q8h
5-49 ml/min	0.25 g-1 g q12h
less than 5 ml/min	0.25-0.5 g q24h or 0.5 g-1 g q48h

AVAILABLE FORMS
- *Intravenous Solution:* 1 g/50 ml, 2 g/50 ml.
- *Powder for Injection:* 500 mg, 1 g, 2 g, 10 g.

CONTRAINDICATIONS: History of anaphylactic reaction to penicillins or hypersensitivity to cephalosporins

PREGNANCY AND LACTATION: Pregnancy category B; excreted in human milk in low concentrations

SIDE EFFECTS
Frequent
Discomfort with IM administration, oral candidiasis, mild diarrhea, mild abdominal cramping, vaginal candidiasis
Occasional
Nausea, serum sickness–like reaction (fever, joint pain; usually occurs after the second course of therapy and resolves after the drug is discontinued)
Rare
Allergic reaction (rash, pruritus, urticaria), thrombophlebitis (pain, redness, swelling at injection site)

SERIOUS REACTIONS
- Antibiotic-associated colitis manifested and other superinfections may result from altered bacterial balance.
- Nephrotoxicity may occur, especially in patients with preexisting renal disease.
- Patients with a history of allergies, especially to penicillin, are at increased risk for developing a severe hypersensitivity reaction, marked by severe pruritus, angioedema, bronchospasm, and anaphylaxis.

INTERACTIONS
Drugs
3 *Aminoglycosides:* Additive nephrotoxicity
3 *Loop diuretics:* Increased nephrotoxicity

SPECIAL CONSIDERATIONS
PATIENT/FAMILY EDUCATION
- IM injections may cause discomfort

MONITORING PARAMETERS
- Signs and symptoms of superinfection, including abdominal pain or cramping, moderate to severe diarrhea, severe anal or genital pruritus or discharge, and severe mouth or tongue soreness
- Daily bowel activity and stool consistency
- Intake and output, renal function

ceftriaxone sodium

(sef-try-ax′-one soe′-dee-um)

Rx: Rocephin, Rocephin IM Convenience Kit

Chemical Class: Cephalosporin (3rd generation)

Therapeutic Class: Antibiotic

CLINICAL PHARMACOLOGY

Mechanism of Action: A third-generation cephalosporin that binds to bacterial cell membranes and inhibits cell wall synthesis. ***Therapeutic Effect:*** Bactericidal.

Pharmacokinetics

Widely distributed (including to CSF). Protein binding: 83%-96%. Primarily excreted unchanged in urine. Not removed by hemodialysis. ***Half-life:*** 4.3-4.6 hr IV; 5.8-8.7 hr IM (increased in impaired renal function).

INDICATIONS AND DOSAGES

Mild to moderate infections

IV, IM

Adults, Elderly. 1-2 g as a single dose or in 2 divided doses.

Serious infections

IV, IM

Adults, Elderly. Up to 4 g/day in 2 divided doses.

Children. 50-75 mg/kg/day in divided doses q12h. Maximum: 2 g/day.

Skin and skin-structure infections

IV, IM

Children. 50-75 mg/kg/day as a single dose or in 2 divided doses. Maximum: 2 g/day

Meningitis

IV

Children. Initially, 75 mg/kg, then 100 mg/kg/day as a single dose or in divided doses q12h. Maximum: 4 g/day.

Lyme disease

IV

Adults, Elderly. 2-4 g a day for 10-14 days.

Acute bacterial otitis media

IM

Children. 50 mg/kg once a day for 3 days. Maximum: 1 g/day

Perioperative prophylaxis

IV, IM

Adults, Elderly. 1 g 0.5-2 hrs before surgery.

Uncomplicated gonorrhea

IM

Adults. 250 mg plus doxycycline one time.

Dosage in renal impairment

Dosage modification is usually unnecessary, but liver and renal function test results should be monitored in those with both renal and liver impairment or severe renal impairment.

AVAILABLE FORMS

• *Kit (Intramuscular [Rocephin IM Convenience Kit]):* 500 mg, 1 g.

• *Intravenous Solution (Rocephin):* 1 g/50 ml, 2 g/50 ml.

• *Powder for Injection (Rocephin):* 250 mg, 500 mg, 1 g, 2 g, 10 g.

CONTRAINDICATIONS: History of anaphylactic reaction to penicillins or hypersensitivity to cephalosporins

PREGNANCY AND LACTATION: Pregnancy category B; excreted in breast milk

SIDE EFFECTS

Frequent

Discomfort with IM administration, oral candidiasis, mild diarrhea, mild abdominal cramping, vaginal candidiasis

Occasional

Nausea, serum sickness–like reaction (marked by fever and joint pain; usually occurs after the second course of therapy and resolves after the drug is discontinued)

Rare
Allergic reaction (rash, pruritus, urticaria), thrombophlebitis (pain, redness, swelling at injection site)

SERIOUS REACTIONS

• Antibiotic-associated colitis and other superinfections may result from altered bacterial balance.
• Nephrotoxicity may occur, especially in patients with preexisting renal disease.
• Patients with a history of allergies, especially to penicillin, are at increased risk for developing a severe hypersensitivity reaction, marked by severe pruritus, angioedema, bronchospasm, and anaphylaxis.

INTERACTIONS

Drugs

3 *Aminoglycosides:* Additive nephrotoxicity
3 *Loop diuretics:* Increased nephrotoxicity
2 *Warfarin:* Hypoprothrombinemic response enhanced

SPECIAL CONSIDERATIONS

• Meningitis the only indication requiring bid dosing; qd sufficient for all other indications in adults
• Often administered in acute care settings for dubious indications due to long $t_{1/2}$, avoid overuse

PATIENT/FAMILY EDUCATION

• IM injections may cause discomfort

MONITORING PARAMETERS

• Intake and output
• Renal function
• Daily bowel activity
• Signs and symptoms of superinfection

cefuroxime axetil/ cefuroxime sodium

(sef-yoor-ox'-eem)
Rx: Zinacef, Kefurox (as sodium), Ceftin (as axetil)
Chemical Class: Cephalosporin (2nd generation)
Therapeutic Class: Antibiotic

CLINICAL PHARMACOLOGY

Mechanism of Action: A second-generation cephalosporin that binds to bacterial cell membranes and inhibits cell wall synthesis. ***Therapeutic Effect:*** Bactericidal.

Pharmacokinetics

Rapidly absorbed from the GI tract. Protein binding: 33%-50%. Widely distributed (including to CSF). Primarily excreted unchanged in urine. Moderately removed by hemodialysis. ***Half-life:*** 1.3 hr (increased in impaired renal function).

INDICATIONS AND DOSAGES

Ampicillin-resistant influenza; bacterial meningitis; early Lyme disease; GU tract, gynecologic, skin, and bone infections; septicemia; gonorrhea, and other gonococcal infections

IV, IM

Adults, Elderly. 750 mg-1.5 g q8h.
Children. 75-100 mg/kg/day divided q8h. Maximum: 8 g/day.
Neonates. 50-100 mg/kg/day divided q12h.

PO

Adults, Elderly. 125-500 mg twice a day, depending on the infection.

Pharyngitis, tonsillitis

PO

Children 3 mo-12 yr. 125 mg (tablets) q12h or 20 mg/kg/day (suspension) in 2 divided doses.

Acute otitis media, acute bacterial maxillary sinusitis, impetigo

PO

Children 3 mo-12 yr. 250 mg (tablets) q12h or 30 mg/kg/day (suspension) in 2 divided doses.

Bacterial meningitis

IV

Children 3 mo-12 yr. 200-240 mg/kg/day in divided doses q6-8h.

Perioperative prophylaxis

IV

Adults, Elderly. 1.5 g 30-60 min before surgery and 750 mg q8h after surgery.

Usual neonatal dosage

IV, IM

Neonates. 20-100 mg/kg/day in divided doses q12h.

Dosage in renal impairment

Adult dosage and frequency are modified based on creatinine clearance and the severity of the infection.

Creatinine Clearance	*Dosage*
greater than 20 ml/min	750 mg-1 g q8h
10-20 ml/min	750 mg q12h
less than 10 ml/min	750 mg q24h

AVAILABLE FORMS

- *Oral Suspension (axetil):* 125 mg/5 ml, 250 mg/5 ml.
- *Tablets (Ceftin):* 125 mg, 250 mg, 500 mg.
- *Powder for Injection (Zinacef):* 750 mg, 1.5 g, 7.5 g.
- *Powder for Injection (ADD-Vantage Vial [Zinacef]):* 750 mg, 1.5 g.
- *Powder for Injection (Infusion Pack [Zinacef]):* 750 mg, 1.5 g.
- *Intravenous Solution (Zinacef):* 750 mg/50 ml, 1.5 g/50 ml.

CONTRAINDICATIONS: History of anaphylactic reaction to penicillins or hypersensitivity to cephalosporins

PREGNANCY AND LACTATION: Pregnancy category B; excreted in breast milk

SIDE EFFECTS

Frequent

Discomfort with IM administration, oral candidiasis, mild diarrhea, mild abdominal cramping, vaginal candidiasis

Occasional

Nausea, serum sickness–like reaction (marked by fever and joint pain; usually occurs after the second course of therapy and resolves after the drug is discontinued)

Rare

Allergic reaction (rash, pruritus, urticaria), thrombophlebitis (pain, redness, swelling at injection site)

SERIOUS REACTIONS

- Antibiotic-associated colitis and other superinfections may result from altered bacterial balance.
- Nephrotoxicity may occur, especially in patients with preexisting renal disease.
- Patients with a history of allergies, especially to penicillin, are at increased risk for developing a severe hypersensitivity reaction, marked by severe pruritus, angioedema, bronchospasm, and anaphylaxis.

INTERACTIONS

Drugs

3 *Aminoglycosides:* Additive nephrotoxicity

3 *Antacids, H_2-blockers, omeprazole, lansoprazole:* Decreased absorption of cefuroxime axetil

3 *Loop diuretics:* Increased nephrotoxicity

SPECIAL CONSIDERATIONS

- Oral tabs and oral susp not bioequivalent
- Take with food
- Alternative to amoxicillin or co-trimoxazole for resistant upper respiratory pathogens; expensive, but bid dosing

celecoxib

(sel-eh-cox'-ib)

Rx: Celebrex

Chemical Class: Cyclooxygenase-2 (COX-2) inhibitor

Therapeutic Class: COX-2 specific inhibitor; NSAID; nonnarcotic analgesic

CLINICAL PHARMACOLOGY

Mechanism of Action: An NSAID that inhibits cyclooxygenase-2, the enzyme responsible for prostaglandin synthesis. Mechanism of action in treating familial adenomatous polyposis is unknown. ***Therapeutic Effect:*** Reduces inflammation and relieves pain.

Pharmacokinetics

Widely distributed. Protein binding: 97%. Metabolized in the liver. Primarily eliminated in feces. ***Half-life:*** 11.2 hr.

INDICATIONS AND DOSAGES

Osteoarthritis

PO

Adults, Elderly. 200 mg/day as a single dose or 100 mg twice a day.

Rheumatoid arthritis

PO

Adults, Elderly. 100-200 mg twice a day.

Acute pain

PO

Adults, Elderly. Initially, 400 mg with additional 200 mg on day 1, if needed. Maintenance: 200 mg twice a day as needed.

Familial adenomatous polyposis

PO

Adults, Elderly. 400 mg twice daily (with food).

Primary dysmenorrhea

PO

Adults. 200 mg twice a day as needed (with food).

Ankylosing spondylitis

PO

Adults, Elderly. 200 mg/day as a single dose or in 2 divided doses. May increase to 400 mg/day if no effect is seen after 6 wks.

AVAILABLE FORMS

- *Capsules:* 100 mg, 200 mg, 400 mg.

CONTRAINDICATIONS: Hypersensitivity to aspirin, NSAIDs, or sulfonamides

PREGNANCY AND LACTATION: Pregnancy category C (D if used in third trimester or near delivery); breast milk secretion unknown

SIDE EFFECTS

Frequent (greater than 5%)

Diarrhea, dyspepsia, headache, upper respiratory tract infection

Occasional (5%-1%)

Abdominal pain, flatulence, nausea, back pain, peripheral edema, dizziness, rash

SERIOUS REACTIONS

- There is an increased risk of cardiovascular events, including MI and cerebrovascular accident, and serious, potentially life-threatening, GI bleeding.

INTERACTIONS

Drugs

3 *Diuretics:* Potential reduction of both diuretic and antihypertensive effects of loop and thiazide diuretics

3 *ACE inhibitors:* May reduce antihypertensive effect of ACE inhibitors

3 *Fluconazole:* Two-fold increase in celecoxib plasma concentration due to inhibition of CYP2C9

3 *Lithium:* Steady-state lithium plasma levels increased 18%

3 *Warfarin:* Bleeding events reported, predominantly in elderly; increases in PT possible

SPECIAL CONSIDERATIONS

• COX-2 specific inhibition good choice for patients with inflammatory conditions who are at high risk of gastrointestinal adverse effects (e.g., older than 60 years, history of peptic ulcer disease, prolonged, high-dose NSAID therapy, concurrent use of corticosteroids or anticoagulants)

PATIENT/FAMILY EDUCATION

• Take celecoxib with food if GI upset occurs
• Avoid alcohol and aspirin during celecoxib therapy because these substances increase the risk of GI bleeding

MONITORING PARAMETERS

• Rheumatoid arthritis—Decreased acute phase reactants (ESR, C-reactive protein), pain relief, reduction in number of swollen joints, improved range of motion, less fatigue, functional capacity, structural damage, maintenance of normal lifestyle
• Osteoarthritis—Decreased pain and stiffness of affected joints
• Toxicity—Initial hemogram, fecal occult blood, then q6-12 mo; electrolytes and renal function tests q6-12 mo; LFTs q6-12 mo in high-risk patients; query patient for dyspepsia, nausea, vomiting, right upper abdominal pain, anorexia, fatigue, jaundice, edema, weight gain, decreased urine output

cellulose sodium phosphate

(sell'u-lose so'dee-um fos'fate)

Rx: Calcibind
Chemical Class: Phosphorylated cellulose
Therapeutic Class: Hypercalciuria

CLINICAL PHARMACOLOGY

Mechanism of Action: A nonabsorbable compound that alters urinary composition of calcium, magnesium, phosphate, and oxalate. Calcium binds to cellulose sodium phosphate, therefore preventing intestinal absorption of it. ***Therapeutic Effect:*** Prevents the formation of kidney stones.

Pharmacokinetics

Not absorbed from gastrointestinal (GI) tract. Eliminated in the feces.

INDICATIONS AND DOSAGES

Absorptive hypercalciuria Type I

Acute bleeding

PO

Adults, Elderly. Initially, 15 g/day (5 g with each meal). Decrease dosage to 10 g/day when urinary calcium is less than 150 mg/day.

AVAILABLE FORMS

• *Powder for Reconstitution:* 300 g (Calcibind).

UNLABELED USES: Absorptive hypercalciuria Type II

CONTRAINDICATIONS: Primary or secondary hyperparathyroidism, including renal hypercalciuria (renal calcium leak), hypomagnesemic states (serum magnesium <1.5 mg/dl), bone disease (osteoporosis, osteomalacia, osteitis), hypocalcemic states (e.g., hypoparathyroidism, intestinal malabsorption), normal or low intestinal absorption and renal excretion of calcium, enteric hyperoxaluria, and patients with high fasting urinary calcium or hypophosphatemia.

PREGNANCY AND LACTATION: Pregnancy category C

SIDE EFFECTS

Occasional

GI disturbance, manifested by poor taste of the drug, loose bowel movements, diarrhea, dyspepsia

SERIOUS REACTIONS

• Hyperoxaluria and hypomagnesiuria, which negate the beneficial effect of hypocalciuria on new stone formation, magnesium depletion, and depletion of trace metals (copper, zinc, iron) may occur.

INTERACTIONS

Drugs

3 *Calcium-containing medications:* May decrease effectiveness of cellulose sodium phosphate

3 *Foods high in oxalate (spinach, rhubarb, chocolate, brewed tea):* May increase risk of hyperoxaluria, which decreases the effect of cellulose sodium phosphate

3 *Magnesium:* May decrease effectiveness of magnesium

3 *Milk, dairy products:* May decrease effectiveness of cellulose sodium phosphate

SPECIAL CONSIDERATIONS

PATIENT/FAMILY EDUCATION

• Suspend each dose of CSP powder in glass of water, soft drink, or fruit juice
• Ingest within 30 min of a meal
• Avoid high-sodium foods, vitamin C, and dairy products
• Reduce intake of foods high in oxalate content such as spinach, chocolate, rhubarb, and brewed tea

MONITORING PARAMETERS

• Serum Ca, Mg, copper, zinc, iron, parathyroid hormone, CBC every 3-6 mo
• Serum parathyroid hormone should be obtained at least once between the first 2 wk to 3 mo of treatment

cephalexin

(sef-a-lex'-in)

Rx: Biocef, Keflex, Keftab

Chemical Class: Cephalosporin (1st generation)

Therapeutic Class: Antibiotic

CLINICAL PHARMACOLOGY

Mechanism of Action: A first-generation cephalosporin that binds to bacterial cell membranes and inhibits cell wall synthesis. ***Therapeutic Effect:*** Bactericidal.

Pharmacokinetics

Rapidly absorbed from the GI tract. Protein binding: 10%-15%. Widely distributed. Primarily excreted unchanged in urine. Moderately removed by hemodialysis. ***Half-life:*** 0.9-1.2 hr (increased in impaired renal function).

INDICATIONS AND DOSAGES

Bone infections, prophylaxis of rheumatic fever, follow-up to parenteral therapy

PO

Adults, Elderly. 250-500 mg q6h up to 4 g/day.

Streptococcal pharyngitis, skin and skin-structure infections, uncomplicated cystitis

PO

Adults, Elderly. 500 mg q12h.

Usual pediatric dosage

Children. 25-100 mg/kg/day in 2-4 divided doses.

Otitis media

PO

Children. 75-100 mg/kg/day in 4 divided doses.

Dosage in renal impairment

After usual initial dose, dosing frequency is modified based on creatinine clearance and the severity of the infection.

Creatinine Clearance	*Dosage Interval*
10-40 ml/min	Usual dose q8-12h
less than 10 ml/min	Usual dose q12-24h

AVAILABLE FORMS

• *Capsules:* 250 mg (Keflex), 500 mg (Biocef, Keflex).

• *Powder for Oral Suspension (Biocef, Keflex):* 125 mg/5 ml, 250 mg/5 ml.

• *Tablets:* 250 mg, 500 mg.

CONTRAINDICATIONS: History of anaphylactic reaction to penicillins or hypersensitivity to cephalosporins

PREGNANCY AND LACTATION: Pregnancy category B; excreted in breast milk

SIDE EFFECTS

Frequent

Oral candidiasis, mild diarrhea, mild abdominal cramping, vaginal candidiasis

Occasional

Nausea, serum sickness–like reaction (marked by fever and joint pain; usually occurs after the second course of therapy and resolves after the drug is discontinued)

Rare

Allergic reaction (rash, pruritus, urticaria)

SERIOUS REACTIONS

• Antibiotic-associated colitis and other superinfections may result from altered bacterial balance.

• Nephrotoxicity may occur, especially in patients with preexisting renal disease.

• Patients with a history of allergies, especially to penicillin, are at increased risk for developing a severe hypersensitivity reaction, marked by severe pruritus, angioedema, bronchospasm, and anaphylaxis.

INTERACTIONS

Drugs

3 *Aminoglycosides:* Additive nephrotoxicity

3 *Loop diuretics:* Increased nephrotoxicity

Labs

• *Increase:* Urinary amino acids

• *False positive:* Urine glucose with Benedict's, Fehlings, Clinitest

• *Decrease:* Urine leukocytes

SPECIAL CONSIDERATIONS

• First-generation oral cephalosporin of choice

PATIENT/FAMILY EDUCATION

• Space doses evenly around the clock and continue therapy for the full course of treatment

• Take the drug with food or milk if GI upset occurs

• Refrigerate oral suspension

MONITORING PARAMETERS

• Signs and symptoms of superinfection, including abdominal pain or cramping, moderate to severe diarrhea, severe anal or genital pruritus or discharge, and severe mouth or tongue soreness

• Daily bowel activity and stool consistency

• Intake and output, renal function

cephradine

(sef'-ra-deen)

Rx: Velosef

Chemical Class: Cephalosporin (1st generation)

Therapeutic Class: Antibiotic

CLINICAL PHARMACOLOGY

Mechanism of Action: A first-generation cephalosporin that binds to bacterial cell membranes. Inhibits synthesis of bacterial cell wall. ***Therapeutic Effect:*** Bactericidal.

Pharmacokinetics

Well absorbed from the gastrointestinal (GI) tract. Protein binding: 18%-20%. Widely distributed. Primarily excreted unchanged in urine. Removed by hemodialysis. ***Half-life:*** 1-2 hrs (half-life is increased with impaired renal function).

INDICATIONS AND DOSAGES

Mild, moderate, or severe infections of the respiratory and genitourinary (GU) tracts; bone, joint, and skin infections; prostatitis; otitis media

PO

Adults, Elderly. 250-500 mg q6h. Maximum: 8 g/day.

Children older than 9 mo. 25-50 mg/kg/day in divided doses q6-12h. Maximum: 4 g/day.

Dosage in renal impairment

Dosage and frequency are based on the degree of renal impairment and the severity of infection. After initial 1-g dose:

Creatinine Clearance	Dosage Interval
10-50 ml/min	250 mg q6h
0-10 ml/min	125 mg q6h

AVAILABLE FORMS

• *Capsules:* 250 mg, 500 mg (Velosef).

• *Oral Suspension:* 125 mg/5 ml, 250 mg/5ml (Velosef).

CONTRAINDICATIONS: History of hypersensitivity to penicillins and cephalosporins

PREGNANCY AND LACTATION: Pregnancy category B; excreted into breast milk in low concentrations; no adverse effects have been observed

SIDE EFFECTS

Frequent

Diarrhea, mild abdominal cramping, vaginal candidiasis (discharge, itching)

Occasional

Nausea, headache, unusual bruising or bleeding, serum sickness–like reaction (fever, joint pain)

Rare

Allergic reaction (rash, pruritus, urticaria)

SERIOUS REACTIONS

• Antibiotic-associated colitis as evidenced by severe abdominal pain and tenderness, fever, and watery and severe diarrhea, and other superinfections may result from altered bacterial balance.

• Nephrotoxicity may occur, especially in patients with preexisting renal disease.

• Severe hypersensitivity reaction, including severe pruritus, angioedema, bronchospasm, and anaphylaxis, particularly in patients with history of allergies, especially penicillin, may occur.

INTERACTIONS

Drugs

3 *Aminoglycosides:* Additive nephrotoxicity

3 *Loop diuretics:* Increased nephrotoxicity

3 *Other antibacterial agents:* May interfere with the bactericidal action of cephradine

3 *Probenecid:* Increased and prolonged blood levels of cephalosporins

SPECIAL CONSIDERATIONS

• No advantage over cephalexin; cost should be major consideration for selection of first-generation cephalosporins

PATIENT/FAMILY EDUCATION

• Continue therapy for the full length of treatment

• Space doses evenly around the clock

MONITORING PARAMETERS

• Daily bowel activity and stool consistency

• Signs and symptoms of superinfection including anal or genital pruritus, changes or ulceration of the oral mucosa, moderate to severe diarrhea, and new or increased fever

cetirizine hydrochloride

(se-ti'-ra-zeen hye-droe-klor'-ide)

Rx: Zyrtec

Combinations

Rx: with pseudoephedrine (Zyrtec-D 12 Hour Tablets)

Chemical Class: Piperazine derivative

Therapeutic Class: Antihistamine

CLINICAL PHARMACOLOGY

Mechanism of Action: A second-generation piperazine that competes with histamine for H_1-receptor sites on effector cells in the GI tract, blood vessels, and respiratory tract. ***Therapeutic Effect:*** Prevents allergic response, produces mild bronchodilation, blocks histamine-induced bronchitis.

Pharmacokinetics

Route	*Onset*	*Peak*	*Duration*
PO	less than 1 hr	4-8 hr	less than 24 hr

Rapidly and almost completely absorbed from the GI tract (absorption not affected by food). Protein binding: 93%. Undergoes low first-pass metabolism; not extensively metabolized. Primarily excreted in urine (more than 80% as unchanged drug). ***Half-life:*** 6.5-10 hr.

INDICATIONS AND DOSAGES

Allergic rhinitis, urticaria

PO

Adults, Elderly, Children older than 5 yr. Initially, 5-10 mg/day as a single or in 2 divided doses.

Children 2-5 yr. 2.5 mg/day. May increase up to 5 mg/day as a single or in 2 divided doses.

Children 12-23 mo. Initially, 2.5 mg/day. May increase up to 5 mg/day in 2 divided doses.

Children 6-11 mo. 2.5 mg once a day.

Dosage in renal or hepatic impairment

For adult and elderly patients with renal impairment (creatinine clearance of 11-31 ml/min), those receiving hemodialysis (creatinine clearance of less than 7 ml/min), and those with hepatic impairment, dosage is decreased to 5 mg once a day.

AVAILABLE FORMS

• *Syrup:* 5 mg/5 ml.

• *Tablets:* 5 mg, 10 mg.

• *Tablets (Chewable):* 5 mg, 10 mg.

UNLABELED USES: Treatment of bronchial asthma

CONTRAINDICATIONS: Hypersensitivity to cetirizine or hydroxyzine

PREGNANCY AND LACTATION: Pregnancy category B; excreted into breast milk

SIDE EFFECTS

Occasional (10%-2%)

Pharyngitis; dry mucous membranes, nose, or throat; nausea and vomiting; abdominal pain; headache; dizziness; fatigue; thickening of mucus; somnolence; photosensitivity; urine retention

SERIOUS REACTIONS

• Children may experience paradoxical reactions, including restlessness, insomnia, euphoria, nervousness, and tremor.

• Dizziness, sedation, and confusion are more likely to occur in elderly patients.

INTERACTIONS

Drugs

3 *Alcohol, other CNS depressants:* May increase CNS depression

SPECIAL CONSIDERATIONS

• H_1-antagonist with minimal effect on CNS; no affinity for other receptors
• Very potent antihistamine
• Kinetics allow qd dosing and do not have cytochrome P-450 drug interactions
• Effective against itching

PATIENT/FAMILY EDUCATION

• Avoid performing tasks that require alertness or motor skills until response to the drug has been established; cetirizine may cause drowsiness
• Avoid alcohol during cetirizine therapy
• Avoid prolonged exposure to sunlight

MONITORING PARAMETERS

• Ensure that the patient with upper respiratory allergies increases fluid intake to maintain thin secretions and offset thirst
• Monitor the patient's symptoms for a therapeutic response

cevimeline hydrochloride

(se-vim'-e-leen hye-droe-klor'-ide)

Rx: Evoxac

Chemical Class: Oxathiolane derivative

Therapeutic Class: Salivation stimulant

CLINICAL PHARMACOLOGY

Mechanism of Action: A cholinergic agonist that binds to muscarinic receptors of effector cells, thereby increasing secretion of exocrine glands, such as salivary glands. ***Therapeutic Effect:*** Relieves dry mouth.

Pharmacokinetics

Rapidly absorbed following PO administration. Protein binding: Less than 20%. Metabolized in liver. Primarily excreted in urine; minimal elimination in feces. ***Half-life:*** 5 hr.

INDICATIONS AND DOSAGES

Dry mouth

PO

Adults. 30 mg 3 times a day.

AVAILABLE FORMS

• *Capsules:* 30 mg.

CONTRAINDICATIONS: Acute iritis, angle-closure glaucoma, uncontrolled asthma

PREGNANCY AND LACTATION: Pregnancy category C; excretion into breast milk unknown, use caution in nursing mothers

SIDE EFFECTS

Frequent (19%-11%)

Diaphoresis, headache, nausea, sinusitis, rhinitis, upper respiratory tract infection, diarrhea

Occasional (10%-3%)

Dyspepsia, abdominal pain, cough, UTI, vomiting, back pain, rash, dizziness, fatigue

Rare (2%-1%)
Skeletal pain, insomnia, hot flashes, excessive salivation, rigors, anxiety

SERIOUS REACTIONS

• Cevimeline use may result in decreased visual acuity, especially at night, and impaired depth perception.

INTERACTIONS

Drugs

3 *Amiodarone, diltiazem, erythromycin, fluoxetine, itraconazole, ketoconazole, paroxetine, quinidine, ritonavir, verapamil:* May increase the effects of cevimeline

3 *Atropine, phenothiazines, tricyclic antidepressants:* May decrease the effects of cevimeline

3 *β-blockers:* Increased possibility of cardiac conduction disturbances

3 *Parasympathomimetics:* Additive pharmacologic effects

3 *Antimuscarinics:* Potential interference with desirable antimuscarinic effects

SPECIAL CONSIDERATIONS

PATIENT/FAMILY EDUCATION

• May cause visual disturbance, use caution driving at night or performing hazardous activities in reduced lighting

• Ensure adequate fluid intake to prevent dehydration, especially if drug causes excessive sweating

MONITORING PARAMETERS

• Monitor patients with a cardiovascular disease for an increase in the frequency, duration, or severity of angina or changes in blood pressure or heart rate

charcoal, activated

Combinations

OTC: with simethicone (Charcoal Plus, Flatulex); with sorbitol (Actidose with sorbitol)

Chemical Class: Carbon
Therapeutic Class: Antidiarrheal; antidote; antiflatulent

CLINICAL PHARMACOLOGY

Mechanism of Action: An antidote that adsorbs (detoxifies) ingested toxic substances, irritants, intestinal gas. ***Therapeutic Effect:*** Inhibits gastrointestinal (GI) absorption and absorbs intestinal gas.

Pharmacokinetics

Not orally absorbed from the GI tract. Not metabolized. Excreted in feces as charcoal. ***Half-life:*** Unknown.

INDICATIONS AND DOSAGES

Acute poisoning

PO

Adults, Elderly, Children 12 yrs and older. Give 30-100 g as slurry (30 g in at least 8 oz H_2O) or 12.5-50 g in aqueous or sorbitol suspension. Usually given as single dose.

Children more than 1 yr and less than 12 yrs. 25-50 g as a single dose. Smaller doses (10-25 g) may be used in children 1-5 yrs due to smaller gut lumen capacity.

AVAILABLE FORMS

• *Capsules, activated:* 260 mg (Charcocaps).

• *Granules, activated:* 15 g (CharcoAid-G).

• *Liquid, activated:* 15 g (Actidose-Aqua, Liqui-Char), 25 g (Actidose-Aqua, Kerr Insta-Char, Liqui-Char), 50 g (Actidose-Aqua, Kerr Insta-Char).

• *Liquid, activated:* 25 g (Actidose with Sorbitol, Liqui-Char, Kerr Insta-Char), 50 g (Actidose with Sorbitol, Liqui-Char, Kerr Insta-Char).
• *Pellets, activated:* 25 g (EZ-Char).
• *Powder for Suspension, activated:* 30 g, 240 g.
• *Tablets, activated:* 250 mg (Charcol Plus DS).

CONTRAINDICATIONS: Intestinal obstruction, GI tract not anatomically intact; patients at risk of hemorrhage or GI perforation, if use would increase risk and severity of aspiration; not effective for cyanide, mineral acids, caustic alkalis, organic solvents, iron, ethanol, methanol poisoning, lithium; do not use charcoal with sorbitol in patients with fructose intolerance; charcoal with sorbitol not recommended in children <1 year of age, hypersensitivity to charcoal or any component of the formation

PREGNANCY AND LACTATION: Pregnancy category C

SIDE EFFECTS

Occasional

Diarrhea, GI discomfort, intestinal gas

SERIOUS REACTIONS

• Hypernatremia, hypokalemia, and hypermagnesemia may occur with coadministration of cathartics.

INTERACTIONS

Drugs

❷ *Digitalis glycosides:* Reduced digoxin levels; less effect on digitoxin

❸ *Ipecac:* May decrease the effect of ipecac

❸ *Oral medications:* May decrease absorption of orally administered medication

SPECIAL CONSIDERATIONS

• Administer activated charcoal for adsorption in emergency management of poisonings as a slurry with water, a saline cathartic, or sorbitol

PATIENT/FAMILY EDUCATION

• Charcoal causes stool to turn black

MONITORING PARAMETERS

• Vital signs
• Electrolytes

chloral hydrate

(klor-al hye′-drate)

Rx: Aquachloral Supprettes, Somnote

Chemical Class: Halogenated alcohol

Therapeutic Class: Sedative/hypnotic

DEA Class: Schedule IV

CLINICAL PHARMACOLOGY

Mechanism of Action: A nonbarbiturate chloral derivative that produces CNS depression. ***Therapeutic Effect:*** Induces quiet, deep sleep, with only a slight decrease in respiratory rate and BP.

Pharmacokinetics

Readily absorbed from the GI tract following PO administration. Well absorbed following rectal administration. Protein binding: 70%-80%. Metabolized in liver and erythrocytes to the active metabolite, trichloroethanol, which may be further metabolized to inactive metabolites. Excreted in urine. ***Half-life:*** 7-10 hr (trichloroethanol).

INDICATIONS AND DOSAGES

Premedication for dental or medical procedures

PO, Rectal

Adults. 0.5-1 g.

Children. 75 mg/kg up to 1 g total.

Premedication for EEG

PO, Rectal

Adults. 0.5-1.5 g.

Children. 25-50 mg/kg/dose 30-60 min prior to EEG. May repeat in 30 min. Maximum: 1 g for infants, 2 g for children.

AVAILABLE FORMS
- *Capsules (Somnote):* 500 mg.
- *Syrup:* 500 mg/5 ml.
- *Suppositories (Aquachloral Supprettes):* 324 mg, 648 mg.

CONTRAINDICATIONS: Gastritis, marked hepatic or renal impairment, severe cardiac disease

PREGNANCY AND LACTATION: Pregnancy category C; excreted into breast milk; may cause mild drowsiness in infant, otherwise compatible with breast-feeding

SIDE EFFECTS

Occasional

Gastric irritation (nausea, vomiting, flatulence, diarrhea), rash, sleepwalking

Rare

Headache, paradoxical CNS hyperactivity or nervousness in children, excitement or restlessness in the elderly (particularly in patients with pain)

SERIOUS REACTIONS
- Overdose may produce somnolence, confusion, slurred speech, severe incoordination, respiratory depression, and coma.
- Allergic-type reaction may occur in those with tartrazine sensitivity.

INTERACTIONS

Drugs

3 *Ethanol:* Additive CNS-depressant effects

3 *Warfarin:* Transient increase in the hypoprothrombinemic response to warfarin

Labs
- *Interference:* Urine catecholamines, urinary 17-hydroxycorticosteroids
- *False positive:* Urine glucose (Benedict's reagent)
- *False increase:* Serum urea nitrogen, vitamin B_{12}

SPECIAL CONSIDERATIONS
- Not as effective as benzodiazepines, loses much of effectiveness for inducing and maintaining sleep after 2 weeks of use
- Frequently used preoperatively or preprocedurally in children because less paradoxical excitement (not confirmed by well-controlled studies)

PATIENT/FAMILY EDUCATION
- May cause GI upset, recommend administration with full glass of water or fruit juice, dilute syrup in a half glass of water or fruit juice

chloramphenicol

(klor-am-fen'-i-kole)

Rx: *Systemic:* AK-Chlor, Chloromycetin, Chloromycetin Ophthalmic, Chloromycetin Sodium Succinate, Chloroptic, Chloroptic S.O.P.

Combinations

Rx: Ophthalmic: Hydrocortisone acetate and polymixin B sulfate (Opthocort); hydrocortisone acetate (Chloromycetin Hydrocortisone)

Chemical Class: Dichloroacetic acid derivative

Therapeutic Class: Antibiotic

CLINICAL PHARMACOLOGY

Mechanism of Action: A dichloroacetic acid derivative that inhibits bacterial protein synthesis by binding to bacterial ribosomal receptor sites. ***Therapeutic Effect:*** Bacteriostatic (may be bactericidal in high concentrations).

Pharmacokinetics

Rapidly and completely absorbed from the GI tract following PO administration. Well absorbed after IM administration. Some systemic absorption following ophthalmic and otic administration. Protein binding: 50%-80%. Metabolized in liver. Excreted in urine. ***Half-life:*** 1.5-3.5 hr.

INDICATIONS AND DOSAGES

Mild to moderate infections caused by organisms resistant to other less toxic antibiotics

IV

Adults, Elderly. 50-100 mg/kg/day in divided doses q6h. Maximum: 4 g/day.

Children older than 1 mo. 50-75 mg/kg/day in divided doses q6h. Maximum: 4 g/day.

Meningitis

IV

Children older than 1 mo. 50-100 mg/kg/day in divided doses q6h.

Usual ophthalmic dosage

Adults, Elderly, Children. 1-2 drops 4-6 times/day.

AVAILABLE FORMS

- *Powder for Injection (Chloromycetin Sodium Succinate):* 1 g.
- *Powder for Reconstitution (Ophthalmic [Chloromycetin Ophthalmic]):* 25 mg.
- *Ophthalmic Ointment (AK-Chlor, Chloroptic S.O.P., Ocu-Chlor):* 1%.
- *Ophthalmic Solution (Chloroptic, AK-Chlor, Ocu-Chlor):* 0.5%.

CONTRAINDICATIONS: Hypersensitivity to chloramphenicol

PREGNANCY AND LACTATION: Pregnancy category C; use caution at term due to potential for "gray baby syndrome" toxicity; excreted into breast milk; milk levels are too low to precipitate the "gray baby syndrome," but a theoretical risk does exist for bone marrow depression

SIDE EFFECTS

Occasional

Systemic: Nausea, vomiting, diarrhea

Ophthalmic: Blurred vision, burning, stinging, hypersensitivity reaction

Otic: Hypersensitivity reaction

Rare

Peripheral neuritis (numbness and weakness in feet and hands), rash, shortness of breath, confusion, headache, optic neuritis (blurred vision, eye pain)

SERIOUS REACTIONS

Alert: Be aware that "gray baby" syndrome (characterized as abdominal distention, progressive cyanosis, vasomotor collapse, unresponsiveness) may occur if chloramphenicol is given to children younger than 2 years or to neonates.

- Superinfection due to bacterial or fungal overgrowth may occur.
- There is a narrow margin between effective therapy and toxic levels producing blood dyscrasias.
- Myelosuppression, with resulting aplastic anemia, hypoplastic anemia, and pancytopenia, may occur weeks or months later.

INTERACTIONS

Drugs

3 *Barbiturates:* Increased serum barbiturate concentrations; reduced serum chloramphenicol concentrations

3 *Ceftazidime:* Inhibited antibacterial activity

3 *Cimetidine:* Increased risk of myelosuppression

3 *Penicillins:* Inhibited antibacterial activity of penicillins

3 *Phenytoin:* Predictable increases in serum phenytoin concentrations, toxicity has occurred

3 *Rifampin:* Reduced chloramphenicol concentrations

3 *Sulfonylureas:* Increased hypoglycemic effects of tolbutamide and chlorpropamide

❷ *Warfarin:* Enhanced hypoprothrombinemic response to warfarin and possibly other oral anticoagulants

Labs

- *False positive:* Urine glucose (copper reduction)
- *False decrease:* Serum folate, serum urea nitrogen, serum uric acid
- *False increase:* 17-ketosteroids, CSF protein, serum protein, serum urea nitrogen

SPECIAL CONSIDERATIONS

- Because of severe adverse effects (e.g., aplastic anemia) not indicated for less serious infections; aplastic anemia reported with topical use

PATIENT/FAMILY EDUCATION

- Space doses evenly around the clock

MONITORING PARAMETERS

- CBC with platelets and reticulocytes before and frequently during therapy (discontinue drug if bone marrow depression occurs); serum iron and iron-binding globulin saturation may also be useful
- Serum drug level (peak 10-20 mcg/ml, trough 5-10 mcg/ml) weekly (more often in impaired hepatic, renal systems)
- Early signs of "gray baby syndrome" (cyanosis, abdominal distension, irregular respiration, failure to feed), ***drug should be discontinued immediately***
- Daily bowel activity and stool consistency

chlordiazepoxide hydrochloride

(klor-dye-az-e-pox'-ide hye-droe-klor'-ide)

Rx: Libritabs, Librium, Mitran, Reposaus-10

Combinations

Rx: with amitriptyline (Limbitrol DS 10-25); with clidinium (Clindex, Librax)

Chemical Class: Benzodiazepine

Therapeutic Class: Anxiolytic

DEA Class: Schedule IV

CLINICAL PHARMACOLOGY

Mechanism of Action: A benzodiazepine that enhances the action of the inhibitory neurotransmitter gamma-aminobutyric acid in the CNS. ***Therapeutic Effect:*** Produces anxiolytic effect.

Pharmacokinetics

Well absorbed from the GI tract following PO administration. Poor absorption following IM administration. Protein binding: 90%-98%. Extensively metabolized in liver. Excreted in urine. Not removed by hemodialysis. ***Half-life:*** 10-48 hr.

INDICATIONS AND DOSAGES

Alcohol withdrawal symptoms

PO

Adults, Elderly. 50-100 mg. May repeat q2-4h. Maximum: 300 mg/24 hr.

Anxiety

PO

Adults. 15-100 mg/day in 3-4 divided doses.

Elderly. 5 mg 2-4 times a day.

IV, IM

Adults. Initially, 50-100 mg, then 25-50 mg 3-4 times a day as needed.

Preoperative anxiety

IM

Adults, Elderly. 50-100 mg once.

AVAILABLE FORMS

- *Capsules:* 5 mg (Librium), 10 mg (Libritabs, Librium), 25 mg (Librium).
- *Injection Powder for Reconstitution (Librium):* 100 mg.

UNLABELED USES: Treatment of panic disorder, tension headache, tremors

CONTRAINDICATIONS: Acute alcohol intoxication, acute angle-closure glaucoma

PREGNANCY AND LACTATION: Pregnancy category D; excreted into breast milk; drug and metabolites may accumulate to toxic levels in nursing infant

SIDE EFFECTS

Frequent

Pain at IM injection site; somnolence, ataxia, dizziness, confusion with oral dose (particularly in elderly or debilitated patients)

Occasional

Rash, peripheral edema, GI disturbances

Rare

Paradoxical CNS reactions, such as hyperactivity or nervousness in children and excitement or restlessness in the elderly (generally noted during first 2 weeks of therapy, particularly in presence of uncontrolled pain)

SERIOUS REACTIONS

- IV administration may produce pain, swelling, thrombophlebitis, and carpal tunnel syndrome.
- Abrupt or too-rapid withdrawal may result in pronounced restlessness, irritability, insomnia, hand tremors, abdominal or muscle cramps, diaphoresis, vomiting, and seizures.
- Overdose results in somnolence, confusion, diminished reflexes, and coma.

INTERACTIONS

Drugs

3 *Cimetidine:* Increased plasma levels of chlordiazepoxide and/or active metabolites

3 *Disulfiram:* Increased serum chlordiazepoxide concentrations

3 *Ethanol:* Enhanced adverse psychomotor side effects of benzodiazepines

3 *Fluconazole, itraconazole, ketoconazole:* Increased chlordiazepoxide concentrations

3 *Levodopa:* Potential for exacerbation of parkinsonism in patients taking levodopa

Labs

- *False increase:* Urine 5-HIAA, urine 17-ketogenic steroids
- *False decrease:* Urine 17-ketogenic steroids
- *False positive:* Urine pregnancy tests

SPECIAL CONSIDERATIONS

- No advantage over diazepam; poor choice for elderly patients
- Do not use for everyday stress or use longer than 4 mo
- Do not discontinue medication abruptly after long-term use

PATIENT/FAMILY EDUCATION

- Change positions slowly—from recumbent to sitting before standing—to prevent dizziness
- Avoid alcohol while taking this drug

chloroquine/ chloroquine phosphate

(klor'-oh-kwin)

Rx: Aralen hydrochloride, Aralen phosphate

Chemical Class: 4-aminoquinoline derivative

Therapeutic Class: Amebicide; antimalarial

CLINICAL PHARMACOLOGY

Mechanism of Action: An amebecide that concentrates in parasite acid vesicles and may interfere with parasite protein synthesis. ***Therapeutic Effect:*** Increases pH and inhibits parasite growth.

Pharmacokinetics

Rate of absorption is variable. Chloroquine is almost completely absorbed from the gastrointestinal (GI) tract. Protein binding: 50%-65%. Widely distributed into body tissues such as eyes, heart, kidneys, liver, and lungs. Partially metabolized to active de-ethylated metabolites (principal metabolite is desethylchloroquine). Excreted in urine. Removed by hemodialysis. ***Half-life:*** 1-2 mos.

INDICATIONS AND DOSAGES

Chloroquine phosphate

Treatment of malaria (acute attack): Dose (mg base)

Dose	Time	Adults	Children
Initial	Day 1	600 mg	10 mg/kg
Second	6 hr later	300 mg	5 mg/kg
Third	Day 2	300 mg	5 mg/kg
Fourth	Day 3	300 mg	5 mg/kg

Suppression of malaria

PO

Adults. 300 mg (base)/wk on same day each week beginning 2 wks before exposure; continue for 6-8 wks after leaving endemic area.

Children. 5 mg (base)/kg/wk.

Malaria prophylaxis

PO

Adults. 600 mg base initially given in 2 divided doses 6 hrs apart.

Children. 10 mg base/kg.

Amebiasis

PO

Adults. 1 g (600 mg base) daily for 2 days; then, 500 mg (300 mg base)/day for at least 2-3 wks.

Chloroquine HCL

Treatment of malaria IM

Adults. Initially, 160-200 mg base (4-5 ml), repeat in 6 hrs. Maximum: 800 mg base in first 24 hrs. Begin oral therapy as soon as possible and continue for 3 days until approximately 1.5 g base given.

Children. Initially, 5 mg base/kg, repeat in 6 hrs. Do not exceed 10 mg base/kg/24 hrs.

Amebiasis

IM

Adults. 160-200 mg base (4-5 ml) daily for 10-12 days. Change to oral therapy as soon as possible.

AVAILABLE FORMS

• *Tablets:* 250 mg, 500 mg (Aralen).

UNLABELED USES: Treatment of sarcoid-associated hypercalcemia, juvenile arthritis, rheumatoid arthritis, systemic lupus erythematosus, solar urticaria, chronic cutaneous vasculitis

CONTRAINDICATIONS: Hypersensitivity to 4-aminoquinoline compounds, retinal or visual field changes

PREGNANCY AND LACTATION: Pregnancy category C; excreted into

breast milk; average infant consumption considered safe
NOTE: Does not protect infant against malaria

SIDE EFFECTS

Frequent
Discomfort with IM administration, mild transient headache, anorexia, nausea, vomiting

Occasional
Visual disturbances (blurring, difficulty focusing); nervousness, fatigue, pruritus, esp. of palms, soles, scalp; bleaching of hair, irritability, personality changes, diarrhea, skin eruptions

Rare
Phlebitis or thrombophlebitis at IV injection site, abdominal cramps, headache, hypotension

SERIOUS REACTIONS

- Ocular toxicity and ototoxicity have been reported.
- Prolonged therapy: peripheral neuritis and neuromyopathy, hypotension, ECG changes, agranulocytosis, aplastic anemia, thrombocytopenia, convulsions, psychosis.
- Overdosage includes symptoms of headache, vomiting, visual disturbance, drowsiness, convulsions, hypokalemia followed by cardiovascular collapse, and death.

INTERACTIONS

Drugs

3 *Chlorpromazine:* Increased chlorpromazine concentrations
3 *Cyclosporine:* Elevates cyclosporine levels, toxicity possible
3 *Methotrexate:* Decreased methotrexate levels
3 *Praziquantel:* Decreased praziquantel absorption

SPECIAL CONSIDERATIONS

- Certain strains of *P. falciparum* have become resistant to chloroquine

MONITORING PARAMETERS

- Ophthalmic examinations (visual acuity, slit lamp, funduscopic, visual fields) and CBC if long-term treatment or drug dosage >150 mg/day

chlorothiazide

(klor-oh-thye'-a-zide)

Rx: Diuril, Diuril Sodium
Combinations
Rx: with methyldopa (Aldoclor); with reserpine (Chloroserp, Diaserp, Diupres)

Chemical Class: Sulfonamide derivative
Therapeutic Class: Antihypertensive; diuretic, thiazide

CLINICAL PHARMACOLOGY

Mechanism of Action: A sulfonamide derivative that acts as a thiazide diuretic and antihypertensive. As a diuretic blocks reabsorption of water, the electrolytes sodium and potassium at cortical diluting segment of distal tubule. As an antihypertensive reduces plasma, extracellular fluid volume, decreases peripheral vascular resistance (PVR) by direct effect on blood vessels. ***Therapeutic Effect:*** Promotes diuresis, reduces blood pressure (BP).

Pharmacokinetics
Poorly absorbed from the gastrointestinal (GI) tract. Not metabolized. Primarily excreted unchanged in urine. Not removed by hemodialysis. ***Half-life:*** 45-120 min.

INDICATIONS AND DOSAGES

Edema, hypertension
PO
Adults. 0.5-1 g 1-2 times/day. May give every other day or 3-5 days/wk.

Children 12 yrs and older. 10-20 mg/kg/dose in divided doses q8-12h. Maximum: 2 g/day.
Children 2-12 yrs. 1 g/day.
Children 6 mos-2 yrs. 10-20 mg/kg/day in divided doses q12-24h. Maximum: 375 mg/day.
Children younger than 6 mos. 20-30 mg/kg/day in divided doses q12h. Maximum: 375 mg/day.

Hypertension

IV

Adults. 0.5-1 g in divided doses q12-24h.

AVAILABLE FORMS

• *Powder for Injection, lyophilized:* 0.5 g.
• *Oral Suspension:* 250 mg/5 ml (Diuril).
• *Tablets:* 250 mg, 500 mg (Diuril).

UNLABELED USES: Treatment of diabetes insipidus, prevention of calcium-containing renal stones

CONTRAINDICATIONS: Anuria, history of hypersensitivity to sulfonamides or thiazide diuretics, renal decompensation

PREGNANCY AND LACTATION: Pregnancy category C; therapy for preexisting hypertension can be continued throughout pregnancy with minimal risk; initiating for simple edema not recommended; few unequivocal indications for diuretic therapy in pregnancy except for pulmonary edema or congestive heart failure; excreted in low concentrations in breast milk; compatible with breast-feeding

SIDE EFFECTS

Expected

Increase in urine frequency and volume

Frequent

Potassium depletion

Occasional

Postural hypotension, headache, gastrointestinal (GI) disturbances, photosensitivity reaction, muscle spasms, alopecia, rash, urticaria

SERIOUS REACTIONS

• Vigorous diuresis may lead to profound water loss and electrolyte depletion, resulting in hypokalemia, hyponatremia, and dehydration.
• Acute hypotensive episodes may occur.
• Hyperglycemia may be noted during prolonged therapy.
• GI upset, pancreatitis, dizziness, paresthesias, headache, blood dyscrasias, pulmonary edema, allergic pneumonitis, and dermatologic reactions occur rarely.
• Overdosage can lead to lethargy and coma without changes in electrolytes or hydration.

INTERACTIONS

Drugs

❷ *Angiotensin-converting enzyme inhibitors:* Risk of postural hypotension when added to ongoing diuretic therapy; more common with loop diuretics; first-dose hypotension possible in patients with sodium depletion or hypovolemia caused by diuretics or sodium restriction; hypotensive response is usually transient; hold diuretic day of first dose

③ *Calcium (high doses):* Risk of milk-alkali syndrome; monitor for hypercalcemia

③ *Carbenoxolone:* Additive potassium wasting; severe hypokalemia

③ *Cholestyramine/colestipol:* Reduced serum concentrations of thiazide diuretics

③ *Corticosteroids:* Concomitant therapy may result in excessive potassium loss

③ *Diazoxide:* Hyperglycemia

③ *Digitalis glycosides:* Diuretic-induced hypokalemia may increase the risk of digitalis toxicity

3 *Hypoglycemic agents:* Thiazide diuretics tend to increase blood glucose, may increase dosage requirements of antidiabetic drugs

3 *Lithium:* Increases serum lithium concentrations; toxicity may occur

3 *Methotrexate:* Increased bone marrow suppression

3 *Nonsteroidal antiinflammatory drugs:* Concurrent use may reduce diuretic and antihypertensive effects

Labs

- *Interference:* Urine 17-hydroxycorticosteroids
- *False decrease:* Urine estriol

SPECIAL CONSIDERATIONS

- Doses above 250 mg provide no further blood pressure reduction, but are more likely to induce metabolic disturbance (i.e., hypokalemia, hyperuricemia.)
- May protect against osteoporotic hip fractures
- Loop diuretics or metolazone more effective if CrCl <40-50 ml/min

PATIENT/FAMILY EDUCATION

- Will increase urination temporarily (approximately 3 wk); take early in the day to prevent sleep disturbance
- May cause sensitivity to sunlight; avoid prolonged exposure to the sun and other ultraviolet light
- May cause gout attacks; notify clinician if sudden joint pain occurs

MONITORING PARAMETERS

- Weight, urine output, serum electrolytes, BUN, creatinine, CBC, uric acid, glucose, lipids

chloroxine

(klor-ox´-ine)

Rx: Capitrol

Chemical Class: Hydroxyquinoline derivative

Therapeutic Class: Antiseborrheic

CLINICAL PHARMACOLOGY

Mechanism of Action: An antifungal that reduces scaling of the epidermis by slowing down mitotic activity. ***Therapeutic Effect:*** Reduces the excess scaling in patients with dandruff or seborrheic dermatitis.

Pharmacokinetics

No studies have investigated the absorption/pharmacokinetics of chloroxine.

INDICATIONS AND DOSAGES

Dandruff, seborrheic dermatitis

Adults. Shampoo affected area twice weekly.

AVAILABLE FORMS

- *Shampoo:* 2% (Capitrol).

UNLABELED USES: Not known

CONTRAINDICATIONS: Acutely inflamed lesions, hypersensitivity to chloroxine or any one of its components

PREGNANCY AND LACTATION: Pregnancy category C; excretion into breast milk unknown

SIDE EFFECTS

Discoloration of light hair, skin irritation, burning

SERIOUS REACTIONS

- None known.

SPECIAL CONSIDERATIONS

PATIENT/FAMILY EDUCATION

- Improvement may not occur for 14 days
- Hair may be discolored after use
- Avoid contact with eyes

MONITORING PARAMETERS

- Skin for irritation
- Hair for discoloration

chlorpheniramine maleate

(klor-fen-ir'-a-meen mal'-ee-ate)

OTC: Aller-Chlor, Chlor-Trimeton, Chlor-Trimeton Allergy, Chlor-Trimeton Allergy 12 Hour, Chlor-Trimeton Allergy 8 Hour, Chlorate, Chlorphen, Diabetic Tussin Allergy Relief

Combinations

Rx: with codeine (Codeprex); with hydrocodone (Tussionex); with phenylephrine and pyrilamine (Rynaton); with phenylpropanolamine (Ornade, Resaid S.R.); with pseudoephedrine (Deconamine, Fedahist)

OTC: with pseudoephedrine (Chlor-Trimeton, Dorcol Children's Cold Formula Liquid, Fedahist)

Chemical Class: Alkylamine derivative

Therapeutic Class: Antihistamine

CLINICAL PHARMACOLOGY

Mechanism of Action: A propylamine derivative antihistamine that competes with histamine for histamine receptor sites on cells in the blood vessels, gastrointestinal (GI) tract, and respiratory tract. ***Therapeutic Effect:*** Inhibits symptoms associated with seasonal allergic rhinitis such as increased mucus production and sneezing.

Pharmacokinetics

Well absorbed after PO and parenteral administration. Food delays absorption. Widely distributed. Metabolized in liver. Primarily excreted in urine. Not removed by dialysis. ***Half-life:*** 20 hrs.

INDICATIONS AND DOSAGES

Allergic rhinitis, common cold

PO

Adults, Elderly. 4 mg q6-8h or 8-12 mg (sustained-release) q8-12h. Maximum: 24 mg/day.

Children 12 yrs and older. 4 mg q6-8h or 8 mg (sustained-release) q12h. Maximum: 24 mg/day.

Children 6-11 yrs. 2 mg q4-6h. Maximum: 12 mg/day.

IM/IV/SC

Adults, Elderly. 5-40 mg as a single dose. Maximum: 40 mg/day.

SC

Children 6 yrs and older. 87.5 mcg/kg or 2.5 mg/m^2 4 times/day.

AVAILABLE FORMS

- *Injection:* 10 mg/ml, 100 mg/ml.
- *Syrup:* 2 mg/5 ml (Aller-Chlor, Diabetic Tussin Allergy Relief [sugar free]).
- *Tablets:* 4 mg (Aller-Chlor, Chlor-Trimeton, Chlorate, Chlorphen).
- *Tablets (Sustained-Release):* 8 mg (Chlor-Trimeton Allergy 8 Hour), 12 mg (Chlor-Trimeton Allergy 12 Hour).

CONTRAINDICATIONS: Hypersensitivity to chlorpheniramine or its components

PREGNANCY AND LACTATION: Pregnancy category C

SIDE EFFECTS

Frequent

Drowsiness, dizziness, muscular weakness, hypotension, dry mouth, nose, throat, and lips, urinary retention, thickening of bronchial secretions

Elderly: Sedation, dizziness, hypotension

Occasional

Epigastric distress, flushing, visual or hearing disturbances, paresthesia, diaphoresis, chills

SERIOUS REACTIONS

- Children may experience dominant paradoxical reactions, including restlessness, insomnia, euphoria, nervousness, and tremors.
- Overdosage in children may result in hallucinations, seizures, and death.
- Hypersensitivity reaction, such as eczema, pruritus, rash, cardiac disturbances, and photosensitivity, may occur.
- Overdosage may vary from CNS depression, including sedation, apnea, hypotension, cardiovascular collapse, or death to severe paradoxical reaction, such as hallucinations, tremor, and seizures.

SPECIAL CONSIDERATIONS

- More potent antihistamine than nonsedating agents (e.g., fexofenidine), good first-line choice for allergic rhinitis

PATIENT/FAMILY EDUCATION

- Tolerance develops to sedation with chronic use
- Dizziness, drowsiness, and dry mouth are expected responses to the drug
- Avoid tasks that require mental alertness or motor skills until response to the drug is established

chlorpromazine

(klor-proe'-ma-zeen)

Rx: Thorazine

Chemical Class: Aliphatic phenothiazine derivative

Therapeutic Class: Antiemetic; antipsychotic

CLINICAL PHARMACOLOGY

Mechanism of Action: A phenothiazine that blocks dopamine neurotransmission at postsynaptic dopamine receptor sites. Possesses strong anticholinergic, sedative, and antiemetic effects; moderate extrapyramidal effects; and slight antihistamine action. ***Therapeutic Effect:*** Relieves nausea and vomiting; improves psychotic conditions; controls intractable hiccups and porphyria.

Pharmacokinetics

Rapidly absorbed after oral or IM administration. Protein binding: 92%-97%. Metabolized in the liver. Excreted in urine. ***Half-life:*** 6 hr.

INDICATIONS AND DOSAGES

Severe nausea or vomiting

PO

Adults, Elderly. 10-25 mg q4-6h.

Children. 0.5-1 mg/kg q4-6h.

IV, IM

Adults, Elderly. 25-50 mg q4-6h.

Children. 0.5-1 mg/kg q6-8h.

Rectal

Adults, Elderly. 50-100 mg q6-8h.

Children. 1 mg/kg q6-8h.

Psychotic disorders

PO

Adults, Elderly. 30-800 mg/day in 1-4 divided doses.

Children older than 6 mo. 0.5-1 mg/kg q4-6h.

IV, IM

Adults, Elderly. Initially, 25 mg; may repeat in 1-4 hr. May gradually increase to 400 mg q4-6h. Usual dose: 300-800 mg/day.

Children older than 6 mo. 0.5-1 mg/kg q6-8h. Maximum: 75 mg/day for children 5-12 yr; 40 mg/day for children younger than 5 yr.

Intractable hiccups

PO, IV, IM

Adults. 25-50 mg 3 times a day.

Porphyria

PO

Adults. 25-50 mg 3-4 times a day.

IM

Adults, Elderly. 25 mg 3-4 times a day.

AVAILABLE FORMS
• *Oral Concentrate:* 30 mg/ml, 100 mg/ml.
• *Syrup:* 10 mg/5 ml.
• *Tablets:* 10 mg, 25 mg, 50 mg, 100 mg, 200 mg.
• *Capsules (Sustained-Release):* 30 mg, 75 mg, 150 mg.
• *Injection:* 25 mg/ml.
• *Suppositories:* 25 mg, 100 mg.

UNLABELED USES: Treatment of choreiform movement of Huntington's disease

CONTRAINDICATIONS: Comatose states, myelosuppression, severe cardiovascular disease, severe CNS depression, subcortical brain damage

PREGNANCY AND LACTATION: Pregnancy category C; enters breast milk in small concentrations; report of drowsy and lethargic infant who consumed milk with 92 ng/ml concentration

SIDE EFFECTS

Frequent

Somnolence, blurred vision, hypotension, color vision or night vision disturbances, dizziness, decreased sweating, constipation, dry mouth, nasal congestion

Occasional

Urinary retention, photosensitivity, rash, decreased sexual function, swelling or pain in breasts, weight gain, nausea, vomiting, abdominal pain, tremors

SERIOUS REACTIONS
• Extrapyramidal symptoms appear to be dose related and are divided into three categories: akathisia (including inability to sit still, tapping of feet), parkinsonian symptoms (such as masklike face, tremors, shuffling gait, hypersalivation), and acute dystonias (including torticollis, opisthotonos, and oculogyric crisis). A dystonic reaction may also produce diaphoresis and pallor.
• Tardive dyskinesia, including tongue protrusion, puffing of the cheeks, and puckering of the mouth is a rare reaction that may be irreversible.
• Abrupt discontinuation after long-term therapy may precipitate nausea, vomiting, gastritis, dizziness, and tremors.
• Blood dyscrasias, particularly agranulocytosis and mild leukopenia, may occur.
• Chlorpromazine may lower the seizure threshold.

INTERACTIONS

Drugs

3 *Amodiaquine, chloroquine, sulfadoxine-pyrimethamine:* Increased chlorpromazine concentrations

3 *Anticholinergics:* May inhibit neuroleptic response; excess anticholinergic effects

3 *Antidepressants:* Potential for increased therapeutic and toxic effects from increased levels of both drugs

3 *Antithyroid agents:* May increase the risk of agranulocytosis

3 *Barbiturates:* Decreased neuroleptic levels

3 *Cigarette smoking:* Reduces drowsiness and hypotension associated with chlorpromazine

3 *Clonidine, guanadrel, guanethidine:* Severe hypotensive episodes possible

3 *Epinephrine:* Blunted pressor response to epinephrine

3 *Ethanol:* Additive CNS depression

2 *Levodopa:* Inhibited antiparkinsonian effect of levodopa

3 *Lithium:* Lowered levels of both drugs, rarely neurotoxicity in acute mania

3 *Narcotic analgesics:* Hypotension and increased CNS depression

3 *Orphenadrine:* Lower neuroleptic concentrations, excessive anticholinergic effects

3 *Propranolol:* Increased plasma levels of both drugs with accentuated responses

Labs

- *False decrease:* 5-HIAA, vitamin B_{12}
- *Interference:* 17-ketogenic steroids
- *False increase:* Urine bilirubin, cholesterol, urine porphobilinogen, CSF protein, urine protein
- *False positive:* Ferric chloride test, guiacols spot test, phenylketones

SPECIAL CONSIDERATIONS

PATIENT/FAMILY EDUCATION

- Orthostasis on rising, especially in elderly
- Avoid hot tubs, hot showers, tub baths
- Meticulous oral hygiene; frequent rinsing of mouth, sugarless gum for dry mouth
- Use a sunscreen and sunglasses
- Urine may turn pink or red
- Drowsiness generally subsides with continued therapy
- Avoid tasks that require mental alertness or motor skills until response to the drug is established
- Avoid alcohol

MONITORING PARAMETERS

- Blood pressure
- CBC
- Therapeutic serum level for chlorpromazine is 50-300 mcg/ml, and the toxic serum level is greater than 750 mcg/ml

chlorpropamide

(klor-proe′-pa-mide)

Rx: Diabinese

Chemical Class: Sulfonylurea (1st generation)

Therapeutic Class: Antidiabetic; hypoglycemic

CLINICAL PHARMACOLOGY

Mechanism of Action: A first-generation sulfonylurea that promotes release of insulin from beta cells of pancreas. ***Therapeutic Effect:*** Lowers blood glucose concentration.

Pharmacokinetics

Rapidly absorbed from the gastrointestinal (GI) tract. Protein binding: 60%-90%. Extensively metabolized in liver. Excreted primarily in urine. Removed by hemodialysis. ***Half-life:*** 30-42 hrs.

INDICATIONS AND DOSAGES

Diabetes mellitus, combination therapy

PO

Adults. Initially, 250 mg once a day. Maintenance: 250-500 mg once a day. Maximum: 750 mg/day.

Elderly. Initially, 100-125 mg once a day. Maintenance: 100-250 mg once a day. Increase or decrease by 50-125 mg a day for 3-5 day intervals.

Renal function impairment

Not recommended.

AVAILABLE FORMS

- *Tablets:* 100 mg, 250 mg (Diabenese).

UNLABELED USES: Neurogenic diabetes insipidus

CONTRAINDICATIONS: Diabetic complications, such as ketosis, acidosis, and diabetic coma, severe liver or renal impairment, sole therapy for type 1 diabetes mellitus, or hypersensitivity to sulfonylureas

PREGNANCY AND LACTATION: Pregnancy category C; inappropriate for use during pregnancy due to inadequate blood glucose control, potential for prolonged neonatal hypoglycemia, and risk of congenital abnormalities; insulin is the drug of choice for control of blood sugars during pregnancy; breast milk reported at 17% of plasma; the potential for neonatal hypoglycemia dictates caution in nursing mothers

SIDE EFFECTS

Frequent

Headache, upper respiratory tract infection

Occasional

Sinusitis, myalgia (muscle aches), pharyngitis, aggravated diabetes mellitus

SERIOUS REACTIONS

• Possible increased risk of cardiovascular mortality with this class of drugs.

• Overdosage can cause severe hypoglycemia prolonged by extended half-life.

INTERACTIONS

Drugs

3 *Anabolic steroids, β-blockers, chloramphenicol, fibric acid derivatives, MAOIs, salicylates, sulfonamides:* Enhanced hypoglycemic effect

▲ *Ethanol:* Altered glycemic control, most commonly hypoglycemia; disulfiram-like reaction may occur

3 *Erythromycin:* Hepatic toxicity has occurred during concomitant administration of erythromycin ethylsuccinate and chlorpropamide

3 *Halofenate:* Increased sulfonylurea concentrations

2 *NSAIDs:* Enhanced hypoglycemic effect

3 *Oral contraceptives:* May increase blood glucose

3 *Thiazide diuretics:* Increased glucose concentrations, may increase dose requirements

Labs

• *False increase:* Serum calcium

SPECIAL CONSIDERATIONS

• Due to potential for prolonged hypoglycemia, other sulfonylureas should be considered before trying chlorpropamide (especially in the elderly)

PATIENT/FAMILY EDUCATION

• Multiple drug interactions, including alcohol and salicylates

• Symptoms of hypoglycemia: tingling lips/tongue, nausea, confusion, fatigue, sweating, hunger, visual changes (spots)

• Carry candy, sugar packets, or other sugar supplements for immediate response to hypoglycemia

• Notify the physician if abdominal or chest pain, dark urine or light stool, hypoglycemia reactions, fever, nausea, palpitations, rash, vomiting, or yellowing of eyes or skin occurs

MONITORING PARAMETERS

• Self-monitored blood glucose; glycosolated hemoglobin q3-6 mo

• Liver function

chlorthalidone

(klor-thal'-i-doan)

Rx: Hygroton, Thalitone

Combinations

Rx: with atenolol (Tenoretic); with clonidine (Combipres, Chlorpres); with reserpine (Demi-Regroton, Regroton)

Chemical Class: Phthalimidine derivative

Therapeutic Class: Antihypertensive; diuretic, thiazide

CLINICAL PHARMACOLOGY

Mechanism of Action: A thiazide diuretic that blocks reabsorption of sodium, potassium, and water at the distal convoluted tubule; also decreases plasma and extracellular fluid volume and peripheral vascular resistance. ***Therapeutic Effect:*** Produces diuresis; lowers BP.

Pharmacokinetics

Route	*Onset*	*Peak*	*Duration*
PO (diuretic)	2 hr	2-6 hr	Up to 36 hr

Rapidly absorbed from the GI tract. Excreted unchanged in urine. ***Half-life:*** 35-50 hr. Onset of antihypertensive effect: 3-4 days; optimal therapeutic effect: 3-4 wk.

INDICATIONS AND DOSAGES

Hypertension, edema

PO

Adults. 25-100 mg/day or 100 mg 3 times a week.

Elderly. Initially, 12.5-25 mg/day or every other day.

AVAILABLE FORMS

• *Tablets (Hygroton, Thalitone):* 15 mg, 25 mg, 50 mg, 100 mg.

CONTRAINDICATIONS: Anuria, history of hypersensitivity to sulfonamides or thiazide diuretics, renal decompensation

PREGNANCY AND LACTATION: Pregnancy category B (D if used in pregnancy-induced hypertension); therapy for preexisting hypertension can be continued throughout pregnancy with minimal risk; initiating for simple edema not recommended; few unequivocal indications for diuretic therapy in pregnancy except for pulmonary edema or congestive heart failure; compatible with breast-feeding.

SIDE EFFECTS

Expected

Increase in urinary frequency and urine volume

Frequent

Potassium depletion (rarely produces symptoms)

Occasional

Anorexia, impotence, diarrhea, orthostatic hypotension, GI disturbances, photosensitivity

Rare

Rash

SERIOUS REACTIONS

• Vigorous diuresis may lead to profound water and electrolyte depletion, resulting in hypokalemia, hyponatremia, and dehydration.

• Acute hypotensive episodes may occur.

• Hyperglycemia may occur during prolonged therapy.

• Overdose can lead to lethargy and coma without changes in electrolytes or hydration.

INTERACTIONS

Drugs

❷ *Angiotensin-converting enzyme inhibitors:* Risk of postural hypotension when added to ongoing diuretic therapy; more common with loop diuretics; first-dose hypotension possible in patients with sodium depletion or hypovolemia due to diuretics or sodium restriction;

hypotensive response is usually transient; hold diuretic day of first dose

3 *Calcium:* Increased risk of milk-alkali syndrome

3 *Carbenoxolone:* Additive potassium wasting, severe hypokalemia

3 *Cholestyramine, colestipol:* Reduced absorption

3 *Corticosteroids:* Concomitant therapy may result in excessive potassium loss

3 *Diazoxide:* Hyperglycemia

3 *Digitalis glycosides:* Diuretic-induced hypokalemia increases risk of digitalis toxicity

3 *Hypoglycemic agents:* Increased dosage requirements due to increased glucose levels

3 *Lithium:* Increased lithium levels, potential toxicity

3 *Methotrexate:* Increased risk of bone marrow depression

3 *Nonsteroidal antiinflammatory drugs:* Concurrent use may reduce diuretic and antihypertensive effects

Labs

• *False decrease:* urine esriol

SPECIAL CONSIDERATIONS

• Doses above 25 mg provide no further blood pressure reduction, but are more likely to induce metabolic disturbance (i.e., hypokalemia, hyperuricemia)

• May protect against osteoporotic hip fractures

• Loop diuretics or metolazone more effective if CrCl <40-50 ml/min

PATIENT/FAMILY EDUCATION

• Will increase urination temporarily (approximately 3 wk); take early in the day to prevent sleep disturbance

• May cause sensitivity to sunlight; avoid prolonged exposure to the sun and other ultraviolet light

• May cause gout attacks; notify clinician if sudden joint pain occurs

• Take chlorthalidone with food to avoid GI distress, preferably early in the morning to avoid nighttime urination

• Change positions slowly to reduce the drug's hypotensive effect

MONITORING PARAMETERS

• Weight, urine output, serum electrolytes, BUN, creatinine, CBC, uric acid, glucose, lipids

chlorzoxazone

(klor-zox′-a-zone)

Rx: Parafon Forte DSC, Remular, Remular-S

Chemical Class: Benzoxazole derivative

Therapeutic Class: Skeletal muscle relaxant

CLINICAL PHARMACOLOGY

Mechanism of Action: A skeletal muscle relaxant that inhibits transmission of reflexes at the spinal cord level. ***Therapeutic Effect:*** Relieves muscle spasticity.

Pharmacokinetics

Readily absorbed from the gastrointestinal (GI) tract. Metabolized in liver. Primarily excreted in urine. ***Half-life:*** 1.1 hrs.

INDICATIONS AND DOSAGES

Musculoskeletal pain

PO

Adults, Elderly. 250-500 mg 3-4 times/day. Maximum: 750 mg 3-4 times/day.

Children. 20 mg/kg/day in 3-4 divided doses.

AVAILABLE FORMS

• *Caplets:* 500 mg (Parafon Forte DSC).

• *Tablets:* 250 mg.

CONTRAINDICATIONS: Hypersensitivity to chlorzoxazone or any one of its components

PREGNANCY AND LACTATION: Pregnancy category C

SIDE EFFECTS

Frequent

Drowsiness, fever, headache

Occasional

Nausea, vomiting, stomach cramps, rash

SERIOUS REACTIONS

• Overdosage results in nausea, vomiting, diarrhea, and hypotension.

SPECIAL CONSIDERATIONS

PATIENT/FAMILY EDUCATION

• Potential for psychologic dependency

• Drowsiness usually diminishes with continued therapy

MONITORING PARAMETERS

• CBC

• Liver and renal function

cholestyramine resin

(koe-less-tir'-a-meen)

Rx: Questran, Questran Light, LoCHOLEST, LoCHOLEST Light, Prevalite

Chemical Class: Bile acid sequestrant

Therapeutic Class: Antilipemic; bile acid sequestrant

CLINICAL PHARMACOLOGY

Mechanism of Action: An antihyperlipoproteinemic that binds with bile acids in the intestine, forming an insoluble complex. Binding results in partial removal of bile acid from enterohepatic circulation. ***Therapeutic Effect:*** Removes LDL cholesterol from plasma.

Pharmacokinetics

Not absorbed from the GI tract. Decreases in serum LDL apparent in 5-7 days and in serum cholesterol in 1 mo. Serum cholesterol returns to baseline levels about 1 mo after drug is discontinued.

INDICATIONS AND DOSAGES

Hypercholesterolemia

PO

Adults, Elderly. Initially, 4 g 1-2 times a day. Maintenance: 8-16 g/day in divided doses. Maximum: 24 g/day.

Children. 80 mg/kg 3 times a day.

Pruritis

PO

Adults, Elderly. Initially, 4 g 1-2 times a day. Maintenance: 8-16 g/day in divided doses. Maximum: 24 g/day.

AVAILABLE FORMS

• *Powder for Oral Suspension:* 4 g/5 g (Questran Light), 4 g/9 g (Prevalite, Questran).

UNLABELED USES: Treatment of diarrhea (due to bile acids), hyperoxaluria

CONTRAINDICATIONS: Complete biliary obstruction, hypersensitivity to cholestyramine or tartrazine (frequently seen in aspirin hypersensitivity)

PREGNANCY AND LACTATION: Pregnancy category C

SIDE EFFECTS

Frequent

Constipation (may lead to fecal impaction), nausea, vomiting, abdominal pain, indigestion

Occasional

Diarrhea, belching, bloating, headache, dizziness

Rare

Gallstones, peptic ulcer disease, malabsorption syndrome

SERIOUS REACTIONS

• GI tract obstruction, hyperchloremic acidosis, and osteoporosis secondary to calcium excretion may occur.

• High dosage may interfere with fat absorption, resulting in steatorrhea.

INTERACTIONS

Drugs

3 *Acetaminophen, amiodarone, corticosteroids, diclofenac, digitalis glycosides, furosemide, methotrexate, metronidazole, thiazide diuretics, thyroid hormones, valproic acid:* Cholestyramine reduces interacting drug concentrations and probably subsequent therapeutic response

3 *Fat-soluble vitamins (A, D, E, and K):* May prevent absorption of fat-soluble vitamins

3 *Oral anticoagulants:* Inhibition of hypoprothrombinemic response; colestipol might be less likely to interact

3 *Oral vancomycin:* Binds and decreases the effects of oral vancomycin

SPECIAL CONSIDERATIONS

• Avoid use in patients with elevated triglycerides

PATIENT/FAMILY EDUCATION

• Give all other medications 1 hr before or 4 hr after cholestyramine to avoid poor absorption

• Mix drug with applesauce or noncarbonated beverage (2-6 oz), let stand for 2 min; do not take dry

• Take cholestyramine before meals and drink several glasses of water between meals

MONITORING PARAMETERS

• Daily bowel activity and stool consistency

choline magnesium trisalicylate

(koe'-leen mag-nees'-ee-um trye-sal'-eh-si-late)

Rx: Tricosal, Trilisate

Chemical Class: Salicylate derivative

Therapeutic Class: NSAID; nonnarcotic analgesic

CLINICAL PHARMACOLOGY

Mechanism of Action: A nonsteroidal salicylate that inhibits prostaglandin synthesis and acts on the hypothalamus heat-regulating center. ***Therapeutic Effect:*** Reduces inflammatory response and intensity of pain stimulus reaching sensory nerve endings.

Pharmacokinetics

Rapidly absorbed from gastrointestinal (GI) tract Oral route onset 1 hr, peak 2 hrs and duration 9-17 hrs. Protein binding: High. Widely distributed. Excreted in the urine. ***Half-life:*** 2-3 hrs.

INDICATIONS AND DOSAGES

Analgesic, acute painful shoulder, antiinflammatory, antipyretic

PO

Adults, Elderly. Initially, 500 mg-1500 mg q8-12h, then 1-4.5 g/day.

Children weighing less than 37 kg. 50 mg/kg/day in divided doses.

AVAILABLE FORMS

• *Tablets:* 500 mg, 750 mg, 1000 mg (Tricosal, Trilisate).

• *Liquid:* 500 mg/5 ml (Trilisate).

CONTRAINDICATIONS: Allergy to tartrazine dye, bleeding disorders, GI bleeding or ulceration, history of hypersensitivity to choline magnesium trisalicylate, aspirin, or NSAIDs

PREGNANCY AND LACTATION: Pregnancy category C; excreted into breast milk

SIDE EFFECTS

Side effects appear less frequently with short-term treatment.

Occasional

Nausea, dyspepsia (heartburn, indigestion, epigastric pain), tinnitus

Rare

Anorexia, headache, vomiting, flatulence, dizziness, somnolence, insomnia, fatigue, hearing impairment

SERIOUS REACTIONS

• High doses may produce GI bleeding.

• Overdosage may be characterized by ringing in ears, generalized pruritus (may be severe), headache, dizziness, flushing, tachycardia, hyperventilation, sweating, and thirst.

INTERACTIONS

Drugs

3 *Corticosteroids:* May reduce plasma salicylate levels by increasing renal elimination

3 *Drugs that alter urine pH:* May enhance renal salicylate clearance and diminish plasma salicylate concentration; urine acidification can decrease urinary salicylate excretion and increase plasma levels

3 *Methotrexate:* May increase the toxic effects of methotrexate

Labs

• *False increase:* Serum bicarbonate, CSF protein, serum theophylline

• *False decrease:* Urine cocaine, urine estrogen, serum glucose, urine 17-hydroxycorticosteroids, urine opiates

• *False positive:* Ferric chloride test

SPECIAL CONSIDERATIONS

• Consider for patients with GI intolerance to aspirin or patients in whom interference with normal platelet function by aspirin or other NSAIDs is undesirable

PATIENT/FAMILY EDUCATION

• Solution may be mixed with fruit juice just before administration; do not mix with antacid

• Report any ringing in the ears or persistent GI pain

MONITORING PARAMETERS

• Liver and renal function studies, stool for occult blood and Hct if long-term therapy

---

ciclopirox

(sye-kloe-peer′-ox)

Rx: Loprox, Penlac

Chemical Class: N-hydroxypyridinone derivative

Therapeutic Class: Antifungal

CLINICAL PHARMACOLOGY

Mechanism of Action: An antifungal that inhibits the transport of essential elements in the fungal cell, thereby interfering with biosynthesis in fungi. ***Therapeutic Effect:*** Results in fungal cell death.

Pharmacokinetics

Absorbed through intact skin. Distributed to epidermis, dermis, including hair, hair follicles, and sebaceous glands. Protein binding: 98%. Primarily excreted in urine and to a lesser extent in feces. ***Half-life:*** 1.7 hrs.

INDICATIONS AND DOSAGES

Tinea pedis

Topical

Adults, Elderly, Children 10 yrs and older. Apply 2 times a day until signs and symptoms significantly improve.

Tinea cruris, Tinea corporis

Topical

Adults, Elderly, Children 10 yrs and older. Apply 2 times a day until signs and symptoms significantly improve.

Onychomycosis

Topical (solution)

Adults, Elderly, Children 10 yrs and older. Apply to the affected area (nails) daily. Remove with alcohol every 7 days.

Seborrheic dermatitis

Shampoo

Adults, Elderly, Children 10 yrs and older. Apply to affected scalp areas 2 times a day, in the morning and evening for 4 wks.

AVAILABLE FORMS

- *Cream:* 0.77% (Loprox).
- *Gel:* 0.77% (Loprox).
- *Lotion:* 0.77% (Loprox TS).
- *Shampoo:* 0.77% (Loprox).
- *Topical Solution, nail lacquer:* 8% (Penlac).

CONTRAINDICATIONS: Hypersensitivity to ciclopirox or any one of its components

PREGNANCY AND LACTATION: Pregnancy category B; excretion into breast milk unknown

SIDE EFFECTS

Rare

Topical: Irritation, burning, redness, pain at the site of application

SERIOUS REACTIONS

- None known.

SPECIAL CONSIDERATIONS

- Use of nail lacquer requires monthly removal of the unattached, infected nails by a health care professional; in clinical trials <12% of patients achieved a clear or almost clear nail

PATIENT/FAMILY EDUCATION

Cream/gel/lotion:

- Continue medication for several days after condition clears
- Consult prescriber if no improvement after 4 wk of treatment
- Avoid contact with eyes and mouth

Nail lacquer:

- 48 wks of daily applications considered full treatment, may take 6 mo before see improvement

cidofovir

(si-dof′-o-veer)

Rx: Vistide

Chemical Class: Acyclic purine nucleoside analog

Therapeutic Class: Antiviral

CLINICAL PHARMACOLOGY

Mechanism of Action: An anti-infective that inhibits viral DNA synthesis by incorporating itself into the growing viral DNA chain. ***Therapeutic Effect:*** Suppresses replication of cytomegalovirus (CMV).

Pharmacokinetics

Protein binding: less than 6%. Excreted primarily unchanged in urine. Effect of hemodialysis unknown. ***Elimination half-life:*** 1.4-3.8 hr.

INDICATIONS AND DOSAGES

CMV retinitis in patients with AIDS (in combination with probenecid)

IV infusion

Adults. Induction: Usual dosage, 5 mg/kg at constant rate over 1 hr once weekly for 2 consecutive wk. Give 2 g of PO probenecid 3 hr before cidofovir dose, and then give 1 g 2 hr and 8 hr after completion of the 1-hr cidofovir infusion (total of 4 g). In addition, give 1 L of 0.9% NaCl over 1-2 hr immediately before the cidofovir infusion. If tolerated, a second liter may be infused over 1-3 hr at the start of the infusion or immediately afterward. Maintenance: 5 mg/kg cidofovir at constant rate over 1 hr once every 2 wk.

Dosage in renal impairment

Changes during therapy. If creatinine increases by 0.3-0.4 mg/dl, reduce dose to 3 mg/kg; if creatinine increases by 0.5 mg/dl or greater or development of 3+ or greater proteinuria, discontinue therapy.

Preexisting renal impairment. Do not use with serum creatinine greater than 1.5 mg/dl, creatinine clearance less than 55 ml/min or urine protein 100 mg/dl or greater (2+ or greater proteinuria).

AVAILABLE FORMS

- *Injection:* 75 mg/ml (5-ml ampule).

UNLABELED USES: Treatment of acyclovir-resistant herpes simplex virus, adenovirus, foscarnet-resistant CMV, ganciclovir-resistant CMV, varicella-zoster virus

CONTRAINDICATIONS: Direct intraocular injection, history of clinically severe hypersensitivity to probenecid or other sulfa-containing drugs, renal function impairment (serum creatinine level greater than 1.5 mg/dl, creatinine clearance of 55 ml/min or less, or urine protein level greater than 100 mg/dl)

PREGNANCY AND LACTATION: Pregnancy category C

SIDE EFFECTS

Frequent

Nausea, vomiting (65%), fever (57%), asthenia (46%), rash (30%), diarrhea (27%), headache (27%), alopecia (25%), chills (24%), anorexia (22%), dyspnea (22%), abdominal pain (17%)

SERIOUS REACTIONS

- Serious adverse reactions may include proteinuria (80%), nephrotoxicity (53%), neutropenia (31%), elevated serum creatinine levels (29%), infection (24%), anemia (20%), ocular hypotony (a decrease in intraocular pressure, 12%), and pneumonia (9%).
- Concurrent use of probenecid may produce a hypersensitivity reaction characterized by a rash, fever, chills, and anaphylaxis.
- Acute renal failure occurs rarely.

INTERACTIONS

Drugs

3 *Aminoglycosides:* Additive nephrotoxicity

3 *Amphotericin B:* Additive nephrotoxicity

3 *Foscarnet:* Additive nephrotoxicity

3 *Pentamidine:* Additive nephrotoxicity (IV route only)

SPECIAL CONSIDERATIONS

- Concurrent high-dose PO probenecid plus saline hydration reduces nephrotoxicity; procedure: probenecid 2 g 3 hr prior to INF, then 1 g at 2 and 8 hr after INF; normal saline 1000 ml over 1 hr immediately prior to INF

PATIENT/FAMILY EDUCATION

- Complete the full course of probenecid with each dose of cidofovir
- Female patients of childbearing age should use effective contraception during and for 1 mo after cidofovir treatment; avoid pregnancy because cidofovir is harmful to the embryo
- Male patients should practice barrier contraceptive methods during and for 3 mos after treatment
- Do not breast-feed while taking cidofovir
- It is important to have regular follow-up ophthalmologic exams

MONITORING PARAMETERS

- Renal function, urinalysis (especially serum creatinine and urine protein prior to each dose), and blood chemistry (to include serum uric acid, phosphate, and bicarbonate), white counts with differential during intravenous therapy

• Periodically evaluate the patient's visual acuity and check for ocular symptoms

cilostazol

(sil-oh'-sta-zol)

Rx: Pletal

Chemical Class: Quinolinone derivative

Therapeutic Class: Hemorrheologic agent

CLINICAL PHARMACOLOGY

Mechanism of Action: A phosphodiesterase III inhibitor that inhibits platelet aggregation. Dilates vascular beds with greatest dilation in femoral beds. ***Therapeutic Effect:*** Improves walking distance in patients with intermittent claudication.

Pharmacokinetics

Moderately absorbed from the GI tract. Protein binding: 95%-98%. Extensively metabolized in the liver. Excreted primarily in the urine and, to a lesser extent, in the feces. Not removed by hemodialysis. ***Half-life:*** 11-13 hr. Therapeutic effect is usually noted in 2-4 wk but may take as long as 12 wk.

INDICATIONS AND DOSAGES

Intermittent claudication

PO

Adults, Elderly. 100 mg twice a day at least 30 min before or 2 hr after meals. 50 mg twice a day during concurrent therapy with clarithromycin, diltiazem, erythromycin, fluconazole, fluoxetine, omeprazole, or sertraline.

AVAILABLE FORMS

• *Tablets:* 50 mg, 100 mg.

CONTRAINDICATIONS: CHF of any severity; hemostatic disorders or active pathologic bleeding, such as bleeding peptic ulcer and intracranial bleeding

PREGNANCY AND LACTATION: Pregnancy category C; excreted in breast milk

SIDE EFFECTS

Frequent (34%-10%)

Headache, diarrhea, palpitations, dizziness, pharyngitis

Occasional (7%-3%)

Nausea, rhinitis, back pain, peripheral edema, dyspepsia, abdominal pain, tachycardia, cough, flatulence, myalgia

Rare (2%-1%)

Leg cramps, paresthesia, rash, vomiting

SERIOUS REACTIONS

• Signs and symptoms of overdose are noted by severe headache, diarrhea, hypotension, and cardiac arrhythmias.

INTERACTIONS

Drugs

3 *Aspirin:* May potentiate inhibition of platelet aggregation

3 *Diltiazam:* Increases cilostazol concentrations

3 *Erythromycin, azole antifungals, fluoxetine, nefazadone, and sertraline:* As CYP3A4 or CYP2C19 inhibitors, may increase cilostazol levels; clinical effects unknown

3 *Omeprazole:* Increases cilostazol concentrations

3 *Foods: Grapefruit juice:* Increases cilostazol levels; *High fat:* Increases absorption of cilostazol (80% increase of Cmax, 25% increase of AUC)

SPECIAL CONSIDERATIONS

• Cilostazol has been shown, in a multicenter, randomized, double-blind study (DPPARA 2), to be superior to pentoxifylline for treatment of claudication symptoms

PATIENT/FAMILY EDUCATION

• Take ½ hr before meal or 2 hr after meal

• Avoid taking cilostazol with grapefruit juice because it may increase the drug's blood concentration and risk of toxicity

MONITORING PARAMETERS

• Beneficial effects usually seen in 2 to 4 wk, may take up to 12 wk

• Assess for relief of cramping in the feet, calf muscles, thighs, and buttocks during exercise

cimetidine

(sye-met'-i-deen)

Rx: Tagamet

OTC: Tagamet HB

Chemical Class: Imidazole derivative

Therapeutic Class: Antiulcer agent

CLINICAL PHARMACOLOGY

Mechanism of Action: An antiulcer agent and gastric acid secretion inhibitor that inhibits histamine action at histamine 2 receptor sites of parietal cells. ***Therapeutic Effect:*** Inhibits gastric acid secretion during fasting, at night, or when stimulated by food, caffeine, or insulin.

Pharmacokinetics

Well absorbed from the GI tract. Protein binding: 15%-20%. Widely distributed. Metabolized in the liver. Primarily excreted in urine. Not removed by hemodialysis. ***Half-life:*** 2 hr; increased with impaired renal function.

INDICATIONS AND DOSAGES

Active ulcer

PO

Adults, Elderly. 300 mg 4 times a day or 400 mg twice a day or 800 mg at bedtime.

IV, IM

Adults, Elderly. 300 mg q6h or 150 mg as single dose followed by 37.5 mg/hr continuous infusion.

Prevention of duodenal ulcer

PO

Adults, Elderly. 400-800 mg at bedtime.

Gastric hypersecretory secretions

PO, IV, IM

Adults, Elderly. 300-600 mg q6h. Maximum: 2400 mg/day.

Children. 20-40 mg/kg/day in divided doses q6h.

Infants. 10-20 mg/kg/day in divided doses q6-12h.

Neonates. 5-10 mg/kg/day in divided doses q8-12h.

Gastrointestinal reflux disease

PO

Adults, Elderly. 800 mg twice a day or 400 mg 4 times a day for 12 wks.

OTC use

PO

Adults, Elderly. 100 mg up to 30 min before meals. Maximum: 2 doses/day.

Prevention of upper GI bleeding

IV Infusion

Adults, Elderly. 50 mg/hr.

Dosage in renal impairment

Dosage is based on a 300-mg dose in adults. Dosage interval is modified based on creatinine clearance.

Creatinine Clearance	*Dosage Interval*
greater than 40 ml/min	q6h
20-40 ml/min	q8h or decrease dose by 25%
less than 20 ml/min	q12h or decrease dose by 50%

Give after hemodialysis and q12h between dialysis sessions.

AVAILABLE FORMS

• *Tablets (Tagamet HB):* 100 mg, 200 mg.

• *Tablets (Tagamet):* 200 mg, 300 mg, 400 mg, 800 mg.

• *Liquid (Tagamet):* 300 mg/5 ml.

• *Liquid (Tagamet HB):* 200 mg/20 ml.

• *Injection (Tagamet):* 150 mg/ml.

UNLABELED USES: Prevention of aspiration pneumonia; treatment of acute urticaria, chronic warts, upper GI bleeding

CONTRAINDICATIONS: Hypersensitivity to other H_2-antagonists

PREGNANCY AND LACTATION: Pregnancy category B; excreted into breast milk and may accumulate; theoretically, adversely affects the nursing infant's gastric acidity, inhibits drug metabolism, and produces CNS stimulation—all not reported; compatible with breast-feeding

SIDE EFFECTS

Occasional (4%-2%)

Headache

Elderly and severely ill patients, patients with impaired renal function: Confusion, agitation, psychosis, depression, anxiety, disorientation, hallucinations. Effects reverse 3-4 days after discontinuance.

Rare (less than 2%)

Diarrhea, dizziness, somnolence, nausea, vomiting, gynecomastia, rash, impotence

SERIOUS REACTIONS

• Rapid IV administration may produce cardiac arrhythmias and hypotension.

INTERACTIONS

Drugs

3 *Amiodarone, benzodiazepines; calcium channel blockers; amiodarone; cyclic antidepressants; carbamazepine; carmustine; chloramphenicol; cisapride; citalopram; clozapine; diltiazem; femoxidine; flecanide; glyburide; glipizide; labetolol; lidocaine; lomustine; melphalan; metoprolol; narcotic analgesics; moricizine; N-acetylprocainamide; nicotine; phenytoin; peridolol; praziquantel; procainamide; propafinone; propranolol; quinidine; tacrine; theophylline; tolbutamide:* Increased concentrations of interacting drugs with potential for toxicity

3 *Antacids:* May decrease the absorption of cimetidine

3 *Ketoconazole, cefpodoxime, cefuroxime:* Reduced concentrations of interacting drugs

2 *Warfarin:* Increased concentrations of interacting drugs with potential for toxicity

Labs

• *False positive:* Hemoccult

SPECIAL CONSIDERATIONS

• Generic formulations offer less costly alternative for patients not at risk for drug interactions

PATIENT/FAMILY EDUCATION

• Stagger doses of cimetidine and antacids

• IM injection may produce transient discomfort at injection site

• Avoid tasks that require mental alertness or motor skills until response to the drug is established

• Avoid smoking

• Notify the physician if blood in vomitus or stool, or dark, tarry stool occurs

MONITORING PARAMETERS

• Blood pressure for hypotension during IV infusion

• Blood in stool

• Mental status in the elderly or those with impaired renal function

cinacalcet hydrochloride

(sin-a-cal'-set hye-droe-klor'-ide)

Rx: Sensipar

Chemical Class: Calcimimetic agent

Therapeutic Class: Hyperparathyroidism (secondary)

CLINICAL PHARMACOLOGY

Mechanism of Action: A calcium receptor agonist that increases the sensitivity of the calcium-sensing receptor on the parathyroid gland to extracellular calcium, thus lowering the parathyroid hormone (PTH) levels. ***Therapeutic Effect:*** Decreases serum calcium and PTH levels.

Pharmacokinetics

Extensively distributed after PO administration. Protein binding: 93%-97%. Rapidly and extensively metabolized by multiple enzymes. Primarily eliminated in urine with a lesser amount excreted in feces. ***Half-life:*** 30-40 hr.

INDICATIONS AND DOSAGES

Hypercalcemia in parathyroid carcinoma

PO

Adults, Elderly. Initially, 30 mg twice a day. Titrate dosage sequentially (60 mg twice a day, 90 mg twice a day, and 90 mg 3-4 times a day) every 2-4 wk as needed to normalize serum calcium levels.

Secondary hyperparathyroidism in patients on dialysis

PO

Adults, Elderly. Initially, 30 mg once a day. Titrate dosage sequentially (60, 90, 120, and 180 mg once a day) every 2-4 wk.

AVAILABLE FORMS

• *Tablets:* 30 mg, 60 mg, 90 mg.

UNLABELED USES: Primary hyperthyroidism

CONTRAINDICATIONS: None known.

PREGNANCY AND LACTATION: Pregnancy category C; unknown if excreted into human milk, but excreted with high milk-to-plasma ratio in rats; not recommended in breast-feeding

SIDE EFFECTS

Frequent (31%-21%)

Nausea, vomiting, diarrhea

Occasional (15%-10%)

Myalgia, dizziness

Rare (7%-5%)

Asthenia, hypertension, anorexia, non-cardiac chest pain

SERIOUS REACTIONS

• Overdose may lead to hypocalcemia.

INTERACTIONS

Drugs

3 *Erythromycin:* Increases cinacalcet plasma concentration

3 *Flecainide, vinblastine, thioridazine, tricyclic antidepressants:* Inhibited metabolism by cinacalcet inhibition of CYP2D6, may require dosage reduction

3 *Ketoconazole:* Increased cinacalcet levels by ketoconazole inhibition of CYP3A4, monitor PTH and calcium levels to determine if dosage adjustment indicated

SPECIAL CONSIDERATIONS

• Can be used alone or in combination with vitamin D sterols and/or phosphate binders

PATIENT/FAMILY EDUCATION

• Take with food or shortly after a meal. Do not divide tablets

• Notify the health care provider immediately if diarrhea or vomiting occurs

MONITORING PARAMETERS

• Serum calcium and phosphorus within 1 wk

• iPTH 1-4 wk after initiation or dose adjustment

• Once maintenance dose established, serum calcium and phosphorus qmonth, iPTH q1-3 mos to target of 150-300 pg/ml
• Pattern of daily bowel activity and stool consistency

ciprofloxacin hydrochloride

(sip-ro-floks'-a-sin hye-droe-klor'-ide)

Rx: Ciloxan (ophthalmic), Cipro, Cipro I.V., Cipro XR
Chemical Class: Fluoroquinolone derivative
Therapeutic Class: Antibiotic

CLINICAL PHARMACOLOGY
Mechanism of Action: A fluoroquinolone that inhibits the enzyme DNA gyrase in susceptible bacteria, interfering with bacterial cell replication. ***Therapeutic Effect:*** Bactericidal.
Pharmacokinetics
Well absorbed from the GI tract (food delays absorption). Protein binding: 20%-40%. Widely distributed (including to CSF). Metabolized in the liver to active metabolite. Primarily excreted in urine. Minimal removal by hemodialysis. ***Half-life:*** 4-6 hr (increased in impaired renal function and the elderly).

INDICATIONS AND DOSAGES
Bone, joint infections
IV
Adults, Elderly. 400 mg q12h for 4-6 wk.
PO
Adults, Elderly. 500 mg q12h for 4-6 wk.
Conjunctivitis
Ophthalmic
Adults, Elderly. 1-2 drops q2h for 2 days, then 2 drops q4h for next 5 days.
Corneal ulcer
Ophthalmic
Adults, Elderly. 2 drops q15min for 6 hr, then 2 drops q30min for the remainder of first day, 2 drops q1h on second day, and 2 drops q4h on days 3-14.
Cystic fibrosis
IV
Children.. 30 mg/kg/day in 2-3 divided doses. Maximum: 1.2 g/day.
PO
Children. 40 mg/kg/day. Maximum: 2 g/day.
Febrile neutropenia
IV
Adults, Elderly. 400 mg q8h for 7-14 days (in combination).
Gonorrhea
PO
Adults, Elderly. 250 mg as a single dose.
Infectious diarrhea
PO
Adults, Elderly. 500 mg q12h for 5-7 days.
Intraabdominal infections (with metronidazole)
IV
Adults, Elderly. 400 mg q12h for 7-14 days.
PO
Adults, Elderly. 500 mg q12h for 7-14 days.
Lower respiratory tract infections
IV
Adults, Elderly. 400 mg q12h for 7-14 days.
PO
Adults, Elderly. 500 mg q12h for 7-14 days (750 mg q12h for 7-14 days for severe or complicated infections).
Nosocomial pneumonia
IV
Adults, Elderly. 400 mg q8h for 10-14 days.

Prostatitis
IV
Adults, Elderly. 400 mg q12h for 28 days.
PO
Adults, Elderly. 500 mg q12h for 28 days.
Sinusitis
IV
Adults, Elderly. 400 mg q12h for 10 days.
PO
Adults, Elderly. 500 mg q12h for 10 days.
Skin and skin structure infections
IV
Adults, Elderly. 400 mg q12h for 7-14 days.
PO
Adults, Elderly. 500 mg q12h for 7-14 days (750 mg q12h for severe or complicated infections).
Susceptible infections
IV
Adults, Elderly. 400 mg q8-12h.
PO
Adults, Elderly. 500-750 mg q12h.
Typhoid fever
PO
Adults, Elderly. 500 mg q12h for 10 days.
UTIs
IV
Adults, Elderly. 200 mg q12h for 7-14 days (400 mg q12h for severe or complicated infections).
PO
Adults, Elderly. 100-250 mg q12h for 3 days for acute uncomplicated infections; 250 mg q12h for 7-14 days for mild to moderate infections; 500 mg q12h for 7-14 days for severe or complicated infections.
Dosage in renal impairment
Dosage and frequency are modified based on creatinine clearance and the severity of the infection.

Creatinine Clearance	*Dosage Interval*
less than 30 ml/min	Usual dose q18-24h

Hemodialysis
Adults, Elderly. 250-500 mg q24h (after dialysis).
Peritoneal dialysis
Adults, Elderly. 250-500 mg q24h (after dialysis).

AVAILABLE FORMS
- *Tablets (Cipro):* 100 mg, 250 mg, 500 mg, 750 mg.
- *Tablets (Extended-Release [Cipro XR]):* 500 mg, 1000 mg.
- *Infusion (Cipro I.V.):* 200 mg/100 ml, 400 mg/200 ml.
- *Intravenous Solution (Cipro I.V.):* 10 mg/ml.
- *Ophthalmic Ointment (Ciloxan):* 0.3%.
- *Ophthalmic Suspension (Ciloxan):* 0.3%.
- *Oral Suspension, Powder for Reconstitution (Cipro):* 250 mg/5 ml, 500 mg/5 ml.

UNLABELED USES: Treatment of chancroid

CONTRAINDICATIONS: Hypersensitivity to ciprofloxacin or other quinolones; for ophthalmic administration: vaccinia, varicella, epithelial herpes simplex, keratitis, mycobacterial infection, fungal disease of ocular structure, use after uncomplicated removal of a foreign body

PREGNANCY AND LACTATION: Pregnancy category C; appears in breast milk at levels similar to serum; allow 48 hr to elapse after last dose before resuming breast-feeding

SIDE EFFECTS
Frequent (5%-2%)
Nausea, diarrhea, dyspepsia, vomiting, constipation, flatulence, confusion, crystalluria
Ophthalmic: Burning, crusting in corner of eye

Occasional (less than 2%)
Abdominal pain or discomfort, headache, rash
Ophthalmic: Bad taste, sensation of something in eye, eyelid redness or itching
Rare (less than 1%)
Dizziness, confusion, tremors, hallucinations, hypersensitivity reaction, insomnia, dry mouth, paresthesia

SERIOUS REACTIONS

• Superinfection (especially enterococcal or fungal), nephropathy, cardiopulmonary arrest, chest pain, and cerebral thrombosis may occur.
• Hypersensitivity reactions, including photosensitivity (as evidenced by rash, pruritus, blisters, edema, and burning skin), have occurred in patients receiving fluoroquinolones.
• Arthropathy may occur if the drug is given to children younger than 18 years.
• Sensitization to the ophthalmic form of the drug may contraindicate later systemic use of ciprofloxacin.

INTERACTIONS

Drugs

3 *Aluminum:* Reduced absorption of ciprofloxacin; do not take within 4 hr of dose
3 *Antacids:* Reduced absorption of ciprofloxacin; do not take within 4 hr of dose
3 *Antipyrine:* Inhibits metabolism of antipyrine; increased plasma antipyrine level
3 *Caffeine:* Inhibits metabolism of caffeine; increased plasma caffeine level
3 *Antidiabetic agents:* May cause changes in blood glucose and increase the risk of hypoglycemia or hyperglycemia
3 *Calcium:* Reduced absorption of ciprofloxacin; do not take within 4 hr of dose
3 *Clozapine:* Increases clozapine concentrations
3 *Corticosteroids:* May increase the risk of tendon rupture
3 *Diazepam:* Inhibits metabolism of diazepam; increased plasma diazepam level
3 *Didanosine:* Markedly reduced absorption of ciprofloxacin; take ciprofloxacin 2 hr before didanosine
3 *Foscarnet:* Coadministration increases seizure risk
3 *Iron:* Reduced absorption of ciprofloxacin; do not take within 4 hr of dose
3 *Magnesium:* Reduced absorption of ciprofloxacin; do not take within 4 hr of dose
3 *Metoprolol:* Inhibits metabolism of metoprolol; increased plasma metoprolol level
3 *Pentoxifylline:* Inhibits metabolism of pentoxifylline; increased plasma pentoxifylline level
3 *Phenytoin:* Inhibits metabolism of phenytoin; increased plasma phenytoin level
3 *Probenecid:* May increase the serum levels of ciprofloxacin
3 *Propranolol:* Inhibits metabolism of propranolol; increased plasma propranolol level
3 *Ropinirole:* Inhibits metabolism of ropinirole; increased plasma ropinirole level
3 *Sodium bicarbonate:* Reduced absorption of ciprofloxacin; do not take within 4 hr of dose
3 *Sucralfate:* Reduced absorption of ciprofloxacin; do not take within 4 hr of dose
3 *Theobromine:* Inhibits metabolism of theobromine; increased plasma theobromine level
3 *Theophylline:* Inhibits metabolism of theophylline; cut maintenance theophylline dose in half during therapy with ciprofloxacin

3 *Warfarin:* Inhibits metabolism of warfarin; increases hypoprothrombinemic response to warfarin
3 *Zinc:* Reduced absorption of ciprofloxacin; do not take within 4 hr of dose
Labs
• *False increase:* Urine coproporphyrin I, coproporphyrin III, urine porphyrins

SPECIAL CONSIDERATIONS

• Reserve use for UTI to documented pseudomonal infection or complicated UTI
• Considered first-line therapy for otitis externa in diabetic patients

PATIENT/FAMILY EDUCATION

• Do not skip drug doses; take for the full course of therapy
• Take with meals and an 8-oz glass of water
• Shake oral suspension well before taking
• Do not take antacids within 2 hrs of taking ciprofloxacin

MONITORING PARAMETERS

• Daily bowel activity and stool consistency
• Therapeutic response to medication

citalopram hydrobromide

(sye-tal'-oh-pram hye-droe-broe'-mide)
Rx: Celexa
Chemical Class: Bicyclic phthalane derivative
Therapeutic Class: Antidepressant, selective serotonin reuptake inhibitor (SSRI)

CLINICAL PHARMACOLOGY

Mechanism of Action: A selective serotonin reuptake inhibitor that blocks the uptake of the neurotransmitter serotonin at CNS presynaptic neuronal membranes, increasing its availability at postsynaptic receptor sites. ***Therapeutic Effect:*** Relieves depression.

Pharmacokinetics

Well absorbed after PO administration. Protein binding: 80%. Primarily metabolized in the liver. Primarily excreted in feces with a lesser amount eliminated in urine. ***Half-life:*** 35 hr.

INDICATIONS AND DOSAGES

Depression

PO

Adults. Initially, 20 mg once a day in the morning or evening. May increase in 20-mg increments at intervals of no less than 1 wk. Maximum: 60 mg/day.

Elderly, Patients with hepatic impairment. 20 mg/day. May titrate to 40 mg/day only for nonresponding patients.

AVAILABLE FORMS

• *Oral Solution:* 10 mg/5 ml.
• *Tablets:* 10 mg, 20 mg, 40 mg.

UNLABELED USES: Treatment of alcohol abuse, dementia, diabetic neuropathy, obsessive-compulsive disorder, panic disorder, smoking cessation

CONTRAINDICATIONS: Sensitivity to citalopram, use within 14 days of MAOIs

PREGNANCY AND LACTATION: Pregnancy category C; breast-feeding: unknown, 2 cases of infants experiencing excessive somnolence, decreased feeding, and weight loss have been reported

SIDE EFFECTS

Frequent (21%-11%)

Nausea, dry mouth, somnolence, insomnia, diaphoresis

Occasional (8%-4%)

Tremor, diarrhea, abnormal ejaculation, dyspepsia, fatigue, anxiety, vomiting, anorexia

Rare (3%-2%)
Sinusitis, sexual dysfunction, menstrual disorder, abdominal pain, agitation, decreased libido

SERIOUS REACTIONS

• Overdose is manifested as dizziness, drowsiness, tachycardia, somnolence, confusion, and seizures.

INTERACTIONS

Drugs

3 *Antifungals, macrolide antibiotics:* May increase the citalopram plasma level

❷ *Buspirone:* Increased risk of serotonin syndrome

3 *Carbamazepine:* May decrease the citalopram plasma level

3 *Cimetidine:* Increased levels of desmethylcitalopram via inhibition of CYP2D6 by cimetidine

3 *Imipramine:* Increased bioavailability and half-life of desipramine (the major metabolite of imipramine) via inhibition of CYP2D6 by citalopram

3 *Ginkgo biloba, St. John's wort:* May increase the risk of serotonin syndrome

3 *Lithium:* May increase lithium concentration and/or increase the risk of serotonin syndrome

⚠ *MAOIs, dexfenfluramine, sibutramine:* Increased risk of sertonin syndrome

3 *Metoprolol:* May increase levels of metoprolol, but no clinically significant changes in blood pressure or heart rate have been observed

❷ *Moclobemide:* Increased risk of developing serotonin syndrome

3 *Naratriptan, rizatriptan, sumatriptan, zolmatriptan:* Increased risk of weakness, hyperreflexia, and incoordination

SPECIAL CONSIDERATIONS

• No clinical advantage over other SSRIs

PATIENT/FAMILY EDUCATION

• Therapeutic response may take 5 to 6 wk; most commonly taken once daily in the afternoon or evening
• Do not discontinue citalopram abruptly or increase the dosage
• Avoid alcohol while taking citalopram
• Avoid tasks that require mental alertness or motor skills until response to the drug has been established
• Take sips of tepid water and chew sugarless gum to help relieve dry mouth

MONITORING PARAMETERS

• Closely supervise the suicidal patient during early therapy; as depression lessens, the patient's energy level improves, increasing the risk of suicide
• Assess the patient's appearance, behavior, level of interest, mood, and sleep pattern to determine the drug's therapeutic effect

---

clarithromycin

(clare-i-thro-mye'-sin)

Rx: Biaxin, Biaxin XL, Biaxin XL-Pak

Chemical Class: Macrolide derivative

Therapeutic Class: Antibiotic

CLINICAL PHARMACOLOGY

Mechanism of Action: A macrolide that binds to ribosomal receptor sites of susceptible organisms, inhibiting protein synthesis of the bacterial cell wall. ***Therapeutic Effect:*** Bacteriostatic; may be bactericidal with high dosages or very susceptible microorganisms.

Pharmacokinetics

Well absorbed from the GI tract. Protein binding: 65%-75%. Widely distributed. Metabolized in the liver to active metabolite. Primarily excreted in urine. Not removed by hemodialysis. ***Half-life:*** 3-7 hr; metabolite 5-7 hr (increased in impaired renal function).

INDICATIONS AND DOSAGES

Bronchitis

PO

Adults, Elderly. 250-500 mg q12h for 7-14 days.

PO (Extended-Release)

Adults, Elderly. 1 g once daily for 7 days.

Skin, soft tissue infections

PO

Adults, Elderly. 250 mg q12h for 7-14 days.

Children. 7.5 mg/kg q12h for 10 days. Maximum: 1 g/day.

Myobacterium avium complex (MAC) prophylaxis

PO

Adults, Elderly. 500 mg twice a day.

Children. 7.5 mg/kg q12h. Maximum: 500 mg twice a day.

MAC treatment

PO

Adults, Elderly. 500 mg twice a day in combination.

Children. 7.5 mg/kg q12h in combination. Maximum: 500 mg twice a day.

Pharyngitis, tonsillitis

PO

Adults, Elderly. 250 mg q12h for 10 days.

Children. 7.5 mg/kg q12h for 10 days. Maximum: 1 g/day.

Pneumonia

PO

Adults, Elderly. 250 mg q12h for 7-14 days.

Children. 7.5 mg/kg q12h.

PO (Extended-Release)

Adults, Elderly. 1 g/day.

Maxillary sinusitis

PO

Adults, Elderly. 500 mg q12h or 1000 mg (2×500 mg extended-release) once daily for 14 days.

Children. 7.5 mg/kg q12h. Maximum: 500 mg twice a day.

H. pylori

PO

Adults, Elderly. 500 mg q8-12h for 10-14 days in combination.

Acute otitis media

PO

Children. 7.5 mg/kg q12h for 10 days.

Dosage in renal impairment

For patients with creatinine clearance less than 30 ml/min, reduce dose by 50% and administer once or twice a day.

AVAILABLE FORMS

- *Oral Suspension (Biaxin):* 125 mg/5 ml, 250 mg/5 ml.
- *Tablets (Biaxin):* 250 mg, 500 mg.
- *Tablets (Extended-Release [Biaxin XL, Biaxin XL Pak]):* 500 mg.

CONTRAINDICATIONS: Hypersensitivity to other macrolide antibiotics

PREGNANCY AND LACTATION: Pregnancy category C; excretion into breast milk unknown; use caution in nursing mothers

SIDE EFFECTS

Occasional (6%-3%)

Diarrhea, nausea, altered taste, abdominal pain

Rare (2%-1%)

Headache, dyspepsia

SERIOUS REACTIONS

- Antibiotic-associated colitis and other superinfections may result from altered bacterial balance.
- Hepatotoxicity and thrombocytopenia occur rarely.

INTERACTIONS

Drugs

3 *Alfentanil:* Prolonged anesthesia and respiratory depression

3 *Alprazolam:* Increased plasma alprazolam concentration

3 *Amprenavir:* Plasma concentrations of clarithromycin may be increased by amprenavir; plasma concentrations of amprenavir may be increased by clarithromycin

3 *Atorvastatin:* Increased plasma atorvastatin concentration with risk of rhabdomyolysis

3 *Bromocriptine:* Increased bromocriptine concentration with toxicity

3 *Buspirone:* Increased plasma buspirone concentration

3 *Carbamazepine:* Markedly increased plasma carbamazepine concentrations

▲ *Cisapride:* QT prolongation and life-threatening dysrhythmia

❷ *Clozapine:* Increased plasma clozapine concentrations

3 *Colchicine:* Potential colchicine toxicity

3 *Cyclosporine:* Increased plasma cyclosporine concentrations

3 *Diazepam:* Increased plasma concentration of diazepam

3 *Digoxin:* Reduced bacterial flora may increase plasma digoxin concentrations

3 *Disopyramide:* Increased plasma disopyramide concentrations

❷ *Ergotamine:* Potential for ergotism

3 *Ethanol:* Ethanol reduces plasma clarithromycin concentration

3 *Felodipine:* Increased plasma felodipine concentrations

3 *Food:* Food may increase or decrease the bioavailability of clarithromycin

3 *Indinavir:* Plasma concentrations of clarithromycin may be increased by indinavir; plasma concentrations of indinavir may be increased by clarithromycin

3 *Itraconazole:* Increased plasma itraconazole concentration

3 *Lovastatin:* Increased plasma lovastatin concentration with risk of rhabdomyolysis

3 *Methylprednisolone:* Increased plasma methylprednisolone concentrations

3 *Midazolam:* Increased plasma concentration of midazolam

3 *Nelfinavir:* Plasma concentrations of clarithromycin may be increased by nelfinavir; plasma concentrations of nelfinavir may be increased by clarithromycin

3 *Penicillin:* Decreased activity of penicillin

▲ *Pimozide:* QT prolongation and life-threatening dysrhythmia

3 *Phenytoin:* Increased plasma phenytoin concentrations

3 *Prednisone:* Increased plasma prednisone concentrations

3 *Quinidine:* Increased plasma concentration of quinidine

3 *Repaglinide:* Increased serum repaglinide concentrations and insulin response to repaglinide

▲ *Rifabutin:* Increased plasma rifabutin concentrations and increases its toxicity; rifabutin reduces the concentration of clarithromycin and may result in loss of efficacy

3 *Rifampin:* Reduces plasma clarithromycin concentrations

3 *Ritonavir:* Plasma concentrations of clarithromycin may be increased by ritonavir; plasma concentrations of ritonavir may be increased by clarithromycin

3 *Saquinavir:* Plasma concentrations of clarithromycin may be increased by saquinavir; plasma concentrations of saquinavir may be increased by clarithromycin

3 *Sildenafil:* Increased plasma sildenafil concentration

❷ *Simvastatin:* Increased plasma simvastatin concentration with risk of rhabdomyolysis

❸ *Tacrolimus:* Increased plasma tacrolimus concentration

⚠ *Terfenadine:* QT prolongation and life-threatening dysrhythmia

❸ *Theophylline:* Increased plasma theophylline concentration

❸ *Triazolam:* Increased plasma triazolam concentration

❸ *Valproic acid:* Increased plasma valproic acid concentration

❸ *Warfarin:* Increased hypoprothrombinemic response to warfarin

❸ *Zafirlukast:* Reduced plasma zafirlukast concentration probably by reducing bioavailability

❸ *Zopiclone:* Increased plasma zopiclone concentration

SPECIAL CONSIDERATIONS

PATIENT/FAMILY EDUCATION

- Take Sus Action TAB with food, immediate release and granules without regard to food
- Do NOT refrigerate suspension
- Take clarithromycin tablets with 8 oz of water; the tablets and oral suspension may be taken with or without food
- Space doses evenly around the clock and continue taking clarithromycin for the full course of treatment

MONITORING PARAMETERS

- Pattern of daily bowel activity and stool consistency; mild GI effects may be tolerable, but severe symptoms may indicate the onset of antibiotic-associated colitis
- Be alert for signs and symptoms of superinfection, including abdominal pain, anal or genital pruritus, moderate to severe diarrhea, and mouth soreness

clemastine fumarate

(klem'-as-teen)

Rx: Contac 12 Hour Allergy, Dayhistol Allergy, Tavist Allergy

Combinations

OTC: with pseudoephedrine and acetaminophen (Tavist Allergy/Sinus/Headache Tablets)

Chemical Class: Ethanolamine derivative

Therapeutic Class: Antihistamine

CLINICAL PHARMACOLOGY

Mechanism of Action: An ethanolamine that competes with histamine on effector cells in the GI tract, blood vessels, and respiratory tract. ***Therapeutic Effect:*** Relieves allergy symptoms, including urticaria, rhinitis, and pruritus.

Pharmacokinetics

Route	Onset	Peak	Duration
PO	15-60 min	5-7 hr	10-12 hr

Well absorbed from the GI tract. Metabolized in the liver. Excreted primarily in urine. ***Half-life:*** 21 hr.

INDICATIONS AND DOSAGES

Allergic rhinitis, urticaria

PO

Adults, Children older than 11 yr. 1.34 mg twice a day up to 2.68 mg 3 times a day. Maximum: 8.04 mg/day.

Children 6-11 yr. 0.67-1.34 mg twice a day. Maximum: 4.02 mg/day.

Children younger than 6 yr. 0.05 mg/kg/day divided into 2-3 doses per day. Maximum: 1.34 mg/day.

Elderly. 1.34 mg 1-2 times a day.

AVAILABLE FORMS

- *Syrup (Tavist):* 0.67 mg/5 ml.

• *Tablets:* 1.34 mg (Contac 12 Hour Allergy), 2.68 mg (Tavist).

CONTRAINDICATIONS: Angle-closure glaucoma, hypersensitivity to clemastine, use within 14 days of MAOIs

PREGNANCY AND LACTATION: Pregnancy category C; excreted into breast milk; may cause drowsiness and irritability in nursing infant; use with caution during breast-feeding

SIDE EFFECTS

Frequent

Somnolence, dizziness, urine retention, thickening of bronchial secretions, dry mouth, nose, or throat; in elderly, sedation, dizziness, hypotension

Occasional

Epigastric distress, flushing, blurred vision, tinnitus, paresthesia, diaphoresis, chills

SERIOUS REACTIONS

• A hypersensitivity reaction, marked by eczema, pruritus, rash, cardiac disturbances, angioedema, and photosensitivity, may occur.

• Overdose symptoms may vary from CNS depression, including sedation, apnea, cardiovascular collapse, and death to severe paradoxical reaction, such as hallucinations, tremor, and seizures.

• Children may experience paradoxical reactions, such as restlessness, insomnia, euphoria, nervousness, and tremors.

• Overdose in children may result in hallucinations, seizures, and death.

INTERACTIONS

Drugs

3 *Alcohol, other CNS depressants:* May increase CNS depression

3 *MAOIs:* May increase the anticholinergic and CNS depressant effects of clemastine

SPECIAL CONSIDERATIONS

• No advantage over loratadine or cetirizine; lower doses associated with less sedation and efficacy

PATIENT/FAMILY EDUCATION

• Dizziness, drowsiness, and dry mouth are expected side effects of clemastine

• Avoid performing tasks that require mental alertness or motor skills until response to the drug has been established

• Avoid alcohol during clemastine therapy

---

clindamycin

(klin-da-mye'-sin)

Rx: Cleocin HCl, Cleocin Ovules, Cleocin Pediatric, Cleocin Phosphate, Cleocin T, Cleocin Vaginal, Clinda-Derm, Clindagel, Clindamax, Clindesse, Clindets Pledget

Chemical Class: Lincomycin derivative

Therapeutic Class: Antibiotic

CLINICAL PHARMACOLOGY

Mechanism of Action: A lincosamide antibiotic that inhibits protein synthesis of the bacterial cell wall by binding to bacterial ribosomal receptor sites. Topically, it decreases fatty acid concentration on the skin. ***Therapeutic Effect:*** Bacteriostatic. Prevents outbreaks of acne vulgaris.

Pharmacokinetics

Rapidly absorbed from the GI tract. Protein binding: 92%-94%. Widely distributed. Metabolized in the liver to some active metabolites. Primarily excreted in urine. Not removed by hemodialysis. ***Half-life:*** 2.4-3 hr (increased in impaired renal function and premature infants).

INDICATIONS AND DOSAGES

Susceptible infections

IV, IM

Adults, Elderly. 600-2700 mg/day in 2-4 divided doses.

Children 1 mo-16 yr. 20-40 mg/kg/day in 2-4 divided doses. Maximum: 4.8 g/day.

Children younger than 1 mo. 15-20 mg/kg/day in 2-3 divided doses.

PO

Adults, Elderly. 150-450 mg q6h.

Children. 8-20 mg/kg/day in 3-4 divided doses.

Bacterial vaginosis

PO

Adults, Elderly. 300 mg twice a day for 7 days.

Intravaginal

Adults. One applicatorful at bedtime for 3-7 days or 1 suppository at bedtime for 3 days.

Intravaginal (Clindesse cream)

Adults. One applicatorful once at any time of the day.

Acne vulgaris

Topical

Adults. Apply thin layer to affected area twice a day.

AVAILABLE FORMS

- *Capsules (Cleocin HCl):* 75 mg, 150 mg, 300 mg.
- *Powder for Reconstitution (Cleocin Pediatric):* 75 mg/5 ml.
- *Intravenous Solution (Cleocin Phosphate):* 150 mg/ml, 300 mg-5%/50 ml, 600 mg-5%/50 ml, 900 mg-5%/50 ml.
- *Topical Gel (Cleocin T, Clindagel, Clindamax):* 1%.
- *Topical Lotion (Cleocin T):* 1%.
- *Topical Solution (Cleocin T, Clinda-Derm):* 1%.
- *Topical Swab (Cleocin T, Clindets Pledget):* 1%.
- *Vaginal Cream (Cleocin Vaginal):* 2%.
- *Vaginal Suppository (Cleocin Ovules):* 100 mg.

UNLABELED USES: Treatment of actinomycosis, babesiosis, erysipelas, malaria, otitis media, *Pneumocystis carinii* pneumonia, sinusitis, toxoplasmosis

CONTRAINDICATIONS: History of antibiotic-associated colitis, regional enteritis, or ulcerative colitis; hypersensitivity to clindamycin or lincomycin; known allergy to tartrazine dye

PREGNANCY AND LACTATION: Pregnancy category B; excreted into breast milk; compatible with breast-feeding

SIDE EFFECTS

Frequent

Systemic: Abdominal pain, nausea, vomiting, diarrhea

Topical: Dry scaly skin

Vaginal: Vaginitis, pruritus

Occasional

Systemic: Phlebitis or thrombophlebitis with IV administration, pain and induration at IM injection site, allergic reaction, urticaria, pruritus

Topical: Contact dermatitis, abdominal pain, mild diarrhea, burning or stinging

Vaginal: Headache, dizziness, nausea, vomiting, abdominal pain

Rare

Vaginal: Hypersensitivity reaction

SERIOUS REACTIONS

- Antibiotic-associated colitis and other superinfections may occur during and several weeks after clindamycin therapy (including the topical form).
- Blood dyscrasias (leukopenia, thrombocytopenia) and nephrotoxicity (proteinuria, azotemia, oliguria) occur rarely.

INTERACTIONS

Drugs

3 *Absorbent antidiarrheals:* May delay absorption of clindamycin

❷ *Chloramphenicol, erythromycin:* May antagonize the effects of clindamycin

❸ *Food:* Decreased clindamycin concentrations with diet foods containing sodium cyclamate

❷ *Kaolin-pectin:* Decreased clindamycin concentrations

❸ *Neuromuscular blockers:* May increase the effects of these drugs

Labs

• *False increase:* Serum theophylline

SPECIAL CONSIDERATIONS

• Most active antibiotic against anaerobes

• Preferred topical antiacne antibiotic

PATIENT/FAMILY EDUCATION

• Avoid intercourse and use of vaginal products (tampons, douches) when using the vag cream or suppositories

• Vag cream contains mineral oil and vag suppositories contain an oleaginous base that may weaken rubber or latex products such as condoms or diaphragms, avoid use within 72 hr following treatment with vag cream or suppositories

• Space doses evenly around the clock and continue taking clindamycin for the full course of treatment

• Do not apply topical preparations near the eyes

MONITORING PARAMETERS

• Daily bowel activity and stool consistency

• Skin for dryness, irritation, and rash with topical application

• Signs and symptoms of superinfection, such as anal or genital pruritus, a change in oral mucosa, increased fever, and severe diarrhea

clioquinol; hydrocortisone

(klye-oh-kwin′-ole)

OTC: Ala-Quin, Dek-Quin, Vioform-Hydrocortisone Cream, Vioform-Hydrocortisone Mild Cream, Vioform-Hydrocortisone Mild Ointment, Vioform-Hydrocortisone Ointment

Chemical Class: Hydroxyquinoline derivative

Therapeutic Class: Topical antiinfective

CLINICAL PHARMACOLOGY

Mechanism of Action: Clioquinol is a broad-spectrum antibacterial agent but the mechanism of action is unknown. Hydrocotisone is a corticosteroid that diffuses across cell membranes, forms complexes with specific receptors and further binds to DNA, and stimulates transcription of mRNA (messenger RNA) and subsequent protein synthesis of various enzymes thought to be ultimately responsible for the antiinflammatory effects of corticosteroids applied topically to the skin. ***Therapeutic Effect:*** Alters membrane function and produces antibacterial activity.

Pharmacokinetics

Clioquinol may be absorbed through the skin in sufficient amounts.

INDICATIONS AND DOSAGES

Antibacterial, antifungal skin conditions

Topical

Adults, Elderly, Children 12 yrs and older. Apply to skin 3-4 times/day.

AVAILABLE FORMS

- *Cream:* 3% clioquinol and 0.5% hydrocortisone (Ala-QuinVioform-Hydrocortisone Mild Cream), 3% clioquinol and 1% hydrocortisone (Vioform-Hydrocortisone Cream, Dek-Quin).
- *Ointment:* 3% clioquinol and 1% hydrocortisone (Vioform-Hydrocortisone Mild Ointment).

CONTRAINDICATIONS: Lesions of the eye, tuberculosis of skin, diaper rash, hypersensitivity to clioquinol or hydrocortisone or any other component of the formulation

PREGNANCY AND LACTATION: Pregnancy category C; excretion into breast milk unknown

SIDE EFFECTS

Occasional

Blistering, burning, itching, peeling, skin rash, redness, swelling

SERIOUS REACTIONS

- Thinning of skin with easy bruising may occur with prolonged use.

SPECIAL CONSIDERATIONS

- Potential neurotoxicity with absorption (with occlusion); since other agents without this toxicity exist, questionable utility

PATIENT/FAMILY EDUCATION

- Avoid contact with eyes
- Rub the topical form well into affected areas
- Medication may stain fabrics, skin, hair, and nails yellow

MONITORING PARAMETERS

- Skin for irritation
- Therapeutic response

clobetasol propionate

(klo-bet'-a-sol proe'-pi-on-ate)

Rx: Cormax, Olux, Temovate

Chemical Class: Corticosteroid, synthetic

Therapeutic Class: Corticosteroid, topical

CLINICAL PHARMACOLOGY

Mechanism of Action: A corticosteroid that inhibits accumulation of inflammatory cells at inflammation sites, phagocytosis, lysosomal enzyme release, and synthesis or release of mediators of inflammation. ***Therapeutic Effect:*** Decreases or prevents tissue response to inflammatory process.

Pharmacokinetics

May be absorbed from intact skin. Metabolized in liver. Excreted in the urine.

INDICATIONS AND DOSAGES

Antiinflammatory, corticosteroid replacement therapy

Topical

Adults, Elderly, Children 12 yrs and older. Apply 2 times/day for 2 wks.

Foam

Adults, Elderly, Children 12 yrs and older. Apply 2 times/day for 2 wks.

AVAILABLE FORMS

- *Cream:* 0.05% (Cormax, Temovate).
- *Cream, in emollient base:* 0.05% (Temovate).
- *Foam:* 0.05% (Olux).
- *Gel:* 0.05% (Temovate).
- *Ointment:* 0.05% (Cormax, Temovate).
- *Topical Solution:* 0.05% (Cormax, Temovate).

CONTRAINDICATIONS: Hypersensitivity to clobetasol or other corticosteroids

PREGNANCY AND LACTATION: Pregnancy category C; unknown whether top application could result in sufficient systemic absorption to produce detectable amounts in breast milk (systemic corticosteroids are secreted into breast milk in quantities not likely to have detrimental effects on infant)

SIDE EFFECTS

Frequent

Local irritation, dry skin, itching, redness

Occasional

Allergic contact dermatitis

Rare

Cushing's syndrome, numbness of fingers, skin atrophy

SERIOUS REACTIONS

- Overdosage can occur from topically applied clobetasol propionate absorbed in sufficient amounts to produce systemic effects producing reversible adrenal suppression, manifestations of Cushing's syndrome, hyperglycemia, and glucosuria in some patients.

SPECIAL CONSIDERATIONS

- No demonstrated superiority over other high-potency agents; cost should govern use

PATIENT/FAMILY EDUCATION

- Apply sparingly only to affected area
- Avoid contact with the eyes
- Do not put bandages or dressings over treated area unless directed by clinician
- Do not use on weeping, denuded, or infected areas
- Discontinue drug, notify clinician if local irritation or fever develops

MONITORING PARAMETERS

- Therapeutic response to medication

clocortolone pivalate

(kloe-kor′-toe-lone piv′-a-late)

Rx: Cloderm

Chemical Class: Corticosteroid, synthetic

Therapeutic Class: Corticosteroid, topical

CLINICAL PHARMACOLOGY

Mechanism of Action: A topical corticosteroid that inhibits accumulation of inflammatory cells at inflammation sites, suppresses mitotic activity, and causes vasoconstriction. ***Therapeutic Effect:*** Decreases or prevents tissue response to inflammatory process.

Pharmacokinetics

Absorption is variable and dependent upon many factors, including integrity of skin, dose, vehicle used, and use of occlusive dressings. Small amounts may be absorbed from the skin. Metabolized in liver. Excreted in the urine and feces.

INDICATIONS AND DOSAGES

Dermatoses

Topical

Adults, Elderly, Children 12 yrs and older. Apply 1-4 times/day.

AVAILABLE FORMS

- *Cream:* 0.1%.

CONTRAINDICATIONS: Hypersensitivity to clocortolone pivalate or other corticosteroids; viral, fungal, or tubercular skin lesions

PREGNANCY AND LACTATION: Pregnancy category C; unknown whether top application could result in sufficient systemic absorption to produce detectable amounts in breast milk (systemic corticosteroids are secreted into breast milk in quantities not likely to have detrimental effects on infant)

SIDE EFFECTS

Occasional

Local irritation, burning, itching, redness

Allergic contact dermatitis

Rare

Hypertrichosis, hypopigmentation, maceration of skin, miliaria, perioral dermatitis, skin atrophy, striae

SERIOUS REACTIONS

• Overdosage can occur from topically applied clocortolone pivalate absorbed in sufficient amounts to produce systemic effects in some patients.

SPECIAL CONSIDERATIONS

• No demonstrated superiority over other low-potency agents; cost should govern use

PATIENT/FAMILY EDUCATION

• Apply sparingly only to affected area

• Avoid contact with the eyes

• Do not put bandages or dressings over treated area unless directed by clinician

• Discontinue drug, notify clinician if local irritation or fever develops

• Do not use on weeping, denuded, or infected areas

MONITORING PARAMETERS

• Therapeutic response to medication

clofazimine

(kloe-faz'-i-meen)

Rx: Lamprene

Chemical Class: Iminophenazine dye

Therapeutic Class: Leprostatic; mycobacterium avium complex

CLINICAL PHARMACOLOGY

Mechanism of Action: An antibiotic that binds to mycobacterial DNA. ***Therapeutic Effect:*** Inhibits mycobacterial growth and produces antiinflammatory action.

Pharmacokinetics

Variable absorption following PO administration. Due to its high lipophilicity, clofazimine is deposited primarily in fatty tissue. Metabolized in liver. Primarily excreted in feces and minimal elimination in urine. ***Half-life:*** 70 days (following long-term therapy).

INDICATIONS AND DOSAGES

Leprosy

PO

Adults, Elderly. 100 mg/day in combination with dapsone and rifampin for 3 yr then 100 mg/day as monotherapy.

Children. 1 mg/kg/day in combination with dapsone and rifampin.

Erythema nodosum

PO

Adults, Elderly. 100-200 mg/day for up to 3 mo, then 100 mg/day.

AVAILABLE FORMS

• *Capsules:* 50 mg.

CONTRAINDICATIONS: None known.

PREGNANCY AND LACTATION: Pregnancy category C; excreted into breast milk; do not administer to nursing mother unless clearly indicated

SIDE EFFECTS

Frequent (greater than 10%)

Dry skin, abdominal pain, nausea, vomiting, diarrhea, skin discoloration (pink to brownish-black)

Occasional (10%-1%)

Rash; pruritus; eye irritation; discoloration of sputum, sweat, and urine

SERIOUS REACTIONS

• Severe abdominal pain and bleeding have been reported.

INTERACTIONS

Drugs

3 *Aluminum/magnesium containing antacids:* May decrease plasma concentrations of clofazimine

3 *Dapsone:* May decrease plasma concentrations of clofazimine

Labs

• *Increase:* Albumin, bilirubin, AST

SPECIAL CONSIDERATIONS

• Use in conjunction with other antileprosy agents to prevent development of resistance

PATIENT/FAMILY EDUCATION

• May discolor skin from pink to brownish black, as well as discoloring the conjunctivae, lacrimal fluid, sweat, sputum, urine, and feces; skin discoloration may take several mo or yr to disappear after discontinuation of therapy

• Take with meals to decrease GI discomfort

clomiphene citrate

(kloe'-mi-feen sye'-trate)

Rx: Clomid, Milophene, Serophene

Chemical Class: Estrogen agonist-antagonist; triarylethylene compound

Therapeutic Class: Ovulation stimulant

CLINICAL PHARMACOLOGY

Mechanism of Action: An ovulation stimulator that promotes release of pituitary gonadotropins. ***Therapeutic Effect:*** Stimulates ovulation.

Pharmacokinetics

Readily absorbed. Time to peak occurs within 6.5 hr. Undergoes enterohepatic recirculation. Primarily excreted in feces. ***Half-life:*** 5-7 days.

INDICATIONS AND DOSAGES

Ovulatory failure, females

PO

Adults. 50 mg/day for 5 days (first course); start the regimen on the fifth day of cycle. Increase dose only if unresponsive to cyclic 50 mg. Maximum: 100 mg/day for 5 days.

AVAILABLE FORMS

• *Tablets:* 50 mg (Clomid, Milophene, Serophene).

UNLABELED USES: Infertility in males

CONTRAINDICATIONS: Liver dysfunction, abnormal uterine bleeding, enlargement or development of ovarian cyst, uncontrolled thyroid or adrenal dysfunction in the presence of an organic intracranial lesion such as pituitary tumor, pregnancy, hypersensitivity to clomiphene

PREGNANCY AND LACTATION: Pregnancy category X; each new course of drug should be started only after pregnancy has been excluded

SIDE EFFECTS

Frequent (13%-10%)

Hot flashes, ovarian enlargement

Occasional (5%-2%)

Abdominal/pelvic discomfort, bloating, nausea, vomiting, breast discomfort (females)

Rare (less than 1%)

Vision disturbances, abnormal menstrual flow, breast enlargement (males), headache, mental depression, ovarian cyst formation, thromboembolism, uterine fibroid enlargement

SERIOUS REACTIONS

• Thrombophlebitis, alopecia, and polyuria occur rarely.

SPECIAL CONSIDERATIONS

• Though gonadotropin therapy is more effective for inducing ovulation, expense and time requirements warrant clomiphene trial

PATIENT/FAMILY EDUCATION

• Risk of multiple births increased—is approx 8% (7% twins, <1% triplets or greater)

• Record basal body temperature to determine whether ovulation has oc-

curred; if ovulation can be determined (there is a slight decrease in temperature, then a sharp increase for ovulation), attempt coitus 3 days before and qod until after ovulation
• Prolonged use may increase the risk of ovarian cancer
• Stop clomiphene immediately and notify the physician if pregnancy is a possibility

MONITORING PARAMETERS
• Ovulatory response

clomipramine hydrochloride

(kloe-mi'-pra-meen hye-droe-klor'-ide)

Rx: Anafranil

Chemical Class: Dibenzocycloheptene derivative; tertiary amine

Therapeutic Class: Antidepressant, tricyclic; antiobsessional

CLINICAL PHARMACOLOGY

Mechanism of Action: A tricyclic antidepressant that blocks the reuptake of neurotransmitters, such as norepinephrine and serotonin, at CNS presynaptic membranes, increasing their availability at postsynaptic receptor sites. ***Therapeutic Effect:*** Reduces obsessive-compulsive behavior.

Pharmacokinetics

Well absorbed from GI tract. Protein binding: 97%. Principally bound to albumin. Distributed into cerebrospinal fluid. Metabolized in the liver. Undergoes extensive first-pass effect. Excreted in urine and feces. ***Half-life:*** 19-37 hr.

INDICATIONS AND DOSAGES

Obsessive-compulsive disorder

PO

Adults, Elderly. Initially, 25 mg/day. May gradually increase to 100 mg/day in the first 2 wk. Maximum: 250 mg/day.

Children 10 yr and older. Initially, 25 mg/day. May gradually increase up to maximum of 200 mg/day.

AVAILABLE FORMS
• *Capsules:* 25 mg, 50 mg, 75 mg.

UNLABELED USES: Treatment of bulimia nervosa, cataplexy associated with narcolepsy, mental depression, neurogenic pain, panic disorder, ejaculatory disorders, pervasive developmental disorder

CONTRAINDICATIONS: Acute recovery period after MI, use within 14 days of MAOIs

PREGNANCY AND LACTATION: Pregnancy category C

SIDE EFFECTS

Frequent

Somnolence, fatigue, dry mouth, blurred vision, constipation, sexual dysfunction (42%), ejaculatory failure (20%), impotence, weight gain (18%), delayed micturition, orthostatic hypotension, diaphoresis, impaired concentration, increased appetite, urine retention

Occasional

GI disturbances (such as nausea, GI distress, and metallic taste), asthenia, aggressiveness, muscle weakness

Rare

Paradoxical reactions (agitation, restlessness, nightmares, insomnia), extrapyramidal symptoms, (particularly fine hand tremor), laryngitis, seizures

SERIOUS REACTIONS
• Overdose may produce seizures; cardiovascular effects, such as severe orthostatic hypotension, dizziness, tachycardia, palpitations, and arrhythmias; and altered temperature regulation, including hyperpyrexia or hypothermia.
• Abrupt discontinuation after prolonged therapy may produce head-

ache, malaise, nausea, vomiting, and vivid dreams.

• Anemia and agranulocytosis have been noted.

INTERACTIONS

3 *Antithyroid agents:* May increase risk of agranulocytosis

3 *Barbiturates:* Reduced serum concentrations of cyclic antidepressants

2 *Bethanidine:* Reduced antihypertensive effect of bethanidine

3 *Carbamazepine:* Reduced cyclic antidepressant serum concentrations

3 *Cimetidine:* May increase concentration and risk of toxicity

2 *Clonidine:* Reduced antihypertensive response to clonidine; enhanced hypertensive response with abrupt clonidine withdrawal

3 *Debrisoquin:* Inhibited antihypertensive response of debrisoquin

2 *Epinephrine:* Markedly enhanced pressor response to IV epinephrine

3 *Ethanol:* Additive impairment of motor skills; abstinent alcoholics may eliminate cyclic antidepressants more rapidly than nonalcoholics

3 *Fluoxetine, fluvoxamine, grapefruit juice:* Marked increases in cyclic antidepressant plasma concentrations

3 *Guanethidine:* Inhibited antihypertensive response to guanethidine

3 *Ibuprofen, other NSAIDs:* Increased risk of GI bleeding

⚠ *MAOIs:* Excessive sympathetic response, mania, or hyperpyrexia possible

2 *Moclobemide:* Potential association with fatal or non-fatal serotonin syndrome

3 *Neuroleptics:* Increased therapeutic and toxic effects of both drugs

2 *Norepinephrine:* Markedly enhanced pressor response to norepinephrine

3 *Phenothiazines:* May increase sedative and anticholinergic effects

2 *Phenylephrine:* Enhanced pressor response to IV phenylephrine

3 *Propoxyphene:* Enhanced effect of cyclic antidepressants

3 *Quinidine:* Increased cyclic antidepressant serum concentrations

SPECIAL CONSIDERATIONS

PATIENT/FAMILY EDUCATION

• Beneficial effects may take 2-3 wk

• Use caution while driving or during other activities requiring alertness; may cause drowsiness

• Avoid alcohol and other CNS depressants

• Do not discontinue abruptly

• Tolerance to postural hypotension, sedative, and anticholinergic effects usually develops during early therapy

MONITORING PARAMETERS

• Supervise suicidal risk patient closely during early therapy (as depression lessens, energy level improves, increasing suicidal potential)

• Assess appearance, behavior, speech pattern, level of interest, and mood

clonazepam

(kloe-na'-zi-pam)

Rx: Klonopin, Klonopin Wafer

Chemical Class: Benzodiazepine

Therapeutic Class: Anticonvulsant; anxiolytic

DEA Class: Schedule IV

CLINICAL PHARMACOLOGY

Mechanism of Action: A benzodiazepine that depresses all levels of the CNS; inhibits nerve impulse transmission in the motor cortex and suppresses abnormal discharge in petit mal seizures. ***Therapeutic Effect:*** Produces anxiolytic and anticonvulsant effects.

Pharmacokinetics

Well absorbed from the GI tract. Protein binding: 85%. Metabolized in the liver. Excreted in urine. Not removed by hemodialysis. ***Half-life:*** 18-50 hr.

INDICATIONS AND DOSAGES

Adjunctive treatment of Lennox-Gastaut syndrome (petit mal variant) and akinetic, myoclonic, and absence (petit mal) seizures

PO

Adults, Elderly, Children 10 yr and older. 1.5 mg/day; may be increased in 0.5- to 1-mg increments every 3 days until seizures are controlled. Do not exceed maintenance dosage of 20 mg/day.

Infants, Children younger than 10 yr or weighing less than 30 kg. 0.01-0.03 mg/kg/day in 2-3 divided doses; may be increased by up to 0.5 mg every 3 days until seizures are controlled. Do not exceed maintenance dosage of 0.2 mg/kg/day.

Panic disorder

PO

Adults, Elderly. Initially, 0.25 mg twice a day; increased in increments of 0.125-0.25 mg twice a day every 3 days. Maximum: 4 mg/day.

AVAILABLE FORMS

- *Tablets (Klonopin):* 0.5 mg, 1 mg, 2 mg.
- *Tablets (Disintegrating [Klonopin Wafer]):* 0.125 mg, 0.25 mg, 0.5 mg, 1 mg, 2 mg.

UNLABELED USES: Adjunctive treatment of seizures; treatment of simple, complex partial, and tonic-clonic seizures

CONTRAINDICATIONS: Narrow-angle glaucoma, significant hepatic disease, hypersensitivity to benzodiazepines

PREGNANCY AND LACTATION: Pregnancy category D; increased risk of congenital malformations, episodes of prolonged apnea, hypothermia in newborn reported; excreted into breast milk, breast-feeding not recommended

SIDE EFFECTS

Frequent

Mild, transient drowsiness; ataxia; behavioral disturbances (aggression, irritability, agitation), especially in children

Occasional

Rash, ankle or facial edema, nocturia, dysuria, change in appetite or weight, dry mouth, sore gums, nausea, blurred vision

Rare

Paradoxical CNS reactions, including hyperactivity or nervousness in children and excitement or restlessness in the elderly (particularly in the presence of uncontrolled pain)

SERIOUS REACTIONS

- Abrupt withdrawal may result in pronounced restlessness, irritability, insomnia, hand tremors, abdominal or muscle cramps, diaphoresis, vomiting, and status epilepticus.

• Overdose results in somnolence, confusion, diminished reflexes, and coma.

INTERACTIONS

Drugs

3 *CNS depressants:* Alcohol, narcotics, barbiturates, anxiolytics, phenothiazine, thioxanthene and butyrophenone antipsychotics, MAOIs, tricyclic antidepressants; CNS depression potentiated

3 *CYP3A inducers:* Phenytoin, carbamazepine, phenobarbital; decreased serum clonazepam concentrations

3 *Disulfiram:* Increased serum clonazepam concentrations

3 *Kava kava:* May increase sedation

3 *Oral antifungals:* Increased serum clonazepam concentrations, use cautiously

3 *St. John's Wort:* May decrease the effectiveness of clonazepam

3 *Valproic acid:* Increased occurrence of absence seizures

SPECIAL CONSIDERATIONS

• Up to 30% of patients have shown a loss of anticonvulsant activity, often within 3 mo of administration; dosage adjustment may reestablish efficacy

PATIENT/FAMILY EDUCATION

• Do not take more than prescribed amount, may be habit-forming

• Avoid driving, activities that require alertness; drowsiness may occur

• Avoid alcohol ingestion or other CNS depressants

• Do not discontinue medication abruptly after long-term use

MONITORING PARAMETERS

• Although relationship between serum concentrations and seizure control is not well established, proposed therapeutic concentrations are 20-80 ng/ml; potentially toxic concentrations >80 ng/ml

• Close attention to seizure frequency is important in order to detect the emergence of tolerance

• CBC and blood chemistry tests periodically to assess hepatic and renal function for patients on long-term therapy

---

clonidine

(kloe'-ni-deen)

Rx: Catapres, Catapres-TTS-1, Catapres-TTS-2, Catapres-TTS-3, Clonidine TTS-1, Clonidine TTS-2, Clonidine TTS-3, Duraclon

Combinations

Rx: with chlorthalidone (Chlorpres, Combipress)

Chemical Class: Imidazoline derivative

Therapeutic Class: Antihypertensive; centrally acting sympathoplegic

CLINICAL PHARMACOLOGY

Mechanism of Action: An antiadrenergic, sympatholytic agent that prevents pain signal transmission to the brain and produces analgesia at pre- and post-alpha-adrenergic receptors in the spinal cord. ***Therapeutic Effect:*** Reduces peripheral resistance; decreases BP and heart rate.

Pharmacokinetics

Route	Onset	Peak	Duration
PO	0.5-1 hr	2-4 hr	Up to 8 hr

Well absorbed from the GI tract. Transdermal best absorbed from the chest and upper arm; least absorbed from the thigh. Protein binding: 20%-40%. Metabolized in the liver.

Primarily excreted in urine. Minimally removed by hemodialysis. ***Half-life:*** 12-16 hr (increased with impaired renal function).

INDICATIONS AND DOSAGES

Hypertension

PO

Adults. Initially, 0.1 mg twice a day. Increase by 0.1-0.2 mg q2-4 days. Maintenance: 0.2-1.2 mg/day in 2-4 divided doses up to maximum of 2.4 mg/day.

Elderly. Initially, 0.1 mg at bedtime. May increase gradually.

Children. Initially, 5-10 mcg/kg/day in divided doses q8-12h. Increase at 5- to 7-day intervals up to 25 mcg/kg/day in divided doses q6h. Maximum: 0.9 mg/day.

Transdermal

Adults, Elderly. System delivering 0.1 mg/24 hr up to 0.6 mg/24 hr q7 days.

Attention deficit hyperactivity disorder (ADHD)

PO

Children. Initially, 0.05 mg/day. May increase by 0.05 mg/day q3-7 days up to 3-5 mcg/kg/day in divided doses 3-4 times a day. Maximum: 0.3-0.4 mg/day.

Severe pain

Epidural

Adults, Elderly. 30-40 mcg/hr.

Children. Initially, 0.5 mcg/kg/hr, not to exceed adult dose.

AVAILABLE FORMS

- *Tablets (Catapres):* 0.1 mg, 0.2 mg, 0.3 mg.
- *Transdermal Patch:* 2.5 mg (release at 0.1 mg/24 hr) (Catapres-TTS-1, Clonidine TTS-1), 5 mg (release at 0.2 mg/24 hr) (Catapres-TTS-2, Clonidine TTS-2), 7.5 mg (release at 0.3 mg/24 hr) (Catapres-TTS-3, Clonidine TTS-3).
- *Injection (Duraclon):* 100 mcg/ml, 500 mcg/ml.

UNLABELED USES: ADHD, diagnosis of pheochromocytoma, opioid withdrawal, prevention of migraine headaches, treatment of diarrhea in diabetes mellitus, treatment of dysmenorrhea, menopausal flushing

CONTRAINDICATIONS: Epidural contraindicated in those patients with bleeding diathesis or infection at the injection site, those receiving anticoagulation therapy

PREGNANCY AND LACTATION: Pregnancy category C; secreted into breast milk; hypotension has not been observed in nursing infants, although clonidine was found in the serum of the infants

SIDE EFFECTS

Frequent

Dry mouth (40%), somnolence (33%), dizziness (16%), sedation, constipation (10%)

Occasional (5%-1%)

Tablets, injection: Depression, swelling of feet, loss of appetite, decreased sexual ability, itching eyes, dizziness, nausea, vomiting, nervousness

Transdermal: Itching, reddening or darkening of skin

Rare (less than 1%)

Nightmares, vivid dreams, cold feeling in fingers and toes

SERIOUS REACTIONS

- Overdose produces profound hypotension, irritability, bradycardia, respiratory depression, hypothermia, miosis (pupillary constriction), arrhythmias, and apnea.
- Abrupt withdrawal may result in rebound hypertension associated with nervousness, agitation, anxiety, insomnia, hand tingling, tremor, flushing, and diaphoresis.

INTERACTIONS

Drugs

3 *β-blockers:* Rebound hypertension from clonidine withdrawal exacerbated by noncardioselective β-blockers

❷ *Cyclic antidepressants:* Cyclic antidepressants may inhibit the antihypertensive response to clonidine

3 *Cyclosporine, tacrolimus:* Increased cyclosporine or tacrolimus concentrations

3 *Insulin:* Diminished symptoms of hypoglycemia

❷ *Mirtazepine:* Severe hypertensive reaction

3 *Neuroleptics, nitroprusside:* Severe hypotension possible

3 *Yohimbine:* May decrease the effectiveness of clonidine

SPECIAL CONSIDERATIONS

PATIENT/FAMILY EDUCATION

- Avoid hazardous activities, since drug may cause drowsiness
- Do not discontinue oral drug abruptly or withdrawal symptoms may occur (anxiety, increased BP, headache, insomnia, increased pulse, tremors, nausea, sweating)
- Response may take 2-3 days if drug is given transdermally
- Do not use OTC (cough, cold, or allergy) products unless directed by clinician
- Rise slowly to sitting or standing position to minimize orthostatic hypotension, especially elderly
- Dizziness, fainting, lightheadedness may occur during first few days of therapy
- May cause dry mouth; use hard candy, saliva product, or frequent rinsing of mouth

MONITORING PARAMETERS

- Blood pressure (posturally), blood glucose in patients with diabetes mellitus, confusion, mental depression
- Daily bowel activity and stool consistency

clopidogrel bisulfate

(kloh-pid′-oh-grel bye-sul′-fate)

Rx: Plavix

Chemical Class: Thienopyridine derivative

Therapeutic Class: Antiplatelet agent

CLINICAL PHARMACOLOGY

Mechanism of Action: A thienopyridine derivative that inhibits binding of the enzyme adenosine phosphate (ADP) to its platelet receptor and subsequent ADP-mediated activation of a glycoprotein complex. ***Therapeutic Effect:*** Inhibits platelet aggregation.

Pharmacokinetics

Route	*Onset*	*Peak*	*Duration*
PO	1 hr	2 hr	N/A

Rapidly absorbed. Protein binding: 98%. Extensively metabolized by the liver. Eliminated equally in the urine and feces. ***Half-life:*** 8 hr.

INDICATIONS AND DOSAGES

MI, stroke reduction

PO

Adults, Elderly. 75 mg once a day.

Acute coronary syndrome

PO

Adults, Elderly. Initially, 300 mg loading dose, then 75 mg once a day (in combination with aspirin).

AVAILABLE FORMS

- *Tablets:* 75 mg.

UNLABELED USES: Graft patency (saphenous vein), mitral regurgitation, mitral stenosis, noncardioembolic stroke, percutaneous coronary intervention

CONTRAINDICATIONS: Active bleeding, coagulation disorders, severe hepatic disease

PREGNANCY AND LACTATION: Pregnancy category B; excreted into breast milk in rats

SIDE EFFECTS

Frequent (15%)

Skin disorders

Occasional (8%-6%)

Upper respiratory tract infection, chest pain, flu-like symptoms, headache, dizziness, arthralgia

Rare (5%-3%)

Fatigue, edema, hypertension, abdominal pain, dyspepsia, diarrhea, nausea, epistaxis, dyspnea, rhinitis

SERIOUS REACTIONS

• Agranulocytosis, aplastic anemia/pancytopenia, and thrombotic thrombocytopenic purpura (TTP) occur rarely.

• Cases of bleeding with fatal outcome (especially intracranial, GI, and retroperitoneal hemorrhage) have been reported.

• Hepatitis, hypersensitivity reactions, anaphylactoid reactions, and angioedema have also been reported.

INTERACTIONS

Drugs

3 *Fluvastatin:* Inhibition of hepatic metabolism (CYP2C9) of fluvastatin with increased risk of myositis; *in vitro* data

3 *Ginger, ginkgo biloba:* May increase the risk of bleeding

3 *Nonsteroidal antiinflammatory agents:* Increased bleeding risk

3 *Phenytoin:* Inhibition of hepatic metabolism (CYP2C9) of phenytoin and increased risk of toxicity; *in vitro* data

3 *Tamoxifen:* Inhibition of hepatic metabolism (CYP2C9) and increased tamoxifen effects; *in vitro* data

3 *Tolbutamide:* Inhibition of hepatic metabolism (CYP2C9) of tolbutamide with increased risk of hypoglycemia; *in vitro* data

3 *Torsemide:* Inhibition of hepatic metabolism (CYP2C9) of torsemide with enhanced diuretic effects; *in vitro* data; increased bleeding risk

3 *Warfarin:* Inhibition of hepatic metabolism (CYP2C9) of warfarin with enhanced hypoprothrombinemic effects; *in vitro* data; increased bleeding risk

SPECIAL CONSIDERATIONS

• Comparative studies indicate that the drug is at least effective as aspirin; comparisons with ticlopidine lacking, however, no frequent CBC monitoring necessary

• Should probably replace ticlopidine as an aspirin alternative

• 28 × the cost of an equivalent supply of aspirin

PATIENT/FAMILY EDUCATION

• Inform clinician of signs and symptoms of bleeding, prior to surgery, dental work; inform clinician of sore throat, fever, etc. (consider neutropenia)

• Notify the dentist and other physicians of clopidogrel therapy before surgery is scheduled or new drugs are prescribed

MONITORING PARAMETERS

• Platelet count for thrombocytopenia

• Hgb, WBC count, and BUN, serum bilirubin, creatinine, AST(SGOT) and ALT(SGPT) levels

• Evaluate for signs and symptoms of hepatic insufficiency during clopidogrel therapy

clorazepate dipotassium

(klor-az'-e-pate)

Rx: Gen-Xene, Tranxene, Tranxene-SD

Chemical Class: Benzodiazepine

Therapeutic Class: Anxiolytic

DEA Class: Schedule IV

CLINICAL PHARMACOLOGY

Mechanism of Action: A benzodiazepine that depresses all levels of the CNS, including limbic and reticular formation, by binding to benzodiazepine receptor sites on the gamma-aminobutyric acid (GABA) receptor complex. Modulates GABA, a major inhibitory neurotransmitter in the brain. ***Therapeutic Effect:*** Produces anxiolytic effect, suppresses seizure activity.

INDICATIONS AND DOSAGES

Anxiety

PO (Regular-Release)

Adults, Elderly. 7.5-15 mg 2-4 times a day.

PO (Sustained-Release)

Adults, Elderly. 11.25 mg or 22.5 mg once a day at bedtime.

Anticonvulsant

PO

Adults, Elderly, Children older than 12 yr. Initially, 7.5 mg 2-3 times a day. May increase by 7.5 mg at weekly intervals. Maximum: 90 mg/day.

Children 9-12 yr. Initially, 3.75-7.5 mg twice a day. May increase by 2.75 mg at weekly intervals. Maximum: 60 mg/day in 2-3 divided doses.

Alcohol withdrawal

PO

Adults, Elderly. Initially, 30 mg, then 15 mg 2-4 times a day on first day. Gradually decrease dosage over subsequent days. Maximum: 90 mg/day.

AVAILABLE FORMS

- *Tablets (Tranxene T-Tab):* 3.75 mg, 7.5 mg, 15 mg.
- *Tablets (Sustained-Release):* 11.25 mg (Tranxene SD Half-Strength), 22.5 mg (Tranxene SD).

CONTRAINDICATIONS: Acute narrow-angle glaucoma

PREGNANCY AND LACTATION: Pregnancy category D; excreted into breast milk; drug and metabolites may accumulate to toxic levels in nursing infant

SIDE EFFECTS

Frequent

Somnolence

Occasional

Dizziness, GI disturbances, nervousness, blurred vision, dry mouth, headache, confusion, ataxia, rash, irritability, slurred speech

Rare

Paradoxical CNS reactions, such as hyperactivity or nervousness in children and excitement or restlessness in the elderly or debilitated (generally noted during first 2 wks of therapy, particularly in presence of uncontrolled pain)

SERIOUS REACTIONS

- Abrupt or too-rapid withdrawal may result in pronounced restlessness, irritability, insomnia, hand tremors, abdominal or muscle cramps, diaphoresis, vomiting, and seizures.
- Overdose results in somnolence, confusion, diminished reflexes, and coma.

INTERACTIONS

Drugs

❷ *Azole antifungals:* May increase the serum concentrations of clorazepate and increase the risk of potential toxicity

3 *Cimetidine:* Increased plasma levels of clorazepate and/or active metabolites

3 *Disulfiram:* Increased serum clorazepate concentrations

3 *Ethanol:* Enhanced adverse psychomotor side effects of benzodiazepines

3 *Kava kava, valerian:* May increase CNS depression

3 *Rifampin:* Reduced serum clorazepate concentrations

3 *St. John's Wort:* May decrease the effectiveness of clorazepate

SPECIAL CONSIDERATIONS

- Do not use for everyday stress or for longer than 4 mo
- No advantage over diazepam

PATIENT/FAMILY EDUCATION

- Do not discontinue medication abruptly after long-term use
- Avoid tasks that require mental alertness or motor skills until response to the drug has been established
- Change positions slowly—from recumbent to sitting before standing—to prevent dizziness
- The female patient should notify the physician immediately if she becomes or may be pregnant
- Avoid smoking and consuming alcoholic beverages during therapy

MONITORING PARAMETERS

- Therapeutic response, characterized by a calm facial expression and decreased restlessness in anxious patients and a decrease in intensity or frequency of seizures in patients with seizure disorder
- Therapeutic peak serum level is 0.12-1.5 mcg/ml; the toxic serum level is greater than 5 mcg/ml

clotrimazole

(kloe-trim'-a-zole)

OTC: Mycelex, Mycelex OTC, Lotrimin, Gyne-Lotrimin, Trivagizole 3

Combinations

Rx: with betamethasone dipropionate (Lotrisone)

Chemical Class: Imidazole derivative

Therapeutic Class: Topical antifungal

CLINICAL PHARMACOLOGY

Mechanism of Action: An antifungal that binds with phospholipids in fungal cell membrane. ***Therapeutic Effect:*** Inhibits yeast growth.

Pharmacokinetics

Poorly, erratically absorbed from GI tract. Bound to oral mucosa. Absorbed portion metabolized in liver. Eliminated in feces. Topical: Minimal systemic absorption (highest concentration in stratum corneum). Intravaginal: Small amount systemically absorbed. ***Half-life:*** 3.5-5 hrs.

INDICATIONS AND DOSAGES

Oropharyngeal candidiasis treatment

PO

Adults, Elderly. 10 mg 5 times/day for 14 days.

Oropharyngeal candidiasis prophylaxis

PO

Adults, Elderly. 10 mg 3 times/day.

Dermatophytosis, cutaneous candidiasis

Topical

Adults, Elderly. 2 times/day. Therapeutic effect may take up to 8 wks.

Vulvovaginal candidiasis
Vaginal (Tablets)
Adults, Elderly. 1 tablet (100 mg) at bedtime for 7 days; 2 tablets (200 mg) at bedtime for 3 days; or 500 mg tablet one time.
Vaginal (Cream)
Adults, Elderly. 1 applicatorful at bedtime for 7-14 days.

AVAILABLE FORMS
• *Combination pack:* Vaginal tablet 100 mg and vaginal cream 1% (Mycelex-7).
• *Lotion:* 1% (Lotrimin).
• *Topical Cream:* 1% (Lotrimin, Lotrimin AF, Mycelex, Mycelex OTC).
• *Topical Solution:* 1% (Lotrimin, Lotrimin AF, Mycelex, Mycelex OTC).
• *Troches:* 10 mg (Mycelex).
• *Vaginal Cream:* 1% (Gyne-Lotrimin, Mycelex-7), 2% (Gyne-Lotrimin 3, Mycelex-3, Trivagizole 3).
• *Vaginal Tablets:* 100 mg, 500 mg (Gyne-Lotrimin, Mycelex-7).

UNLABELED USES: *Topical:* Treatment of paronychia, tinea barbae, tinea capitas

CONTRAINDICATIONS: Hypersensitivity to clotrimazole or any component of the formulation, children <3 yrs

PREGNANCY AND LACTATION: Pregnancy category B; excretion in breast milk unknown

SIDE EFFECTS
Frequent
Oral: Nausea, vomiting, diarrhea, abdominal pain
Occasional
Topical: Itching, burning, stinging, erythema, urticaria
Vaginal: Mild burning (tablets/cream); irritation, cystitis (cream)
Rare
Vaginal: Itching, rash, lower abdominal cramping, headache

SERIOUS REACTIONS
• None reported.

INTERACTIONS
Drugs
3 *Cyclosporine, tacrolimus:* Clotrimazole troche administration may increase cyclosporine or tacrolimus concentrations

SPECIAL CONSIDERATIONS

PATIENT/FAMILY EDUCATION
• Continue for the full length of therapy
• Avoid contact with eyes
• Refrain from sexual intercourse or advise partner to use a condom during therapy

MONITORING PARAMETERS
• Skin for blistering or urticaria
• With vaginal therapy, evaluate for vulvovaginal irritation, abdominal cramping, urinary frequency, and discomfort

clozapine
(klo′-za-peen)
Rx: Clozaril, FazaClo
Chemical Class: Dibenzodiazepine derivative
Therapeutic Class: Antipsychotic

CLINICAL PHARMACOLOGY
Mechanism of Action: A dibenzodiazepine derivative that interferes with the binding of dopamine at dopamine receptor sites; binds primarily at nondopamine receptor sites. ***Therapeutic Effect:*** Diminishes schizophrenic behavior.
Pharmacokinetics
Absorbed rapidly and almost completely. Distributed rapidly and extensively. Crosses the blood-brain

barrier. Protein binding: 95%. Metabolized in the liver. Excreted in urine and feces. ***Half-life:*** 8 hr.

INDICATIONS AND DOSAGES

Schizophrenic disorders, reduce suicidal behavior

PO

Adults. Initially, 25 mg once or twice a day. May increase by 25-50 mg/day over 2 wk until dosage of 300-450 mg/day is achieved. May further increase by 50-100 mg/day no more than once or twice a week, Range: 200-600 mg/day. Maximum: 900 mg/day.

Elderly. Initially, 25 mg/day. May increase by 25 mg/day. Maximum: 450 mg/day.

AVAILABLE FORMS

- *Tablets (Clozaril):* 12.5 mg, 25 mg, 100 mg.
- *Tablets (Oral-Disintegrating-[FazaClo]):* 25 mg, 100 mg.

CONTRAINDICATIONS: Coma, concurrent use of other drugs that may suppress bone marrow function, history of clozapine-induced agranulocytosis or severe granulocytopenia, myeloproliferative disorders, severe CNS depression

PREGNANCY AND LACTATION: Pregnancy category B

SIDE EFFECTS

Frequent

Somnolence (39%), salivation (31%), tachycardia (25%), dizziness (19%), constipation (14%)

Occasional

Hypotension (9%); headache (7%); tremor, syncope, diaphoresis, dry mouth (6%); nausea, visual disturbances (5%); nightmares, restlessness, akinesia, agitation, hypertension, abdominal discomfort or heartburn, weight gain (4%)

Rare

Rigidity, confusion, fatigue, insomnia, diarrhea, rash

SERIOUS REACTIONS

- *Alert:* Blood dyscrasias, particularly agranulocytosis and mild leukopenia, may occur.
- Seizures occur in about 3% of patients.
- Overdose produces CNS depression (including sedation, coma, and delirium), respiratory depression, and hypersalivation.

INTERACTIONS

Drugs

3 *Alcohol, CNS depressants:* May increase CNS depressant effects

3 *Bone marrow depressants:* May increase myelosuppression

3 *Carbamazepine, phenytoin, primadone, valproic acid:* Considerable reduction in plasma clozapine concentrations

3 *Cigarette smoking:* Serious clozapine toxicity has occurred following smoking cessation

3 *Cimetidine, clarithromycin, troleandomycin:* Increased serum clozapine concentrations

3 *Digitoxin:* Increased serum digitoxin concentrations due to protein-binding displacement

3 *Diazepam:* Isolated cases of cardiorespiratory collapse have been reported

3 *Epinephrine:* Reversed pressor effects of epinephrine

❷ *Erythromycin:* Increased serum clozapine concentrations

3 *Fluoxetine:* Modest elevation of serum clozapine concentrations

❷ *Fluvoxamine:* Marked increase in plasma clozapine concentrations and side effects; increased risk of leukocytosis

3 *Lithium:* May increase risk of seizures, confusion, dyskinesias

3 *Lorazepam:* Cardiovascular and respiratory collapse has been reported

3 *Paroxetine:* Modest elevation of serum clozapine concentrations

3 *Quinidine:* Increased serum clozapine concentrations possible

3 *Sertraline:* Modest elevation of serum clozapine concentrations

3 *Type 1C antiarrhythmics:* Propafenone, flecainide, encainide; increased serum clozapine concentration possible

3 *Warfarin:* Increased serum warfarin concentrations due to protein-binding displacement

SPECIAL CONSIDERATIONS

- The risk of agranulocytosis and seizures limits use to patients who have failed to respond or were unable to tolerate treatment with appropriate courses of standard antipsychotics.
- Advise patients to report immediately the appearance of lethargy, weakness, fever, sore throat, malaise, mucous membrane ulceration, or other possible signs of infection.
- Patients cannot be reinitiated on clozapine if WBC counts fall below $2000/mm^3$ or ANC falls below $1000/mm^3$ during clozapine therapy.

PATIENT/FAMILY EDUCATION

- Do not abruptly withdraw from long-term drug therapy.
- Drowsiness generally subsides during continued therapy.
- Avoid tasks that require mental alertness or motor skills until response to the drug is established.
- Avoid alcohol.

MONITORING PARAMETERS

- WBC at baseline and then qwk for first 6 mo, every other week thereafter if WBC counts maintained (WBC $\geq 3000/mm^3$, ANC $\geq 1500/mm^3$); WBC counts qwk for at least 4 weeks after discontinuation.
- Blood pressure, LFTs
- Pulse for tachycardia
- Supervise suicidal risk patient closely during early therapy (as depression lessens, energy level improves, increasing suicide potential)
- Assess for therapeutic response (interest in surroundings, improvement in self-care, increased ability to concentrate, relaxed facial expression)

codeine phosphate/ codeine sulfate

(koe'-deen foss'-fate/koe'-deen sul'-fate)

Rx: Codeine Phosphate, Codeine Sulfate

Combinations

Rx: with acetaminophen (Tylenol no. 2, Tylenol no. 3, Tylenol no. 4); with aspirin (Empirin no. 3, Empirin no. 4); with chlorpheniramine (Codeprex); with guaifenesin (Robitussin AC); with APAP (Capital, Aceta); with APAP butalbital, caffeine (Fioricet, Phenaphen); with aspirin (Fiorinal)

Chemical Class: Natural opium alkaloid; phenanthrene derivative

Therapeutic Class: Antitussive; narcotic analgesic

DEA Class: Schedule II

CLINICAL PHARMACOLOGY

Mechanism of Action: An opioid agonist that binds to opioid receptors at many sites in the CNS, particularly in the medulla. This action inhibits the ascending pain pathways. ***Therapeutic Effect:*** Alters the perception of and emotional response to pain, suppresses cough reflex.

Pharmacokinetics

Well absorbed following PO administration. Protein binding: Very low. Metabolized in liver. Excreted in urine. ***Half-life:*** 2.5-3.5 hr.

INDICATIONS AND DOSAGES

Analgesia

PO, IM, Subcutaneous

Adults, Elderly. 30 mg q4-6h. Range: 15-60 mg.

Children. 0.5-1 mg/kg q4-6h. Maximum: 60 mg/dose.

Cough

PO

Adults, Elderly, Children 12 yr and older. 10-20 mg q4-6h.

Children 6-11 yr. 5-10 mg q4-6h.

Children 2-5 yr. 2.5-5 mg q4-6h.

Dosage in renal impairment

Dosage is modified based on creatinine clearance.

Creatinine Clearance	*Dosage*
10-50 ml/min	75% of usual dose
less than 10 ml/min	50% of usual dose

AVAILABLE FORMS

- *Tablets (phosphate):* 30 mg, 60 mg.
- *Tablets (sulfate):* 15 mg, 30 mg, 60 mg.
- *Oral Solution:* 15 mg/5 ml.
- *Injection:* 15 mg/ml, 30 mg/ml, 60 mg/ml.

UNLABELED USES: Treatment of diarrhea

CONTRAINDICATIONS: Premature infants

PREGNANCY AND LACTATION: Pregnancy category C (category D if used for prolonged periods or in high doses at term); use during labor produces neonatal respiratory depression; passes into breast milk in very small amounts; compatible with breast-feeding

Controlled Substance: Schedule II (analgesic), III (fixed-combination form)

SIDE EFFECTS

Frequent

Constipation, somnolence, nausea, vomiting

Occasional

Paradoxical excitement, confusion, palpitations, facial flushing, decreased urination, blurred vision, dizziness, dry mouth, headache, hypotension (including orthostatic hy-

potension), decreased appetite, injection site redness, burning, or pain
Rare
Hallucinations, depression, abdominal pain, insomnia
SERIOUS REACTIONS
- Too-frequent use may result in paralytic ileus.
- Overdose may produce cold and clammy skin, confusion, seizures, decreased BP, restlessness, pinpoint pupils, bradycardia, respiratory depression, decreased LOC, and severe weakness.
- The patient who uses codeine repeatedly may develop a tolerance to the drug's analgesic effect as well as physical dependence.

INTERACTIONS
Drugs
3 *Barbiturates:* Additive respiratory and CNS depressant effects
3 *Antihistamines, chloral hydrate, glutethimide, methocarbamol:* Enhanced depressant effects
3 *Cimetidine:* Increased respiratory and CNS depression
3 *Ethanol, other CNS depressants:* Additive CNS effects
❷ *MAOIs:* May produce a severe, sometimes fatal reaction; plan to administer a test dose, which is one-quarter of usual codeine dose
❷ *Quinidine:* Inhibited analgesic effect of codeine
Labs
- *Increase:* Urine morphine
- False elevatons of amylase and lipase

SPECIAL CONSIDERATIONS
PATIENT/FAMILY EDUCATION
- Minimize nausea by administering with food and remain lying down following dose
- Do not administer agonist/antagonist analgesics (i.e., pentazocine, nalbuphine, butorphanol, dezocine, buprenorphine) to patient who has received a prolonged course of codeine (a pure agonist). In opioid-dependent patients, mixed agonist/antagonist analgesics may precipitate withdrawal symptoms
- Change positions slowly to avoid orthostatic hypotension
- Avoid tasks that require mental alertness or motor skills until response to the drug has been established
- Avoid alcohol during codeine therapy

MONITORING PARAMETERS
- Clinical improvement and onset of pain or cough relief
- Bowel activity and stool consistency

---

colchicine
(kol'-chi-seen)
Rx: Colchicine
Combinations
Rx: with probenicid (Proben-C, Colbenemid)
Chemical Class: Colchicum autumnale alkaloid
Therapeutic Class: Antigout agent

CLINICAL PHARMACOLOGY
Mechanism of Action: An alkaloid that decreases leukocyte motility, phagocytosis, and lactic acid production. ***Therapeutic Effect:*** Decreases urate crystal deposits and reduces inflammatory process.
Pharmacokinetics
Rapidly absorbed from the GI tract. Highest concentration is in the liver, spleen, and kidney. Protein binding: 30%-50%. Reenters the intestinal tract by biliary secretion and is reabsorbed from the intestines. Partially metabolized in the liver. Eliminated primarily in feces.

INDICATIONS AND DOSAGES
Acute gouty arthritis
PO
Adults, Elderly. Initially, 0.6-1.2 mg; then 0.6 mg q1-2h until pain is relieved or nausea, vomiting, or diarrhea occurs. Total dose: 6 mg.
IV
Adults, Elderly. Initially, 1-2 mg; then 0.5 mg q6h until satisfactory response. Maximum: 4 mg/wk or 4 mg/one course of treatment. If pain recurs, may give 1-2 mg/day for several days but no sooner than 7 days after a full course of IV therapy (total of 4 mg).
Chronic gouty arthritis
PO
Adults, Elderly. 0.6 mg every other day up to 3 times a day.
AVAILABLE FORMS
- *Tablets:* 0.5 mg, 0.6 mg.
- *Injection:* 0.5 mg/ml.

UNLABELED USES: To reduce frequency of recurrence of familial Mediterranean fever; treatment of acute calcium pyrophosphate deposition, amyloidosis, biliary cirrhosis, recurrent pericarditis, sarcoid arthritis
CONTRAINDICATIONS: Blood dyscrasias; severe cardiac, GI, hepatic, or renal disorders
PREGNANCY AND LACTATION: Pregnancy category D (known teratogen)
SIDE EFFECTS
Frequent
PO: Nausea, vomiting, abdominal discomfort
Occasional
PO: Anorexia
Rare
Hypersensitivity reaction, including angioedema
Parenteral: Nausea, vomiting, diarrhea, abdominal discomfort, pain or redness at injection site, neuritis in injected arm
SERIOUS REACTIONS
- Bone marrow depression, including aplastic anemia, agranulocytosis, and thrombocytopenia, may occur with long-term therapy.
- Overdose initially causes a burning feeling in the skin or throat, severe diarrhea, and abdominal pain. The patient then experiences fever, seizures, delirium, and renal impairment, marked by hematuria and oliguria. The third stage of overdose causes hair loss, leukocytosis, and stomatitis.

INTERACTIONS
Drugs
3 *Bone marrow depressants:* May increase the risk of blood dyscrasias
3 *Cyclosporine, tacrolimus:* Increased serum level of cyclosporine or tacrolimus
3 *Erythromycin, clarithromycin, troleandomycin:* Potential for severe colchicine toxicity
3 *NSAIDs:* May increase the risk of bone marrow depression, neutropenia, and thrombocytopenia
Labs
- *Interference:* Urinary 17-hydroxycorticosteroids

SPECIAL CONSIDERATIONS
PATIENT/FAMILY EDUCATION
- Limit intake of high-purine foods, such as fish and organ meats, and drink 8-10 eight-ounce glasses of fluid daily while taking colchicine
- Notify the physician if fever, numbness, skin rash, sore throat, fatigue, unusual bleeding or bruising, or weakness occurs
- Discontinue colchicine as soon as gout pain is relieved, or at the first appearance of diarrhea, nausea, or vomiting

MONITORING PARAMETERS
- CBC, platelets, reticulocytes before and during therapy (q3mo)
- Fluid intake and output
- Serum uric acid level

• Therapeutic response, including improved joint range of motion and reduced joint tenderness, redness, and swelling

colesevelam

(koh-le-sev′-e-lam hye-droe-klor′-ide)

Rx: WelChol

Chemical Class: Hydrophilic nonabsorbed polymer

Therapeutic Class: Antilipemic; bile acid sequestrant

CLINICAL PHARMACOLOGY

Mechanism of Action: A bile acid sequestrant and nonsystemic polymer that binds with bile acids in the intestines, preventing their reabsorption and removing them from the body. ***Therapeutic Effect:*** Decreases LDL cholesterol.

Pharmacokinetics

Not absorbed. Primarily eliminated in feces.

INDICATIONS AND DOSAGES

To decrease LDL cholesterol level in primary hypercholesterolemia (Fredrickson type IIa)

PO

Adults, Elderly. 3 tablets with meals twice a day or 6 tablets once a day with a meal. May increase daily dose to 7 tablets a day.

AVAILABLE FORMS

• *Tablets:* 625 mg.

CONTRAINDICATIONS: Complete biliary obstruction

PREGNANCY AND LACTATION: Pregnancy category B (no harm in animal studies, but no adequate and well-controlled studies in pregnant women; no expected excretion into breast milk

SIDE EFFECTS

Frequent (12%-8%)

Flatulence, constipation, infection, dyspepsia (heartburn, epigastric distress)

SERIOUS REACTIONS

• GI tract obstruction may occur.

INTERACTIONS

Drugs

• Although no drug interactions have been documented, binding to drugs given concomitantly may be significantly impacted; drug where small differences in serum level may be significant should be monitored closely

SPECIAL CONSIDERATIONS

• Combination colesevelam and an HMG-CoA reductase inhibitor is effective in further lowering serum total cholesterol and LDL cholesterol levels beyond that achieved by either agent alone

PATIENT/FAMILY EDUCATION

• Tablets should be taken with a liquid, and with a meal
• Follow the prescribed diet
• Periodic laboratory tests are an essential part of therapy
• Do not take any medications, including OTC drugs, without physician approval

MONITORING PARAMETERS

• Plasma lipids
• Pattern of daily bowel activity and stool consistency

colestipol hydrochloride

(koe-les'-ti-pole hye-droe-klor'-ide)

Rx: Colestid

Chemical Class: Bile acid sequestrant

Therapeutic Class: Antilipemic; bile acid sequestrant

CLINICAL PHARMACOLOGY

Mechanism of Action: An antihyperlipoproteinemic that binds with bile acids in the intestine, forming an insoluble complex. Binding results in partial removal of bile acid from enterohepatic circulation. ***Therapeutic Effect:*** Removes low-density lipoproteins (LDL) and cholesterol from plasma.

Pharmacokinetics

Not absorbed from the gastrointestinal (GI) tract. Excreted in the feces.

INDICATIONS AND DOSAGES

Primary hypercholesterolemia

PO, granules

Adults, Elderly. Initially, 5 g 1-2 times/day. Range: 5-30 g/day once or in divided doses.

PO, tablets

Adults, Elderly. Initially, 2 g 1-2 times/day. Range: 2-16 g/day.

AVAILABLE FORMS

• *Granules:* 5-g packet (Colestid).
• *Tablet:* 1 g (Colestid).

UNLABELED USES: Treatment of diarrhea (due to bile acids); hyperoxaluria

CONTRAINDICATIONS: Complete biliary obstruction, hypersensitivity to bile acid sequestering resins

PREGNANCY AND LACTATION: Pregnancy category C

SIDE EFFECTS

Frequent

Constipation (may lead to fecal impaction), nausea, vomiting, stomach pain, indigestion

Occasional

Diarrhea, belching, bloating, headache, dizziness

Rare

Gallstones, peptic ulcer, malabsorption syndrome

SERIOUS REACTIONS

• GI tract obstruction, hyperchloremic acidosis, and osteoporosis secondary to calcium excretion may occur.
• High dosage may interfere with fat absorption, resulting in steatorrhea.

INTERACTIONS

Drugs

3 *Acetaminophen, amiodarone, corticosteroids, diclofenac, digitalis glycosides, furosemide, gemfibrozil, methotrexate, metronidazole, oral vancomycin, tetracycline, thiazide diuretics, thyroid hormones, valproic acid:* Colestipol reduces interacting drug concentrations and probably subsequent therapeutic response

3 *Oral anticoagulants:* Inhibition of hypoprothrombinemic response; colestipol might be less likely to interact

SPECIAL CONSIDERATIONS

• Bile acid sequestrant choice should be based on cost and patient acceptability
• Give all other medications 1 hr before colestipol or 4 hr after colestipol to avoid poor absorption

PATIENT/FAMILY EDUCATION

• Mix the powder with 3-6 oz fruit juice, milk, soup, or water; place the powder on the surface of a liquid for 1-2 min to prevent lumping and then mix the powder into liquid; never take colestipol in its dry form
• Take colestipol before meals and drink several glasses of water between meals

• Eat high-fiber foods such as fruits, whole grain cereals, and vegetables to reduce the risk of constipation

MONITORING PARAMETERS

• Daily bowel activity and stool consistency

• Blood chemistry test

cortisone acetate

(kor'-ti-sone)

Rx: Cortone

Chemical Class: Glucocorticoid

Therapeutic Class: Corticosteroid, systemic

CLINICAL PHARMACOLOGY

Mechanism of Action: An adrenocortical steroid that inhibits the accumulation of inflammatory cells at inflammation sites, phagocytosis, lysosomal enzyme release and synthesis, and release of mediators of inflammation. ***Therapeutic Effect:*** Prevents or suppresses cell-mediated immune reactions. Decreases or prevents tissue response to inflammatory process.

Pharmacokinetics

Rapidly and almost completely absorbed after PO administration. Protein binding: 90%. Metabolized in liver. Excreted in urine. ***Half-life:*** Unknown.

INDICATIONS AND DOSAGES

Adrenocortical insufficiency

PO

Adults, Elderly. 12-15 mg/m^2 divided as two-thirds in the morning and one-third in the afternoon.

Children. 0.5-0.75 mg/kg/day in 3 divided doses.

IM

Children. 0.25-0.35 mg/kg/day.

Dosage is dependent on the condition being treated and patient response.

Inflammatory conditions

PO

Adults, Elderly. 25-300 mg/day.

Children. 2.5-10 mg/kg/day in 3-4 divided doses.

IM

Adults, Elderly. 25-300 mg/day.

Children. 1-5 mg/kg/day in 1-2 doses/day.

AVAILABLE FORMS

• *Tablets:* 5 mg, 10 mg, 25 mg.

• *Injectable Suspension:* 25 mg/ml, 50 mg/ml.

CONTRAINDICATIONS: Hypersensitivity to corticosteroids, administration of live virus vaccine, peptic ulcers (except in life-threatening situations), systemic fungal infection

PREGNANCY AND LACTATION: Pregnancy category C (D if used in the first trimester); excreted in breast milk

SIDE EFFECTS

Frequent

Insomnia, heartburn, anxiety, abdominal distention, increased diaphoresis, acne, mood swings, increased appetite, facial flushing, delayed wound healing, increased susceptibility to infection, diarrhea or constipation

Occasional

Headache, edema, change in skin color, frequent urination

Rare

Tachycardia, allergic reaction (such as rash and hives), psychologic changes, hallucinations, depression

SERIOUS REACTIONS

• Long-term therapy may cause hypocalcemia, hypokalemia, muscle wasting in arms and legs, osteoporosis, spontaneous fractures, amenorrhea, cataracts, glaucoma, peptic ulcer disease, and CHF.

• Abrupt withdrawal following long-term therapy may cause anorexia, nausea, fever, headache, joint pain, rebound inflammation, fatigue, weakness, lethargy, dizziness, and orthostatic hypotension.

INTERACTIONS

Drugs

3 *Aminoglutethamide:* Enhanced elimination of corticosteroids; marked reduction in corticosteroid response; doubling of dose may be necessary

3 *Amphotericin:* May increase hypokalemia

3 *Antidiabetics:* Increased blood glucose

3 *Barbiturates, carbamazepine:* Reduced serum concentrations of corticosteroids

❷ *Bupropion:* May lower the seizure threshold

3 *Cholestyramine, colestipol:* Possible reduced absorption of corticosteroids

3 *Cyclosporine:* Possible increased concentration of both drugs, seizures

3 *Digoxin:* May increase digoxin toxicity caused by hypokalemia

3 *Diuretics:* May decrease the effects of diuretics

3 *Erythromycin, troleandomycin, clarithromycin, ketoconazole:* Possible enhanced steroid effect

3 *Estrogens, oral contraceptives:* Enhanced effects of corticosteroids

3 *Fluoroquinolones:* May increase the risk for tendon rupture

3 *Isoniazid:* Reduced plasma concentrations of isoniazid

3 *IUDs:* Inhibition of inflammation may decrease contraceptive effect

3 *Live-virus vaccines:* May decrease the patient's antibody response to vaccine, increase vaccine side effects, and potentiate virus replication

3 *NSAIDs:* Increased risk GI ulceration

3 *Potassium supplements:* May decrease the effects of potassium supplements

3 *Rifampin:* Reduced therapeutic effect of corticosteroids

3 *Salicylates:* Subtherapeutic salicylate concentrations possible

SPECIAL CONSIDERATIONS

- Increased dose of rapidly acting corticosteroids may be necessary in patient subjected to unusual stress
- May mask infections
- Do not give live virus vaccines to patients on prolonged therapy
- Patients on chronic steroid therapy should wear medical bracelet
- Drug-induced adrenocorticoid insufficiency may be minimized by gradual systemic dosage reduction; relative insufficiency may exist for up to 1 yr after discontinuation
- Symptoms of adrenal insufficiency include nausea, fatigue, anorexia, hypotension, hypoglycemia, and fever

PATIENT/FAMILY EDUCATION

- Report fever, muscle aches, sore throat, and sudden weight gain or swelling

MONITORING PARAMETERS

- Serum K and glucose
- Growth in children on prolonged therapy
- Edema, blood pressure, CHF, mental status, weight
- For patients on long-term therapy, signs and symptoms of hypocalcemia (such as muscle twitching, cramps, and positive Chvostek's or Trousseau's signs), or hypokalemia (such as EKG changes, nausea and vomiting, irritability, weakness and muscle cramps, and numbness or tingling, especially in the lower extremities)

cosyntropin

(kos-syn-troe'-pin)

Rx: Cortrosyn

Chemical Class: ACTH derivative

Therapeutic Class: Corticosteroid, adrenal

CLINICAL PHARMACOLOGY

Mechanism of Action: A glucocorticoid that stimulates initial reaction in synthesis of adrenal steroids from cholesterol. ***Therapeutic Effect:*** Increases endogenous corticoid synthesis.

Pharmacokinetics

None reported.

INDICATIONS AND DOSAGES

Screening test for adrenal function

IM

Adults, Elderly, Children 2 yrs and older. 0.25-0.75 mg one time.

Children less than 2 yrs. 0.125 mg one time.

Neonates. 0.015 mg/kg/dose.

IV infusion

Adults. 0.25 mg in D5W or 0.9% NaCl infused at rate of 0.04 mg/hr.

AVAILABLE FORMS

• *Powder for reconstitution:* 0.25 mg (Cortrosyn).

CONTRAINDICATIONS: Hypersensitivity to cosyntropin or corticotropin

PREGNANCY AND LACTATION: Pregnancy category C

SIDE EFFECTS

Occasional

Nausea, vomiting

Rare

Hypersensitivity reaction (fever, pruritus)

SERIOUS REACTIONS

• None reported.

SPECIAL CONSIDERATIONS

PATIENT/FAMILY EDUCATION

• Explain procedure and purpose of test to the patient

MONITORING PARAMETERS

• Check plasma cortisol levels at baseline and 30-60 min after drug is administered; normal adrenal function indicated by an increase of at least 70 mcg/L or a measured level of 20 mcg

co-trimoxazole (sulfamethoxazole and trimethoprim)

(sul-fa-meth-ox'-a-zole; trye-meth'-oh-prim)

Rx: Bactrim, Bactrim DS, Bactrim Pediatric, Bethaprim, Bethaprim Pediatric, Septra, Septra DS, Sulfatrim Pediatric, Sulfatrim Suspension, Uroplus, Uroplus DS

Chemical Class: Dihydrofolate reductase inhibitor (trimethoprim); sulfonamide derivative (sulfamethoxazole)

Therapeutic Class: Antibiotic

CLINICAL PHARMACOLOGY

Mechanism of Action: A sulfonamide and folate antagonist that blocks bacterial synthesis of essential nucleic acids. ***Therapeutic Effect:*** Bactericidal in susceptible microorganisms.

Pharmacokinetics

Rapidly and well absorbed from the GI tract. Protein binding: 45%-60%. Widely distributed. Metabolized in the liver. Excreted in urine. Minimally removed by hemodialysis. ***Half-life:*** sulfamethoxazole 6-12 hr, trimethoprim 8-10 hr (increased in impaired renal function).

INDICATIONS AND DOSAGES

Chronic bronchitis

PO

Adults, Elderly. 1 double-strength or 2 single-strength tablets or 20-ml suspension q12h for 14 days.

Pneumocystis carinii pneumonia (PCP) prophylaxis

PO

Adults, Elderly. 1 double-strength tablet daily or 3 times a week or 1 single-strength tablet daily.

Children 1 mo and older. 150 mg/m^2 as trimethoprim each day in 2 divided doses 3 times a week on consecutive days.

PCP treatment

PO, IV

Adults, Elderly, Children 2 mo and older. 15-20 mg/kg as trimethoprim a day in 4 divided doses for 14-21 days.

Shigellosis

PO

Adults, Elderly. 1 double-strength tablet or 2 single-strength tablets or 20-ml suspension q12h for 5 days.

IV

Children. 8-10 mg/kg as trimethoprim a day in 2-4 divided doses for up to 5 days.

Otitis media

PO

Children 2 mo and older. 8 mg/kg trimethoprim a day q12h for 10 days.

UTIs

PO

Adults, Elderly. 1 double-strength or 2 single-strength tablets or 20-ml suspension q12h for 10-14 days.

Children 2 mo and older. 8 mg/kg as trimethoprim a day in 2 divided doses for 10 days.

Travelers' diarrhea

PO

Adults, Elderly. 1 double-strength or 2 single-strength tablets or 20-ml suspension q12h for 5 days.

Dosage in renal impairment

Dosage and frequency are modified based on creatinine clearance, the severity of the infection, and the serum concentration of the drug. For those with creatinine clearance of 15-30 ml/min, a 50% dosage reduction is recommended.

AVAILABLE FORMS

- **Alert:** All dosage forms have same 5:1 ratio of sulfamethoxazole (SMX) to trimethoprim (TMP).
- *Oral Suspension (Bactrim Pediatric, Bethaprim Pediatric, Septra, Sulfatrim, Sulfatrim Pediatric):* SMX 200 mg and TMP 40 mg per 5 ml.
- *Tablets (Bactrim, Septra, Uroplus):* SMX 400 mg and TMP 80 mg.
- *Tablets (Double Strength [Bactrim DS, Septra DS, Uroplus DS]):* SMX 800 mg and TMP 160 mg.
- *Injection:* SMX 80 mg and TMP 16 mg per ml.

UNLABELED USES: Treatment of bacterial endocarditis; gonorrhea; meningitis; septicemia; sinusitis; and biliary tract, bone, joint, chancroid, chlamydial, intraabdominal, skin, and soft-tissue infections

CONTRAINDICATIONS: Hypersensitivity to trimethoprim or any sulfonamides, infants younger than 2 months old, megaloblastic anemia due to folate deficiency.

PREGNANCY AND LACTATION: Pregnancy category C; **do not use at term,** may cause kernicterus in the neonate; not recommended in the neonatal nursing period because sulfonamides excreted in breast milk may cause kernicterus

SIDE EFFECTS

Frequent

Anorexia, nausea, vomiting, rash (generally 7-14 days after therapy begins), urticaria

Occasional
Diarrhea, abdominal pain, pain or irritation at the IV infusion site
Rare
Headache, vertigo, insomnia, seizures, hallucinations, depression

SERIOUS REACTIONS

- Rash, fever, sore throat, pallor, purpura, cough, and shortness of breath may be early signs of serious adverse reactions.
- Fatalities have occasionally occurred after Stevens-Johnson syndrome, toxic epidermal necrolysis, fulminant hepatic necrosis, agranulocytosis, aplastic anemia, and other blood dyscrasias in patients taking sulfonamides.
- Myelosuppression, decreased platelet count, and severe dermatologic reactions may occur, especially in the elderly.

INTERACTIONS

Drugs

3 *Dapsone:* Increased dapsone and trimethoprim concentrations

3 *Disulfiram, metronidazole:* Co-trimoxazole contains 10% ethanol, disulfiram reaction possible

3 *Hemolytics:* May increase the risk of toxicity

3 *Hepatotoxic medications:* May increase the risk of hepatotoxicity

3 *Methenamine:* May form a precipitate

3 *Methotrexate:* Elevated methotrexate concentrations and toxicity

3 *Oral anticoagulants:* Enhanced hypoprothrombinemic response to warfarin and possibly other oral anticoagulants

3 *Oral hypoglycemics:* Increased potential for hypoglycemia

3 *Phenytoin:* Increased phenytoin concentrations

Labs

- *False increase:* Creatinine (due to interference with assay), urobilinogen, urine protein, plasma α-amino-nitrogen
- *False positive:* Urinary glucose test
- *False decrease:* Serum creatine kinase

SPECIAL CONSIDERATIONS

- Pay special attention to complaints of skin rash, especially those involving mucous membranes (could signify early Stevens-Johnson syndrome), sore throat, mouth sores, fever, or unusual bruising or bleeding

PATIENT/FAMILY EDUCATION

- Take oral doses with 8 oz of water and drink several extra glasses of water each day
- Space drug doses evenly around the clock and continue taking for the full course of treatment
- Notify the physician immediately if any new symptom, especially bleeding, bruising, fever, sore throat, and a rash or other skin changes, occurs

MONITORING PARAMETERS

- Baseline and periodic CBC for patients on long-term or high-dose therapy
- Intake and output
- Pattern of daily bowel activity and stool consistency
- Skin for pallor, purpura, and rash
- Renal and liver function
- Vital signs

cromolyn sodium

(kroe'-moe-lin)

Rx: *Inhalation:* Intal

Rx: *Opthalmic:* Crolom, Opticrom

Rx: *Oral:* Gastrocrom

Rx: *Nasal:* Nasalcrom

Chemical Class: Mast cell stabilizer

Therapeutic Class: Antiasthmatic; inhaled antiinflammatory; nasal antiinflammatory; ophthalmic antiinflammatory

CLINICAL PHARMACOLOGY

Mechanism of Action: An antiasthmatic and antiallergic agent that prevents mast cell release of histamine, leukotrienes, and slow-reacting substances of anaphylaxis by inhibiting degranulation after contact with antigens. ***Therapeutic Effect:*** Helps prevent symptoms of asthma, allergic rhinitis, mastocytosis, and exercise-induced bronchospasm.

Pharmacokinetics

Minimal absorption after PO, inhalation, or nasal administration. Absorbed portion excreted in urine or by biliary system. ***Half-life:*** 80-90 min.

INDICATIONS AND DOSAGES

Asthma

Inhalation (nebulization)

Adults, Elderly, Children older than 2 yr. 20 mg 3-4 times a day.

Aerosol Spray

Adults, Elderly, Children 12 yr and older. Initially, 2 sprays 4 times a day. Maintenance: 2-4 sprays 3-4 times a day.

Children 5-11 yr. Initially, 2 sprays 4 times a day, then 1-2 sprays 3-4 times a day.

Prevention of bronchospasm

Inhalation (nebulization)

Adults, Elderly, Children older than 2 yr. 20 mg within 1 hr before exercise or exposure to allergens.

Aerosol Spray

Adults, Elderly, Children older than 5 yr. 2 sprays within 1 hr before exercise or exposure to allergens.

Food allergy, inflammatory bowel disease

PO

Adults, Elderly, Children older than 12 yr. 200-400 mg 4 times a day.

Children 2-12 yr. 100-200 mg 4 times a day. Maximum: 40 mg/kg/day.

Allergic rhinitis

Intranasal

Adults, Elderly, Children older than 6 yr. 1 spray each nostril 3-4 times a day. May increase up to 6 times a day.

Systemic mastocytosis

PO

Adults, Elderly, Children older than 12 yr. 200 mg 4 times a day.

Children 2-12 yr. 100 mg 4 times a day. Maximum: 40 mg/kg/day.

Children younger than 2 yr. 20 mg/kg/day in 4 divided doses. Maximum: 30 mg/kg/day (children 6 mo-2 yr).

Conjunctivitis

Ophthalmic

Adults, Elderly, Children older than 4 yr. 1-2 drops in both eyes 4-6 times a day.

AVAILABLE FORMS

- *Oral Concentrate (Gastrocrom):* 100 mg/5 ml.
- *Oral Capsules (Gastrocrom):* 100 mg.
- *Nasal Spray (Nasalcrom):* 40 mg/ml.
- *Solution for Nebulization (Intal):* 10 mg/ml.
- *Solution for Oral Inhalation (Intal):* 800 mcg/inhalation.

• *Ophthalmic Solution (Crolom, Opticrom):* 4%.

CONTRAINDICATIONS: Status asthmaticus

PREGNANCY AND LACTATION: Pregnancy category B; excretion in breast milk unknown

SIDE EFFECTS

Frequent

PO: Headache, diarrhea

Inhalation: Cough, dry mouth and throat, stuffy nose, throat irritation, unpleasant taste

Nasal: Nasal burning, stinging, or irritation; increased sneezing

Ophthalmic: Eye burning or stinging

Occasional

PO: Rash, abdominal pain, arthralgia, nausea, insomnia

Inhalation: Bronchospasm, hoarseness, lacrimation

Nasal: Cough, headache, unpleasant taste, postnasal drip

Ophthalmic: Lacrimation and itching of eye

Rare

Inhalation: Dizziness, painful urination, arthralgia, myalgia, rash

Nasal: Epistaxis, rash

Ophthalmic: Chemosis or edema of conjunctiva, eye irritation

SERIOUS REACTIONS

• Anaphylaxis occurs rarely when cromolyn is given by the inhalation, nasal, or oral route.

SPECIAL CONSIDERATIONS

PATIENT/FAMILY EDUCATION

• Therapeutic effect in asthma may take up to 4 wk

• Administer cromolyn at regular intervals

• Explain to the patient how to use a Spinhaler if he or she is to receive cromolyn by nebulization or inhalation capsules

• Rinse mouth with water immediately after inhalation to prevent mouth and throat dryness

• Drink plenty of fluids to decrease the thickness of lung secretions

MONITORING PARAMETERS

• Pulse rate and quality and respiratory rate, depth, rhythm, and type

• Observe the patient for cyanosis manifested as lips and fingernails with a blue or dusky color in light-skinned patients; a gray color in dark-skinned patients

• Auscultate the patient's breath sounds for crackles, rhonchi, and wheezing

---

crotamiton

(kroe-tam'-i-ton)

Rx: Eurax

Chemical Class: Chloroformate salt

Therapeutic Class: Scabicide

CLINICAL PHARMACOLOGY

Mechanism of Action: A scabicidal agent whose exact mechanism is unknown. ***Therapeutic Effect:*** Scabicidal activity against *Sarcoptes scabiei.*

Pharmacokinetics

Not known.

INDICATIONS AND DOSAGES

Treatment of scabies

Topical

Adults, Elderly, Children. Wash and scrub away loose scales and towel dry. Apply a thin layer and massage into skin over the entire body with special attention to skin folds, creases, and interdigital spaces. Repeat application in 24 hrs. Take a cleansing bath 48 hrs after the final application. Treatment may be repeated after 7-10 days if live mites are still present.

Pruritus

Topical

Adults, Elderly, Children. Massage into affected areas until medication is completely absorbed. Repeat as needed.

AVAILABLE FORMS

- *Cream:* 10% (Eurax).
- *Lotion:* 10% (Eurax).

UNLABELED USES: Folliculitis, pediculosis

CONTRAINDICATIONS: Hypersensitivity to crotamiton or any one of its components

PREGNANCY AND LACTATION: Pregnancy category C

SIDE EFFECTS

Occasional

Itching, burning, irritation, warm sensation, contact dermatitis

SERIOUS REACTIONS

- None known.

SPECIAL CONSIDERATIONS

PATIENT/FAMILY EDUCATION

- 60 g is sufficient for 2 applications/adult
- Reapply locally during 48-hr treatment period after handwashing, etc.
- A cleansing bath should be taken 48 hr after the last application
- After treatment, use topical corticosteroids to decrease contact dermatitis, antihistamines for pruritus; pruritus may continue for 4-6 wk
- Wash all contaminated clothing and bed linens to avoid reinfestation
- It is important to massage into the skin, especially to skin folds, digits, and creases

MONITORING PARAMETERS

- Check the skin for local burning, itching, and irritation

cyanocobalamin (vitamin B_{12})

(sye-an-oh-koe-bal'-a-min)

Rx: Cobal-1000, Cobolin-M, Crystal B-12, Cyomin, Depo-Cobalin, LA-12, Liver, Neuroforte-R, Vita #12, Vitabee 12, Vitamin B-12

Chemical Class: Vitamin B complex

Therapeutic Class: Hematinic; vitamin

CLINICAL PHARMACOLOGY

Mechanism of Action: Acts as a coenzyme for various metabolic functions, including fat and carbohydrate metabolism and protein synthesis. ***Therapeutic Effect:*** Necessary for cell growth and replication, hematopoiesis, and myelin synthesis.

Pharmacokinetics

In the presence of calcium, absorbed systemically in lower half of ileum. Initially, bound to intrinsic factor; this complex passes down intestine, binding to receptor sites on ileal mucosa. Protein binding: High. Metabolized in the liver. Primarily eliminated unchanged in urine. ***Half-life:*** 6 days.

INDICATIONS AND DOSAGES

Pernicious anemia

IM, Subcutaneous

Adults, Elderly. 100 mcg/day for 7 days, then every other day for 7 days, then every 3-4 days for 2-3 wks. Maintenance: 100 mcg/mo (oral 1000-2000 mcg/day).

Children. 30-50 mcg/day for 2 or more wks. Maintenance: 100 mcg/mo.

Neonates. 1000 mcg/day for 2 or more wks. Maintenance: 50 mcg/mo.

Intranasal

Adults, Elderly. 500 mcg once a week.

Uncomplicated vitamin B_{12} deficiency

PO

Adults, Elderly. 1000-2000 mcg/day.

IM, Subcutaneous

Adults, Elderly. 100 mcg/day for 5-10 days, followed by 100-200 mcg/mo.

Complicated vitamin B_{12} deficiency

IM, Subcutaneous

Adults, Elderly. 1000 mcg (with IM or IV folic acid 15 mg) as a single dose, then 1000 mcg/day plus oral folic acid 5 mg/day for 7 days.

AVAILABLE FORMS

- *Tablets:* 50 mcg, 100 mcg, 250 mcg, 500 mcg, 1000 mcg, 5000 mcg.
- *Tablets (Extended-Release):* 1500 mcg.
- *Injection:* 1000 mcg/ml.
- *Nasal Gel (Nascobal):* 500 mcg/0.1 ml.

CONTRAINDICATIONS: Folic acid deficiency anemia, hereditary optic nerve atrophy, history of allergy to cobalamins

PREGNANCY AND LACTATION: Pregnancy category C; excreted in breast milk in concentrations that approximate the mother's serum; compatible with breast-feeding

SIDE EFFECTS

Occasional

Diarrhea, pruritus

SERIOUS REACTIONS

- Impurities in preparation may cause a rare allergic reaction.
- Peripheral vascular thrombosis, pulmonary edema, hypokalemia, and CHF may occur.

INTERACTIONS

Drugs

3 *Alcohol, colchicine:* May decrease absorption of cyanocobalamin

3 *Ascorbic acid:* May destroy cyanocobalamin

3 *Folic acid (large doses):* May decrease cyanocobalamin blood concentration

SPECIAL CONSIDERATIONS

- Recommended dietary allowance: 0.5-2.6 mcg/day depending on age and status (i.e., more during pregnancy and lactation)
- Nutritional sources: egg yolks, fish, organ meats, dairy products, clams, oysters

PATIENT/FAMILY EDUCATION

- Lifetime treatment may be necessary with pernicious anemia
- Report symptoms of infection
- Eat foods rich in vitamin B_{12}, including clams, dairy products, egg yolks, fermented cheese, herring, muscle and organ meats, oysters, and red snapper

MONITORING PARAMETERS

- CBC with reticulocyte count after first wk of therapy
- Serum potassium level, which normally ranges from 3.5-5 mEq/L, and serum cyanocobalamin level, which normally ranges from 200-800 mcg/ml
- Evaluate the patient for reversal of deficiency symptoms (anorexia, ataxia, fatigue, hyporeflexia, insomnia, irritability, loss of positional sense, pallor, and palpitations on exertion); a therapeutic response to treatment usually occurs within 48 hrs

cyclobenzaprine hydrochloride

(sye-kloe-ben′-za-preen)

Rx: Flexeril

Chemical Class: Tricyclic amine

Therapeutic Class: Skeletal muscle relaxant

CLINICAL PHARMACOLOGY

Mechanism of Action: A centrally acting skeletal muscle relaxant that reduces tonic somatic muscle activity at the level of the brainstem. ***Therapeutic Effect:*** Relieves local skeletal muscle spasm.

Pharmacokinetics

Route	*Onset*	*Peak*	*Duration*
PO	1 hr	3-4 hr	12-24 hr

Well but slowly absorbed from the GI tract. Protein binding: 93%. Metabolized in the GI tract and the liver. Primarily excreted in urine. ***Half-life:*** 1-3 days.

INDICATIONS AND DOSAGES

Acute, painful musculoskeletal conditions

PO

Adults. Initially, 5 mg 3 times a day. May increase to 10 mg 3 times a day.

Elderly. 5 mg 3 times a day.

Dosage in hepatic impairment

Mild: 5 mg 3 times a day.

Moderate and severe: Not recommended.

AVAILABLE FORMS

• *Tablets:* 5 mg, 10 mg.

UNLABELED USES: Treatment of fibromyalgia

CONTRAINDICATIONS: Acute recovery phase of MI, arrhythmias, CHF, heart block, conduction disturbances, hyperthyroidism, use within 14 days of MAOIs

PREGNANCY AND LACTATION: Pregnancy category B; no data available, but closely related tricyclic antidepressants are excreted into breast milk

SIDE EFFECTS

Frequent

Somnolence (39%), dry mouth (27%), dizziness (11%)

Rare (3%-1%)

Fatigue, asthenia, blurred vision, headache, nervousness, confusion, nausea, constipation, dyspepsia, unpleasant taste

SERIOUS REACTIONS

• Overdose may result in visual hallucinations, hyperactive reflexes, muscle rigidity, vomiting, and hyperpyrexia.

INTERACTIONS

Drugs

3 *Alcohol, other CNS depression-producing medications:* May increase CNS depression

3 *Droperidol, fluoxetine:* A patient receiving cyclobenzaprine and fluoxetine developed ventricular tachycardia and fibrillation after droperidol was added; relative contribution of each drug to the adverse effect unclear

❷ *MAOIs:* Hyperpyretic crisis, severe convulsions, and deaths have occurred in patients receiving closely related tricyclic antidepressants and MAOIs; separate use by 14 days

❷ *Tramadol:* May increase the risk of seizures

Labs

• *Interference:* Serum amitriptyline assay

SPECIAL CONSIDERATIONS

• Avoid use in elderly due to anticholinergic side effects

PATIENT/FAMILY EDUCATION

• Use caution with alcohol, other CNS depressants

- Avoid with hazardous activities if drowsiness or dizziness occur
- Drowsiness usually diminishes with continued therapy
- Change positions slowly to help avoid the drug's hypotensive effects
- Sip tepid water and chew sugarless gum to relieve dry mouth

MONITORING PARAMETERS

- Evidence of a therapeutic response, such as decreased skeletal muscle pain, stiffness, and tenderness and improved mobility

---

cyclophosphamide

(sye-kloe-fos'-fa-mide)

Rx: Cytoxan, Cytoxan Lyophilized, Neosar

Chemical Class: Nitrogen mustard, synthetic

Therapeutic Class: Antineoplastic

CLINICAL PHARMACOLOGY

Mechanism of Action: An alkylating agent that inhibits DNA and RNA protein synthesis by cross-linking with DNA and RNA strands, preventing cell growth. Cell cycle-phase nonspecific. ***Therapeutic Effect:*** Potent immunosuppressant.

Pharmacokinetics

Well absorbed from the GI tract. Protein binding: Low. Crosses the blood-brain barrier. Metabolized in the liver to active metabolites. Primarily excreted in urine. Removed by hemodialysis. ***Half-life:*** 3-12 hr.

INDICATIONS AND DOSAGES

Ovarian adenocarcinoma, breast carcinoma, Hodgkin's disease, non-Hodgkin's lymphoma, multiple myeloma, leukemia (acute lymphoblastic, acute myelogenous, acute monocytic, chronic granulocytic, chronic lymphocytic), mycosis fungoides, disseminated neuroblastoma, retinoblastoma

PO

Adults. 1-5 mg/kg/day.

Children. Initially, 2-8 mg/kg/day. Maintenance: 2-5 mg/kg twice a week.

IV

Adults. 40-50 mg/kg in divided doses over 2-5 days; or 10-15 mg/kg every 7-10 days or 3-5 mg/kg twice a week.

Children. 2-8 mg/kg/day for 6 days or total dose for 7 days once a week.

Biopsy-proven minimal-change nephrotic syndrome

PO

Adults, Children. 2.5-3 mg/kg/day for 60-90 days.

AVAILABLE FORMS

- *Tablets (Cytoxan):* 25 mg, 50 mg.
- *Powder for Injection (Neosar):* 100 mg, 200 mg, 500 mg, 1 g, 2 g.
- *Powder for Injection (Lyophilized [Cytoxan Lyophilized]):* 100 mg, 200 mg, 500 mg, 1 g, 2 g.

UNLABELED USES: Adrenocortical, bladder, cervical, endometrial, prostatic, testicular carcinomas; Ewing's sarcoma; multiple sclerosis: non-small cell, small cell lung cancer; organ transplant rejection; osteosarcoma; ovarian germ cell, primary brain, trophoblastic tumors; rheumatoid arthritis; soft-tissue sarcomas, systemic dermatomyositis, systemic lupus erythematosus, Wilms' tumor

CONTRAINDICATIONS: Severe bone marrow suppression

PREGNANCY AND LACTATION: Pregnancy category D; excreted in breast milk; contraindicated because of potential for adverse effects relating to immune suppression, growth, and carcinogenesis

SIDE EFFECTS

Expected

Marked leukopenia 8-15 days after initial therapy

Frequent

Nausea, vomiting (beginning about 6 hr after administration and lasting about 4 hr); alopecia (33%)

Occasional

Diarrhea, darkening of skin and fingernails, stomatitis, headache, diaphoresis

Rare

Pain or redness at injection site

SERIOUS REACTIONS

- Cyclophosphamide's major toxic effect is myelosuppression resulting in blood dyscrasias, such as leukopenia, anemia, thrombocytopenia, and hypoprothrombinemia.
- Expect leukopenia to resolve in 17-28 days. Anemia generally occurs after large doses or prolonged therapy. Thrombocytopenia may occur 10-15 days after drug initiation.
- Hemorrhagic cystitis occurs commonly in long-term therapy, especially in pediatric patients.
- Pulmonary fibrosis and cardiotoxicity have been noted with high doses.
- Amenorrhea, azoospermia, and hyperkalemia may also occur.

INTERACTIONS

Drugs

3 *Allopurinol:* Increased cyclophosphamide toxicity

3 *Antigout medications:* May decrease the effects of these drugs

3 *Bone marrow depressants:* May increase myelosuppression

3 *Cytarabine:* May increase the risk of cardiomyopathy

3 *Digoxin:* Decreased digoxin absorption from tablets; Lanoxicaps and elixir not affected

❷ *Immunosuppressants:* May increase the risk of infection and development of neoplasms

3 *Live-virus vaccines:* May potentiate virus replication, increase vaccine side effects, and decrease the patient's antibody response to the vaccine

3 *Succinylcholine:* Prolonged neuromuscular blockade

3 *Warfarin:* Inhibited hypoprothrombinemic response to warfarin

SPECIAL CONSIDERATIONS

PATIENT/FAMILY EDUCATION

- Drink plenty of fluids before, during, and after therapy and void frequently to prevent cystitis
- Avoid receiving vaccinations without the physician's approval and avoid contact with anyone who has recently received a live-virus vaccine because cyclophosphamide lowers the body's resistance
- Report easy bruising, fever, signs of local infection, sore throat, or unusual bleeding from any site
- Hair loss is reversible, but new hair may have a different color or texture

MONITORING PARAMETERS

- CBC, differential, platelet count qwk; withhold drug if WBC is <4000 or platelet count is <75,000
- Renal function studies: BUN, UA, serum uric acid; urine CrCl before, during therapy
- I&O; report fall in urine output ≤30 ml/hr

cycloserine

(sye-kloe-ser′-een)

Rx: Seromycin

Chemical Class: Streptomyces orchidaceus product

Therapeutic Class: Antituberculosis agent

CLINICAL PHARMACOLOGY

Mechanism of Action: An antitubercular that inhibits cell wall synthesis by competing with the amino acid, D-alanine, for incorporation into the bacterial cell wall. ***Therapeutic Effect:*** Causes disruption of bacterial cell wall. Bactericidal or bacteriostatic.

Pharmacokinetics

Readily absorbed from the gastrointestinal (GI) tract. No protein binding. Widely distributed (including cerebrospinal fluid [CSF]). Metabolized in liver. Primarily excreted in urine. Removed by hemodialysis. ***Half-life:*** 10 hrs.

INDICATIONS AND DOSAGES

Tuberculosis

Adults, Elderly. 250 mg q12h for 14 days, then 500 mg to 1g/day in 2 divided doses for 18-24 mos. Maximum: 1 g as a single daily dose.

Children. 10-20 mg/kg/day in 2 divided doses. Maximum: 1000 mg/day for 18-24 mos.

Dosage in renal impairment

Creatinine Clearance	Dosage Interval
10-50 ml/min	q24h
less than 10 ml/min	q36-48h

AVAILABLE FORMS

• *Capsules:* 250 mg (Seromycin).

UNLABELED USES: Gaucher's disease, acute urinary tract infections

CONTRAINDICATIONS: Epilepsy, depression, severe anxiety, psychosis, severe renal insufficiency, excessive concurrent use of alcohol, history of hypersensitivity reactions with previous cycloserine therapy

PREGNANCY AND LACTATION: Pregnancy category C; excreted into breast milk (72% of serum levels); compatible with breast-feeding

SIDE EFFECTS

Occasional

Drowsiness, headache, dizziness, vertigo, seizures, confusion, psychosis, paresis, tremor, vitamin B_{12} deficiency, folate deficiency, cardiac arrhythmias, increased liver enzymes

SERIOUS REACTIONS

• Neurotoxicity, as evidenced by confusion, agitation, CNS depression, psychosis, coma, and seizures, occurs rarely.

• Neurotoxic effects of cycloserine may be treated and prevented with the administration of 200-300 mg of pyridoxine daily.

INTERACTIONS

Drugs

3 *Alcohol:* May increase CNS effects

3 *Folic acid:* May decrease folic acid

3 *Isoniazid:* Increased risk of CNS toxicity

3 *Phenytoin:* May increase the risk of epileptic seizures

3 *Vitamin B_{12}:* May decrease vitamin B_{12}

SPECIAL CONSIDERATIONS

• L-enantiomer (1-cycloserine) in Gaucher's disease (Orphan Drug)

• Pyridoxine may prevent neurotoxicity (200-300 mg/day)

PATIENT/FAMILY EDUCATION

• Avoid concurrent alcohol

• Cycloserine may cause drowsiness, mental confusion, dizziness, or tremors

• Do not skip doses

MONITORING PARAMETERS

• Mental status closely and liver function tests qwk

• Monitor cycloserine concentrations; toxicity is greatly increased at levels more than 30 mcg/ml

cyclosporine

(sye-kloe-spor'-in)

Rx: Gengraf, Neoral, Restasis, Sandimmune

Chemical Class: Cyclic peptide

Therapeutic Class: Immunosuppressant

CLINICAL PHARMACOLOGY

Mechanism of Action: A cyclic polypeptide that inhibits both cellular and humoral immune responses by inhibiting interleukin-2, a proliferative factor needed for T-cell activity. ***Therapeutic Effect:*** Prevents organ rejection and relieves symptoms of psoriasis and arthritis.

Pharmacokinetics

Variably absorbed from the GI tract. Protein binding: 90%. Widely distributed. Metabolized in the liver. Eliminated primarily by biliary or fecal excretion. Not removed by hemodialysis. ***Half-life:*** Adults, 10-27 hr; children, 7-19 hr.

INDICATIONS AND DOSAGES

Transplantation, prevention of organ rejection

PO

Adults, Elderly, Children. 10-18 mg/kg/dose given 4-12 hr prior to organ transplantation. Maintenance: 5-15 mg/kg/day in divided doses then tapered to 3-10 mg/kg/day.

IV

Adults, Elderly, Children. Initially, 5-6 mg/kg/dose given 4-12 hr prior to organ transplantation. Maintenance: 2-10 mg/kg/day in divided doses.

Rheumatoid arthritis

PO

Adults, Elderly. Initially, 2.5 mg/kg a day in 2 divided doses. May increase by 0.5-0.75 mg/kg/day. Maximum: 4 mg/kg/day.

Psoriasis

PO

Adults, Elderly. Initially, 2.5 mg/kg/day in 2 divided doses. May increase by 0.5 mg/kg/day. Maximum: 4 mg/kg/day.

Dry eye

Ophthalmic

Adults, Elderly. Instill 1 drop in each affected eye q12h.

AVAILABLE FORMS

- *Capsules (Softgel [Gengraf, Neoral, Sandimmune]):* 25 mg, 100 mg.
- *Oral Solution (Sandimmune):* 50-ml bottle with calibrated liquid-measuring device.
- *Injection (Sandimmune):* 50 mg/ml.
- *Ophthalmic Emulsion (Restasis):* 0.05%.

UNLABELED USES: Treatment of alopecia areata, aplastic anemia, atopic dermatitis, Behçet's disease, biliary cirrhosis, prevention of corneal transplant rejection

CONTRAINDICATIONS: History of hypersensitivity to cyclosporine or polyoxyethylated castor oil

PREGNANCY AND LACTATION: Pregnancy category C; excreted into breast milk; avoid nursing

SIDE EFFECTS

Frequent

Mild to moderate hypertension (26%), hirsutism (21%), tremor (12%)

Occasional (4%-2%)

Acne, leg cramps, gingival hyperplasia (marked by red, bleeding, and tender gums), paresthesia, diarrhea, nausea, vomiting, headache

Rare (less than 1%)

Hypersensitivity reaction, abdominal discomfort, gynecomastia, sinusitis

SERIOUS REACTIONS

• Mild nephrotoxicity occurs in 25% of renal transplant patients, 38% of cardiac transplant patients, and 37% of liver transplant patients, generally 2-3 mos after transplantation (more severe toxicity is generally occurs soon after transplantation). Hepatotoxicity occurs in 4% of renal transplant patients, 7% of cardiac transplant patients, and 4% of liver transplant patients, generally within the first month after transplantation. Both toxicities usually respond to dosage reduction.

• Severe hyperkalemia and hyperuricemia occur occasionally.

INTERACTIONS

Drugs

3 *Allopurinol, amiodarone, chloroquine, clarithromycin, clonidine, clotrimazole, oral contraceptives, erythromycin, fluconazole, griseofulvin, itraconazole, ketoconazole, miconazole, ticlopidine:* Increased cyclosporine levels, potential for toxicity

3 *Aminoglycosides, amphotericin B, colchicine, enalapril, melphalan, sulfonamides:* Additive nephrotoxicity with cyclosporine

2 *Anabolic steroids:* Increased cyclosporine levels, potential for toxicity

3 *Barbiturates, carbamazepine, nafcillin, pyrazinamide, phenytoin, sulfonamides:* Reduced cyclosporine levels, potential for therapeutic failure

3 *Calcium channel blockers:* Diltiazem, verapamil increase cyclosporine levels; isradipine, nifedipine, nitrendipine do not interact

3 *Cisapride, metoclopramide:* Increased bioavailability and serum levels of single-dose cyclosporine

3 *Digitalis glycosides:* Cyclosporine in patients stabilized on digitalis leads to increased levels and potential toxicity

3 *Doxorubicin, imipenem:* CNS toxicity

3 *Grapefruit juice:* May increase absorption and risk of toxicity

3 *HMG-CoA reductase inhibitors:* Increased risk of reversible myopathy

3 *Methotrexate:* Increased toxicity of both agents

3 *NSAIDs:* Increased risk of cyclosporine nephrotoxicity

2 *Rifampin:* Reduced cyclosporine levels, potential for therapeutic failure

3 *St. John's Wort:* May alter absorption

SPECIAL CONSIDERATIONS

• Neoral has increased bioavailability compared to Sandimmune (do NOT use interchangeably)

PATIENT/FAMILY EDUCATION

• Oral sol may be mixed with milk, chocolate milk, or orange juice to improve palatability. Do not mix with grapefruit juice (increased cyclosporine levels).

• Ophth product may be used with artificial tears—allow 15 min interval between products

• Essential to repeat blood testing on a routine basis while receiving medication

• Headache and tremor may occur as a response to medication

MONITORING PARAMETERS

• Renal function studies: BUN, creatinine qmo during treatment, 3 mo after treatment

• Liver function studies and serum levels during treatment

• Blood level monitoring: maintenance of 24-hr trough levels of 250-800 ng/ml (whole blood, RIA) or 50-

300 ng/ml (plasma, RIA) should minimize side effects and rejection events
• Potassium level for evidence of hyperkalemia
• Blood pressure

cyproheptadine hydrochloride

(si-proe-hep′-ta-deen hye-droe-klor′-ide)
Rx: Periactin
Chemical Class: Piperidine derivative
Therapeutic Class: Antihistamine

CLINICAL PHARMACOLOGY
Mechanism of Action: An antihistamine that competes with histamine at histaminic receptor sites. Anticholinergic effects cause drying of nasal mucosa. ***Therapeutic Effect:*** Relieves allergic conditions (urticaria, pruritus).
Pharmacokinetics
Well absorbed from GI tract. Metabolized in liver. Primarily eliminated in feces. ***Half-life:*** 16 hrs.
INDICATIONS AND DOSAGES
Allergic condition
PO
Adults, Children older than 15 yrs. 4 mg 3 times/day. May increase dose but do not exceed 0.5 mg/kg/day.
Children 7-14 yrs. 4 mg 2-3 times/day, or 0.25 mg/kg daily in divided doses.
Children 2-6 yrs. 2 mg 2-3 times/day, or 0.25 mg/kg daily in divided doses.
Usual elderly dosage
PO
Initially, 4 mg 2 times/day.
AVAILABLE FORMS
• *Syrup:* 2 mg/5 ml (Periactin).
• *Tablets:* 4 mg (Periactin).

CONTRAINDICATIONS: Acute asthmatic attack, patients receiving MAO inhibitors, history of hypersensitivity to antihistamines
PREGNANCY AND LACTATION: Pregnancy category B; excreted in breast milk
SIDE EFFECTS
Frequent
Drowsiness, dizziness, muscular weakness, dry mouth/nose/throat/lips, urinary retention, thickening of bronchial secretions
Frequent
Elderly: Sedation, dizziness, hypotension
Occasional
Epigastric distress, flushing, visual disturbances, hearing disturbances, paresthesia, sweating, chills
SERIOUS REACTIONS
• Children may experience dominant paradoxical reaction (restlessness, insomnia, euphoria, nervousness, tremors).
• Overdosage in children may result in hallucinations, convulsions, death.
• Hypersensitivity reaction (eczema, pruritus, rash, cardiac disturbances, angioedema, photosensitivity) may occur.
• Overdosage may vary from CNS depression (sedation, apnea, cardiovascular collapse, death) to severe paradoxical reaction (hallucinations, tremor, seizures).
INTERACTIONS
Drugs
3 *Alcohol, CNS depressants:* May increase CNS depression
3 *Fluoxetine:* Potential for worsening of depression when cyproheptadine added to fluoxetine therapy
2 *MAOIs:* May increase anticholinergic and CNS depressant effects
3 *Paroxetine:* Potential for worsening of depression when cyproheptadine added to paroxetine therapy

3 *Protirelin:* May decrease TSH response

Labs

• *False positive:* Urine tricyclic antidepressant assay

SPECIAL CONSIDERATIONS

PATIENT/FAMILY EDUCATION

• Dry mouth, drowsiness, and dizziness are expected responses to the drug

• Avoid tasks that require mental alertness or motor skills until response to the drug is established

MONITORING PARAMETERS

• Blood pressure, especially in the elderly

dalteparin sodium

(dal-te-pa'-rin soe'-dee-um)

Rx: Fragmin

Chemical Class: Heparin derivative, depolymerized; low-molecular-weight heparin

Therapeutic Class: Anticoagulant

CLINICAL PHARMACOLOGY

Mechanism of Action: An antithrombin that inhibits factor Xa and thrombin in the presence of low-molecular-weight heparin. Only slightly influences platelet aggregation, PT, and aPTT. ***Therapeutic Effect:*** Produces anticoagulation.

Pharmacokinetics

Route	Onset	Peak	Duration
Subcutaneous	N/A	4 hr	N/A

Protein binding: Less than 10%. ***Half-life:*** 3-5 hr.

INDICATIONS AND DOSAGES

Low- to moderate-risk abdominal surgery

Subcutaneous

Adults, Elderly. 2500 international units 1-2 hr before surgery, then daily for 5-10 days.

High-risk abdominal surgery

Subcutaneous

Adults, Elderly. 5000 international units 1-2 hr before surgery, then daily for 5-10 days.

Total hip surgery

Subcutaneous

Adults, Elderly. 2500 international units 1-2 hr before surgery, then 2500 units 6 hr after surgery, then 5000 units/day for 7-10 days.

Unstable angina, non-Q-wave MI

Subcutaneous

Adults, Elderly. 120 international units/kg q12h (maximum: 10,000 international units/dose) given with aspirin until clinically stable.

Prevention of deep vein thrombosis (DVT) or pulmonary edema in the acutely ill patient

Subcutaneous

Adults, Elderly. 5000 international units once a day.

AVAILABLE FORMS

• *Syringe:* 2500 international units/0.2 ml, 5000 international units/0.2 ml, 7500 international units/0.3 ml, 10,000 international units/ml.

• *Vial:* 10,000 international units/ml, 25,000 international units/ml.

CONTRAINDICATIONS: Active major bleeding; concurrent heparin therapy; hypersensitivity to dalteparin, heparin, or pork products; thrombocytopenia associated with positive in vitro test for antiplatelet antibody

PREGNANCY AND LACTATION: Pregnancy category B

SIDE EFFECTS

Occasional (7%-3%)

Hematoma at injection site

Rare (less than 1%)

Hypersensitivity reaction (chills, fever, pruritus, urticaria, asthma, rhinitis, lacrimation, headache); mild, local skin irritation

SERIOUS REACTIONS

• Overdose may lead to bleeding complications ranging from local ecchymoses to major hemorrhage.

• Thrombocytopenia occurs rarely.

INTERACTIONS

Drugs

3 *Aspirin:* Increased risk of hemorrhage

3 *Oral anticoagulants:* Additive anticoagulant effects

SPECIAL CONSIDERATIONS

• Cannot be used interchangeably (unit for unit) with unfractionated heparin or other low-molecular-weight heparins

PATIENT/FAMILY EDUCATION

• Usual length of dalteparin therapy is 5-10 days

• Notify the physician of signs of bleeding, breathing difficulty, bruising, dizziness, fever, itching, lightheadedness, rash, and swelling

• Rotate injection sites daily

• Perform an ice massage at the injection site shortly before injection, to prevent excessive bruising

MONITORING PARAMETERS

• CBC with platelets, stool occult blood, urinalysis

• Monitoring aPTT is not required

• Assess for signs of bleeding, including bleeding at surgical or injection sites or from gums, hematuria, blood in stool, bruising, and petechiae

danazol

(da'-na-zole)

Rx: Danocrine

Chemical Class: Androgen; ethisterone derivative

Therapeutic Class: Androgen

D

CLINICAL PHARMACOLOGY

Mechanism of Action: A testosterone derivative that suppresses the pituitary-ovarian axis by inhibiting the output of pituitary gonadotropins. Causes atrophy of both normal and ectopic endometrial tissue in endometriosis. Follicle-stimulating hormone (FSH) and luteinizing hormone (LH) are depressed in fibrocystic breast disease. Inhibits steroid synthesis and binding of steroids to their receptors in breast tissues. Increases serum levels of esterase inhibitor. ***Therapeutic Effect:*** Produces anovulation and amenorrhea, reduces the production of estrogen, corrects biochemical deficiency as seen in hereditary angioedema.

Pharmacokinetics

Well absorbed from gastrointestinal (GI) tract. Metabolized in liver, primarily to 2-hydroxymethylethisterone. Excreted in urine. ***Half-life:*** 4.5 hrs.

INDICATIONS AND DOSAGES

Endometriosis

PO

Adults. 200-800 mg/day in 2 divided doses for 3-9 mos.

Fibrocystic breast disease

PO

Adults. 100-400 mg/day in 2 divided doses.

Hereditary angioedema

PO

Adults. Initially, 200 mg 2-3 times/day. Decrease dose by 50% or less at 1-3 mo intervals. If attack occurs, increase dose by up to 200 mg/day.

AVAILABLE FORMS

• *Capsules:* 50 mg, 100 mg, 200 mg (Danocrine).

UNLABELED USES: Treatment of gynecomastia, menorrhagia, precocious puberty

CONTRAINDICATIONS: Cardiac impairment, hypercalcemia, pregnancy, prostatic or breast cancer in males, severe liver or renal disease

PREGNANCY AND LACTATION: Pregnancy category X; may result in androgenic effects in the fetus; initiate therapy during menstruation or rule out pregnancy prior to initiating therapy in women of child-bearing potential; contraindicated during breast-feeding

SIDE EFFECTS

Frequent

Females: Amenorrhea, breakthrough bleeding/spotting, decreased breast size, increased weight, irregular menstrual period

Occasional

Males/females: Edema, rhabdomyolysis (muscle cramps, unusual fatigue), virilism (acne, oily skin), flushed skin, altered moods

Rare

Males/females: Hematuria, gingivitis, carpal tunnel syndrome, cataracts, severe headache, vomiting, rash, photosensitivity

Females: Enlarged clitoris, hoarseness, deepening voice, hair growth, monilial vaginitis

Males: Decreased testicle size

SERIOUS REACTIONS

• Jaundice may occur in those receiving 400 mg/day or more. Liver dysfunction, eosinophilia, thrombocytopenia, pancreatitis occur rarely.

INTERACTIONS

Drugs

❷ *Carbamazepine:* Predictably increases serum carbamazepine concentrations, toxicity possible

❷ *Cyclosporine:* Increased serum cyclosporine concentrations, toxicity possible

❸ *HMG-CoA reductase inhibitors (lovastatin, pravastatin):* Myositis risk increased

❷ *Oral anticoagulants:* Enhanced hypoprothrombinemic response

❷ *Tacrolimus:* Increased tacrolimus concentrations, toxicity possible

Labs

• *False decrease:* Plasma cortisol, serum testosterone, serum thyroxine

• *False increase:* Plasma cortisol, serum testosterone

SPECIAL CONSIDERATIONS

• Useful for palliative treatment of moderate to severe endometriosis or infertility due to endometriosis and for those whom alternative hormonal therapy is ineffective, intolerable, or contraindicated

• Drug of choice for treating all types of hereditary angioedema except for children or pregnant women where fibrolytic inhibitors (aminocaproic acid) may be preferred

• Breast pain should be treated conservatively (analgesics, supportive bra). Hormonal therapy is not innocuous. Symptoms usually return after discontinuation

• Ovarian function usually returns within 60-90 days after discontinuation

PATIENT/FAMILY EDUCATION

• Use nonhormonal contraceptive measures during therapy; discontinue use if pregnancy is suspected

• Essential to repeat blood testing on a routine basis while receiving medication

• Notify physician promptly of masculinizing effects (may not be reversible), weight gain, muscle cramps, or fatigue
• Spotting or bleeding may occur in first months of therapy for endometriosis (does not mean lack of efficacy)
• In fibrocystic breast disease, irregular menstrual periods and amenorrhea may occur with or without ovulation

MONITORING PARAMETERS

• Potassium, blood sugar, urine glucose during long-term therapy
• Weight 2-3 times/wks; report more than 5 lbs/wks gain or swelling of fingers or feet
• Blood pressure
• Check for jaundice

dantrolene sodium

(dan'-troe-leen)

Rx: Dantrium

Chemical Class: Hydantoin derivative

Therapeutic Class: Antidote, malignant hyperthermia; skeletal muscle relaxant

CLINICAL PHARMACOLOGY

Mechanism of Action: A skeletal muscle relaxant that reduces muscle contraction by interfering with release of calcium ion. Reduces calcium ion concentration. ***Therapeutic Effect:*** Dissociates excitation-contraction coupling. Interferes with catabolic process associated with malignant hyperthermic crisis.

Pharmacokinetics

Poorly absorbed from the GI tract. Protein binding: High. Metabolized in the liver. Primarily excreted in urine. ***Half-life:*** IV: 4-8 hr; PO: 8.7 hr.

INDICATIONS AND DOSAGES

Spasticity

PO

Adults, Elderly. Initially, 25 mg/day. Increase to 25 mg 2-4 times a day, then by 25-mg increments up to 100 mg 2-4 times a day.

Children. Initially, 0.5 mg/kg twice a day. Increase to 0.5 mg/kg 3-4 times a day, then in increments of 0.5 mg/kg/day up to 3 mg/kg 2-4 times a day. Maximum: 400 mg/day.

Prevention of malignant hyperthermic crisis

PO

Adults, Elderly, Children. 4-8 mg/kg/day in 3-4 divided doses 1-2 days before surgery; give last dose 3-4 hr before surgery.

IV

Adults, Elderly, Children. 2.5 mg/kg about 1.25 hr before surgery.

Management of malignant hyperthermic crisis

IV

Adults, Elderly, Children. Initially, a minimum of 1 mg/kg rapid IV; may repeat up to total cumulative dose of 10 mg/kg. May follow with 4-8 mg/kg/day PO in 4 divided doses up to 3 days after crisis.

AVAILABLE FORMS

• *Capsules (Dantrium):* 25 mg, 50 mg, 100 mg.
• *Powder for Injection (Dantrium Intravenous):* 20-mg vial.

UNLABELED USES: Relief of exercise-induced pain in patients with muscular dystrophy, treatment of flexor spasms and neuroleptic malignant syndrome

CONTRAINDICATIONS: Active hepatic disease

PREGNANCY AND LACTATION: Pregnancy category C; do not use in nursing women

SIDE EFFECTS

Frequent

Drowsiness, dizziness, weakness, general malaise, diarrhea (mild)

Occasional

Confusion, diarrhea (may be severe), headache, insomnia, constipation, urinary frequency

Rare

Paradoxical CNS excitement or restlessness, paresthesia, tinnitus, slurred speech, tremor, blurred vision, dry mouth, nocturia, impotence, rash, pruritus

SERIOUS REACTIONS

- There is a risk of hepatotoxicity, most notably in females, those 35 years of age and older, and those taking other medications concurrently.
- Overt hepatitis noted most frequently between third and twelfth month of therapy.
- Overdosage results in vomiting, muscular hypotonia, muscle twitching, respiratory depression, and seizures.

INTERACTIONS

Drugs

3 *Calcium channel blockers:* Rare cases of CV collapse with concomitant use of dantrolene and verapamil; calcium channel blockers and dantrolene use not recommended during management of malignant hyperthermia

3 *CNS depressants:* Increased drowsiness

3 *Estrogen:* Possible increased hepatotoxicity in females >35 yr on estrogen therapy

3 *Liver toxic medications:* May increase the risk of liver toxicity with chronic use

3 *Vecuronium:* Dantrium may potentiate vecuronium-induced neuromuscular block

SPECIAL CONSIDERATIONS

- Use carefully where spasticity is utilized to sustain upright posture and balance in locomotion or to obtain or maintain increased function
- Discontinue after 6 wk if improvement does not occur
- Use lowest dose possible (hepatotoxicity dose-related)

PATIENT/FAMILY EDUCATION

- IV therapy may decrease grip strength and increase weakness of leg muscles, especially walking down stairs
- Caution driving or operating hazardous machinery
- Avoid tasks that require mental alertness or motor skills until response to the drug is established
- Notify the physician if bloody or tarry stools, continued weakness, diarrhea, fatigue, itching, nausea, or skin rash occurs

MONITORING PARAMETERS

- Baseline and periodic LFTs (AST, ALT, alk phosphatase, total bilirubin)

---

dapsone

(dap′-sone)

Rx: Dapsone

Chemical Class: Sulfone

Therapeutic Class: Antiprotozoal; leprostatic

CLINICAL PHARMACOLOGY

Mechanism of Action: An antibiotic that is a competitive antagonist of para-aminobenzoic acid (PABA); it prevents normal bacterial utilization of PABA for synthesis of folic acid. ***Therapeutic Effect:*** Inhibits bacterial growth.

Pharmacokinetics

Slowly absorbed from the GI tract. Protein binding: 70%-90%. Metabolized in liver. Excreted in urine. *Half-life:* 10-50 hr.

INDICATIONS AND DOSAGES

Leprosy

PO

Adults, Elderly. 50-100 mg/day for 3-10 yr.

Children. 1-2 mg/kg/24 hr. Maximum: 100 mg/day.

Dermatitis herpetiformis

PO

Adults, Elderly. Initially, 50 mg/day. May increase up to 300 mg/day.

Pneumocystis carinii pneumonia (PCP)

PO

Adults, Elderly. 100 mg/day in combination with trimethoprim for 21 days.

Prevention of PCP

PO

Adults, Elderly. 100 mg/day.

Children older than 1 mo. 2 mg/kg/day. Maximum: 100 mg/day.

AVAILABLE FORMS

- *Tablets:* 25 mg, 100 mg.

UNLABELED USES: Treatment of inflammatory bowel disorders, malaria

CONTRAINDICATIONS: None known.

PREGNANCY AND LACTATION: Pregnancy category C; extensive, but uncontrolled, experience and 2 published surveys in pregnant women have not shown increases in the risk for fetal abnormalities if administered during all trimesters; excreted in breast milk, hemolytic reactions can occur in neonates, discontinue nursing or discontinue drug; alternatively, some authors have suggested infants should be kept with mothers infected with leprosy, and breast-feeding during drug therapy encouraged

SIDE EFFECTS

Frequent (greater than 10%)

Hemolytic anemia, methemoglobinemia, rash

Occasional (10%-1%)

Hemolysis, photosensitivity reaction

SERIOUS REACTIONS

- Agranulocytosis and blood dyscrasias may occur.

INTERACTIONS

Drugs

3 *Didanosine:* Higher failure rate in pneumocystis infections, possibly due to inhibited dissolution of dapsone in stomach; administer dapsone 2-3 hr before didanosine

3 *Methotrexate:* May increase hematologic reactions

3 *Probenecid:* Increased serum dapsone concentrations, clinical importance not established

3 *Protease inhibitors:* May increase dapsone blood concentration

3 *Rifampin:* Reduced serum dapsone concentrations; increased methemoglobin concentrations

3 *St. John's Wort:* May decrease dapsone blood concentration

3 *Trimethoprim:* Increased serum dapsone concentrations; increased trimethoprim concentrations

SPECIAL CONSIDERATIONS

- Use in conjunction with either rifampin or clofazimine to prevent development of drug resistance and reduce infectiousness of patient with leprosy more quickly

PATIENT/FAMILY EDUCATION

- Full therapeutic effects on leprosy may not occur for several mo; compliance with dosage schedule, duration is necessary
- Frequent blood tests are necessary, especially during early dapsone therapy
- Notify the physician and discontinue if a rash occurs

• Report persistent fatigue, fever, or sore throat
• Avoid overexposure to sun or ultraviolet light

MONITORING PARAMETERS

• CBC weekly for the first mo, qmo for 6 mo, and semiannually thereafter
• Periodic LFTs
• Skin for a dermatologic reaction
• Signs and symptoms of hemolysis, such as jaundice

daptomycin

(dap'-toe-mye-sin)

Rx: Cubicin

Chemical Class: Lipopeptide, cyclic

Therapeutic Class: Antibiotic

CLINICAL PHARMACOLOGY

Mechanism of Action: A lipopeptide antibacterial agent that binds to bacterial membranes and causes a rapid depolarization of the membrane potential. The loss of membrane potential leads to inhibition of protein, DNA, and RNA synthesis. ***Therapeutic Effect:*** Bactericidal.

Pharmacokinetics

Widely distributed. Protein binding: 90%. Primarily excreted unchanged in urine. Moderately removed by hemodialysis. ***Half-life:*** 7-8 hr (increased in impaired renal function).

INDICATIONS AND DOSAGES

Complicated skin and skin-structure infections

IV

Adults, Elderly. 4 mg/kg every 24 hr for 7-14 days.

Dosage in renal impairment

For patients with creatinine clearance of less than 30 ml/min, dosage is 4 mg/kg q48h for 7-14 days.

AVAILABLE FORMS

• *Powder for Injection:* 250 mg/vial, 500 mg/vial.

CONTRAINDICATIONS: None known.

PREGNANCY AND LACTATION: Pregnancy category B; breast milk excretion unknown

SIDE EFFECTS

Frequent (6%-5%)

Constipation, nausea, peripheral injection site reactions, headache, diarrhea

Occasional (4%-3%)

Insomnia, rash, vomiting

Rare (less than 3%)

Pruritus, dizziness, hypotension

SERIOUS REACTIONS

• Skeletal muscle myopathy, characterized by muscle pain and weakness, particularly of the distal extremities, occurs rarely.
• Antibiotic-associated colitis and other superinfections may result from altered bacterial balance.

INTERACTIONS

Drugs

3 *HMG-CoA reductase inhibitors:* May cause myopathy

3 *Tobramycin:* Increases the serum concentration of daptomycin

SPECIAL CONSIDERATIONS

• Experience with coadministration of HMG-CoA reductase inhibitors and daptomycin is limited; consider holding HMG-CoA reductase inhibitors in patients receiving daptomycin
• Not effective for pneumonia even due to susceptible organisms

PATIENT/FAMILY EDUCATION

• Notify the physician if headache, nausea, rash, severe diarrhea, new muscle weakness, or any other new symptoms occurs

MONITORING PARAMETERS

• CPK (weekly; discontinue in symptomatic patients with CPK elevation >1000 U/L (~5× ULN), or in asymptomatic patients with CPK >10× ULN

• Check for white patches on the mucous membranes and tongue
• Pattern of daily bowel activity and stool consistency; mild GI effects may be tolerable, but severe symptoms may indicate the onset of antibiotic-associated colitis
• Be alert for signs and symptoms of superinfection, including abdominal pain, moderate to severe diarrhea, severe anal or genital pruritus, and severe mouth soreness

darbepoetin alfa

(dar-be-poe′-e-tin al′-fa)

Rx: Aranesp

Chemical Class: Amino acid glycoprotein

Therapeutic Class: Hematopoietic agent

CLINICAL PHARMACOLOGY

Mechanism of Action: A glycoprotein that stimulates formation of RBCs in bone marrow; increases serum half-life of epoetin. ***Therapeutic Effect:*** Induces erythropoiesis and release of reticulocytes from bone marrow.

Pharmacokinetics

Well absorbed after subcutaneous administration. ***Half-life:*** 48.5 hr.

INDICATIONS AND DOSAGES

Anemia in chronic renal failure

IV Bolus, Subcutaneous

Adults, Elderly. Initially, 0.45 mcg/kg once weekly. Adjust dosage to achieve and maintain a target Hgb not to exceed 12 g/dl. Do not increase dosage more frequently than once monthly. Limit increases in Hgb by less than 1 g/dl over any 2-wk period.

Anemia associated with chemotherapy

IV, Subcutaneous

Adults, Elderly. 2.25 mcg/kg/dose once a week. May increase up to 4.5 mcg/kg/dose once a week.

AVAILABLE FORMS

• *Injection:* 25 mcg/ml, 40 mcg/ml, 60 mcg/ml, 100 mcg/ml, 150 mcg/ml, 200 mcg/ml, 300 mcg/ml.
• *Prefilled syringe:* 25 mcg/0.42 ml, 40 mcg/0.4 ml, 60 mcg/0.3 ml, 100 mcg/0.5 ml, 200 mcg/0.4 ml, 300 mcg/0.6 ml, 500 mcg/ml.

CONTRAINDICATIONS: History of sensitivity to mammalian cell-derived products or human albumin, uncontrolled hypertension

PREGNANCY AND LACTATION: Pregnancy category C; unknown if excreted in human milk

SIDE EFFECTS

Frequent

Myalgia, hypertension or hypotension, headache, diarrhea

Occasional

Fatigue, edema, vomiting, reaction at administration site, asthenia, dizziness

SERIOUS REACTIONS

• Vascular access thrombosis, CHF, sepsis, arrhythmias, and anaphylactic reaction occur rarely.

SPECIAL CONSIDERATIONS

• Two formulations available, one containing polysorbate 80, the other containing human albumin; a theoretical risk for Creutzfeldt-Jakob disease exists with the albumin formulation but is considered extremely remote
• Advantage over erythropoietin is decreased frequency of dosing

PATIENT/FAMILY EDUCATION

• Educate about blood pressure monitoring

• Proper instruction for home administration if deemed appropriate
• Report severe headache
• Avoid tasks that require mental alertness or motor skills until response to the drug is established

MONITORING PARAMETERS
• Hematocrit/hemoglobin weekly for 4 wks or until stable; if Hb increases >1.0 g/dL in any 2-wk period, decrease dose (possible increased seizure risk); target Hb level to not exceed 12 g/L
• Serum ferritin, transferrin saturation; supplemental iron recommended if ferritin <100 mcg/L or transferrin saturation <20%
• If lack of response or failure to maintain response occur, check for causative factors (e.g., folate or vitamin B_{12} deficiency, occult blood loss, malignancy)
• Blood pressure aggressively for an increase because 25% of patients taking darbepoietin alfa require antihypertensive therapy and dietary restrictions

deferoxamine mesylate

(de-fer-ox'-a-meen mes'-sil-ate)
Rx: Desferal
Chemical Class: Siderochrome
Therapeutic Class: Antidote, heavy metal

CLINICAL PHARMACOLOGY
Mechanism of Action: An antidote that binds with iron to form complex. ***Therapeutic Effect:*** Promotes urine excretion of acute iron poisoning.
Pharmacokinetics
Well absorbed after IM, SC administration. Widely distributed. Rapidly metabolized in tissues, plasma. Excreted in urine, eliminated in feces via biliary excretion. Removed by hemodialysis. ***Half-life:*** 6 hrs.

INDICATIONS AND DOSAGES
Acute iron intoxication
IM
Adults: Initially, 90 mg/kg, then 45 mg/kg up to 1 g q4-12h. Maximum: 6 g/day.
IV
Adults: 15 mg/kg/hr up to 90 mg/kg q8hrs. Maximum: 6 g/day.
Children: 15 mg/kg/hr.
Chronic iron overload
Subcutaneous
Adults: 1-2 g/day (20-40 mg/kg) over 8-24 hrs.
Children: 10 mg/kg/day.
IM
Adults: 0.5-1 g/day. In addition to IM, 2 g infused at rate not to exceed 15 mg/kg/hr.

AVAILABLE FORMS
• *Injection:* 500 mg (Desferal Mesylate).

CONTRAINDICATIONS: Severe renal disease, anuria, primary hemochromatosis, hypersensitivity to deferoxamine mesylate or any component of the formulation

PREGNANCY AND LACTATION: Pregnancy category C; excretion into breast milk unknown; use caution in nursing mothers

SIDE EFFECTS
Frequent
Pain, induration at injection site, urine color change (to orange-rose)
Occasional
Abdominal discomfort, diarrhea, leg cramps, impaired vision

SERIOUS REACTIONS
• Neurotoxicity, including high-frequency hearing loss, has been reported.

INTERACTIONS
Drugs
3 *Vitamin C:* May increase the effect of deferoxamine

SPECIAL CONSIDERATIONS
- Acute iron intoxication
- Deferoxamine indicated if:
  - Free serum iron present
  - Patient symptomatic
  - Serum iron >350 mcg/dL

PATIENT/FAMILY EDUCATION
- May turn urine red
- Discomfort may occur at site of injection

MONITORING PARAMETERS
- Visual acuity tests, slit-lamp examinations, funduscopy, and audiometry are recommended periodically in patients treated for prolonged periods of time
- BUN, creatinine, CrCl
- Serum iron levels

delavirdine mesylate

(de-la-vir'-deen mes'-sil-ate)

Rx: Rescriptor

Chemical Class: Arylpiperazine derivative; non-nucleoside reverse transcriptase inhibitor

Therapeutic Class: Antiretroviral

CLINICAL PHARMACOLOGY

Mechanism of Action: A non-nucleoside reverse transcriptase inhibitor that binds directly to HIV-1 reverse transcriptase and blocks RNA- and DNA-dependent DNA polymerase activities. ***Therapeutic Effect:*** Interrupts HIV replication, slowing the progression of HIV infection.

Pharmacokinetics

Rapidly absorbed after PO administration. Protein binding: 98%. Primarily distributed in plasma. Metabolized in the liver. Eliminated in feces and urine. ***Half-life:*** 2-11 hr.

INDICATIONS AND DOSAGES

HIV infection (in combination with other antiretrovirals)

PO

Adults. 400 mg 3 times a day.

AVAILABLE FORMS
- *Tablets:* 100 mg, 200 mg.

CONTRAINDICATIONS: None known.

PREGNANCY AND LACTATION: Pregnancy category C; teratogenic in rats; excreted in breast milk at high concentrations

SIDE EFFECTS

Frequent (18%)

Rash, pruritus

Occasional (greater than 2%)

Headache, nausea, diarrhea, fatigue, anorexia

SERIOUS REACTIONS
- Hepatic failure, severe rash, hemolytic anemia, rhabdomyolysis, erythema multiforme, Stevens-Johnson syndrome, and acute kidney failure have been reported.

INTERACTIONS

Drugs

3 *Aluminum:* Antacids reduce GI absorption of delavirdine by 50% if taken at same time; separate doses by at least 1 hr

3 *Antacids:* Antacids reduce GI absorption of delavirdine by 50% if taken at same time; separate doses by at least 1 hr

3 *Barbiturates:* Barbiturates decrease plasma delavirdine levels

3 *Benzodiazepines:* Delavirdine increases benzodiazepine plasma levels by inhibiting hepatic metabolism

3 *Calcium:* Antacids reduce GI absorption of delavirdine by 50% if taken at same time; separate doses by at least 1 hr

3 *Carbamazepine:* Carbamazepine decreases plasma delavirdine levels

❷ *Cimetidine:* Cimetidine reduces GI absorption of delavirdine; coadministration not recommended
❷ *Cisapride:* Delavirdine increases cisapride plasma level; coadministration not recommended
❸ *Clarithromycin:* Delavirdine increases clarithromycin plasma levels; clarithromycin increases delavirdine plasma levels
❸ *Dapsone:* Delavirdine increases dapsone plasma level
❸ *Didanosine:* Delavirdine reduces didanosine absorption; didanosine reduces delavirdine absorption; separate doses by at least 1 hr
❷ *Ergotamines:* Delavirdine increases ergotamine plasma level; coadministration not recommended
❷ *Famotidine:* Famotidine reduces GI absorption of delavirdine; coadministration not recommended
❸ *Fluoxetine:* Fluoxetine increases delavirdine levels by inhibiting hepatic metabolism
❸ *Indinavir:* Delavirdine increases indinavir AUC by 40%; reduce indinavir dose to 600 mg tid
❷ *Lansoprazole:* Lansoprazole reduces GI absorption of delavirdine; coadministration not recommended
❷ *Lovastatin:* Delavirdine increases lovastatin plasma level; coadministration not recommended
❸ *Magnesium:* Antacids reduce GI absorption of delavirdine by 50% if taken at same time; separate doses by at least 1 hr
❷ *Midazolam:* Delavirdine increases midazolam plasma level; coadministration not recommended
❸ *Nelfinavir:* Delavirdine increases nelfinavir AUC by 100%; nelfinavir reduces delavirdine AUC by 50%; no data on dose adjustment
❷ *Nizatidine:* Nizatidine reduces GI absorption of delavirdine; coadministration not recommended
❸ *Nifedipine:* Delavirdine increases nifedipine plasma level
❷ *Omeprazole:* Omeprazole reduces GI absorption of delavirdine; coadministration not recommended
❸ *Paclitaxel:* Increased risk of paclitaxel toxicity
❸ *Phenytoin:* Phenytoin decreases plasma delavirdine level
❷ *Quinidine:* Delavirdine increases quinidine plasma level
❷ *Ranitidine:* Ranitidine reduces GI absorption of delavirdine; coadministration not recommended
❷ *Rifabutin:* Rifabutin decreases plasma delavirdine level; coadministration not recommended
▲ *Rifampin:* Rifampin decreases plasma delavirdine level; coadministration contraindicated
❸ *Ritonavir:* Delavirdine increases ritonavir AUC by 70%; no data on dose adjustment
❷ *Saquinavir:* Delavirdine increases saquinavir AUC by 5-fold; additive hepatic toxicity possible; adjust Fortovase dose to 800 mg tid
❷ *Simvastatin:* Delavirdine increases simvastatin plasma level; coadministration not recommended
❸ *Sodium bicarbonate:* Antacids reduce GI absorption of delavirdine by 50% if taken at same time; separate doses by at least 1 hr
▲ *Terfenadine:* Delavirdine increases terfenadine plasma level; coadministration contraindicated
❷ *Triazolam:* Delavirdine increases triazolam plasma level; coadministration not recommended
❸ *Warfarin:* Delavirdine increases warfarin effect

SPECIAL CONSIDERATIONS

PATIENT/FAMILY EDUCATION

• May take without regard to food; patients with achlorhydria should take with acidic beverage (orange or cranberry juice); may cause alcohol intolerance

• Do not take any other medications, including OTC drugs, without notifying the physician
• Delavirdine is not a cure for HIV infection, nor does it reduce the risk of transmitting HIV to others

MONITORING PARAMETERS

• CBC, hepatic, and renal function
• Skin for rash
• Daily pattern of bowel activity and stool consistency
• Assess eating pattern, and monitor for nausea and weight loss

demeclocycline hydrochloride

(dem-e-kloe-sye'-kleen hye-droe-klor'-ide)

Rx: Declomycin
Chemical Class: Tetracycline derivative
Therapeutic Class: Antibiotic

CLINICAL PHARMACOLOGY

Mechanism of Action: A tetracycline antibiotic that inhibits bacterial protein synthesis by binding to ribosomal receptor sites; also inhibits ADH-induced water reabsorption. ***Therapeutic Effect:*** Bacteriostatic; also produces water diuresis.

Pharmacokinetics

Food and dairy products interfere with absorption. Protein binding: 41%-91%. Metabolized in liver. Excreted in urine. Removed by hemodialysis. ***Half-life:*** 10-15 hr.

INDICATIONS AND DOSAGES

Mild to moderate infections, including acne, pertussis, chronic bronchitis, and UTIs

PO

Adults, Elderly. 150 mg 4 times a day or 300 mg 2 times a day.

Children older than 8 yr. 8-12 mg/kg/day in 2-4 divided doses.

Uncomplicated gonorrhea

PO

Adults. Initially, 600 mg, then 300 mg q12h for 4 days for total of 3 g.

Syndrome of inappropriate ADH secretion (SIADH)

PO

Adults, Elderly. Initially, 900-1200 mg/day in 3-4 divided doses, then decrease dose to 600-900 mg/day in divided doses.

AVAILABLE FORMS

• *Tablets:* 150 mg, 300 mg.

CONTRAINDICATIONS: Children 8 yrs and younger, last half of pregnancy

PREGNANCY AND LACTATION: Pregnancy category D; problems associated with use of the tetracyclines during or around pregnancy include adverse effects on fetal teeth and bones, maternal liver toxicity, and congenital defects; excreted into breast milk in low concentrations; use caution in nursing mothers

SIDE EFFECTS

Frequent

Anorexia, nausea, vomiting, diarrhea, dysphagia, possibly severe photosensitivity, (with moderate to high demeclocycline dosage).

Occasional

Urticaria, rash; diabetes insipidus syndrome, marked by polydipsia, polyuria, and weakness (with long-term therapy).

SERIOUS REACTIONS

• Superinfection (especially fungal), anaphylaxis, and benign intracranial hypertension occur rarely.
• Bulging fontanelles occur rarely in infants.

INTERACTIONS

Drugs

3 *Antacids:* Reduced serum concentration of demeclocycline; take 2 hr before or 6 hr after antacids containing aluminum, calcium, or magnesium

❷ *Bismuth:* Reduced serum concentration of demeclocycline; do not coadminister

❸ *Calcium:* See antacids

❸ *Cholestyramine:* Reduced serum concentration of demeclocycline; take 2 hr before or 3 hr after cholestyramine

❸ *Colestipol:* Reduced serum concentration of demeclocycline; take 2 hr before or 3 hr after colestipol

❸ *Digoxin:* Demeclocycline may increase serum digoxin levels

❸ *Food:* Reduced serum concentration of demeclocycline; take 2 hr before or 3 hr after food

❸ *Iron:* Reduced serum concentration of demeclocycline; take 2 hr before or 3 hr after iron

❸ *Magnesium:* See antacids

❷ *Methoxyflurane:* Demeclocycline enhances nephrotoxicity of methoxyflurane

❸ *Oral contraceptives:* Contraceptive failure may occur rarely; mechanism unknown

❸ *Penicillins:* Demeclocycline may reduce penicillin efficacy

❸ *Warfarin:* Demeclocycline may increase effect of warfarin

❸ *Zinc:* Reduced serum concentration of demeclocycline; take 2 hr before or 3 hr after zinc

Labs

- *False increase:* Urinary catecholamines

SPECIAL CONSIDERATIONS

- No advantages over other tetracyclines as antiinfective; higher incidence of phototoxicity; active against water intoxication and SIADH

PATIENT/FAMILY EDUCATION

- Sunscreen does not seem to decrease photosensitivity
- Avoid milk products; take with full glass of water on an empty stomach 1 hr before meals or 2 hr after meals
- Space drug doses evenly around the clock and continue taking demeclocycline for the full course of treatment

MONITORING PARAMETERS

- LFTs during prolonged administration
- Skin for rash
- Signs and symptoms of superinfection, such as anal or genital pruritus, diarrhea, and ulceration or changes of the oral mucosa or tongue

desipramine hydrochloride

(dess-ip′-ra-meen)

Rx: Norpramin

Chemical Class: Dibenzazepine derivative; secondary amine

Therapeutic Class: Antidepressant, tricyclic

CLINICAL PHARMACOLOGY

Mechanism of Action: A tricyclic antidepressant that blocks the reuptake of neurotransmitters, such as norepinephrine and serotonin, at presynaptic membranes, increasing their availability at postsynaptic receptor sites. Also has strong anticholinergic activity. ***Therapeutic Effect:*** Relieves depression.

Pharmacokinetics

Rapidly and well absorbed from the GI tract. Protein binding: 90%. Metabolized in the liver. Primarily excreted in urine. Minimally removed by hemodialysis. ***Half-life:*** 12-27 hr.

INDICATIONS AND DOSAGES

Depression

PO

Adults. 75 mg/day. May gradually increase to 150-200 mg/day. Maximum: 300 mg/day.

Elderly. Initially, 10-25 mg/day. May gradually increase to 75-100 mg/day. Maximum: 300 mg/day.
Children older than 12 yr. Initially, 25-50 mg/day. May gradually increase to 100 mg/day. Maximum: 150 mg/day.
Children 6-12 yr. 1-3 mg/kg/day. Maximum: 5 mg/kg/day.

AVAILABLE FORMS

- *Tablets:* 10 mg, 25 mg, 50 mg, 75 mg, 100 mg, 150 mg.

UNLABELED USES: Treatment of attention deficit hyperactivity disorder, bulimia nervosa, cataplexy associated with narcolepsy, cocaine withdrawal, neurogenic pain, panic disorder

CONTRAINDICATIONS: Angle-closure glaucoma, use within 14 days of MAOIs

PREGNANCY AND LACTATION: Pregnancy category C; excreted into breast milk; effect on the nursing infant unknown, but may be of concern

SIDE EFFECTS

Frequent

Somnolence, fatigue, dry mouth, blurred vision, constipation, delayed micturition, orthostatic hypotension, diaphoresis, impaired concentration, increased appetite, urine retention

Occasional

GI disturbances (such as nausea, GI distress, metallic taste)

Rare

Paradoxical reactions (agitation, restlessness, nightmares, insomnia), extrapyramidal symptoms (particularly fine hand tremor)

SERIOUS REACTIONS

- Overdose may produce confusion, seizures, somnolence, arrhythmias, fever, hallucinations, dyspnea, vomiting, and unusual fatigue or weakness.
- Abrupt discontinuation after prolonged therapy may produce severe headache, malaise, nausea, vomiting, and vivid dreams.

INTERACTIONS

Drugs

3 *Antithyroid agents:* May increase risk of agranulocytosis
3 *Barbiturates:* Reduced serum concentrations of cyclic antidepressants
2 *Bethanidine:* Reduced antihypertensive effect of bethanidine
3 *Carbamazepine:* Reduced serum concentrations of cyclic antidepressants
3 *Cimetidine:* Increased serum concentrations of cyclic antidepressants
2 *Clonidine:* Reduced antihypertensive effect of clonidine; enhanced hypertensive response with abrupt clonidine withdrawal
3 *Debrisoquin:* Reduced antihypertensive effect of debrisoquin
3 *Diltiazem:* Increased serum concentrations of cyclic antidepressants
2 *Epinephrine:* Markedly enhanced pressor response to IV epinephrine
3 *Ethanol:* Additive impairment of motor skills; abstinent alcoholics may eliminate cyclic antidepressants faster than nonalcoholics
3 *Fluoxetine:* Marked increases in serum concentrations of cyclic antidepressants
3 *Fluvoxamine:* Marked increases in serum concentrations of cyclic antidepressants
2 *Guanabenz, guanethidine:* Reduced antihypertensive effect
3 *Guanadrel, guanfacine:* Reduced antihypertensive effect
3 *Indinavir:* Increase in serum concentrations of cyclic antidepressants
3 *Lithium:* Increased risk of neurotoxicity

❷ *Moclobemide:* Potential association with fatal or nonfatal serotonin syndrome
❷ *MAOIs:* Excessive sympathetic response, manias, or hyperpyrexia possible
❸ *Neuroleptics:* Increased therapeutic and toxic effects of both drugs
❷ *Norepinephrine:* Markedly enhanced pressor response to IV norepinephrine
❸ *Paroxetine:* Marked increases in serum concentrations of cyclic antidepressants
❸ *Phenytoin:* May decrease desipramine concentration
❸ *Propoxyphene:* Increased serum concentrations of cyclic antidepressants
❸ *Quinidine:* Increased serum concentrations of cyclic antidepressants
❸ *Rifampin:* Reduced serum concentrations of cyclic antidepressants
❸ *Ritonavir:* Marked increases in serum concentrations of cyclic antidepressants
❸ *St. John's Wort:* May have additive effects
❸ *Sulfonylureas:* Cyclic antidepressants may increase hypoglycemic effect

SPECIAL CONSIDERATIONS

• Equally effective as other tricyclic antidepressants for depression; fewer anticholinergic effects than tertiary amines, less orthostasis, and mild stimulatory property

PATIENT/FAMILY EDUCATION

• Therapeutic effects may take 4-6 wk
• Use caution in driving or other activities requiring alertness
• Avoid alcohol and other CNS depressants
• Do not discontinue abruptly after long-term use
• Change positions slowly to avoid hypotensive effect

MONITORING PARAMETERS

• Determination of desipramine plasma concentrations is not routinely recommended but may be useful in identifying toxicity, drug interactions, or noncompliance (adjustments in dosage should be made according to clinical response not plasma concentrations); therapeutic level is 50-200 ng/ml
• Supervise suicidal risk patient closely during early therapy (as depression lessens, energy level improves, increasing suicide potential)
• Assess appearance, behavior, speech pattern, level of interest, mood

---

desirudin

(deh-seer'-ew-din)

Rx: Iprivask

Chemical Class: Hirudin derivative; thrombin inhibitor

Therapeutic Class: Anticoagulant

CLINICAL PHARMACOLOGY

Mechanism of Action: An anticoagulant that binds specifically and directly to thrombin, inhibiting free circulating and clot-bound thrombin. ***Therapeutic Effect:*** Prolongs the clotting time of human plasma.

Pharmacokinetics

Completely absorbed. Distributed in extracellular space. Metabolized and eliminated by the kidney. ***Half-life:*** 2-3 hr.

INDICATIONS AND DOSAGES

Prevention of deep vein thrombosis (DVT) in patients undergoing hip replacement surgery

Subcutaneous

Adults, Elderly. Initially, 15 mg q12h given 5-15 min before surgery

but following induction of regional block anesthesia, if used. May administer up to 12 days post surgery.
Moderate renal impairment (creatinine clearance 31-60 ml/min or higher)
Subcutaneous
Adults, Elderly. 5 mg q12h.
Severe renal impairment (creatinine clearance less than 31 ml/min)
Subcutaneous
Adults, Elderly. 1.7 mg q12h.

AVAILABLE FORMS

• *Powder for Injection:* 15-mg vial with diluent (diluent includes 0.6 ml mannitol [3%] in water for injection).

CONTRAINDICATIONS: Hypersensitivity to natural or recombinant hirudins (anticoagulation factors), active bleeding, irreversible coagulation disorders

PREGNANCY AND LACTATION: Pregnancy category C; teratogenic in animal studies; excretion into breast milk unknown, use caution in nursing mothers

SIDE EFFECTS

Frequent (6%)
Hematoma
Occasional (4%-2%)
Injection site mass, wound secretion, nausea, hypersensitivity reaction

SERIOUS REACTIONS

Alert: When neuraxial anesthesia (epidural/spinal anesthesia) or spinal puncture is employed, patients anticoagulated or scheduled to be anticoagulated with selective inhibitors of thrombin such as desirudin may be at risk of developing an epidural or spinal hematoma, which can result in long-term or permanent paralysis.

• Serious or major hemorrhage and anaphylactic reaction occur rarely.

INTERACTIONS

Drugs

3 *Dextran 40, systemic glucocorticoids, thrombolytics, and anticoagulants:* Increased risk of bleeding
3 *Salicylates, NSAIDS, aspirin, ticlopidine, dipyridamole, sulfinpyrazone, clopidogrel, glycoprotein IIb/IIIa antagonists:* Increased risk of bleeding

D

SPECIAL CONSIDERATIONS

PATIENT/FAMILY EDUCATION

• Use an electric razor and soft toothbrush to prevent bleeding during therapy
• Do not take other medications, including OTC drugs (especially aspirin), without physician approval
• Report black or red stool, coffee-ground vomitus, dark or red urine, or red-speckled mucus from cough
• Tell the female patient that her menstrual flow may be heavier than usual

MONITORING PARAMETERS

• If CrCl <60 ml/min, monitor aPTT and serum Cr at least daily; if aPTT exceeds 2× control, interrupt therapy until the value returns to less than 2× control and then resume therapy at a reduced dose guided by the initial degree of aPTT abnormality
• Assess for abdominal or back pain, a decrease in blood pressure and Hct, an increase in pulse rate, and severe headache because these signs may indicate hemorrhage
• Determine the amount of the female patient's menstrual discharge and monitor for an increase
• Assess the patient's gums for erythema and gingival bleeding, skin for bruises, and urine for hematuria
• Examine the patient for excessive bleeding from minor cuts and scratches

desloratadine

(des-lor-at'-a-deen)

Rx: Clarinex, Clarinex RediTabs

Chemical Class: Piperidine derivative

Therapeutic Class: Antihistamine

CLINICAL PHARMACOLOGY

Mechanism of Action: A nonsedating antihistamine that exhibits selective peripheral histamine H_1-receptor blocking action. Competes with histamine at receptor sites. ***Therapeutic Effect:*** Prevents allergic responses mediated by histamine, such as rhinitis and urticaria.

Pharmacokinetics

Rapidly and almost completely absorbed from the GI tract. Distributed mainly in liver, lungs, GI tract, and bile. Metabolized in the liver to active metabolite and undergoes extensive first-pass metabolism. Eliminated in urine and feces. ***Half-life:*** 27 hr (increased in the elderly and in renal or hepatic impairment).

INDICATIONS AND DOSAGES

Allergic rhinitis, urticaria

PO

Adults, Elderly, Children older than 12 yr. 5 mg once a day.

Children 6-12 yr. 2.5 mg once a day.

Children 1-5 yr. 1.25 mg once a day.

Children 6-11 mo. 1 mg once a day.

Dosage in hepatic or renal impairment

Dosage is decreased to 5 mg every other day.

AVAILABLE FORMS

- *Tablets (Clarinex):* 5 mg.
- *Tablets (Orally Disintegrating [Clarinex Reditabs]):* 2.5 mg, 5 mg.
- *Syrup (Clarinex):* 2.5 mg/5 ml.

CONTRAINDICATIONS: None known.

PREGNANCY AND LACTATION: Pregnancy category C; passes into breast milk, use caution in nursing mothers

SIDE EFFECTS

Frequent (12%)

Headache

Occasional (3%)

Dry mouth, somnolence

Rare (less than 3%)

Fatigue, dizziness, diarrhea, nausea

SERIOUS REACTIONS

- None known.

INTERACTIONS

Drugs

3 *Erythromycin, ketoconazole:* May increase desloratidine blood concentration

SPECIAL CONSIDERATIONS

- No advantage over loratadine (parent compound), which is now available OTC
- Intranasal corticosteroids are preferred therapy unless allergy symptoms are mild and infrequent
- Reserve for patients unable to tolerate sedating antihistamines such as chlorpheniramine

PATIENT/FAMILY EDUCATION

- May be taken without regard to meals
- Take orally disintegrating tabs immediately after opening the blister packet
- Desloratidine does not cause drowsiness
- Avoid alcohol during therapy

MONITORING PARAMETERS

- Therapeutic response

desmopressin

(des-moe-press'-in)

Rx: DDAVP, DDAVP Nasal, DDAVP Rhinal Tube, Minirin, Stimate

Chemical Class: Arginine vasopressin analog

Therapeutic Class: Antidiuretic; antihemophilic; hemostatic

CLINICAL PHARMACOLOGY

Mechanism of Action: A synthetic pituitary hormone that increases reabsorption of water by increasing permeability of collecting ducts of the kidneys. Also serves as a plasminogen activator. ***Therapeutic Effect:*** Increases plasma factor VIII (antihemophilic factor). Decreases urinary output.

Pharmacokinetics

Route	*Onset*	*Peak*	*Duration*
PO	1 hr	2-7 hr	6-8 hr
IV	15-30 min	1.5-3 hr	N/A
Intranasal	15 min-1 hr	1-5 hr	5-21 hr

Poorly absorbed after oral or nasal administration. Metabolism: Unknown. ***Half-life:*** Oral: 1.5-2.5 hr. Intranasal: 3.3-3.5 hr. IV: 0.4-4 hr.

INDICATIONS AND DOSAGES

Primary nocturnal enuresis

PO

Children 12 yr and older. 0.2-0.6 mg once before bedtime.

Intranasal

Children 6 yr and older. Initially, 20 mcg (0.2 ml) at bedtime; use one-half dose in each nostril. Adjust to maximum of 40 mcg/day. Range: 10-40 mcg.

Central cranial diabetes insipidus

PO

Adults, Elderly, Children 12 yr and older. Initially, 0.05 mg twice a day. Range: 0.1-1.2 mg/day in 2-3 divided doses.

Children younger than 12 yr. Initially, 0.05 mg; then twice a day. Range: 0.1-0.8 mg daily.

IV, Subcutaneous

Adults, Elderly, Children 12 yr and older. 2-4 mcg/day in 2 divided doses or 1⁄10 of maintenance intranasal dose.

Intranasal (use 100 mcg/ml concentration)

Adults, Elderly, Children older than 12 yr. 5-40 mcg (0.05-0.4 ml) in 1-3 doses/day.

Children 3 mo-12 yr. Initially, 5 mcg (0.05 ml)/day. Range: 5-30 mcg (0.05–0.3 ml)/day.

Hemophilia A, von Willebrand's disease (Type I)

IV Infusion

Adults, Elderly, Children weighing more than 10 kg. 0.3 mcg/kg diluted in 50 ml 0.9% NaCl.

Children weighing 10 kg and less. 0.3 mcg/kg diluted in 10 ml 0.9% NaCl.

Intranasal (use 1.5 mg/ml concentration providing 150 mcg/spray)

Adults, Elderly, Children 12 yr and older weighing more than 50 kg. 300 mcg; use 1 spray in each nostril.

Adults, Elderly, Children 12 yr and older weighing 50 kg or less. 150 mcg as a single spray.

AVAILABLE FORMS

- *Tablets (DDAVP):* 0.1 mg, 0.2 mg.
- *Injection (DDAVP):* 4 mcg/ml.
- *Nasal Solution (DDAVP):* 0.01%.
- *Nasal Spray:* 0.01 mg/inhalation (DDAVP Nasal), 0.15 mg/inhalation (Stimate).

UNLABELED USES: Prophylaxis and treatment of central diabetes insipidus, treatment of hemophilia A, primary nocturnal enuresis, von Willebrand's disease

CONTRAINDICATIONS: Hemophilia A with factor VIII levels less than 5%; hemophilia B; severe type I, type IIB, or platelet-type von Willebrand's disease

PREGNANCY AND LACTATION: Pregnancy category B (no uterotonic action at antidiuretic doses); compatible with breast-feeding

SIDE EFFECTS

Occasional

IV: Pain, redness, or swelling at injection site; headache; abdominal cramps; vulval pain; flushed skin; mild BP elevation; nausea with high dosages

Nasal: Rhinorrhea, nasal congestion, slight BP elevation

SERIOUS REACTIONS

• Water intoxication or hyponatremia, marked by headache, somnolence, confusion, decreased urination, rapid weight gain, seizures, and coma, may occur in overhydration. Children, elderly patients, and infants are especially at risk.

INTERACTIONS

3 *Carbamazepine, chlorpropamide, clofibrate:* May increase the effects of desmopressin

3 *Demeclocycline, lithium, norepinephrine:* May decrease effects of desmopressin

SPECIAL CONSIDERATIONS

• Though useful in the treatment of children with enuresis, relapse following discontinuation is common; conservative therapy preferred long-term; desmopressin best used intermittently (e.g., overnight with friend)

PATIENT/FAMILY EDUCATION

• Nasal tube delivery system is supplied with a flexible calibrated plastic tube (rhinyle); draw sol into the rhinyle, insert 1 end of tube into nostril, blow on the other end to deposit sol deep into nasal cavity

• Ingest only enough water to satisfy thirst (especially elderly and children)

• Report abdominal cramps, headache, heartburn, nausea, or shortness of breath

MONITORING PARAMETERS

• Diabetes insipidus: Urine volume and osmolality, plasma osmolality, child's sleep pattern

• Hemophilia A: Determine factor VIII coagulant activity before injecting desmopressin for hemostasis; if activity is <5% of normal, do not rely on desmopressin

• von Willebrand's disease: Assess levels of factor VIII coagulant, factor VIII antigen, and ristocetin cofactor; skin bleeding time may also be helpful

desonide

(dess'-oh-nide)

Rx: Delonide, DesOwen, Tridesilon

Chemical Class: Corticosteroid, synthetic

Therapeutic Class: Corticosteroid, topical

CLINICAL PHARMACOLOGY

Mechanism of Action: A topical corticosteroid that has antiinflammatory, antipruritic, and vasoconstrictive properties. The exact mechanism of the antiinflammatory process is unclear. ***Therapeutic Effect:*** Reduces or prevents tissue response to the inflammatory process.

Pharmacokinetics

Large variation in absorption determined by many factors. Metabolized in the liver. Primarily excreted by the kidneys and small amounts in the bile.

INDICATIONS AND DOSAGES

Dermatoses

Topical

Adults, Elderly. Apply sparingly 2-3 times/day.

Otitis externa

Aural

Adults, Elderly, Children. Instill 3-4 drops into the ear 3-4 times/day.

AVAILABLE FORMS

- *Lotion:* 0.05% (DesOwen).
- *Cream:* 0.05% (DesOwen).
- *Ointment:* 0.05% (DesOwen, Tridesilon).

CONTRAINDICATIONS: Perforated eardrum, history of hypersensitivity to desonide or other corticosteroids

PREGNANCY AND LACTATION: Pregnancy category C; unknown whether top application could result in sufficient systemic absorption to produce detectable amounts in breast milk (systemic corticosteroids are secreted into breast milk in quantities not likely to have detrimental effects on infant)

SIDE EFFECTS

Occasional

Burning and stinging at site of application, dryness, skin peeling, contact dermatitis

SERIOUS REACTIONS

- The serious reactions of long-term therapy and the addition of occlusive dressings are reversible hypothalamic-pituitary-adrenal (HPA) axis suppression, manifestations of Cushing's syndrome, hyperglycemia, and glucosuria.

INTERACTIONS

Drugs

❷ *Bupropion:* May lower the seizure threshold

SPECIAL CONSIDERATIONS

PATIENT/FAMILY EDUCATION

- Apply sparingly only to affected area
- Avoid contact with the eyes
- Do not put bandages or dressings over treated area unless directed by clinician
- Discontinue drug and notify clinician if local irritation or fever develops
- Do not use on weeping, denuded, or infected areas

MONITORING PARAMETERS

- Skin for rash

desoximetasone

(des-ox-i-met'-a-sone)

Rx: Topicort, Topicort LP

Chemical Class: Corticosteroid, synthetic

Therapeutic Class: Corticosteroid, topical

CLINICAL PHARMACOLOGY

Mechanism of Action: A high potency, fluoronated topical corticosteroid that has antiinflammatory, antipruritic, and vasoconstrictive properties. The exact mechanism of the antiinflammatory process is unclear. ***Therapeutic Effect:*** Reduces tissue response to the inflammatory process.

Pharmacokinetics

Large variation in absorption among sites. Protein binding in varying degrees. Metabolized in liver. Primarily excreted in urine.

INDICATIONS AND DOSAGES

Dermatoses

Topical

Adults, Elderly. Apply sparingly 2 times/day.

Children. Apply sparingly 1-2 times/day.

AVAILABLE FORMS

- *Cream:* 0.25% (Topicort), 0.05% (Topicort-LP).
- *Gel:* 0.05% (Topicort).
- *Ointment:* 0.25% (Topicort).

UNLABELED USES: Eczema, psoriasis vulgaris

CONTRAINDICATIONS: History of hypersensitivity to desoximetasone or other corticosteroids

PREGNANCY AND LACTATION: Pregnancy category C; it is unknown whether topical application could result in sufficient systemic absorption to produce detectable amounts in breast milk (systemic corticosteroids are secreted into breast milk in quantities not likely to have any detrimental effects on infant)

SIDE EFFECTS

Frequent

Itching, redness, irritation, burning at site of application

Occasional

Dryness, folliculitis, hypertrichosis, acneiform eruptions, hypopigmentation, perioral dermatitis

Rare

Allergic contact dermatitis, adrenal suppression, atrophy, striae, miliaria, photosensitivity

SERIOUS REACTIONS

- Serious reactions of long-term therapy and addition of occlusive dressings are reversible hypothalamic-pituitary-adrenal (HPA) axis suppression, manifestations of Cushing's syndrome, hyperglycemia, and glucosuria.
- Abruptly withdrawing the drug after long-term therapy may require supplemental systemic corticosteroids.

SPECIAL CONSIDERATIONS

- Potent, fluorinated topical corticosteroid with comparable efficacy to fluocinonide, diflorasone, amcinonide, betamethasone, dipropionate, and halcinonide; cost should govern use

PATIENT/FAMILY EDUCATION

- Apply sparingly only to affected area
- Avoid contact with the eyes
- Do not put bandages or dressings over treated area unless directed by clinician
- Discontinue drug, notify clinician if local irritation or fever develops
- Do not use on weeping, denuded, or infected areas

MONITORING PARAMETERS

- Be alert for signs and symptoms of infection such as fever and sore throat that indicate reduced immune response

dexamethasone

(dex-a-meth'-a-sone)

Rx: Adrenocot, Cortastat, Cortastat 10, Cortastat LA, Dalalone, Dalalone D.P., Dalalone L.A., Decadron, Decadron 5-12 Pak, Decadron Phosphate Injectable, Decaject, De-Sone LA, Dexacen-4, Dexamethasone Intensol, Dexasone, Dexasone LA, Dexpak Taperpak, Hexadrol, Hexadrol Phosphate, Maxidex, Solurex, Solurex LA

Combinations

Rx: with neomycin, (Neo-Decadron, Ak-Neo-Dex); with neomycin and polymixin B (Dexacidin, Maxitrol, Dexasporin); with tobramycin (Tobradex); with lidocaine (Decadron with Xylocaine)

Chemical Class: Glucocorticoid, synthetic

Therapeutic Class: Corticosteroid, ophthalmic; corticosteroid, systemic

CLINICAL PHARMACOLOGY

Mechanism of Action: A long-acting glucocorticoid that inhibits accumulation of inflammatory cells at inflammation sites, phagocytosis, lysosomal enzyme release and synthesis, and release of mediators of inflammation. ***Therapeutic Effect:*** Prevents and suppresses cell and tissue immune reactions and inflammatory process.

Pharmacokinetics

Rapidly, completely absorbed from the GI tract after oral administration. Widely distributed. Protein binding: High. Metabolized in the liver. Primarily excreted in urine. Minimally removed by hemodialysis. ***Half-life:*** 3-4.5 hr.

INDICATIONS AND DOSAGES

Antiinflammatory

PO, IV, IM

Adults, Elderly. 0.75-9 mg/day in divided doses q6-12h.

Children. 0.08-0.3 mg/kg/day in divided doses q6-12h.

Cerebral edema

IV

Adults, Elderly. Initially, 10 mg, then 4 mg (IV or IM) q6h.

PO, IV, IM

Children. Loading dose of 1-2 mg/kg, then 1-1.5 mg/kg/day in divided doses q4-6h.

Nausea and vomiting in chemotherapy patients

IV

Adults, Elderly. 8-20 mg once, then 4 mg (PO) q4-6h or 8 mg q8h.

Children. 10 mg/m^2/dose (Maximum: 20 mg), then 5 mg/m^2/dose q6h.

Usual topical dosage

Topical

Adults, Elderly, Children. Apply to affected area 3-4 times a day.

Physiologic replacement

PO, IV, IM

Children. 0.03-0.15 mg/kg/day in divided doses q6-12h.

Usual ophthalmic dosage, ocular inflammatory conditions

Ointment

Adults, Elderly, Children. Thin coating 3-4 times/day.

Suspension

Adults, Elderly, Children. Initially, 2 drops q1h while awake and q2h at night for 1 day, then reduce to 3-4 times/day.

AVAILABLE FORMS

- *Nasal Aerosol:* 100 mcg.
- *Ophthalmic Ointment (Decadron, Maxidex):* 0.05%.

• *Ophthalmic Solution (Decadron):* 0.1%.
• *Ophthalmic Suspension (Maxidex):* 0.1%.
• *Oral Concentrate (Dexamethasone Intensol):* 1 mg/ml.
• *Oral Solution:* 0.5 mg/5 ml, 1 mg/ml.
• *Tablets:* 0.25 mg, 0.5 mg (Decadron), 0.75 mg (Decadron, Decadron 5-12 Pak), 1 mg, 1.5 mg (Dexpak Taperpak), 2 mg, 4 mg (Decadron, Hexadrol), 6 mg.
• *Topical Aerosol:* 0.01%, 0.04%.
• *Topical Cream (Decadron):* 0.1%,
• *Topical Gel:* 0.1%.
• *Injectable Solution:* 4 mg/ml (Adrenocot, Cortastat, Dalalone, Decadron Phosphate Injectable, Decaject, Dexacen-4, Dexasone, Hexadrol Phosphate, Solurex), 10 mg/ml (Cortastat 10, Dexasone, Hexadrol Phosphate).
• *Injectable Suspension:* 8 mg/ml (Cortastat LA, Dalalone LA, De-Sone LA, Dexasone LA, Solurex LA), 16 mg/ml (Dalalone D.P.).

UNLABELED USES: Antiemetic, croup

CONTRAINDICATIONS: Active untreated infections, fungal, tuberculosis, or viral diseases of the eye

PREGNANCY AND LACTATION: Pregnancy category C (D if used in the first trimester); used in patients with premature labor at about 24-36 wk gestation to stimulate fetal lung maturation; excreted in breast milk; could suppress infant's growth and interfere with endogenous corticosteroid production

SIDE EFFECTS

Frequent

Inhalation: Cough, dry mouth, hoarseness, throat irritation

Intranasal: Burning, mucosal dryness

Ophthalmic: Blurred vision

Systemic: Insomnia, facial swelling or cushingoid appearance, moderate abdominal distention, indigestion, increased appetite, nervousness, facial flushing, diaphoresis

Occasional

Inhalation: Localized fungal infection, such as thrush

Intranasal: Crusting inside nose, nosebleed, sore throat, ulceration of nasal mucosa.

Ophthalmic: Decreased vision, watering of eyes, eye pain, burning, stinging, redness of eyes, nausea, vomiting

Systemic: Dizziness, decreased or blurred vision

Topical: Allergic contact dermatitis, purpura or blood-containing blisters, thinning of skin with easy bruising, telangiectasis or raised dark red spots on skin

Rare

Inhalation: Increased bronchospasm, esophageal candidiasis

Intranasal: Nasal and pharyngeal candidiasis, eye pain

Systemic: General allergic reaction (such as rash and hives); pain, redness, or swelling at injection site; psychologic changes; false sense of well-being; hallucinations; depression

SERIOUS REACTIONS

• Long-term therapy may cause muscle wasting (especially in the arms and legs), osteoporosis, spontaneous fractures, amenorrhea, cataracts, glaucoma, peptic ulcer disease, and CHF.
• The ophthalmic form may cause glaucoma, ocular hypertension, and cataracts.
• Abrupt withdrawal following long-term therapy may cause severe joint pain, severe headache, anorexia, nausea, fever, rebound inflam-

mation, fatigue, weakness, lethargy, dizziness, and orthostatic hypotension.

INTERACTIONS

Drugs

3 *Aminoglutethamide:* Enhanced elimination of corticosteroids; marked reduction in corticosteroid response; increased clearance of dexamethasone; doubling of dose may be necessary

3 *Amphotericin:* May increase hypokalemia

3 *Antidiabetics:* Increased blood glucose

3 *Barbiturates, carbamazepine:* Reduced serum concentrations of corticosteroids; increased clearance of dexamethasone

3 *Cholestyramine, colestipol:* Possible reduced absorption of corticosteroids

3 *Cyclosporine:* Possible increased concentration of both drugs, seizures

3 *Digoxin:* May increase digoxin toxicity caused by hypokalemia

3 *Diuretics, potassium supplements:* May decrease the effects of these drugs

3 *Erythromycin, troleandomycin, clarithromycin, ketoconazole:* Possible enhanced steroid effect

3 *Estrogens, oral contraceptives:* Enhanced effects of corticosteroids

3 *Isoniazid:* Reduced plasma concentrations of isoniazid

3 *IUDs:* Inhibition of inflammation may decrease contraceptive effect

3 *Live virus vaccines:* May decrease the patient's antibody response to vaccine, increase vaccine side effects, and potentiate virus replication

3 *NSAIDs:* Increased risk GI ulceration

3 *Rifampin:* Reduced therapeutic effect of corticosteroids

3 *Salicylates:* Subtherapeutic salicylate concentrations possible

Labs

- *False negative:* Skin allergy tests

SPECIAL CONSIDERATIONS

- Signs of adrenal insufficiency include fatigue, anorexia, nausea, vomiting, diarrhea, weight loss, weakness, dizziness, and low blood sugar; drug-induced secondary adrenocorticoid insufficiency and low blood sugar; drug-induced adrenocorticoid insufficiency may be minimized by gradual systemic dosage reduction; relative insufficiency may exist for up to 1 yr after discontinuation, therefore, be prepared to supplement in situations of stress
- May mask infections
- Do not give live-virus vaccines to patients on prolonged therapy
- Patients on chronic steroid therapy should wear medical alert bracelet

PATIENT/FAMILY EDUCATION

- Do not abruptly discontinue the drug or change the dosage or schedule; the drug must be withdrawn gradually under medical supervision
- Report fever, muscle aches, sore throat, and sudden weight gain or swelling. Severe stress, including serious infection, surgery, or trauma, may require an increase in dexamethasone dosage
- Inform the dentist and other physicians if patient is taking dexamethasone or has taken it within the past 12 mos
- Use the topical form after a bath or shower for best absorption
- Steroids often cause mood swings, ranging from euphoria to depression

MONITORING PARAMETERS

- Potassium and blood sugar during long-term therapy

D

• Observe growth and development of children on prolonged therapy
• Check lens and intraocular pressure frequently during prolonged use of ophthalmic preparations

dexchlorpheniramine maleate

(dex'-klor-fen-eer'-a-meen mal'-ee-ate)

Rx: Polaramine, Polaramine Repetabs

Combinations

Rx: with guaifenesin, pseudoephedrine (Polaramine Expectorant)

Chemical Class: Alkylamine derivative

Therapeutic Class: Antihistamine

CLINICAL PHARMACOLOGY

Mechanism of Action: A propylamine derivative that competes with histamine for H_1-receptor sites on effector cells in the gastrointestinal (GI) tract, blood vessels, and respiratory tract. Dexchlorpheniramine is the dextro-isomer of chlorpheniramine and is approximately two times more active. ***Therapeutic Effect:*** Prevents allergic response, produces mild bronchodilation, blocks histamine-induced bronchitis.

Pharmacokinetics

Route	*Onset*	*Peak*	*Duration*
PO	0.5 hr	1-2 hr	3-6 hr

Well absorbed from the GI tract. Protein binding: 70%. Widely distributed. Metabolized in liver to active metabolite, undergoes extensive first-pass metabolism. Excreted primarily in urine. Not removed by hemodialysis. ***Half-life:*** 20 hrs.

INDICATIONS AND DOSAGES

Allergic rhinitis, common cold

PO

Adults, Elderly, Children 12 yrs or older. 2 mg q4-6h or 4-6 mg timed release at bedtime or q8-10h.

Children 6-11 yrs. 4 mg timed release at bedtime or 1 mg q4-6h.

Children 2-5 yrs. 0.5 mg q4-6h. Do not use timed release.

AVAILABLE FORMS

• *Tablets:* 2 mg (Polaramine [DSC]).
• *Extended-Release Tablets:* 4 mg, 6 mg (Polaramine Repetabs).
• *Syrup:* 2 mg/5 ml (Polaramine).

UNLABELED USES: Asthma, chemotherapy-induced stomatitis, dermographia, familial immunodeficiency disease, malaria, mastocytosi, Meniere's disease, nausea, neurocysticercosis, otitis media, psoriasis, radiocontrast media reactions, urticaria

CONTRAINDICATIONS: History of hypersensitivity to antihistamines, newborn or premature infants, nursing mothers, third trimester of pregnancy

PREGNANCY AND LACTATION: Pregnancy category B

SIDE EFFECTS

Frequent

Drowsiness, dizziness, headache, dry mouth, nose, or throat, urinary retention, thickening of bronchial secretions, sedation, hypotension

Occasional

Epigastric distress, flushing, blurred vision, tinnitus, paresthesia, sweating, chills

SERIOUS REACTIONS

• Children may experience dominant paradoxical reactions, including restlessness, insomnia, euphoria, nervousness, and tremors.

• Hypersensitivity reaction, such as eczema, pruritus, rash, cardiac disturbances, and photosensitivity, may occur.

• Overdosage may vary from CNS depression, including sedation, apnea, hypotension, cardiovascular collapse, or death to severe paradoxical reaction, such as hallucinations, tremor, and seizures.

INTERACTIONS

Drugs

3 *Alcohol, CNS depressants:* May increase CNS depression

3 *Methacholine:* May interfere with interpretation of pulmonary function tests after a methacholine bronchial challenge

3 *Procarbazine:* May increase CNS depression

Labs

• *False negative:* Skin allergy tests

SPECIAL CONSIDERATIONS

• Active dextro-isomer of chlorpheniramine

PATIENT/FAMILY EDUCATION

• The patient may develop tolerance to the drug's sedative effect

• Avoid performing tasks that require mental alertness or motor skills until response to the drug is established

• Notify the physician if he or she experiences visual disturbances

• Dizziness, drowsiness, and dry mouth are expected side effects of dexchlorpheniramine

• Avoid alcohol

D

dexmethylphenidate hydrochloride

(dex-meth-ill-fen'-i-date hye-droe-klor'-ide)

Rx: Focalin, Focalin XR

Chemical Class: Piperidine derivative of amphetamine

Therapeutic Class: Central nervous system stimulant

CLINICAL PHARMACOLOGY

Mechanism of Action: A CNS stimulant that blocks the reuptake of norepinephrine and dopamine into presynaptic neurons, increasing the release of these neurotransmitters into the synaptic cleft. ***Therapeutic Effect:*** Decreases motor restlessness and fatigue; increases motor activity, mental alertness, and attention span; elevates mood.

Pharmacokinetics

Route	*Onset*	*Peak*	*Duration*
PO	N/A	N/A	4-5 hr

Readily absorbed from the GI tract. Plasma concentrations increase rapidly. Metabolized in the liver. Excreted unchanged in urine. ***Half-life:*** 2.2 hr.

INDICATIONS AND DOSAGES

Attention deficit hyperactivity disorder (ADHD)

PO (Patients new to dexmethylphenidate or methylphenidate)

Adults, Elderly. 2.5 mg twice a day (5 mg/day). May adjust dosage in 2.5- to 5-mg increments. Maximum: 20 mg/day.

PO (Patients currently taking methylphenidate)

Adults, Elderly. Half the methylphenidate dosage. Maximum: 20 mg/day.

PO (Exended-Release [Patients new to dexmethylphenidate or methylphenidate])

Adults, Elderly. Initially, 10 mg/day.

Children. Initially, 5 mg/day. May increase dosage at weekly intervals. Maximum: 20 mg/day.
PO (Extended-Release [Patients currently taking methylphenidate])
Adults, Elderly. Half the methylphenidate dosage. Maximum: 20 mg/day. Patients using Focalin may be switched to the same daily dose for Focalin XR.

AVAILABLE FORMS

- *Tablets (Focalin):* 2.5 mg, 5 mg, 10 mg.
- *Capsules (Extended-Release [Focalin XR]):* 5 mg, 10 mg, 20 mg.

CONTRAINDICATIONS: Diagnosis or family history of Tourette syndrome; glaucoma; history of marked agitation, anxiety, or tension; motor tics; use within 14 days of MAOIs

PREGNANCY AND LACTATION: Pregnancy category C; excretion into breast milk unknown; use caution in nursing mothers
Controlled Substance: Schedule II

SIDE EFFECTS

Frequent
Abdominal pain, nausea, anorexia, fever
Occasional
Tachycardia, arrhythmias, palpitations, insomnia, twitching
Rare
Blurred vision, rash, arthralgia

SERIOUS REACTIONS

- Withdrawal after prolonged therapy may unmask symptoms of the underlying disorder.
- Dexmethylphenidate may lower the seizure threshold in those with a history of seizures.
- Overdose produces excessive sympathomimetic effects, including vomiting, tremor, hyperreflexia, seizures, confusion, hallucinations, and diaphoresis.
- Prolonged administration to children may delay growth.
- Neuroleptic malignant syndrome occurs rarely.

INTERACTIONS

Drugs
3 *Clonidine:* Serious adverse effects have been reported but no causality has been established
2 *MAOIs:* Hypertensive crisis
3 *Phenytoin, phenobarbital, primidone:* Increased levels and risk of toxicity
3 *SSRIs:* Increased serum concentrations
3 *Tricyclic antidepressants:* Increased serum concentrations
3 *Warfarin:* Increased PT and bleeding risk; inhibits warfarin metabolism
Labs
- *False positive:* Urine amphetamine

SPECIAL CONSIDERATIONS

- No clinical data to support use of this agent over racemic methylphenidate

PATIENT/FAMILY EDUCATION

- Take last dose late afternoon or early evening to prevent insomnia
- Reinforce habit-forming potential of medication; caution against taking more than required dose
- Avoid tasks that require mental alertness or motor skills until response to the drug has been established
- Potential for growth retardation

MONITORING PARAMETERS

- Improvement of clinical symptoms, lack of adverse effects; periodic complete blood count with differential, routine blood chemistry; growth determinations (body weight and height), blood pressure, pulse rate

dextroamphetamine sulfate

(dex-troe-am-fet'-a-meen sul'-fate)

Rx: Dexamphetamine [AUS], Dexedrine, Dexedrine Spansule, Dextrostat

Chemical Class: D-β-phenyl-isopropylamine

Therapeutic Class: Central nervous system stimulant

DEA Class: Schedule II

CLINICAL PHARMACOLOGY

Mechanism of Action: An amphetamine that enhances the action of dopamine and norepinephrine by blocking their reuptake from synapses; also inhibits monoamine oxidase and facilitates the release of catecholamines. ***Therapeutic Effect:*** Increases motor activity and mental alertness; decreases motor restlessness, drowsiness, and fatigue; suppresses appetite.

Pharmacokinetics

Well absorbed following PO administration. Metabolized in liver. Excreted in urine. Removed by hemodialysis. ***Half-life:*** 7-34 hr.

INDICATIONS AND DOSAGES

Narcolepsy

PO

Adults, Children older than 12 yr. Initially, 10 mg/day. Increase by 10 mg/day at weekly intervals until therapeutic response is achieved.

Children 6-12 yr. Initially, 5 mg/day. Increase by 5 mg/day at weekly intervals until therapeutic response is achieved. Maximum: 60 mg/day.

Attention deficit hyperactivity disorder (ADHD)

PO

Children 6 yr and older. Initially, 5 mg once or twice a day. Increase by 5 mg/day at weekly intervals until therapeutic response is achieved.

Children 3-5 yr. Initially, 2.5 mg/day. Increase by 2.5 mg/day at weekly intervals until therapeutic response is achieved. Range: 0.1-0.5 mg/kg/dose. Maximum: 40 mg/day.

Appetite suppressant

PO

Adults. 5-30 mg daily in divided doses of 5-10 mg each, given 30-60 min before meals; or 1 extended-release capsule in the morning.

AVAILABLE FORMS

- *Capsules (Sustained-Release [Dexedrine Spansule]):* 5 mg, 10 mg, 15 mg.
- *Tablets:* 5 mg (Dexedrine), 10 mg (Dexedrine, Dextrostat).

CONTRAINDICATIONS: Advanced arteriosclerosis, agitated states, glaucoma, history of drug abuse, hypersensitivity to sympathomimetic amines, hyperthyroidism, moderate to severe hypertension, symptomatic cardiovascular disease, use within 14 days of MAOIs

PREGNANCY AND LACTATION: Pregnancy category C; excreted in breast milk

Controlled Substance: Schedule II

SIDE EFFECTS

Frequent

Irregular pulse, increased motor activity, talkativeness, nervousness, mild euphoria, insomnia

Occasional

Headache, chills, dry mouth, GI distress, worsening depression in patients who are clinically depressed, tachycardia, palpitations, chest pain, dizziness, decreased appetite

SERIOUS REACTIONS

- Overdose may produce skin pallor or flushing, arrhythmias, and psychosis.

• Abrupt withdrawal after prolonged use of high doses may produce lethargy lasting for weeks.
• Prolonged administration to children with ADHD may inhibit growth.

INTERACTIONS

Drugs

3 *Antacids:* Decreased urinary excretion of dextroamphetamine
3 *Digoxin:* May increase the risk of arrhythmias
3 *Fluoxetine:* Hallucinations have been reported
3 *Furazolidone:* Hypertensive reactions
3 *Guanadrel, Guanethidine:* Antihypertensive effect inhibited by dextroamphetamine
▲ *MAOIs:* Severe hypertensive reactions possible
3 *Meperidine:* May increase the risk of hypotension, respiratory depression, seizures, and cardiovascular collapse
3 *CNS stimulants:* May increase the effects of dextroamphetamine
❷ *Selegiline:* Severe hypertensive reactions possible
3 *Sodium bicarbonate:* May inhibit dextroamphetamine excretion
3 *Thyroid hormones:* May increase the effects of either drug
3 *Tricyclic antidepressants:* May increase the effect of dextroamphetamine

Labs

• *False positive:* Urine amino acids

SPECIAL CONSIDERATIONS

• Use for obesity should be reserved for patients failing to respond to alternative therapy; weigh the limited benefit against the substantial risk of addiction and dependence

PATIENT/FAMILY EDUCATION

• Tolerance or dependency is common
• Avoid OTC preparations unless approved by clinician
• Do not crush or chew Sus Action dosage forms
• Take dextroamphetamine early in the day
• Avoid performing tasks that require mental alertness or motor skills until response to the drug has been established
• Notify the physician if decreased appetite, dizziness, dry mouth, or pronounced nervousness occurs

MONITORING PARAMETERS

• Blood pressure
• Weight
• CNS for overstimulation

dextromethorphan hydrobromide

(dex-troe-meth-or′-fan hye-droe-broe′-mide)

Rx: Babee Cof Syrup, Benylin Adult, Benylin Pediatric, Creomulsion Cough, Creomulsion for Children, Creo-Terpin, Delsym, Dexalone, ElixSure Cough, Hold DM, Scot-Tussin DM Cough Chasers, Silphen DM, Simply Cough

OTC: PediaCare Infants' Long-Acting Cough, Robitussin CoughGels, Robitussin Honey Cough, Robitussin Maximum Strength Cough, Robitussin Pediatric Cough, Vicks 44 Cough Relief

Combinations

OTC: with benzocaine (Spec T, Vicks Formula 44 cough control discs, Vicks cough silencers); with guaifenesin (Robitussin DM)

Chemical Class: Levorphanol derivative

Therapeutic Class: Antitussive

CLINICAL PHARMACOLOGY

Mechanism of Action: A chemical relative of morphine without the narcotic properties that acts on the cough center in the medulla oblongata by elevating the threshold for coughing. ***Therapeutic Effect:*** Suppresses cough.

Pharmacokinetics

Rapidly absorbed from the gastrointestinal (GI) tract. Distributed into cerebrospinal fluid (CSF). Extensively and poorly metabolized in liver to dextrorphan (active metabolite). Excreted unchanged in urine. ***Half-life:*** 1.4-3.9 hrs (parent compound), 3.4-5.6 hrs. (dextrorphan).

INDICATIONS AND DOSAGES

Cough

PO

Adults, Elderly, Children 12 yrs and older. 10-20 mg q4h. Maximum: 120 mg/day.

Children 6-12 yrs. 5-10 mg q4h. Maximum: 60 mg/day.

Children 2-5 yrs. 2.5-5 mg q4h. Maximum: 30 mg/day.

AVAILABLE FORMS

- *Gelcap:* 15 mg (Robitussin CoughGels), 30 mg (Dexalone).
- *Liquid:* 5 mg/5ml (Simply Cough), 10 mg/5 ml (Vicks Cough Relief), 10 mg/15 ml (Creo-Terpin).
- *Liquid drops:* 7.5 mg/0.8 ml (PediaCare Infants' Long-Acting Cough).
- *Lozenges:* 5 mg (Hold DM, Scot-Tussin DM Cough Chasers).
- *Suspension (Extended-Release):* 30 mg/5 ml (Delsym).
- *Syrup:* 7.5 mg/5 ml (Babee Cof Syrup, Benylin Pediatric, ElixSure, Robitussin Pediatric Cough), 10 mg/5 ml (Robitussin Honey Cough, Silphen DM), 15 mg/5 ml (Benylin Adult, Robitussin Maximum Strength Cough), 20 mg/15 ml (Creomulsion Cough, Creomulsion for Children).

UNLABELED USES: N-methyl-D-aspartate (NMDA) antagonist in cerebral injury

CONTRAINDICATIONS: Coadministration with monoamine oxidase inhibitors (MAOIs), hypersensitivity to dextromethorphan or its components

PREGNANCY AND LACTATION: Pregnancy category C

SIDE EFFECTS

Rare

Abdominal discomfort, constipation, dizziness, drowsiness, GI upset, nausea

SERIOUS REACTIONS

• Overdosage may result in muscle spasticity, increase or decrease in blood pressure (BP), blurred vision, blue fingernails and lips, nausea, vomiting, hallucinations, and respiratory depression.

INTERACTIONS

Drugs

▲ *Isocarboxazid, MAOIs, phenelzine:* Increased risk of toxicity due to dextromethorphan

3 *Quinidine, terbinafine:* Reduced hepatic metabolism of dextromethorphan

3 *Fluoxetine:* Case report of a patient on fluoxetine developing visual hallucinations when she began to take dextromethorphan; causality not established

❷ *Sibutramine:* Increased risk of serotonin syndrome

SPECIAL CONSIDERATIONS

PATIENT/FAMILY EDUCATION

• Avoid performing tasks that require mental alertness or motor skills until response to the drug is established

• Do not take dextromethorphan for chronic cough

• Maintain adequate hydration by drinking plenty of fluids

• Notify the physician if cough persists or if fever, rash, headache, or sore throat is present with cough

MONITORING PARAMETERS

• Clinical improvement and onset of relief of cough

diazepam

(dye-az'-e-pam)

Rx: Diastat, Diastat Pediatric, Dizac, Valium

Chemical Class: Benzodiazepine

Therapeutic Class: Anesthesia adjunct; anticonvulsant; anxiolytic; sedative/hypnotic; skeletal muscle relaxant

DEA Class: Schedule IV

CLINICAL PHARMACOLOGY

Mechanism of Action: A benzodiazepine that depresses all levels of the CNS by enhancing the action of gamma-aminobutyric acid, a major inhibitory neurotransmitter in the brain. ***Therapeutic Effect:*** Produces anxiolytic effect, elevates the seizure threshold, produces skeletal muscle relaxation.

Pharmacokinetics

Route	*Onset*	*Peak*	*Duration*
PO	30 min	1-2 hr	2-3 hr
IV	1-5 min	15 min	15-60 min
IM	15 min	30-90 min	30-90 min

Well absorbed from the GI tract. Widely distributed. Protein binding: 98%. Metabolized in the liver to active metabolite. Excreted in urine. Minimally removed by hemodialysis. ***Half-life:*** 20-70 hr (increased in hepatic dysfunction and the elderly).

INDICATIONS AND DOSAGES

Anxiety, skeletal muscle relaxation

PO

Adults. 2-10 mg 2-4 times a day.

Elderly. 2-5 mg 2-4 times a day.

Children. 0.12-0.8 mg/kg/day in divided doses q6-8h.

IV, IM

Adults. 2-10 mg repeated in 3-4 hr.

Children. 0.04-0.3 mg/kg/dose q2-4h. Maximum: 0.6 mg/kg in an 8-hr period.

Preanesthesia

IV

Adults, Elderly. 5-15 mg 5-10 min before procedure.

Children. 0.2-0.3 mg/kg. Maximum: 10 mg.

Alcohol withdrawal

PO

Adults, Elderly. 10 mg 3-4 times during first 24 hr, then reduced to 5-10 mg 3-4 times a day as needed.

IV, IM

Adults, Elderly. Initially, 10 mg, followed by 5-10 mg q3-4h.

Status epilepticus

IV

Adults, Elderly. 5-10 mg q10-15min up to 30 mg/8 hr.

Children 5 yr and older. 0.05-0.3 mg/kg/dose q15-30min. Maximum: 10 mg/dose.

Children 1 mo to younger than 5 yr. 0.05-0.3 mg/kg/dose q15-30min. Maximum: 5 mg/dose.

Control of increased seizure activity in patients with refractory epilepsy who are on stable regimens of anticonvulsants

Rectal Gel

Adults, Children 12 yr and older. 0.2 mg/kg; may be repeated in 4-12 hr.

Children 6-11 yr. 0.3 mg/kg; may be repeated in 4-12 hr.

Children 2-5 yr. 0.5 mg/kg; may be repeated in 4-12 hr.

AVAILABLE FORMS

- *Oral Concentrate (Diazepam Intensol):* 5 mg/ml.
- *Oral Solution:* 5 mg/5 ml.
- *Tablets (Valium):* 2 mg, 5 mg, 10 mg.
- *Injection:* 5 mg/ml.
- *Rectal Gel (Diastat):* 5 mg/ml.

UNLABELED USES: Treatment of panic disorder, tension headache, tremors

CONTRAINDICATIONS: Angle-closure glaucoma, coma, preexisting CNS depression, respiratory depression, severe, uncontrolled pain

PREGNANCY AND LACTATION: Pregnancy category D; drug and metabolite enter breast milk; lethargy and loss of weight in nursing infant have been reported

Controlled Substance: Schedule IV

SIDE EFFECTS

Frequent

Pain with IM injection, somnolence, fatigue, ataxia

Occasional

Slurred speech, orthostatic hypotension, headache, hypoactivity, constipation, nausea, blurred vision

Rare

Paradoxical CNS reactions, such as hyperactivity or nervousness in children and excitement or restlessness in the elderly or debilitated (generally noted during first 2 weeks of therapy, particularly in presence of uncontrolled pain)

SERIOUS REACTIONS

- IV administration may produce pain, swelling, thrombophlebitis, and carpal tunnel syndrome.
- Abrupt or too-rapid withdrawal may result in pronounced restlessness, irritability, insomnia, hand tremor, abdominal or muscle cramps, diaphoresis, vomiting, and seizures.
- Abrupt withdrawal in patients with epilepsy may produce an increase in the frequency or severity of seizures.
- Overdose results in somnolence, confusion, diminished reflexes, and coma.

INTERACTIONS

Drugs

3 *Carbamazepine:* Markedly reduces effect of oral diazepam; parenteral diazepam less affected

3 *Cimetidine:* Inhibits hepatic metabolism of diazepam
3 *Ciprofloxacin:* Inhibits hepatic metabolism of diazepam; may also competitively inhibit gamma-aminobutyric acid receptors
❷ *Clarithromycin:* Inhibits hepatic metabolism of diazepam
3 *Clozapine:* Additive respiratory and cardiovascular depression
3 *Delavirdine:* Inhibits hepatic metabolism of diazepam
3 *Disulfiram:* Inhibits hepatic metabolism of diazepam
3 *Erythromycin:* Inhibits hepatic metabolism of diazepam
3 *Ethanol:* Additive CNS effects
3 *Fluconazole:* Inhibits hepatic metabolism of diazepam
3 *Fluoxetine:* Inhibits hepatic metabolism of diazepam
3 *Fluvoxamine:* Inhibits hepatic metabolism of diazepam
3 *Isoniazid:* Inhibits hepatic metabolism of diazepam
3 *Itraconazole:* Inhibits hepatic metabolism of diazepam
3 *Kava kava, valerian:* May increase CNS depression
3 *Ketoconazole:* Inhibits hepatic metabolism of diazepam
3 *Levodopa:* May reduce antiparkinsonian effect
3 *Metoprolol:* Inhibits hepatic metabolism of diazepam
3 *Omeprazole:* Inhibits hepatic metabolism of diazepam
3 *Phenytoin:* Markedly reduces effect of oral diazepam; parenteral diazepam less affected
3 *Quinolones:* Inhibits hepatic metabolism of diazepam; may also competitively inhibit gamma-aminobutyric acid receptors
3 *Rifampin:* Markedly reduces effect of diazepam
3 *Troleandomycin:* Inhibits hepatic metabolism of diazepam

Labs

- *Increase:* Urine 5-HIAA

SPECIAL CONSIDERATIONS

- Flumazenil (Mazicon), a benzodiazepine receptor antagonist is indicated for complete or partial reversal of the sedative effects of benzodiazepines

PATIENT/FAMILY EDUCATION

- Avoid driving, activities that require alertness; drowsiness may occur
- Avoid alcohol, other psychotropic medications unless prescribed by clinician
- Urge the female patient on long-term therapy to use effective contraception during therapy and to notify the physician immediately if she becomes or may be pregnant
- Do not take the rectal form of the drug more than once every 5 days or more than 5 times a month

MONITORING PARAMETERS

- Blood pressure, heart rate, respiratory rate. Therapeutic response in patients with seizure disorder, a decrease in the frequency or intensity of seizures; in patients with anxiety, a calm facial expression and decreased restlessness; in patients with musculoskeletal spasm, decreased intensity of skeletal muscle pain
- The therapeutic serum level for diazepam is 0.5-2 mcg/ml, and the toxic serum level is greater than 3 mcg/ml

diclofenac

(dye-kloe'-fen-ak)

Rx: Cataflam, Solaraze, Voltaren, Voltaren Ophthalmic, Voltaren XR

Combinations

Rx: with misoprostol (Arthotec)

Chemical Class: Phenylacetic acid derivative

Therapeutic Class: NSAID; antipyretic; nonnarcotic analgesic

CLINICAL PHARMACOLOGY

Mechanism of Action: An NSAID that inhibits prostaglandin synthesis, reducing the intensity of pain. Also constricts the iris sphincter. May inhibit angiogenesis (the formation of blood vessels) by inhibiting substance P or blocking the angiogenic effects of prostaglandin E.

Therapeutic Effect: Produces analgesic and antiinflammatory effects. Prevents miosis during cataract surgery. May reduce angiogenesis in inflamed tissue.

Pharmacokinetics

Route	*Onset*	*Peak*	*Duration*
PO	30 min	2-3 hr	Up to 8 hr

Completely absorbed from the GI tract; penetrates cornea after ophthalmic administration (may be systemically absorbed). Protein binding: Greater than 99%. Widely distributed. Metabolized in the liver. Primarily excreted in urine. Minimally removed by hemodialysis.

Half-life: 1.2-2 hr.

INDICATIONS AND DOSAGES

Osteoarthritis

PO (Cataflam, Voltaren)

Adults, Elderly. 50 mg 2-3 times a day.

PO (Voltaren XR)

Adults, Elderly. 100-200 mg/day as a single dose.

Rheumatoid arthritis

PO (Cataflam, Voltaren)

Adults, Elderly. 50 mg 2-4 times a day. Maximum: 225 mg/day.

PO (Voltaren XR)

Adults, Elderly. 100 mg once a day. Maximum: 100 mg twice a day.

Ankylosing spondylitis

PO (Voltaren)

Adults, Elderly. 100-125 mg/day in 4-5 divided doses.

Analgesia, primary dysmenorrhea

PO (Cataflam)

Adults, Elderly. 50 mg 3 times a day.

Usual pediatric dosage

Children. 2-3 mg/kg/day in 2-4 divided doses.

Actinic keratoses

Topical

Adults, Adolescents. Apply twice a day to lesion for 60-90 days.

Cataract surgery

Ophthalmic

Adults, Elderly. Apply 1 drop to eye 4 times a day commencing 24 hr after cataract surgery. Continue for 2 wk afterward.

Pain, relief of photophobia in patients undergoing corneal refractive surgery

Ophthalmic

Adults, Elderly. Apply 1-2 drops to affected eye 1 hr before surgery, within 15 min after surgery, then 4 times a day for up to 3 days.

AVAILABLE FORMS

- *Topical Gel (Solaraze):* 3%.
- *Tablets (Immediate-Release [Cataflam]):* 50 mg.
- *Tablets (Delayed-Release [Voltaren]):* 25 mg, 50 mg, 75 mg.
- *Tablets (Extended-Release [Voltaren XR]):* 100 mg.
- *Ophthalmic Solution (Voltaren Ophthalmic):* 0.1%.

UNLABELED USES: Treatment of vascular headaches (oral); to reduce the occurrence and severity of cystoid macular edema after cataract surgery (ophthalmic form)

CONTRAINDICATIONS: Hypersensitivity to aspirin, diclofenac, and other NSAIDs; porphyria

PREGNANCY AND LACTATION: Pregnancy category B (D if used in third trimester or near delivery; C for ophthalmic solution); excreted in breast milk

SIDE EFFECTS

Frequent (9%-4%)

PO: Headache, abdominal cramps, constipation, diarrhea, nausea, dyspepsia

Ophthalmic: Burning or stinging on instillation, ocular discomfort

Occasional (3%-1%)

PO: Flatulence, dizziness, epigastric pain

Ophthalmic: Ocular itching or tearing

Rare (less than 1%)

PO: Rash, peripheral edema or fluid retention, visual disturbances, vomiting, drowsiness

SERIOUS REACTIONS

• Overdose may result in acute renal failure.

• Rare reactions with long-term use include peptic ulcer disease, GI bleeding, gastritis, a severe hepatic reaction (jaundice), nephrotoxicity (hematuria, dysuria, proteinuria), and a severe hypersensitivity reaction (bronchospasm or angioedema).

INTERACTIONS

Drugs

3 *Acetylcholine, carbachol:* May decrease the effects of these drugs (with ophthalmic diclofenac)

3 *Aminoglycosides:* Reduced clearance with elevated aminoglycoside levels and potential for toxicity (especially indomethacin in premature infants; other NSAIDs probably)

3 *Anticoagulants:* Excessive hypoprothrombinemia, decreased platelet aggregation with increased risk of GI bleeding

3 *Antihypertensives (α-blockers, angiotension-converting enzyme inhibitors, angiotensin II receptor blockers, β-blockers, diuretics):* Inhibition of antihypertensive and other favorable hemodynamic effects

3 *Aspirin, other salicylates:* May increase the risk of GI side effects such as bleeding

3 *Corticosteroids:* Increased risk of GI ulceration

3 *Cyclosporine:* Increased nephrotoxicity risk

3 *Digoxin:* Increased serum digoxin concentrations

3 *Epinephrine, other antiglaucoma medications:* May decrease the antiglaucoma effect of these drugs

3 *Lithium:* Decreased clearance of lithium (mediated via prostaglandins) resulting in elevated serum lithium levels and risk of toxicity

2 *Methotrexate:* Decreased renal secretion of methotrexate resulting in elevated methotrexate levels and risk of toxicity

3 *Phenylpropanolamine:* Possible acute hypertensive reaction

3 *Potassium-sparing diuretics:* Additive hyperkalemia potential

3 *Probenecid:* May increase diclofenac blood concentration

2 *Triamterene:* Acute renal failure reported with addition of indomethacin; caution with other NSAIDs

Labs

• *Increase:* Serum AST, plasma cortisol, plasma glucose (oxidase-peroxidase method)

SPECIAL CONSIDERATIONS

- No significant advantage over other NSAIDs; cost should govern use

PATIENT/FAMILY EDUCATION

- Swallow diclofenac tablets whole and do not crush or chew them
- Take diclofenac with food or milk if GI upset occurs
- Avoid alcohol and aspirin during diclofenac therapy because these substances increase the risk of GI bleeding
- Notify the physician if a persistent headache, black stools, changes in vision, pruritus, rash, or weight gain occurs
- Do not use hydrogel soft contact lenses during ophthalmic diclofenac therapy
- Notify the physician if rash occurs while using topical diclofenac

MONITORING PARAMETERS

- Initial hemogram and fecal occult blood test within 3 mo of starting regular chronic therapy; repeat every 6-12 mo (more frequently in high-risk patients (>65 years, peptic ulcer disease, concurrent steroids or anticoagulants); electrolytes, creatinine, and BUN within 3 mo of starting regular chronic therapy; repeat every 6-12 mo
- Complete healing of actinic keratoses may not be evident for up to 30 days post cessation of therapy
- Daily bowel activity and stool consistency
- Therapeutic response, such as improved grip strength, increased joint mobility, and decreased joint pain, tenderness, stiffness, and swelling

dicloxacillin sodium

(dye-klox'-a-sill-in soe'-dee-um)

Rx: Dycil, Pathocil

Chemical Class: Penicillin derivative, penicillinase-resistant

Therapeutic Class: Antibiotic

D

CLINICAL PHARMACOLOGY

Mechanism of Action: A penicillin that acts as a bactericidal in susceptible microorganisms. ***Therapeutic Effect:*** Inhibits bacterial cell wall synthesis.

Pharmacokinetics

Well absorbed from gastrointestinal (GI) tract. Rate and extent reduced by food. Distributed throughout body including CSF. Protein binding: 96%. Partially metabolized in liver. Primarily excreted in feces and urine. Not removed by hemodialysis. ***Half-life:*** 0.7 hr.

INDICATIONS AND DOSAGES

Respiratory tract infection, staphylococcal and streptococcal infections

PO

Adults, Elderly, Children weighing more than 40 kg. 125-250 mg q6h.

Children weighing less than 40 kg. 12.5-25 mg/kg/day q6h.

AVAILABLE FORMS

- *Capsules:* 250 mg, 500 mg (Dycil, Pathocil).

CONTRAINDICATIONS: Hypersensitivity to any penicillin

PREGNANCY AND LACTATION: Pregnancy category B

SIDE EFFECTS

Frequent

Gastrointestinal (GI) disturbances (mild diarrhea, nausea, or vomiting), headache

Occasional
Generalized rash, urticaria

SERIOUS REACTIONS

- Altered bacterial balance may result in potentially fatal superinfections and antibiotic-associated colitis as evidenced by abdominal cramps, watery or severe diarrhea, and fever.
- Severe hypersensitivity reactions, including anaphylaxis and acute interstitial nephritis occur rarely.

INTERACTIONS

Drugs

3 *Allopurinol:* May increase the incidence of rash

3 *Aminoglycosides:* May decrease aminoglycoside efficacy

3 *Macrolide antibiotics, chloramphenicol, tetracyclines:* Possible inhibition of antibacterial activity of penicillins

3 *Methotrexate:* Potentiation of methotrexate toxicity

3 *Oral contraceptives:* Possible impaired contraceptive efficacy

3 *Probenecid:* May increase dicloxacillin blood concentration and risk for dicloxacillin toxicity

3 *Warfarin:* Reduced hypoprothrombinemic response

Labs

- *False increase:* Nafcillin level

SPECIAL CONSIDERATIONS

PATIENT/FAMILY EDUCATION

- Should be taken with water 1 hr before or 2 hr after meals on an empty stomach
- Continue dicloxacillin for the full length of treatment
- Notify the physician if diarrhea, rash, or other new symptoms occur

MONITORING PARAMETERS

- CBC
- Renal function
- Urinalysis

dicyclomine hydrochloride

(dye-sye'-kloe-meen hye-droe-klor'-ide)

Rx: Bentyl, Dicyclocot

Chemical Class: Tertiary amine

Therapeutic Class: Anticholinergic; antispasmodic; gastrointestinal

CLINICAL PHARMACOLOGY

Mechanism of Action: A GI antispasmodic and anticholinergic agent that directly acts as a relaxant on smooth muscle. ***Therapeutic Effect:*** Reduces tone and motility of GI tract.

Pharmacokinetics

Route	*Onset*	*Peak*	*Duration*
PO	1-2 hr	N/A	4 hr

Readily absorbed from the GI tract. Widely distributed. Metabolized in the liver. ***Half-life:*** 9-10 hr.

INDICATIONS AND DOSAGES

Functional disturbances of GI motility

PO

Adults. 10-20 mg 3-4 times a day up to 40 mg 4 times/day.

Children older than 2 yr. 10 mg 3-4 times a day.

Children 6 mos-2 yr. 5 mg 3-4 times a day.

Elderly. 10-20 mg 4 times a day. May increase up to 160 mg/day.

IM

Adults. 20 mg q4-6h.

AVAILABLE FORMS

- *Capsules (Bentyl):* 10 mg.
- *Tablets (Bentyl):* 20 mg.
- *Syrup (Bentyl):* 10 mg/5 ml.
- *Injection (Bentyl, Dicyclocot):* 10 mg/ml.

CONTRAINDICATIONS: Bladder neck obstruction due to prostatic hyperplasia, coronary vasospasm, intestinal atony, myasthenia gravis in patients not treated with neostigmine, narrow-angle glaucoma, obstructive disease of the GI tract, paralytic ileus, severe ulcerative colitis, tachycardia secondary to cardiac insufficiency or thyrotoxicosis, toxic megacolon, unstable cardiovascular status in acute hemorrhage

PREGNANCY AND LACTATION: Pregnancy category B; single case report of apnea in nursing infant; avoid in nursing women

SIDE EFFECTS

Frequent

Dry mouth (sometimes severe), constipation, diminished sweating ability

Occasional

Blurred vision; photophobia; urinary hesitancy; somnolence (with high dosage); agitation, excitement, confusion, or somnolence noted in elderly (even with low dosages); transient lightheadedness (with IM route), irritation at injection site (with IM route)

Rare

Confusion, hypersensitivity reaction, increased IOP, nausea, vomiting, unusual fatigue

SERIOUS REACTIONS

- Overdose may produce temporary paralysis of ciliary muscle; pupillary dilation; tachycardia; palpitations; hot, dry, or flushed skin; absence of bowel sounds; hyperthermia; increased respiratory rate; EKG abnormalities; nausea; vomiting; rash over face or upper trunk; CNS stimulation; and psychosis (marked by agitation, restlessness, rambling speech, visual hallucinations, paranoid behavior, and delusions, followed by depression).

D

INTERACTIONS

Drugs

3 *Amantadine, tricyclic antidepressants, MAOIs, H_1-antihistamines:* Increased anticholinergic effects

3 *Antacids, antidiarrheals:* May decrease the absorption of dicyclomine

3 *Other anticholinergics:* May increase the effects of dicyclomine

3 *Potassium chloride:* May increase the severity of GI lesions with the wax matrix formulation of potassium chloride

3 *Phenothiazines, levodopa, ketoconazole:* Decreased therapeutic effects of these drugs

SPECIAL CONSIDERATIONS

• Not for intravenous use

PATIENT/FAMILY EDUCATION

• Avoid becoming overheated while exercising in hot weather because this may cause heat stroke
• Avoid hot baths and saunas
• Avoid tasks that require mental alertness or motor skills until response to the drug has been established
• Do not take antacids or antidiarrheals within 1 hr of taking dicyclomine because these drugs decrease dicyclomine's effectiveness

MONITORING PARAMETERS

• Evaluate the patient for urine retention
• Blood pressure, body temperature
• Bowel sounds for peristalsis, and mucous membranes and skin turgor for hydration status
• Daily bowel activity and stool consistency

didanosine

(dye-dan'-o-seen)

Rx: Videx, Videx-EC

Chemical Class: Nucleoside analog

Therapeutic Class: Antiretroviral

CLINICAL PHARMACOLOGY

Mechanism of Action: A purine nucleoside analog that is intracellularly converted into a triphosphate, which interferes with RNA-directed DNA polymerase (reverse transcriptase). ***Therapeutic Effect:*** Inhibits replication of retroviruses, including HIV.

Pharmacokinetics

Variably absorbed from the GI tract. Protein binding: Less than 5%. Rapidly metabolized intracellularly to active form. Primarily excreted in urine. Partially (20%) removed by hemodialysis. ***Half-life:*** 1.5 hr; metabolite: 8-24 hr.

INDICATIONS AND DOSAGES

HIV infection (in combination with other antiretrovirals)

PO (Chewable Tablets)

Adults, Children 13 yr and older weighing 60 kg and more. 200 mg q12h or 400 mg once a day.

Adults, Children 13 yr and older weighing less than 60 kg. 125 mg q12h or 250 mg once a day.

Children 3 mo-12 yr. 180-300 mg/m^2/day in divided doses q12h.

Children younger than 3 mo. 50 mg/m^2/day in divided doses q12h.

PO (Delayed-Release Capsules)

Adults, Children 13 yr and older weighing 60 kg and more. 400 mg once a day.

Adults, Children 13 yr and older weighing less than 60 kg. 250 mg once a day.

PO (Oral Solution)
Adults, Children 13 yr and older weighing 60 kg and more. 250 mg q12h.
Adults, Children 13 yr and older weighing less than 60 kg. 167 mg q12h.
PO (Pediatric Powder for Oral Solution)
Children 3 mo-12 yr. 180-300 $mg/m^2/day$ in divided doses q12h.
Children younger than 3 mo. $50mg/m^2/day$ in divided doses q12h.

Dosage in renal impairment
Patients weighing less than 60 kg:

CrCl	*Tablets*	*Oral Solution*	*Delayed-Release Capsules*
30-59 ml/min	75 mg twice a day	100 mg twice a day	125 mg once a day
10-29 ml/min	100 mg once a day	100 mg once a day	125 mg once a day
less than 10 ml/min	75 mg once a day	100 mg once a day	N/A

CrCl = creatinine clearance

Patients weighing 60 kg or more:

CrCl	*Tablets*	*Oral Solution*	*Delayed-Release Capsules*
30-59 ml/ min	100 mg twice a day	100 mg twice a day	200 mg once a day
10-29 ml/ min	150 mg once a day	167 mg once a day	125 mg once a day
less than 10 ml/ min	100 mg once a day	100 mg once a day	125 mg once a day

CrCl = creatinine clearance

AVAILABLE FORMS
• *Capsules (Delayed-Release):* 125 mg (Videx), 200 mg (Videx-EC), 250 mg (Videx-EC), 400 mg (Videx-EC).
• *Pediatric Powder for Oral Solution (Videx):* 10 mg/ml.
• *Powder for Oral Solution (Videx):* 100 mg, 167 mg, 250 mg.
• *Tablets (Chewable [Videx]):* 25 mg, 50 mg, 100 mg, 150 mg, 200 mg.

CONTRAINDICATIONS: Hypersensitivity to didanosine or any of its components

PREGNANCY AND LACTATION: Pregnancy category B; unknown if excreted in breast milk; discontinuation of breast-feeding recommended

SIDE EFFECTS
Frequent
Adults (greater than 10%): Diarrhea, neuropathy, chills and fever
Children (greater than 25%): Chills, fever, decreased appetite, pain, malaise, nausea, vomiting, diarrhea, abdominal pain, headache, nervousness, cough, rhinitis, dyspnea, asthenia, rash, pruritus
Occasional
Adults (9%-2%): Rash, pruritus, headache, abdominal pain, nausea, vomiting, pneumonia, myopathy, decreased appetite, dry mouth, dyspnea
Children (25%-10%): Failure to thrive, weight loss, stomatitis, oral thrush, ecchymosis, arthritis, myalgia, insomnia, epistaxis, pharyngitis

SERIOUS REACTIONS
• Pneumonia and opportunistic infections occur occasionally.
• Peripheral neuropathy, potentially fatal pancreatitis, retinal changes, and optic neuritis are the major toxic effects.

INTERACTIONS
Drugs
▲ *Allopurinol:* Increased plasma didanosine concentrations; coadministration not recommended
3 *Dapsone:* Buffering compound may inhibit dissolution of dapsone in the stomach
3 *Delavirdine:* Decreased plasma delavirdine concentrations; give ddI 1 hr after delavirdine

3 *Food:* Reduced bioavailability
3 *Ganciclovir:* Increased ddI concentrations
3 *Indinavir:* Decreased plasma indinavir concentrations; give ddI 1 hr after indinavir
3 *Itraconazole, ketoconazole:* Alkalinization of stomach by didanosine reduces the solubility and absorption of antifungal
3 *Methadone:* Decreased plasma didanosine concentrations
3 *Quinolones:* Decreased concentrations after binding to the aluminum and magnesium ions in the didanosine buffering compound
2 *Stavudine:* Increased risk of pancreatitis
3 *Tenofovir:* Increases didanosine plasma concentrations; increased didanosine toxicity may occur
3 *Tetracyclines:* Decreased antibiotic concentrations after binding to calcium ions in ddI buffering compound

SPECIAL CONSIDERATIONS

PATIENT/FAMILY EDUCATION

- Administer on empty stomach
- Shake the oral suspension well before using it, keep it refrigerated, and discard the solution after 30 days and obtain a new supply
- Avoid consuming alcohol
- Notify the physician if nausea or vomiting, numbness, or persistent, severe abdominal pain occurs
- Didanosine is not a cure for HIV infection, nor does it reduce the risk of transmitting HIV to others

MONITORING PARAMETERS

- Amylase, lipase, ophthalmologic examinations
- Suspend use until pancreatitis excluded if patient develops nausea, abdominal pain
- Tablets contain 264.5 mg sodium, packets 1380 mg sodium
- Weight
- Pattern of daily bowel activity and stool consistency
- Signs and symptoms of peripheral neuropathy, including burning feet, restless leg syndrome (inability to find a comfortable position for legs and feet), and lack of coordination
- Skin for eruptions and a rash
- Signs and symptoms of opportunistic infections, including cough or other respiratory symptoms, fever, and oral mucosa changes

diethylpropion hydrochloride

(die-ethyl-prop′-ion hye-droe-klor′-ide)

Rx: Tenuate, Teunate Dospan

Chemical Class: Phenethylamine derivative
Therapeutic Class: Anorexiant
DEA Class: Schedule IV

CLINICAL PHARMACOLOGY

Mechanism of Action: A sympathomimetic amine that stimulates the release of norepinephrine and dopamine. ***Therapeutic Effect:*** Decreases appetite.

Pharmacokinetics

Rapidly absorbed from the gastrointestinal (GI) tract. Widely distributed. Metabolized in liver to active metabolite and undergoes extensive first-pass metabolism. Excreted in urine. Unknown if removed by hemodialysis. ***Half-life:*** 4-6 hrs.

INDICATIONS AND DOSAGES

Obesity

PO

Adults. 25 mg 3 times/day before meals. (Extended-release) 75 mg at midmorning.

AVAILABLE FORMS

- *Tablets:* 25 mg (Tenuate).

• *Tablets (extended-release):* 75 mg (Tenuate Dospan).

UNLABELED USES: Migraines

CONTRAINDICATIONS: Agitated states, use of MAOIs within 14 days, glaucoma, history of drug abuse, hyperthyroidism, advanced arteriosclerosis or severe cardiovascular disease, severe hypertension, and hypersensitivity to sympathomimetic amines

PREGNANCY AND LACTATION: Pregnancy category B; excreted in breast milk; no reports of adverse effects

Controlled Substance: Schedule IV

SIDE EFFECTS

Frequent

Elevated blood pressure, nervousness, insomnia

Occasional

Dizziness, drowsiness, tremor, headache, nausea, stomach pain, fever, rash

Rare

Agranulocytosis, leukopenia, blurred vision, psychosis, CVA, seizure

SERIOUS REACTIONS

• Overdose may produce agitation, tachycardia, palpitations, cardiac irregularities, chest pain, psychotic episode, seizures, and coma.

• Hypersensitivity reactions and blood dyscrasias occur rarely.

INTERACTIONS

Drugs

❷ *Anesthetics:* May increase the risk of arrhythmias

❸ *Antidiabetic agents, insulin:* May alter blood glucose concentrations

❸ *Guanethidine:* May decrease the effects of guanethidine

⚠ *MAOIs, amphetamines:* May increase the risk of hypertensive crisis

❷ *Sibutramine:* Increased risk of hypertension and tachycardia

❸ *Tricyclic antidepressants:* May increase the cardiac and CNS effects of diethylpropion

Labs

• *False positive:* Urine cocaine, diazepam, methaqualone, phencyclidine

SPECIAL CONSIDERATIONS

• Tolerance to anorectic effects may develop within weeks; cross-tolerance is almost universal

• Measure the limited usefulness against the inherent risks (habituation) of this agent

• Most patients will eventually regain weight lost during use of this product

PATIENT/FAMILY EDUCATION

• Notify the physician if any increase in seizures, fever, nervousness, palpitations, skin rash, or vomiting occurs

• Avoid alcohol

• Take the last dose of diethylpropion in the early morning to avoid insomnia

• Avoid consuming caffeine during diethylpropion therapy

• Do not abruptly discontinue the drug after prolonged use

MONITORING PARAMETERS

• Blood pressure

• CBC

diflorasone diacetate

(die-floor′-a-sone dye-as′-uh-tate)

Rx: Maxiflor, Psorcon, Psorcon-e

Chemical Class: Corticosteroid, synthetic

Therapeutic Class: Corticosteroid, topical

CLINICAL PHARMACOLOGY

Mechanism of Action: A high-potency, fluorinated corticosteroid that decreases inflammation by suppression of migration of polymorphonuclear leukocytes and reversal of increased capillary permeability. The exact mechanism of the antiinflammatory process is unclear. ***Therapeutic Effect:*** Decreases or prevents tissue response to the inflammatory process.

Pharmacokinetics

Poor absorption; occlusive dressings increase absorption. Metabolized in liver. Primarily excreted in urine.

INDICATIONS AND DOSAGES

Dermatoses

Topical

Adults, Elderly. (Cream) Apply sparingly 2-4 times/day. (Ointment) Apply sparingly 1-3 times/day.

AVAILABLE FORMS

• *Cream:* 0.05% (Maxiflor, Psorcon).

• *Ointment:* 0.05% (Maxiflor, Psorcon).

• *Ointment, emollient:* 0.05% (Psorcon-e).

UNLABELED USES: Psoriasis

CONTRAINDICATIONS: History of hypersensitivity to diflorasone or other corticosteroids

PREGNANCY AND LACTATION: Pregnancy category C; unknown whether topical application could result in sufficient systemic absorption to produce detectable amounts in breast milk (systemic corticosteroids are secreted into breast milk in quantities not likely to have detrimental effects on infant)

SIDE EFFECTS

Rare

Itching, redness, dryness, irritation, burning at site of application, arthralgia, folliculitis, maceration, muscle atrophy, secondary infection

SERIOUS REACTIONS

• Overdosage symptoms include moon face, central obesity, hypertension, diabetes, hyperlipidemia, peptic ulcer, increased susceptibility to infection, electrolyte and fluid imbalance, psychosis, and hallucinations.

• The serious reactions of long-term therapy and the addition of occlusive dressings are reversible hypothalamic-pituitary-adrenal (HPA) axis suppression, manifestations of Cushing's syndrome, hyperglycemia, and glucosuria.

SPECIAL CONSIDERATIONS

• No demonstrated superiority over other high-potency agents; cost should govern use

PATIENT/FAMILY EDUCATION

• Apply sparingly only to affected area

• Avoid contact with the eyes

• Do not put bandages or dressings over treated area unless directed by clinician

• Discontinue drug, notify clinician if local irritation or fever develops

• Do not use on weeping, denuded, or infected areas

• Notify the physician if fever or rash occurs

• Avoid exposure to sunlight

MONITORING PARAMETERS
- Skin for rash
- Discontinue the use of diflorasone if no improvement is seen; reassess diagnosis

diflunisal
(dye-floo'-ni-sal)
Rx: Dolobid
Chemical Class: Salicylate derivative
Therapeutic Class: NSAID; antipyretic; nonnarcotic analgesic

CLINICAL PHARMACOLOGY
Mechanism of Action: A nonsteroidal antiinflammatory that inhibits prostaglandin synthesis, reducing inflammatory response and intensity of pain stimulus reaching sensory nerve endings. ***Therapeutic Effect:*** Produces analgesic and antiinflammatory effect.
Pharmacokinetics

Route	*Onset*	*Peak*	*Duration*
PO	1 hr	2-3 hr	8-12 hr

Completely absorbed from the GI tract. Widely distributed. Protein binding: greater than 99%. Metabolized in liver. Primarily excreted in urine. Not removed by hemodialysis. ***Half-life:*** 8-12 hr.

INDICATIONS AND DOSAGES
Mild to moderate pain
PO
Adults, Elderly. Initially, 0.5-1 g, then 250-500 mg q8-12h. Maximum: 1.5 g/day.
Osteoarthritis
PO
Adults, Elderly. 500-750 mg/day in divided doses.
Rheumatoid arthritis
PO
Adults, Elderly. 0.5-1 g/day in 2 divided doses. Maximum: 1.5 g/day.

AVAILABLE FORMS
- *Tablets:* 250 mg, 500 mg.

UNLABELED USES: Treatment of psoriatic arthritis, vascular headache

CONTRAINDICATIONS: Active GI bleeding, factor VII or factor IX deficiencies, hypersensitivity to aspirin or NSAIDs

PREGNANCY AND LACTATION: Pregnancy category C (D if used in third trimester or near delivery); use during third trimester not recommended due to effects on fetal cardiovascular system (closure of ductus arteriosus); excreted into breast milk in concentrations 2%-7% those in maternal plasma; use caution in nursing mothers

SIDE EFFECTS
Side effects are less common with short-term treatment.
Occasional (9%-3%)
Nausea, dyspepsia (heartburn, indigestion, epigastric pain), diarrhea, headache, rash
Rare (3%-1%)
Vomiting, constipation, flatulence, dizziness, somnolence, insomnia, fatigue, tinnitus

SERIOUS REACTIONS
- Overdosage may produce drowsiness, vomiting, nausea, diarrhea, hyperventilation, tachycardia, diaphoresis, stupor, and coma.
- Peptic ulcer, GI bleeding, gastritis, and severe hepatic reaction, including cholestasis, jaundice occur rarely.
- Nephrotoxicity, including dysuria, hematuria, proteinuria, and nephrotic syndrome, and severe hypersensitivity reaction, marked by bronchospasm and angioedema, occur rarely.

INTERACTIONS
Drugs
3 *Aminoglycosides:* Reduced clearance with elevated aminogly-

coside levels and potential for toxicity

3 *Anticoagulants:* Excessive hypoprothrombinemia, decreased platelet aggregation with increased risk of GI bleeding

3 *Antihypertensives (α-blockers, angiotensin-converting enzyme inhibitors, angiotensin II receptor blockers, β-blockers, diuretics):* Inhibition of antihypertensive and other favorable hemodynamic effects

3 *Aspirin, salicylates:* May increase the risk of GI bleeding and side effects

3 *Corticosteroids:* Increased risk of GI ulceration

3 *Cyclosporine:* Increased nephrotoxicity risk

3 *Lithium:* Decreased clearance of lithium (mediated via prostaglandins) resulting in elevated serum lithium levels and risk of toxicity

3 *Methotrexate:* Decreased renal secretion of methotrexate resulting in elevated methotrexate levels and risk of toxicity

3 *Phenylpropanolamine:* Possible acute hypertensive reaction

3 *Potassium-sparing diuretics:* Additive hyperkalemia potential

3 *Triamterene:* Acute renal failure reported with addition of indomethacin; caution with other NSAIDs

3 *Probenecid:* May increase diflunisal blood concentration

Labs

- *False increase:* Serum salicylate
- *False decrease:* T_4, T_3 uptake

SPECIAL CONSIDERATIONS

- No significant advantage over other NSAIDs; cost should govern use

PATIENT/FAMILY EDUCATION

- Swallow tablets whole; do not chew or crush
- Take diflunisal with food or milk if GI upset occurs
- Notify the physician if GI distress, headache, or rash occurs
- The female patient should notify the physician if she is or plans to become pregnant

MONITORING PARAMETERS

- Initial hemogram and fecal occult blood test within 3 mo of starting regular chronic therapy; repeat every 6-12 mo (more frequently in high-risk patients (> 65 years, peptic ulcer disease, concurrent steroids or anticoagulants); electrolytes, creatinine, and BUN within 3 mo of starting regular chronic therapy; repeat every 6-12 mo
- Skin for rash
- Daily bowel activity and stool consistency
- Therapeutic response for improved grip strength, increased joint mobility, reduced joint tenderness, and relief of pain, stiffness, and swelling

digoxin

(di-jox'-in)

Rx: Digitek, Lanoxicaps, Lanoxin

Chemical Class: Digitalis glycoside

Therapeutic Class: Antiarrhythmic; cardiac glycoside

CLINICAL PHARMACOLOGY

Mechanism of Action: A cardiac glycoside that increases the influx of calcium from extracellular to intracellular cytoplasm. ***Therapeutic Effect:*** Potentiates the activity of the contractile cardiac muscle fibers and increases the force of myocardial contraction. Slows the heart rate by decreasing conduction through the SA and AV nodes.

Pharmacokinetics

Route	Onset	Peak	Duration
PO	0.5-2 hr	28 hr	3-4 days
IV	5-30 min	1-4 hr	3-4 days

Readily absorbed from the GI tract. Widely distributed. Protein binding: 30%. Partially metabolized in the liver. Primarily excreted in urine. Minimally removed by hemodialysis. ***Half-life:*** 36-48 hr (increased with impaired renal function and in the elderly).

INDICATIONS AND DOSAGES

Rapid loading dose for the management and treatment of CHF; control of ventricular rate in patients with atrial fibrillation; treatment and prevention of recurrent paroxysmal atrial tachycardia

PO

Adults, Elderly. Initially, 0.5-0.75 mg, additional doses of 0.125-0.375 mg at 6- to 8-hr intervals. Range: 0.75-1.25 mg.

Children 10 yr and older. 10-15 mcg/kg.

Children 5-9 yr. 20-35 mcg/kg.

Children 2-4 yr. 30-40 mcg/kg.

Children 1-23 mo. 35-60 mcg/kg.

Neonate, full-term. 25-35 mcg/kg.

Neonate, premature. 20-30 mcg/kg.

IV

Adults, Elderly. 0.6-1 mg.

Children 10 yr and older. 8-12 mcg/kg.

Children 5-9 yr. 15-30 mcg/kg.

Children 2-4 yr. 25-35 mcg/kg.

Children 1-23 mo. 30-50 mcg/kg

Neonates, full-term. 20-30 mcg/kg.

Neonates, premature. 15-25 mcg/kg.

Maintenance dosage for CHF; control of ventricular rate in patients with atrial fibrillation; treatment and prevention of recurrent paroxysmal atrial tachycardia

PO, IV

Adults, Elderly. 0.125-0.375 mg/day.

Children. 25%-35% loading dose (20%-30% for premature neonates).

Dosage in renal impairment

Dosage adjustment is based on creatinine clearance. Total digitalizing dose: decrease by 50% in end-stage renal disease.

Creatinine Clearance	Dosage
10-50 ml/min	25%-75% usual
less than 10 ml/min	10%-25% usual

AVAILABLE FORMS

- *Capsules (Lanoxicaps):* 50 mcg, 100 mcg, 200 mcg.
- *Elixir (Lanoxin):* 50 mcg/ml.
- *Tablets (Digitek, Lanoxin):* 125 mcg, 250 mcg.
- *Injection (Lanoxin):* 100 mcg/ml, 250 mcg/ml.

CONTRAINDICATIONS: Ventricular fibrillation, ventricular tachycardia unrelated to CHF

PREGNANCY AND LACTATION: Pregnancy category C; passes readily to fetus; excreted into breast milk; considered compatible with breast-feeding

SIDE EFFECTS

None known. However, there is a very narrow margin of safety between a therapeutic and toxic result. Long-term therapy may produce mammary gland enlargement in women but is reversible when drug is withdrawn.

SERIOUS REACTIONS

- The most common early manifestations of digoxin toxicity are GI disturbances (anorexia, nausea, vomiting) and neurologic abnormalities (fatigue, headache, depression, weakness, drowsiness, confusion, nightmares).

• Facial pain, personality change, and ocular disturbances (photophobia, light flashes, halos around bright objects, yellow or green color perception) may be noted.

INTERACTIONS

Drugs

3 *Alprazolam, amiodarone, diltiazem, verapamil, bepridil, nitrendipine, quinidine, carvedilol, cyclosporine, erythromycin and tetracyclines (change in bacterial flora causing effect may persist for months), hydroxychloroquine, NSAIDs, azole antifungals, omeprazole, lansoprazole, propafenone, quinine, spironolactone, tacrolimus:* Increased digoxin levels

3 *Amphotericin B diuretics, glucocorticoids, potassium-depleting:* Enhanced digitalis toxicity secondary to drug-induced hypokalemia

3 *β-blockers:* Potentiation of bradycardia

3 *Calcium (IV):* Digitalis toxicity

2 *Charcoal:* Reduced digitalis levels

3 *Cholestyramine, kaolo-pectin (digoxin tablets only) neomycin, penicillamine, rifampin, sulfasalazine:* Reduced digitalis levels

3 *Cyclophosphamide:* Impaired digoxin (especially tablets) absorption; digitoxin not affected

3 *Magnesium (parenteral):* May cause cardiac conduction changes and heart block

3 *Metoclopramide, cisapride:* Reduced digitalis levels by slowly dissolving digoxin tablets only (Lanoxin tablets and capsules not affected)

3 *Siberian ginseng:* May increase serum digoxin levels

3 *St. John's Wort:* May reduce digoxin efficacy

3 *Succinylcholine:* Increased arrhythmias

3 *Sympathomimetics:* May increase risk of arrhythmias

Labs

• *False increase:* Urine 17-hydroxycorticosteroids

SPECIAL CONSIDERATIONS

• Preferred digitalis glycoside

• Rule out digitalis toxicity if nausea, vomiting, arrhythmias develop

• Listed adverse effects are mostly signs of toxicity

PATIENT/FAMILY EDUCATION

• Take apical pulse and notify the physician of a pulse rate of 60 beats/minute or less or a rate less than that indicated by the physician

• Carry or wear identification that the patient is receiving digoxin and to inform dentists and other physicians about digoxin therapy

• Do not take OTC medications without physician approval

• Notify the physician if decreased appetite, diarrhea, nausea, visual changes, or vomiting occurs

MONITORING PARAMETERS

• Heart rate and rhythm, periodic ECGs

• Serum potassium, magnesium, calcium, creatinine

• Serum digoxin levels when compliance, effectiveness, or systemic availability is questioned or toxicity suspected

• Obtain serum drug concentrations at least 8-12 hr after a dose (preferably prior to next scheduled dose); therapeutic range 0.5-2.0 ng/ml

digoxin immune Fab

(di-jox'-in)

Rx: Digibind, DigiFab

Chemical Class: Antibody fragment

Therapeutic Class: Antidote, digitalis

CLINICAL PHARMACOLOGY

Mechanism of Action: An antidote that binds molecularly to digoxin in the extracellular space. ***Therapeutic Effect:*** Makes digoxin unavailable for binding at its site of action on cells in the body.

Pharmacokinetics

Route	*Onset*	*Peak*	*Duration*
IV	30 min	N/A	3-4 days

Widely distributed into extracellular space. Excreted in urine. ***Half-life:*** 15-20 hr.

INDICATIONS AND DOSAGES

Potentially life-threatening digoxin overdose

IV

Adults, Elderly, Children. Dosage varies according to amount of digoxin to be neutralized. Refer to manufacturer's dosing guidelines.

AVAILABLE FORMS

- *Powder for Injection:* 38-mg vial (Digibind), 40-mg vial (DigiFab).

CONTRAINDICATIONS: None known.

PREGNANCY AND LACTATION: Pregnancy category C; excretion into breast milk unknown; use caution in nursing mothers

SIDE EFFECTS

Rare

Allergic reaction

SERIOUS REACTIONS

- Hyperkalemia may occur as a result of digitalis toxicity. Signs and symptoms of hyperkalemia include diarrhea, paresthesia of extremities, heaviness of legs, decreased BP, cold skin, grayish pallor, hypotension, mental confusion, irritability, flaccid paralysis, tented T waves, widening QRS interval, and ST depression.
- Hypokalemia may develop rapidly when the effect of digitalis is reversed. Signs and symptoms of hypokalemia include muscle cramping, nausea, vomiting, hypoactive bowel sounds, abdominal distention, difficulty breathing, and orthostatic hypotension.
- Low cardiac output and CHF may occur rarely.

INTERACTIONS

Labs

- *Interference:* Immunoassay digoxin

SPECIAL CONSIDERATIONS

PATIENT/FAMILY EDUCATION

- Before discharge, review the digoxin dosages carefully with the patient, and make sure he or she knows how to take the drug as prescribed
- Follow-up care, including monitoring serum digoxin level, is important to maintain
- Notify the physician if anorexia, nausea, vomiting, or visual changes occurs

MONITORING PARAMETERS

- Potassium, serum digoxin level prior to therapy
- Continuous ECG monitoring
- Blood pressure
- Signs and symptoms of an arrhythmia (such as palpitations), or heart failure (such as dyspnea and edema) if the digoxin level falls below the therapeutic level

dihydroergotamine mesylate

(dye-hye-droe-er-got'-a-meen mes'-sil-ate)

Chemical Class: Ergot alkaloid

Therapeutic Class: Antimigraine agent

CLINICAL PHARMACOLOGY

Mechanism of Action: An ergotamine derivative, alpha-adrenergic blocker that directly stimulates vascular smooth muscle. May also have antagonist effects on serotonin. ***Therapeutic Effect:*** Peripheral and cerebral vasoconstriction.

Pharmacokinetics

Slow, incomplete absorption from the gastrointestinal (GI) tract; rate of absorption of intranasal varies. Protein binding: Greater than 90%. Undergoes extensive first-pass metabolism in liver. Metabolized to active metabolite. Eliminated in feces via biliary system. ***Half-life:*** 7-9 hrs.

INDICATIONS AND DOSAGES

Migraine headaches, cluster headaches

IM/Subcutaneous

Adults, Elderly. 1 mg at onset of headache; repeat hourly. Maximum: 3 mg/day; 6 mg/wk.

IV

Adults, Elderly. 1 mg at onset of headache; repeat hourly. Maximum: 2 mg/day; 6 mg/wk.

Intranasal

Adults, Elderly. 1 spray (0.5 mg) into each nostril; repeat in 15 min. Maximum: 4 sprays/day; 8 sprays/wk.

AVAILABLE FORMS

- *Injection:* 1 mg/ml (D.H.E. 45).
- *Nasal spray:* 4 mg/ml [0.5mg/spray] (Migranal).

CONTRAINDICATIONS: Coronary artery disease, hypertension, impaired liver or renal function, malnutrition, peripheral vascular diseases, such as thromboangiitis obliterans, syphilitic arteritis, severe arteriosclerosis, thrombophlebitis, Raynaud's disease, sepsis, severe pruritus

PREGNANCY AND LACTATION: Pregnancy category X; likely excreted into breast milk; ergotamine has caused symptoms of ergotism (e.g., vomiting, diarrhea) in the infant; excessive dosage or prolonged administration may inhibit lactation

SIDE EFFECTS

Occasional

Cough, dizziness, rhinitis, altered taste, throat and nose irritation

Rare

Muscle pain, fatigue, diarrhea, upper respiratory infection, dyspepsia

SERIOUS REACTIONS

- Prolonged administration or excessive dosage may produce ergotamine poisoning manifested as nausea, vomiting, weakness of legs, pain in limb muscles, numbness and tingling of fingers or toes, precordial pain, tachycardia or bradycardia, and hypertension or hypotension.
- Localized edema and itching due to vasoconstriction of peripheral arteries and arterioles may occur.
- Feet or hands will become cold, pale, and numb.
- Muscle pain will occur when walking and later, even at rest.
- Gangrene may occur.
- Occasionally confusion, depression, drowsiness, and seizures appear.

INTERACTIONS

Drugs

3 β-*blockers:* May increase the risk of vasospasm

❷ *Clarithromycin, erythromycin (not azithromycin or dirithromycin), fluoxetine:* Increased ergotism (hypertention and ischemia)

❷ *Nitroglycerin:* Enhanced ergot effect, decreased antianginal effects

❷ *Protease inhibitors:* May increase the risk of toxicity of dihydroergotamine

❷ *Sibutramine:* Increased risk of serotonin syndrome

⚠ *Systemic vasoconstrictors:* May increase pressor effect

SPECIAL CONSIDERATIONS

• Considered alternative abortive acute migraine agent; nasal spray less effective than triptans

PATIENT/FAMILY EDUCATION

• Initiate therapy at first sign of attack

• Prolonged use may lead to withdrawal headaches

• Notify the physician if the dihydroergotamine dosage does not relieve vascular headaches, or if irregular heartbeat, nausea, numbness or tingling of the fingers and toes, pain or weakness of the extremities, or vomiting occurs

• Avoid pregnancy and report any suspected pregnancy immediately to the physician

MONITORING PARAMETERS

• Determine if the female patient is pregnant before initiating therapy

• Therapeutic response to medication

dihydrotachysterol

(dye-hye-droe-tak-iss′-ter-ole)

Rx: DHT, DHT Intensol, Hytakerol

Chemical Class: Sterol derivative

Therapeutic Class: Antiosteoporotic; vitamin D analog

CLINICAL PHARMACOLOGY

Mechanism of Action: A fat-soluble vitamin that is essential for absorption, utilization of calcium phosphate, and normal calcification of bone. ***Therapeutic Effect:*** Stimulates calcium and phosphate absorption from small intestine, promotes secretion of calcium from bone to blood, promotes renal tubule phosphate resorption, acts on bone cells to stimulate skeletal growth and on parathyroid gland to suppress hormone synthesis and secretion.

Pharmacokinetics

Well absorbed from small intestine. Metabolized in liver. Eliminated via biliary system; excreted in urine. ***Half-life:*** Unknown.

INDICATIONS AND DOSAGES

Hypoparathyroidism

PO

Adults, Elderly, Older Children. Initially, 0.8-2.4 mg/day for several days. Maintenance: 0.2-1 mg/day.

Infants, Young Children. Initially, 1-5 mg/day for 4 days, then 0.1-0.5 mg/day.

Nutritional rickets

PO

Adults, Elderly, Children. 0.5 mg as a single dose or 13-50 mcg/day until healing occurs.

Renal osteodystorphy

PO

Adults, Elderly. 0.25-0.6 mg/24 hrs adjusted as necessary to achieve normal serum calcium levels and promote bone healing.

AVAILABLE FORMS

- *Oral Solution:* 0. 2 mg/ml (DHT Intensol).
- *Capsule:* 0. 125 mg (Hytakerol).
- *Tablets:* 0. 125 mg, 0. 2 mg, 0. 4 mg (DHT).

CONTRAINDICATIONS: Hypercalcemia, malabsorption syndrome, vitamin D toxicity, hypersensitivity to vitamin D products or analogs

PREGNANCY AND LACTATION: Pregnancy category A (category D if used in doses above the recommended daily allowance); excretion into breast milk unknown; vitamin D is excreted into breast milk in limited amounts; considered compatible with breast-feeding, however, serum calcium levels of the infant should be monitored if the mother is receiving pharmacologic doses

SIDE EFFECTS

Occasional

Nausea, vomiting

SERIOUS REACTIONS

- Early signs of overdosage are manifested as weakness, headache, somnolence, nausea, vomiting, dry mouth, constipation, muscle and bone pain, and metallic taste sensation.
- Later signs of overdosage are evidenced by polyuria, polydipsia, anorexia, weight loss, nocturia, photophobia, rhinorrhea, pruritus, disorientation, hallucinations, hyperthermia, hypertension, and cardiac arrhythmias.

INTERACTIONS

Drugs

3 *Aluminum-containing antacids:* May increase aluminum concentration and risk of aluminum bone toxicity

3 *Calcium-containing preparations, thiazide diuretics:* May increase the risk of hypercalcemia

3 *Magnesium-containing antacids:* May increase magnesium concentration

SPECIAL CONSIDERATIONS

- Vitamin D analog of choice for prevention and treatment of renal osteodystrophy; less expensive than calcitriol

PATIENT/FAMILY EDUCATION

- Compliance with dosage instructions, diet (evaluate vitamin D ingested in fortified foods, maintain adequate calcium intake) is essential
- Drink plenty of fluids

MONITORING PARAMETERS

- Serum Ca^{++} and phosphate
- If adverse reactions occur rule out hypercalcemia, worsening renal function
- BUN, serum alkaline phosphatase, serum creatinine
- Fluid intake

diltiazem hydrochloride

(dil-tye'-a-zem hye-droe-klor'-ide)

Rx: Cardizem, Cardizem CD, Cardizem LA, Cardizem SR, Cartia, Dilacor XR, Diltia XT, Taztia XT, Tiazac

Combinations

Rx: with enalapril (Teczem)

Chemical Class: Benzothiazepine

Therapeutic Class: Antianginal; antiarrhythmic, class IV; antihypertensive; calcium channel blocker

CLINICAL PHARMACOLOGY

Mechanism of Action: An antianginal, antihypertensive, and antiarrhythmic agent that inhibits calcium movement across cardiac and vascular smooth-muscle cell membranes. This action causes the dilation of coronary arteries, peripheral arteries, and arterioles. ***Therapeutic Effect:*** Decreases heart rate and myocardial contractility, slows SA and AV conduction and decreases total peripheral vascular resistance by vasodilation.

Pharmacokinetics

Route	Onset	Peak	Duration
PO	0.5-1 hr	N/A	N/A
PO (extended-release)	2-3 hr	N/A	N/A
IV	3 min	N/A	N/A

Well absorbed from the GI tract. Protein binding: 70%-80%. Undergoes first-pass metabolism in the liver to active metabolite. Primarily excreted in urine. Not removed by hemodialysis. ***Half-life:*** 3-8 hr.

INDICATIONS AND DOSAGES

Angina

PO (Cardizem)

Adults, Elderly. Initially, 30 mg 4 times a day. Range: 180-360 mg/day.

PO (Cardizem CD, Cartia XT, Dilacor XR, Diltia XT, Tiazac)

Adults, Elderly. Initially, 120-180 mg/day. Maximum: 480 mg/day.

PO (Cardizem LA)

Adults, Elderly. Initially, 180 mg/day. May increase at intervals of 7-14-day intervals. Maximum: 360 mg/day.

Hypertension

PO (Cardizem CD, Cartia XT, Dilacor XR, Diltia XT, Tiazac)

Adults, Elderly. Initially, 180-240 mg/day. Range: 180-420 mg/day, Tiazac: 120-540 mg/day.

PO (Cardizem SR)

Adults, Elderly. Initially, 60-120 mg twice a day. May increase at 14-day intervals. Maintenance: 240-360 mg/day.

PO (Cardizem LA)

Adults, Elderly. Initially, 180-240 mg/day. May increase at 14-day intervals. Range: 120-540 mg/day.

Temporary control of rapid ventricular rate in atrial fibrillation or flutter, rapid conversion of paroxysmal supraventricular tachycardia to normal sinus rhythm.

IV push

Adults, Elderly. Initially, 0.25 mg/kg actual body weight over 2 min. May repeat in 15 min at dose of 0.35 mg/kg actual body weight. Subsequent doses individualized.

IV Infusion

Adults, Elderly. After initial bolus injection, may begin infusion at 5-10 mg/hr; may increase by 5 mg/hr up to a maximum of 15 mg/hr. Infusion duration should not exceed 24 hr.

AVAILABLE FORMS

- *Capsules (Sustained-Release [Cardizem SR]):* 60 mg, 90 mg, 120 mg.
- *Capsules (Extended-Release [Cardizem CD]):* 120 mg (Cardizem CD, Cartia XT, Dilacor XR, Diltia XT, Taztia XT, Tiazac), 180 mg (Cardizem CD, Cartia XT, Dilacor XR, Diltia XT, Taztia XT, Tiazac), 240 mg (Cardizem CD, Cartia XT, Dilacor XR, Diltia XT, Taztia XT, Tiazac), 300 mg (Cardizem CD, Cartia XT, Taztia XT, Tiazac), 360 mg (Cardizem CD, Taztia XT, Tiazac), 420 mg (Tiazac).
- *Tablets (Cardizem):* 30 mg, 60 mg, 90 mg, 120 mg.
- *Tablets (Extended-Release[Cardizem LA]):* 120 mg, 180 mg, 240 mg, 300 mg, 360 mg, 420 mg.
- *Injection (Ready-to-Hang Infusion):* 1 mg/ml.

CONTRAINDICATIONS: Acute MI, pulmonary congestion, hypersensitivity to diltiazem or other calcium channel blockers, second- or third-degree AV block (except in the presence of a pacemaker), severe hypotension (less than 90 mm Hg, systolic), sick sinus syndrome

PREGNANCY AND LACTATION: Pregnancy category C; excreted into breast milk in concentrations that may approximate those in maternal serum; use caution in nursing mothers

SIDE EFFECTS

Frequent (10%-5%)

Peripheral edema, dizziness, lightheadedness, headache, bradycardia, asthenia (loss of strength, weakness)

Occasional (5%-2%)

Nausea, constipation, flushing, EKG changes

Rare (less than 2%)

Rash, micturition disorder (polyuria, nocturia, dysuria, frequency of urination), abdominal discomfort, somnolence

SERIOUS REACTIONS

- Abrupt withdrawal may increase frequency or duration of angina.
- CHF and second- and third-degree AV block occur rarely.
- Overdose produces nausea, somnolence, confusion, slurred speech, and profound bradycardia.

INTERACTIONS

Drugs

3 *α-blockers:* Additive increased antihypertensive effect

3 *Amiodarone:* Cardiotoxicity with bradycardia and decreased cardiac output

3 *Antipyrine:* Increased antipyrine concentrations

3 *Aspirin:* Enhanced antiplatelet activity

3 *Azole antifungals:* Possible increased calcium channel blocker effects

3 *β-blockers:* Inhibition of metabolism of propranolol and metoprolol (not atenolol); additive effects on cardiac conduction and hypotension

2 *Carbamazepine:* Increase in carbamazepine toxicity

3 *Cyclosporine, tacrolimus:* Increased blood concentrations, renal toxicity

3 *Digitalis glycosides:* Reduced elimination, increased digitalis levels, toxicity

3 *Ecainide:* Increased ecainide levels

3 *Erythromycin, troleandomycin:* Increased levels calcium channel blocker

3 *Fentanyl:* Severe hypotension or increased fluid volume requirements

3 *H_2-receptor antagonists:* Serum diltiazem concentrations increased

3 *Lithium:* Neurotoxicity

3 *Neuromuscular blockers:* Prolonged blockade by vecuronium and pancuronium

3 *Nitroprusside:* Enhanced hypotension

3 *Phenobarbital:* Reduced calcium channel blocker concentration

3 *Phenytoin:* Increased phenytoin levels

3 *Procainamide, quinidine:* May increase the risk of QT-interval prolongation

3 *Rifampin:* Decreased diltiazem concentrations

3 *Tricyclic antidepressants:* Increased TCA levels

Labs

- *False positive:* Urine ketones

SPECIAL CONSIDERATIONS

PATIENT/FAMILY EDUCATION

- Do not abruptly discontinue diltiazem

• Rise slowly from a lying position to a sitting position and wait momentarily before standing to avoid diltiazem's hypotensive effect
• Avoid tasks that require mental alertness or motor skills until response to the drug has been established
• Notify the physician if constipation, irregular heartbeat, nausea, pronounced dizziness, or shortness of breath occurs

MONITORING PARAMETERS

• Blood pressure
• EKG
• Liver and renal function
• Assess the patient for peripheral edema behind the medial malleolus in ambulatory patients or in the sacral area in bedridden patients

dimenhydrinate

(dye-men-hye'-dri-nate)

Rx: Motion-Aid

Chemical Class: Ethanolamine derivative

Therapeutic Class: Antihistamine; antivertigo agent

CLINICAL PHARMACOLOGY

Mechanism of Action: An antihistamine and anticholinergic that competes for H_1 receptor sites on effector cells of the GI tract, blood vessels, and respiratory tract. The anticholinergic action diminishes vestibular stimulation and depresses labyrinthine function. ***Therapeutic Effect:*** Prevents symptoms of motion sickness.

Pharmacokinetics

Well absorbed following PO administration. Metabolized in liver. Excreted in urine. ***Half-life:*** Unknown.

INDICATIONS AND DOSAGES

Motion sickness

PO

Adults, Elderly, Children older than 12 yr. 50-100 mg q4-6h. Maximum: 400 mg/day.

Children 6-12 yr. 25-50 mg q6-8h. Maximum: 150 mg/day.

Children 2-5 yr. 12.5-25 mg q6-8h. Maximum: 75 mg/day.

IM

Adults, Elderly. 50-100 mg q4-6h as needed.

Children older than 2 yr. 1.25 mg/kg or 37.5 mg/m^2 q6h. Maximum: 300 mg/day.

IV

Adults. 50 mg over 2 min.

AVAILABLE FORMS

• *Tablets (Chewable [Dramamine]):* 50 mg.
• *Tablets (Dramamine):* 50 mg.
• *Injectable Solution (Motion-Aid):* 50 mg/ml.

CONTRAINDICATIONS: Hypersensitivity to diphenhydramine

PREGNANCY AND LACTATION: Pregnancy category B; has been used for the treatment of hyperemesis gravidarum; small amounts are excreted into breast milk; use caution in nursing mothers

SIDE EFFECTS

Frequent

Dry mouth

Occasional

Hypotension, palpitations, tachycardia, headache, somnolence, dizziness, paradoxical stimulation (especially in children), anorexia, constipation, dysuria, blurred vision, tinnitus, wheezing, chest tightness

Rare

Photosensitivity, rash, urticaria

SERIOUS REACTIONS

• None significant.

INTERACTIONS

Drugs

3 *Alcohol, other CNS depressants:* May increase CNS depression

3 *Aminoglycosides:* Masks signs and symptoms of ototoxicity associated with aminoglycosides

3 *Other anticholinergics:* Increases anticholinergic effect

SPECIAL CONSIDERATIONS

PATIENT/FAMILY EDUCATION

• For prevention of motion sickness administer at least 30 min before exposure to motion

• May cause drowsiness, dizziness, and dry mouth

• Avoid tasks requiring mental alertness or motor skills until response to the drug has been established

• Avoid prolonged sun exposure

MONITORING PARAMETERS

• Blood pressure

• Signs and symptoms of motion sickness

dimercaprol

(dye-mer-kap'-role)

Rx: BAL in Oil

Chemical Class: Dithiol derivative

Therapeutic Class: Antidote, heavy metal

CLINICAL PHARMACOLOGY

Mechanism of Action: A chelating agent that contains two sulfhydryl groups that form a stable, nontoxic chelate 5-membered heterocyclic ring with heavy metals. ***Therapeutic Effect:*** Prevents the metal from combining with sulfhydryl groups on physiologic proteins and keeps them inactive until they can be excreted.

Pharmacokinetics

Time to peak after IM administration occurs in 30-60 min. Widely distributed to all tissues including the brain and, mainly, intracellular space. Rapidly metabolized by the liver to inactive metabolites. Excreted in the urine and bile. Removed by hemodialysis. ***Half-life:*** 4 hrs.

INDICATIONS AND DOSAGES

Poisoning, arsenic (mild)

IM

Adults, Elderly, Children. 2.5 mg/kg 4 times/day for 2 days, 2 times on day 3, then once daily for 10 days or recovery.

Poisoning, arsenic (severe)

IM

Adults, Elderly, Children. 3 mg/kg q4h for 2 days, 4 times on day 3, then twice daily for 10 days or recovery.

Poisoning, gold (mild)

IM

Adults, Elderly, Children. 2.5 mg/kg 4 times/day for 2 days, 2 times on day 3, then once daily for 10 days or recovery.

Poisoning, lead (mild)

IM

Adults, Elderly, Children. Initially, 4 mg/kg, then 3 mg/kg q4h for 2-7 days in combination with edetate calcium disodium injection at different injection sites.

Poisoning, lead (severe)

IM

Adults, Elderly, Children. 4 mg/kg q4h for 2-7 days in combination with edetate calcium disodium injection at different injection sites.

Poisoning, mercury
IM
Adults, Elderly, Children. 5 mg/kg for 1 day, followed by 2.5 mg/kg 1 or 2 times/day for 10 days.
Dosage in renal impairment
Adults, Elderly. 2 mg/kg q12h during dialysis.

AVAILABLE FORMS
- *Injection, oil:* 100 mg/ml (BAL in Oil).

UNLABELED USES: Antimony poisoning, bismuth poisoning, selenium poisoning, silver poisoning, vanadium poisoning

CONTRAINDICATIONS: Acute renal impairment, alkyl mercuring poisoning, G6PD deficiency (unless a life-threatening situation exists), hepatic insufficiency (unless due to arsenic poisoning), use of iron, cadmium or selenium poisoning, hypersensitivity to dimercaprol or any component of the formulations

PREGNANCY AND LACTATION: Pregnancy category C; use only in life-threatening poisoning

SIDE EFFECTS
Frequent
Hypertension, dose-related tachycardia, headache
Occasional
Nausea, vomiting
Rare
Burning eyes, lips, mouth, throat, and penis; nervousness; pain at injection site; salivation; fever; dysuria

SERIOUS REACTIONS
- Abscess formation at injection site, blepharospasm, convulsions, thrombocytopenia, and transient neutropenia occur rarely.

SPECIAL CONSIDERATIONS
- Administer by deep IM injection only

PATIENT/FAMILY EDUCATION
- Frequent blood and urine tests are required

MONITORING PARAMETERS
- Blood pressure, pulse
- BUN, Cr, urine pH (alkaline urinary pH decreases renal damage)
- Specific heavy metal levels

---

dinoprostone
(dye-noe-prost'-one)
Rx: Cervidil, Prepidil, Prostin E_2
Chemical Class: Prostaglandin E_2
Therapeutic Class: Abortifacient; uterine stimulant

CLINICAL PHARMACOLOGY
Mechanism of Action: A prostaglandin that directly acts on the myometrium, causing softening and dilation effect of the cervix. ***Therapeutic Effect:*** Stimulates myometrial contractions in gravid uterus.
Pharmacokinetics
Undergoes rapid enzymatic deactivation primarily in maternal lungs. Protein binding: 73%. Primarily excreted in urine. ***Half-life:*** Less than 5 min.

INDICATIONS AND DOSAGES
Abortifacient
Intravaginal
Adults. 20 mg (or one suppository) high into vagina. May repeat at 3- to 5-hr intervals until abortion occurs. Do not administer for longer than 2 days. Maximum: 240 mg.
Ripening of unfavorable cervix
Intracervical (Prepidil)
Adults. Initially, 0.5 mg (2.5 ml); if no cervical or uterine response, may

repeat 0.5-mg dose in 6 hr. Maximum: 1.5 mg (7.5 ml) for a 24-hr period.

Intracervical (Cervidil)

Adults. 10 mg over 12-hr period; remove upon onset of active labor or 12 hr after insertion.

AVAILABLE FORMS

- *Vaginal Gel (Prepidil):* 0.5 mg.
- *Vaginal Inserts (Cervidil):* 10 mg.
- *Vaginal Suppositories (Prostin E_2 Vaginal Cream):* 20 mg.

CONTRAINDICATIONS: Gel: Active cardiac, hepatic, pulmonary, or renal disease; acute pelvic inflammatory disease (PID); fetal malpresentation; grand multiparae with 6 or more previous term pregnancy cases with non-vertex presentation; history of cesarean section or major uterine surgery; history of difficult labor and/or traumatic delivery; hypersensitivity to other prostaglandins; placenta previa or unexplained vaginal bleeding during this pregnancy; patients for whom vaginal delivery is not indicated, such as vasa previa or active herpes genitalia; significant cephalopelvic disproportion

Vaginal suppository: Active cardiac, hepatic, pulmonary, or renal disease; acute PID

PREGNANCY AND LACTATION: Pregnancy category C; complete any failed attempts at pregnancy termination by some other means

SIDE EFFECTS

Frequent

Vomiting (66%), diarrhea (40%), nausea (33%)

Occasional

Headache (10%), chills or shivering (10%), hives, bradycardia, increased uterine pain accompanying abortion, peripheral vasoconstriction

Rare

Flushing, vulvae edema

SERIOUS REACTIONS

- Overdose may cause uterine hypertonicity with spasm and tetanic contraction, leading to cervical laceration or perforation, and uterine rupture or hemorrhage.

INTERACTIONS

Drugs

- *Oxytoxin:* Augmented activity, use sequentially not concurrently (6-12 hr after gel, 30 min after removal of insert)

SPECIAL CONSIDERATIONS

- Do not place gel above level of internal os; use 20-mm endocervical catheter if no effacement present; 10-mm catheter if cervix 50% effaced
- May use small amount water-soluble lubricant with insert; do not use insert without retrieval system

PATIENT/FAMILY EDUCATION

- Remain supine for 10-15 min (vag supp), 15-30 min (gel), 2 h (insert)
- The patient receiving the suppository form should notify the physician if chills, fever, foul-smelling or increased vaginal discharge, or uterine cramps or pain occurs

MONITORING PARAMETERS

- Blood pressure, fetal monitor (for cervical ripening)
- Check the duration, frequency, and strength of contractions in the patient receiving the suppository form
- Vital signs of the patient receiving the suppository form every 15 mins until stable, and then hourly until abortion is complete
- Resting uterine tone of the patient receiving the suppository form
- Record vital signs of the patient receiving the vaginal gel at least hourly in the presence of uterine activity
- Reassess the Bishop score of the patient receiving the vaginal gel

diphenhydramine hydrochloride

(dye-fen-hye'-dra-meen hye-droe-klor'-ide)

Rx: Banaril, Benadryl, Diphedryl

OTC: Allermax, Banophen, Banophen Caplets, Belix, Benadryl 25, Benylin Cough, Bydramine Cough, Diphen Cough, Dormarex 2, Genahist, Gen-D-phen, Hydramine Cough, Nidryl, Nordryl Cough, Phendry, Uni-Bent Cough

Combinations

OTC: with acetaminophen (Excedrin PM, Extra Strength Tylenol PM, Sominex Pain Relief, Unisom with Pain Relief); with calamine (Caladryl)

Chemical Class: Ethanolamine derivative

Therapeutic Class: Anti-Parkinson's agent; antianaphylactic (adjunct); antihistamine; antipruritic; antivertigo agent; hypnotic

CLINICAL PHARMACOLOGY

Mechanism of Action: An ethanolamine that competitively blocks the effects of histamine at peripheral H_1 receptor sites. ***Therapeutic Effect:*** Produces anticholinergic, antipruritic, antitussive, antiemetic, antidyskinetic, and sedative effects.

Pharmacokinetics

Route	*Onset*	*Peak*	*Duration*
PO	15-30 min	1-4 hr	4-6 hr
IV, IM	less than 15 min	1-4 hr	4-6 hr

Well absorbed after PO or parenteral administration. Protein binding: 98%-99%. Widely distributed. Metabolized in the liver. Primarily excreted in urine. ***Half-life:*** 1-4 hr.

INDICATIONS AND DOSAGES

Moderate to severe allergic reaction

PO, IV, IM

Adults, Elderly. 25-50 mg q4h. Maximum: 400 mg/day.

Children. 5 mg/kg/day in divided doses q6-8h. Maximum: 300 mg/day.

Motion sickness

PO

Adults, Elderly, Children 12 yr and older. 25-50 mg q4-6h. Maximum: 300 mg/day.

Children 6-11 yr. 12.5-25 mg q4-6h. Maximum: 150 mg/day.

Children 2-5 yr. 6.25 mg q4-6h. Maximum: 37.5 mg/day.

Parkinson's disease

PO

Adults, Elderly. 25-50 mg 3-4 times a day.

Antitussive

PO

Adults, Elderly, Children 12 yr and older. 2-5 mg q4h. Maximum: 150 mg/day.

Children 6-11 yr. 12.5 mg q4h. Maximum: 75 mg/day.

Children 2-5 yr. 6.25 mg q4h. Maximum: 37.5 mg/day.

Nighttime sleep aid

PO

Adults, Elderly, Children 12 yr and older. 50 mg at bedtime.

Children 2-11 yr. 1 mg/kg/dose. Maximum: 50 mg.

Pruritus

Topical

Adults, Elderly, Children 12 yr and older. Apply 1% or 2% cream or spray 3-4 times a day.

Children 2-11 yr. Apply 1% cream or spray 3-4 times a day.

AVAILABLE FORMS
- *Capsules:* 25 mg (Banophen, Diphen, Genahist), 50 mg (Nytol).
- *Syrup (Diphen, Diphenhist):* 12.5 mg/5 ml.
- *Tablets (Banophen, Benadryl, Genahist, Nytol):* 25 mg, 50 mg.
- *Injection (Benadryl):* 50 mg/ml.
- *Cream (Benadryl):* 1%, 2%.
- *Spray (Benadryl):* 1%, 2%.

CONTRAINDICATIONS: Acute exacerbation of asthma, use within 14 days of MAOIs

PREGNANCY AND LACTATION: Pregnancy category C; excreted into breast milk; although levels are not thought to be sufficiently high after therapeutic doses to affect the infant, the manufacturer considers the drug contraindicated in nursing mothers due to the increased sensitivity of newborn or premature infants to antihistamines

SIDE EFFECTS

Frequent

Somnolence, dizziness, muscle weakness, hypotension, urine retention, thickening of bronchial secretions, dry mouth, nose, throat, or lips; in elderly, sedation, dizziness, hypotension

Occasional

Epigastric distress, flushing, visual or hearing disturbances, paresthesia, diaphoresis, chills

SERIOUS REACTIONS
- Hypersensitivity reactions, such as eczema, pruritus, rash, cardiac disturbances, and photosensitivity, may occur.
- Overdose symptoms may vary from CNS depression, including sedation, apnea, hypotension, cardiovascular collapse, and death, to severe paradoxical reactions, such as hallucinations, tremor, and seizures.
- Children and neonates may experience paradoxical reactions, including restlessness, insomnia, euphoria, nervousness, and tremors.
- Overdosage in children may result in hallucinations, seizures, and death.

INTERACTIONS

Drugs

3 *Alcohol, other CNS depressants:* May increase CNS depressant effects

3 *Anticholinergics:* Possible enhanced anticholinergic, CNS effects

3 *MAOIs:* May increase the anticholinergic and CNS depressant effects of diphenhydramine

3 *Metoprolol:* May increase the plasma concentration of metoprolol

3 *Thioridazine:* May increase thioridazine serum concentrations

Labs
- *False negative:* Skin allergy tests
- *False positive:* Urine methadone, serum and urine tricyclic antidepressant

SPECIAL CONSIDERATIONS

PATIENT/FAMILY EDUCATION
- Dizziness, drowsiness, and dry mouth are expected side effects of diphenhydramine but the patient may develop a tolerance to the drug's sedative effects
- Avoid performing tasks that require mental alertness or motor skills until response to the drug has been established
- Avoid alcohol

MONITORING PARAMETERS
- Blood pressure, especially in the elderly
- Children for paradoxical reactions

dipyridamole

(dye-peer-id'-a-mole)

Rx: Persantine

Combinations

Rx: with aspirin (Aggrenox)

Chemical Class: Pyrimidine derivative

Therapeutic Class: Antiplatelet agent; coronary vasodilator

CLINICAL PHARMACOLOGY

Mechanism of Action: A blood modifier and platelet aggregation inhibitor that inhibits the activity of adenosine deaminase and phosphodiesterase, enzymes causing accumulation of adenosine and cyclic adenosine monophosphate. ***Therapeutic Effect:*** Inhibits platelet aggregation; may cause coronary vasodilation.

Pharmacokinetics

Slowly, variably absorbed from the GI tract. Widely distributed. Protein binding: 91%-99%. Metabolized in the liver. Primarily eliminated via biliary excretion. ***Half-life:*** 10-15 hr.

INDICATIONS AND DOSAGES

Prevention of thromboembolic disorders

PO

Adults, Elderly. 75-100 mg 4 times a day in combination with other medications.

Children. 3-6 mg/kg/day in 3 divided doses.

Diagnostic aid

IV

Adults, Elderly (based on weight). 0.142 mg/kg/min infused over 4 min; although a maximum hasn't been determined, doses greater than 60 mg have been determined to be unnecessary for any patient.

AVAILABLE FORMS

- *Tablets:* 25 mg, 50 mg, 75 mg.
- *Injection:* 5 mg/ml.

UNLABELED USES: Reduces risk of reinfarction in patients recovering from MI, treatment of transient ischemic attacks (TIAs)

CONTRAINDICATIONS: None known.

PREGNANCY AND LACTATION: Pregnancy category B; excreted in breast milk

SIDE EFFECTS

Frequent (14%)

Dizziness

Occasional (6%-2%)

Abdominal distress, headache, rash

Rare (less than 2%)

Diarrhea, vomiting, flushing, pruritus

SERIOUS REACTIONS

- Overdose produces peripheral vasodilation, resulting in hypotension.

INTERACTIONS

Drugs

3 *Adenosine:* Increased concentrations of adenosine, potentiates adenosine's pharmacologic effects

3 *Anticoagulants, heparin, salicylates, thrombolytics:* Increased risk of bleeding with these drugs

3 *β-blockers:* Additive bradycardia

3 *Ginkgo biloba:* Increased risk of bleeding

SPECIAL CONSIDERATIONS

PATIENT/FAMILY EDUCATION

- Avoid alcohol; drinking 3 or more alcoholic beverages a day increases the risk of stomach bleeding and dizziness, possibly resulting in a fall
- Try dry toast or unsalted crackers to relieve nausea
- Therapeutic response may not be achieved before 2-3 mos of continuous therapy
- Use caution when rising suddenly from lying or sitting position

MONITORING PARAMETERS
- Blood pressure for hypotension
- Skin for rash

dirithromycin

(dye-rith-roe-mye'-sin)

Rx: Dynabac, Dynabac D5-Pak

Chemical Class: Macrolide derivative

Therapeutic Class: Antibiotic

CLINICAL PHARMACOLOGY

Mechanism of Action: A macrolide that binds to ribosomal receptor sites of susceptible organisms, inhibiting bacterial protein synthesis. ***Therapeutic Effect:*** Bactericidal or bacteriostatic, depending on drug dosage.

Pharmacokinetics

Rapidly absorbed from the GI tract. Protein binding: 15%-30%.Widely distributed into tissues and within cells. Eliminated primarily unchanged by biliary excretion. Not removed by hemodialysis. ***Half-life:*** 30-44 hr.

INDICATIONS AND DOSAGES

Pharyngitis, tonsillitis

PO

Adults, Elderly, Children 12 yr and older. 500 mg once a day for 10 days.

Acute or chronic bronchitis, skin and skin-structure infections

PO

Adults, Elderly, Children 12 yr and older. 500 mg once a day for 7 days.

Community-acquired pneumonia

PO

Adults, Elderly, Children 12 yr and older. 500 mg once a day for 14 days.

AVAILABLE FORMS
- *Tablets (Enteric-Coated [Dynabac, Dynabac D5-Pak]):* 250 mg.

CONTRAINDICATIONS: Hypersensitivity to other macrolide antibiotics

PREGNANCY AND LACTATION: Pregnancy category C; excreted into rodent breast milk; no human data

SIDE EFFECTS

Frequent (10%-8%)

Abdominal pain, headache, nausea, diarrhea

Occasional (3%-2%)

Vomiting, dyspepsia, dizziness, nonspecific pain, asthenia

Rare (less than 2%)

Increased cough, flatulence, rash, dyspnea, pruritus and urticaria, insomnia

SERIOUS REACTIONS
- Antibiotic-associated colitis and other superinfections may result from altered bacterial balance.

INTERACTIONS

Drugs

3 *Aluminum- and magnesium-containing antacids:* May decrease dirithromycin blood concentration

3 *H2 antagonists:* Increase dirithromycin absorption

3 *Penicillins:* Dirithromycin may inhibit antibacterial activity of penicillins

SPECIAL CONSIDERATIONS
- Long $t_{1/2}$ and higher tissue concentrations allow qd dosing; however, the improved antimicrobial activity against *H. influenzae* and lower incidence of GI adverse effects have not been realized with this agent; azithromycin probably best choice pending further comparisons

PATIENT/FAMILY EDUCATION
- Take with food or within 1 hr of having eaten
- Continue therapy for the full length of treatment
- If the patient must take an antacid containing aluminum or magnesium, take the drug 1 hr before or 2 hrs after the antacid

MONITORING PARAMETERS
- WBC count to determine if the infection is improving

• Evaluate for diarrhea, GI discomfort, headache, and nausea
• Pattern of daily bowel activity and stool consistency
• Evaluate for signs and symptoms of superinfection, including anal or genital pruritus, moderate to severe diarrhea, abdominal cramps, fever, and sore mouth or tongue

disopyramide phosphate

(dye-soe-peer'-a-mide foss'-fate)
Rx: Norpace, Norpace CR
Chemical Class: Pyramide derivative
Therapeutic Class: Antiarrhythmic, class IA

CLINICAL PHARMACOLOGY
Mechanism of Action: An antiarrhythmic that prolongs the refractory period of the cardiac cell by direct effect, decreasing myocardial excitability and conduction velocity. ***Therapeutic Effect:*** Depresses myocardial contractility. Has anticholinergic and negative inotropic effects.
Pharmacokinetics
Rapidly and almost completely absorbed from the GI tract. Protein binding: 50%-65%. Metabolized in liver. Excreted in urine. Removed by hemodialysis. ***Half-life:*** 4-10 hr.
INDICATIONS AND DOSAGES
Suppression and prevention of ventricular ectopy, unifocal or multifocal premature ventricular contractions, paired ventricular contractions (couplets), and episodes of ventricular tachycardia
PO
Adults, Elderly weighing 50 kg and more. 150 mg q6h (300 mg ql2h with extended-release).
Adults, Elderly weighing less than 50 kg. 100 mg q6h (200 mg q12h with extended-release).
Usual pediatric dosage
PO (Immediate-Release Capsules)
Children 12-18 yr. 6-15 mg/kg/day in divided doses q6h.
Children 5-11 yr. 10-15 mg/kg/day in divided doses q6h.
Children 1-4 yr. 10-20 mg/kg/day in divided doses q6h.
Children younger than 1 yr. 10-30 mg/kg/day in divided doses q6h.
Dosage in renal impairment
With or without loading dose of 150 mg:

Creatinine Clearance	*Dosage*
40 ml/min and higher	100 mg q6h (extended-release 200 mg q12h)
30-39 ml/min	100 mg q8h
15-29 ml/min	100 mg q12h
less than 15 ml/min	100 mg q24h

Dosage in liver impairment
Adults, Elderly weighing 50 kg and more. 100 mg q6h (200 mg q12h with extended-release).
Dosage in cardiomyopathy, cardiac decompensation
Adults, Elderly weighing 50 kg and more. No loading dose; 100 mg q6-8h with gradual dosage adjustments.
AVAILABLE FORMS
• *Capsules (Norpace):* 100 mg, 150 mg.
• *Capsules (Extended-Release [Norpace CR]):* 100 mg, 150 mg.
UNLABELED USES: Prophylaxis and treatment of supraventricular tachycardia
CONTRAINDICATIONS: Cardiogenic shock, congenital QT prolon-

gation, narrow-angle glaucoma (unless patient is undergoing cholinergic therapy), preexisting second- or third-degree AV block, preexisting urinary retention

PREGNANCY AND LACTATION: Pregnancy category C; excreted in breast milk

SIDE EFFECTS

Frequent (greater than 9%)

Dry mouth (32%), urinary hesitancy, constipation

Occasional (9%-3%)

Blurred vision, dry eyes, nose, or throat, urinary retention, headache, dizziness, fatigue, nausea

Rare (less than 1%)

Impotence, hypotension, edema, weight gain, shortness of breath, syncope, chest pain, nervousness, diarrhea, vomiting, decreased appetite, rash, itching

SERIOUS REACTIONS

- May produce or aggravate CHF.
- May produce severe hypotension, shortness of breath, chest pain, syncope (especially in patients with primary cardiomyopathy or CHF).
- Hepatotoxicity occurs rarely.

INTERACTIONS

Drugs

3 *Barbiturates, phenytoin, rifampin:* Reduced disopyramide level via induction

3 *β-blockers:* Enhanced negative inotropy

3 *Clarithromycin, erythromycin, troleandromycin:* Macrolide increased disopyramide-serum concentration resulting in dysrhythmias

3 *Diltiazem,verapamil:* May prolong cardiac conduction and decrease cardiac output

3 *Lidocaine:* Arrhythmias or heart failure in predisposed patients

3 *Pimozide:* Increased risk of cardiac arrhythmias

3 *Potassium, potassium-sparing diuretics:* Increased potassium concentration can enhance disopyramide effects on myocardial conduction

Labs

- *Increase:* Liver enzymes, lipids, BUN, creatinine
- *Decrease:* Hgb/Hct, blood glucose

SPECIAL CONSIDERATIONS

- Due to potential for prodysrhythmic effects, use for asymptomatic PVCs or lesser dysrhythmias should be avoided

PATIENT/FAMILY EDUCATION

- Notify the physician if productive cough or shortness of breath occurs
- Do not take nasal decongestants or OTC cold preparations, especially those containing stimulants, without consulting the physician for approval
- Limit alcohol and salt consumption

MONITORING PARAMETERS

- Monitor ECG closely; if PR, QRS, or QT interval increases by 25%, stop drug
- Therapeutic plasma levels are 2-4 mcg/ml
- Blood glucose, liver enzymes, and serum alkaline phosphatase, bilirubin, and potassium, AST (SGOT), and ALT (SGPT) levels
- Intake and output
- Signs and symptoms of CHF, including cough, dyspnea (particularly on exertion), fatigue, and rales at the base of the lungs

dobutamine hydrochloride

(doe-byoo′-ta-meen hye-droe-klor′-ide)

Chemical Class: Catecholamine, synthetic

Therapeutic Class: Sympathomimetic; β-adrenergic agonist

CLINICAL PHARMACOLOGY

Mechanism of Action: A direct-acting inotropic agent acting primarily on $beta_1$-adrenergic receptors. ***Therapeutic Effect:*** Decreases preload and afterload, and enhances myocardial contractility, stroke volume, and cardiac output. Improves renal blood flow and urine output.

Pharmacokinetics

Route	Onset	Peak	Duration
IV	1-2 min	10 min	Length of infusion

Metabolized in the liver. Primarily excreted in urine. Not removed by hemodialysis. ***Half-life:*** 2 min.

INDICATIONS AND DOSAGES

Short-term management of cardiac decompensation

IV Infusion

Adults, Elderly, Children. 2.5-20 mcg/kg/min. Rarely, drug can be infused at a rate of up to 40 mcg/kg/min to increase cardiac output.

Neonates. 2-15 mcg/kg/min.

AVAILABLE FORMS

- *Infusion (Ready-to-Use):* 1 mg/ml, 2 mg/ml, 4 mg/ml.
- *Injection:* 12.5-mg/ml vial.

CONTRAINDICATIONS: Hypovolemia patients, idiopathic hypertrophic subaortic stenosis, sulfite sensitivity

PREGNANCY AND LACTATION: Pregnancy category B; excreted in breast milk

SIDE EFFECTS

Frequent (greater than 5%)

Increased heart rate, increased BP

Occasional (5%-3%)

Pain at injection site

Rare (3%-1%)

Nausea, headache, anginal pain, shortness of breath, fever

SERIOUS REACTIONS

- Overdose may produce a marked increase in heart rate (by 30 beats/minute or higher) marked increase in BP (by 50 mm Hg or higher), anginal pain, and premature ventricular contractions (PVCs).

INTERACTIONS

Drugs

3 *β-blockers:* May antagonize the effects of dobutamine

3 *Digoxin:* May increase the risk of arrhythmias and enhance the inotropic effect of both drugs

3 *Entacapone:* May increase the risk of tachycardia, hypertension, and arrhythmias

3 *MAOIs, oxytocics, tricyclic antidepressants:* May increase the adverse effects of dobutamine, such as arrhythmias and hypertension

3 *Sodium bicarbonate:* Alkalinizing substances inactivate dobutamine

SPECIAL CONSIDERATIONS

PATIENT/FAMILY EDUCATION

- Report chest pain or palpitations during the infusion or pain or burning at the IV site

MONITORING PARAMETERS

- Continuously monitor ECG, BP, and PCWP
- Signs and symptoms of infiltration of the IV solution, which can cause local inflammatory changes and possible dermal necrosis
- Intake and output
- Serum potassium levels
- Dobutamine plasma levels; dobutamine's therapeutic range is 40-190 ng/ml

docusate

(dok'-yoo-sate)

OTC: *Docusate Sodium:* Colace, Dioeze, Diocto, DOK, DOSS DSS, Modane Soft, Regulax SS

OTC: *Docusate Calcium:* Sulfolax, Surfak Stool Softener

Combinations

OTC: with senna concentrate (Senokot-S); with phenolphthalein (Doxidan); with casanthranol (Peri-Colace); with cascara sagrada (Nature's Remedy)

Chemical Class: Anionic surfactant

Therapeutic Class: Laxative, stool softener

CLINICAL PHARMACOLOGY

Mechanism of Action: A bulk-producing laxative that decreases surface film tension by mixing liquid and bowel contents. ***Therapeutic Effect:*** Increases infiltration of liquid to form a softer stool.

Pharmacokinetics

Minimal absorption from the GI tract. Acts in small and large intestines. Results usually occur 1-2 days after first dose, but may take 3-5 days.

INDICATIONS AND DOSAGES

Stool softener

PO

Adults, Elderly, Children 12 yr and older. 50-500 mg/day in 1-4 divided doses.

Children 6-11 yr. 40-150 mg/day in 1-4 divided doses.

Children 3-5 yr. 20-60 mg/day in 1-4 divided doses.

Children younger than 3 yr. 10-40 mg in 1-4 divided doses.

AVAILABLE FORMS

- *Capsules:* 50 mg (Colace), 100 mg (Colace, Ducosoft-S), 240 mg (Surfak).
- *Liquid (Colace):* 50 mg/5 ml (sodium).
- *Syrup (Colace, Diocto):* 60 mg/15 ml.

CONTRAINDICATIONS: Acute abdominal pain, concomitant use of mineral oil, intestinal obstruction, nausea, vomiting

PREGNANCY AND LACTATION: Pregnancy category C; no reports linking use of docusate with congenital defects have been located; diarrhea has been reported in 1 infant exposed to docusate while breast-feeding, but relationship between symptom and drug is unknown

SIDE EFFECTS

Occasional

Mild GI cramping, throat irritation (with liquid preparation)

Rare

Rash

SERIOUS REACTIONS

- None known.

INTERACTIONS

Drugs

3 *Danthron, mineral oil:* May increase the absorption of danthron or mineral oil

SPECIAL CONSIDERATIONS

PATIENT/FAMILY EDUCATION

- Drink plenty of water during administration
- Institute measures to promote defecation, such as increasing fluid intake, exercising, and eating a high-fiber diet
- Notify the physician if unrelieved constipation, dizziness, muscle cramps or pain, rectal bleeding, or weakness occurs
- Notify the physician of sudden changes in bowel habits or over 2 wks duration

MONITORING PARAMETERS
• Daily bowel activity and stool consistency
• Bowel sounds for peristalsis

dofetilide

(doe-fet'-il-ide)
Rx: Tikosyn
Chemical Class: Methanesulfonanilide derivative
Therapeutic Class: Antiarrhythmic, class III

CLINICAL PHARMACOLOGY
Mechanism of Action: A selective potassium channel blocker that prolongs repolarization without affecting conduction velocity by blocking one or more time-dependent potassium currents. Dofetilide has no effect on sodium channels or adrenergic alpha or beta receptors. ***Therapeutic Effect:*** Terminates reentrant tachyarrhythmias, preventing reinduction.
Pharmacokinetics
Well absorbed from the GI tract. Protein binding: 60%-70%. Metabolized in liver. Primarily excreted in urine; minimal elimination in feces. ***Half-life:*** 7.5-10 hr.
INDICATIONS AND DOSAGES
Maintain normal sinus rhythm after conversion from atrial fibrillation or flutter
PO
Adults, Elderly. Individualized using a seven-step dosing algorithm dependent upon calculated creatinine clearance and QT interval measurements.
AVAILABLE FORMS
• *Capsules:* 125 mcg, 250 mcg, 500 mcg.
CONTRAINDICATIONS: Concurrent use of drugs that prolong the QT interval; concurrent use of amiodarone, megestrol, prochlorperazine, or verapamil; congenital or acquired prolonged QT syndrome; paroxysmal atrial fibrillation; severe renal impairment
PREGNANCY AND LACTATION: Pregnancy category C; no information on the presence of dofetilide in breast milk; breast-feeding while on dofetilide not advised
SIDE EFFECTS
Occasional (less than 5%)
Headache, chest pain, dizziness, dyspnea, nausea, insomnia, back and abdominal pain, diarrhea, rash
SERIOUS REACTIONS
• Angioedema, bradycardia, cerebral ischemia, facial paralysis, and serious ventricular arrhythmias or various forms of heart block may be noted.
INTERACTIONS
Drugs
3 *Amiloride:* May compete with dofetilide for renal cationic secretion and subsequently increase dofetilide levels
2 *Cimetidine:* Increases dofetilide levels by 13%-58%, dose dependent
2 *Ketoconazole and other azole antifungals:* Increases dofetilide levels by 53%-97% by inhibition of CYP3A4
3 *Metformin:* May compete with dofetilide for renal cationic secretion and subsequently increase dofetilide levels
2 *Sulfamethoxazole:* Increases dofetilide AUC by 93% and Cmax by 103%
3 *Triamterene:* May compete with dofetilide for renal cationic secretion and subsequently increase dofetilide levels
2 *Trimethoprim:* Increases dofetilide AUC by 93% and Cmax by 103%

❷ *Verapamil:* Increases dofetilide levels by 42% and increased risk of torsade de pointes

❸ *Other potential drug interactions:* Macrolide antibiotics, protease inhibitors, serotonin reuptake inhibitors, amiodarone, cannabinoids, diltiazem, grapefruit juice, nefazadone, norfloxacin, quinine, zafirlukast: potential to increase dofetilide concentrations via inhibition of CYP3A4

SPECIAL CONSIDERATIONS

PATIENT/FAMILY EDUCATION

- Take without regard to food
- Dofetilide therapy compliance is essential and dosing instructions must be followed diligently
- Notify the physician if dizziness, severe diarrhea, or other adverse effects occur

MONITORING PARAMETERS

- ECG, QTc intervals, renal function

---

dolasetron

(dol-a'-se-tron)

Rx: Anzemat

Chemical Class: Nonbenzamide

Therapeutic Class: Antiemetic

CLINICAL PHARMACOLOGY

Mechanism of Action: A 5-HT_3 receptor antagonist that acts centrally in the chemoreceptor trigger zone and peripherally at the vagal nerve terminals. ***Therapeutic Effect:*** Prevents nausea and vomiting.

Pharmacokinetics

Readily absorbed from the GI tract after PO administration. Protein binding: 69%-77%. Metabolized in the liver. Primarily excreted in urine. Unknown if removed by hemodialysis. ***Half-life:*** 5-10 hr.

INDICATIONS AND DOSAGES

Prevention of chemotherapy-induced nausea and vomiting

PO

Adults. 100 mg within 1 hr of chemotherapy.

Children 2-16 yr. 1.8 mg/kg within 1 hr of chemotherapy. Maximum: 100 mg.

IV

Adults, Children 1-16 yr. 1.8 mg/kg as a single dose 30 min before chemotherapy. Maximum: 100 mg.

Treatment or prevention of postoperative nausea or vomiting

PO

Adults. 100 mg within 2 hr of surgery.

Children 2-16 yr. 1.2 mg/kg within 2 hr of surgery. Maximum: 100 mg.

IV

Adults. 12.5 mg 15 min before cessation of anesthesia or as soon as nausea occurs.

Children 2-16 yr. 0.35 mg/kg 15 min before cessation of anesthesia or as soon as nausea occurs. Maximum: 12.5 mg.

AVAILABLE FORMS

- *Tablets:* 50 mg, 100 mg.
- *Injection:* 20 mg/ml in single-use 0.625-ml amps, 0.625 ml fill in 2-ml Carpuject and 5-ml vials.

UNLABELED USES: Radiation therapy–induced nausea and vomiting

CONTRAINDICATIONS: None known.

PREGNANCY AND LACTATION: Pregnancy category B; excretion in breast milk unknown; use caution in nursing mothers

SIDE EFFECTS

Frequent (10%-5%)

Headache, diarrhea, fatigue

Occasional (5%-1%)

Fever, dizziness, tachycardia, dyspepsia

SERIOUS REACTIONS

• Overdose may produce a combination of CNS stimulant and depressant effects.

SPECIAL CONSIDERATIONS

• No obvious advantage over other agents in this class (ondansetron, granisetron)

PATIENT/FAMILY EDUCATION

• Do not cut, break, or chew film-coated tablets

• The postoperative patient should report nausea as soon as it occurs because prompt administration of the drug increases its effectiveness

• The patient should try other methods of reducing nausea, such as lying quietly and avoiding strong odors

MONITORING PARAMETERS

• Relief of nausea and vomiting

• EKG

donepezil hydrochloride

(doe-nep'-e-zil hye-droe-klor'-ide)

Rx: Aricept, Aricept ODT

Chemical Class: Cholinesterase inhibitor; piperidine derivative

Therapeutic Class: Antidementia agent; cholinergic

CLINICAL PHARMACOLOGY

Mechanism of Action: A cholinesterase inhibitor that inhibits the enzyme acetylcholinesterase, thus increasing the concentration of acetylcholine at cholinergic synapses and enhancing cholinergic function in the CNS. ***Therapeutic Effect:*** Slows the progression of Alzheimer's disease.

Pharmacokinetics

Well absorbed after PO administration. Protein binding: 96%. Extensively metabolized. Eliminated in urine and feces. ***Half-life:*** 70 hr.

INDICATIONS AND DOSAGES

Alzheimer's disease

PO

Adults, Elderly. Initially, 5 mg/day at bedtime. May increase at 4-6 wk interval to 10 mg/day at bedtime.

AVAILABLE FORMS

• *Tablets (Aricept):* 5 mg, 10 mg.

• *Tablets (Orally Disintegrating [Aricept ODT]):* 5 mg, 10 mg.

UNLABELED USES: Treatment of attention deficit hyperactivity disorder, autism, behavioral syndromes in dementia

CONTRAINDICATIONS: History of hypersensitivity to piperidine derivatives

PREGNANCY AND LACTATION: Pregnancy category C

SIDE EFFECTS

Frequent (11%-8%)

Nausea, diarrhea, headache, insomnia, nonspecific pain, dizziness

Occasional (6%-3%)

Mild muscle cramps, fatigue, vomiting, anorexia, ecchymosis

Rare (3%-2%)

Depression, abnormal dreams, weight loss, arthritis, somnolence, syncope, frequent urination

SERIOUS REACTIONS

• Overdose may result in cholinergic crisis, characterized by severe nausea, increased salivation, diaphoresis, bradycardia, hypotension, flushed skin, abdominal pain, respiratory depression, seizures, and cardiorespiratory collapse. Increasing muscle weakness may result in death if respiratory muscles are involved. The antidote is 1-2 mg IV atropine sulfate with subsequent doses based on therapeutic response.

INTERACTIONS

Drugs

3 *Anticholinergics:* May decrease the effect of anticholinergics

3 *Cholinergic agonists, neuromuscular blockers, succinylcholine:* May increase the synergistic effects of these drugs

3 *Ketoconazole, quinidine:* May inhibit the metabolism of donepezil

3 *NSAIDs:* May increase gastric acid secretion of NSAIDs

3 *Paroxetine:* May decrease the metabolism and increase the blood concentration of donepezil

SPECIAL CONSIDERATIONS

- Clinicians were unable to notice improvement in the majority of patients in clinical trials; advantages over tacrine include qd dosing and apparent lack of liver toxicity

PATIENT/FAMILY EDUCATION

- May be taken with or without food
- Notify the physician if abdominal pain, diarrhea, excessive sweating or salivation, dizziness, or nausea and vomiting occur
- Donepezil is not a cure for Alzheimer's disease but may slow the progression of its symptoms

MONITORING PARAMETERS

- Close monitoring for clinical improvement and periodic reassessment of need for continued therapy
- Monitor the patient's behavioral, cognitive, and functional status
- Monitor the patient for cholinergic reactions, such as diaphoresis, dizziness, excessive salivation, facial warmth, abdominal cramps or discomfort, lacrimation, pallor, and urinary urgency
- Monitor the patient for diarrhea, headache, insomnia, and nausea

dopamine hydrochloride

(doe'-pa-meen)

Chemical Class: Catecholamine, synthetic

Therapeutic Class: Vasopressor; α- and β-adrenergic sympathomimetic

CLINICAL PHARMACOLOGY

Mechanism of Action: A sympathomimetic (adrenergic agonist) that stimulates adrenergic receptors. Effects are dose dependent. Low dosages (less than 5 mcg/kg/min) stimulate dopaminergic receptors, causing renal vasodilation. Low to moderate dosages (10 mcg/kg/min or less) have a positive inotropic effect by direct action and release of norepinephrine. High dosages (greater than 10 mcg/kg/min) stimulate alpha-receptors. ***Therapeutic Effect:*** With low dosages, increases renal blood flow, urine flow, and sodium excretion. With low to moderate dosages, increases myocardial contractility, stroke volume, and cardiac output. With high dosages, increases peripheral resistance, renal vasoconstriction, and systolic and diastolic BP.

Pharmacokinetics

Route	*Onset*	*Peak*	*Duration*
IV	1-2 min	N/A	less than 10 min

Widely distributed. Does not cross blood-brain barrier. Metabolized in the liver, kidney, and plasma. Primarily excreted in urine. Not removed by hemodialysis. ***Half-life:*** 2 min.

INDICATIONS AND DOSAGES

Treatment and prevention of acute hypotension, shock (associated with cardiac decompensation, MI, open heart surgery, renal failure,

or trauma); treatment of low cardiac output; treatment of CHF

IV

Adults, Elderly. 1 mcg/kg/min up to 50 mcg/kg/min titrated to desired response.

Children. 1-20 mcg/kg/min. Maximum: 50 mcg/kg/min.

Neonates. 1-20 mcg/kg/min.

AVAILABLE FORMS

• *Injection:* 40 mg/ml, 80 mg/ml, 160 mg/ml.

• *Injection (Premix with dextrose):* 80 mg/100 ml, 160 mg/100 ml, 320 mg/100 ml.

CONTRAINDICATIONS: Pheochromocytoma, sulfite sensitivity, uncorrected tachyarrhythmias, ventricular fibrillation

PREGNANCY AND LACTATION: Pregnancy category C; because dopamine is indicated only in life-threatening situations, chronic use would not be expected; no data available regarding use in breast-feeding

SIDE EFFECTS

Frequent

Headache, ectopic beats, tachycardia, anginal pain, palpitations, vasoconstriction, hypotension, nausea, vomiting, dyspnea

Occasional

Piloerection or goose bumps, bradycardia, widening of QRS complex

SERIOUS REACTIONS

• High doses may produce ventricular arrhythmias.

• Patients with occlusive vascular disease are at high risk for further compromise of circulation to the extremities, which may result in gangrene.

• Tissue necrosis with sloughing may occur with extravasation of IV solution.

INTERACTIONS

Drugs

3 *β-blockers:* May decrease the effects of dopamine

3 *Ergot alkaloids:* Gangrene has been reported

2 *MAOIs:* May increase cardiac stimulation and vasopressor effects

3 *Phenytoin:* Increased risk of hypotension with IV phenytoin administration

3 *Tricyclic antidepressants:* May increase cardiovascular effects

Labs

• *False increase:* Urine amino acids, urine catecholamines, serum creatinine

• *False decrease:* Serum creatinine

SPECIAL CONSIDERATIONS

• Dilute before use if not prediluted; antidote for extravasation: infiltrate area as soon as possible with 10-15 ml NS containing 5-10 mg phentolamine

PATIENT/FAMILY EDUCATION

• Report chest pain or palpitations during the infusion or pain or burning at the IV site

MONITORING PARAMETERS

• Urine flow, cardiac output, blood pressure, pulmonary wedge pressure

• Immediately notify the physician if the patient experiences arrhythmias, decreased peripheral circulation (marked by cold, pale, or mottled extremities), decreased urine output, or significant changes in BP or heart rate. Also notify the physician if the patient fails to respond to increase or decrease in infusion rate

• Taper the dopamine dosage before discontinuing the drug because abrupt cessation of dopamine therapy may result in marked hypotension

• Be alert to excessive vasoconstriction as evidenced by decreased urine output, disproportionate increase in diastolic BP, and increased arrhythmias or heart rate. Slow or temporarily stop the dopamine infusion and notify the physician if excessive vasoconstriction occurs

dornase alfa

(door'-nace al'-fa)

Rx: Pulmozyme

Chemical Class: Recombinant human deoxyribonuclease I

Therapeutic Class: Mucolytic

CLINICAL PHARMACOLOGY

Mechanism of Action: An enzyme that selectively splits and hydrolyzes DNA in sputum. ***Therapeutic Effect:*** Reduces sputum viscosity and elasticity.

Pharmacokinetics

Minimal absorption occurs via inhalation.

INDICATIONS AND DOSAGES

To improve management of pulmonary function in patients with cystic fibrosis

Nebulization

Adults, Children older than 5 yr. 2.5 mg (1 ampule) once daily by recommended nebulizer. May increase to 2.5 mg twice daily.

AVAILABLE FORMS

• *Inhalation:* 2.5 mg/2.5 ml ampules for nebulization.

CONTRAINDICATIONS: Sensitivity to epoetin alfa

PREGNANCY AND LACTATION: Pregnancy category B; excretion into breast milk unknown; however, since serum levels of DNase have not been shown to increase above endogenous levels, little drug would be expected to be excreted into breast milk

SIDE EFFECTS

Frequent (greater than 10%)

Pharyngitis, chest pain or discomfort, voice changes

Occasional (10%-3%)

Conjunctivitis, hoarseness, rash

SERIOUS REACTIONS

• None significant.

SPECIAL CONSIDERATIONS

• Safety and efficacy have been demonstrated only with the following nebulizers and compressors: disposable jet nebulizer *Hudson T Updraft II,* disposable jet nebulizer *Marquest Acorn II* in conjunction with a *Pulmo-Aide* compressor, and reusable *PARI LC Jet+* nebulizer in conjunction with the *PARI PRONEB* compressor

PATIENT/FAMILY EDUCATION

• Must be stored in refrigerator at 2-8°C and protected from strong light (keep refrigerated when transporting and do not leave at room temp for >24 hr)

• Do not dilute or mix with other drugs in nebulizer

• Hoarseness, chest pain, or sore throat may occur during dornase alfa therapy

• Drink plenty of fluids

MONITORING PARAMETERS

• Check for decreased viscosity of pulmonary secretions

• Assess for relief of dyspnea and fatigue

doxapram hydrochloride

(dox'-a-pram)

Rx: Dopram

Chemical Class: Pyrrolidinone derivative

Therapeutic Class: Analeptic

CLINICAL PHARMACOLOGY

Mechanism of Action: A central nervous system stimulant that directly stimulates the respiratory center in the medulla or indirectly by effects on the carotid. ***Therapeutic Effect:*** Increases pulmonary ventilation by increasing resting minute ventilation, tidal volume, respiratory frequency, and inspiratory neuromuscular drive, and enhances the ventilatory response to carbon dioxide.

Pharmacokinetics

IV onset 20-40 sec, peak 1-2 min, duration 5-12 min. Metabolized in the liver to metabolites, ketodoxapram (active) and desethyldoxapram (inactive). Partially excreted in the urine. Not removed by hemodialysis. ***Half-life:*** 2.4-9.9 hrs.

INDICATIONS AND DOSAGES

Chronic obstructive pulmonary disease (COPD)

IV infusion

Adults, Elderly, Children older than 12 yrs. Initially, 1-2 mg/min. Maximum: 3 g/day for no more than 2 hrs.

Drug-induced CNS depression

IV injection

Adults, Elderly, Children older than 12 yrs. Initially, 1-2 mg/kg, repeat after 5 min. May repeat at 1-2 hour intervals, until sustained consciousness. Maximum: 3 g/day.

IV infusion

Adults, Elderly, Children older than 12 yrs. Initially, bolus dose of 2 mg/kg, repeat after 5 min. If no response, wait 1-2 hrs and repeat. If stimulation is noted, initiate infusion at 1-3 mg/min. Infusion should not be continued for more than 2 hrs. Maximum: 3 g/day.

Respiratory depression

IV injection

Adults, Elderly, Children older than 12 yrs. Initially, 0.5-1 mg/kg. May repeat at 5-min intervals in patients who demonstrate initial response. Maximum: 2 mg/kg.

IV infusion

Adults, Elderly, Children older than 12 yrs. Initially, 5 mg/min until adequate response or adverse effects are seen. Decrease to 1-3 mg/min. Maximum: 4 mg/kg.

AVAILABLE FORMS

- *Injection:* 20 mg/ml (Dopram).

UNLABELED USES: Apnea of prematurity, sleep apnea, congenital central hypoventilation syndrome, obesity-hypoventilation syndrome, post-anesthetic respiratory depression, shivering

CONTRAINDICATIONS: Convulsive disorders, cardiovascular impairment, head injury or cerebral vascular accident, severe hypertension, mechanical ventilation disorders, newborns, hypersensitivity to doxapram

PREGNANCY AND LACTATION: Pregnancy category B; excretion into breast milk unknown

SIDE EFFECTS

Occasional

Flushing, sweating, pruritus, disorientation, headache, dizziness, hyperactivity, convulsions, dyspnea, cough, tachypnea, hiccough, rebound hypoventilation, phlebitis, variations in heart rate, arrhythmias, chest pain, nausea, vomiting, diarrhea, stimulation of urinary bladder with spontaneous voiding

SERIOUS REACTIONS

- Overdosage may produce extensions of the pharmacologic effects of the drug. Excessive pressor effect, skeletal muscle hyperactivity, tachycardia, and enhanced deep tendon reflexes may be early signs of overdosage.

INTERACTIONS

Drugs

3 *Anesthetics, inhalation:* Sensitized myocardium at risk of arrhythmia; delay administration of doxapram 10 min

3 *CNS stimulant medications:* May increase the risk of stimulation to excessive levels, causing nervousness, insomnia, irritability, or possible cardiac arrhythmias or seizures

❷ *MAOIs:* Additive pressor effect

SPECIAL CONSIDERATIONS

PATIENT/FAMILY EDUCATION

- Notify the nurse on duty immediately of trouble breathing

MONITORING PARAMETERS

- Baseline ABG then q30 min (for use in COPD)
- Blood pressure, heart rate, deep tendon reflexes

doxazosin mesylate

(dox-ay'-zoe-sin)

Rx: Cardura, Cardura XL

Chemical Class: Quinazoline derivative

Therapeutic Class: Antihypertensive; α_1-adrenergic blocker

CLINICAL PHARMACOLOGY

Mechanism of Action: An antihypertensive that selectively blocks alpha$_1$-adrenergic receptors, decreasing peripheral vascular resistance. ***Therapeutic Effect:*** Causes peripheral vasodilation and lowers BP. Also relaxes smooth muscle of bladder and prostate.

Pharmacokinetics

Route	Onset	Peak	Duration
PO	N/A	2-6 hr	24 hr

Well absorbed from the GI tract. Protein binding: 98%-99%. Metabolized in the liver. Primarily eliminated in feces. Not removed by hemodialysis. ***Half-life:*** 19-22 hr.

INDICATIONS AND DOSAGES

Mild to moderate hypertension

PO

Adults. Initially, 1 mg once a day. May increase to a maximum of 16 mg/day.

Elderly. Initially, 0.5 mg once a day.

Benign prostatic hyperplasia, alone or in combination with finasteride (Proscar)

PO

Adults, Elderly. Initially, 1 mg/day. May increase q1-2 wk. Maximum: 8 mg/day.

AVAILABLE FORMS

- *Tablets:* 1 mg, 2 mg, 4 mg, 8 mg.

CONTRAINDICATIONS: Hypersensitivity to other quinazolines

PREGNANCY AND LACTATION: Pregnancy category C; may accumulate in breast milk; use caution in nursing mothers

SIDE EFFECTS

Frequent (20%-10%)

Dizziness, asthenia, headache, edema

Occasional (9%-3%)

Nausea, pharyngitis, rhinitis, pain in extremities, somnolence

Rare (3%-1%)

Palpitations, diarrhea, constipation, dyspnea, myalgia, altered vision, dizziness, nervousness

SERIOUS REACTIONS

• First-dose syncope (hypotension with sudden loss of consciousness) may occur 30-90 mins following initial dose of 2 mg or greater, a too-rapid increase in dosage, or addition of another antihypertensive agent to therapy. First-dose syncope may be preceded by tachycardia (pulse rate of 120-160 beats/minute).

INTERACTIONS

Drugs

3 *ACE inhibitors:* Increased potential for first-dose hypotension

3 *Estrogen, NSAIDs:* May decrease the effect of doxazosin

3 *Hypotension-producing medications:* May increase the effect of doxazosin

3 *Indomethacin:* Decreased hypotensive effect of doxazosin

3 *Sildenafil, tadalafil, vardenafil:* May potentiate hypotensive effects

3 *Verapamil, nifedipine:* Enhanced hypotensive effects of both drugs

3 *β-adrenergic blockers:* Exaggerated first-dose response

Labs

• False positive urinary metabolites of norepinephrine and VMA

• No effect on prostate specific antigen (PSA)

SPECIAL CONSIDERATIONS

• The doxazosin arm of the ALLHAT study was stopped early; the doxazosin group had a 25% greater risk of combined cardiovascular disease events, which was primarily accounted for by a doubled risk of CHF vs the chlorthalidone group; doxazosin was also found to be less effective at controlling systolic BP an average of 3 mm Hg; may want to consider primary antihypertensives in addition to α-blockers for BPH symptoms

• Use as a single antihypertensive agent limited by tendency to cause sodium and water retention and increased plasma volume

PATIENT/FAMILY EDUCATION

• Alert patient to the possibility of syncopal and orthostatic symptoms, especially with first dose ("first-dose syncope")

• Initial dose should be administered at bedtime in the smallest possible dose

• Full therapeutic effect may not appear for 3-4 wks

• Avoid performing tasks that require mental alertness or motor skills until response to doxazosin has been established

MONITORING PARAMETERS

• Pulse

• Assess for edema and headache

doxepin hydrochloride

(dox'-eh-pin hye-droe-klor'-ide)

Rx: Prudoxin, Sinequan, Zonalon

Chemical Class: Dibenzoxepin derivative; tertiary amine

Therapeutic Class: Antidepressant, tricyclic; antipruritic, topical

CLINICAL PHARMACOLOGY

Mechanism of Action: A tricyclic antidepressant, antianxiety agent, antineuralgic agent, antipruritic, and antiulcer agent that increases synaptic concentrations of norepinephrine and serotonin. ***Therapeutic Effect:*** Produces antidepressant and anxiolytic effects.

Pharmacokinetics

Rapidly and well absorbed from the GI tract. Protein binding: 80%-85%. Metabolized in the liver to active metabolite. Primarily excreted in urine. Not removed by hemodialysis. ***Half-life:*** 6-8 hr. Topical: Absorbed through the skin. Distributed to body tissues. Metabolized to active metabolite. Excreted in urine.

INDICATIONS AND DOSAGES

Depression, anxiety

PO

Adults. 30-150 mg/day at bedtime or in 2-3 divided doses. May increase to 300 mg/day.

Elderly. Initially, 10-25 mg at bedtime. May increase by 10-25 mg/day every 3-7 days. Maximum: 75 mg/day.

Adolescents. Initially, 25-50 mg/day as a single dose or in divided doses. May increase to 100 mg/day.

Children 12 yr and younger. 1-3 mg/kg/day.

Pruritus associated with eczema

Topical

Adults, Elderly. Apply thin film 4 times a day.

AVAILABLE FORMS

- *Capsules (Sinequan):* 10 mg, 25 mg, 50 mg, 75 mg, 100 mg, 150 mg.
- *Oral Concentrate (Sinequan):* 10 mg/ml.
- *Cream (Prudoxin, Zonalon):* 5%.

UNLABELED USES: Treatment of neurogenic pain, panic disorder; prevention of vascular headache, pruritus in idiopathic urticaria

CONTRAINDICATIONS: Angle-closure glaucoma, hypersensitivity to other tricyclic antidepressants, urine retention

PREGNANCY AND LACTATION: Pregnancy category C (topical formulation is category B); paralytic ileus has been observed in an infant exposed to doxepin and chlorpromazine at term; excreted into breast milk (as well as active metabolite); effect on nursing infant unknown, but may be of concern

SIDE EFFECTS

Frequent

Oral: Orthostatic hypotension, somnolence, dry mouth, headache, increased appetite, weight gain, nausea, unusual fatigue, unpleasant taste

Topical: Edema; increased pruritus and eczema; burning, tingling, or stinging at application site; altered taste; dizziness; drowsiness; dry skin; dry mouth; fatigue; headache; thirst

Occasional

Oral: Blurred vision, confusion, constipation, hallucinations, difficult urination, eye pain, irregular heartbeat, fine muscle tremors, nervousness, impaired sexual function, diarrhea, diaphoresis, heartburn, insomnia

Topical: Anxiety, skin irritation or cracking, nausea

Rare

Oral: Allergic reaction, alopecia, tinnitus, breast enlargement

Topical: Fever, photosensitivity

SERIOUS REACTIONS

- Abrupt or too-rapid withdrawal may result in headache, malaise, nausea, vomiting, and vivid dreams.
- Overdose may produce seizures, dizziness, and cardiovascular effects, such as severe orthostatic hypotension, tachycardia, palpitations, and arrhythmias.

INTERACTIONS

Drugs

3 *Barbiturates:* Reduced serum concentrations of cyclic antidepressants

2 *Bethanidine:* Reduced antihypertensive effect of bethanidine

3 *Carbamazepine:* Reduced cyclic antidepressant serum concentrations

3 *Cimetidine:* May increase doxepin blood concentration and risk of toxicity

❷ *Clonidine:* Reduced antihypertensive response to clonidine; enhanced hypertensive response with abrupt clonidine withdrawal
❸ *Debrisoquin:* Inhibited antihypertensive response of debrisoquin
❷ *Epinephrine:* Markedly enhanced pressor response to IV epinephrine
❸ *Ethanol:* Additive impairment of motor skills; abstinent alcoholics may eliminate cyclic antidepressants more rapidly than non-alcoholics
❸ *Fluoxetine, fluvoxamine, grapefruit juice:* Marked increases in cyclic antidepressant plasma concentrations
❸ *Guanethidine:* Inhibited antihypertensive response to guanethidine
❷ *Moclobemide:* Potential association with fatal or non-fatal serotonin syndrome
⚠ *MAOIs:* Excessive sympathetic response, mania, or hyperpyrexia possible
❸ *Neuroleptics:* Increased therapeutic and toxic effects of both drugs
❷ *Norepinephrine:* Markedly enhanced pressor response to norepinephrine
❷ *Phenylephrine:* Enhanced pressor response to IV phenylephrine
❸ *Propoxyphene:* Enhanced effect of cyclic antidepressants
❸ *Quinidine:* Increased cyclic antidepressant serum concentrations
❸ *Tolazamide:* May enhance the hypoglycemic effects of tolazamide
❷ *Sympathomimetics:* May increase cardiac effects

SPECIAL CONSIDERATIONS
- Equally effective as other tricyclic antidepressants for depression; distinguishing characteristics include: sedative, anxiolytic, antihistaminic properties

PATIENT/FAMILY EDUCATION
- Therapeutic effects may take 4-6 wk
- Do not discontinue abruptly after long-term use
- If drowsiness occurs with top application, decrease surface area being treated or number of daily applications
- Change positions slowly to avoid hypotensive effect
- Tolerance to postural hypotension, sedative and anticholinergic effects usually develops during early therapy
- Avoid tasks that require mental alertness or motor skills until response to the drug has been established

MONITORING PARAMETERS
- CBC; ECG; mental status: mood, sensorium, affect, suicidal tendencies
- Supervise the suicidal risk patient closely during early therapy (as depression lessens, energy level improves, increasing suicidal potential)
- Assess appearance, behavior, speech pattern, level of interest, and mood

doxercalciferol

(docks-er-kal-sif'-e-role)

Rx: Hectorol

Chemical Class: Vitamin D analog

Therapeutic Class: Hyperparathyroidism

CLINICAL PHARMACOLOGY

Mechanism of Action: A fat-soluble vitamin that is essential for absorption, utilization of calcium phosphate, and normal calcification of bone. ***Therapeutic Effect:*** Stimulates calcium and phosphate absorption from small intestine, promotes secretion of calcium from bone to blood, promotes renal tubule phosphate resorption, acts on bone cells to stimulate skeletal growth and on parathyroid gland to suppress hormone synthesis and secretion.

Pharmacokinetics

Readily absorbed from small intestine. Metabolized in liver. Partially eliminated in urine. Not removed by hemodialysis. ***Half-life:*** up to 96 hrs.

INDICATIONS AND DOSAGES

Secondary hyperparathyroidism, dialysis patients

IV

Adults, Elderly. Titrate dose to lower iPTH to 150-300 pg/ml. Adjust dose at 8-wk intervals to a maximum dose of 18 mcg/wk. Initially, if iPTH level is more than 400 pg/ml, give 4 mcg 3 times/wk after dialysis, administered as a bolus dose.

Dose titration

iPTH level decreased by 50% and more than 300 pg/ml: Dose may be increased by 1-2 mcg at 8-wk intervals as needed.

iPTH level 150-300 pg/ml: Maintain the current dose.

iPTH level <100 pg/ml: Suspend drug for 1 wk and resume at a reduced dose of at least 1 mcg lower.

PO

Adults, Elderly. Dialysis patients: Titrate dose to lower iPTH to 150-300 pg/ml. Adjust dose at 8-wk intervals to a maximum dose of 20 mcg 3 times/wk. Initially, if iPTH is more than 400 pg/ml, give 10 mcg 3 times/wk at dialysis.

Dose titration

iPTH level decreased by 50% and more than 300 pg/ml: Increase dose to 12.5 mcg 3 times/wk for 8 more wks. This titration process may continue at 8-wk intervals. Each increase should be by 2.5 mcg/dose.

iPTH level 150-300 pg/ml: Maintain current dose.

iPTH level less than 100 pg/ml: Suspend drug for 1 wk and resume at a reduced dose. Decrease each dose by at least 2.5 mcg.

Secondary hyperparathyroidism, predialysis patients

PO

Adults, Elderly. Titrate dose to lower iPTH to 35-70 pg/ml with stage 3 disease or to 70-110 pg/ml with stage 4 disease. Dose may be adjusted at 2-wk intervals with a maximum dose of 3.5 mcg/day. Begin with 1 mcg/day.

Dose titration

iPTH level more than 70 pg/ml with stage 3 disease or more than 110 pg/ml with stage 4 disease: Increase dose by 0.5 mcg every 2 wks as needed.

iPTH level 35-70 pg/ml with stage 3 disease or 70-110 pg/ml with stage 4 disease: Maintain current dose.

iPTH level is less than 35 pg/ml with stage 3 disease or less than 70 pg/ml with stage 4 disease: Suspend drug for 1 wk, then resume at a reduced dose of at least 0.5 mcg lower.

AVAILABLE FORMS

- *Capsule:* 2.5 mcg (Hectorol).
- *Injection:* 2 mcg/ml (Hectorol).

CONTRAINDICATIONS: Hypercalcemia, malabsorption syndrome, vitamin D toxicity, hypersensitivity to doxercalciferol or other vitamin D analogs

PREGNANCY AND LACTATION: Pregnancy category B; excretion into breast milk unknown; use caution in nursing mothers

SIDE EFFECTS

Occasional

Edema, headache, malaise, dizziness, nausea, vomiting, dyspnea

Rare

Bradycardia, sleep disorder, pruritus, anorexia, constipation

SERIOUS REACTIONS

• Early signs of overdosage are manifested as weakness, headache, somnolence, nausea, vomiting, dry mouth, constipation, muscle and bone pain, and metallic taste sensation.

• Later signs of overdosage are evidenced by polyuria, polydipsia, anorexia, weight loss, nocturia, photophobia, rhinorrhea, pruritus, disorientation, hallucinations, hyperthermia, hypertension, and cardiac arrhythmias.

INTERACTIONS

Drugs

3 *Cholestyramine:* Possible impaired intestinal absorption of fat-soluble vitamins

3 *Magnesium:* Possible hypermagnesemia, use not recommended

3 *Phenytoin:* Inhibits doxercalciferol synthesis

SPECIAL CONSIDERATIONS

• Do not take Ca supplements; vitamin D, or Mg containing antacids

PATIENT/FAMILY EDUCATION

• Avoid magnesium-containing antacids

• Notify the physician if weakness, loss of appetite, nausea, vomiting, excessive thirst, dry mouth, or muscle or bone pain occurs

MONITORING PARAMETERS

• iPTH, serum Ca and serum phosphate qwk during titration

• D/C drug if hypercalcemia, hyperphosphatemia, or serum Ca × serum phosphate product >70, resume when parameters decreased, at a dose ≤2.5 mcg

• Urinary Ca, alkaline phosphatase, renal function tests

doxycycline

(dox-i-sye′-kleen)

Rx: Adoxa, Atridox, Doryx, Doxy-100, Doxy Caps, Doxychel Hyclate, Monodox, Periostat, Vibramycin, Vibra-Tabs

Chemical Class: Tetracycline derivative

Therapeutic Class: Antibiotic

CLINICAL PHARMACOLOGY

Mechanism of Action: A tetracycline antibiotic that inhibits bacterial protein synthesis by binding to ribosomes. ***Therapeutic Effect:*** Bacteriostatic.

Pharmacokinetics

Rapidly and almost completely absorbed after PO administration. Protein binding: Greater than 90%. Metabolized in liver. Partially excreted in urine; partially eliminated in bile. ***Half-life:*** 15-24 hr.

INDICATIONS AND DOSAGES

Respiratory, skin, and soft-tissue infections; UTIs; pelvic inflammatory disease (PID); brucellosis; trachoma; Rocky Mountain spotted fever; typhus; Q fever; rickettsia; severe acne (Adoxa); smallpox; psittacosis; ornithosis; granuloma inguinale; lymphogranuloma venereum; intestinal amebiasis (adjunctive treatment); prevention of rheumatic fever

PO

Adults, Elderly. Initially, 100 mg q12h, then 100 mg/day as single dose or 50 mg q12h for severe infections.

Children 8 yr and older and weighing more than 45 kg. 2-4 mg/kg/day divided q12-24h. Maximum: 200 mg/day.

IV

Adults, Elderly. Initially, 200 mg as 1-2 infusions; then 100-200 mg/day in 1-2 divided doses.

Children 8 yr and older. 2-4 mg/kg/day divided q12-24h. Maximum: 200 mg/day.

Acute gonococcal infections

PO

Adults. Initially, 200 mg, then 100 mg at bedtime on first day; then 100 mg twice a day for 14 days.

Syphilis

PO, IV

Adults. 200 mg/day in divided doses for 14-28 days.

Traveler's diarrhea

PO

Adults, Elderly. 100 mg/day during a period of risk (up to 14 days) and for 2 days after returning home.

Periodontitis

PO

Adults. 20 mg twice a day.

AVAILABLE FORMS

- *Capsules:* 50 mg (Monodox), 75 mg (Doryx), 100 mg (Doryx, Monodox, Vibramycin).
- *Oral Suspension (Vibramycin):* 25 mg/5 ml.
- *Syrup (Vibramycin):* 50 mg/5 ml.
- *Tablets:* 20 mg (Periostat), 50 mg (Adoxa), 75 mg (Adoxa), 100 mg (Adoxa, Vibra-Tabs).
- *Injection, Powder for Reconstitution (Doxy-100):* 100 mg.

UNLABELED USES: Treatment of atypical mycobacterial infections, gonorrhea, malaria, rheumatoid arthritis; prevention of Lyme disease; prevention or treatment of traveler's diarrhea

CONTRAINDICATIONS: Children 8 years and younger, hypersensitivity to tetracyclines or sulfites, last half of pregnancy, severe hepatic dysfunction

PREGNANCY AND LACTATION: Pregnancy category D; excreted into breast milk; theoretical possibility for dental staining seems remote because serum levels in infant undetectable

SIDE EFFECTS

Frequent

Anorexia, nausea, vomiting, diarrhea, dysphagia, possibly severe photosensitivity

Occasional

Rash, urticaria

SERIOUS REACTIONS

- Superinfection (especially fungal) and benign intracranial hypertension (headache, visual changes) may occur.
- Hepatoxicity, fatty degeneration of the liver, and pancreatitis occur rarely.

INTERACTIONS

Drugs

3 *Antacids:* Reduced serum concentration and efficacy of doxycycline

3 *Barbiturates:* Reduced serum doxycycline concentrations

3 *Bismuth:* Reduced bioavailability of doxycycline

3 *Calcium:* See antacids

3 *Carbamazepine:* Reduced serum doxycycline concentrations

3 *Cholestyramine; colestipol:* Reduced serum concentration of doxycycline; take 2 hr before or 3 hr after resin dose

3 *Ethanol:* Chronic ethanol ingestion may reduce the serum concentrations of doxycycline

3 *Iron:* Reduced serum concentration and efficacy of doxycycline

3 *Methotrexate:* Increases methotrexate concentrations and risk of toxicity

3 *Magnesium:* See antacids

3 *Oral contraceptives:* Potential for decreased efficacy of oral contraceptives

3 *Penicillins:* Doxycycline may reduce penicillin efficacy

3 *Phenytoin:* Reduced serum doxycycline concentrations

3 *Warfarin:* Potential for enhanced hypoprothrombinenic response to warfarin

3 *Zinc:* Reduced serum concentration of doxycycline; take 2 hr before or 3 hr after zinc

SPECIAL CONSIDERATIONS

- Tetracycline of choice due to broad spectrum, long $t_{1/2}$, superior tissue penetration, and excellent oral absorption

PATIENT/FAMILY EDUCATION

- Do not take with antacids, iron products
- Take with food
- Continue taking doxycycline for the full course of therapy
- Avoid overexposure to sun or ultraviolet light to prevent photosensitivity reactions

MONITORING PARAMETERS

- Daily bowel activity and stool consistency
- Skin for rash
- Monitor the patient's LOC because of the potential for benign intracranial hypertension
- Signs and symptoms of superinfection, such as anal or genital pruritus, diarrhea, and ulceration or changes of the oral mucosa

dronabinol

(droe-nab'-i-nol)

Rx: Marinol

Chemical Class: Cannabinoid derivative

Therapeutic Class: Antiemetic; appetite stimulant

DEA Class: Schedule II; Schedule III

CLINICAL PHARMACOLOGY

Mechanism of Action: An antiemetic and appetite stimulant that may act by inhibiting vomiting control mechanisms in the medulla oblongata. ***Therapeutic Effect:*** Inhibits vomiting and stimulates appetite.

Pharmacokinetics

Well absorbed after PO administration. Protein binding: 97%. Undergoes first-pass metabolism. Is highly lipid soluble. Primarily excreted in feces. ***Half-life:*** 4 hr.

INDICATIONS AND DOSAGES

Prevention of chemotherapy-induced nausea and vomiting

PO

Adults, Children. Initially, 5 mg/m^2 1-3 hr before chemotherapy, then q2-4h after chemotherapy for total of 4-6 doses a day. May increase by 2.5 mg/m^2 up to 15 mg/m^2 per dose.

Appetite stimulant

PO

Adults. Initially, 2.5 mg twice a day (before lunch and dinner). Range: 2.5-20 mg/day.

AVAILABLE FORMS

- *Capsules (Gelatin [Marinol]):* 2.5 mg, 5 mg, 10 mg.

UNLABELED USES: Postoperative nausea and vomiting

CONTRAINDICATIONS: Treatment of nausea and vomiting not caused by chemotherapy, hypersensitivity to sesame oil or tetrahydrocannabinol products

PREGNANCY AND LACTATION: Pregnancy category C; excreted in breast milk; Controlled Substance Schedule III

SIDE EFFECTS

Frequent (24%-3%)

Euphoria, dizziness, paranoid reaction, somnolence

Occasional (3%-1%)

Asthenia, ataxia, confusion, abnormal thinking, depersonalization

Rare (less than 1%)

Diarrhea, depression, nightmares, speech difficulties, headache, anxiety, tinnitus, flushed skin

SERIOUS REACTIONS

- Mild intoxication may produce increased sensory awareness (including taste, smell, and sound), altered time perception, reddened conjunctiva, dry mouth, and tachycardia.
- Moderate intoxication may produce memory impairment and urine retention.
- Severe intoxication may produce lethargy, decreased motor coordination, slurred speech, and orthostatic hypotension.

INTERACTIONS

Drugs

3 *Alcohol, other CNS depressants:* May increase CNS depression

SPECIAL CONSIDERATIONS

- May have additive sedative or behavioral effects with CNS depressants
- Use caution escalating the dose because of increased frequency of adverse reactions at higher doses

PATIENT/FAMILY EDUCATION

- Drowsiness usually disappears with continued therapy
- Change positions slowly—from recumbent, to sitting, before standing—to prevent dizziness
- Avoid tasks that require mental alertness or motor skills until response to the drug has been established
- Do not use other medications, including OTC drugs, without consulting the physician
- Avoid alcohol

MONITORING PARAMETERS

- Monitor patients with history of psychiatric illness

droperidol

(droe-per'-i-dole)

Rx: Inapsine

Combinations

Rx: with fentanyl (Innovar)

Chemical Class: Butyrophenone derivative

Therapeutic Class: Anesthesia adjunct; antiemetic; sedative

CLINICAL PHARMACOLOGY

Mechanism of Action: A general anesthetic and antiemetic agent that antagonizes dopamine neurotransmission at synapses by blocking postsynaptic dopamine receptor sites; partially blocks adrenergic receptor binding sites. ***Therapeutic Effect:*** Produces tranquilization, antiemetic effect.

Pharmacokinetics

Onset of action occurs within 30 mins. Well absorbed. Metabolized in liver. Excreted in urine and feces. ***Half-life:*** 2.3 hrs.

INDICATIONS AND DOSAGES

Preoperative

IM/IV

Adults, Elderly, Children 12 yrs and older. 2.5-10 mg 30-60 mins before induction of general anesthesia.

Children 2-12 yrs. 0.088-0.165 mg/kg.

Adjunct for induction of general anesthesia

IV

Adults, Elderly, Children 12 yrs and older. 0.22-0.275 mg/kg.

Children 2-12 yrs. 0.088-0.165 mg/kg.

Adjunct for maintenance of general anesthesia

IV

Adults, Elderly. 1.25-2.5 mg.

Diagnostic procedures w/o general anesthesia

IM

Adults, Elderly. 2.5-10 mg 30-60 min before procedure. If needed, may give additional doses of 1.25-2.5 mg (usually by IV injection).

AVAILABLE FORMS

• *Injection:* 2.5 mg/ml (Inapsine).

CONTRAINDICATIONS: Known or suspected QT prolongation, hypersensitivity to droperidol or any component of the formulation

PREGNANCY AND LACTATION: Pregnancy category C; has been used to promote analgesia for cesarean section patients without affecting respiration of the newborn; excretion into breast milk unknown; use caution in nursing mothers

NOTE: Has been used as a continuous IV infusion for hyperemesis gravidarum during the second and third trimesters without apparent fetal harm

SIDE EFFECTS

Frequent

Mild to moderate hypotension

Occasional

Tachycardia, postop drowsiness, dizziness, chills, shivering

Rare

Postop nightmares, facial sweating, bronchospasm

SERIOUS REACTIONS

• Extrapyramidal symptoms may appear as akathisia (motor restlessness) and dystonias: torticollis (neck muscle spasm), opisthotonos (rigidity of back muscles), and oculogyric crisis (rolling back of eyes).

• Overdosage includes symptoms of hypotension, tachycardia, hallucinations, and extrapyramidal symptoms.

• Prolonged QT interval, seizures, and arrhythmias have been reported.

INTERACTIONS

Drugs

⚠ *Arrhythmogenic agents:* Any drug known to prolong QT interval should not be used with droperidol; class I or III antiarrhythmics, antimalarials, calcium channel blockers (bepridil, isradipine, nicardipine), neuroleptics (haloperidol, pimozide, thioridazine), antidepressants (desimipramine, venlafaxine)

❷ *Diuretics, laxatives:* Hypokalemia or hypomagnesemia may precipitate QT prolongation

❸ *CNS depressants:* Additive or potentiating effects with droperidol; barbiturates, tranquilizers, opioids

SPECIAL CONSIDERATIONS

PATIENT/FAMILY EDUCATION

• Change positions slowly to avoid orthostatic hypotension

• Avoid tasks that require mental alertness or motor skills until response to the drug is established

MONITORING PARAMETERS

• QT prolongation has occurred in patients with no known CV disease and with doses at or below recommended doses, reserve use for patients who fail to show response to other adequate treatments

• Baseline ECG, blood pressure, heart rate, respiratory rate; if QT >440 msec for males or >450 msec for females, do not use droperidol

• Therapeutic response from anxiety

• Monitor for extrapyramidal symptoms

drotrecogin alfa

(droe-tre-koe'-jin al'-fa)

Rx: Xigris

Chemical Class: Glycoprotein

Therapeutic Class: Antisepsis syndrome agent

CLINICAL PHARMACOLOGY

Mechanism of Action: A recombinant form of human-activated protein C that exerts an antithrombotic effect by inhibiting factors Va and VIIIa and may exert an indirect profibrinolytic effect by inhibiting plasminogen activator inhibitor-1 and limiting the generation of activated thrombin-activatable-fibrinolysis-inhibitor. The drug may also exert an antiinflammatory effect by inhibiting tumor necrosis factor (TNF) production by monocytes, by blocking leukocyte adhesion to selectins, and by limiting thrombin-induced inflammatory responses. ***Therapeutic Effect:*** Produces antiinflammatory, antithrombotic, and profibrinolytic effects.

Pharmacokinetics

Inactivated by endogenous plasma protease inhibitors. Clearance occurs within 2 hr of initiating infusion. ***Half-life:*** 1.6 hr.

INDICATIONS AND DOSAGES

Severe sepsis

IV Infusion

Adults, Elderly. 24 mcg/kg/hr for 96 hr. Immediately stop infusion if clinically significant bleeding is identified.

AVAILABLE FORMS

• *Powder for Infusion:* 5 mg, 20 mg.

CONTRAINDICATIONS: Active internal bleeding, evidence of cerebral herniation, intracranial neoplasm or mass lesion, presence of an epidural catheter, recent (within the past 3 mo) hemorrhagic stroke, recent (within the past 2 mo) intracranial or intraspinal surgery or severe head trauma, trauma with an increased risk of life-threatening bleeding

PREGNANCY AND LACTATION: Pregnancy category C; excretion into breast milk unknown

SIDE EFFECTS

None known.

SERIOUS REACTIONS

• Bleeding (intrathoracic, retroperitoneal, GI, GU, intraabdominal, intracranial) occurs in about 2% of patients.

INTERACTIONS

Labs

• *aPTT:* Drotrecogin alfa affects the aPTT assay, and one-stage coagulation assays based on the aPTT (such as factor VIII, IX, and XI assays); this interference may result in an apparent factor concentration that is less than the true concentration; drotrecogin alfa present in plasma samples does not interfere with one-stage factor assays based on the PT (such as factor II, V, VII, and X assays)

SPECIAL CONSIDERATIONS

• The efficacy of drotrecogin alfa was studied in an international, multi-center, randomized, double-blind, placebo-controlled trial (PROWESS) of 1690 patients with severe sepsis (Bernard GR, et al. Efficacy and Safety of Recombinant Human Activated Protein C for Severe Sepsis. N Engl J Med. 2001;344:699-709); entry criteria included a systemic inflammatory response presumed due to infection and at least one associated acute organ dysfunction; acute organ dysfunction was defined as one of the following: cardiovascular dysfunction (shock, hypotension, or the need for vasopressor support despite adequate fluid resuscitation); respiratory dysfunction [relative hypox-

emia (PaO_2/FiO_2 ratio <250); renal dysfunction (oliguria despite adequate fluid resuscitation); thrombocytopenia (platelet count <80,000/mm^3 or 50% decrease from the highest value the previous 3 days); or metabolic acidosis with elevated lactic acid concentrations
• The primary efficacy endpoint was all-cause mortality assessed 28 days after the start of study drug administration; prospectively defined subsets for mortality analyses included groups defined by APACHE II score (a score designed to assess risk of mortality based on acute physiology and chronic health evaluation, see http://www.sfar.org/scores2/scores2.html); the APACHE II score was calculated from physiologic and laboratory data obtained within the 24-hr period immediately preceding the start of study drug administration irrespective of the preceding length of stay in the Intensive Care Unit; the study was terminated after a planned interim analysis due to significantly decrease mortality in patients on drotrecogin alfa than in patients on placebo (210/850, 25% vs 259/840, 31% p=0.005); the observed mortality difference between drotrecogin alfa and placebo was limited to the half of patients with higher risk of death, i.e., APACHE II score >25, the third and fourth quartile APACHE II scores (mortality 31% with treatment, 44% with placebo); the efficacy of drotrecogin alfa has not been established in patients with lower risk of death, e.g., APACHE II score <25

PATIENT/FAMILY EDUCATION
• Inform the patient that bleeding may occur for up to 28 days after treatment; warn the patient to immediately notify the physician if signs or symptoms of unusual bleeding occur

MONITORING PARAMETERS
• CBC with platelets, INR
• Monitor the patient closely for hemorrhagic complications

duloxetine hydrochloride

(du-lox′-uh-teen hye-droe-klor′-ide)

Rx: Cymbalta
Chemical Class: Aryloxypropylamine
Therapeutic Class: Antidepressant (SSNRI or NE/5-HT reuptake inhibitor)

CLINICAL PHARMACOLOGY
Mechanism of Action: An antidepressant that appears to inhibit serotonin and norepinephrine reuptake at CNS neuronal presynaptic membranes; is a less potent inhibitor of dopamine reuptake. ***Therapeutic Effect:*** Relieves depression.
Pharmacokinetics
Well absorbed from the GI tract. Protein binding: Greater than 90%. Extensively metabolized to active metabolites. Excreted primarily in urine and, to a lesser extent, in feces. ***Half-life:*** 8-17 hr.

INDICATIONS AND DOSAGES
Major depressive disorder
PO
Adults. 20 mg twice a day, increased up to 60 mg/day as a single dose or in 2 divided doses.
Diabetic neuropathy pain
PO
Adults. 60 mg once a day.

AVAILABLE FORMS
• *Capsules:* 20 mg, 30 mg, 60 mg.

UNLABELED USES: Treatment of chronic pain syndromes, fibromyalgia, stress incontinence, urinary incontinence

CONTRAINDICATIONS: End-stage renal disease (creatinine clearance less than 30 ml/min), severe hepatic impairment, uncontrolled angle-closure glaucoma, use within 14 days of MAOIs

PREGNANCY AND LACTATION: Pregnancy category C; neonates exposed to SSRIs or SNRIs late in the third trimester have developed serious complications, sometimes requiring prolonged hospitalization, respiratory support, and tube feeding: respiratory distress, cyanosis, apnea, seizures, temperature instability, feeding difficulty, vomiting, hypoglycemia, hypotonia, hypertonia, hyperreflexia, tremor jitteriness, irritability, and constant crying. This clinical picture is consistent with a toxic effect of SSRIs and SNRIs or, possibly, a drug discontinuation syndrome. Human breast milk excretion unknown; there is excretion into breast milk of lactating rats; breast-feeding not recommended at this time

SIDE EFFECTS

Frequent (20%-11%)

Nausea, dry mouth, constipation, insomnia

Occasional (9%-5%)

Dizziness, fatigue, diarrhea, somnolence, anorexia, diaphoresis, vomiting

Rare (4%-2%)

Blurred vision, erectile dysfunction, delayed or failed ejaculation, anorgasmia, anxiety, decreased libido, hot flashes

SERIOUS REACTIONS

- Duloxetine use may slightly increase the patient's heart rate.
- Colitis, dysphagia, gastritis, and irritable bowel syndrome occur rarely.

INTERACTIONS

Drugs

Duloxetine: Substrate for CYP1A2, CYP2D6; moderate inhibitor of CYP2D6

3 *Amitriptylline, desipramine, tricyclic antidepressants:* Inhibits CYP2D6-mediated tricyclic agent metabolism, increased bioavailability of tricyclics, increasing risk of adverse events (anticholinergic effects, sedation, confusion, cardiac arrhythmias)

3 *Class I-C antiarrhythmic agents:* Inhibits CYP2D6-mediated metabolism of class I-C antiarrhythmic agents (flecainide, propafenone, moricizine); increased risk of cardiotoxicity (QT prolongation, torsades de points, cardiac arrest)

3 *Fluoroquinolone antibiotics (ciprofloxacin, enoxacin):* Inhibit CYP1A2-mediated duloxetine metabolism, increased risk of adverse effects

3 *Fluoxetine:* Moderately potent inhibitor of CYP2D6-mediated metabolism of duloxetine; increased serum levels, increased risk of adverse effects

3 *Fluvoxamine:* Inhibits CYYP1A2-mediated duloxetine metabolism, increased risk of adverse effects

▲ *Monoamine oxidase inhibitors:* Duloxetine inhibitor effects on both norepinephrine and serotonin reuptake set up overlapping therapy with monoamine oxidase inhibitor to cause CNS toxicity or serotonin syndrome

3 *Paroxetine:* Moderately potent inhibitor of CYP2D6-mediated metabolism of duloxetine; increased serum levels, increased risk of adverse effects

3 *Phenothiazines:* Duloxetine inhibition of CYP2D6-mediated phenothiazine metabolism leads to increased phenothiazine concentrations and potential toxicity
2 *Quinidine:* Quinidine inhibition of CYP2D6-mediated duloxetine metabolism; increased adverse effects
3 *St. John's Wort:* May increase adverse effects
3 *Warfarin:* May increase the warfarin plasma concentration

SPECIAL CONSIDERATIONS

• Place in therapy: Similar to venlafaxine, with far less experience and comparative data; alternative in major depression in poor responders to other agents; at least as effective as tricyclics, but with lower toxicity; more efficacious than SSRIs

PATIENT/FAMILY EDUCATION

• Therapeutic response may take 4-6 wks; be alert for emergence of anxiety, agitation, panic, mania, or worsening of depressive state
• Do not abruptly discontinue duloxetine
• Avoid tasks that require mental alertness or motor skills until response to the drug has been established
• The female patient should inform the physician if she becomes or intends to become pregnant
• Do not consume large amounts of alcohol to prevent liver damage

MONITORING PARAMETERS

• *Efficacy:* Resolution/improvement in symptoms of depression
• *Toxicity:* Blood pressure and pulse in patients prior to initiating treatment and periodically thereafter; signs of toxicity: somnolence, sleep disturbances, persistent GI symptoms
• Liver function test results for patients on long-term duloxetine therapy

---

dyphylline

(dye′-fi-lin)

Rx: Dilor, Lufyllin

Combinations

Rx: with guaifenesin (Dilex-G, Dilor-G, Lufyllin-GG); with ephedrine, guaifenesin, phenobarbital (Lufyllin-EPG)

Chemical Class: Xanthine derivative

Therapeutic Class: COPD agent; antiasthmatic; bronchodilator

CLINICAL PHARMACOLOGY

Mechanism of Action: A xanthine derivative that acts as a bronchodilator by directly relaxing smooth muscle of the bronchial airway and pulmonary blood vessels similar to theophylline. ***Therapeutic Effect:*** Relieves bronchospasm, increases vital capacity, produces cardiac and skeletal muscle stimulation.

Pharmacokinetics

Rapid absorption after PO administration. Excreted in urine. ***Half-life:*** 2 hrs.

INDICATIONS AND DOSAGES

Chronic bronchospasm, asthma

PO

Adults, Elderly. 15 mg/kg 4 times/day.

IM

Adults, Elderly. 250-500 mg. Maximum: 15 mg/kg q6h.

Children. 4.4-6.6 mg/kg/day in divided doses.

Dosage in renal impairment

Creatinine Clearance	*Dosage Percent*
50-80 ml/min	Administer 75% of dose
10-50 ml/min	Administer 50% of dose
<10 ml/min	Administer 25% of dose

AVAILABLE FORMS

• *Elixir:* 100 mg/15 ml (Lufyllin).
• *Injection:* 250 mg/ml (Dilor).
• *Tablet:* 200 mg, 400 mg (Dilor, Lufyllin).

CONTRAINDICATIONS: Uncontrolled arrhythmias, hyperthyroidism, history of hypersensitivity to dyphylline, related xanthine derivatives, or any component of the formulation

PREGNANCY AND LACTATION: Pregnancy category C; excreted into breast milk, compatible with breast-feeding

SIDE EFFECTS

Frequent

Tachycardia, nervousness, restlessness

Occasional

Heartburn, vomiting, headache, mild diuresis, insomnia, nausea

SERIOUS REACTIONS

• Ventricular arrhythmias, hypotension, circulatory failure, seizures, hyperglycemia, and syndrome of inappropriate antidiuretic hormone (SIADH) have been reported.

INTERACTIONS

Drugs

3 *Ephedrine:* Toxic synergism may occur

3 *Probenecid:* Increased serum dyphylline concentrations

SPECIAL CONSIDERATIONS

• Though better tolerated, significantly less bronchodilating activity vs theophylline. Serious dosing errors possible if dyphylline monitored with theophylline serum assays

MONITORING PARAMETERS

• Minimal effective serum concentration 12 mcg/ml
• Signs of clinical improvement such as cessation of clavicular retractions, quieter and slower respirations, and a relaxed facial expression
• Examine the patient's lips and fingernails for evidence of oxygen depletion such as blue or gray lips, blue or dusky colored fingernails in light-skinned patients; and gray fingernails in dark-skinned patients

econazole nitrate

(e-kone'-a-zole nye'-trate)

Rx: Spectazole

Chemical Class: Imidazole derivative

Therapeutic Class: Antifungal

CLINICAL PHARMACOLOGY

Mechanism of Action: An imidazole derivative that changes the permeability of the fungal cell wall. ***Therapeutic Effect:*** Inhibits fungal biosynthesis of triglycerides, phospholipids. Fungistatic.

Pharmacokinetics

Low systemic absorption. Protein binding: 98%. Metabolized in liver to more than 20 metabolites. Primarily excreted in urine; minimal excretion in feces. Not removed by hemodialysis.

INDICATIONS AND DOSAGES

Treatment of tinea pedis, tinea cruris, tinea corporis, tinea versicolor

Topical

Adults, Elderly, Children. Apply once daily to affected area for 2-4 wks.

AVAILABLE FORMS

- *Cream:* 1% (Spectazole).

UNLABELED USES: Cutaneous candidiasis, otomycosis

CONTRAINDICATIONS: Hypersensitivity to econazole

PREGNANCY AND LACTATION: Pregnancy category C; excretion into breast milk unknown; limited systemic absorption would minimize possibility of exposure to nursing infant

SIDE EFFECTS

Occasional (10%-1%)

Vulvar/vaginal burning

Rare (less than 1%)

Itching and burning of sexual partner, polyuria, vulvar itching, soreness, edema, discharge

SERIOUS REACTIONS

- None known.

SPECIAL CONSIDERATIONS

PATIENT/FAMILY EDUCATION

- For external use only; avoid contact with eyes; cleanse skin with soap and water and dry thoroughly prior to application
- Use medication for full treatment time outlined by clinician, even though symptoms may have improved
- Notify clinician if no improvement after 2 wk (jock itch, ringworm) or 4 wk (athlete's foot)

MONITORING PARAMETERS

- Evaluate the patient's skin for itching, irritation, or rash

edetate calcium disodium (calcium EDTA)

(ed'-eh-tate kal'-see-um dye-soe'-dee-um)

Rx: Calcium Disodium Versenate

Chemical Class: Chelating agent

Therapeutic Class: Antidote, heavy metal

CLINICAL PHARMACOLOGY

Mechanism of Action: A chelating agent that reduces blood concentration of heavy metals, especially lead, forming stable complexes. ***Therapeutic Effect:*** Allows heavy metal excretion in urine.

Pharmacokinetics

Well absorbed after parenteral administration; poorly absorbed from the gastrointestinal (GI) tract. Penetrates to extracellular fluid and slowly diffuses into cerebrospinal fluid (CSF). No metabolism occurs. Excreted in the urine either unchanged or as the metal chelates. ***Half-life:*** 20-60 min (IV), 1.5 hrs (IM).

INDICATIONS AND DOSAGES

Diagnosis of lead poisoning

IM/IV

Adults, Elderly. 500 mg/m^2. Maximum: 1 g/m^2/day divided in equal doses 8-12 hr apart for 5 days, skip 2-4 days and repeat course if needed.

IM

Children. 500 mg/m^2 as single dose or 500 mg/m^2 each at 12-hr intervals.

IV

Children. 1 g/m^2/day IV infusion over 8-12 hr for 5 days, skip 2-4 days and repeat course as needed. Maximum: 75 mg/kg/day.

Lead poisoning (without encephalopathy)
IM/IV
Adults, Elderly, Children. 1-1.5 g/m^2 daily for 3-5 days (if blood lead concentration >100 mcg/dl, calcium edetate usually given with dimercaprol.) Allow at least 2-4 days, up to 2-3 wks between courses of therapy. Adults should not be given more than 2 courses of therapy.
Lead poisoning (with encephalopathy)
IM
Adults, elderly, children. Initially, dimercaprol 4 mg/kg; then give dimercaprol 4 mg/kg and calcium EDTA 250 mg/m^2; then 4 hrs later and q4h for 5 days.

AVAILABLE FORMS
• *Injection:* 200 mg/ml (Calcium Disodium Verchate).

CONTRAINDICATIONS: Anuria, severe renal disease, hypersensitivity to EDTA or any component of the formulation

PREGNANCY AND LACTATION: Pregnancy category B; excretion into breast milk unknown; use caution in nursing mothers

SIDE EFFECTS
Frequent
Chills, fever, anorexia, headache, histamine-like reaction (sneezing, stuffy nose, watery eyes), decreased blood pressure (BP), nausea, vomiting, thrombophlebitis
Rare
Frequent urination, secondary gout (severe pain in feet, knees, elbows).

SERIOUS REACTIONS
• Drug may produce same signs of renal damage as severe acute lead poisoning (proteinuria, microscopic hematuria). Transient anemia/bone marrow depression, hypercalcemia (constipation, drowsiness, dry mouth, metallic taste) occurs occasionally.

SPECIAL CONSIDERATIONS

PATIENT/FAMILY EDUCATION
• Notify clinician immediately if no urine output in a 12-hr period

MONITORING PARAMETERS
• Urinalysis and urine sediment daily during therapy to detect signs of progressive renal tubular damage
• Renal function tests, liver function tests, and serum electrolytes before and periodically during therapy
• ECG during IV therapy
• BUN

edetate disodium

(ed′-eh-tate dye-soe′-dee-um)
Rx: Disotate, Endrate
Chemical Class: Chelating agent
Therapeutic Class: Antidote, digitalis; antihypercalcemic

CLINICAL PHARMACOLOGY
Mechanism of Action: A chelating agent that forms a soluble chelate with calcium, resulting in rapid decrease in plasma calcium concentrations. ***Therapeutic Effect:*** Allows calcium to be excreted in urine.
Pharmacokinetics
Distributed in extracellular fluid and does not appear in red blood cells. No metabolism occurs. Rapidly excreted in the urine. ***Half-life:*** 1.4-3 hrs.

INDICATIONS AND DOSAGES
Digitalis toxicity, hypercalcemia
IV
Adults, Elderly. 500 mg/kg/day over 3 hrs or more, daily for 5 days, skip 2 days, repeat as needed up to 15 doses. Maximum: 3 g/day.

Children. 40 mg/kg/day over 3 hrs or more, daily for 5 days, skip 5 days, repeat as needed. Maximum: 70 mg/kg/day.

AVAILABLE FORMS

• *Injection:* 150 mg/ml (Disotate, Endrate).

CONTRAINDICATIONS: Anuria, renal impairment, hypersensitivity to EDTA or any component of the formulation

PREGNANCY AND LACTATION: Pregnancy category C; excretion into breast milk unknown; use caution in nursing mothers

SIDE EFFECTS

Frequent

Abdominal cramps or pain, diarrhea, nausea, vomiting, circumoral paresthesia, headache, numbness, postural hypotension

Rare

Exfoliative dermatitis, toxic skin and mucous membrane reactions, thrombophlebitis (at injection site)

SERIOUS REACTIONS

• Nephrotoxicity may occur with excessive dosages.

• Hypomagnesemia may occur with prolonged use.

SPECIAL CONSIDERATIONS

• Have patient remain supine for a short time after INF due to the possibility of orthostatic hypotension

• Additives may be incompatible with the reconstituted (diluted) solution required for IV infusion

MONITORING PARAMETERS

• ECG, blood pressure during INF

• Renal function before and during therapy

• Serum calcium, magnesium, potassium levels

• BUN

edrophonium chloride

(ed-roe-foe′-nee-um klor′-ide)

Rx: Enlon, Reversol, Tensilon

Combinations

Rx: with atropine (Enlon-Plus)

Chemical Class: Cholinesterase inhibitor; quaternary ammonium derivative

Therapeutic Class: Antidote, curare; cholinergic

CLINICAL PHARMACOLOGY

Mechanism of Action: A parasympathetic, anticholinesterase agent that inhibits destruction of acetylcholine by acetylcholinesterase, thus causing accumulation of acetylcholine at cholinergic synapses. Results in an increase in cholinergic responses such as miosis, increased tonus of intestinal and skeletal muscles, bronchial and ureteral constriction, bradycardia, and increased salivary and sweat gland secretions. ***Therapeutic Effect:*** Diagnosis of myasthenia gravis.

Pharmacokinetics

Onset of action occurs within 30-60 secs and has duration of 10 mins. Rapid absorption after IV administration. Exact method of metabolism is unknown. Rapidly excreted in urine. ***Half-life:*** 1.8 hrs.

INDICATIONS AND DOSAGES

Diagnosis of myasthenia gravis

IV

Adults, Elderly. 2-mg test dose over 15-30 secs. If no reaction in 45 secs, give additional dose of 8 mg. Test dose may be repeated after 30 mins.

Children more than 34 kg. Initially, 2 mg over 1 min. If no reaction in 45 secs, may repeat at a rate of 1 mg every 30-45 secs. Maximum cumulative dose: 10 mg.

Children less than 34 kg. Initially, 1 mg over 1 min. If no reaction in 45 secs, may repeat at a rate of 1 mg every 30-45 secs. Maximum cumulative dose: 5 mg.
Infants. 0.5 mg infused over 1 min.
IM/SC
Adults, Elderly, Children. Initially, 10 mg as a single dose. If no cholinergic reaction occurs, give 2 mg 30 mins later to rule out false-negative reaction.
Children more than 34 kg. 5 mg as a single dose.
Children less than 34 kg. 2 mg as a single dose.
Infants. 0.5-1 mg as a single dose.
Neuromuscular blockade antagonism
IV
Adults, Elderly. 10 mg over 30-45 secs. May be repeated as needed until a cholinergic response is detected. Maximum: 40 mg.
IM
Children. 233 mcg/kg as a single dose.
Infants. 145 mcg/kg as a single dose.
Dosage in renal impairment
Dose may need to be reduced in patients with chronic renal failure.

AVAILABLE FORMS

• *Injection:* 10 mg/ml (Enlon, Reversol, Tensilon).

CONTRAINDICATIONS: Gastrointestinal (GI); or genitourinary (GU) obstruction, hypersensitivity to edrophonium, sulfites, or any component of the formulation

PREGNANCY AND LACTATION: Pregnancy category C; because it is ionized at physiologic pH, would not be expected to cross placenta in significant amounts; may cause premature labor; because it is ionized at physiologic pH, would not be expected to be excreted into breast milk

SIDE EFFECTS

Frequent
Increase salivation, intestinal secretions, lacrimation, urinary urgency, hyperperistalsis, sweating
Occasional
Bradycardia, hypotension, convulsions, dysphagia, nausea, vomiting, diarrhea
Rare
Bronchoconstriction, cardiac arrest, central respiratory paralysis

SERIOUS REACTIONS

• Overdosage causes symptoms of cholinergic crisis such as muscle weakness, nausea, vomiting, miosis, bronchospasm, and respiratory paralysis.

INTERACTIONS

Drugs

3 *Procainamide:* Edrophonium tests in patients with myasthenia gravis may be unreliable in procainamide-treated patients

3 *Tacrine:* Increased cholinergic effects of edrophonium

SPECIAL CONSIDERATIONS

• Because symptoms of anticholinesterase overdose (cholinergic crisis) may mimic underdosage (myasthenic weakness), their condition may be worsened by the use of this drug

PATIENT/FAMILY EDUCATION

• Notify the physician or healthcare advisor of difficulty breathing, dizziness, muscle cramps and spasms, or vomiting

• Side effects of the drug should not last long because the effects of the drug are short-lived

MONITORING PARAMETERS

• Preinjection and postinjection strength

• Heart rate, respiratory rate, blood pressure

efalizumab

(e-fa-li-zoo'-mab)

Rx: Raptiva

Chemical Class: Monoclonal antibody

Therapeutic Class: Antipsoriatic; immunomodulatory agent

CLINICAL PHARMACOLOGY

Mechanism of Action: A monoclonal antibody that interferes with lymphocyte activation by binding to the lymphocyte antigen, inhibiting the adhesion of leukocytes to other cell types. ***Therapeutic Effect:*** Prevents the release of cytokines and the growth and migration of circulating total lymphocytes, predominant in psoriatic lesions.

Pharmacokinetics

Clearance is affected by body weight, not by gender or race, after subcutaneous injection. Serum concentration reaches steady state at 4 wk. Mean time to elimination: 25 days.

INDICATIONS AND DOSAGES

Psoriasis

Subcutaneous

Adults, Elderly. Initially, 0.7 mg/kg followed by weekly doses of 1 mg/kg. Maximum: 200 mg (single dose).

AVAILABLE FORMS

• *Powder for Injection:* 150 mg, designed to deliver 125 mg/1.25 ml.

CONTRAINDICATIONS: Concurrent use of immunosuppressive agents, hypersensitivity to any murine or humanized monoclonal antibody preparation

PREGNANCY AND LACTATION: Pregnancy category C; breast milk excretion unknown

SIDE EFFECTS

Frequent (32%-10%)

Headache, chills, nausea, injection site pain

Occasional (8%-7%)

Myalgia, flu-like symptoms, fever

Rare (4%)

Back pain, acne

SERIOUS REACTIONS

• Hypersensitivity reaction, malignancies, serious infections (abscess, cellulitis, postoperative wound infection, pneumonia), thrombocytopenia, and worsening of psoriasis occur rarely.

INTERACTIONS

Drugs

▲ *Immunosuppressives:* Efalizumab should not be given with other immunosuppressive drugs

▲ *Acellular, live and live-attenuated vaccines:* Administration during efalizumab therapy is not recommended

Labs

• Increased lymphocyte counts related to pharmacologic mechanism of action

SPECIAL CONSIDERATIONS

• Evaluate for latent tuberculosis infection with a tuberculin skin test before initiation of therapy

PATIENT/FAMILY EDUCATION

• Intended for use under the guidance and supervision of clinician; patients may self-inject if appropriate and with medical follow-up, after proper training in injection technique, including proper syringe and needle disposal

• Efalizumab treatment increases the risk of developing an infection

• Notify the health care provider if bleeding from the gums, bruising or petechiae of the skin, or signs of infection occur

• Do not undergo phototherapy treatments

MONITORING PARAMETERS
• *Efficacy:* Improvement of clinical signs/symptoms of psoriasis (e.g., itching, redness, scaling, psoriatic body surface area coverage); PASI scores are based on plaque thickness, scaling, and redness, adjusted for percentage of affected body surface area; quality of life assessments
• *Toxicity:* CBC with differential periodically, particularly platelets; vital signs in patients with a history of hypersensitivity to any medication (first injection); temperature periodically (infection)

efavirenz

(e-fa-veer'-ens)
Rx: Sustiva
Chemical Class: Benzoxazinone, substituted; nonnucleoside reverse transcriptase inhibitor
Therapeutic Class: Antiretroviral

CLINICAL PHARMACOLOGY
Mechanism of Action: A nonnucleoside reverse transcriptase inhibitor that inhibits the activity of HIV reverse transcriptase of HIV-1 and the transcription of HIV-1 RNA to DNA. ***Therapeutic Effect:*** Interrupts HIV replication, slowing the progression of HIV infection.
Pharmacokinetics
Rapidly absorbed after PO administration. Protein binding: 99%. Metabolized to major isoenzymes in the liver. Eliminated in urine and feces. ***Half-life:*** 40-55 hr.

INDICATIONS AND DOSAGES
HIV infection (in combination with other antiretrovirals)
PO
Adults, Elderly, Children 3 yr and older weighing 40 kg or more. 600 mg once a day at bedtime.
Children 3 yr and older weighing 32.5 kg-less than 40 kg. 400 mg once a day.
Children 3 yr and older weighing 25 kg-less than 32.5 kg. 350 mg once a day.
Children 3 yr and older weighing 20 kg-less than 25 kg. 300 mg once a day.
Children 3 yr and older weighing 15 kg-less than 20 kg. 250 mg once a day.
Children 3 yr and older weighing 10 kg-less than 15 kg. 200 mg once a day.

AVAILABLE FORMS
• *Capsules:* 50 mg, 100 mg, 200 mg.
• *Tablets:* 600 mg.

CONTRAINDICATIONS: Concurrent use with ergot derivatives, midazolam, or triazolam; efavirenz as monotherapy

PREGNANCY AND LACTATION: Pregnancy category D (fetal malformations observed in monkeys); breast-feeding not recommended

SIDE EFFECTS
Frequent (52%)
Mild to severe: Dizziness, vivid dreams, insomnia, confusion, impaired concentration, amnesia, agitation, depersonalization, hallucinations, euphoria, somnolence (mild symptoms do not interfere with daily activities; severe symptoms interrupt daily activities)
Occasional
Mild to moderate: Maculopapular rash (27%); nausea, fatigue, headache, diarrhea, fever, cough (less than 26%) (moderate symptoms may interfere with daily activities)

SERIOUS REACTIONS
• Serious psychiatric adverse experiences (aggressive reactions, agitation, delusions, emotional lability,

mania, neurosis, paranoia, psychosis, suicide) have been reported.

INTERACTIONS

Drugs

❷ *Amprenavir:* Efavirenz decreases amprenavir plasma level; amprenavir dose adjustment recommended

❸ *Barbiturates:* Barbiturates decrease plasma efavirenz levels; dose adjustment not recommended

❸ *Carbamazepine:* Carbamazepine decreases plasma efavirenz levels; dose adjustment not recommended

❷ *Cisapride:* Efavirenz increases cisapride plasma level; coadministration not recommended

❸ *Clarithromycin:* Efavirenz decreases clarithromycin plasma levels; coadministration not recommended

❷ *Ergotamines:* Efavirenz increases ergotamine plasma level; coadministration not recommended

❸ *Ethinyl estradiol:* Efavirenz increases ethinyl estradiol plasma levels; dose adjustment not recommended

❸ *High-fat meals:* May increase drug absorption

❸ *Indinavir:* Efavirenz reduces indinavir AUC by 31%; increase indinavir dose to 1000 mg q8h

❸ *Lopinavir:* Decreased plasma lopinavir concentrations; consider increase dose of lopinavir/ritonavir combination to 533 mg lopinavir and 133 mg ritonavir

❸ *Lovastatin:* Efavirenz increases lovastatin plasma level; dose adjustment not recommended

❸ *Methadone:* Reduces methadone plasma concentrations

❷ *Midazolam:* Efavirenz increases midazolam plasma level; coadministration not recommended

❸ *Nelfinavir:* Efavirenz increases nelfinavir AUC by 20%; dose adjustment not recommended

❸ *Phenobarbital:* Decreased plasma efavirenz concentrations

❸ *Phenytoin:* Phenytoin decreases plasma efavirenz level; dose adjustment not recommended

❸ *Psychoactive drugs:* Potential for additive CNS effects

❷ *Rifabutin:* Efavirenz decreases plasma rifabutin level by 35%; no change in plasma efavirenz level; increase rifabutin dose to 450 mg qd

❸ *Rifampin:* Rifampin decreases plasma efavirenz level by 25%; dose adjustment not recommended

❸ *Ritonavir:* Ritonavir increases efavirenz AUC by 21%; efavirenz increases ritonavir AUC by 18%; dose adjustment not recommended

❸ *St. John's Wort (Hypericum perforatum):* Substantial decrease in plasma efavirenz concentrations likely; coadministration not recommended

❷ *Saquinavir:* Saquinavir reduces efavirenz AUC by 12%; efavirenz reduces saquinavir AUC by 62%; coadministration not recommended

❸ *Simvastatin:* Efavirenz increases simvastatin plasma level; dose adjustment not recommended

❷ *Triazolam:* Efavirenz increases triazolam plasma level; coadministration not recommended

❸ *Warfarin:* Efavirenz potentially increases or decreases plasma warfarin concentrations

Labs

• *False positive:* Cannabinoid screening test by CEDIA DAU Multi-level THC assay

SPECIAL CONSIDERATIONS

PATIENT/FAMILY EDUCATION

• May be taken without regard for meals; absorption increased by a

high-fat meal, which should be avoided
• Take at bedtime for first 2-4 wk of therapy; may continue at bedtime if desired
• Use caution in driving or other activities requiring alertness
• Avoid alcohol ingestion
• CNS and psychological side effects, such as delusions, depression, dizziness, and impaired concentration, occur in more than half of patients taking this drug; notify the physician if these symptoms continue or become problematic

MONITORING PARAMETERS
• ALT, AST, CBC, cholesterol, triglycerides
• Monitor the patient for adverse CNS and psychological effects, such as abnormal dreams, dizziness, impaired concentration, insomnia, severe acute depression (including suicidal ideation or attempts), and somnolence. Be aware that insomnia may begin during the first or second day of therapy and generally resolves in 2-4 wks
• Assess skin for rash

eflornithine

(ee-flor′-ni-theen)
Rx: Vaniqa
Chemical Class: Ornithine decarboxylase inhibitor
Therapeutic Class: Antiprotozoal

CLINICAL PHARMACOLOGY
Mechanism of Action: A topical antiprotozoal that inhibits ornithine deczarboxylase cell division and synthetic function in the skin. ***Therapeutic Effect:*** Reduces rate of hair growth.

Pharmacokinetics
Absorption is less than 1% from intact skin. Not metabolized. Primarily excreted as unchanged drug in urine. ***Half life:*** 8 hrs.

INDICATIONS AND DOSAGES
For reduction of unwanted facial hair in women
Topical
Adults, Elderly. Apply thin layer to affected area of face and adjacent involved areas under chin; rub in thoroughly. Use twice daily at least 8 hrs apart. Do not wash area for at least 4 hrs.

AVAILABLE FORMS
• *Cream:* 13.9% (Vaniqa).

CONTRAINDICATIONS: Hypersensitivity to eflornithine or any component of the formulation

PREGNANCY AND LACTATION: Pregnancy category C; excretion into breast milk unknown; use caution in nursing mothers

SIDE EFFECTS
Frequent
Acne
Occasional
Headache, stinging/burning skin, dry skin, pruritus, erythema
Rare
Tingling skin, rash, dyspepsia (heartburn, GI distress)

SERIOUS REACTIONS
• Bleeding skin, cheilitis, contact dermatitis, herpes simplex, lip swelling, nausea, numbness, rosacea, and weakness have been reported.

SPECIAL CONSIDERATIONS
• The most frequent, serious, toxic effect of eflornithine is myelosuppression, which may be unavoidable if successful treatment is to be completed; decisions to modify dosage or to interrupt or cease treatment depend on the severity of the observed adverse event(s) and the availability of support facilities

PATIENT/FAMILY EDUCATION

• Take for the full length of treatment

• Notify the physician of rash, skin irritation or intolerance

MONITORING PARAMETERS

• Serial audiograms if feasible

• CBC with platelets before and twice weekly during therapy and qwk after completion of therapy until hematologic values return to baseline levels

• Follow-up for at least 24 mo is advised to ensure further therapy should relapses occur

eletriptan

(el-ih-trip′-tan)

Rx: Relpax

Chemical Class: Serotonin derivative

Therapeutic Class: Antimigraine agent

CLINICAL PHARMACOLOGY

Mechanism of Action: A serotonin receptor agonist that binds selectively to vascular receptors, producing a vasoconstrictive effect on cranial blood vessels. ***Therapeutic Effect:*** Relieves migraine headache.

Pharmacokinetics

Well absorbed after PO administration. Metabolized by the liver to inactive metabolite. Eliminated in urine. ***Half-life:*** 4.4 hr (increased in hepatic impairment and the elderly [older than 65 yr]).

INDICATIONS AND DOSAGES

Acute migraine headache

PO

Adults, Elderly. 20-40 mg. If headache improves but then returns, dose may be repeated after 2 hr. Maximum: 80 mg/day.

AVAILABLE FORMS

• *Tablets:* 20 mg, 40 mg.

CONTRAINDICATIONS: Arrhythmias associated with conduction disorders, cerebrovascular syndrome including strokes and transient ischemic attacks (TIAs), coronary artery disease, hemiplegic or basilar migraine, ischemic heart disease, peripheral vascular disease including ischemic bowel disease, severe hepatic impairment, uncontrolled hypertension; use within 24 hr of treatment with another 5-HT1 agonist, an ergotamine-containing or ergot-type medication such as dihydroergotamine (DHE) or methysergide

PREGNANCY AND LACTATION: Pregnancy category C; excreted in human breast milk—approximately 0.02% of the administered dose; breast milk to plasma ratio 1:4, with great variability; caution should be exercised when eletriptan hydrobromide is administered to nursing women

SIDE EFFECTS

Occasional (6%-5%)

Dizziness, somnolence, asthenia, nausea

Rare (3%-2%)

Paresthesia, headache, dry mouth, warm or hot sensation, dyspepsia, dysphagia

SERIOUS REACTIONS

• Cardiac reactions (including ischemia, coronary artery vasospasm, and MI) and noncardiac vasospasm-related reactions (such as hemorrhage and cerebrovascular accident [CVA]) occur rarely, particularly in patients with hypertension, diabetes, or a strong family history of coronary artery disease; obese patients; smokers; males older than 40 years; and postmenopausal women.

INTERACTIONS

Drugs

❷ *Ergot-containing drugs (dihydroergotamine, methysergide):* Additive vasospastic effects; avoid use within 24 hrs of each other

❷ *Clarithromycin, erythromycin, troleandomycin:* Avoid use within 72 hrs of treatment with potent CYP3A4 inhibitors

❸ *Fluconazole:* 1.4-fold increase in C_{max}, 2-fold increase in AUC of eletriptan

❷ *Itraconazole, ketoconazole:* Avoid use within 72 hrs of treatment with potent CYP3A4 inhibitors

❷ *Nefazodone:* Avoid use within 72 hrs of treatment with potent CYP3A4 inhibitors

❷ *Nelfinavir, ritonavir:* Avoid use within 72 hrs of treatment with potent CYP3A4 inhibitors

❸ *Sibutramine:* May produce serotonin syndrome (marked by altered LOC, CNS irritability, motor weakness, myoclonus, and shivering)

❸ *Verapamil:* 2-fold increase in C_{max}, 3-fold increase in AUC of eletriptan

SPECIAL CONSIDERATIONS

• First dose should be administered under medical supervision, particularly in patients with risk factors for coronary artery disease

PATIENT/FAMILY EDUCATION

• Use for treatment of migraines, not prophylaxis
• Swallow the tablets whole; do not to crush or break them
• Take a single dose of eletriptan as soon as migraine symptoms appear
• Avoid tasks that require mental alertness or motor skills until response to the drug has been established
• Notify the physician immediately if palpitations, pain or tightness in the chest or throat, pain or weakness in the extremities, or sudden or severe abdominal pain occurs
• Female patients who are planning pregnancy should understand that the drug may suppress ovulation
• Lie down in a dark, quiet room for additional benefit after taking eletriptan

MONITORING PARAMETERS

• *Efficacy:* Headache response 1-4 hrs after a dose (reduction from moderate or severe pain to minimal or no pain); headache recurrence within 24 hrs
• *Toxicity:* Vital signs (pulse blood pressure), electrocardiogram particularly in patient with coronary artery disease risk factors

emtricitabine

(em-tri-sit′-uh-bean)

Rx: Emtriva

Combinations

Rx: with tenofovir (Truvada)

Chemical Class: Nucleoside analog

Therapeutic Class: Antiretroviral

CLINICAL PHARMACOLOGY

Mechanism of Action: An antiretroviral that inhibits HIV-1 reverse transcriptase by incorporating itself into viral DNA, resulting in chain termination. ***Therapeutic Effect:*** Interrupts HIV replication, slowing the progression of HIV infection.

Pharmacokinetics

Rapidly and extensively absorbed from the GI tract. Excreted primarily in urine (86%) and, to a lesser extent, in feces (14%); 30% removed by hemodialysis. Unknown if removed by peritoneal dialysis. ***Half-life:*** 10 hr.

INDICATIONS AND DOSAGES

HIV infection (in combination with other antiretrovirals)

PO

Adults, Elderly. 200 mg once a day.

Dosage in renal impairment

Dosage and frequency are modified based on creatinine clearance.

Creatinine Clearance	*Dosage*
30-49 ml/min	200 mg q48h
15-29 ml/min	200 mg q72h
less than 15 ml/min, hemodialysis patients	200 mg q96h

AVAILABLE FORMS

- *Capsules:* 200 mg.

CONTRAINDICATIONS: None known.

PREGNANCY AND LACTATION: Pregnancy category B; breast milk excretion unknown (breast-feeding not advised for HIV-infected women)

SIDE EFFECTS

Frequent (23%-13%)

Headache, rhinitis, rash, diarrhea, nausea

Occasional (14%-4%)

Cough, vomiting, abdominal pain, insomnia, depression, paresthesia, dizziness, peripheral neuropathy, dyspepsia, myalgia

Rare (3%-2%)

Arthralgia, abnormal dreams

SERIOUS REACTIONS

- Lactic acidosis and hepatomegaly with steatosis occur rarely and may be severe.

SPECIAL CONSIDERATIONS

- Current treatment guidelines use emtricitabine as an alternative to lamivudine in the nucleoside reverse transcriptase "backbone" that is part of combination antiretroviral therapy; it has no known advantages over lamivudine
- Reduced susceptibility to emtricitabine is associated with HIV reverse transcriptase gene mutation M184V/I
- Always check updated treatment guidelines before initiating or changing antiretroviral therapy (http://AIDSinfo.nih.gov)

PATIENT/FAMILY EDUCATION

- Success of an antiretroviral regimen requires >95% adherence to dosing schedule
- Emtricitabine use may cause a redistribution of body fat
- Continue taking the drug for the full course of treatment
- Emtricitabine is not a cure for HIV infection, nor does it reduce the risk of transmitting HIV to others

MONITORING PARAMETERS

- CBC, renal function, ALT, AST, triglycerides, HIV RNA, CD4 count
- Daily pattern of bowel activity and stool consistency
- Skin for rash and urticaria

E

enalapril maleate

(e-nal′-a-pril mal′-ee-ate)

Rx: Enalaprilat, Enalaprit Novaplus, Vasotec

Combinations

Rx: with diltiazem (Teczem); with felodipine (Lexxel); with hydrochlorothiazide (Vaseretic)

Chemical Class: Angiotensin-converting enzyme (ACE) inhibitor, nonsulfhydryl

Therapeutic Class: Antihypertensive

CLINICAL PHARMACOLOGY

Mechanism of Action: This angiotensin-converting enzyme (ACE) inhibitor suppresses the renin-angiotensin-aldosterone system, and prevents conversion of angiotensin I to angiotensin II, a potent vasoconstrictor; may inhibit angiotensin II at local vascular, renal sites. Decreases plasma angiotensin II, increases plasma renin activity, decreases aldosterone secretion. ***Therapeutic Effect:*** In hypertension, reduces peripheral arterial resistance. In congestive heart failure (CHF), increases cardiac output; decreases peripheral vascular resistance, BP, pulmonary capillary wedge pressure, heart size.

Pharmacokinetics

Route	Onset	Peak	Duration
PO	1 hr	4-6 hr	24 hr
IV	15 min	1-4 hr	6 hr

Readily absorbed from the GI tract (not affected by food). Protein binding: 50%-60%. Converted to active metabolite. Primarily excreted in urine. Removed by hemodialysis. ***Half-life:*** 11 hr (half-life is increased in those with impaired renal function).

INDICATIONS AND DOSAGES

Hypertension alone or in combination with other antihypertensives

PO

Adults, Elderly. Initially, 2.5-5 mg/day. May increase at 1-2-wk intervals. Range: 10-40 mg/day in 1-2 divided doses.

Children. 0.1 mg/kg/day in 1-2 divided doses. Maximum: 0.5 mg/kg/day.

Neonates. 0.1 mg/kg/day q24h.

IV

Adults, Elderly. 0.625-1.25 mg q6h up to 5 mg q6h.

Children, Neonates. 5-10 mcg/kg/dose q8-24h.

Adjunctive therapy for CHF

PO

Adults, Elderly. Initially, 2.5-5 mg/day. Range: 5-20 mg/day in 2 divided doses.

Dosage in renal impairment

Dosage is modified based on creatinine clearance.

Creatinine Clearance	% Usual Dose
10-50 ml/min	75-100
less than 10 ml/min	50

AVAILABLE FORMS

• *Tablets:* 2.5 mg, 5 mg, 10 mg, 20 mg.

• *Injection:* 1.25 mg/ml.

UNLABELED USES: Diabetic nephropathy, hypertension due to scleroderma renal crisis, hypertensive crisis, idiopathic edema, renal artery stenosis, rheumatoid arthritis, post MI for prevention of ventricular failure

CONTRAINDICATIONS: History of angioedema from previous treatment with ACE inhibitors

PREGNANCY AND LACTATION: Pregnancy category C (first trimester), category D (second and third trimesters); ACE inhibitors can cause fetal and neonatal morbidity and death when administered to pregnant women; when pregnancy is detected, discontinue ACE inhibitors as soon as possible; detectable in breast milk in trace amounts; effect on nursing infant has not been determined; use with caution in nursing mothers

SIDE EFFECTS

Frequent (7%-5%)

Headache, dizziness

Occasional (3%-2%)

Orthostatic hypotension, fatigue, diarrhea, cough, syncope

Rare (less than 2%)

Angina, abdominal pain, vomiting, nausea, rash, asthenia (loss of strength, energy), syncope

SERIOUS REACTIONS

- Excessive hypotension ("first-dose syncope") may occur in patients with CHF and in those who are severely salt or volume depleted.
- Angioedema (swelling of face, lips) and hyperkalemia occur rarely.
- Agranulocytosis and neutropenia may be noted in patients with collagen vascular diseases, including scleroderma and systemic lupus erythematosus, and impaired renal function.
- Nephrotic syndrome may be noted in those with history of renal disease.

INTERACTIONS

Drugs

3 *Alcohol:* May increase the effects of enalapril

2 *Allopurinol:* Predisposition to hypersensitivity reactions to ACE inhibitors

3 *Aspirin, NSAIDs:* Inhibition of the antihypertensive response to ACE inhibitors

3 *Azathioprine:* Increased myelosuppression

3 *Insulin:* Enhanced insulin sensitivity

3 *Iron:* Increased risk of anaphylaxis with administration of parenteral (IV) iron

3 *Lithium:* Increased risk of serious lithium toxicity

3 *Loop diuretics:* Initiation of ACE inhibitor therapy in the presence of intensive diuretic therapy results in a precipitous fall in blood pressure in some patients; ACE inhibitors may induce renal insufficiency in the presence of diuretic-induced sodium depletion

3 *Potassium:* Increased risk for hyperkalemia

3 *Potassium-sparing diuretics:* Increased risk for hyperkalemia

3 *Prazosin, terazosin, doxazosin:* Exaggerated first-dose hypotensive response to α-blockers

3 *Rofecoxib:* Increased risk for hyperkalemia

3 *Trimethoprim:* Additive risk of hyperkalemia, especially in patient predisposed to renal insufficiency

Labs

- ACE inhibition can account for approximately 0.5 mEq/L rise in serum potassium

SPECIAL CONSIDERATIONS

PATIENT/FAMILY EDUCATION

- Caution with salt substitutes containing potassium chloride
- Rise slowly to sitting/standing position to minimize orthostatic hypotension
- Dizziness, fainting, lightheadedness may occur during first few days of therapy
- May cause altered taste perception or cough; persistent dry cough usually does not subside unless medication is stopped; notify clinician if these symptoms persist
- Noncompliance with drug therapy or skipping drug doses may produce severe, rebound hypertension

• Notify the physician if diarrhea, difficulty breathing, excessive perspiration, vomiting, or swelling of the face, lips, or tongue occurs

MONITORING PARAMETERS

• BUN, creatinine, potassium within 2 wk after initiation of therapy (increased levels may indicate acute renal failure)
• Blood pressure
• Daily bowel activity and stool consistency

enfuvirtide

(en-fyoo'-vir-tide)

Rx: Fuzeon

Chemical Class: Fusion inhibitor, HIV; polypeptide, synthetic

Therapeutic Class: Antiretroviral

CLINICAL PHARMACOLOGY

Mechanism of Action: A fusion inhibitor that interferes with the entry of HIV-1 into CD4+ cells by inhibiting the fusion of viral and cellular membranes. ***Therapeutic Effect:*** Impairs HIV replication, slowing the progression of HIV infection.

Pharmacokinetics

Comparable absorption when injected into subcutaneous tissue of abdomen, arm, or thigh. Protein binding: 92%. Undergoes catabolism to amino acids. ***Half-life:*** 3.8 hr.

INDICATIONS AND DOSAGES

HIV infection (in combination with other antiretrovirals)

Subcutaneous

Adults, Elderly. 90 mg (1 ml) twice a day.

Children 6-16 yr. 2 mg/kg twice a day. Maximum 90 mg twice a day.

Pediatric Dosing Guidelines	
Weight: kg (lb)	*Dose: mg (ml)*
11-15.5 (24-34)	27 (0.3)
15.6-20 (35-44)	36 (0.4)
20.1-24.5 (45-54)	45 (0.5)
24.6-29 (55-64)	54 (0.6)
29.1-33.5 (65-74)	63 (0.7)
33.6-38 (75-84)	72 (0.8)
38.1-42.5 (85-94)	81 (0.9)
greater than 42.5 (greater than 94)	90 (1)

AVAILABLE FORMS

• *Powder for Injection:* 108-mg (approximately 90 mg/ml when reconstituted) vials.

CONTRAINDICATIONS: None known.

PREGNANCY AND LACTATION: Pregnancy category B; breast milk excretion unknown (breast-feeding not advised for HIV-infected women)

SIDE EFFECTS

Expected (98%)

Local injection site reactions (pain, discomfort, induration, erythema, nodules, cysts, pruritus, ecchymosis)

Frequent (26%-16%)

Diarrhea, nausea, fatigue

Occasional (11%-4%)

Insomnia, peripheral neuropathy, depression, cough, decreased appetite or weight loss, sinusitis, anxiety, asthenia, myalgia, cold sores

Rare (3%-2%)

Constipation, influenza, upper abdominal pain, anorexia, conjunctivitis

SERIOUS REACTIONS

• Enfuvirtide use may potentiate bacterial pneumonia.
• Hypersensitivity (rash, fever, chills, rigors, hypotension), thrombocytopenia, neutropenia, and renal insufficiency or failure may occur rarely.

SPECIAL CONSIDERATIONS

• Not active against HIV-2

• In heavily pretreated patients, randomized to receiving an "optimized" backbone regimen (based on treatment history and resistance testing) versus an optimized backbone regimen plus enfuvirtide, changes in HIV RNA at 24 wks were $-0.73 \log_{10}$ copies/ml and $-1.52 \log_{10}$ copies/ml, respectively; CD4 cell count changes from baseline were 35 and 71 cells/mm^3, respectively; clinical outcomes were not improved by enfuvirtide during this study

PATIENT/FAMILY EDUCATION

• Injection site reactions occur commonly

• Hypersensitivity reactions have included individually and in combination: rash, fever, nausea and vomiting, chills, rigors, hypotension

• Increased rate of bacterial pneumonia was observed in subjects treated with enfuvirtide in clinical trials (4.68 pneumonia events per 100 patient-years in the treatment group versus 0.61 events per 100 patient-years in the control group)

• More information is available for patients at www.FUZEON.com, or 877-438-9366

• Take for the full course of treatment

• Enfuvirtide is not a cure for HIV infection, nor does it reduce the risk of transmitting HIV to others; continue practices to prevent transmission of HIV

MONITORING PARAMETERS

• CBC with differential (eosinophilia), ALT, AST, triglycerides

• Skin for a hypersensitivity reaction and local injection site reactions

• Observe for evidence of fatigue or nausea

• Signs and symptoms of depression

enoxaparin sodium

(ee-nox-a-pa'-rin soe'-dee-um)

Rx: Lovenox

Chemical Class: Heparin derivative, depolymerized; low-molecular-weight heparin

Therapeutic Class: Anticoagulant

CLINICAL PHARMACOLOGY

Mechanism of Action: A low-molecular-weight heparin that potentiates the action of antithrombin III and inactivates coagulation factor Xa. ***Therapeutic Effect:*** Produces anticoagulation. Does not significantly influence bleeding time, PT, or aPTT.

Pharmacokinetics

Route	*Onset*	*Peak*	*Duration*
Subcutaneous	N/A	3-5 hr	12 hr

Well absorbed after subcutaneous administration. Eliminated primarily in urine. Not removed by hemodialysis. ***Half-life:*** 4.5 hr.

INDICATIONS AND DOSAGES

Prevention of deep vein thrombosis (DVT) after hip and knee surgery

Subcutaneous

Adults, Elderly. 30 mg twice a day, generally for 7-10 days.

Prevention of DVT after abdominal surgery

Subcutaneous

Adults, Elderly. 40 mg a day for 7-10 days.

Prevention of long-term DVT in nonsurgical acute illness

Subcutaneous

Adults, Elderly. 40 mg once a day for 3 wk.

Prevention of ischemic complications of unstable angina and non-Q-wave MI (with oral aspirin therapy)

Subcutaneous

Adults, Elderly. 1 mg/kg q12h.

Acute DVT
Subcutaneous
Adults, Elderly. 1 mg/kg q12h or 1.5 mg/kg once daily.
Usual pediatric dosage
Subcutaneous
Children. 0.5 mg/kg q12h (prophylaxis); 1 mg/kg q12h (treatment).
Dosage in renal impairment
Clearance of enoxaparin is decreased when creatinine clearance is less than 30 ml/min. Monitor patient and adjust dosage as necessary. When enoxaparin is used in abdominal, hip, or knee surgery or acute illness, the dosage in renal impairment is 30 mg once a day. When enoxaparin is used to treat DVT, angina, or MI the dosage in renal impairment is 1 mg/kg once a day.

AVAILABLE FORMS
- *Injection:* 30 mg/0.3 ml, 40 mg/0.4 ml, 60 mg/0.6 ml, 80 mg/0.8 ml, 100 mg/ml, 120 mg/0.8 ml, 150 mg/ml in prefilled syringes.

UNLABELED USES: Prevention of DVT following general surgical procedures

CONTRAINDICATIONS: Active major bleeding, concurrent heparin therapy, hypersensitivity to heparin or pork products, thrombocytopenia associated with positive *in vitro* test for antiplatelet antibodies

PREGNANCY AND LACTATION: Pregnancy category B; reports of congenital anomalies and fetal death, cause and effect relationship has not been determined; excretion into breast milk unknown; use caution in nursing mothers

SIDE EFFECTS
Occasional (4%-1%)
Injection site hematoma, nausea, peripheral edema

SERIOUS REACTIONS
- Overdose may lead to bleeding complications ranging from local ecchymoses to major hemorrhage. Antidote: Protamine sulfate (1% solution) equal to the dose of enoxaparin injected. One mg protamine sulfate neutralizes 1 mg enoxaparin. A second dose of 0.5 mg protamine sulfate per 1 mg enoxaparin may be given if aPTT tested 2-4 hr after first injection remains prolonged.

INTERACTIONS
Drugs
3 *Aspirin:* Increased risk of hemorrhage
3 *Oral anticoagulants:* Additive anticoagulant effects

SPECIAL CONSIDERATIONS
- Cannot be used interchangeably with unfractionated heparin or other low-molecular-weight heparins
- 1.5 mg/kg qd dosing should not be used in patients with cancer or obese patients
- Recent labeling changes regarding use in patients with mechanical prosthetic heart valves based on study involving a small number of pregnant women with mechanical valves; other evidence exists to substantiate cautious use in non-pregnant patients with mechanical valves

PATIENT/FAMILY EDUCATION
- Administer by deep SC inj into abdominal wall; alternate inj sites
- Report any unusual bruising or bleeding to clinician
- The usual length of therapy is 7-10 days
- Use an electric razor and soft toothbrush to prevent bleeding during therapy
- Do not take other medications, including OTC drugs (especially aspirin), without physician approval
- The female patient should know her menstrual flow may be heavier than usual

MONITORING PARAMETERS
- CBC with platelets, stool occult blood, urinalysis

• Monitoring aPTT is not required
• Assess for signs of bleeding, including bleeding at injection or surgical sites or from gums, blood in stool, bruising, hematuria, and petechiae

entacapone

(en-ta'-ka-pone)

Rx: Comtan

Chemical Class: Catechol-O-methyl-tranferase (COMT) inhibitor; nitrocatechol

Therapeutic Class: Antiparkinson's agent

CLINICAL PHARMACOLOGY

Mechanism of Action: An antiparkinson agent that inhibits the enzyme, catechol-*O*-methyl-transferase (COMT), potentiating dopamine activity and increasing the duration of action of levodopa. ***Therapeutic Effect:*** Decreases signs and symptoms of Parkinson's disease.

Pharmacokinetics

Rapidly absorbed after PO administration. Protein binding: 98%. Metabolized in the liver. Primarily eliminated by biliary excretion. Not removed by hemodialysis. ***Half-life:*** 2.4 hr.

INDICATIONS AND DOSAGES

Adjunctive treatment of Parkinson's disease

PO

Adults, Elderly. 200 mg concomitantly with each dose of carbidopa and levodopa up to a maximum of 8 times a day (1600 mg).

AVAILABLE FORMS

• *Tablets:* 200 mg.

CONTRAINDICATIONS: Hypersensitivity, use within 14 days of MAOIs

PREGNANCY AND LACTATION: Pregnancy category C; use caution in nursing mothers

SIDE EFFECTS

Frequent (greater than 10%)

Dyskinesia, nausea, dark yellow or orange urine and sweat, diarrhea

Occasional (9%-3%)

Abdominal pain, vomiting, constipation, dry mouth, fatigue, back pain

Rare (less than 2%)

Anxiety, somnolence, agitation, dyspepsia, flatulence, diaphoresis, asthenia, dyspnea

SERIOUS REACTIONS

• Hallucinations have been reported.

INTERACTIONS

Drugs

❷ *Nonselective MAO inhibitors (phenelzine, tranylcypromine):* Inhibition of the majority of the pathways responsible for normal catecholamine metabolism

❸ *Iron:* Decreased absorption of iron via chelation

❸ *Isoproterenol, epinephrine, norepinephrine, dopamine, dobutamine, α-methyldopa, apomorphine, isoetherine, and bitolterol:* Decreased metabolism of these drugs

SPECIAL CONSIDERATIONS

PATIENT/FAMILY EDUCATION

• Take entacapone with carbidopa and levodopa for best results
• Avoid tasks that require mental alertness or motor skills until response to the drug has been established
• Entacapone may cause sweat or urine to turn dark yellow or orange
• Notify the physician if uncontrolled movement of the hands, arms, legs, eyelids, face, mouth, or tongue occurs

MONITORING PARAMETERS

• Blood pressure

• Monitor for dyskinesia, diarrhea, and orthostatic hypotension
• Assess for relief of symptoms, including improvement of masklike facial expression, muscular rigidity, shuffling gait, and resting tremors of the hands and head

ephedrine

(eh-fed'-rin)

OTC: Pretz-D, Kondon's Nasal

Combinations

Rx: with potassium iodide, phenobarbital, theophylline (Quadrinal), with hydroxyine, theophylline (Hydrophed DF, Marax-DF); with guaifenesin (Broncholate, Ephex SR)

Chemical Class: Catecholamine

Therapeutic Class: Bronchodilator; decongestant; vasopressor

CLINICAL PHARMACOLOGY

Mechanism of Action: An adrenergic agonist that stimulates alpha-adrenergic receptors causing vasoconstriction and pressor effects, $beta_1$-adrenergic receptors, resulting in cardiac stimulation, and $beta_2$-adrenergic receptors, resulting in bronchial dilation and vasodilation. ***Therapeutic Effect:*** Increases blood pressure (BP) and pulse rate.

Pharmacokinetics

Well absorbed after nasal and parenteral absorption. Metabolized in liver. Excreted in urine. ***Half-life:*** 3-6 hrs.

INDICATIONS AND DOSAGES

Asthma

PO

Adults. 25-50 mg q3-4h as needed.

Children. 3 mg/kg/day in 4 divided doses.

Hypotension

IM

Adults. 25-50 mg as a single dose. Maximum 150 mg/day.

Children. 0.2-0.3 mg/kg/dose q4-6h.

IV

Adults. 5 mg/dose slow IVP as prevention. 10-25 mg/dose slow IVP repeated q5-10min as treatment. Maximum: 150 mg/day.

Children. 0.2-0.3 mg/kg/dose slow IVP q4-6h.

SC

Adults. 25-50 q4-6h. Maximum 150 mg/day.

Children. 3 mg/kg/day q4-6h.

Nasal congestion

PO

Adults. 25-50 mg q6h as needed.

Children. 3 mg/kg/day in 4 divided doses.

Nasal

Adults, Children 12 yrs and older. 2-3 sprays into each nostril q4h.

Children 6-12 yrs. 1-2 sprays into each nostril q4h.

AVAILABLE FORMS

• *Capsules:* 25 mg.
• *Injection:* 50 mg/ml.
• *Intranasal spray:* 0.25% (Pretz-D).

UNLABELED USES: Obesity, propofol-induced pain, radiocontrast media reactions

CONTRAINDICATIONS: Anesthesia with cyclopropane or halothane, diabetes (ephedrine injection), hypersensitivity to ephedrine or other sympathomimetic amines, hypertension or other cardiovascular disorders, pregnancy with maternal blood pressure above 130/80, thyrotoxicosis

PREGNANCY AND LACTATION: Pregnancy category C; routinely used to treat or prevent maternal hypotension following spinal anesthesia; may cause fetal heart rate changes; excretion into breast milk unknown; one case report of adverse effects (excessive crying, irritability, and disturbed sleeping patterns) in a 3-month-old nursing infant whose mother consumed disoephedrine

SIDE EFFECTS

Frequent

Hypertension, anxiety

Occasional

Nausea, vomiting, palpitations, tremor

Nasal: Burning, stinging, runny nose

Rare

Psychosis, decreased urination, necrosis at injection site from repeated injections

SERIOUS REACTIONS

- Excessive doses may cause hypertension, intracranial hemorrhage, anginal pain, and fatal arrhythmias.
- Prolonged or excessive use may result in metabolic acidosis due to increased serum lactic acid concentrations.
- Observe for disorientation, weakness, hyperventilation, headache, nausea, vomiting, and diarrhea.

INTERACTIONS

Drugs

3 *Antacids:* Increased ephedrine serum concentrations

3 *Furazolidone:* Hypertensive response possible

3 *Guanadrel:* Inhibits antihypertensive response

3 *Guanethidine:* Inhibits antihypertensive response

2 *MAOIs:* Substantially enhanced pressor response to ephedrine, severe hypertension

3 *Moclobemide:* Enhances the pressor response to ephedrine and increases the risk of palpitations, headache, and lightheadedness

3 *Sodium bicarbonate:* Increased ephedrine serum concentrations

Labs

- *False increase:* Urine amino acids, urine 5-HIAA

SPECIAL CONSIDERATIONS

- Found in many OTC weight-loss products containing mahuang; use should be avoided

PATIENT/FAMILY EDUCATION

- May cause wakefulness or nervousness; take last dose 4-6 hr prior to bedtime
- Do not use nasal products for >3-5 days
- Avoid consuming an excessive amount of caffeine derivatives such as chocolate, cocoa, coffee, cola, or tea
- Report any unusual side effects including headaches, dizziness, and fast heart beat

MONITORING PARAMETERS

- Heart rate, ECG, blood pressure (when using for vasopressor effect)
- Urine output
- Mental status changes

epinephrine

(ep-i-nef'-rin)

Rx: Adrenalin, Adrenalin Topical, EpiPen, EpiPen 2-Pak, EpiPen Auto Injector, EpiPen Jr. Auto Injector, Sus-Phrine Injection

OTC: Adrenalin, AsthmaHaler Mist, Asthma-Nefrin, microNefrin, Nephron, Primatene Mist, S-2

Combinations

Rx: with etidocaine (Duranest with Epinephrine); with prilocaine (Citanest Forte); with lidocaine (Xylocaine with Epinephrine); with pilocarpine (E-Pilo Ophthalmic)

Chemical Class: Catecholamine

Therapeutic Class: Antiglaucoma agent; bronchodilator; decongestant; vasopressor

CLINICAL PHARMACOLOGY

Mechanism of Action: A sympathomimetic, adrenergic agonist that stimulates alpha-adrenergic receptors causing vasoconstriction and pressor effects, $beta_1$-adrenergic receptors, resulting in cardiac stimulation, and $beta_2$-adrenergic receptors, resulting in bronchial dilation and vasodilation. With ophthalmic form, increases outflow of aqueous humor from anterior eye chamber. ***Therapeutic Effect:*** Relaxes smooth muscle of the bronchial tree, produces cardiac stimulation, and dilates skeletal muscle vasculature. The ophthalmic form dilates pupils and constricts conjunctival blood vessels.

Pharmacokinetics

Route	*Onset*	*Peak*	*Duration*
IM	5-10 min	20 min	1-4 hr
Subcutaneous	5-10 min	20 min	1-4 hr
Inhalation	3-5 min	20 min	1-3 hr
Ophthalmic	1 hr	4-8 hr	12-24 hr

Well absorbed after parenteral administration; minimally absorbed after inhalation. Metabolized in the liver, other tissues, and sympathetic nerve endings. Excreted in urine. The ophthalmic form may be systemically absorbed as a result of drainage into nasal pharyngeal passages. Mydriasis occurs within several min and persists several hr; vasoconstriction occurs within 5 min, and lasts less than 1 hr.

INDICATIONS AND DOSAGES

Anaphylaxis

IM

Adults, Elderly. 0.3 mg (0.3 ml of 1:1000 solution). May repeat if anaphylaxis persists.

Children. 0.15-0.3 mg or 0.01 mg/kg for patients weighing less than 30 kg. May repeat if anaphylaxis persists.

Asthma

Subcutaneous

Adults, Elderly. 0.2-0.5 mg (0.2-0.5 ml of 1:1000 solution) q2h as needed. In severe attacks, may repeat q20min times 3 doses.

Children. 0.01 ml/kg/dose (1:1000 solution). Maximum: 0.4-0.5 ml/dose. May repeat q15-20min for 3-4 doses or q4h as needed.

Inhalation

Adults, Elderly, Children 4 yr and older. 1 inhalation, wait at least 1 min. May repeat once. Do not use again for at least 3 hr.

Cardiac arrest
IV
Adults, Elderly. Initially, 1 mg. May repeat q3-5min as needed.
Children. Initially, 0.01 mg/kg (0.1 ml/kg of a 1:10,000 solution). May repeat q3-5min as needed.
Endotracheal
Children. 0.1 mg/kg (0.1 ml/kg of a 1:1000 solution. May repeat q3-5min as needed.
Hypersensitivity reaction
IM, Subcutaneous
Adults, Elderly. 0.3-0.5 mg q15-20min
Subcutaneous
Children. 0.01 mg/kg q15min for 2 doses, then q4h. Maximum single dose: 0.5 mg.
Inhalation
Adults, Elderly, Children 4 yr and older. 1 inhalation, may repeat in at least 1 min. Give subsequent doses no sooner than 3 hr.
Nebulizer
Adults, Elderly, Children 4 yr and older. 1-3 deep inhalations. Give subsequent doses no sooner than 3 hr.
Glaucoma
Ophthalmic
Adults, Elderly. 1-2 drops 1-2 times a day.

AVAILABLE FORMS
- *Injection (Adrenalin):* 0.1 mg/ml, 1 mg/ml.
- *Injection:* 0.3 mg/0.3 ml (EpiPen Auto Injector), 0.15 mg/0.3 ml (EpiPen Jr Auto-Injector, EpiPen 2-Pak).
- *Inhalation (Aerosol [Primatene Mist]):* 0.2 mg/inhalation.
- *Inhalation Solution:* 1%, 2.25%.
- *Ophthalmic Solution (Epifrin):* 0.5%, 1%, 2%.
- *Subcutaneous Suspension (Sus-Phrine Injection):* 5 mg/ml.
- *Topical Solution (Adrenalin, Topical):* 1:100.

UNLABELED USES: *Systemic:* Treatment of gingival or pulpal hemorrhage, priapism
Ophthalmic: Treatment of conjunctival congestion during surgery, secondary glaucoma

CONTRAINDICATIONS: Cardiac arrhythmias, cerebrovascular insufficiency, hypertension, hyperthyroidism, ischemic heart disease, narrow-angle glaucoma, shock

PREGNANCY AND LACTATION: Pregnancy category C; excreted into breast milk; use caution in nursing mothers

SIDE EFFECTS
Frequent
Systemic: Tachycardia, palpitations, nervousness
Ophthalmic: Headache, eye irritation, watering of eyes
Occasional
Systemic: Dizziness, lightheadedness, facial flushing, headache, diaphoresis, increased BP, nausea, trembling, insomnia, vomiting, fatigue
Ophthalmic: Blurred or decreased vision, eye pain
Rare
Systemic: Chest discomfort or pain, arrhythmias, bronchospasm, dry mouth or throat

SERIOUS REACTIONS
- Excessive doses may cause acute hypertension or arrhythmias.
- Prolonged or excessive use may result in metabolic acidosis due to increased serum lactic acid concentrations. Metabolic acidosis may cause disorientation, fatigue, hyperventilation, headache, nausea, vomiting, and diarrhea.

INTERACTIONS
Drugs
3 *Antihistamines:* Effects of epinephrine may be potentiated by certain antihistamines; diphenhy-

dramine, tripelennamine, d-chlorpheniramine
3 *β-blockers:* Noncardioselective β-blockers enhance pressor response to epinephrine, resulting in hypertension and bradycardia
3 *Chlorpromazine, clozaril, thioridazine:* Reversal of epinephrine pressor response
❷ *Cyclic antidepressants:* Pressor response to IV epinephrine markedly enhanced
3 *Digoxin, sympathomimetics:* May increase risk of arrhythmias
3 *Ergonovine, methergine, oxytocin:* May increase vasoconstriction
3 *Levothyroxine:* Effects of epinephrine may be potentiated

SPECIAL CONSIDERATIONS

PATIENT/FAMILY EDUCATION

- Do not exceed recommended doses
- Wait at least 3-5 min between inhalations with MDI
- Notify clinician of dizziness or chest pain
- Do not use nasal preparations for >3-5 days to prevent rebound congestion
- To avoid contamination of ophth preparations, do not touch tip of container to any surface
- Do not use ophth preparations while wearing soft contact lenses
- Transitory stinging may occur on instillation of ophth preparations
- Report any decrease in visual acuity immediately
- Use of OTC asthma preparations containing epinephrine should be discouraged
- Avoid consuming excessive amounts of caffeine derivatives such as chocolate, cocoa, coffee, cola, and tea

MONITORING PARAMETERS

- Blood pressure, heart rate
- Intraocular pressure
- Breath sounds for crackles, rhonchi, and wheezing
- ECG and patient's condition, especially in the patient with cardiac arrest

eplerenone

(e-pler′-en-one)

Rx: Inspra

Chemical Class: Pregnene methyl ester

Therapeutic Class: Selective aldosterone receptor antagonist

CLINICAL PHARMACOLOGY

Mechanism of Action: An aldosterone receptor antagonist that binds to the mineralocorticoid receptors in the kidney, heart, blood vessels, and brain, blocking the binding of aldosterone. ***Therapeutic Effect:*** Reduces BP.

Pharmacokinetics

Absorption unaffected by food. Protein binding: 50%. No active metabolites. Excreted in the urine with a lesser amount eliminated in the feces. Not removed by hemodialysis. ***Half-life:*** 4-6 hr.

INDICATIONS AND DOSAGES

Hypertension

PO

Adults, Elderly. 50 mg once a day. If 50 mg once a day produces an inadequate BP response, may increase dosage to 50 mg twice a day. If patient is concurrently receiving erythromycin, saquinavir, verapamil, or fluconazole, reduce initial dose to 25 mg once a day.

CHF following MI

PO

Adults, Elderly. Initially, 25 mg once a day. If tolerated, titrate up to 50 mg once a day within 4 wk.

AVAILABLE FORMS

• *Tablets:* 25 mg, 50 mg.

CONTRAINDICATIONS: Concurrent use of potassium supplements or potassium-sparing diuretics (such as amiloride, spironolactone, and triamterene), or strong inhibitors of the cytochrome P450 3A4 enzyme system (including ketoconazole and itraconazole), creatinine clearance less than 50 ml/min, serum creatinine level greater than 2 mg/dl in males or 1.8 mg/dl in females, serum potassium level greater than 5.5 mEq/L, type 2 diabetes mellitus with microalbuminuria

PREGNANCY AND LACTATION: Pregnancy category B; excreted into breast milk of lactating rabbits; human information unknown

SIDE EFFECTS

Rare (3%-1%)

Dizziness, diarrhea, cough, fatigue, flu-like symptoms, abdominal pain

SERIOUS REACTIONS

• Hyperkalemia may occur, particularly in patients with type 2 diabetes mellitus and microalbuminuria.

INTERACTIONS

Drugs

❷ *Angiotensin-converting enzyme inhibitors, and angiotensin II receptor antagonists:* Increased risk of hyperkalemia

❷ *Azole antifungal agents (fluconazole [less significant], itraconazole, ketoconazole, miconazole, voriconazole):* Inhibition of hepatic metabolism (CYP3A4) leads to increased eplerenone levels (2-6 times)

3 *Grapefruit, grapefruit juice:* Produces small increase in serum potassium level

3 *Lithium:* Increased risk of lithium toxicity

3 *Macrolide antibiotics (erythromycin, clarithromycin):* Caution, up to 2-fold increases in eplerenone levels due to inhibition of hepatic metabolism (CYP3A4)

3 *Nonsteroidal antiinflammatory drugs:* Reduction in antihypertensive effect of eplerenone

3 *Saquinavir:* Caution, up to two-fold increases in eplerenone levels due to inhibition of hepatic metabolism (CYP3A4)

3 *St. John's Wort:* Decreases eplerenone effectiveness

3 *Verapamil:* Caution, up to 2-fold increases in eplerenone levels due to inhibition of hepatic metabolism (CYP3A4)

SPECIAL CONSIDERATIONS

• Primary advantage of eplerenone over spironolactone is a potentially decreased incidence of endocrine-related adverse effects, such as gynecomastia or sexual dysfunction

PATIENT/FAMILY EDUCATION

• Avoid tasks that require mental alertness or motor skills until response to the drug has been established

• Do not break, crush, or chew film-coated tablets

• Avoid exercising outside during hot weather because of the risks of dehydration and hypotension

MONITORING PARAMETERS

• *Efficacy:* Blood pressure, heart rate, ECG, urine output, cardiac output, improvement in symptoms of heart failure

• *Toxicity:* Serum electrolytes (especially potassium), renal function tests, BP, ECG (hyperkalemia), signs and symptoms of toxicity

E

epoetin alfa

(eh-poh'-ee-tin al'-fa)

Rx: Epogen, Procrit

Chemical Class: Amino acid glycoprotein

Therapeutic Class: Hematopoietic agent

CLINICAL PHARMACOLOGY

Mechanism of Action: A glycoprotein that stimulates division and differentiation of erythroid progenitor cells in bone marrow. ***Therapeutic Effect:*** Induces erythropoiesis and releases reticulocytes from bone marrow.

Pharmacokinetics

Well absorbed after subcutaneous administration. Following administration, an increase in reticulocyte count occurs within 10 days, and increases in Hgb, Hct, and RBC count are seen within 2-6 wk. ***Half-life:*** 4-13 hr.

INDICATIONS AND DOSAGES

Treatment of anemia in chemotherapy patients

IV, Subcutaneous

Adults, Elderly, Children. 150 units/kg/dose 3 times a wk. Maximum: 1200 units/kg/wk.

Reduction of allogenic blood transfusions in elective surgery

Subcutaneous

Adults, Elderly. 300 units/kg/day 10 days before day of, and 4 days after surgery.

Chronic renal failure

IV Bolus, Subcutaneous

Adults, Elderly. Initially, 50-100 units/kg 3 times a wk. Target Hct range: 30%-36%. Adjust dosage no earlier than 1-mo intervals unless prescribed. Decrease dosage if Hct is increasing and approaching 36%. Plan to temporarily withhold doses if Hct continues to rise and to reinstate lower dosage when Hct begins to decrease. If Hct increases by more than 4 points in 2 wk, monitor Hct twice a wk for 2-6 wk. Increase dose if Hct does not increase 5-6 points after 8 wk (with adequate iron stores) and if Hct is below target range. Maintenance: *For patients on dialysis:* 75 units/kg 3 times a wk. Range: 12.5-525 units/kg. *For patients not on dialysis:* 75-150 units/kg/wk.

HIV infection in patients treated with AZT

IV, Subcutaneous

Adults. Initially, 100 units/kg 3 times a wk for 8 wk; may increase by 50-100 units/kg 3 times a wk. Evaluate response q4-8wk thereafter. Adjust dosage by 50-100 units/kg 3 times a wk. If dosages larger than 300 units/kg 3 times a wk are not eliciting response, it is unlikely patient will respond. Maintenance: Titrate to maintain desired Hct.

AVAILABLE FORMS

- *Injection (Epogen, Procrit):* 2000 units/ml, 3000 units/ml, 4000 units/ml, 10,000 units/ml, 20,000 units/ml, 40,000 units/ml.

UNLABELED USES: Anemia associated with frequent blood donations, anemia in critically ill patients, malignancy, management of hepatitis C, myelodysplastic syndromes

CONTRAINDICATIONS: History of sensitivity to mammalian cell-derived products or human albumin, uncontrolled hypertension

PREGNANCY AND LACTATION: Pregnancy category C; excretion into breast milk unknown; use caution in nursing mothers

SIDE EFFECTS

Patients receiving chemotherapy

Frequent (20%-17%)

Fever, diarrhea, nausea, vomiting, edema

Occasional (13%-11%)

Asthenia, shortness of breath, paresthesia

Rare (5%-3%)

Dizziness, trunk pain

Patients with chronic renal failure

Frequent (24%-11%)

Hypertension, headache, nausea, arthralgia

Occasional (9%-7%)

Fatigue, edema, diarrhea, vomiting, chest pain, skin reactions at administration site, asthenia, dizziness

Patients with HIV infection treated with AZT

Frequent (38%-15%)

Fever, fatigue, headache, cough, diarrhea, rash, nausea

Occasional (14%-9%)

Shortness of breath, asthenia, skin reaction at injection site, dizziness

SERIOUS REACTIONS

- Hypertensive encephalopathy, thrombosis, cerebrovascular accident, MI, and seizures have occurred rarely.
- Hyperkalemia occurs occasionally in patients with chronic renal failure, usually in those who do not conform to medication regimen, dietary guidelines, and frequency of dialysis regimen.

INTERACTIONS

Drugs

3 *Heparin:* An increase in RBC volume may enhance blood clotting; heparin dosage may need to be increased

SPECIAL CONSIDERATIONS

- Iron supplementation should be given during therapy to provide for increased requirements during expansion of red cell mass secondary to marrow stimulation by erythropoietin
- Use prior to elective surgery should be limited to patients with presurgery hemoglobin of >10 but ≤13 g/dl undergoing noncardiac, nonvascular procedures

PATIENT/FAMILY EDUCATION

- Do not shake vials as this may denature the glycoprotein, rendering the drug inactive
- Notify clinician if severe headache develops
- Frequent blood tests required to determine optimal dose
- Avoid potentially hazardous activities during the first 90 days of therapy; there is an increased risk of seizure development in patients with chronic renal failure during the first 90 days of therapy

MONITORING PARAMETERS

- Hct (target range 30%-33%, max 36%), serum iron, ferritin (keep >100 ng/dl)
- Baseline erythropoietin level (treatment of patients with erythropoietin levels >200 mU/ml is not recommended)
- Blood pressure
- BUN, uric acid, creatinine, phosphorus, potassium on a regular basis
- Body temperature, especially in patients receiving chemotherapy and in patients with HIV infection treated with zidovudine

epoprostenol sodium, prostacyclin

(e-poe-pros'-ten-ol soe'-dee-um)

Rx: Flolan

Chemical Class: Prostaglandin I_2

Therapeutic Class: Vasodilator

CLINICAL PHARMACOLOGY

Mechanism of Action: An antihypertensive that directly dilates pulmonary and systemic arterial vascular beds and inhibits platelet aggregation. ***Therapeutic Effect:*** Reduces right and left ventricular afterload; increases cardiac output and stroke volume.

Pharmacokinetics

Extensively metabolized by rapid hydrolysis at neutral pH in blood and by enzymatic degradation. The metabolites are excreted in urine. ***Half-life:*** 3-5 min.

INDICATIONS AND DOSAGES

Long-term treatment of New York Heart Association Class III and IV primary pulmonary hypertension

IV Infusion

Adults, Elderly. Procedure to determine dose range: Initially, 2 ng/kg/min, increased in increments of 2 ng/kg/min q15min until dose-limiting adverse effects occur. Chronic infusion: Start at 4 ng/kg/min less than the maximum dose rate tolerated during acute dose ranging (or one half of the maximum rate if rate was less than 5 ng/kg/min).

AVAILABLE FORMS

• *Injection, Powder for Reconstitution:* 0.5 mg, 1.5 mg.

UNLABELED USES: Cardiopulmonary bypass surgery; hemodialysis; pulmonary hypertension associated with acute respiratory distress syndrome, systemic lupus erythematosus, or congenital heart disease; neonatal pulmonary hypertension, refractory CHF; severe community-acquired pneumonia

CONTRAINDICATIONS: Long-term use in patients with CHF (severe ventricular systolic dysfunction)

PREGNANCY AND LACTATION: Pregnancy category B; women with pulmonary hypertension should avoid pregnancy; unknown if excreted in breast milk

SIDE EFFECTS

Frequent

Acute phase: Flushing (58%), headache (49%), nausea (32%), vomiting (32%), hypotension (16%), anxiety (11%), chest pain (11%), dizziness (8%)

Chronic phase: (greater than 20%): Dyspnea, asthenia, dizziness, headache, chest pain, nausea, vomiting, palpitations, edema, jaw pain, tachycardia, flushing, myalgia, nonspecific muscle pain, paresthesia, diarrhea, anxiety, chills, fever, or flu-like symptoms

Occasional

Acute phase (5%-2%): Bradycardia, abdominal pain, muscle pain, dyspnea, back pain

Chronic phase (20%-10%): Rash, depression, hypotension, pallor, syncope, bradycardia, ascites

Rare

Acute phase: Paresthesia

Chronic phase (less than 2%): Diaphoresis, dyspepsia, tachycardia

SERIOUS REACTIONS

• Overdose may cause hyperglycemia or ketoacidosis manifested as increased urination, thirst, and fruit-like breath odor.

• Angina, MI, and thrombocytopenia occur rarely.

• Abrupt withdrawal, including a large reduction in dosage or interruption in drug delivery, may produce rebound pulmonary hypertension as evidenced by dyspnea, dizziness, and asthenia.

INTERACTIONS

Drugs

3 *Anticoagulants:* May increase the risk of bleeding

3 *Antihypertensives, diuretics, vasodilators:* Additive effects on blood pressure

3 *Digoxin:* Possible elevations of plasma digoxin concentrations

3 *Vasoconstrictors:* May decrease the effects of epoprostenol

SPECIAL CONSIDERATIONS

- Clinically shown to improve exercise capacity, dyspnea, and fatigue as early as first week of therapy
- Drug is administered chronically on an ambulatory basis with a portable infusion pump through a permanent central venous cathether; peripheral IV infusions may be used temporarily until central venous access obtained
- Patients must be taught sterile technique, drug reconstitution, and care of catheter
- Do not interrupt infusion or decrease rate abruptly, may cause rebound symptoms (dyspnea, dizziness, asthenia, death)
- Unless contraindicated, patients should be anticoagulated to reduce risk of pulmonary thromboembolism or systemic embolism through a patent foramen ovale

PATIENT/FAMILY EDUCATION

- Therapy will be necessary for a prolonged period, possibly years
- Brief interruptions in drug delivery may result in rapidly, worsening symptoms

MONITORING PARAMETERS

- Postural BP and heart rate for several hr following dosage adjustments
- Assess for a therapeutic response as evidenced by decreased chest pain, dyspnea on exertion, fatigue, pulmonary arterial pressure, pulmonary vascular resistance, and syncope, and improved pulmonary function

eprosartan mesylate

(ep-roe-sar'-tan mes'-sil-ate)

Rx: Teveten

Chemical Class: Angiotensin II receptor antagonist

Therapeutic Class: Antihypertensive

CLINICAL PHARMACOLOGY

Mechanism of Action: An angiotensin II receptor antagonist that blocks the vasoconstrictor and aldosterone-secreting effects of angiotensin II, inhibiting the binding of angiotensin II to the AT_1 receptors. ***Therapeutic Effect:*** Causes vasodilation, decreases peripheral resistance, and decreases BP.

Pharmacokinetics

Rapidly absorbed after PO administration. Protein binding: 98%. Undergoes first-pass metabolism in the liver to active metabolites. Excreted in urine and biliary system. Minimally removed by hemodialysis. ***Half-life:*** 5-9 hr.

INDICATIONS AND DOSAGES

Hypertension

PO

Adults, Elderly. Initially, 600 mg/day. Range: 400-800 mg/day.

AVAILABLE FORMS

- *Tablets:* 400 mg, 600 mg.

CONTRAINDICATIONS: Bilateral renal artery stenosis, hyperaldosteronism

PREGNANCY AND LACTATION: Pregnancy category C (D if used in second or third trimester); drugs acting directly on the renin-angiotensin-aldosterone system are documented to cause fetal harm (hypotension, oligohydramnios, neonatal anemia, hyperkalemia, neonatal skull hypoplasia, anuria, and renal failure; neonatal limb contractures, craniofacial deformities, and hypoplastic lung development)

SIDE EFFECTS

Occasional (5%-2%)

Headache, cough, dizziness

Rare (less than 2%)

Muscle pain, fatigue, diarrhea, upper respiratory tract infection, dyspepsia

SERIOUS REACTIONS

• Overdosage may manifest as hypotension and tachycardia. Bradycardia occurs less often.

SPECIAL CONSIDERATIONS

• Potentially as or more effective than angiotensin-converting enzyme inhibitors, without cough; no evidence for reduction in morbidity and mortality as first-line agents in hypertension, yet; whether they provide the same cardiac and renal protection also still tentative; like ACE inhibitors, less effective in black patients

PATIENT/FAMILY EDUCATION

• Call your clinician immediately if note following side effects: wheezing; lip, throat, or face swelling; hives or rash

• Female patients should be aware of the consequences of second- and third-trimester exposure to eprosartan

• Avoid tasks that require mental alertness or motor skills until response to the drug has been established

• Restrict alcohol and sodium consumption while taking eprosartan, adhere to the provided diet, and control weight

• Do not exercise outside during hot weather because of the risks of dehydration and hypotension

MONITORING PARAMETERS

• Baseline electrolytes, urinalysis, blood urea nitrogen, and creatinine with recheck at 2-4 wk after initiation (sooner in volume-depleted patients); monitor sitting blood pressure; watch for symptomatic hypotension, particularly in volume-depleted patients

eptifibatide

(ep-tih-fib′-ah-tide)

Rx: Integrilin

Chemical Class: Glycoprotein (GP) IIb/IIIa inhibitor

Therapeutic Class: Antiplatelet agent

CLINICAL PHARMACOLOGY

Mechanism of Action: A glycoprotein IIb/IIIa inhibitor that rapidly inhibits platelet aggregation by preventing binding of fibrinogen to receptor sites on platelets. ***Therapeutic Effect:*** Prevents closure of treated coronary arteries. Also prevents acute cardiac ischemic complications.

Pharmacokinetics

Protein binding: 25%. Excreted in urine. ***Half-life:*** 2.5 hr.

INDICATIONS AND DOSAGES

Adjunct to percutaneous coronary intervention (PCI)

IV Bolus, IV Infusion

Adults, Elderly. 180 mcg/kg before PCI initiation; then continuous drip of 2 mcg/kg/min and a second 180 mcg/kg bolus 10 min after the first. Maximum: 15 mg/h. Continue until hospital discharge or for up to 18-24 hrs. Minimum 12 hrs is recommended. Concurrent aspirin and heparin therapy is recommended.

Acute coronary syndrome

IV Bolus, IV Infusion

Adults, Elderly. 180 mcg/kg bolus then 2 mcg/kg/min until discharge or coronary artery bypass graft, up to

72 hr. Maximum: 15 mg/h. Concurrent aspirin and heparin therapy is recommended.

Dosage in renal impairment

Creatinine clearance less than 50 ml/min. Use 180 mcg/kg bolus (maximum 22.6 mg) and 1 mcg/kg/min infusion (maximum: 7.5 mg/h).

AVAILABLE FORMS

- *Injection solution:* 0.75 mg/ml, 2 mg/ml.

CONTRAINDICATIONS: Active internal bleeding, AV malformation or aneurysm, history of cerebrovascular accident (CVA) within 2 yrs or CVA with residual neurologic defect, history of vasculitis, intracranial neoplasm, oral anticoagulant use within last 7 days unless PT is less than 1.22 times the control, recent (6 wk or less) GI or GU bleeding, recent (6 wk or less) surgery or trauma, prior IV dextran use before or during percutaneous transluminal coronary angioplasty (PTCA), severe uncontrolled hypertension, thrombocytopenia (less than 100,000 cells/mcL)

PREGNANCY AND LACTATION: Pregnancy category B; use caution in nursing mothers

SIDE EFFECTS

Occasional (7%)

Hypotension

SERIOUS REACTIONS

- Minor to major bleeding complications may occur, most commonly at arterial access site for cardiac catheterization.

INTERACTIONS

Drugs

3 *Anticoagulants (heparin, warfarin), antiplatelet agents (ticlopidine, clopidogrel, dipyridamole), thrombolytics (alteplase, streptokinase), NSAIDs, aspirin:* Increased risk of bleeding

SPECIAL CONSIDERATIONS

- When bleeding cannot be controlled with pressure, discontinue INF
- Most major bleeding occurs at arterial access site for cardiac catheterization; prior to pulling femoral artery sheath, discontinue heparin for 3-4 hr and document activated clotting time (ACT) <150 sec or aPTT <45 sec; achieve sheath hemostasis 2-4 hr before discharge
- In patients who undergo CABG, discontinue eptifibatide INF prior to surgery
- Eptifibatide, tirofiban, and abciximab can all decrease the incidence of cardiac events associated with acute coronary syndromes; direct comparisons are needed to establish which, if any, is superior; for angioplasty, until more data become available, abciximab appears to be the drug of choice

PATIENT/FAMILY EDUCATION

- Report bleeding from surgical site, chest pain, or dyspnea
- Use an electric razor and soft toothbrush, to prevent bleeding during eptifibatide therapy
- Do not take other medications, including OTC drugs (especially aspirin), without physician approval
- Report black or red stool, coffee-ground emesis, dark or red urine, or red-speckled mucus from cough
- The female patient should understand that her menstrual flow may be heavier than usual

MONITORING PARAMETERS

- Platelet count, hemoglobin, hematocrit, PT/aPTT (baseline, within 6 hr following bolus dose, then daily thereafter)
- In patients undergoing PCI, also measure ACT; maintain aPTT between 50 and 70 sec unless PCI is to be performed; during PCI, maintain ACT between 300 and 350 sec

ergoloid mesylates

(er'-goe-loid mess'-i-lates)

Rx: Gerimal, Hydergine

Chemical Class: Ergot alkaloid

Therapeutic Class: Cerebral metabolic enhancer

CLINICAL PHARMACOLOGY

Mechanism of Action: An ergot alkaloid that centrally acts and decreases vascular tone, slows heart rate. Peripheral action blocks alpha adrenergic receptors. ***Therapeutic Effect:*** Improved O_2 uptake and improves cerebral metabolism.

Pharmacokinetics

Rapidly, incompletely absorbed from GI tract. Metabolized in liver. Eliminated primarily in feces. ***Half-life:*** 2-5 hrs.

INDICATIONS AND DOSAGES

Age-related decline in mental capacity

PO

Adults, Elderly. Initially, 1 mg 3 times/day. Range: 1.5-12 mg/day.

AVAILABLE FORMS

- *Capsules:* 1 mg (Hydergine).
- *Oral solution:* 1 mg/ml (Hydergine).
- *Tablets:* 1 mg (Germinal, Hydergine).
- *Tablets, sublingual:* 1 mg (Germinal, Hydergine).

CONTRAINDICATIONS: Acute or chronic psychosis (regardless of etiology), hypersensitivity to ergoloid mesylates or any component of the formulation

PREGNANCY AND LACTATION: Pregnancy category C

SIDE EFFECTS

Occasional

GI distress, transient nausea, sublingual irritation

SERIOUS REACTIONS

- Overdose may produce blurred vision, dizziness, syncope, headache, flushed face, nausea, vomiting, decreased appetite, stomach cramps, and stuffy nose.

SPECIAL CONSIDERATIONS

PATIENT/FAMILY EDUCATION

- Results may not be observed for 3-4 wk
- May cause transient GI disturbances; allow sublingual tablets to completely dissolve under tongue; do not chew or crush sublingual tablets

MONITORING PARAMETERS

- Before prescribing, exclude the possibility that the patient's signs and symptoms arise from a potentially reversible and treatable condition
- Periodically reassess the diagnosis and the benefit of current therapy to the patient; discontinue if no benefit
- Pulse
- Therapeutic response and improvement

ergonovine maleate

(er-goe-noe'-veen mal'-ee-ate)

OTC: Ergotrate Maleate

Chemical Class: Ergot alkaloid

Therapeutic Class: Oxytocic

CLINICAL PHARMACOLOGY

Mechanism of Action: An oxytoxic agent that directly stimulates uterine muscle. Stimulates alpha-adrenergic, serotonin receptors producing arterial vasoconstriction. Causes vasospasm of coronary arteries. ***Therapeutic Effect:*** Increases force and frequency of contractions. Induces cervical contractions.

Pharmacokinetics

None reported.

INDICATIONS AND DOSAGES
Oxytocic
IM/IV
Adults. Initially, 0.2 mg. May repeat no more than q2-4h for no more than 5 doses total.
AVAILABLE FORMS
• *Injection:* 0.2 mg/ml (Ergotrate).
UNLABELED USES: Treatment of incomplete abortion, diagnosis of angina pectoris
CONTRAINDICATIONS: Induction of labor, threatened spontaneous abortions, hypersensitivity to ergonovine maleate or any component of the formulation
PREGNANCY AND LACTATION: Pregnancy category X; Not recommended for routine use prior to delivery of the placenta; may lower prolactin levels, which may decrease lactation
SIDE EFFECTS
Frequent
Uterine cramping
Occasional
Diarrhea, dizziness, nasal congestion, sweating, ringing in ears
Rare
Headache, nausea, vomiting, allergic reaction
SERIOUS REACTIONS
• Severe hypertensive episodes may result in cerebrovascular accident, serious arrhythmias, seizures; hypertensive effects more frequent with rapid IV administration, concurrent regional anesthesia or vasoconstrictors.
• Peripheral ischemia may lead to gangrene.
• Overdose includes symptoms of angina; bradycardia; confusion; drowsiness; fast, weak pulse; miosis; severe peripheral vasoconstriction (numbness in arms or legs, blue skin color); seizures; tachycardia; thirst; and severe uterine cramping.

INTERACTIONS
Drugs
3 *Dopamine:* Excessive vasoconstriction
SPECIAL CONSIDERATIONS
• Symptoms of ergotism occur with overdosage (nausea, vomiting, diarrhea, seizure, hallucinations, delirium, numb/gangrenous extremities)
PATIENT/FAMILY EDUCATION
• Report any chest pain
MONITORING PARAMETERS
• Blood pressure, pulse, and uterine response

ergotamine tartrate/ dihydroergotamine
(er-got'-a-meen tar'-trate)
Combinations
Rx: with caffeine (Cafergot, Ercaf, Wigraine); with belladonna alkaloids, phenobarbital (Bellergal-S)
Chemical Class: Ergot alkaloid
Therapeutic Class: Antimigraine agent

CLINICAL PHARMACOLOGY
Mechanism of Action: An ergotamine derivative and alpha-adrenergic blocker that directly stimulates vascular smooth muscle, resulting in peripheral and cerebral vasoconstriction. May also have antagonist effects on serotonin. ***Therapeutic Effect:*** Suppresses vascular headaches.
Pharmacokinetics
Slowly and incompletely absorbed from the GI tract; rapidly and extensively absorbed after rectal administration. Protein binding: greater than 90%. Undergoes extensive first-pass metabolism in the liver to

active metabolite. Eliminated in feces by the biliary system. ***Half-life:*** 21 hr.

INDICATIONS AND DOSAGES

Vascular headaches

PO (Cafergot [fixed-combination of ergotamine and caffeine])

Adults, Elderly. 2 mg at onset of headache, then 1-2 mg q30min. Maximum: 6 mg/episode; 10 mg/wk.

PO, Sublingual

Children. 1 mg at onset of headache, then 1 mg q30min. Maximum: 3 mg/episode.

IV

Adults, Elderly. 1 mg at onset of headache; may repeat hourly. Maximum: 2 mg/day; 6 mg/wk.

Sublingual

Adults, Elderly. 1 tablet at onset of headache, then 1 tablet q30min. Maximum: 3 tablets/24 hr; 5 tablets/wk.

IM, Subcutaneous (dihydroergotamine)

Adults, Elderly. 1 mg at onset of headache; may repeat hourly. Maximum: 3 mg/day; 6 mg/wk.

Intranasal

Adults, Elderly. 1 spray (0.5 mg) into each nostril; may repeat in 15 min. Maximum: 4 sprays/day; 8 sprays/wk.

Rectal

Adults, Elderly. 1 suppository at onset of headache; may repeat dose in 1 hr. Maximum: 2 suppositories/episode; 5 suppositories/wk.

AVAILABLE FORMS

- *Tablets (Sublingual [Ergomar]):* 2 mg.
- *Injection (DHE 45):* 1 mg/ml.
- *Nasal Spray (Migranal):* 0.5 mg/spray.
- *Suppositories (ergotamine and caffeine):* 2 mg, with 100 mg caffeine.

UNLABELED USES: Prevention of deep venous thrombosis, prevention and treatment of orthostatic hypotension, pulmonary thromboembolism

CONTRAINDICATIONS: Coronary artery disease, hypertension, impaired hepatic or renal function, malnutrition, peripheral vascular diseases (such as thromboangiitis obliterans, syphilitic arteritis, severe arteriosclerosis, thrombophlebitis, and Raynaud's disease), sepsis, severe pruritus

PREGNANCY AND LACTATION: Pregnancy category X; excreted into breast milk; has caused symptoms of ergotism (e.g., vomiting, diarrhea) in the infant; excessive dosage or prolonged administration may inhibit lactation

SIDE EFFECTS

Occasional (5%-2%)

Cough, dizziness

Rare (less than 2%)

Myalgia, fatigue, diarrhea, upper respiratory tract infection, dyspepsia

SERIOUS REACTIONS

- Prolonged administration or excessive dosage may produce ergotamine poisoning, manifested as nausea and vomiting; paresthesia, muscle pain or weakness; precordial pain; tachycardia or bradycardia; and hypertension or hypotension. Vasoconstriction of peripheral arteries and arterioles may result in localized edema and pruritus. Muscle pain will occur when walking and later, even at rest. Other rare effects include confusion, depression, drowsiness, seizures, and gangrene.

INTERACTIONS

Drugs

❷ *Azithromycin, dirithromycin, erythromycin:* Coadministration may result in ergotism

3 *β-blockers:* May increase the risk of vasospasm

3 *Ergot alkaloids, systemic vasoconstrictors:* May increase the pressor effect

❷ *Indinavir:* Increases the plasma concentrations of ergotamine, possibly leading to toxicity including vasospasm and cyanosis

❷ *Nitroglycerin:* Decreased antianginal effects of nitroglycerin

❷ *Voriconazole:* Elevated ergotamine concentrations and toxicity may occur if voriconazole and ergotamine are coadministered

SPECIAL CONSIDERATIONS

PATIENT/FAMILY EDUCATION

- Initiate therapy at first sign of attack
- DO NOT exceed recommended dosage
- Notify clinician of irregular heart beat, nausea, vomiting, numbness or tingling of fingers or toes, pain or weakness of extremities
- Regular use may lead to withdrawal headaches
- Avoid pregnancy during therapy and notify the physician immediately if pregnant; teach the patient methods of contraception if needed

MONITORING PARAMETERS

- Monitor the patient closely for evidence of ergotamine overdose from prolonged administration or excessive dosage

---

ertapenem

(er-ta-pen′-em)

Rx: Invanz

Chemical Class: Carbapenem

Therapeutic Class: Antibiotic

CLINICAL PHARMACOLOGY

Mechanism of Action: A carbapenem that penetrates the bacterial cell wall of microorganisms and binds to penicillin-binding proteins, inhibiting cell wall synthesis. ***Therapeutic Effect:*** Produces bacterial cell death.

Pharmacokinetics

Almost completely absorbed after IM administration. Protein binding: 85%-95%. Widely distributed. Primarily excreted in urine with smaller amount eliminated in feces. Removed by hemodialysis. ***Half-life:*** 4 hr.

INDICATIONS AND DOSAGES

Intraabdominal infection

IV, IM

Adults, Elderly. 1 g/day for 5-14 days.

Skin and skin structure infection

IV, IM

Adults, Elderly. 1 g/day for 7-14 days.

Pneumonia, UTI

IV, IM

Adults, Elderly. 1 g/day for 10-14 days.

Pelvic infection

IV, IM

Adults, Elderly. 1 g/day for 3-10 days.

Dosage in renal impairment

For adults and elderly patients with creatinine clearance less than 30 ml/min, dosage is 500 mg once a day.

AVAILABLE FORMS

- *Injection Powder for Reconstitution:* 1 g/vial.

CONTRAINDICATIONS: History of hypersensitivity to beta-lactams (imipenem and cilastin, meropenem), hypersensitivity to amide-type local anesthetics (IM)

PREGNANCY AND LACTATION: Pregnancy category B; excreted into breast milk; bottle feeding recommended during and for 5 days after therapy

SIDE EFFECTS

Frequent (10%-6%)

Diarrhea, nausea, headache

Occasional (5%-2%)
Altered mental status, insomnia, rash, abdominal pain, constipation, vomiting, edema, fever
Rare (less than 2%)
Dizziness, cough, oral candidiasis, anxiety, tachycardia, phlebitis at IV site

SERIOUS REACTIONS

- Antibiotic-associated colitis and other superinfections may occur.
- Anaphylactic reactions have been reported.
- Seizures may occur in those with CNS disorders (including patients with brain lesions or a history of seizures), bacterial meningitis, or severe renal impairment.

INTERACTIONS

Drugs

3 *Probenecid:* Increased ertapenem half-life

SPECIAL CONSIDERATIONS

- Daily dosing is advantage over imipenem or meropenem

PATIENT/FAMILY EDUCATION

- Notify the physician if diarrhea, a rash, seizures, tremors, or any other new symptoms occur

MONITORING PARAMETERS

- Skin for rash
- Hydration status, check for nausea and vomiting
- IV injection site for inflammation
- Mental status, and watch for seizures and tremors
- Sleep pattern for evidence of insomnia
- Pattern of daily bowel activity and stool consistency

erythromycin

(er-ith-roe-mye′-sin)
Rx: (A/T/S, Akne-Mycin, EES, Emgel, E-Mycin, Eryc, Erycette, EryDerm, Erygel, EryPed, Erymax, Ery-Tab, Erythra-Derm, Erythrocin, PCE Dispertab, Romycin, Roymicin, Staticin, Theramycin, Theramycin Z, T-Stat)
Combinations
Rx: with sulfisoxazole (Pediazole); with benzoyl peroxide (Benzamycin)
Chemical Class: Macrolide derivative
Therapeutic Class: Antibiotic

CLINICAL PHARMACOLOGY

Mechanism of Action: A macrolide that reversibly binds to bacterial ribosomes, inhibiting bacterial protein synthesis. ***Therapeutic Effect:*** Bacteriostatic.

Pharmacokinetics

Variably absorbed from the GI tract (depending on dosage form used). Protein binding: 70%-90%. Widely distributed. Metabolized in the liver. Primarily eliminated in feces by bile. Not removed by hemodialysis. ***Half-life:*** 1.4-2 hr (increased in impaired renal function).

INDICATIONS AND DOSAGES

Mild to moderate infections of the upper and lower respiratory tract, pharyngitis, skin infections

PO

Adults, Elderly. 250 mg q6h, 500 mg q12h, or 333 mg q8h. Maximum: 4 g/day.

Children. 30-50 mg/kg/day in divided doses up to 60-100 mg/kg/day for severe infections.

Neonates. 20-40 mg/kg/day in divided doses q6-12h.

IV

Adults, Elderly, Children. 15-20 mg/kg/day in divided doses. Maximum: 4 g/day.

Preoperative intestinal antisepsis

PO

Adults, Elderly. 1 g at 1 p.m., 2 p.m., and 11 p.m. on day before surgery (with neomycin).

Children. 20 mg/kg at 1 p.m., 2 p.m., and 11 p.m. on day before surgery (with neomycin).

Acne vulgaris

Topical

Adults. Apply thin layer to affected area twice a day.

Gonococcal ophthalmia neonatorum

Ophthalmic

Neonates. 0.5-2 cm no later than 1 hr after delivery.

AVAILABLE FORMS

- *Topical Gel (A/T/S, Emgel, Erygel):* 2%.
- *Injection Powder for Reconstitution (Erythrocin):* 500 mg, 1 g.
- *Ophthalmic Ointment (Roymicin):* 0.5%.
- *Oral Suspension (EryPed, EES):* 200 mg/5 ml, 400 mg/5 ml.
- *Topical Ointment (Akne-Mycin):* 2%.
- *Topical Solution:* 1.5% (Staticin), 2% (A/T/S, Erymax, EryDerm, Erythra-Derm, Romycin, Theramycin Z, T-Stat).
- *Topical Swab (Erycette, T-Stat):* 2%.
- *Tablets (Chewable [Ery-Ped]):* 200 mg.
- *Tablets:* 250 mg (E-Mycin, Ery-Tab, Erythrocin), 333 mg (Ery-Tab, E-Mycin, PCE Dispertab), 400 mg (EES), 500 mg (E-Mycin, Ery-Tab, Erythrocin, PCE Dispertab).
- *Capsules (Enteric-Coated [Eryc]):* 250 mg.

UNLABELED USES: *Systemic:* Treatment of acne vulgaris, chancroid, *Campylobacter* enteritis, gastroparesis, Lyme disease

Topical: Treatment of minor bacterial skin infections

Ophthalmic: Treatment of blepharitis, conjunctivitis, keratitis, chlamydial trachoma

CONTRAINDICATIONS: Administration of fixed-combination product, Pediazole, to infants younger than 2 months; history of hepatitis due to macrolides; hypersensitivity to macrolides; preexisting hepatic disease.

PREGNANCY AND LACTATION: Pregnancy category B; excreted into breast milk; compatible with breastfeeding

SIDE EFFECTS

Frequent

IV: Abdominal cramping or discomfort, phlebitis or thrombophlebitis

Topical: Dry skin (50%)

Occasional

Nausea, vomiting, diarrhea, rash, urticaria

Rare

Ophthalmic: Sensitivity reaction with increased irritation, burning, itching, and inflammation

Topical: Urticaria

SERIOUS REACTIONS

- Antibiotic-associated colitis and other superinfections may occur.
- High dosages in patients with renal impairment may lead to reversible hearing loss.
- Anaphylaxis and hepatotoxicity occur rarely.
- Ventricular arrhythmias and prolonged QT interval occur rarely with the IV drug form.

INTERACTIONS

Drugs

3 *Alfentanil:* Prolonged anesthesia and respiratory depression

3 *Alprazolam:* Increased plasma alprazolam concentration

3 *Amprenavir:* Plasma concentrations of erythromycin may be increased by amprenavir; plasma concentrations of amprenavir may be increased by erythromycin

3 *Atorvastatin:* Increased plasma atorvastatin concentration with risk of rhabdomyolysis

3 *Bromocriptine:* Increased bromocriptine concentration with toxicity

3 *Buspirone:* Increased plasma buspirone concentration

3 *Carbamazepine:* Markedly increased plasma carbamazepine concentrations

❷ *Cisapride:* QT prolongation and dysrhythmia

❷ *Clozapine:* Increased plasma clozapine concentrations

3 *Colchicine:* Potential colchicine toxicity

3 *Cyclosporine:* Increased plasma cyclosporine concentrations

3 *Diazepam:* Increased plasma concentration of diazepam

3 *Digoxin:* Reduced bacterial flora may increase plasma digoxin concentrations

3 *Disopyramide:* Increased plasma disopyramide concentrations

❷ *Ergotamine:* Potential for ergotism

3 *Ethanol:* Ethanol reduces plasma erythromycin concentration

3 *Felodipine:* Increased plasma felodipine concentrations

3 *Food:* Food may increase or decrease the bioavailability of erythromycin

3 *Indinavir:* Plasma concentrations of erythromycin may be increased by indinavir; plasma concentrations of indinavir may be increased by erythromycin

3 *Itraconazole:* Increased plasma itraconazole concentration

3 *Lovastatin:* Increased plasma lovastatin concentration with risk of rhabdomyolysis

3 *Methylprednisolone:* Increased plasma methylprednisolone concentrations

3 *Midazolam:* Increased plasma concentration of midazolam

3 *Nelfinavir:* Plasma concentrations of erythromycin may be increased by nelfinavir; plasma concentrations of nelfinavir may be increased by erythromycin

3 *Penicillin:* Decreased activity of penicillin

3 *Quetiapine:* Increases quetiapine plasma concentrations

3 *Quinidine:* Increased plasma concentration of quinidine

3 *Ritonavir:* Plasma concentrations of erythromycin may be increased by ritonavir; plasma concentrations of ritonavir may be increased by erythromycin

3 *Saquinavir:* Plasma concentrations of erythromycin may be increased by saquinavir; plasma concentrations of saquinavir may be increased by erythromycin

3 *Sertraline:* Increased risk of developing serotonin syndrome

3 *Sildenafil:* Increased plasma sildenafil concentration

❷ *Simvastatin:* Increased plasma simvastatin concentration with risk of rhabdomyolysis

3 *Tacrolimus:* Increased plasma tacrolimus concentration

3 *Theophylline:* Increased plasma theophylline concentration

3 *Triazolam:* Increased plasma triazolam concentration

3 *Valproic acid:* Increased plasma valproic acid concentration

3 *Warfarin:* Markedly increased hypoprothrombinemic response to warfarin

3 *Zafirlukast:* Reduced plasma zafirlukast concentration, probably by reducing bioavailability

3 *Zopiclone:* Increased plasma zopiclone concentration

Labs

- *False decrease:* Folate assay
- *False increase:* Urine 17-ketosteroids, AST, urine amino acids

SPECIAL CONSIDERATIONS

PATIENT/FAMILY EDUCATION

- Take with food to minimize GI discomfort
- Take each dose with 180-240 ml of water
- Wash, rinse, and dry affected area prior to top application
- Keep top preparations away from eyes, nose, and mouth
- Ophth ointments may cause temporary blurring of vision following administration
- Space doses evenly around the clock and continue erythromycin therapy for the full course of treatment
- Wait at least 1 hr before using other topical acne preparations containing abrasive or peeling agents, such as medicated soaps, and cosmetics or aftershave containing alcohol

MONITORING PARAMETERS

- LFTs if hepatotoxicity suspected
- Check daily for vein irritation and phlebitis in patients receiving IV forms
- Daily bowel activity and stool consistency
- Skin for rash
- Signs and symptoms of superinfection, such as genital and anal pruritus, sore mouth or tongue, abdominal cramps, and moderate to severe diarrhea
- Signs of hearing loss because high dosages can cause hearing loss in patients with hepatic or renal dysfunction

escitalopram oxalate

(es-sye-tal'-oh-pram ok'-sal-ate)

Rx: Lexapro

Chemical Class: Bicyclic phthalane derivative

Therapeutic Class: Antidepressant, selective serotonin reuptake inhibitor (SSRI)

E

CLINICAL PHARMACOLOGY

Mechanism of Action: A selective serotonin reuptake inhibitor that blocks the uptake of the neurotransmitter serotonin at neuronal presynaptic membranes, increasing its availability at postsynaptic receptor sites. ***Therapeutic Effect:*** Relieves depression.

Pharmacokinetics

Well absorbed after PO administration. Primarily metabolized in the liver. Primarily excreted in feces with a lesser amount eliminated in urine. ***Half-life:*** 35 hr.

INDICATIONS AND DOSAGES

Depression, general anxiety disorder (GAD)

PO

Adults. Initially, 10 mg once a day in the morning or evening. May increase to 20 mg after a minimum of 1 wk.

Elderly, Patients with hepatic impairment. 10 mg/day.

AVAILABLE FORMS

- *Oral Solution:* 5 mg/5 ml.
- *Tablets:* 5 mg, 10 mg, 20 mg.

UNLABELED USES: Mixed anxiety and depressive disorder

CONTRAINDICATIONS: Breastfeeding, use within 14 days of MAOIs

PREGNANCY AND LACTATION: Pregnancy category C; excreted in human breast milk; reports of infants experiencing excessive somnolence, decreased feeding, and weight loss in association with breast-feeding from a citalopram-treated mother

SIDE EFFECTS

Frequent (21%-11%)

Nausea, dry mouth, somnolence, insomnia, diaphoresis

Occasional (8%-4%)

Tremor, diarrhea, abnormal ejaculation, dyspepsia, fatigue, anxiety, vomiting, anorexia

Rare (3%-2%)

Sinusitis, sexual dysfunction, menstrual disorder, abdominal pain, agitation, decreased libido

SERIOUS REACTIONS

• Overdose is manifested as dizziness, drowsiness, tachycardia, somnolence, confusion, and seizures.

INTERACTIONS

Drugs

3 *Alcohol, other CNS depressants:* May increase CNS depression

3 *Antifungals, macrolide antibiotics:* May increase plasma level of escitalopram

3 *Carbamazepine:* May decrease plasma level of escitalopram

3 *Cimetidine:* Increased citalopram levels

3 *Ginkgo biloba, St. John's wort:* May increase the risk of serotonin syndrome

3 *Lithium:* May increase lithium concentrations and/or increase the risk of serotonin syndrome

▲ *MAOIs:* See Precautions

3 *Metoprolol:* Increases plasma level of metoprolol

3 *Sumatriptan:* Syndrome of weakness, hyperreflexia, and incoordination following combination (rarely)

SPECIAL CONSIDERATIONS

• Patent extension for a useful agent; not different from citalopram

PATIENT/FAMILY EDUCATION

• Do not discontinue escitalopram or increase the dosage

• Avoid alcohol while taking escitalopram

• Avoid tasks that require mental alertness or motor skills until response to the drug has been established

MONITORING PARAMETERS

• Improvement of symptoms of depression or anxiety/depression, suicidal ideation, signs of toxicity (e.g., somnolence, sleep disturbances, persistent GI symptoms)

esmolol hydrochloride

(ess'-moe-lol hye-droe-klor'-ide)

Rx: Brevibloc

Chemical Class: β_1-adrenergic blocker, cardioselective

Therapeutic Class: Antiarrhythmic, class II

CLINICAL PHARMACOLOGY

Mechanism of Action: An antiarrhythmic that selectively blocks beta$_1$-adrenergic receptors. ***Therapeutic Effect:*** Slows sinus heart rate, decreases cardiac output, reducing BP.

Pharmacokinetics

Rapidly metabolized primarily by esterase in the cytosol of red blood cells. Protein binding: 55%. Less than 1%-2% excreted in urine. ***Half-life:*** 9 min.

INDICATIONS AND DOSAGES

Arrhythmias

IV

Adults, Elderly. Initially, loading dose of 500 mcg/kg/min for 1 min, followed by 50 mcg/kg/min for 4 min. If optimum response is not attained in 5 min, give second loading dose of 500 mcg/kg/min for 1 min, followed by infusion of 100 mcg/kg/min for 4 min. Additional loading doses can be given and infusion increased by 50 mcg/kg/min, up to 200 mcg/kg/min, for 4 min. Once desired response is attained, cease loading dose and increase infusion by no more than 25 mcg/kg/min. Interval between doses may be increased to 10 min. Infusion usually administered over 24-48 hr in most patients. Range: 50-200 mcg/kg/min, with average dose of 100 mcg/kg/min.

Intraoperative tachycardia or hypertension (immediate control)

IV

Adults, Elderly. Initially, 80 mg over 30 secs, then 150 mcg/kg/min infusion up to 300 mcg/kg/min.

AVAILABLE FORMS

• *Injection:* 10 mg/ml, 20 mg/ml, 250 mg/ml.

CONTRAINDICATIONS: Cardiogenic shock, overt cardiac failure, second- and third-degree heart block, sinus bradycardia

PREGNANCY AND LACTATION: Pregnancy category C; potential for hypotension and subsequent decreased uterine blood flow and fetal hypoxia should be considered; excretion into breast milk unknown; use caution in nursing mothers

SIDE EFFECTS

Frequent

Esmolol is generally well tolerated, with transient and mild side effects. Hypotension (systolic BP less than 90 mm Hg) manifested as dizziness, nausea, diaphoresis, headache, cold extremities, fatigue

Occasional

Anxiety, drowsiness, flushed skin, vomiting, confusion, inflammation at injection site, fever

SERIOUS REACTIONS

• Overdose may produce profound hypotension, bradycardia, dizziness, syncope, drowsiness, breathing difficulty, bluish fingernails or palms of hands, and seizures.

• Esmolol administration may potentiate insulin-induced hypoglycemia in diabetic patients.

INTERACTIONS

Drugs

3 *α_1-adrenergic blockers:* Potential enhanced first-dose response (marked initial drop in blood pressure, particularly on standing [especially prazocin])

3 *Amiodarone:* Symptomatic bradycardia and sinus arrest; AV node refractory period is prolonged and sinus node automaticity is decreased by amiodarone. The sinus rate can be further slowed or AV block worsened in patients with bradycardia, sick sinus syndrome, or partial AV block

3 *Dihydropyridine calcium channel blockers:* Severe hypotension or impaired cardiac performance; most prevalent with impaired left ventricular function, cardiac arrhythmias, or aortic stenosis

3 *Digoxin:* Additive prolongation of atrioventricular (AV) conduction time

3 *Diltiazem:* Potentiates β-adrenergic effects; hypotension, left ventricular failure, and AV conduction disturbances problematic in elderly, patients with left ventricular dysfunction, aortic stenosis, or with large doses of either drug

3 *Hypoglycemic agents:* Masked hypoglycemia, hyperglycemia

3 *MAOIs:* May cause significant hypertension

3 *Sympathomimetics, xanthines:* May mutually inhibit effects

3 *Verapamil:* Potentiates β-adrenergic effects; hypotension, left ventricular failure, and AV conduction disturbances problematic in elderly, patients with left ventricular dysfunction, aortic stenosis, or with large doses of either drug

SPECIAL CONSIDERATIONS

- Transfer to alternative agent (e.g., propranolol, digoxin, verapamil): ½ hr after first dose of alternative agent, reduce esmolol INF rate by 50%; following second dose of alternative agent, monitor patient's response and, if satisfactory control is maintained for the first hr, discontinue esmolol INF
- Do not discontinue abruptly; may require taper; rapid withdrawal may produce rebound hypertension or angina

PATIENT/FAMILY EDUCATION

- Blood pressure and heart rate should be continuously monitored during esmolol therapy
- Report cold extremities, dizziness, faintness, or nausea

MONITORING PARAMETERS

- *Angina:* Reduction in nitroglycerin usage; frequency, severity, onset, and duration of angina pain; heart rate
- *Arrhythmias:* Heart rate
- *Hypertension:* Blood pressure
- *Postmyocardial infarction:* Left ventricular function, lower resting heart rate
- *Toxicity:* Blood glucose, bronchospasm, hypotension, bradycardia, depression, confusion, hallucination, sexual dysfunction

esomeprazole

(es-om-eh-pray'-zole)

Rx: Nexium, Nexium IV

Chemical Class: Benzimidazole derivative

Therapeutic Class: Antiulcer agent; gastrointestinal antisecretory agent

CLINICAL PHARMACOLOGY

Mechanism of Action: A proton pump inhibitor that is converted to active metabolites that irreversibly bind to and inhibit hydrogen-potassium adenosine triphosphates, an enzyme on the surface of gastric parietal cells. Inhibits hydrogen ion transport into gastric lumen. ***Therapeutic Effect:*** Increases gastric pH, reducing gastric acid production.

Pharmacokinetics

Well absorbed after oral administration. Protein binding: 97%. Extensively metabolized by the liver. Primarily excreted in urine. ***Half-life:*** 1-1.5 hrs.

INDICATIONS AND DOSAGES

Erosive esophagitis

PO

Adults, Elderly. 20-40 mg once daily for 4-8 wk.

IV

Adults, Elderly. 20 or 40 mg once daily by IV injection over at least 3 mins or IV infusion over 10-30 mins.

To maintain healing of erosive esophagitis

PO

Adults, Elderly. 20 mg/day.

Gastroesophageal reflux disease, to reduce the risk of NSAID-induced gastric ulcer

PO

Adults, Elderly. 20 mg once a day for 4 wk.

***Duodenal ulcer caused by** Helicobacter pylori*
PO
Adults, Elderly. 40 mg (esomeprazole) once a day, with amoxicillin 1000 mg and clarithromycin 500 mg twice a day for 10 days.

AVAILABLE FORMS

• *Capsules (Delayed-Release, Magnesium [Nexium]):* 20 mg, 40 mg.
• *Powder for Solution (Sodium [Nexium IV]):* 20 mg, 40 mg.

CONTRAINDICATIONS: Hypersensitivity to benzimidazoles

PREGNANCY AND LACTATION: Pregnancy category B; likely to be excreted into breast milk, use caution in nursing mothers (suppression of gastric acid secretion is potential effect in nursing infant, clinical significance unknown)

SIDE EFFECTS

Frequent (7%)
Headache
Occasional (3%-2%)
Diarrhea, abdominal pain, nausea
Rare (less than 2%)
Dizziness, asthenia or loss of strength, vomiting, constipation, rash, cough

SERIOUS REACTIONS

• None known.

INTERACTIONS

Drugs

3 *Ketoconazole, iron salts, digoxin:* Reduced gastric acidity may result in decreased absorption of these and other drugs where gastric pH is an important determinant of bioavailability

SPECIAL CONSIDERATIONS

• S-isomer of omeprazole (racemate)
• No advantage over other proton-pump inhibitors, cost should govern choice
• Notify the physician if headache occurs during therapy

PATIENT/FAMILY EDUCATION

• Take at least 1 hr before meals
• Capsules may be opened, mixed with cold applesauce, and swallowed immediately without chewing for patients who cannot swallow capsules whole

MONITORING PARAMETERS

• Therapeutic response (relief of GI symptoms)

---

estazolam

(es-ta'-zoe-lam)
Rx: ProSom
Chemical Class: Benzodiazepine
Therapeutic Class: Sedative/hypnotic
DEA Class: Schedule IV

CLINICAL PHARMACOLOGY

Mechanism of Action: A benzodiazepine that enhances action of gamma aminobutyric acid (GABA) neurotransmission in the central nervous system (CNS). ***Therapeutic Effect:*** Produces depressant effect at all levels of CNS.

Pharmacokinetics

Rapidly absorbed from gastrointestinal (GI) tract. Protein binding: 93%. Metabolized in liver. Primarily excreted in urine, minimal in feces. ***Half-life:*** 10-24 hrs.

INDICATIONS AND DOSAGES

Insomnia
PO
Adults (older than 18 yrs). 1-2 mg at bedtime.
Elderly, debilitated, liver disease, low serum albumin. 0.5-1 mg at bedtime.

AVAILABLE FORMS

• *Tablets:* 1 mg, 2 mg (ProSom).

CONTRAINDICATIONS: Pregnancy, hypersensitivity to other benzodiazepines

PREGNANCY AND LACTATION: Pregnancy category X; may cause fetal damage when administered during pregnancy; excreted into breast milk; may accumulate in breast-fed infants and is therefore not recommended

Controlled Substance: Schedule IV

SIDE EFFECTS

Frequent

Drowsiness, sedation, rebound insomnia (may occur for 1-2 nights after drug is discontinued), dizziness, confusion, euphoria

Occasional

Weakness, anorexia, diarrhea

Rare

Paradoxical CNS excitement, restlessness (particularly noted in elderly/debilitated)

SERIOUS REACTIONS

- Overdosage results in somnolence, confusion, diminished reflexes, and coma.

INTERACTIONS

Drugs

3 *Cimetidine:* Increased serum benzodiazepine concentrations

3 *Disulfiram:* May increase benzodiazepine serum concentrations

3 *Erythromycin:* Increased estazolam sedative effects

3 *Ethanol:* Enhanced adverse psychomotor effects of benzodiazepines

3 *Rifampin:* Reduced serum benzodiazepine concentrations

3 *Smoking:* Reduces the drug's effectiveness

SPECIAL CONSIDERATIONS

PATIENT/FAMILY EDUCATION

- Do not discontinue abruptly after prolonged therapy
- May experience disturbed sleep for the first or second night after discontinuing the drug
- Avoid alcohol
- Smoking decreases the drug's effectiveness

MONITORING PARAMETERS

- Therapeutic response: decrease in number of nocturnal awakenings, increase in length of sleep

estradiol

(ess-tra-dye'-ole)

Rx: Alora, Climara, Delestrogen, Depo-Estradiol, Esclim, Estrace, Estraderm, Estrasorb, Estrogel, Estring, Femring, Menostar, Vagifem, Vivelle, Vivelle Dot

Chemical Class: Estrogen derivative

Therapeutic Class: Antineoplastic; antiosteoporotic; estrogen

CLINICAL PHARMACOLOGY

Mechanism of Action: An estrogen that increases synthesis of DNA, RNA, and proteins in target tissues; reduces release of gonadotropin-releasing hormone from the hypothalamus; and reduces follicle-stimulating hormone and luteinizing hormone (LH) release from the pituitary. ***Therapeutic Effect:*** Promotes normal growth, promotes development of female sex organs, and maintains GU function and vasomotor stability. Prevents accelerated bone loss by inhibiting bone resorption, restoring balance of bone resorption and formation. Inhibits LH and decreases serum testosterone concentration.

Pharmacokinetics

Well absorbed from the GI tract. Widely distributed. Protein binding: 50%-80%. Metabolized in the liver. Primarily excreted in urine. ***Half-life:*** Unknown.

INDICATIONS AND DOSAGES

Prostate cancer

IM (estradiol valerate)

Adults, Elderly. 30 mg or more q1-2 wk.

PO

Adults, Elderly. 10 mg 3 times a day for at least 3 mo.

Breast cancer

PO

Adults, Elderly. 10 mg 3 times a day for at least 3 mo.

Osteoporosis prophylaxis in postmenopausal females

PO

Adults, Elderly. 0.5 mg/day cyclically (3 weeks on, 1 week off).

Transdermal (Climara)

Adults, Elderly. Initially, 0.025 mg weekly, adjust dose as needed.

Transdermal (Alora, Vivelle, Vivelle-Dot)

Adults, Elderly. Initially, 0.025 mg patch twice weekly, adjust dose as needed.

Transdermal (Estraderm)

Adults, Elderly. 0.05 mg twice weekly.

Transdermal (Menostar)

Adults, Elderly. 1 mg weekly.

Female hypoestrogenism

PO

Adults, Elderly. 1-2 mg/day, adjust dose as needed.

IM (estradiol cypionate)

Adults, Elderly. 1.5-2 mg monthly.

IM (estradiol valerate)

Adults, Elderly. 10-20 mg q4wk.

Vasomotor symptoms associated with menopause

PO

Adults, Elderly. 1-2 mg/day cyclically (3 weeks on, 1 week off), adjust dose as needed.

IM (estradiol cypionate)

Adults, Elderly. 1-5 mg q3-4wk.

IM (estradiol valerate)

Adults, Elderly. 10-20 mg q4wk.

Topical emulsion (Estrasorb)

Adults, Elderly. 3.84 g once a day in the morning.

Topical gel (Estrogel)

Adults, Elderly. 1.25 g/day.

Transdermal (Climara)

Adults, Elderly. 0.025 mg weekly. Adjust dose as needed.

Transdermal (Alora, Esclim, Estrader, Vivelle-Dot)

Adults, Elderly. 0.05 mg twice a week.

Transdermal (Vivelle)

Adults, Elderly. 0.0375 mg twice a week.

Vaginal ring (Femring)

Adults, Elderly. 0.05 mg. May increase to 0.1 mg if needed.

Vaginal atrophy

Vaginal ring (Estring)

Adults, Elderly. 2 mg.

Atrophic vaginitis

Vaginal tablet (Vagifem)

Adults, Elderly. Initially, 1 tablet/day for 2 weeks. Maintenance: 1 tablet twice a week.

AVAILABLE FORMS

- *Tablets (Estrace):* 0.5 mg, 1 mg, 2 mg.
- *Emulsion (Topical [Estrasorb]):* 2.5 mg/g.
- *Injection (Cypionate [Depo-Estradiol]):* 5 mg/ml.
- *Injection (Valerate [Delestrogen]):* 10 mg/ml.
- *Topical Gel (EstroGel):* 1.25 g.
- *Transdermal System (Alora):* twice weekly: 0.025 mg, 0.05 mg, 0.075 mg, 0.1 mg.
- *Transdermal System (Climara):* once weekly: 0.025 mg, 0.0375 mg, 0.05 mg, 0.06 mg, 0.075 mg, 0.1 mg.
- *Transdermal System (Esclim):* twice weekly: 0.025 mg, 0.0375 mg, 0.05 mg, 0.075 mg, 0.1 mg.
- *Transdermal System (Estraderm):* twice weekly: 0.05 mg, 0.1 mg.
- *Transdermal System (Menostar):* once a week: 1 mg.

• *Transdermal System (Vivelle):* twice weekly: 0.025 mg, 0.0375 mg, 0.05 mg, 0.075 mg, 0.1 mg.
• *Transderamal System (Vivelle Dot):* twice weekly: 0.0375 mg, 0.05 mg, 0.075 mg, 0.1 mg.
• *Vaginal Cream (Estrace):* 0.1 mg/g.
• *Vaginal Ring (Estring):* 2 mg.
• *Vaginal Ring (Femring):* 0.05 mg.
• *Vaginal Tablet (Vagifem):* 25 mcg.

UNLABELED USES: Treatment of Turner's syndrome

CONTRAINDICATIONS: Abnormal vaginal bleeding, active arterial thrombosis, blood dyscrasias, estrogen-dependent cancer, known or suspected breast cancer, pregnancy, thrombophlebitis or thromboembolic disorders, thyroid dysfunction

PREGNANCY AND LACTATION: Pregnancy category X

SIDE EFFECTS

Frequent

Anorexia, nausea, swelling of breasts, peripheral edema marked by swollen ankles and feet

Transdermal: Skin irritation, redness

Occasional

Vomiting, especially with high doses; headache that may be severe; intolerance to contact lenses; hypertension; glucose intolerance; brown spots on exposed skin

Vaginal: Local irritation, vaginal discharge, changes in vaginal bleeding, including spotting, and breakthrough or prolonged bleeding

Rare

Chorea or involuntary movements, hirsutism or abnormal hairiness, loss of scalp hair, depression

SERIOUS REACTIONS

• Estrogen therapy may increase the risk of developing coronary heart disease, hypercalcemia, gallbladder disease, cerebrovascular disease, and breast cancer.
• Prolonged administration increases the risk of gallbladder disease, thromboembolic disease, and breast, cervical, vaginal, endometrial, and hepatic carcinoma.
• Cholestatic jaundice occurs rarely.

INTERACTIONS

Drugs

3 *Bromocriptine:* May interfere with the effects of bromocriptine

3 *P450 inducers (e.g., rifampin, barbiturates):* Decreased estrogen levels

3 *Corticosteroids:* Increased steroid effect

3 *Cyclosporine:* May increase blood cyclosporine concentration and the risk of hepatotoxicity and nephrotoxicity

3 *Phenytoin:* Loss of seizure control, decreased estrogen levels

3 *Warfarin:* Theoretical increased risk thromboembolism

SPECIAL CONSIDERATIONS

• Progestins recommended in nonhysterectomized women. Estring may have minimal systemic absorption

PATIENT/FAMILY EDUCATION

• Limit alcohol and caffeine intake
• Stop smoking tobacco
• Report calf or chest pain, depression, numbness or weakness of an extremity, severe abdominal pain, shortness of breath, speech or vision disturbance, sudden headache, unusual bleeding, or vomiting

MONITORING PARAMETERS

• Blood pressure, weight, blood glucose, liver function, and serum calcium levels

estrogens, conjugated

(ess'-troe-jens, kon'-joo-gay-ted)

Rx: Cenestin, Enjuvia, Premarin, Premarin Intravenous, Premarin Vaginal

Combinations

Rx: with medroxyprogesterone (Prempro [daily product], Premphase [cycled product]); with meprobamate (PMB); with methyltestosterone (Premarin with methyltestosterone)

Chemical Class: Estrogen derivative

Therapeutic Class: Antineoplastic; antiosteoporotic; estrogen

CLINICAL PHARMACOLOGY

Mechanism of Action: An estrogen that increases synthesis of DNA, RNA, and various proteins in target tissues; reduces release of gonadotropin-releasing hormone from the hypothalamus; and reduces follicle-stimulating hormone (FSH) and luteinizing hormone (LH) release from the pituitary gland. ***Therapeutic Effect:*** Promotes normal growth, promotes development of female sex organs, and maintains GU function and vasomotor stability. Prevents accelerated bone loss by inhibiting bone resorption, restoring balance of bone resorption and formation. Inhibits LH and decreases serum concentration of testosterone.

Pharmacokinetics

Well absorbed from the GI tract. Widely distributed. Protein binding: 50%-80%. Metabolized in the liver. Primarily excreted in urine.

INDICATIONS AND DOSAGES

Vasomotor symptoms associated with menopause, atrophic vaginitis, kraurosis vulvae

PO

Adults, Elderly. 0.3-0.625 mg/day cyclically (21 days on, 7 days off) or continuously.

Intravaginal

Adults, Elderly. 0.5-2 g/day cyclically, such as 21 days on and 7 days off.

Female hypogonadism

PO

Adults. 0.3-0.625 mg/day in divided doses for 20 days; then a rest period of 10 days.

Female castration, primary ovarian failure

PO

Adults. Initially, 1.25 mg/day cyclically. Adjust dosage, upward or downward, according to severity of symptoms and patient response. For maintenance, adjust dosage to lowest level that will provide effective control.

Osteoporosis

PO

Adults, Elderly. 0.3-0.625 mg/day, cyclically, such as 25 days on and 5 days off.

Breast cancer

PO

Adults, Elderly. 10 mg 3 times a day for at least 3 mo.

Prostate cancer

PO

Adults, Elderly. 1.25-2.5 mg 3 times a day.

Abnormal uterine bleeding

PO

Adults. 1.25 mg q4h for 24 hr, then 1.25 mg/day for 7-10 days.

IV, IM

Adults. 25 mg; may repeat once in 6-12 hr.

AVAILABLE FORMS

• *Tablets:* 0.3 mg (Cenestin, Premarin), 0.45 mg (Cenestin, Premarin), 0.625 mg (Cenestin, Enjuvia, Premarin), 0.9 mg (Cenestin, Premarin), 1.25 mg (Cenestin, Enjuvia, Premarin), 2.5 mg (Cenestin, Premarin).

• *Injection (Premarin Intravenous):* 25 mg.

• *Vaginal Cream (Premarin Vaginal):* 0.625 mg/g.

UNLABELED USES: Prevention of estrogen deficiency–induced premenopausal osteoporosis

Cream: Prevention of nosebleeds

CONTRAINDICATIONS: Breast cancer with some exceptions, hepatic disease, thrombophlebitis, undiagnosed vaginal bleeding

PREGNANCY AND LACTATION: Pregnancy category X; may decrease quantity and quality of breast milk

SIDE EFFECTS

Frequent

Vaginal bleeding, such as spotting or breakthrough bleeding; breast pain or tenderness; gynecomastia

Occasional

Headache, hypertension, intolerance to contact lenses

High doses: Anorexia, nausea

Rare

Loss of scalp hair, depression

SERIOUS REACTIONS

• Prolonged administration may increase the risk of breast, cervical, endometrial, hepatic, and vaginal carcinoma; cerebrovascular disease, coronary heart disease, gallbladder disease, and hypercalcemia.

INTERACTIONS

Drugs

3 *Bromocriptine:* May interfere with the effects of bromocriptine

3 *P450 inducers (e.g., rifampin, barbiturates):* Decreased estrogen levels

3 *Corticosteroids:* Increased steroid effect

3 *Cyclosporine:* May increase blood cyclosporine concentration and the risk of hepatotoxicity and nephrotoxicity

3 *Phenytoin:* Loss of seizure control, decreased estrogen levels

3 *Warfarin:* Theoretical increased risk thromboembolism

SPECIAL CONSIDERATIONS

• Progestins recommended in nonhysterectomized women

• Premarin is derived from pregnant mare's urine; Cenestin from yams and soy. Although probably therapeutically equivalent, they are not substitutable by the pharmacist

• Consider topical products if treatment is solely for vulvar or vaginal atrophy

• Currently recommended that use of hormone replacement therapy be limited to treating symptomatic women, preferrably for ≤5 yrs. Risk felt to outweigh benefit in asymptomatic women using only for prophylaxis of other conditions

PATIENT/FAMILY EDUCATION

• Avoid smoking because of the increased risk of blood clot formation and MI

• Diet and exercise are important when conjugated estrogens are taken to retard osteoporosis

• Report abnormal vaginal bleeding, depression, or signs and symptoms of blood clots

• Perform breast self-examination monthly

• Report weekly weight gain of more than 5 lbs

• Notify the physician and discontinue the drug, as prescribed, if she suspects she is pregnant

MONITORING PARAMETERS

• Blood pressure periodically

• Weight

• Signs and symptoms of thromboembolic or thrombotic disorders, including loss of coordination, numbness or weakness of an extremity, shortness of breath, speech or vision disturbance, sudden severe headache, and pain in the chest, leg, or groin

estrogens, esterified

(ess'-troe-jens, ess'-ter-i-fyed)

Rx: Estratab, Menest

Combinations

Rx: with methyltestosterone (Estratest, Menogen)

Chemical Class: Estrogen derivative

Therapeutic Class: Antineoplastic; antiosteoporotic; estrogen

CLINICAL PHARMACOLOGY

Mechanism of Action: A combination of sodium salts of sulfate esters of estrogenic substances (principal component is estrone) that increases synthesis of DNA, RNA, and various proteins in responsive tissues. Reduces release of gonadotropin-releasing hormone, reducing follicle-stimulating hormone (FSH) and luteinizing hormone (LH). ***Therapeutic Effect:*** Promotes vasomotor stability, maintains genitourinary (GU) function, normal growth, development of female sex organs. Prevents accelerated bone loss by inhibiting bone resorption, restoring balance of bone resorption and formation.

Pharmacokinetics

Readily absorbed from the gastrointestinal (GI) tract. Widely distributed. Protein binding: 50%-80%. Rapidly metabolized in liver and GI tract to estrone sulfate and conjugated and unconjugated metabolites. Excreted in urine and bile. ***Half-life:*** Unknown.

INDICATIONS AND DOSAGES

Vasomotor symptoms associated with menopause, atrophic vaginitis, kraurosis vulvae

PO

Adults, Elderly. 0.3-1.25 mg/day.

Female hypogonadism

PO

Adults. 2.5-7.5 mg/day in divided doses for 20 days; rest 10 days.

Female castration, primary ovarian failure

PO

Adults. Initially, 1. 25 mg/day cyclically.

Breast cancer

PO

Adults, Elderly. 10 mg 3 times/day for at least 3 mos.

Prostate cancer

PO

Adults, Elderly. 1.25-2.5 mg 3 times/day.

AVAILABLE FORMS

• *Tablets:* 0.3 mg (Menest), 0.625 mg (Estratab).

CONTRAINDICATIONS: Breast cancer with some exceptions, liver disease, thrombophlebitis, undiagnosed vaginal bleeding

PREGNANCY AND LACTATION: Pregnancy category X; may decrease quantity and quality of breast milk

SIDE EFFECTS

Frequent

Change in vaginal bleeding, such as spotting or breakthrough bleeding, breast pain or tenderness, gynecomastia

Occasional

Headache, increased blood pressure (BP), intolerance to contact lenses, nausea

Rare
Loss of scalp hair, clinical depression

SERIOUS REACTIONS

• Prolonged administration may increase risk of gallbladder, thromboembolic disease; breast, cervical, vaginal, endometrial, and liver carcinoma.

INTERACTIONS

Drugs

3 *Bromocriptine:* May interfere with the effects of bromocriptine

3 *P450 inducers (e.g., rifampin, barbiturates):* Decreased estrogen levels

3 *Corticosteroids:* Increased steroid effect

3 *Cyclosporine:* May increase blood cyclosporine concentration and the risk of hepatotoxicity and nephrotoxicity

3 *Phenytoin:* Loss of seizure control, decreased estrogen levels

3 *Warfarin:* Theoretical increased risk thromboembolism

SPECIAL CONSIDERATIONS

• Progestins recommended in nonhysterectomized women

PATIENT/FAMILY EDUCATION

• Avoid smoking because of the increased risk of blood clot formation and MI

• Report abnormal vaginal bleeding, depression, or signs and symptoms of blood clots

• Perform breast self-examination monthly

• Report weekly weight gain of more than 5 lbs

• Notify the physician and discontinue the drug, as prescribed, if she suspects she is pregnant

MONITORING PARAMETERS

• Blood pressure periodically

• Weight

• Signs and symptoms of thromboembolic or thrombotic disorders, including loss of coordination, numbness or weakness of an extremity, shortness of breath, speech or vision disturbance, sudden severe headache, and pain in the chest, leg, or groin

---

estrone

(ess'-trone)

Rx: Estragyn 5, Estro-A, Estrogenic, Estrogens, Kestrone 5

Chemical Class: Estrogen derivative

Therapeutic Class: Antineoplastic; estrogen

CLINICAL PHARMACOLOGY

Mechanism of Action: An estrogen that increases synthesis of DNA, RNA, proteins in target tissues; reduces release of gonadotropin-releasing hormone from hypothalamus; reduces follicle-stimulating hormone (FSH) and luteinizing hormone (LH) release from the pituitary. ***Therapeutic Effect:*** Promotes normal growth, development of female sex organs, maintaining genitourinary (GU) function, vasomotor stability. Prevents accelerated bone loss by inhibiting bone resorption, restoring balance of bone resorption and formation. Inhibits LH, decreases serum concentration of testosterone.

Pharmacokinetics

Well absorbed from the gastrointestinal (GI) tract. Widely distributed. Protein binding: 50%-80%. Metabolized in liver as well as a certain proportion excreted into the bile and reabsorbed from the intestine. Primarily excreted in urine. ***Half-life:*** Unknown.

INDICATIONS AND DOSAGES

Atrophic vaginitis, female castration, female hypogonadism, krau-

rosis vulvae, menopausal symptoms, primary ovarian failure, prostatic carcinoma

IM

Adults. Initially, 0.1 or 0.5 mg 2-3 times weekly cyclically (21 days on; 7 days off or continuously). When progestin is given concomitantly, begin progestin after 10-13 days of each estrogen cycle.

AVAILABLE FORMS

• *Injection:* 2 mg/ml (Estro-A, Estrogenic, Estrogens), 5 mg/ml (Estragyn 5, Kestrone 5).

CONTRAINDICATIONS: Abnormal vaginal bleeding, active arterial thrombosis, blood dyscrasias, estrogen-dependent cancer, known or suspected breast cancer, pregnancy, thrombophlebitis or thromboembolic disorders, hypersensitivity to estrone or any of its components.

PREGNANCY AND LACTATION: Pregnancy category X; may reduce quantity and quality of breast milk

SIDE EFFECTS

Frequent

Transient menstrual abnormalities including spotting, change in menstrual flow or cervical secretions, and amenorrhea at initiation of therapy

Occasional

Edema, weight change, breast tenderness, nervousness, insomnia, fatigue, dizziness

Rare

Alopecia, mental depression, dermatologic changes, headache, fever, nausea

SERIOUS REACTIONS

• Thrombophlebitis, pulmonary or cerebral embolism, and retinal thrombosis occur rarely.

INTERACTIONS

Drugs

3 *Bromocriptine:* May interfere with the effects of bromocriptine

3 *P450 inducers (e.g., rifampin, barbiturates):* Decreased estrogen levels

3 *Corticosteroids:* Increased steroid effect

3 *Cyclosporine:* May increase blood cyclosporine concentration and the risk of hepatotoxicity and nephrotoxicity

3 *Phenytoin:* Loss of seizure control, decreased estrogen levels

3 *Warfarin:* Theoretical increased risk thromboembolism

SPECIAL CONSIDERATIONS

• Progestins recommended in nonhysterectomized women

• Consider topical products if treatment is solely for vulvar or vaginal atrophy

• Currently recommended that use of hormone replacement therapy be limited to treating symptomatic women, preferrably for ≤5 yrs. Risk felt to outweigh benefit in asymptomatic women using only for prophylaxis of other conditions

PATIENT/FAMILY EDUCATION

• Avoid smoking because of the increased risk of blood clot formation and MI

• Report abnormal vaginal bleeding, depression, or signs and symptoms of blood clots

• Perform breast self-examination monthly

• Report weekly weight gain of more than 5 lbs

• Notify the physician and discontinue the drug, as prescribed, if she suspects she is pregnant

MONITORING PARAMETERS

• Blood pressure periodically

• Blood glucose levels, hepatic enzymes, serum calcium levels

• Weight

• Signs and symptoms of thromboembolic or thrombotic disorders, including loss of coordination, numbness or weakness of an extremity, shortness of breath, speech or vision disturbance, sudden severe headache, and pain in the chest, leg, or groin

estropipate

(es-troe-pih'-pate)

Rx: Ogen, Ortho-Est

Chemical Class: Estrogen derivative

Therapeutic Class: Antiosteoporotic; estrogen

CLINICAL PHARMACOLOGY

Mechanism of Action: An estrogen that increases synthesis of DNA, RNA, and proteins in target tissues; reduces release of gonadotropin-releasing hormone from the hypothalamus; and reduces follicle-stimulating hormone (FSH) and luteinizing hormone (LH) from the pituitary. ***Therapeutic Effect:*** Promotes normal growth, promotes development of female sex organs, and maintains GU function and vasomotor stability. Prevents accelerated bone loss by inhibiting bone resorption, restoring balance of bone resorption and formation. Inhibits LH and decreases serum testosterone concentration.

Pharmacokinetics

Readily absorbed through the skin, mucous membranes, and GI tract. Widely distributed. Protein binding: 50%-80%. Metabolized in the liver. Primarily excreted in urine. ***Half-life:*** 12-20 hr.

INDICATIONS AND DOSAGES

Vasomotor symptoms, atrophic vaginitis, kraurosis vulvae

PO

Adults, Elderly. 0.625-5 mg/day cyclically.

Atrophic vaginitis, kraurosis vulvae

Intravaginal

Adults, Elderly. 2-4 g/day cyclically.

Female hypogonadism, castration, primary ovarian failure

PO

Adults, Elderly. 1.25-7.5 mg/day for 21 days; then off for 8-10 days. Repeat if bleeding does not occur by end of off cycle.

Prevention of osteoporosis

PO

Adults, Elderly. 0.625 mg/day (25 days of 31-day cycle/mo).

AVAILABLE FORMS

- *Tablets (Ogen, Ortho-Est):* 0.625 mg (0.75 mg estropipate), 1.25 mg (1.5 mg estropipate), 2.5 mg (3 mg estropipate).
- *Vaginal Cream (Ogen):* 1.5 mg/g.

CONTRAINDICATIONS: Abnormal vaginal bleeding, active arterial thrombosis, blood dyscrasias, estrogen-dependent cancer, known or suspected breast cancer, pregnancy, thrombophlebitis or thromboembolic disorders, thyroid dysfunction

PREGNANCY AND LACTATION: Pregnancy category X; may reduce quantity and quality of breast milk

SIDE EFFECTS

Frequent

Anorexia, nausea, swelling of breasts, peripheral edema marked by swollen ankles and feet

Occasional

Vomiting, especially with high doses; headache that may be severe; intolerance to contact lenses; hypertension; glucose intolerance; brown spots on exposed skin

Vaginal: Local irritation, vaginal discharge, changes in vaginal bleeding, including spotting, and breakthrough or prolonged bleeding

Rare
Chorea or involuntary movements, hirsutism or abnormal hairiness, loss of scalp hair, depression

SERIOUS REACTIONS

- Prolonged administration may increase the risk of breast, cervical, endometrial, hepatic, and vaginal carcinoma; cerebrovascular disease, coronary heart disease, gallbladder disease, and hypercalcemia.
- Cholestatic jaundice occurs rarely.

INTERACTIONS

Drugs

3 *Bromocriptine:* May interfere with the effects of bromocriptine

3 *P450 inducers (e.g., rifampin, barbiturates):* Decreased estrogen levels

3 *Corticosteroids:* Increased steroid effect

3 *Cyclosporine:* May increase blood cyclosporine concentration and the risk of hepatotoxicity and nephrotoxicity

3 *Phenytoin:* Loss of seizure control, decreased estrogen levels

3 *Saw palmetto:* Increases the effects of saw palmetto

3 *Warfarin:* Theoretical increased risk thromboembolism

SPECIAL CONSIDERATIONS

- Unopposed estrogen increases risk of endometrial cancer; recommended administration of concurrent progestational agents for nonhysterectomized women

PATIENT/FAMILY EDUCATION

- Avoid smoking because of the increased risk of blood clot formation and MI
- Remain recumbent for at least 30 mins after vaginal application and do not use tampons during estropipate therapy
- Report depression or abnormal vaginal bleeding
- Notify the physician and discontinue the drug, as prescribed, if she suspects she is pregnant

MONITORING PARAMETERS

- Signs and symptoms of thromboembolic or thrombotic disorders, including loss of coordination, numbness or weakness of an extremity, shortness of breath, speech or vision disturbance, sudden severe headache, and pain in the chest, leg, or groin

E

---

etanercept

(eh-tan′-er-sept)

Rx: Enbrel

Chemical Class: Recombinant human fusion protein

Therapeutic Class: Disease-modifying antirheumatic drug (DMARD); immunomodulatory agent

---

CLINICAL PHARMACOLOGY

Mechanism of Action: A protein that binds to tumor necrosis factor (TNF), blocking its interaction with cell surface receptors. Elevated levels of TNF, which is involved in inflammatory and immune responses, are found in the synovial fluid of rheumatoid arthritis patients. ***Therapeutic Effect:*** Relieves symptoms of rheumatoid arthritis.

Pharmacokinetics

Well absorbed after subcutaneous administration. ***Half-life:*** 115 hr.

INDICATIONS AND DOSAGES

Rheumatoid arthritis, psoriatic arthritis, ankylosing spondylitis

Subcutaneous

Adults, Elderly. 25 mg twice weekly given 72-96 hr apart. Alternative weekly dosing: 0.8 mg/kg/dose once a week. Maximum: 50 mg/week. Maximum: 25 mg/dose.

Juvenile rheumatoid arthritis
Subcutaneous
Children 4-17 yrs. 0.4 mg/kg (Maximum: 25 mg dose) twice weekly given 72-96 hrs apart. Alternative weekly dosing: 50 mg once weekly. Maximum: 25 mg/dose.
Plaque psoriasis
Subcutaneous
Adults, Elderly. 50 mg twice a week (give 3-4 days apart) for 3 mo. Maintenance: 50 mg once a week.

AVAILABLE FORMS
- *Powder for Injection:* 25 mg.
- *Prefilled Syringe:* 50 mg.

UNLABELED USES: Treatment of Crohn's disease, reactive arthritis

CONTRAINDICATIONS: Serious active infection or sepsis

PREGNANCY AND LACTATION: Pregnancy category B; information on breast milk excretion is unknown; breast-feeding not advised

SIDE EFFECTS
Frequent (37%)
Injection site erythema, pruritus, pain, and swelling; abdominal pain, vomiting (more common in children than adults)
Occasional (16%-4%)
Headache, rhinitis, dizziness, pharyngitis, cough, asthenia, abdominal pain, dyspepsia
Rare (less than 3%)
Sinusitis, allergic reaction

SERIOUS REACTIONS
- Infections (such as pyelonephritis, cellulitis, osteomyelitis, wound infection, leg ulcer, septic arthritis, diarrhea, bronchitis, and pneumonia) occur in 38%-29% of patients.
- Rare adverse effects include heart failure, hypertension, hypotension, pancreatitis, GI hemorrhage, and dyspnea. The patient also may develop autoimmune antibodies.

SPECIAL CONSIDERATIONS
- Immunizations should be up to date, especially in children prior to starting therapy

PATIENT/FAMILY EDUCATION
- Review injection techniques to ensure safe self-administration
- Avoid receiving live-virus vaccines during treatment
- Notify the physician if bleeding, bruising, pallor, or persistent fever occurs
- Reassure the patient that injection site reactions generally occur in the first month of treatment and decrease in frequency with continued etanercept therapy

MONITORING PARAMETERS
- Efficacy: ESR, C-reactive protein, rheumatoid factor, improvement in tender/painful swollen joints, quality of life
- Temporarily discontinue therapy and expect to treat the patient with varicella-zoster immunoglobulin, as prescribed, if the patient experiences significant exposure to varicella virus during treatment

ethambutol hydrochloride
(e-tham'-byoo-tole hye-droe-klor'-ide)
Rx: Myambutol
Chemical Class: Diisopropylethylene diamide derivative
Therapeutic Class: Antituberculosis agent

CLINICAL PHARMACOLOGY
Mechanism of Action: An isonicotinic acid derivative that interferes with RNA synthesis. ***Therapeutic Effect:*** Suppresses the multiplication of mycobacteria.

Pharmacokinetics
Rapidly and well absorbed from the GI tract. Protein binding: 20%-30%. Widely distributed. Metabolized in the liver. Primarily excreted in urine. Removed by hemodialysis. ***Half-life:*** 3-4 hr (increased in impaired renal function).

INDICATIONS AND DOSAGES
Tuberculosis, other myobacterial diseases
PO
Adults, Elderly. 15-25 mg/kg/day. Maximum: 1.6 g/dose.
Children. 15-20 mg/kg/day. Maximum: 1 g/day.
Dosage in renal impairment
Dosage interval is modified based on creatinine clearance.

Creatinine Clearance	Dosage Interval
10-50 ml/min	q24-36h
less than 10 ml/min	q48h

AVAILABLE FORMS
• *Tablets:* 100 mg, 400 mg.
UNLABELED USES: Treatment of atypical mycobacterial infections such as *Mycobacterium avium* complex (MAC)
CONTRAINDICATIONS: Optic neuritis
PREGNANCY AND LACTATION: Pregnancy category B; compatible with breast-feeding
SIDE EFFECTS
Occasional
Acute gouty arthritis (chills, pain, swelling of joints with hot skin), confusion, abdominal pain, nausea, vomiting, anorexia, headache
Rare
Rash, fever, blurred vision, eye pain, red-green color blindness
SERIOUS REACTIONS
• Optic neuritis (more common with high-dosage or long-term ethambutol therapy), peripheral neuritis, thrombocytopenia, and an anaphylactoid reaction occur rarely.
INTERACTIONS
Drugs
3 *Neurotoxic medications:* May increase the risk of neurotoxicity
SPECIAL CONSIDERATIONS
• Initial therapy in tuberculosis should include 4 drugs: isoniazid, rifampin, pyrazinamide, and ethambutol, until drug susceptibility results available
PATIENT/FAMILY EDUCATION
• Administer with meals to decrease GI symptoms
• Do not skip drug doses and take ethambutol for the full course of therapy, which may be months or years
• Notify the physician immediately of any visual problems; effects are generally reversible after ethambutol is discontinued, but in rare cases they may take up to a year to resolve or may become permanent
• Promptly report burning, numbness, or tingling of the feet or hands, as well as pain and swelling of joints
MONITORING PARAMETERS
• Perform visual acuity testing before beginning therapy and periodically during drug administration (qmo if dose >15 mg/kg/day)
• Serum uric acid levels; assess the patient for signs and symptoms of gout, including hot, painful, or swollen joints, especially in the ankle, big toe, or knee
• Signs and symptoms of peripheral neuritis, as evidenced by burning, numbness, or tingling of the extremities

ethinyl estradiol

(eth′-in-il es-tra-dye′-ole)

Rx: Estinyl

Chemical Class: Estrogen derivative

Therapeutic Class: Contraceptive; estrogen

CLINICAL PHARMACOLOGY

Mechanism of Action: A synthetic derivative of estradiol that increases synthesis of DNA, RNA, proteins in target tissues; reduces release of gonadotropin-releasing hormone from hypothalamus; reduces follicle-stimulating hormone (FSH) and luteinizing hormone (LH) release from the pituitary. ***Therapeutic Effect:*** Promotes normal growth, development of female sex organs, maintaining genitourinary (GU) function, vasomotor stability. Prevents accelerated bone loss by inhibiting bone resorption, restoring balance of bone resorption and formation. Inhibits LH, decreases serum concentration of testosterone.

Pharmacokinetics

Well absorbed from the gastrointestinal (GI) tract. Widely distributed. Protein binding: 50%-80%. Rapidly metabolized in liver to estrone and estriol. Excreted in urine and feces. ***Half-life:*** 8-25 hrs.

INDICATIONS AND DOSAGES

Female hypogonadism

PO

Adults. 0.05 mg 1-3 times/day during the first 2 wks of menstrual cycle, followed by progesterone during the last half of cycle for 3-6 mos.

Menopausal symptoms

PO

Adults. 0.02- 0.05 mg/day cyclically (3 wks on, 1 wk off).

Breast cancer

PO

Adults. 1 mg 3 times/day for at least 3 mos.

Prostate cancer

PO

Adults. 0.15-2 mg/day.

AVAILABLE FORMS

- *Tablets:* 0.02 mg, 0.05, 0.5 mg (Estinyl).

CONTRAINDICATIONS: Abnormal vaginal bleeding, active arterial thrombosis, blood dyscrasias, estrogen-dependent cancer, known or suspected breast cancer, pregnancy, thrombophlebitis or thromboembolic disorders, thyroid dysfunction, hypersensitivity to estrongens

PREGNANCY AND LACTATION: Pregnancy category X; may reduce quantity and quality of breast milk

SIDE EFFECTS

Frequent

Anorexia, nausea, swelling of breasts, peripheral edema, evidenced by swollen ankles, feet

Occasional

Vomiting, especially with high dosages, headache that may be severe, intolerance to contact lenses, increased blood pressure (BP), glucose intolerance, brown spots on exposed skin

Rare

Chorea or involuntary movements, hirsutism or abnormal hairiness, loss of scalp hair, depression

SERIOUS REACTIONS

- Prolonged administration increases risk of gallbladder disease, thromboembolic disease, and breast, cervical, vaginal, endometrial, and liver carcinoma.
- Cholestatic jaundice occurs rarely.

INTERACTIONS

Drugs

3 *Bromocriptine:* May interfere with the effects of bromocriptine

3 *Corticosteroids:* Increased steroid effect

3 *Cyclosporine:* May increase blood cyclosporine concentration and the risk of hepatotoxicity and nephrotoxicity

3 *Grapefruit juice:* Increases ethinyl estradiol serum concentrations

3 *P450 inducers (e.g., rifampin, barbiturates):* Decreased estrogen levels

3 *Phenytoin:* Loss of seizure control, decreased estrogen levels

3 *Warfarin:* Theoretical increased risk of thromboembolism

SPECIAL CONSIDERATIONS

- Unopposed estrogen increases risk of endometrial cancer; recommended administration of concurrent progestational agents for nonhysterectomized women

PATIENT/FAMILY EDUCATION

- Limit alcohol and caffeine intake
- Stop smoking tobacco
- Report calf or chest pain, depression, numbness or weakness of an extremity, severe abdominal pain, shortness of breath, speech or vision disturbance, sudden headache, unusual bleeding, or vomiting

MONITORING PARAMETERS

- Blood pressure periodically
- Weight
- Signs and symptoms of thromboembolic or thrombotic disorders, including loss of coordination, numbness or weakness of an extremity, shortness of breath, speech or vision disturbance, sudden severe headache, and pain in the chest, leg, or groin

ethionamide

(e-thye-on′-am-ide)

Rx: Trecator-SC

Chemical Class: Thiomine derivative

Therapeutic Class: Antituberculosis agent

E

CLINICAL PHARMACOLOGY

Mechanism of Action: An antitubercular agent that inhibits peptide synthesis. ***Therapeutic Effect:*** Suppresses mycobacterial multiplication. Bactericidal.

Pharmacokinetics

Rapidly absorbed from the gastrointestinal (GI) tract. Widely distributed. Protein binding: 10%. Metabolized in liver. Primarily excreted in urine. Removed by hemodialysis. ***Half-life:*** 2-3 hrs (half-life is increased with impaired renal function).

INDICATIONS AND DOSAGES

Tuberculosis

PO

Adults, Elderly. 500-1000 mg/day as a single to 3 divided doses.

Children. 15-20 mg/kg/day. Maximum 1 g/day.

Dosage in renal impairment

Creatinine clearance less than 50 ml/min, reduce dose by 50%.

AVAILABLE FORMS

- *Tablets:* 250 mg (Trecator).

UNLABELED USES: Treatment of atypical mycobacterial infections

CONTRAINDICATIONS: Severe hepatic impairment, hypersensitivity to ethionamide

PREGNANCY AND LACTATION: Pregnancy category C

SIDE EFFECTS

Occasional

Abdominal pain, nausea, vomiting, weakness, postural hypotension, psychiatric disturbances, drowsiness, dizziness, headache, confusion, anorexia, headache, metallic taste, anorexia, diarrhea, stomatitis, peripheral neuritis

Rare

Rash, fever, blurred vision, optic neuritis, seizures, hypothyroidism, hypoglycemia, gynecomastia, thrombocytopenia, jaundice

SERIOUS REACTIONS

• Peripheral neuropathy, anorexia, and joint pain rarely occur.

INTERACTIONS

Labs

• *False decrease:* Urine alkaline phosphatase, urine lactate dehydrogenase

SPECIAL CONSIDERATIONS

• Use only with at least 1 other effective antituberculous agent

MONITORING PARAMETERS

• Serum transaminases (AST, ALT) biweekly during therapy

ethosuximide

(eth-oh-sux'-i-mide)

Rx: Zarontin

Chemical Class: Succinimide derivative

Therapeutic Class: Anticonvulsant

CLINICAL PHARMACOLOGY

Mechanism of Action: An anticonvulsant that increases the seizure threshold and suppresses paroxysmal spike-and-wave pattern in absence seizures; depresses nerve transmission in the motor cortex. ***Therapeutic Effect:*** Produces anticonvulsant activity.

Pharmacokinetics

Well absorbed from the gastrointestinal (GI) tract. Metabolized in liver. Excreted in urine. Removed by hemodialysis. ***Half-life:*** 50-60 hrs (in adults); 30 hrs (in children).

INDICATIONS AND DOSAGES

Absence seizures

PO

Adults, Elderly, Children older than 6 yrs. Initially, 250 mg/day or 15 mg/kg/day in 2 divided doses. Maintenance: 15-40 mg/kg/day in 2 divided doses.

Children 3-6 yrs. Initially, 250 mg in 2 divided doses, increased by 250 mg as needed every 4-7 days. Maintenance: 20-40 mg/kg/day in 2 divided doses.

Use with caution in patients with renal impairment.

AVAILABLE FORMS

• *Capsule:* 250 mg, 100 mg, 150 mg, 200 mg (Zarontin).

• *Syrup:* 250 mg/5 ml (Zarontin).

UNLABELED USES: Treatment of learning problems

CONTRAINDICATIONS: Hypersensitivity to succinimides

PREGNANCY AND LACTATION: Pregnancy category C; freely enters breast milk; no adverse effects on infants reported; compatible with breast-feeding

SIDE EFFECTS

Occasional

Dizziness, drowsiness, double vision, headache, ataxia, nausea, diarrhea, vomiting, somnolence, urticaria

Rare

Arganulocytosis, gum hypertrophy, leucopenia, myopia, swelling of the tongue, systemic lupus erythematosus, vaginal bleeding

SERIOUS REACTIONS

• Abrupt withdrawal may increase seizure frequency.

• Overdosage results in nausea, vomiting, and CNS depression including coma with respiratory depression.

INTERACTIONS

Drugs

3 *Antiepileptic drugs:* May increase or decrease serum levels of these drugs

SPECIAL CONSIDERATIONS

PATIENT/FAMILY EDUCATION

- Take doses at regularly spaced intervals
- OK with food or milk
- Avoid alcohol and tasks that require mental alertness or motor skills until response to the drug is established
- Notify the physician if fever, rash, or swelling of glands occurs

MONITORING PARAMETERS

- Blood counts, renal function tests, liver function tests, urinalysis periodically
- Therapeutic serum concentrations 40-100 mcg/ml
- Evidence of toxicity such as bruising, fever, joint pain, mouth ulcerations, sore throat, and unusual bleeding

etidronate disodium

(ee-tid'-roe-nate dye-soe'-dee-um)

Rx: Didronel

Chemical Class: Pyrophosphate analog

Therapeutic Class: Bisphosphonate; bone resorption inhibitor

CLINICAL PHARMACOLOGY

Mechanism of Action: A bisphosphonate that decreases mineral release and matrix in bone and inhibits osteocytic osteolysis. ***Therapeutic Effect:*** Decreases bone resorption.

Pharmacokinetics

Variable absorption following PO administration. Not metabolized. Approximately 50% of drug is excreted in urine. Unabsorbed drug is excreted intact in feces. ***Half-life:*** 1-6 hr (oral); 6 hr (IV).

INDICATIONS AND DOSAGES

Paget's disease

PO

Adults, Elderly. Initially, 5-10 mg/kg/day not to exceed 6 mo, or 11-20 mg/kg/day not to exceed 3 mo. Repeat only after drug-free period of at least 90 days.

Heterotopic ossification caused by spinal cord injury

PO

Adult, Elderly. 20 mg/kg/day for 2 wk; then 10 mg/kg/day for 10 wks.

Heterotopic ossification complicating total hip replacement

PO

Adults, Elderly. 20 mg/kg/day for 1 mo before surgery; then 20 mg/kg/day for 3 mo after surgery.

Hypercalcemia associated with malignancy

IV

Adults, Elderly. 7.5 mg/kg/day for 3 days. For retreatment, allow 7 days between treatment courses. Follow with oral therapy on day after last infusion. Begin with 20 mg/kg/day for 30 days; may extend up to 90 days.

AVAILABLE FORMS

- *Tablets (Didronel):* 200 mg, 400 mg.
- *Injection (Didronel I.V.):* 300-mg ampule (50 mg/ml).

CONTRAINDICATIONS: Clinically overt osteomalacia

PREGNANCY AND LACTATION: Pregnancy category C; breast milk excretion not known; problems in humans have not been documented

SIDE EFFECTS

Frequent

Nausea; diarrhea; continuing or more frequent bone pain in patients with Paget's disease

Occasional
Bone fractures, especially of the femur
Parenteral: Metallic, altered taste
Rare
Hypersensitivity reaction
SERIOUS REACTIONS
• Nephrotoxicity, including hematuria, dysuria, and proteinuria, has occurred with parenteral route.
INTERACTIONS
Drugs
3 *Antacids containing aluminum, calcium, magnesium mineral supplements:* May decrease the absorption of etidronate
SPECIAL CONSIDERATIONS
PATIENT/FAMILY EDUCATION
• Administer on empty stomach with H_2O, 2 hr ac
• Exceeding the 2-wk treatment periods for osteoporosis may lead to bone demineralization and osteomalacia
• It may take up to 3 mos for a noticeable therapeutic response
• Consume calcium-rich foods, such as dairy products and milk
MONITORING PARAMETERS
• Electrolytes, BUN, fluid intake and output in patients with impaired renal function
• Assess the patient for diarrhea

etodolac
(e-toe'-doe-lak)
Rx: Lodine, Lodine XL
Chemical Class: Acetic acid derivative
Therapeutic Class: NSAID; antipyretic; nonnarcotic analgesic

CLINICAL PHARMACOLOGY
Mechanism of Action: An NSAID that produces analgesic and antiinflammatory effects by inhibiting prostaglandin synthesis. ***Therapeutic Effect:*** Reduces the inflammatory response and intensity of pain.
Pharmacokinetics

Route	Onset	Peak	Duration
PO (analgesic)	30 min	N/A	4-12 hr

Completely absorbed from the GI tract. Protein binding: greater than 99%. Widely distributed. Metabolized in the liver. Primarily excreted in urine. Not removed by hemodialysis. ***Half-life:*** 6-7 hr.
INDICATIONS AND DOSAGES
Osteoarthritis, rheumatoid arthritis
PO (Immediate-Release)
Adults, Elderly. Initially, 300 mg 2-3 times a day or 400-500 mg twice a day. Maintenance: 600-1000 mg/day in 2-4 divided doses.
PO (Extended-Release)
Adults, Elderly. 400-1000 mg once daily. Maximum: 1200 mg/day.
Juvenile rheumatoid arthritis
PO (Extended-Release)
Children 6-16 yr. 1000 mg in children weighing more than 60 kg, 800 mg once daily in children weighing 46-60 kg, 600 mg once daily in children weighing 31-45 kg, 400 mg once daily in children weighing 20-30 kg.
Analgesia
PO
Adults, Elderly. 200-400 mg q6-8h as needed. Maximum: 1200 mg/day.
AVAILABLE FORMS
• *Capsules (Lodine):* 200 mg, 300 mg.
• *Tablets (Lodine):* 400 mg, 500 mg.
• *Tablets (Extended-Release [Lodine XL]):* 400 mg, 500 mg, 600 mg.
UNLABELED USES: Treatment of acute gouty arthritis, vascular headache

CONTRAINDICATIONS: Active peptic ulcer disease, chronic inflammation of GI tract, GI bleeding or ulceration, history of hypersensitivity to aspirin or NSAIDs

PREGNANCY AND LACTATION: Pregnancy category C (D if used in third trimester or near delivery); breast milk excretion unknown; problems in humans have not been documented

SIDE EFFECTS

Occasional (9%-4%)

Dizziness, headache, abdominal pain or cramps, bloated feeling, diarrhea, nausea, indigestion

Rare (3%-1%)

Constipation, rash, pruritus, visual disturbances, tinnitus

SERIOUS REACTIONS

- Overdose may result in acute renal failure.
- There is an increased risk of cardiovascular events (including MI and CVA) and serious and potentially life-threatening GI bleeding.
- Rare reactions with long-term use include peptic ulcer disease, GI bleeding, gastritis, severe hepatic reactions (jaundice), nephrotoxicity (hematuria, dysuria, proteinuria), and a severe hypersensitivity reaction (bronchospasm, angioedema).

INTERACTIONS

Drugs

3 *Aminoglycosides:* Reduced clearance with elevated aminoglycoside levels and potential for toxicity (especially indomethacin in premature infants; other NSAIDs probably)

3 *Antihypertensives (α-blockers, angiotensin-converting enzyme inhibitors, angiotensin II receptor blockers, β-blockers, diuretics):* Inhibition of antihypertensive and other favorable hemodynamic effects

3 *Corticosteroids:* Increased risk of GI ulceration

3 *Anticoagulants:* Excessive hypoprothrombinemia, decreased platelet aggregation with increased risk of GI bleeding; may be less likely to increase bleeding risk than other NSAIDs due to preferential effects on COX-2

3 *Bone marrow depressants:* May increase the risk of hematologic reactions

3 *Cyclosporine:* Increased nephrotoxicity risk

3 *Feverfew, ginkgo biloba:* May increase the risk of bleeding

3 *Lithium:* Decreased clearance of lithium (mediated via prostaglandins) resulting in elevated serum lithium levels and risk of toxicity

3 *Methotrexate:* Decreased renal secretion of methotrexate resulting in elevated methotrexate levels and risk of toxicity

3 *Phenylpropanolamine:* Possible acute hypertensive reaction

3 *Potassium-sparing diuretics:* Additive hyperkalemia potential

3 *Probenecid:* Probenecid

3 *Triamterene:* Acute renal failure reported with addition of indomethacin; caution with other NSAIDs

SPECIAL CONSIDERATIONS

PATIENT/FAMILY EDUCATION

- Swallow etodolac capsules whole and do not open, chew, or crush them
- Take etodolac with food, milk, or antacids if GI distress occurs
- Notify the physician if edema, GI distress, headache, rash, signs of bleeding, or visual disturbances occurs
- Avoid alcohol and aspirin during etodolac therapy because these substances increase the risk of GI bleeding

E

• Avoid performing tasks that require mental alertness or motor skills until response to the drug has been established
• The female patient should notify the physician if she is or plans to become pregnant

MONITORING PARAMETERS

• Initial hemogram and fecal occult blood test within 3 mo of starting regular chronic therapy; repeat every 6-12 mo (more frequently in high-risk patients [>65 years, peptic ulcer disease, concurrent steroids or anticoagulants]); electrolytes, creatinine, and BUN within 3 mo of starting regular chronic therapy; repeat every 6-12 mo
• Therapeutic response, such as improved grip strength, increased joint mobility, and decreased pain, tenderness, stiffness, and swelling

---

ezetimibe

(ez-et'-i-mibe)
Rx: Zetia
Combinations
Rx: with simvastatin (Vytorin)
Chemical Class: Substituted azetidinone
Therapeutic Class: Selective cholesterol absorption inhibitor

---

CLINICAL PHARMACOLOGY

Mechanism of Action: An antihyperlipidemic that inhibits cholesterol absorption in the small intestine, leading to a decrease in the delivery of intestinal cholesterol to the liver. ***Therapeutic Effect:*** Reduces total serum cholesterol, LDL cholesterol, and triglyceride levels; and increases HDL cholesterol concentration.

Pharmacokinetics

Well absorbed following oral administration. Protein binding: greater than 90%. Metabolized in the small intestine and liver. Excreted by the kidneys and bile. ***Half-life:*** 22 hr.

INDICATIONS AND DOSAGES

Hypercholesterolemia

PO

Adults, Elderly. Initially, 10 mg once a day, given with or without food. If the patient is also receiving a bile acid sequestrant, give ezetimibe at least 2 hr before or at least 4 hr after the bile acid sequestrant.

Sitosterolemia

PO

Adults, Elderly. 10 mg/day.

AVAILABLE FORMS

• *Tablets:* 10 mg.

CONTRAINDICATIONS: Concurrent use of an hydroxamethylglutaryl-CoA (HMG-CoA) reductase inhibitor (atorvastatin, fluvastatin, lovastatin, pravastatin, or simvastatin) in patients with active hepatic disease or unexplained persistent elevations in serum transaminase levels, moderate or severe hepatic insufficiency

PREGNANCY AND LACTATION: Pregnancy category C; human breast milk exposure unknown; up to half of exposure of maternal plasma in animal pups

SIDE EFFECTS

Occasional (4%-3%)

Back pain, diarrhea, arthralgia, sinusitis, abdominal pain

Rare (2%)

Cough, pharyngitis, fatigue

SERIOUS REACTIONS

• Hepatitis, hypersensitivity reactions, myopathy, and rhabdomyolysis occur rarely.

INTERACTIONS
Drugs
3 *Aluminum and magnesium-containing antacids, cyclosporine, fenofibrate, gemfibrozil:* Increase ezetimibe plasma concentration
2 *Cholestyramine:* Decreased ezetimibe plasma levels 55%-80%

SPECIAL CONSIDERATIONS
- Modest cholesterol reductions as monotherapy (15%); primary use in combination with statins to achieve and sustain LDL goals

PATIENT/FAMILY EDUCATION
- Periodic laboratory tests are an essential part of therapy
- Do not discontinue ezetimibe without physician approval

MONITORING PARAMETERS
- Lipid profile, LFTs, serum CPK, electrolytes, blood glucose, signs and symptoms of toxicity (GI symptoms, headache, rash); pattern of daily bowel activity and stool consistency

famciclovir
(fam-sye'-kloe-veer)
Rx: Famvir
Chemical Class: Acyclic purine nucleoside analog
Therapeutic Class: Antiviral

CLINICAL PHARMACOLOGY
Mechanism of Action: A synthetic nucleoside that inhibits viral DNA synthesis. ***Therapeutic Effect:*** Suppresses replication of herpes simplex virus and varicella-zoster virus.
Pharmacokinetics
Rapidly and extensively absorbed after PO administration. Protein binding: 20%-25%. Rapidly metabolized to penciclovir by enzymes in the GI wall, liver, and plasma. Eliminated unchanged in urine. Removed by hemodialysis. ***Half-life:*** 2 hr.

INDICATIONS AND DOSAGES
Herpes zoster
PO
Adults. 500 mg q8h for 7 days.
Genital herpes, first episode
PO
Adults, Elderly. 250 mg 3 times a day for 7-10 days.
Recurrent genital herpes
PO
Adults. 125 mg twice a day for 5 days.
Suppression of recurrent genital herpes
PO
Adults. 250 mg twice a day for up to 1 yr.
Recurrent herpes simplex
PO
Adults. 500 mg twice a day for 7 days.
Dosage in renal impairment
Dosage and frequency are modified based on creatinine clearance.

Creatinine Clearance	*Herpes Zoster*	*Genital Herpes*
40-59 ml/min	500 mg q12h	125 mg q12h
20-39 ml/min	500 mg q24h	125 mg q24h
less than 20 ml/min	250 mg q24h	125 mg q24h

Dosage in hemodialysis patients
For adults with herpes zoster, give 250 mg after each dialysis treatment; for adults with genital herpes, give 125 mg after each dialysis treatment.

AVAILABLE FORMS
- *Tablets:* 125 mg, 250 mg, 500 mg.

CONTRAINDICATIONS: Hypersensitivity to penciclovir cream

PREGNANCY AND LACTATION: Pregnancy category B; excreted in breast milk

SIDE EFFECTS
Frequent
Headache (23%), nausea (12%)

Occasional (10%-2%)
Dizziness, somnolence, numbness of feet, diarrhea, vomiting, constipation, decreased appetite, fatigue, fever, pharyngitis, sinusitis, pruritus
Rare (less than 2%)
Insomnia, abdominal pain, dyspepsia, flatulence, back pain, arthralgia

SERIOUS REACTIONS

• Urticaria, hallucinations, and confusion (including delirium, disorientation, confusional state, occurring predominantly in the elderly) have been reported.

SPECIAL CONSIDERATIONS

• Reserve chronic suppressive therapy for patients without prodromal symptoms who have frequent recurrences

PATIENT/FAMILY EDUCATION

• Drink adequate fluids
• Keep fingernails short and hands clean
• Do not touch the lesions for the duration of an outbreak to prevent cross-contamination and spreading the infection to new sites
• Space doses evenly around the clock and take famciclovir for the full course of treatment
• Notify the physician if the lesions fail to improve or if they recur

MONITORING PARAMETERS

• Assess for signs and symptoms of neurologic effects, including dizziness and headache

famotidine

(fa-moe'-ti-deen)
Rx: Pepcid, Pepcid RPD
OTC: Mylanta AR, Pepcid AC
Combinations
OTC: with calcium carbonate and magnesium hydroxide (Pepcid Complete)
Chemical Class: Thiazole derivative
Therapeutic Class: Antiulcer agent

CLINICAL PHARMACOLOGY

Mechanism of Action: An antiulcer agent and gastric acid secretion inhibitor that inhibits histamine action at histamine$_2$ receptors of parietal cells. ***Therapeutic Effect:*** Inhibits gastric acid secretion when fasting, at night, or when stimulated by food, caffeine, or insulin.

Pharmacokinetics

Route	Onset	Peak	Duration
PO	1 hr	1-4 hr	10-12 hr
IV	1 hr	0.5-3 hr	10-12 hr

Rapidly, incompletely absorbed from the GI tract. Protein binding: 15%-20%. Partially metabolized in the liver. Primarily excreted in urine. Not removed by hemodialysis. ***Half-life:*** 2.5-3.5 hr (increased with impaired renal function).

INDICATIONS AND DOSAGES

Acute treatment of duodenal and gastric ulcers
PO
Adults, Elderly, Children 12 yr and older. 40 mg/day at bedtime.
Children 1-11 yr. 0.5 mg/kg/day at bedtime. Maximum: 40 mg/day.

Duodenal ulcer maintenance
PO
Adults, Elderly. 20 mg/day at bedtime.

Gastroesophageal reflux disease
PO
Adults, Elderly, Children 12 yr and older. 20 mg twice a day.
Children 1-11 yr. 1 mg/kg/day in 2 divided doses.
Children 3-11 mo. 0.5 mg/kg/dose twice a day.
Children younger than 3 mo. 0.5 mg/kg/dose once a day.
Esophagitis
PO
Adults, Elderly, Children 12 yr and older. 2-40 mg twice a day.
Hypersecretory conditions
PO
Adults, Elderly, Children 12 yr and older. Initially, 20 mg q6h. May increase up to 160 mg q6h.
Acid indigestion, heartburn (over-the-counter)
PO
Adults, Elderly, Children 12 yr and older. 10-20 mg 15-60 min before eating. Maximum: 2 doses per day.
Usual parenteral dosage
IV
Adults, Elderly, Children 12 yr and older. 20 mg q12h.
Dosage in renal impairment
Dosing frequency is modified based on creatinine clearance.

Creatinine Clearance	*Dosing Frequency*
10-50 ml/min	q24h
less than 10 ml/min	q36-48h

AVAILABLE FORMS
- *Oral Suspension (Pepcid):* 40 mg/5 ml.
- *Tablets:* 10 mg (Pepcid AC), 20 mg (Pepcid, Pepcid AC), 40 mg (Pepcid).
- *Tablets (Chewable [Pepcid AC]):* 10 mg.
- *Capsules (Pepcid AC):* 10 mg.
- *Injection (Pepcid):* 10 mg/ml.

UNLABELED USES: Autism, prevention of aspiration pneumonitis, *H. pylori* eradication
CONTRAINDICATIONS: None known.
PREGNANCY AND LACTATION: Pregnancy category B; concentrated in breast milk (less than cimetidine or ranitidine); no problems reported with other H_2-histamine receptor antagonists; compatible with breast-feeding

F

SIDE EFFECTS
Occasional (5%)
Headache
Rare (2% or less)
Constipation, diarrhea, dizziness
SERIOUS REACTIONS
- None known.

INTERACTIONS
Drugs
3 *Antacids:* May decrease the absorption of famotidine
3 *Cefpodoxime, cefuroxime, enoxacin, ketoconazole:* Reduction in gastric acidity reduces absorption, decreased plasma levels, potential for therapeutic failure
3 *Glipizide, glyburide, tolbutamide:* Increased absorption of these drugs, potential for hypoglycemia
3 *Nifedipine, nitrendipine, nisoldipine:* Increased concentrations of these drugs

SPECIAL CONSIDERATIONS
- No advantage over other agents in this class, base selection on cost

PATIENT/FAMILY EDUCATION
- Stagger doses of famotidine and antacids
- May take famotidine without regard to meals but it is best taken after meals or at bedtime
- Notify the physician if headache occurs
- Avoid alcohol, aspirin, and coffee, all of which may cause GI distress, during famotidine therapy

• Contact the physician if persistent acid indigestion, heartburn, or sour stomach persists despite the medication

MONITORING PARAMETERS

• Pattern of bowel activity and stool consistency

felodipine

(fell-o'-da-peen)

Rx: Plendil

Combinations

Rx: with enalapril (Lexxel)

Chemical Class: Dihydropyridine

Therapeutic Class: Antianginal; antihypertensive; calcium channel blocker

CLINICAL PHARMACOLOGY

Mechanism of Action: An antihypertensive and antianginal agent that inhibits calcium movement across cardiac and vascular smooth-muscle cell membranes. Potent peripheral vasodilator (does not depress SA or AV nodes). ***Therapeutic Effect:*** Increases myocardial contractility, heart rate, and cardiac output; decreases peripheral vascular resistance and BP.

Pharmacokinetics

Route	Onset	Peak	Duration
PO	2-5 hr	N/A	N/A

Rapidly, completely absorbed from the GI tract. Protein binding: greater than 99%. Undergoes first-pass metabolism in the liver. Primarily excreted in urine. Not removed by hemodialysis. ***Half-life:*** 11-16 hr.

INDICATIONS AND DOSAGES

Hypertension

PO

Adults. Initially, 5 mg/day as single dose.

Elderly, Patients with impaired hepatic function. Initially, 2.5 mg/day. Adjust dosage at no less than 2-wk intervals. Maintenance: 2.5-10 mg/day. Range: 2.5-20 mg/day.

AVAILABLE FORMS

• *Tablets (Extended-Release):* 2.5 mg, 5 mg, 10 mg.

UNLABELED USES: Treatment of CHF, chronic angina pectoris, Raynaud's phenomenon

CONTRAINDICATIONS: None known.

PREGNANCY AND LACTATION: Pregnancy category C

SIDE EFFECTS

Frequent (22%-18%)

Headache, peripheral edema

Occasional (6%-4%)

Flushing, respiratory infection, dizziness, lightheadedness, asthenia (loss of strength, weakness)

Rare (less than 3%)

Paresthesia, abdominal discomfort, nervousness, muscle cramping, cough, diarrhea, constipation

SERIOUS REACTIONS

• Overdose produces nausea, somnolence, confusion, slurred speech, hypotension, and bradycardia.

INTERACTIONS

Drugs

3 *β-blockers:* May have additive effect

3 *Barbiturates:* Decreased felodipine bioavailability

3 *DHEA:* May increase felodipine blood concentration

3 *Digitalis glycosides:* Increased digitalis levels; increased risk of toxicity

3 *Erythromycin:* Increased felodipine concentrations

3 *Fentanyl:* Severe hypotension or increased fluid volume requirements

3 *Grapefruit juice:* Inhibits felodipine metabolism, 200% increase in AUC

3 *Histamine H_2 antagonists:* Increased bioavailability of felodipine
3 *Hydantoins:* Serum felodipine level may be decreased
3 *Hypokalemia-producing agents (such as furosemide and certain other diuretics):* May increase risk of arrhythmias
3 *Itraconazole:* Increases felodipine concentrations and enhances its vasodilatory effects; excessive hypotensive response could result
3 *Nelfinavir:* May increase hypotensive effects of felodipine
3 *Procainamide, quinidine:* May increase risk of QT-interval prolongation
3 *Propranolol:* Enhanced hypotension, increased propranolol concentrations

SPECIAL CONSIDERATIONS

- Results of V-HeFT III indicate felodipine may be used safely in patients with left ventricular dysfunction

PATIENT/FAMILY EDUCATION

- Administer as whole tablet (do not crush or chew)
- Avoid grapefruit juice (see drug interactions)
- Do not abruptly discontinuing felodipine; compliance with the therapy regimen is essential to control hypertension
- Rise slowly from a lying to a sitting position and wait momentarily before standing to avoid felodipine's hypotensive effect
- Avoid tasks that require mental alertness or motor skills until response to the drug has been established
- Notify the physician if an irregular heartbeat, nausea, prolonged dizziness, or shortness of breath

MONITORING PARAMETERS

- Liver function
- Pulse for bradycardia
- Skin for flushing

fenofibrate

(fen-oh-fye'-brate)

Rx: Antara, Lipidil Supra, Lofibra, Tricor, Triglide

Chemical Class: Fibric acid derivative

Therapeutic Class: Antilipemic

CLINICAL PHARMACOLOGY

Mechanism of Action: An antihyperlipidemic that enhances synthesis of lipoprotein lipase and reduces triglyceride-rich lipoproteins and VLDLs. ***Therapeutic Effect:*** Increases VLDL catabolism and reduces total plasma triglyceride levels.

Pharmacokinetics

Well absorbed from the GI tract. Absorption increased when given with food. Protein binding: 99%. Rapidly metabolized in the liver to active metabolite. Excreted primarily in urine; lesser amount in feces. Not removed by hemodialysis. ***Half-life:*** 20 hr.

INDICATIONS AND DOSAGES

Hypertriglyceridemia

PO (Antara)

Adults, Elderly. 43-130 mg/day.

PO (Lofibra)

Adults, Elderly. 67-200 mg/day with meals.

PO (Tricor)

Adults, Elderly. 48-145 mg/day.

PO (Triglide)

Adults, Elderly. 50-160 mg/day.

Hypercholesterolemia

PO (Antara)

Adults, Elderly. 130 mg/day.

PO (Lofibra)

Adults, Elderly. 200 mg/day with meals.

PO (Tricor)

Adults, Elderly. 145 mg/day.

PO (Triglide)

Adults, Elderly. 160 mg/day.

AVAILABLE FORMS

• *Capsules:* 43 mg (Antara), 67 mg (Lofibra), 87 mg (Antara), 130 mg (Antara), 134 mg (Lofibra), 200 mg (Lipidil Supra, Lofibra).

• *Tablets:* 48 mg (Tricor), 50 mg (Triglide), 145 mg (Tricor), 160 mg (Triglide).

CONTRAINDICATIONS: Gallbladder disease, severe renal or hepatic dysfunction (including primary biliary cirrhosis, unexplained persistent liver function abnormality)

PREGNANCY AND LACTATION: Pregnancy category C; embryocidal and teratogenic in rats; no adequate and well-controlled studies in pregnant women; tumorigenicity seen in animal studies; avoid breast-feeding

SIDE EFFECTS

Frequent (8%-4%)

Pain, rash, headache, asthenia or fatigue, flu symptoms, dyspepsia, nausea or vomiting, rhinitis

Occasional (3%-2%)

Diarrhea, abdominal pain, constipation, flatulence, arthralgia, decreased libido, dizziness, pruritus

Rare (less than 2%)

Increased appetite, insomnia, polyuria, cough, blurred vision, eye floaters, earache

SERIOUS REACTIONS

• Fenofibrate may increase excretion of cholesterol into bile, leading to cholelithiasis.

• Pancreatitis, hepatitis, thrombocytopenia, and agranulocytosis occur rarely.

INTERACTIONS

Drugs

3 *β-blockers:* Antagonistic effects; exacerbate hypertriglyceridemia

3 *Cyclosporine:* Increases risk of nephrotoxicity

3 *Estrogens:* Antagonistic effects; exacerbate hypertriglyderidemia

2 *HMG-CoA reductase inhibitors (statins):* Increased risk of markedly elevated creatine kinase (CK), rhabdomyolysis, myoglobinuria, acute renal failure

3 *Resins (bile acid sequestrants):* Decreased absorption if taken concomitantly; separate by 1 hr before or 4 hr after to avoid interaction

3 *Thiazide diuretics:* Antagonistic effects; exacerbate hypertriglyceridemia

3 *Warfarin:* Potentiation leading to prolonged PT/INR; all oral coumarin-type anticoagulants

Labs

• *Uric acid:* Decreased

SPECIAL CONSIDERATIONS

• Plasma concentrations of fenofibric acid after administration of 54-mg and 160-mg tablets are equivalent to 67- and 200-mg capsules

PATIENT/FAMILY EDUCATION

• Signs, symptoms, and resources for management of myositis

• Take with food

• Notify the physician if constipation, diarrhea, or nausea becomes severe

• Notify the physician if dizziness, insomnia, muscle pain, rash, or skin irritation occurs

MONITORING PARAMETERS

• Serum cholesterol, triglycerides, LDL-cholesterol, HDL-cholesterol, LFTs (serum transaminases), periodic CBC, serum CK

fenoldopam mesylate

(fhe-knowl'-doh-pam)

Rx: Corlopam

Chemical Class: Benzazepine derivative

Therapeutic Class: Vasodilator

CLINICAL PHARMACOLOGY

Mechanism of Action: A rapid-acting vasodilator. An agonist for D_1-like dopamine receptors; also produces vasodilation in coronary, renal, mesenteric, and peripheral arteries. ***Therapeutic Effect:*** Reduces systolic and diastolic BP and increases heart rate.

Pharmacokinetics

After IV administration, metabolized in the liver. Primarily excreted in urine. Unknown if removed by hemodialysis. ***Half-life:*** Approximately 5 min.

INDICATIONS AND DOSAGES

Short-term management of severe hypertension when rapid, but quickly reversible emergency reduction of BP is clinically indicated, including malignant hypertension with deteriorating end-organ function

IV Infusion (continuous)

Adults, Elderly. Initially, 0.1 mcg/kg/min. May increase in increments of 0.05-0.1 mcg/kg/min until target BP is achieved. Usual length of treatment is 1-6 hrs with tapering of dose q15-30min. Average rate: 0.25-0.5 mcg/kg/min. Maximum rate: 1.6 mcg/kg/min.

Children. Initially, 0.2 mcg/kg/min. May increase increments of 0.3-0.5 mcg/kg/min q20-30min. Dosage greater than 0.8 mcg/kg/min have resulted in tachycardia with no additional benefit.

AVAILABLE FORMS

- *Injection:* 10 mg/ml.

UNLABELED USES: Prevention of contrast media-induced nephrotoxicity

CONTRAINDICATIONS: Sensitivity to sulfites

PREGNANCY AND LACTATION: Pregnancy category B; animal studies show no evidence of impaired fertility or fetal harm; no human data available; excreted into breast milk of rats; human information unknown

SIDE EFFECTS

Expected

Beta blockers may cause unforeseen hypotension.

Occasional

Headache (7%), flushing (3%), nausea (4%), hypotension (2%)

Rare (2% or less)

Nervousness or anxiety, vomiting, constipation, nasal congestion, diaphoresis, back pain

SERIOUS REACTIONS

- Excessive hypotension occurs occasionally.
- Substantial tachycardia may lead to ischemic cardiac events or worsened heart failure.
- Allergic-type reactions, including anaphylaxis and life-threatening asthmatic exacerbation, may occur in patients with sulfite sensitivity.

INTERACTIONS

Drugs

3 *Acetaminophen:* May increase fenoldopam serum concentrations due to competition for sulfation (especially with oral fenoldopam)

3 *β-blockers:* May produce excessive hypotension

Labs

- Hypokalemia, increased blood urea nitrogen and serum creatinine, elevated liver transaminases, elevated LDH

F

SPECIAL CONSIDERATIONS

- *Preparation of infusion solution:* Contents of ampules must be diluted prior to infusion: 1 ml of 10 mg/ml solution in 250 ml 0.9% sodium chloride or 5% dextrose yields a final concentration of 40 mcg/ml
- *Potential advantage over sodium nitroprusside in hypertensive crisis:* Induction of naturesis, diuresis; ability to increase creatinine clearance, preserve renal function

PATIENT/FAMILY EDUCATION

- Change positions slowly to avoid orthostasis

MONITORING PARAMETERS

- Blood pressure, pulse, serum electrolytes, urine volume, urinary sodium, serum creatinine, blood urea nitrogen, electrocardiogram, hepatic function tests, infusion rate

---

fenoprofen calcium

(fen-oh-proe'-fen kal'-see-um)

Rx: Nalfon

Chemical Class: Propionic acid derivative

Therapeutic Class: NSAID; antipyretic; nonnarcotic analgesic

CLINICAL PHARMACOLOGY

Mechanism of Action: An NSAID that produces analgesic and antiinflammatory effects by inhibiting prostaglandin synthesis. ***Therapeutic Effect:*** Reduces the inflammatory response and intensity of pain.

Pharmacokinetics

Rapidly absorbed following PO administration. Protein binding: 99%. Metabolized in liver. Primarily excreted in urine; small amount excreted in feces. ***Half-life:*** 3 hr.

INDICATIONS AND DOSAGES

Mild to moderate pain

PO

Adults, Elderly. 200 mg q4-6h as needed.

Rheumatoid arthritis, osteoarthritis

PO

Adults, Elderly. 300-600 mg 3-4 times a day.

AVAILABLE FORMS

- *Capsules:* 200 mg, 300 mg.
- *Tablets:* 600 mg.

UNLABELED USES: Treatment of ankylosing spondylitis, psoriatic arthritis, vascular headaches

CONTRAINDICATIONS: Active peptic ulcer disease, chronic inflammation of GI tract, GI bleeding or ulceration, history of hypersensitivity to aspirin or NSAIDs, significant renal impairment

PREGNANCY AND LACTATION: Pregnancy category B (category D, third trimester); excreted in breast milk

SIDE EFFECTS

Frequent (9%-3%)

Headache, somnolence, dyspepsia, nausea, vomiting, constipation

Occasional (2%-1%)

Dizziness, pruritus, nervousness, asthenia, diarrhea, abdominal cramps, flatulence, tinnitus, blurred vision, peripheral edema and fluid retention

SERIOUS REACTIONS

- Overdose may result in acute hypotension and tachycardia.
- Rare reactions with long-term use include peptic ulcer disease, GI bleeding, gastritis, severe hepatic reaction (jaundice), nephrotoxicity (hematuria, dysuria, proteinuria), and a severe hypersensitivity reaction (bronchospasm, angioedema).

INTERACTIONS

Drugs

3 *Aminoglycosides:* Reduced clearance with elevated aminoglycoside levels and potential for toxicity (especially indomethacin in premature infants; other NSAIDs probably)

3 *Antihypertensives (α-blockers, angiotensin-converting enzyme inhibitors, angiotensin II receptor blockers, β-blockers, diuretics):* Inhibition of antihypertensive and other favorable hemodynamic effects

3 *Aspirin, other salicylates:* May increase the risk of GI side effects such as bleeding

3 *Bone marrow depressants:* May increase the risk of hematologic reactions

3 *Corticosteroids:* Increased risk of GI ulceration

3 *Anticoagulants:* Excessive hypoprothrombinemia, decreased platelet aggregation with increased risk of GI bleeding

3 *Cyclosporine:* Increased nephrotoxicity risk

3 *Lithium:* Decreased clearance of lithium (mediated via prostaglandins) resulting in elevated serum lithium levels and risk of toxicity

3 *Methotrexate:* Decreased renal secretion of methotrexate resulting in elevated methotrexate levels and risk of toxicity

3 *Phenylpropranolamine:* Possible acute hypertensive reaction

3 *Potassium-sparing diuretics:* Additive hyperkalemia potential

3 *Probenecid:* May increase fenoprofen blood concentration

3 *Triamterene:* Acute renal failure reported with addition of indomethacin; caution with other NSAIDs

Labs

- *False increase:* Free and total triiodothyronine levels, plasma cortisol
- *False positive:* Urine barbiturate, urine benzodiazepine

SPECIAL CONSIDERATIONS

- No significant advantage over other NSAIDs; cost should govern use

PATIENT/FAMILY EDUCATION

- Swallow fenoprofen capsules whole and do not chew or crush them
- Take with food or milk if GI upset occurs
- Avoid tasks that require mental alertness or motor skills until response to the drug has been established
- Avoid alcohol and aspirin during fenoprofen therapy because these substances increase the risk of GI bleeding

MONITORING PARAMETERS

- Initial hemogram and fecal occult blood test within 3 mo of starting regular chronic therapy; repeat every 6-12 mo (more frequently in high-risk patients [>65 years, peptic ulcer disease, concurrent steroids or anticoagulants]); electrolytes, creatinine, and BUN within 3 mo of starting regular chronic therapy; repeat every 6-12 mo
- Pattern of daily bowel activity and stool consistency
- Therapeutic response, such as improved grip strength, increased joint mobility, and decreased pain, stiffness, and swelling

fentanyl citrate

(fen'-ta-nill sit'-trate)

Rx: *Injection:* Sublimaze

Rx: *Transdermal:* Duragesic

Rx: *Lozenge:* Actiq

Combinations

Rx: with droperidol (Innovar)

Chemical Class: Opiate derivative; phenylpiperidine derivative

Therapeutic Class: Narcotic analgesic

DEA Class: Schedule II

CLINICAL PHARMACOLOGY

Mechanism of Action: An opioid agonist that binds to opioid receptors in the CNS, reducing stimuli from sensory nerve endings and inhibiting ascending pain pathways. ***Therapeutic Effect:*** Alters pain reception and increases the pain threshold.

Pharmacokinetics

Route	Onset	Peak	Duration
IV	1-2 min	3-5 min	0.5-1 hr
IM	7-15 min	20-30 min	1-2 hr
Transdermal	6-8 hr	24 hr	72 hr
Transmucosal	5-15 min	20-30 min	1-2 hr

Well absorbed after IM or topical administration. Transmucosal form absorbed through the buccal mucosa and GI tract. Protein binding: 80%-85%. Metabolized in the liver. Primarily eliminated by biliary system. ***Half-life:*** 2-4 hrs IV; 17 hr transdermal; 6.6 hrs transmucosal.

INDICATIONS AND DOSAGES

Sedation in minor procedures, analgesia

IV, IM

Adults, Elderly, Children 12 yr and older. 0.5-1 mcg/kg/dose; may repeat in 30-60 mins.

Children 1-11 yr. 1-2 mcg/kg/dose.

Children younger than 1 yr. 1-4 mcg/kg/dose.

Preoperative sedation, postoperative pain, adjunct to regional anesthesia

IV, IM

Adults, Elderly, Children 12 yrs and older. 50-100 mcg/dose.

Adjunct to general anesthesia

IV

Adults, Elderly, Children 12 yrs and older. 2-50 mcg/kg.

Usual transdermal dose

Adults, Elderly, Children 12 yrs and older. Initially, 25 mcg/hr. May increase after 3 days.

Usual transmucosal dose

Adults, Children. 200-400 mcg for breakthrough cancer pain.

Usual epidural dose

Adults, Elderly. Bolus dose of 100 mcg, followed by continuous infusion of 10 mcg/ml concentration at 4-12 ml/hr.

Continuous analgesia

IV

Adults, Elderly, Children 1-12 yr. Bolus dose of 1-2 mcg/kg, followed by continuous infusion of 1 mcg/kg/hr. Range: 1-5 mcg/kg/hr.

Children younger than 1 yr. Bolus dose of 1-2 mcg/kg, followed by continuous infusion of 0.5-1 mcg/kg/hr.

Dosage in renal impairment

Dosage is modified based on creatinine clearance.

Creatinine Clearance	Dosage
10-50 ml/min	75% of usual dose
less than 10 ml/min	50% of usual dose

AVAILABLE FORMS

- *Injection (Sublimaze):* 50 mcg/ml.
- *Transdermal Patch (Duragesic):* 12 mcg/hr, 25 mcg/hr, 50 mcg/hr, 75 mcg/hr, 100 mcg/hr.

• *Transmucosal Lozenges (Actiq):* 200 mcg, 400 mcg, 600 mcg, 800 mcg, 1200 mcg, 1600 mcg.

CONTRAINDICATIONS: Increased intracranial pressure, severe hepatic or renal impairment, severe respiratory depression

PREGNANCY AND LACTATION: Pregnancy category C (D if used for prolonged periods or at high dosages at term); excreted in breast milk. Controlled Substance: Schedule II

SIDE EFFECTS

Frequent

IV: Postoperative drowsiness, nausea, vomiting

Transdermal (10%-3%): Headache, pruritus, nausea, vomiting, diaphoresis, dyspnea, confusion, dizziness, somnolence, diarrhea, constipation, decreased appetite

Occasional

IV: Postoperative confusion, blurred vision, chills, orthostatic hypotension, constipation, difficulty urinating

Transdermal (3%-1%): Chest pain, arrhythmias, erythema, pruritus, swelling of skin, syncope, agitation, tingling or burning of skin

SERIOUS REACTIONS

• Overdose or too-rapid IV administration may produce severe respiratory depression and skeletal and thoracic muscle rigidity (which may lead to apnea), laryngospasm, bronchospasm, cold and clammy skin, cyanosis, and coma.

• The patient who uses fentanyl repeatedly may develop a tolerance to the drug's analgesic effect.

INTERACTIONS

Drugs

3 *Antihistamines, chloral hydrate, glutethimide, methocarbamol:* Enhanced depressant effects

3 *Barbiturates:* Additive respiratory and CNS-depressant effects

3 *Buprenorphine:* May decrease the effects of fentanyl

3 *Cimetidine:* Increased respiratory and CNS depression

3 *Diazepam:* Cardiovascular depression

3 *Ethanol:* Additive CNS effects

3 *Nitrous oxide:* Cardiovascular depression

Labs

• False elevations of serum amylase and lipase

SPECIAL CONSIDERATIONS

• Increased skin temperature increases absorption rate of transdermal preparation

• Lozenge should be used only in a monitored anesthesia care setting

• Following removal of transdermal system, 17 hr are required for 50% decrease in serum fentanyl concentrations

• Do not administer agonist/antagonist analgesics (i.e., pentazocine, nalbuphine, butorphanol, dezocine, buprenorphine) to patient who has received a prolonged course of fentanyl (a pure agonist). In opioid-dependent patients, mixed agonist/antagonist analgesics may precipitate withdrawal symptoms

PATIENT/FAMILY EDUCATION

• Use fentanyl as directed to avoid an overdosage; prolonged use of the drug may cause physical dependence

• Discontinue fentanyl slowly after long-term use

• Avoid alcohol during fentanyl therapy and consult the physician before taking any other drugs

• Avoid tasks requiring mental alertness or motor skills until response to the drug has been established

MONITORING PARAMETERS

• Blood pressure, heart rate, respiratory rate, and oxygen saturation

• Relief of pain

ferrous salts

(fer'-rous)
Rx: (ferrous fumarate)
Feostat, Femiron,
Ferro-Sequels, Nephro-Fer
Rx: (ferrous gluconate)
Fergon
Rx: (ferrous sulfate)
Fer-In-Sol, Fer-Iron, Slow-Fe
Chemical Class: Iron preparation
Therapeutic Class: Hematinic

CLINICAL PHARMACOLOGY
Mechanism of Action: An enzymatic mineral that is as an essential component in the formation of Hgb, myoglobin, and enzymes. Promotes effective erythropoiesis and transport and utilization of oxygen (O_2). ***Therapeutic Effect:*** Prevents iron deficiency.
Pharmacokinetics
Absorbed in the duodenum and upper jejunum. Ten percent absorbed in patients with normal iron stores; increased to 20%-30% in those with inadequate iron stores. Primarily bound to serum transferrin. Excreted in urine, sweat, and sloughing of intestinal mucosa and by menses. ***Half-life:*** 6 hr.

INDICATIONS AND DOSAGES
Iron deficiency anemia
PO (ferrous fumarate)
Adults, Elderly. 60-100 mg twice a day.
Children. 3-6 mg/kg/day in 2-3 divided doses.
PO (ferrous gluconate)
Adults, Elderly. 60 mg 2-4 times a day.
Children. 3-6 mg/kg/day in 2-3 divided doses.
PO (ferrous sulfate)
Adults, Elderly. 325 mg 2-4 times a day.
Children. 3-6 mg/kg/day in 2-3 divided doses.
Dosage is expressed in terms of milligrams of elemental iron, degree of anemia, patient weight, and presence of any bleeding. Expect to use periodic hematologic determinations as guide to therapy.
Prevention of iron deficiency
PO (ferrous fumarate)
Adults, Elderly. 60-100 mg/day.
Children. 1-2 mg/kg/day.
PO (ferrous gluconate)
Adults, Elderly. 60 mg/day.
Children. 1-2 mg/kg/day.
PO (ferrous sulfate)
Adults, Elderly. 325 mg/day.
Children. 1-2 mg/kg/day.

AVAILABLE FORMS
Ferrous fumarate
- *Tablets:* 63 mg (20 mg elemental iron) (Femiron), 350 mg (115 mg elemental iron) (Nephro-Fer).
- *Tablets (Chewable [Feostat]):* 100 mg (33 mg elemental iron).
- *Tablets (Time-Release [Ferro-Sequels]):* 150 mg (50 mg elemental iron).

Ferrous gluconate
- *Tablets:* 240 mg (27 mg elemental iron) (Fergon), 325 mg (36 mg elemental iron).

Ferrous sulfate
- *Tablets:* 325 mg (65 mg elemental iron).
- *Tablets (Timed-Release [Slow FE]):* 160 mg (50 mg elemental iron).
- *Elixir:* 220 mg/5 ml (44 mg elemental iron per 5 ml).
- *Oral Drops (Fer-In-Sol, Fer-Iron):* 75 mg/0.6 ml.

CONTRAINDICATIONS: Hemochromatosis, hemosiderosis, hemolytic anemias, peptic ulcer disease, regional enteritis, ulcerative colitis

PREGNANCY AND LACTATION: Pregnancy category A; excreted in breast milk

SIDE EFFECTS

Occasional

Mild, transient nausea

Rare

Heartburn, anorexia, constipation, diarrhea

SERIOUS REACTIONS

- Large doses may aggravate existing GI tract disease, such as peptic ulcer disease, regional enteritis, and ulcerative colitis.
- Severe iron poisoning occurs most often in children and is manifested as vomiting, severe abdominal pain, diarrhea, and dehydration, followed by hyperventilation, pallor or cyanosis, and cardiovascular collapse.

INTERACTIONS

Drugs

3 *Antacids:* Reduce iron absorption

3 *Ciprofloxacin, levodopa, levofloxacin, methyldopa, norfloxacin, penicillamine, tetracyclines, vitamin E:* Absorption reduced by iron

3 *Enalapril:* Three patients on enalapril developed systemic reactions following IV iron; causal relationship not established

Labs

- Urine discoloration black, brown, or dark color
- *Glucose:* Decreased with clinistix, diastix; no effect observed with testape
- *Occult blood:* 25%-65% false positives

SPECIAL CONSIDERATIONS

PATIENT/FAMILY EDUCATION

- Best absorbed on empty stomach, may take with food if GI upset occurs
- Drink liquid iron preparations in water or juice and through a straw to prevent tooth stains
- 4-6 mo of therapy generally required
- Iron changes stools black or dark green

MONITORING PARAMETERS

- Hemoglobin, hematocrit, reticulocyte count, ferritin and serum iron levels, and total iron-binding capacity
- Pattern of daily bowel activity and stool consistency
- Clinical improvement and record relief of iron deficiency symptoms (fatigue, headache, irritability, pallor, and paresthesia of extremities)

fexofenadine hydrochloride

(fex-oh-fen′-eh-deen hye-droe-klor′-ide)

Rx: Allegra

Combinations

Rx: with pseudoephedrine (Allegra-D)

Chemical Class: Piperidine derivative

Therapeutic Class: Antihistamine

CLINICAL PHARMACOLOGY

Mechanism of Action: An anti-infective that inhibits viral DNA synthesis by incorporating itself into the growing viral DNA chain. ***Therapeutic Effect:*** Suppresses replication of cytomegalovirus (CMV).

Pharmacokinetics

Protein binding: less than 6%. Excreted primarily unchanged in urine. Effect of hemodialysis unknown. ***Elimination half-life:*** 1.4-3.8 hr.

INDICATIONS AND DOSAGES

CMV retinitis in patients with AIDS (in combination with probenecid)

IV infusion

Adults. Induction: Usual dosage, 5 mg/kg at constant rate over 1 hr once

F

weekly for 2 consecutive wk. Give 2 g of PO probenecid 3 hr before cidofovir dose, and then give 1 g 2 hr and 8 hr after completion of the 1-hr cidofovir infusion (total of 4 g). In addition, give 1 L of 0.9% NaCl over 1-2 hr immediately before the cidofovir infusion. If tolerated, a second liter may be infused over 1-3 hr at the start of the infusion or immediately afterward. Maintenance: 5 mg/kg cidofovir at constant rate over 1 hr once every 2 wk.

Dosage in renal impairment

Changes during therapy. If creatinine increases by 0.3-0.4 mg/dl, reduce dose to 3 mg/kg; if creatinine increases by 0.5 mg/dl or greater or development of 3+ or greater proteinuria, discontinue therapy.

Preexisting renal impairment. Do not use with serum creatinine greater than 1.5 mg/dl, creatinine clearance less than 55 ml/min or urine protein 100 mg/dl or greater (2+ or greater proteinuria).

AVAILABLE FORMS

- *Injection:* 75 mg/ml (5-ml ampule).

UNLABELED USES: Treatment of acyclovir-resistant herpes simplex virus, adenovirus, foscarnet-resistant CMV, ganciclovir-resistant CMV, varicella-zoster virus

CONTRAINDICATIONS: Direct intraocular injection, history of clinically severe hypersensitivity to probenecid or other sulfa-containing drugs, renal function impairment (serum creatinine level greater than 1.5 mg/dl, creatinine clearance of 55 ml/min or less, or urine protein level greater than 100 mg/dl)

PREGNANCY AND LACTATION: Pregnancy category C; breast milk excretion unknown

SIDE EFFECTS

Frequent

Nausea, vomiting (65%), fever (57%), asthenia (46%), rash (30%), diarrhea (27%), headache (27%), alopecia (25%), chills (24%), anorexia (22%), dyspnea (22%), abdominal pain (17%)

SERIOUS REACTIONS

- Serious adverse reactions may include proteinuria (80%), nephrotoxicity (53%), neutropenia (31%), elevated serum creatinine levels (29%), infection (24%), anemia (20%), ocular hypotony (a decrease in intraocular pressure 12%), and pneumonia (9%).
- Concurrent use of probenecid may produce a hypersensitivity reaction characterized by a rash, fever, chills, and anaphylaxis.
- Acute renal failure occurs rarely.

INTERACTIONS

Drugs

3 *Antacids:* Decreased plasma fexofenadine concentrations; avoid taking aluminum and magnesium containing antacids with fexofenadine

3 *Erythromycin:* Increased plasma fexofenadine concentrations

3 *Ketoconazole:* Increased plasma fexofenadine concentrations

SPECIAL CONSIDERATIONS

- Essentially the same as terfenadine without the potential for QT prolongation; relatively weak antihistamine with minimal sedation
- Consider alternating q hs chlorpeniramine with qam fexofenadine 60 mg to minimize cost

PATIENT/FAMILY EDUCATION

- Avoid performing tasks that require mental alertness or motor skills until response to the drug has been established
- Drinking coffee or tea may help reduce drowsiness

• Avoid alcohol during antihistamine therapy

MONITORING PARAMETERS

• Assess for relief of allergy symptoms including rhinorrhea, sneezing, itching, and red, watery eyes

finasteride

(fin-as'-tur-ide)

Rx: Proscar, Propecia

Chemical Class: 5α-reductase inhibitor

Therapeutic Class: Antiandrogen; hair growth stimulant

CLINICAL PHARMACOLOGY

Mechanism of Action: An androgen hormone inhibitor that inhibits 5-alpha reductase, an intracellular enzyme that converts testosterone into dihydrotestosterone (DHT) in the prostate gland, resulting in a decreased serum DHT level. ***Therapeutic Effect:*** Reduces size of the prostate gland.

Pharmacokinetics

Route	*Onset*	*Peak*	*Duration*
PO	24 hr	1-2 days	5-7 days

Rapidly absorbed from the GI tract. Protein binding: 90%. Widely distributed. Metabolized in the liver. ***Half-life:*** 6-8 hr. Onset of clinical effect: 3-6 mo of continued therapy.

INDICATIONS AND DOSAGES

Benign prostatic hyperplasia (BPH)

PO

Adults, Elderly. 5 mg once a day (for a minimum of 6 mo).

Hair loss

PO

Adults. 1 mg/day.

AVAILABLE FORMS

• *Tablets:* 1 mg (Propecia), 5 mg (Proscar).

UNLABELED USES: Adjuvant monotherapy after radical prostatectomy in treatment of prostate cancer, female hirsutism

CONTRAINDICATIONS: Exposure to the patient's semen or handling of finasteride tablets by those who are or may be pregnant

PREGNANCY AND LACTATION: Pregnancy category X; not indicated for use in women; pregnant women should not handle crushed tablets

SIDE EFFECTS

Rare (4%-2%)

Gynecomastia, sexual dysfunction (impotence, decreased libido, decreased volume of ejaculate)

SERIOUS REACTIONS

• Hypersensitivity reactions, including rash, pruritus, urticaria, circumoral swelling, and testicular pain, have been reported.

SPECIAL CONSIDERATIONS

• Minimal benefit for benign prostatic hypertrophy if the prostate is not very large; response is not immediate

• Combination therapy with α-blocker may be optimal

• Whether long-term treatment can reduce prostate cancer risk is unknown; decreases prostate specific antigen (PSA)

PATIENT/FAMILY EDUCATION

• Condoms should be used if the female partner is at risk of pregnancy

• Women who are or may be pregnant should not handle finasteride tablets or be exposed to semen because of the potential risk to a fetus

• Withdrawal of drug for hair loss leads to reversal within 12 mo

• Finasteride may cause impotence and decrease ejaculate volume

• Take the drug for at least 6 mos

• It is unknown if taking this drug decreases the need for surgery

F

MONITORING PARAMETERS

- 6-12 mo of therapy may be necessary in some patients to assess effectiveness (BPH), 3 or more mo for hair loss
- Fluid intake and output

flavoxate

(fla-vox'-ate)

Rx: Urispas

Chemical Class: Flavone derivative

Therapeutic Class: Genitourinary muscle relaxant

CLINICAL PHARMACOLOGY

Mechanism of Action: An anticholinergic that relaxes detrusor and other smooth muscle by cholinergic blockade, counteracting muscle spasm in the urinary tract. ***Therapeutic Effect:*** Produces anticholinergic, local anesthetic, and analgesic effects, relieving urinary symptoms.

Pharmacokinetics

Unknown absorption, distribution, metabolism. Protein binding: 50%-80%. Excreted in urine. ***Half-life:*** 10-20 hr.

INDICATIONS AND DOSAGES

To relieve symptoms of cystitis, prostatitis, urethritis, urethrocystitis, or urethrotrigonitis

PO

Adults, Elderly, Adolescents. 100-200 mg 3-4 times a day.

AVAILABLE FORMS

- *Tablets:* 100 mg.

CONTRAINDICATIONS: Duodenal or pyloric obstruction, GI hemorrhage or obstruction, ileus, lower urinary tract obstruction

PREGNANCY AND LACTATION: Pregnancy category B; excretion into breast milk unknown; use caution in nursing mothers

SIDE EFFECTS

Frequent

Somnolence, dry mouth and throat

Occasional

Constipation, difficult urination, blurred vision, dizziness, headache, increased light sensitivity, nausea, vomiting, abdominal pain

Rare

Confusion (primarily in elderly), hypersensitivity, increased IOP, leukopenia

SERIOUS REACTIONS

- Overdose may produce anticholinergic effects, including unsteadiness, severe dizziness, somnolence, fever, facial flushing, dyspnea, nervousness, and irritability.

SPECIAL CONSIDERATIONS

- Urinary antispasmodic that is no more effective than propantheline or other similar agents

PATIENT/FAMILY EDUCATION

- Avoid performing tasks that require mental alertness or motor skills until response to the drug has been established
- Be aware of signs and symptoms of flavoxate overdose, including unsteadiness, severe dizziness, drowsiness, fever, flushed face, shortness of breath, nervousness, and irritability

MONITORING PARAMETERS

- Monitor for symptomatic relief
- Observe elderly patients for confusion

flecainide

(fle'-kah-nide)

Rx: Tambocor

Chemical Class: Benzamide derivative

Therapeutic Class: Antiarrhythmic, class IC

CLINICAL PHARMACOLOGY

Mechanism of Action: An antiarrhythmic that slows atrial, AV, His-Purkinje, and intraventricular conduction. Decreases excitability, conduction velocity, and automaticity. ***Therapeutic Effect:*** Controls atrial, supraventricular, and ventricular arrhythmias.

Pharmacokinetics

Almost completely absorbed following PO administration. Protein binding: 40%. Metabolized in liver. Excreted in urine. ***Half-life:*** 19-22 hr.

INDICATIONS AND DOSAGES

Life-threatening ventricular arrhythmias, sustained ventricular tachycardia

PO

Adults, Elderly. Initially, 100 mg q12h, increased by 100 mg (50 mg twice a day) every 4 days until effective dose or maximum of 400 mg/day is attained.

Paroxysmal supraventricular tachycardias (PSVT), paroxysmal atrial fibrillation (PAF)

PO

Adults, Elderly. Initially, 50 mg q12h, increased by 100 mg (50 mg twice a day) every 4 days until effective dose or maximum of 300 mg/day is attained.

AVAILABLE FORMS

- *Tablets:* 50 mg, 100 mg.

CONTRAINDICATIONS: Cardiogenic shock, preexisting second- or third-degree AV block, right bundle-branch block (without presence of a pacemaker)

PREGNANCY AND LACTATION: Pregnancy category C; excreted into breast milk with milk-plasma ratios 1.6:3.7, but considered compatible with breast-feeding

SIDE EFFECTS

Frequent (19%-10%)

Dizziness, dyspnea, headache

Occasional (9%-4%)

Nausea, fatigue, palpitations, chest pain, asthenia (loss of strength, energy), tremor, constipation

SERIOUS REACTIONS

- Flecainide may worsen existing arrhythmias or produce new ones.
- CHF may occur or existing CHF may worsen.
- Overdose may increase QRS duration, prolong QT interval, cause conduction disturbances, reduce myocardial contractility, and cause hypotension.

INTERACTIONS

Drugs

3 *Acetazolamide, ammonium chloride, antacids, sodium bicarbonate:* Increases in urine pH decreases flecainide urinary clearance

3 *Amiodarone:* Reduced flecainide dosage requirements

3 *Cimetidine:* Inhibits metabolism of flecainide

3 *Digoxin:* May increase blood concentration of digoxin

3 *Other antiarrhythmics:* May have additive effects

3 *Propranolol, other β-blockers:* Inhibitors of each other's metabolism; additive negative inotropic effects

3 *Sotalol:* Additive myocardial conduction depression; cardiac arrest reported

3 *Urinary acidifiers:* May increase the excretion of flecainide

3 *Urinary alkalinizers:* May decrease the excretion of flecainide

SPECIAL CONSIDERATIONS

- Not first-line therapy
- Reserve for resistant arrhythmias due to proarrhythmic effects
- Initiate therapy in facilities capable of providing continuous ECG monitoring and managing life-threatening dysrhythmias

PATIENT/FAMILY EDUCATION

- Side effects of flecainide therapy generally disappear with continued use or decreased dosage
- Do not abruptly discontinue the medication
- Do not use nasal decongestants or OTC cold preparations without physician approval
- Use caution when performing tasks that require mental alertness or motor skills
- Notify the physician if chest pain, faintness, or palpitations occurs

MONITORING PARAMETERS

- Monitor trough plasma levels periodically, especially in patients with moderate to severe chronic renal failure or severe hepatic disease and CHF; therapeutic range 0.2-1 mcg/ml
- Pulse for irregular rate and quality
- EKG for changes, particularly widening of the QRS complex or prolongation of the QT interval
- Evidence of CHF, including weight gain, pulmonary crackles, and dyspnea
- Intake and output; a decrease in urine output may indicate CHF

fluconazole

(floo-con′-a-zole)

Rx: Diflucan

Chemical Class: Triazole derivative

Therapeutic Class: Antifungal

CLINICAL PHARMACOLOGY

Mechanism of Action: A fungistatic antifungal that interferes with cytochrome P-450, an enzyme necessary for ergosterol formation. ***Therapeutic Effect:*** Directly damages fungal membrane, altering its function.

Pharmacokinetics

Well absorbed from GI tract. Widely distributed, including to CSF. Protein binding: 11%. Partially metabolized in liver. Excreted unchanged primarily in urine. Partially removed by hemodialysis. ***Half-life:*** 20-30 hr (increased in impaired renal function).

INDICATIONS AND DOSAGES

Oropharyngeal candidiasis

PO, IV

Adults, Elderly. 200 mg once, then 100 mg/day for at least 14 days.

Children. 6 mg/kg/day once, then 3 mg/kg/day.

Esophageal candidiasis

PO, IV

Adults, Elderly. 200 mg once, then 100 mg/day (up to 400 mg/day) for 21 days and at least 14 days following resolution of symptoms.

Children. 6 mg/kg/day once, then 3 mg/kg/day (up to 12 mg/kg/day) for 21 days and at least 14 days following resolution of symptoms.

Vaginal candidiasis

PO

Adults. 150 mg once.

Prevention of candidiasis in patients undergoing bone marrow transplantation

PO
Adults. 400 mg/day
Systemic candidiasis
PO, IV
Adults, Elderly. 400 mg once, then 200 mg/day (up to 400 mg/day) for at least 28 days and at least 14 days following resolution of symptoms.
Children. 6-12 mg/kg/day.
Urinary candidiasis
PO, IV
Adults, Elderly. 50-200 mg/day.
Cryptococcal meningitis
PO, IV
Adults, Elderly. 400 mg once, then 200 mg/day (up to 800 mg/day) for 10-12 wk after CSF becomes negative (200 mg/day for suppression of relapse in patients with AIDS).
Children. 12 mg/kg/day once, then 6-12 mg/kg/day (6 mg/kg/day for suppression of relapse in patients with AIDS).
Onychomycosis
PO
Adults. 150 mg/wk.
Dosage in renal impairment
After a loading dose of 400 mg, the daily dosage is based on creatinine clearance.

Creatinine Clearance	*% of Recommended Dose*
greater than 50 ml/min	100
21-50 ml/min	50
11-20 ml/min	25
Dialysis	Dose after dialysis

AVAILABLE FORMS
• *Tablets:* 50 mg, 100 mg, 150 mg, 200 mg.
• *Powder for Oral Suspension:* 10 mg/ml, 40 mg/ml.
• *Injection:* 2 mg/ml (in 100- or 200-ml containers).

UNLABELED USES: Treatment of coccidioidomycosis, cryptococcosis, fungal pneumonia, onychomycosis, ringworm of the hand, septicemia
CONTRAINDICATIONS: None known.
PREGNANCY AND LACTATION: Pregnancy category C; excreted into breast milk in concentrations similar to plasma; not recommended in nursing mothers

F

SIDE EFFECTS
Occasional (4%-1%)
Hypersensitivity reaction (including chills, fever, pruritus, and rash), dizziness, drowsiness, headache, constipation, diarrhea, nausea, vomiting, abdominal pain
SERIOUS REACTIONS
• Exfoliative skin disorders, serious hepatic effects, and blood dyscrasias (such as eosinophilia, thrombocytopenia, anemia, and leukopenia) have been reported rarely.
INTERACTIONS
Drugs
3 *Alprazolam:* Increased plasma alprazolam concentration
3 *Atevirdine:* Increased plasma atevirdine concentration
3 *Atorvastatin:* Increased plasma atorvastatin concentration with risk of rhabdomyolysis
3 *Buspirone:* Increased plasma buspirone concentration
3 *Caffeine:* Increased plasma caffeine concentration
3 *Chlordiazepoxide:* Increased plasma chlordiazepoxide concentration
2 *Cisapride:* QT prolongation and dysrhythmia
3 *Cyclosporine:* Increased plasma cyclosporine concentration
3 *Diazepam:* Increased plasma diazepam concentration
3 *Felodipine:* Increased plasma felodipine concentration

3 *Fluvastatin:* Increased plasma fluvastatin concentration with risk of rhabdomyolysis
3 *Losartan:* Reduced concentration of losartan's active metabolite may reduce efficacy of losartan
❷ *Lovastatin:* Increased plasma lovastatin concentration with risk of rhabdomyolysis
3 *Methadone:* Increased plasma methadone concentration
3 *Midazolam:* Increased plasma midazolam concentration
3 *Nateglinide:* Increases the serum concentration of nateglinide
❷ *Phenytoin:* Markedly reduced plasma fluconazole concentration
3 *Pravastatin:* Increased plasma pravastatin concentration with risk of rhabdomyolysis
3 *Quinidine:* Increased plasma quinidine concentration
3 *Rifabutin:* Increases rifabutin plasma concentrations; increased side effects including uveitis, rash, and liver or bone marrow toxicity may occur
3 *Rifampin:* Decreased plasma fluconazole concentration; decreased plasma rifampin concentration
❷ *Simvastatin:* Increased plasma simvastatin concentration with risk of rhabdomyolysis
3 *Tacrolimus:* Increased plasma tacrolimus concentration
❷ *Triazolam:* Increased plasma triazolam concentration
3 *Tolbutamide:* Increased plasma tolbutamide concentration
3 *Warfarin:* Increased hypoprothrombinemic response

Labs

• *Benzoylecgonine:* False negative urine results

SPECIAL CONSIDERATIONS

PATIENT/FAMILY EDUCATION

• Do not drive or use machinery until response to the drug is established
• Notify the physician if dark urine, pale stool, rash with or without itching, or yellow skin or eyes develops
• The patient with an oropharyngeal infection should maintain good oral hygiene
• Consult the physician before taking any other medications

MONITORING PARAMETERS

• Periodic liver function tests with prolonged therapy
• CBC, renal function, platelet count, serum potassium levels
• Signs and symptoms of a hypersensitivity reaction, including chills and fever
• Take temperature daily
• Daily pattern of bowel activity and stool consistency

flucytosine

(floo-sye'-toe-seen)

Rx: Ancobon

Chemical Class: Pyrimidine derivative, fluorinated

Therapeutic Class: Antifungal

CLINICAL PHARMACOLOGY

Mechanism of Action: An antifungal that penetrates fungal cells and is converted to fluorouracil, which competes with uracil interfering with fungal RNA and protein synthesis. ***Therapeutic Effect:*** Damages fungal membrane.

Pharmacokinetics

Well absorbed from gastrointestinal (GI) tract. Widely distributed, including cerebrospinal fluid (CSF). Protein binding: 2%-4%. Metabolized in liver. Partially removed by hemodialysis. ***Half-life:*** 3-8 hrs (half-life is increased with impaired renal function).

INDICATIONS AND DOSAGES

Fungal infections, candidiasis, cryptococcosis

PO

Adults, Elderly, Children. 50-150 mg/kg/day in 4 equally divided doses.

Dosage in renal function impairment

Based on creatinine clearance:

Creatinine Clearance	*Dosage Interval*
20-40 ml/min	q12h
10-20 ml/min	q24h
0-10 ml/min	q24-48h

AVAILABLE FORMS

• *Capsule:* 250 mg, 500 mg.

CONTRAINDICATIONS: Hypersensitivity to flucytosine.

PREGNANCY AND LACTATION: Pregnancy category C; 4% of drug metabolized to 5-fluorouracil, an antineoplastic suspected of producing congenital defects in humans; excretion into breast milk unknown; use caution in nursing mothers

SIDE EFFECTS

Occasional

Pruritus, rash, photosensitivity, dizziness, drowsiness, headache, diarrhea, nausea, vomiting, abdominal pain, increased liver enzymes, jaundice, increased BUN and creatinine, weakness, hearing loss

SERIOUS REACTIONS

• Hepatic dysfunction and severe bone marrow suppression occur rarely.

INTERACTIONS

Drugs

3 *Cytosine arabinoside:* Inactivates antifungal activity by competitive inhibition

3 *Drugs that impair glomerular filtration:* May prolong the half-life of flucytosine

Labs

• *False increase:* Serum creatinine (when Ektachem analyzer is used)

SPECIAL CONSIDERATIONS

• Rarely used as monotherapy; generally used in combination with amphotericin B

PATIENT/FAMILY EDUCATION

• Reduce or avoid GI upset by taking caps a few at a time over a 15-min period

• Continue therapy for the full length of treatment and space doses evenly around the clock

• Notify the physician if unexplained fever, sore throat, rash or hives, trouble breathing, yellow skin or eyes, persistent chest pain, or blood urine develops

MONITORING PARAMETERS

• Creatinine, BUN, alk phosphatase, AST, ALT, CBC

• Serum flucytosine concentrations (therapeutic range 25-100 mcg/ml)

• Be alert to bone marrow suppressive symptoms

fludrocortisone

(floo-droe-kor′-tis-sone)

Rx: Florinef Acetate

Chemical Class: Mineralocorticoid, synthetic

Therapeutic Class: Mineralocorticoid

CLINICAL PHARMACOLOGY

Mechanism of Action: A mineralocorticoid that acts at distal tubules. ***Therapeutic Effect:*** Increases potassium and hydrogen ion excretion. Replaces sodium loss and raises blood pressure (with low dosages). Inhibits endogenous adrenal cortical secretion, thymic activity, and secretion of corticotropin by pituitary gland (with higher dosages).

Pharmacokinetics
Well absorbed from the GI tract. Protein binding: 42%. Widely distributed. Metabolized in the liver and kidney. Primarily excreted in urine. ***Half-life:*** 3.5 hr.

INDICATIONS AND DOSAGES
Addison's disease
PO
Adults, Elderly. 0.05-0.1 mg/day. Range: 0.1 mg 3 times a wk to 0.2 mg/day. Administration with cortisone or hydrocortisone preferred.
Salt-losing adrenogenital syndrome
PO
Adults, Elderly. 0.1-0.2 mg/day.
Usual pediatric dosage
Children. 0.05-0.1 mg/day.

AVAILABLE FORMS
• *Tablets:* 0.1 mg.

UNLABELED USES: Treatment of acidosis in renal tubular disorders, idiopathic orthostatic hypotension

CONTRAINDICATIONS: CHF, systemic fungal infection

PREGNANCY AND LACTATION: Pregnancy category C; observe newborn for signs and symptoms of adrenocortical insufficiency; corticosteroids are found in breast milk; use caution in nursing mothers

SIDE EFFECTS
Frequent
Increased appetite, exaggerated sense of well-being, abdominal distention, weight gain, insomnia, mood swings
High dosages, prolonged therapy, too-rapid withdrawal: Increased susceptibility to infection with masked signs and symptoms, delayed wound healing, hypokalemia, hypocalcemia, GI distress, diarrhea or constipation, hypertension
Occasional
Headache, dizziness, menstrual difficulty or amenorrhea, gastric ulcer development
Rare
Hypersensitivity reaction

SERIOUS REACTIONS
• Long-term therapy may cause muscle wasting (especially in the arms and legs), osteoporosis, spontaneous fractures, amenorrhea, cataracts, glaucoma, peptic ulcer disease, and CHF.
• Abruptly withdrawing the drug after long-term therapy may cause anorexia, nausea, fever, headache, joint pain, rebound inflammation, fatigue, weakness, lethargy, dizziness, and orthostatic hypotension.

INTERACTIONS
Drugs
3 *Amphotericin:* Excessive potassium depletion
3 *Diuretics, loop:* Opposite therapeutic effect; excessive potassium loss
3 *Diuretics, thiazide:* Opposite therapeutic effect; excessive potassium loss
3 *Digitalis:* Increased potential for digitalis toxicity associated with hypokalemia
3 *Hepatic enzyme inducers (e.g., phenytoin):* May increase the metabolism of fludrocortisones
3 *Hypokalemia-causing medications:* May increase the effects of fludrocortisones
3 *Sodium-containing medications:* May increase blood pressure, incidence of edema, and serum sodium level

SPECIAL CONSIDERATIONS

PATIENT/FAMILY EDUCATION
• Notify clinician of dizziness, severe headache, swelling of feet or lower legs, unusual weight gain
• Do not discontinue abruptly
• Maintain careful personal hygiene and avoid exposure to disease or trauma

• Severe stress, such as serious infection, surgery, or trauma may require an increase in the fludrocortisone dosage
• Steroids often cause mood swings, ranging from euphoria to depression

MONITORING PARAMETERS

• Serum electrolytes, blood pressure, serum renin
• Taper dosage slowly if fludrocortisones is to be discontinued

flumazenil

(floo-may'-zuh-nil)

Rx: Romazicon

Chemical Class: Imidazobenzodiazepine derivative

Therapeutic Class: Benzodiazepine antagonist

CLINICAL PHARMACOLOGY

Mechanism of Action: An antidote that antagonizes the effect of benzodiazepines on the gamma-aminobutyric acid receptor complex in the CNS. ***Therapeutic Effect:*** Reverses sedative effect of benzodiazepines.

Pharmacokinetics

Route	Onset	Peak	Duration
IV	1-2 min	6-10 min	less than 1 hr

Duration and degree of benzodiazepine reversal depend on dosage and plasma concentration. Protein binding: 50%. Metabolized by the liver; excreted in urine.

INDICATIONS AND DOSAGES

Reversal of conscious sedation or general anesthesia

IV

Adults, Elderly. Initially, 0.2 mg (2 ml) over 15 sec; may repeat dose in 45 sec; then at 60-sec intervals. Maximum: 1 mg (10-ml) total dose.

Children, Neonates. Initially, 0.01 mg/kg; may repeat in 45 sec, then at 60-sec intervals. Maximum: 0.2 mg single dose; 0.05 mg/kg or 1 mg cumulative dose.

Benzodiazepine overdose

IV

Adults, Elderly. Initially, 0.2 mg (2 ml) over 30 sec; if desired level of consciousness (LOC) is not achieved after 30 sec, 0.3 mg (3 ml) may be given over 30 sec. Further doses of 0.5 mg (5 ml) may be administered over 30 sec at 60-sec intervals. Maximum: 3 mg (30 ml) total dose.

Children, Neonates. Initially, 0.01 mg/kg; may repeat in 45 sec, then at 60-sec intervals. Maximum: 0.2 mg single dose; 1 mg cumulative dose.

AVAILABLE FORMS

• *Injection:* 0.1 mg/ml.

CONTRAINDICATIONS: Anticholinergic signs (such as mydriasis, dry mucosa, and hypoperistalsis), arrhythmias, cardiovascular collapse, history of hypersensitivity to benzodiazepines, patients with signs of serious cyclic antidepressant overdose (such as motor abnormalities), patients who have been given a benzodiazepine for control of a potentially life-threatening condition (such as control of status epilepticus or increased intracranial pressure [ICP])

PREGNANCY AND LACTATION: Pregnancy category C; excretion into breast milk unknown; use caution in nursing mothers

SIDE EFFECTS

Frequent (11%-4%)

Agitation, anxiety, dry mouth, dyspnea, insomnia, palpitations, tremors, headache, blurred vision, dizziness, ataxia, nausea, vomiting, pain at injection site, diaphoresis

Occasional (3%-1%)
Fatigue, flushing, auditory disturbances, thrombophlebitis, rash
Rare (less than 1%)
Urticaria, pruritus, hallucinations

SERIOUS REACTIONS

- Toxic effects, such as seizures and arrhythmias, of other drugs taken in overdose, especially tricyclic antidepressants, may emerge with reversal of sedative effect of benzodiazepines.
- Flumazenil may provoke a panic attack in those with a history of panic disorder.

INTERACTIONS

Drugs

3 *Tricyclic antidepressants:* May produce seizures and arrhythmias as flumazenil reverses the sedative effects of tricyclic antidepressants

SPECIAL CONSIDERATIONS

PATIENT/FAMILY EDUCATION

- Resedation may occur; do not engage in any activities requiring complete alertness or operate hazardous machinery or a motor vehicle until at least 18-24 hr after discharge
- Do not use any alcohol or non-prescription drugs for 18-24 hr after flumazenil administration

MONITORING PARAMETERS

- Monitor for seizures, sedation, respiratory depression, or other residual benzodiazepine effects for an appropriate period (up to 120 min) based on dose and duration of effect of the benzodiazepine employed; pharmacokinetics of benzodiazepines are not altered in the presence of flumazenil
- Heart rate and rhythm and blood pressure
- Monitor and maintain a patent airway and prepare to assist with ventilation if flumazenil does not fully reverse the respiratory depressant effects of the benzodiazepine
- Closely monitor for return of unconsciousness or narcosis for at least 1 hr after he or she is fully alert

flunisolide

(floo-niss'-oh-lide)

Rx: AeroBid, AeroBid-M, Nasalide, Nasarel

Chemical Class: Glucocorticoid, synthetic

Therapeutic Class: Antiasthmatic; corticosteroid, antiinflammatory; corticosteroid, nasal

CLINICAL PHARMACOLOGY

Mechanism of Action: An adrenocorticosteroid that controls the rate of protein synthesis, depresses migration of polymorphonuclear leukocytes, reverses capillary permeability, and stabilizes lysosomal membranes. ***Therapeutic Effect:*** Prevents or controls inflammation.

Pharmacokinetics

Rapidly absorbed from lungs and GI tract following inhalation. About 50% of dose is absorbed from the nasal mucosa following intranasal administration. Metabolized in liver. Partially excreted in urine and feces. ***Half-life:*** 1-2 hr.

INDICATIONS AND DOSAGES

Long-term control of bronchial asthma, assists in reducing or discontinuing oral corticosteroid therapy

Inhalation

Adults, Elderly. 2 inhalations twice a day, morning and evening. Maximum: 4 inhalations twice a day.

Children 6-15 yr. 2 inhalations twice a day.

Relief of symptoms of perennial and seasonal rhinitis

Intranasal

Adults, Elderly. Initially, 2 sprays each nostril twice a day, may increase at 4-7-day intervals to 2 sprays 3 times a day. Maximum: 8 sprays in each nostril daily.

Children 6-14 yr. Initially, 1 spray 3 times a day or 2 sprays twice a day. Maximum: 4 sprays in each nostril daily. Maintenance: 1 spray into each nostril each day.

AVAILABLE FORMS

- *Aerosol with Adapter (AeroBid):* 250 mcg/activation.
- *Aerosol (AeroBid-M):* 250 mcg/activation.
- *Nasal Spray (Nasalide, Nasarel):* 25 mcg/activation.

UNLABELED USES: To prevent recurrence of nasal polyps after surgery

CONTRAINDICATIONS: Hypersensitivity to any corticosteroid, persistently positive sputum cultures for *Candida albicans,* primary treatment of status asthmaticus, systemic fungal infections

PREGNANCY AND LACTATION: Pregnancy category C; excretion into breast milk unknown; use caution in nursing mothers

SIDE EFFECTS

Frequent

Inhalation (25%-10%): Unpleasant taste, nausea, vomiting, sore throat, diarrhea, upset stomach, cold symptoms, nasal congestion

Occasional

Inhalation (9%-3%): Dizziness, irritability, nervousness, tremors, abdominal pain, heartburn, oropharynx candidiasis, edema

Nasal: Mild nasopharyngeal irritation or dryness, rebound congestion, bronchial asthma, rhinorrhea, altered taste

SPECIAL CONSIDERATIONS

PATIENT/FAMILY EDUCATION

- To be used on a regular basis, not for acute symptoms
- Use bronchodilators before oral inhaler (for patients using both)
- Nasal sol may cause drying and irritation of nasal mucosa
- Clear nasal passages prior to use of nasal sol
- Maintain fastidious oral hygiene; rinse mouth with water immediately after inhalation to prevent mouth and throat dryness and a fungal infection
- Drink plenty of fluids to decrease the thickness of lung secretions
- Notify the physician if nasal irritation occurs or if symptoms, such as sneezing, fail to improve

MONITORING PARAMETERS

- Monitor children for growth as well as for effects on the HPA axis during chronic therapy
- Monitor patients switched from chronic systemic corticosteroids to avoid acute adrenal insufficiency in response to stress
- Pulse rate and quality and respiratory rate, depth, rhythm, and type
- ABG levels
- Breath sounds for rales, rhonchi, and wheezing

fluocinolone acetonide

(floo-oh-sin'-oh-lone a-seat'-oh-nide)

Rx: Capex, Derma-Smoothe/FS, FS Shampoo, Synalar

Combinations

Rx: with hydroquinone/tretinoin (Tri-Luma)

Chemical Class: Corticosteroid, synthetic

Therapeutic Class: Corticosteroid, topical

CLINICAL PHARMACOLOGY

Mechanism of Action: A fluorinated topical corticosteroid that controls the rate of protein synthesis; depresses migration of polymorphonuclear leukocytes and fibroblasts; reduces capillary permeability; prevents or controls inflammation. ***Therapeutic Effect:*** Decreases tissue response to inflammatory process.

Pharmacokinetics

Use of occlusive dressings may increase percutaneous absorption. Protein binding: more than 90%. Excreted in urine. ***Half-life:*** Unknown.

INDICATIONS AND DOSAGES

Atopic dermatitis

Topical

Adults, Elderly. Apply 3 times/day.

Children 2 yrs and older. Apply 2 times/day.

Scalp psoriasis

Topical

Adults, Elderly. Apply to damp or wet hair and leave on overnight or for at least 4 hrs. Remove by washing hair with shampoo.

Seborrheic dermatitis, scalp

Shampoo

Adults, Elderly. Apply once daily allowing to remain on scalp for at least 5 min.

AVAILABLE FORMS

- *Cream:* 0.01%, 0.025% (Synalar).
- *Oil:* 0.01% (Derma-Smoothe/FS).
- *Ointment:* 0.025% (Synalar).
- *Shampoo:* 0.01% (Capex).
- *Solution:* 0.01% (Synalar).

UNLABELED USES: Vitiligo

CONTRAINDICATIONS: Hypersensitivity to fluocinolone or other corticosteroids

PREGNANCY AND LACTATION: Pregnancy category C; unknown whether topical application could result in sufficient systemic absorption to produce detectable amounts in breast milk (systemic corticosteroids are secreted into breast milk in quantities not likely to have detrimental effects on infant)

SIDE EFFECTS

Occasional

Burning, dryness, itching, stinging

Rare

Allergic contact dermatitis, purpura or blood-containing blisters, thinning of skin with easy bruising, telangiectasis or raised dark red spots on skin

SERIOUS REACTIONS

- When taken in excessive quantities, systemic hypercorticism and adrenal suppression may occur.

SPECIAL CONSIDERATIONS

- Topical oil contains refined peanut oil

PATIENT/FAMILY EDUCATION

- Apply sparingly only to affected area
- Avoid contact with eyes
- Do not put bandages or dressings over treated area unless directed by clinician
- Do not use on weeping, denuded, or infected areas

• Discontinue drug, notify clinician if local irritation or fever develops

MONITORING PARAMETERS

• Assess for improvement of skin conditions, relief of pruritus, and healing of lesions

fluocinonide

(floo-oh-sin′-oh-nide)

Rx: Lidex, Lidex-E

Chemical Class: Corticosteroid, synthetic

Therapeutic Class: Corticosteroid, topical

CLINICAL PHARMACOLOGY

Mechanism of Action: A topical corticosteroid that has anti-inflammatory, antipruritic, and vasoconstrictive properties. The exact mechanism of the antiinflammatory process is unclear. ***Therapeutic Effect:*** Reduces or prevents tissue response to the inflammatory process.

Pharmacokinetics

Well absorbed systemically. Large variation in absorption among sites. Protein binding: varies. Metabolized in liver. Primarily excreted in urine.

INDICATIONS AND DOSAGES

Dermatoses

Topical

Adults, Elderly. Apply sparingly 2-4 times/day.

AVAILABLE FORMS

• *Cream (Anhydrous Emollient):* 0.05% (Lidex).

• *Cream (Aqueous Emollient):* 0.05% (Lidex-E).

• *Gel:* 0.05% (Lidex).

• *Ointment:* 0.05% (Lidex).

• *Solution:* 0.05% (Lidex).

CONTRAINDICATIONS: History of hypersensitivity to fluocinonide or other corticosteroids

PREGNANCY AND LACTATION: Pregnancy category C; unknown whether topical application could result in sufficient systemic absorption to produce detectable amounts in breast milk (systemic corticosteroids are secreted into breast milk in quantities not likely to have detrimental effects on infant)

SIDE EFFECTS

Occasional

Itching, redness, irritation, burning at site of application, dryness, folliculitis, acneiform eruptions, hypopigmentation

Rare

Allergic contact dermatitis, maceration of the skin, secondary infection, skin atrophy

SERIOUS REACTIONS

• The serious reactions of long-term therapy and the addition of occlusive dressings are reversible hypothalamic-pituitary-adrenal (HPA) axis suppression, manifestations of Cushing's syndrome, hyperglycemia, and glucosuria.

SPECIAL CONSIDERATIONS

PATIENT/FAMILY EDUCATION

• Apply sparingly only to affected area

• Avoid contact with eyes

• Do not put bandages or dressings over treated area unless directed by clinician

• Do not use on weeping, denuded, or infected areas

• Discontinue drug, notify clinician if local irritation or fever develops

• Avoid exposure to sunlight

MONITORING PARAMETERS

• Skin for rash or irritation

F

fluorescein

(flure'-e-seen)

Rx: AK-Fluor, Angioscein, Fluorescite, Fluorets, Fluor-I-Strip, Fluor-I-Strip-A.T., Ful-Glo, Ocu-Flur 10

Combinations

Rx: with proparacaine (Fluoracaine)

Chemical Class: Xanthine dye

Therapeutic Class: Ophthalmic diagnostic agent

CLINICAL PHARMACOLOGY

Mechanism of Action: An indicator dye used as a diagnostic agent with a low molecular weight, high water solubility, and fluorescence that penetrates any break in epithelial barrier to permit rapid penetration. Emits light at a wavelength of 520-530 nanometers (green-yellow) when exposed to light in the blue wavelength (465-490 nanometers). ***Therapeutic Effect:*** Diagnosis of corneal and conjunctival abnormalities.

Pharmacokinetics

Rapidly absorbed. Protein binding: 85%. Widely distributed. Metabolized in liver to an active metabolite, fluorescein monoglucuronide. Primarily excreted in urine. ***Half-life:*** 24 min (parent compound), 4 hrs (metabolite).

INDICATIONS AND DOSAGES

Retinal angiography

Injection

Adults, Elderly. Inject contents of ampule or vial of 10% or 25% solution rapidly into the antecubital vein.

Applanation tonometry

Ophthlalmic strips

Adults, Elderly. Place strip, which has been moistened with a drop of sterile water, at the fornix in the lower cul-de-sac close to the punctum. Patient should close lid tightly over strip until desired amount of staining is observed or retract upper lid and touch tip of strip to the bulbar conjunctiva on the temporal side until adequate staining is achieved.

AVAILABLE FORMS

- *Injection, solution:* 10% (AK-Fluor, Angiscein, Fluorescite), 25% (AK-Fluor, Fluorescite).
- *Strip, ophthalmic:* 0.6 mg (Ful-Glo), 1 mg (Fluorets, Fluor-I-Strip-AT), 9 mg (Fluor-I-Strip).

CONTRAINDICATIONS: Concomitant soft contact lens use (ophthalmic strips), hypersensitivity to fluorescein or any component of the formulation

PREGNANCY AND LACTATION: Pregnancy category X; avoid parenteral use, especially in first trimester; excreted into breast milk; use caution in nursing mothers

SIDE EFFECTS

Occasional

Ophthalmic: Burning sensation in the eye

Injection: Stinging, bronchospasm, generalized hives and itching, hypersensitivity, headache gastrointestinal distress, nausea, strong taste, vomiting, hypotension, syncope

Rare

Injection: anaphylaxis, basilar artery ischemia, cardiac arrest, severe shock, convulsions, thrombophlebitis at injection site

SERIOUS REACTIONS

- Anaphylactic reactions have occurred leading to laryngeal edema, bronchospasm, shock, and even death.

SPECIAL CONSIDERATIONS

PATIENT/FAMILY EDUCATION

- May cause temporary yellowish discoloration of skin (fades in 6-12 hr)

• Urine will appear bright yellow (fades in 24-36 hr)
• Soft contact lenses may become stained, wait at least 1 hr after thorough rinsing of eye before replacing lenses
• Take extra caution when driving or operating machinery after this medication has been used

MONITORING PARAMETERS

• Luminescence appears in the retina and choroidal vessels 9-15 min following IV inj; can be observed by standard viewing equipment

fluoxetine hydrochloride

(floo-ox'-e-teen hye-droe-klor'-ide)

Rx: Prozac, Prozac Weekly, Sarafem

Combinations

Rx: with olanzapine (Symbyax)

Chemical Class: Aryloxypropylamine

Therapeutic Class: Antidepressant, selective serotonin reuptake inhibitor (SSRI)

CLINICAL PHARMACOLOGY

Mechanism of Action: A psychotherapeutic agent that selectively inhibits serotonin uptake in the CNS, enhancing serotonergic function. ***Therapeutic Effect:*** Relieves depression; reduces obsessive-compulsive and bulimic behavior.

Pharmacokinetics

Well absorbed from the GI tract. Crosses the blood-brain barrier. Protein binding: 94%. Metabolized in the liver to active metabolite. Primarily excreted in urine. Not removed by hemodialysis. ***Half-life:*** 2-3 days; metabolite 7-9 days.

INDICATIONS AND DOSAGES

Depression

PO

Adults. Initially, 20 mg each morning. If therapeutic improvement does not occur after 2 wk, gradually increase to maximum of 80 mg/day in 2 equally divided doses in morning and at noon. Prozac Weekly: 90 mg/wk, begin 7 days after last dose of 20 mg.

Elderly. Initially, 10 mg/day. May increase by 10-20 mg q2wk.

Children 7-17 yr. Initially, 5-10 mg/day. Titrate upward as needed. Usual dosage is 20 mg/day.

Panic disorder

PO

Adults, Elderly. Initially, 10 mg/day. May increase to 20 mg/day after 1 week. Maximum: 60 mg/day.

Bulimia nervosa

PO

Adults. 60 mg each morning.

Obsessive-compulsive disorder (OCD)

PO

Adults, Elderly. 40-80 mg/day.

Children 7-18 yr. Initially, 10 mg/day. May increase to 20 mg/day after 2 wk. Range: 10-80 mg/day.

Premenstrual dysphoric disorder

PO

Adults. 20 mg/day.

AVAILABLE FORMS

• *Capsules:* 10 mg (Prozac, Sarafem), 20 mg (Prozac, Sarafem), 40 mg (Prozac).
• *Capsules (Delayed-Release [Prozac Weekly]):* 90 mg.
• *Oral Solution (Prozac):* 20 mg/5 ml.
• *Tablets (Prozac, Rapiflux):* 10 mg, 20 mg.

UNLABELED USES: Treatment of body dysmorphic disorder, fibromyalgia, hot flashes, post-traumatic stress disorder, Raynaud's phenomena

F

CONTRAINDICATIONS: Use within 14 days of MAOIs

PREGNANCY AND LACTATION: Pregnancy category C; excreted into breast milk; use caution in nursing mothers

SIDE EFFECTS

Frequent (more than 10%)

Headache, asthenia, insomnia, anxiety, nervousness, somnolence, nausea, diarrhea, decreased appetite

Occasional (9%-2%)

Dizziness, tremor, fatigue, vomiting, constipation, dry mouth, abdominal pain, nasal congestion, diaphoresis, rash

Rare (less than 2%)

Flushed skin, lightheadedness, impaired concentration

SERIOUS REACTIONS

• Overdose may produce seizures, nausea, vomiting, agitation, and restlessness.

INTERACTIONS

Drugs

3 *Alcohol:* May increase CNS depression

3 *Benzodiazepines (alprazolam, diazepam):* Probable inhibition of metabolism (CYP3A4) leading to accumulation of diazepam and alprazolam

3 *β-blockers (metroprolol, propranolol, sotalol):* Inhibition of metabolism (CYP2D6) leads to increased plasma concentrations of selective β-blockers and potential cardiac toxicity; atenolol may be safer choice

3 *Buspirone:* Reduced therapeutic effect of both drugs; possible seizures

3 *Carbamazepine:* Inhibition of hepatic metabolism of carbamazepine, but the formation of carbamazepine epoxide is not inhibited, contributing to increased toxicity

3 *Clozapine:* Increased serum clozapine concentrations

3 *Cyproheptadine:* Serotonin antagonist may partially reverse antidepressant and other effects

3 *Dextromethorphan:* Inhibition of dextromethorphan's metabolism (CYP2D6) by fluoxetine and additive serotonergic effects

3 *Diuretics, loop (bumetanide, furosemide, torsemide):* Possible additive hyponatremia; 2 fatal case reports with furosemide and fluoxetine

❷ *Fenfluramine:* Duplicate effects on inhibition of serotonin reuptake; inhibition of dexfenfluramine metabolism (CYP2D6) exaggerates effect; both mechanisms increase risk of serotonin syndrome

3 *Haloperidol:* Inhibition of haloperidol's metabolism (CYP2D6) may increase risks of extrapyramidal symptoms

❷ *HMG-CoA reductase inhibitors (atorvastatin, lovastatin, simvastatin):* Inhibition of statin metabolism (CYP3A4), by fluoxetine, may lead to rhabdomyolysis

3 *Lithium:* Neurotoxicity (tremor, confusion, ataxia, dizziness, dysarthria, and absence seizures) reported in patients receiving this combination; mechanism unknown

▲ *MAOIs (isocarboxazid, phenelzine, tranylcypromine):* Increased CNS serotonergic effect has been associated with severe or fatal reactions with this combination

3 *Nefazodone:* Increased risk of developing serotonin syndrome

3 *Phenytoin:* Inhibition of metabolism and phenytoin toxicity

3 *Propafenone:* Increases the plasma concentration of propafenone; increased effect on myocardial conduction may occur, including the induction of arrhythmias

3 *Selegiline:* Sporadic cases of mania and hypertension

3 *Sibutramine:* Increased risk of developing serotonin syndrome
3 *St. John's Wort:* May increase fluoxetine's pharmacologic effects and risk of toxicity
⚠ *Thioridazine:* Increased serum thioridazine concentrations resulting in an increased risk of QTc interval prolongation, serious ventricular arrhythmias, and death
3 *Tricyclic antidepressants (clomipramine, desipramine, doxepin, imipramine, nortriptylline, trazodone):* Marked increases in tricyclic antidepressant levels due to inhibition of metabolism (CYP2D6)
❷ *Tryptophan:* Additive serotonergic effects
3 *Warfarin:* Altered anticoagulant effects, including increased bleeding

SPECIAL CONSIDERATIONS

PATIENT/FAMILY EDUCATION

- Therapeutic response may take 4-6 wk
- May cause insomnia, administer in a.m.; sedating antidepressants, in small doses (i.e., trazadone 50 mg), frequently administered hs, concurrently
- Avoid tasks that require mental alertness or motor skills until response to the drug has been established
- Avoid alcohol

MONITORING PARAMETERS

- Closely supervise suicidal patients during early therapy; as depression lessens, the patient's energy level improves, increasing the suicide potential
- Assess the patient's appearance, behavior, level of interest, mood, and sleep pattern before and during therapy
- Pattern of daily bowel activity and stool consistency
- Skin for rash
- Blood glucose level and serum alkaline phosphatase, bilirubin, sodium, AST (SGOT) and ALT (SGPT) levels

---

fluoxymesterone

(floo-ox-i-mes'-te-rone)
Rx: Halotestin
Chemical Class: Testosterone derivative
Therapeutic Class: Androgen; antineoplastic
DEA Class: Schedule III

CLINICAL PHARMACOLOGY

Mechanism of Action: An androgen that suppresses gonadotropin-releasing hormone, LH, and FSH. ***Therapeutic Effect:*** Stimulates spermatogenesis, development of male secondary sex characteristics, and sexual maturation at puberty. Stimulates production of red blood cells (RBCs).

Pharmacokinetics

Rapidly absorbed from the gastrointestinal (GI) tract. Protein binding: 98%. Metabolized in liver. Excreted in urine. ***Half-life:*** 9.2 hrs.

INDICATIONS AND DOSAGES

Males (hypogonadism)

PO

Adults. 5-20 mg/day.

Males (delayed puberty)

PO

Adults. 2.5-20 mg/day for 4-6 mos.

Females (inoperable breast cancer)

PO

Adults. 10-40 mg/day in divided doses for 1-3 mos.

Females (prevent postpartum breast pain/engorgement)

PO

Adults. Initially, 2.5 mg shortly after delivery, then 5-10 mg/day in divided doses for 4-5 days.

AVAILABLE FORMS

• *Tablets:* 2 mg, 5 mg, 10 mg (Halotestin).

CONTRAINDICATIONS: Serious cardiac, renal, or hepatic dysfunction, men with carcinomas of the breast or prostate, hypersensitivity to fluoxymesterone or any component of the formulation including tartrazine

PREGNANCY AND LACTATION: Pregnancy category X; causes virilization of external genitalia of female fetus; excretion into breast milk unknown; use extreme caution in nursing mothers

Controlled Substance: Schedule III

SIDE EFFECTS

Frequent

Females: Amenorrhea, virilism (e.g., acne, decreased breast size, enlarged clitoris, male pattern baldness), deepening voice

Males: UTI, breast soreness, gynecomastia, priapism, virilism (e.g., acne, early pubic hair growth)

Occasional

Edema, nausea, vomiting, mild acne, diarrhea, stomach pain

Males: Impotence, testicular atrophy

SERIOUS REACTIONS

• Peliosis hepatitis (liver, spleen replaced with blood-filled cysts), hepatic neoplasms, and hepatocellular carcinoma have been associated with prolonged high dosage.

INTERACTIONS

Drugs

❷ *Cyclosporine, tacrolimus:* Increased cyclosporine and tacrolimus levels with potential toxicity

❷ *Oral anticoagulants:* Enhanced hypoprothrombinemic response to oral anticoagulants

3 *Oxyphenbutazone:* May result in elevated serum levels of oxyphenbutazone

SPECIAL CONSIDERATIONS

PATIENT/FAMILY EDUCATION

• Weigh oneself each day and report to physician weight gains of 5 lbs or more per week

• Notify the physician of acne, nausea, pedal edema, or vomiting

• The female patient should report deepening of voice, hoarseness, and menstrual irregularities

• The male patient should report difficulty urinating, frequent erections, and gynecomastia

MONITORING PARAMETERS

• Frequent urine and serum calcium determinations (breast cancer)

• Periodic LFTs, Hct, Hgb

• X-ray examinations of bone age q6mo during treatment of prepubertal males

• Electrolytes, cholesterol

• Signs of virilization, such as deepening of voice

• Sleep patterns

fluphenazine hydrochloride

(floo-fen′-a-zeen hye-droe-klor′-ide)

Rx: Permitil, Prolixin

Chemical Class: Piperazine phenothiazine derivative

Therapeutic Class: Antipsychotic

CLINICAL PHARMACOLOGY

Mechanism of Action: A phenothiazine that antagonizes dopamine neurotransmission at synapses by blocking postsynaptic dopaminergic receptors in the brain. ***Therapeutic Effect:*** Decreases psychotic behavior. Also produces weak anticholinergic, sedative, and antiemetic effects and strong extrapyramidal effects.

Pharmacokinetics
Erratic absorption. Protein binding: greater than 90%. Metabolized in liver. Excreted in urine. ***Half-life:*** 33 hr.

INDICATIONS AND DOSAGES
Psychosis
PO
Adults, Elderly. 0.5-10 mg/day in divided doses q6-8h.
IM
Adults, Elderly. 2.5-10 mg/day in divided doses q6-8h or 12.5 mg (decanoate) q2wk.

AVAILABLE FORMS
- *Elixir (Prolixin):* 2.5 mg/5 ml.
- *Oral concentrate (Permitil):* 5 mg/ml.
- *Tablets (Prolixin):* 1 mg, 2.5 mg, 5 mg, 10 mg.
- *Injection:* 2.5 mg/ml (Prolixin), 25 mg/ml (Prolixin Decanoate).

UNLABELED USES: Treatment of neurogenic pain (adjunct to tricyclic antidepressants)

CONTRAINDICATIONS: Angle-closure glaucoma, myelosuppression, severe cardiac or hepatic disease, severe hypertension or hypotension, subcortical brain damage

PREGNANCY AND LACTATION: Pregnancy category C; EPS in the newborn have been attributed to *in utero* exposure; other reports have indicated that phenothiazines are relatively safe during pregnancy; excretion into breast milk unknown; use caution in nursing mothers

SIDE EFFECTS
Frequent
Hypotension, dizziness, and syncope (occur frequently after first injection, occasionally after subsequent injections, and rarely with oral doses)
Occasional
Somnolence (during early therapy), dry mouth, blurred vision, lethargy, constipation or diarrhea, nasal congestion, peripheral edema, urine retention
Rare
Ocular changes, altered skin pigmentation (with prolonged use of high doses)

SERIOUS REACTIONS
- Extrapyramidal symptoms (EPS) appear to be related to high dosages and are divided into 3 categories: akathisia (inability to sit still, tapping of feet), parkinsonian symptoms (such as hypersalivation, masklike facial expression, shuffling gait, and tremors), and acute dystonias (such as torticollis, opisthotonos, and oculogyric crisis).
- Tardive dyskinesia, manifested as tongue protrusion, puffing of the cheeks, and chewing or puckering of the mouth occurs rarely but may be irreversible.
- Abrupt withdrawal after long-term therapy may precipitate dizziness, gastritis, nausea and vomiting, and tremors.
- Blood dyscrasias, particularly agranulocytosis and mild leukopenia, may occur.
- Fluphenzine use may lower the seizure threshold.

INTERACTIONS
Drugs
3 *Alcohol, other CNS depressants:* May increase hypotensive and CNS and respiratory depressant effects
3 *Antithyroid agents:* May increase the risk of agranulocytosis
3 *Anticholinergics:* Inhibition of therapeutic response to neuroleptics, additive anticholinergic effects
3 *Antimalarials (amodiaquine, chloroquine, sulfadoxine-pyrimethamine):* Increased neuroleptic concentrations
3 *Barbiturates:* Reduced serum neuroleptic concentrations

3 *β-blockers:* Potential increases in serum concentrations of both drugs
3 *Bromocriptine:* Reduced effects of both drugs
3 *Clonidine:* Acute organic brain syndrome
3 *Cyclic antidepressants:* Increased serum concentrations of both drugs
3 *Epinephrine:* Reversal of pressor response to epinephrine
3 *Extrapyramidal symptom-producing medications:* May increase extrapyramidal symptoms
3 *Guanadrel:* Inhibits antihypertensive response
2 *Levodopa:* Inhibition of the antiparkinsonian effect of levodopa
3 *Lithium:* Rare cases of severe neurotoxicity have been reported in acute manic patients
3 *MAOIs:* May increase anticholinergic and sedative effects
3 *Meperidine:* Hypotension, excessive CNS depression
3 *Orphenadrine:* Reduced serum neuroleptic concentrations

Labs

- Urine pregnancy test: false positive

SPECIAL CONSIDERATIONS

- Concentrate must be diluted prior to administration; use only the following diluents: water, saline, 7-Up, homogenized milk, carbonated orange beverage, and pineapple, apricot, prune, orange, V-8, tomato, and grapefruit juices; do not mix with beverages containing caffeine, tannics (tea), or pectinates (apple juice), as physical incompatibility may result

PATIENT/FAMILY EDUCATION

- May cause drowsiness; use caution while driving or performing other tasks requiring alertness; drowsiness generally subsides during continued therapy
- Avoid contact with skin when using concentrates
- Avoid prolonged exposure to sunlight
- May discolor urine pink or reddish-brown
- Use caution in hot weather, heatstroke may result
- Arise slowly from a reclining position
- Full therapeutic effect may take up to 6 wks to appear
- Do not abruptly discontinue fluphenazine

MONITORING PARAMETERS

- Monitor closely for the appearance of tardive dyskinesia
- Blood pressure for hypotension
- CBC for blood dyscrasias
- Closely supervise suicidal patients during early therapy
- Therapeutic response, such as improvement in self-care, increased ability to concentrate and interest in surroundings, and relaxed facial expression

flurandrenolide

(flure-an-dren′-oh-lide)

Rx: Cordran, Cordran SP, Cordran Tape

Chemical Class: Corticosteroid, synthetic

Therapeutic Class: Corticosteroid, topical

CLINICAL PHARMACOLOGY

Mechanism of Action: A fluorinated corticosteroid that decreases inflammation by suppressing the migration of polymorphonuclear leukocytes and reversal of increased capillary permeability. ***Therapeutic Effect:*** Decreases tissue response to inflammatory process.

Pharmacokinetics
Repeated applications may lead to percutaneous absorption. Absorption is about 36% from scrotal area, 7% from the forehead, 4% from scalp, and 1% from forearm. Metabolized in liver. Excreted in urine. ***Half-life:*** Unknown.

INDICATIONS AND DOSAGES

Antiinflammatory, immunosuppressant, corticosteroid replacement therapy
Topical
Adults, Elderly. Apply 2-3 times/day.
Children. Apply 1-2 times/day.

AVAILABLE FORMS

- *Cream:* 0.025%, 0.05% (Cordran SP).
- *Lotion:* 0.05% (Cordran).
- *Ointment:* 0.025%, 0.05% (Cordran).
- *Tape, topical:* 4 mcg/cm^2 (Cordran).

CONTRAINDICATIONS: Hypersensitivity to flurandrenolide or any component of the formulation, viral, fungal, or tubercular skin lesions

PREGNANCY AND LACTATION: Pregnancy category C; unknown whether topical application could result in sufficient systemic absorption to produce detectable amounts in breast milk (systemic corticosteroids are secreted into breast milk in quantities not likely to have detrimental effects on infant)

SIDE EFFECTS

Occasional
Itching, dry skin, folliculitis
Rare
Intracranial hemorrhage, acne, striae, miliaria, allergic contact dermatitis, telangiectasis or raised dark red spots on skin

SERIOUS REACTIONS

- When taken in excessive quantities, systemic hypercorticism and adrenal suppression may occur.

SPECIAL CONSIDERATIONS

PATIENT/FAMILY EDUCATION

- Apply sparingly only to affected area
- Avoid contact with the eyes
- Do not put bandages or dressings over treated area unless directed by clinician
- Do not use on weeping, denuded, or infected areas
- Discontinue drug, notify clinician if local irritation or fever develops

MONITORING PARAMETERS

- Assess the patient for clinical signs of improvement

flurazepam hydrochloride

(flure-az'-e-pam hye-droe-klor'-ide)
Rx: Dalmane
Chemical Class: Benzodiazepine
Therapeutic Class: Sedative/hypnotic
DEA Class: Schedule IV

CLINICAL PHARMACOLOGY

Mechanism of Action: A benzodiazepine that enhances action of inhibitory neurotransmitter gamma-aminobutyric acid (GABA). ***Therapeutic Effect:*** Produces hypnotic effect due to CNS depression.

Pharmacokinetics

Route	Onset	Peak	Duration
PO	15-20 min	3-6 hrs	7-8 hrs

Well absorbed from the GI tract. Protein binding: 97%. Crosses the blood-brain barrier. Widely distributed. Metabolized in liver to active metabolite. Primarily excreted in urine. Not removed by hemodialysis. ***Half-life:*** 2.3 hr; metabolite: 40-114 hrs.

F

INDICATIONS AND DOSAGES

Insomnia

PO

Adults. 15-30 mg at bedtime.

Elderly, debilitated, liver disease, low serum albumin, Children 15 yr and older. 15 mg at bedtime.

AVAILABLE FORMS

- *Capsules:* 15 mg, 30 mg.

CONTRAINDICATIONS: Acute alcohol intoxication, acute angle-closure glaucoma, hypersensitivity to other benzodiazepines, pregnancy or breast-feeding

PREGNANCY AND LACTATION: Pregnancy category X; administration to nursing mothers is not recommended

Controlled Substance: Schedule IV

SIDE EFFECTS

Frequent

Drowsiness, dizziness, ataxia, sedation

Morning drowsiness may occur initially.

Occasional

GI disturbances, nervousness, blurred vision, dry mouth, headache, confusion, skin rash, irritability, slurred speech

Rare

Paradoxical CNS excitement or restlessness, particularly noted in elderly or debilitated

SERIOUS REACTIONS

- Abrupt or too-rapid withdrawal after long-term use may result in pronounced restlessness and irritability, insomnia, hand tremors, abdominal or muscle cramps, vomiting, diaphoresis, and seizures.
- Overdose results in somnolence, confusion, diminished reflexes, and coma.

INTERACTIONS

Drugs

3 *Alcohol, other CNS depressants:* May increase CNS depression

2 *Azole antifungals (fulconazole, itraconazole, ketoconazole):* Increased serum concentrations of flurazepam via inhibition of oxidative metabolism (CYP3A4)

3 *β-blockers (labetaolol, metoprolol, propranolol):* Reduces the metabolism of benzodiazepines and may increase the pharmacodynamic effects

3 *Cimetidine:* Increased plasma levels of flurazepam and metabolites via inhibition of hepatic oxidative metabolism

3 *Clozapine:* Isolated cases of cardiorespiratory collapse, but a causal relationship not established

3 *Disulfiram:* May increase serum concentrations of flurazepam via inhibition of oxidative metabolism (CYP3A4)

3 *Isoniazid:* May increase flurazepam serum concentrations via inhibition of metabolism

3 *Kava kava, valerian:* May increase CNS depression

3 *Loxapine:* Isolated cases of respiratory depression, stupor, and hypotension reported; role of drug interaction not established

3 *Macrolide antibiotics (clarithromycin, erythromycin, troleandomycin):* Macrolides increase flurazepam plasma concentrations via inhibition of metabolism (CYP3A4)

3 *Omeprazole:* Increases plasma concentrations of flurazepam via inhibition of hepatic metabolism

3 *Rifampin:* Reduced serum concentrations of flurazepam via enhanced hepatic metabolism (CYP3A4)

3 *Serotonin reuptake inhibitors (fluoxetine, fluvoxamine):* May increase serum concentrations of flurazepam via inhibition of oxidative metabolism (CYP3A4)

SPECIAL CONSIDERATIONS

- Poor choice for elderly patients

PATIENT/FAMILY EDUCATION

- Avoid alcohol and other CNS depressants
- Do not discontinue abruptly after prolonged therapy
- May experience disturbed sleep for the first or second night after discontinuing the drug
- May cause drowsiness or dizziness; use caution while driving or performing other tasks requiring alertness; hangover daytime drowsiness possible secondary to long duration of action
- Inform clinician if you are planning to become pregnant, you are pregnant, or if you become pregnant while taking this medicine

MONITORING PARAMETERS

- Assess patients for paradoxical reaction, such as excitability, particularly during early therapy
- Evaluate the patient for therapeutic response to insomnia, a decrease in number of nocturnal awakenings, and an increase in length of sleep

flurbiprofen

(flure-bi′-proe-fen)

Rx: Ansaid, Ocufen (ophthalmic)

Chemical Class: Propionic acid derivative

Therapeutic Class: NSAID; antipyretic; nonnarcotic analgesic

CLINICAL PHARMACOLOGY

Mechanism of Action: A phenylalkanoic acid that produces analgesic and antiinflammatory effect by inhibiting prostaglandin synthesis. Also relaxes the iris sphincter. ***Therapeutic Effect:*** Reduces the inflammatory response and intensity of pain. Prevents or decreases miosis during cataract surgery.

Pharmacokinetics

Well absorbed from the GI tract; ophthalmic solution penetrates cornea after administration, and may be systemically absorbed. Protein binding: 99%. Widely distributed. Metabolized in the liver. Primarily excreted in urine. ***Half-life:*** 3-4 hr.

INDICATIONS AND DOSAGES

Rheumatoid arthritis, osteoarthritis

PO

Adults, Elderly. 200-300 mg/day in 2-4 divided doses. Maximum: 100 mg/dose or 300 mg/day.

Dysmenorrhea, pain

PO

Adults. 50 mg 4 times a day.

Usual ophthalmic dosage

Adults, Elderly, Children. Apply 1 drop q30min starting 2 hr before surgery for total of 4 doses.

AVAILABLE FORMS

- *Tablets (Ansaid):* 50 mg, 100 mg.
- *Ophthalmic Solution (Ocufen):* 0.03%.

UNLABELED USES: Oral: Ankylosing spondylitis, dental pain, postoperative gynecologic pain

CONTRAINDICATIONS: Active peptic ulcer, chronic inflammation of GI tract, GI bleeding or ulceration, history of hypersensitivity to aspirin or NSAIDs

PREGNANCY AND LACTATION: Pregnancy category B (D if used in third trimester or near delivery; C for ophthalmic solution); excreted into breast milk; use caution in nursing mothers

SIDE EFFECTS

Occasional

PO (9%-3%): Headache, abdominal pain, diarrhea, indigestion, nausea, fluid retention

Ophthalmic: Burning or stinging on instillation, keratitis, elevated intraocular pressure

Rare (less than 3%)
PO: Blurred vision, flushed skin, dizziness, somnolence, nervousness, insomnia, unusual fatigue, constipation, decreased appetite, vomiting, confusion

SERIOUS REACTIONS

• Overdose may result in acute renal failure.

• Rare reactions with long-term use include peptic ulcer disease, GI bleeding, gastritis, severe hepatic reaction (jaundice), nephrotoxicity (hematuria, dysuria, proteinuria), a severe hypersensitivity reaction (angioedema, bronchospasm), and cardiac arrhythmias.

INTERACTIONS

Drugs

3 *Acetylcholine, carbachol:* May decrease the effects of these drugs (with ophthalmic flurbiprofen)

3 *Aminoglycosides:* Reduced clearance with elevated aminoglycoside levels and potential for toxicity (especially indomethacin in premature infants; other NSAIDs probably)

3 *Antihypertensives (α-blockers, angiotensin-converting enzyme inhibitors, angiotensin II receptor blockers, β-blockers, diuretics):* Inhibition of antihypertensive and other favorable hemodynamic effects

3 *Aspirin:* 50% decrease in plasma flurbiprofen concentrations, concurrent use not recommended

3 *Anticoagulants:* Excessive hypoprothrombinemia, decreased platelet aggregation with increased risk of GI bleeding

3 *Bone marrow depressants:* May increase the risk of hematologic reactions

3 *Corticosteroids:* Increased risk of GI ulceration

3 *Cyclosporine:* Increased nephrotoxicity risk

3 *Epinephrine, other antiglaucoma medications:* May decrease the antiglaucoma effect of these drugs

3 *Feverfew:* May decrease the effects of feverfew

3 *Ginkgo biloba:* May increase the risk of bleeding

3 *Lithium:* Decreased clearance of lithium (mediated via prostaglandins) resulting in elevated serum lithium levels and risk of toxicity

3 *Methotrexate:* Decreased renal secretion of methotrexate resulting in elevated methotrexate levels and risk of toxicity

3 *Phenylpropanolamine:* Possible acute hypertensive reaction

3 *Potassium-sparing diuretics:* Additive hyperkalemia potential

3 *Probenecid:* May increase the flurbiprofen blood concentration

3 *Triamterene:* Acute renal failure reported with addition of indomethacin; caution with other NSAIDs

Labs

• *Cortisol:* Increased at high flurbiprofen levels

SPECIAL CONSIDERATIONS

PATIENT/FAMILY EDUCATION

• Avoid aspirin and alcoholic beverages

• Take with food, milk, or antacids to decrease GI upset

• Notify clinician if edema, black stools, or persistent headache occurs

• Swallow flurbiprofen tablets whole and do not chew or crush them

• The eyes may sting momentarily during drug instillation of ophthalmic flurbiprofen

• The female patient should notify the physician if she is or plans to become pregnant

MONITORING PARAMETERS

• Initial hemogram and fecal occult blood test within 3 mo of starting regular chronic therapy; repeat every 6-12 mos (more frequently in high-risk patients (>65 years, peptic ulcer disease, concurrent steroids or anticoagulants); electrolytes, creatinine, and BUN within 3 mos of starting regular chronic therapy; repeat every 6-12 mos

- Pattern of daily bowel activity and stool consistency
- Periodic eye exams on patients using ophthalmic flurbiprofen
- Therapeutic response, such as improved grip strength, increased joint mobility, and decreased pain, stiffness, and swelling

---

flutamide

(floo′-ta-mide)

Rx: Eulexin

Chemical Class: Acetanilid derivative

Therapeutic Class: Anitandrogen; antineoplastic

CLINICAL PHARMACOLOGY

Mechanism of Action: An antiandrogen hormone that inhibits androgen uptake and prevents androgen from binding to androgen receptors in target tissue. Used in conjunction with leuprolide to inhibit the stimulant effects of flutamide on serum testosterone levels. ***Therapeutic Effect:*** Suppresses testicular androgen production and decreases growth of prostate carcinoma.

Pharmacokinetics

Completely absorbed from the GI tract. Protein binding: 94%-96%. Metabolized in the liver to active metabolite. Primarily excreted in urine. Not removed by hemodialysis. ***Half-life:*** 6 hrs (increased in elderly).

INDICATIONS AND DOSAGES

Prostatic carcinoma (in combination with leuprolide)

PO

Adults, Elderly. 250 mg q8h.

AVAILABLE FORMS

- *Capsules:* 125 mg.

UNLABELED USES: Female hirsutism

CONTRAINDICATIONS: Severe hepatic impairment

PREGNANCY AND LACTATION: Pregnancy category D

SIDE EFFECTS

Frequent

Hot flashes (50%); decreased libido, diarrhea (24%); generalized pain (23%); asthenia (17%); constipation (12%); nausea, nocturia (11%)

Occasional (8%-6%)

Dizziness, paresthesia, insomnia, impotence, peripheral edema, gynecomastia

Rare (5%-4%)

Rash, diaphoresis, hypertension, hematuria, vomiting, urinary incontinence, headache, flu-like syndromes, photosensitivity

SERIOUS REACTIONS

- Hepatoxicity, including hepatic encephalopathy, and hemolytic anemia may be noted.

INTERACTIONS

Drugs

3 *Warfarin:* Increased hypoprothrombinemic effect

SPECIAL CONSIDERATIONS

- Begin 8 wks before radiation therapy in Stage B_2-C carcinoma, continue during radiation
- In metastatic carcinoma continue until progression noted

PATIENT/FAMILY EDUCATION

- Feminization may occur during therapy
- Do not discontinue therapy without discussion with clinician

• Urine may become amber or yellow-green during flutamide therapy
• Avoid overexposure to the sun or ultraviolet light and wear protective clothing outdoors until tolerance of ultraviolet light is determined

MONITORING PARAMETERS

• Periodic LFTs during long-term treatment

---

fluticasone propionate

(flu-tic'-a-zone)

Rx: Cutivate, Flonase, Flovent, Flovent Diskus, Flovent HFA, Flovent Rotadisk

Combinations

Rx: with salmeterol (Advair Diskus)

Chemical Class: Corticosteroid, synthetic

Therapeutic Class: Corticosteroid, inhaled; corticosteroid, systemic; corticosteroid, topical

---

CLINICAL PHARMACOLOGY

Mechanism of Action: A corticosteroid that controls the rate of protein synthesis, depresses migration of polymorphonuclear leukocytes, reverses capillary permeability, and stabilizes lysosomal membranes. ***Therapeutic Effect:*** Prevents or controls inflammation.

Pharmacokinetics

Inhalation/intranasal: Protein binding: 91%. Undergoes extensive first-pass metabolism in liver. Excreted in urine. ***Half-life:*** 3-7.8 hrs. Topical: Amount absorbed depends on affected area and skin condition (absorption increased with fever, hydration, inflamed or denuded skin).

INDICATIONS AND DOSAGES

Allergic Rhinitis

Intranasal

Adults, Elderly. Initially, 200 mcg (2 sprays in each nostril once daily or 1 spray in each nostril q12h). Maintenance: 1 spray in each nostril once daily. Maximum: 200 mcg/day.

Children 4 yrs and older. Initially, 100 mcg (1 spray in each nostril once daily). Maximum: 200 mcg/day.

Relief of inflammation and pruritus associated with steroid-responsive disorders, such as contact dermatitis and eczema

Topical

Adults, Elderly, Children 3 mos and older. Apply sparingly to affected area once or twice a day.

Maintenance treatment for asthma for those previously treated with bronchodilators

Inhalation Powder (Flovent Diskus)

Adults, Elderly, Children 12 yrs and older. Initially, 100 mcg q12h. Maximum: 500 mcg/day.

Inhalation (Oral [Flovent])

Adults, Elderly, Children 12 yr and older. 88 mcg twice a day. Maximum: 440 mcg twice a day.

Maintenance treatment for asthma for those previously treated with inhaled steroids

Inhalation Powder (Flovent Diskus)

Adults, Elderly, Children 12 yr and older. Initially, 100-250 mcg q12h. Maximum: 500 mcg q12h.

Inhalation (Oral [Flovent])

Adults, Elderly, Children 12 yr and older. 88-220 mcg twice a day. Maximum: 440 mcg twice a day.

Maintenance treatment for asthma for those previously treated with oral steroids

Inhalation Powder (Flovent Diskus)

Adults, Elderly, Children 12 yr and older. 500-1000 mcg twice a day.

Inhalation (Oral [Flovent])

Adults, Elderly, Children 12 yrs and older. 880 mcg twice a day.

AVAILABLE FORMS

- *Aerosol for Oral Inhalation (Flovent, Flovent HFA):* 44 mcg/inhalation, 110 mcg/inhalation, 220 mcg/ inhalation.
- *Powder for Oral Inhalation (Flovent Diskus):* 50 mcg, 100 mcg, 250 mcg.
- *Intranasal Spray (Flonase):* 50 mcg/inhalation.
- *Topical Cream (Cutivate):* 0.05%.
- *Topical Ointment (Cutivate):* 0.005%.

CONTRAINDICATIONS: Primary treatment of status asthmaticus or other acute asthma episodes (inhalation); untreated localized infection of nasal mucosa

PREGNANCY AND LACTATION: Pregnancy category C; no information on excretion into human breast milk

SIDE EFFECTS

Frequent

Inhalation: Throat irritation, hoarseness, dry mouth, cough, temporary wheezing, oropharyngeal candidiasis (particularly if mouth is not rinsed with water after each administration)

Intranasal: Mild nasopharyngeal irritation; nasal burning, stinging, or dryness; rebound congestion; rhinorrhea; loss of taste

Occasional

Inhalation: Oral candidiasis

Intranasal: Nasal and pharyngeal candidiasis, headache

Topical: Skin burning, pruritus

SERIOUS REACTIONS

- Deaths due to adrenal insufficiency have occurred in asthma patients during and after transfer from use of long-term systemic corticosteroids to less systemically available inhaled corticosteroids.

INTERACTIONS

Drugs

3 *Ketoconazole:* Possible increased plasma fluticasone concentrations

3 *Bupropion:* May lower the seizure threshold

Labs

- *Cholesterol:* Increased

SPECIAL CONSIDERATIONS

- Improvement following inhalation, 24 hr to 1-2 wk
- Systemic corticosteroid effects from inhaled and nasal steroids inadequate to prevent adrenal insufficiency in most patients withdrawn abruptly from corticosteroids
- Observe for evidence of inadequate adrenal response following periods of stress; use caution with extended use in children and adolescents as reduction in growth velocity may occur

PATIENT/FAMILY EDUCATION

- Rinsing the mouth following INH and using a spacer device reduces common EENT adverse effects
- Review proper MDI administration technique regularly
- Do not discontinue the drug abruptly or change the dosage schedule; the dosage must be tapered gradually under medical supervision
- Drink plenty of fluids to decrease the thickness of lung secretions
- If the patient is using a bronchodilator inhaler concomitantly with a steroid inhaler, use the bronchodilator several minutes before using the corticosteroid to help the steroid penetrate into the bronchial tree
- Clear nasal passages before use
- Notify the physician if nasal irritation occurs or if symptoms, such as sneezing, fail to improve
- Symptoms should improve in several days

• The patient using topical fluticasone should rub a thin film gently on the affected area
• Keep the preparation away from the eyes

MONITORING PARAMETERS

• Pulse rate and quality and respiratory depth, rate, rhythm, and type
• ABG levels
• Breath sounds for rales, rhonchi, and wheezing
• Oral mucous membranes for evidence of candidiasis

---

fluvastatin sodium

(floo'-va-sta-tin soe'-dee-um)

Rx: Lescol, Lescol XL

Chemical Class: Substituted hexahydronaphthalene

Therapeutic Class: HMG-CoA reductase inhibitor; antilipemic

CLINICAL PHARMACOLOGY

Mechanism of Action: An antihyperlipidemic that inhibits HMG-CoA reductase, the enzyme that catalyzes the early step in cholesterol synthesis. ***Therapeutic Effect:*** Decreases LDL cholesterol, VLDL, and plasma triglyceride levels. Slightly increases HDL cholesterol concentration.

Pharmacokinetics

Well absorbed from the GI tract and is unaffected by food. Does not cross the blood-brain barrier. Protein binding: greater than 98%. Primarily eliminated in feces. ***Half-life:*** 1.2 hr.

INDICATIONS AND DOSAGES

Hyperlipoproteinemia

PO

Adults, Elderly. Initially, 20 mg/day (capsule) in the evening. May increase up to 40 mg/day. Maintenance: 20-40 mg/day in a single dose or divided doses.

Patients requiring more than a 25% decrease in LDL cholesterol. 40 mg (capsule) 1-2 times a day or 80 mg tablet once a day.

AVAILABLE FORMS

• *Capsules (Lescol):* 20 mg, 40 mg.
• *Tablets (Extended-Release [Lescol XL]):* 80 mg.

CONTRAINDICATIONS: Active hepatic disease, lactation, pregnancy, unexplained increased serum transaminase levels

PREGNANCY AND LACTATION: Pregnancy category X; contraindicated in breast-feeding—present in breast milk (2:1 milk: plasma ratio)

SIDE EFFECTS

Frequent (8%-5%)

Headache, dyspepsia, back pain, myalgia, arthralgia, diarrhea, abdominal cramping, rhinitis

Occasional (4%-2%)

Nausea, vomiting, insomnia, constipation, flatulence, rash, pruritus, fatigue, cough, dizziness

SERIOUS REACTIONS

• Myositis (inflammation of voluntary muscle) with or without increased CK, and muscle weakness, occur rarely. These conditions may progress to frank rhabdomyolysis and renal impairment.

INTERACTIONS

Drugs

3 *Alcohol:* 20 g of alcohol within 1 hr of dosing, increased fluvastatin AUC by 30%

2 *Azole antifungals (fluconazole, itraconazole, ketoconazole, miconazole):* Increased fluvastatin levels via inhibition of metabolism with increased risk of rhabdomyolysis

3 *Cholestyramine, colestipol:* Reduced bioavailability of fluvastatin

3 *Cimetidine, ranitidine, omeprazole:* Coadministration increases fluvastatin Cmax 43%-70% with

18%-23% decrease in plasma clearance

3 *Cyclosporine:* Concomitant administration increases risk of severe myopathy or rhabdomyolysis

3 *Danazol:* Inhibition of metabolism (CYP3A4) thought to yield increased fluvastatin levels with increased risk of rhabdomyolysis

3 *Diclofenac:* Increased plasma diclofenac concentrations

3 *Fluoxetine:* Less likely to inhibit CYP3A4 hepatic metabolism (vs lovastatin) with less risk of rhabdomyolysis

2 *Gemfibrazil:* Small increased risk of myopathy with combination, especially at high doses of statin

3 *Glyburide:* Increased plasma concentrations of glyburide and fluvastatin

3 *Isradipine:* Isradipine probably decreases fluvastatin plasma concentrations minimally

3 *Macrolide antibiotics (clarithromycin, erythromycin, troleandomycin):* Increased fluvastatin levels via inhibition of metabolism with increased risk of rhabdomyolysis

3 *Niacin:* Concomitant administration increases risk of severe hepatotoxicity

3 *Nefazadone:* Less likely to inhibit CYP3A4 hepatic metabolism (vs lovastatin) with less risk of rhabdomyolysis

3 *Phenytoin:* Increased plasma concentrations of phenytoin and fluvastatin

3 *Rifampin:* Coadministration decreases fluvastatin Cmax and AUC

3 *Terbinafine:* Minimal effect on the metabolism of fluvastatin

3 *Warfarin:* Addition of fluvastatin may increase hypoprothrombinemic response to warfarin via inhibition of metabolism (CYP2C9)

SPECIAL CONSIDERATIONS

- Statin selection based on lipid-lowering prowess, cost, and availability

PATIENT/FAMILY EDUCATION

- Report symptoms of myalgia, muscle tenderness, or weakness
- Take daily doses in the evening for increased effect
- May take without regard to food
- Follow the prescribed diet
- Periodic laboratory tests are an essential part of therapy

MONITORING PARAMETERS

- Cholesterol (max therapeutic response 4-6 wks)
- LFT's (AST, ALT) at baseline and at 12 wk of therapy; if no change, nor further monitoring necessary (discontinue if elevations persist at >3 times upper limit of normal)
- CPK in patients complaining of diffuse myalgia, muscle tenderness, or weakness

fluvoxamine maleate

(floo-vox'-a-meen)

Rx: Luvox

Chemical Class: Aralkylketone derivative

Therapeutic Class: Antidepressant, selective serotonin reuptake inhibitor (SSRI)

CLINICAL PHARMACOLOGY

Mechanism of Action: An antidepressant and antiobsessive agent that selectively inhibits neuronal reuptake of serotonin. ***Therapeutic Effect:*** Relieves depression and symptoms of obsessive-compulsive disorder.

Pharmacokinetics

Well absorbed following PO administration. Protein binding: 77%. Metabolized in liver. Excreted in urine. ***Half-life:*** 15.6 hrs.

INDICATIONS AND DOSAGES
Obsessive-compulsive disorder (OCD)
PO
Adults. 50 mg at bedtime; may increase by 50 mg every 4-7 days. Dosages greater than 100 mg/day given in 2 divided doses. Maximum: 300 mg/day.
Children 8-17 yr. 25 mg at bedtime; may increase by 25 mg every 4-7 days. Dosages greater than 50 mg/day given in 2 divided doses. Maximum: 200 mg/day.

AVAILABLE FORMS
- *Tablets:* 25 mg, 50 mg, 100 mg.

UNLABELED USES: Treatment of anxiety disorders in children, depression, panic disorder

CONTRAINDICATIONS: Use within 14 days of MAOIs, coadministration of thioridazine, terfenadine, astemizole, cisapride, or pimozide with fluvoxamine

PREGNANCY AND LACTATION: Pregnancy category C; excreted into breast milk; use caution in nursing mothers

SIDE EFFECTS
Frequent
Nausea (40%), headache, somnolence, insomnia (21%-22%)
Occasional (14%-8%)
Dizziness, diarrhea, dry mouth, asthenia, weakness, dyspepsia, constipation, abnormal ejaculation
Rare (6%-3%)
Anorexia, anxiety, tremor, vomiting, flatulence, urinary frequency, sexual dysfunction, altered taste

SERIOUS REACTIONS
- Overdose may produce seizures, nausea, vomiting, and extreme agitation and restlessness.

INTERACTIONS
Drugs
▲ *Antihistamines, nonsedating (astemizole, terfenadine):* Fluvoxamine inhibits metabolism (CYP3A4) for detoxifying these antihistamines; cardiac rhythm disturbances
③ *Benzodiazepines (alprazolam, midazolam, triazolam, diazepam):* Probable inhibition of metabolism (CYP3A4) leading to accumulation of benzodiazepines, avoid combination
③ *β-blockers (metoprolol, propranolol, sotalol):* Inhibition of metabolism (CYP2D6) leads to increased plasma concentrations of selective β-blockers and potential cardiac toxicity; atenolol may be safer choice
③ *Buspirone:* Reduced therapeutic effect of both drugs; possible seizures
③ *Carbamazepine:* Inhibition of hepatic metabolism of carbamazepine, but the formation of carbamazepine epoxide is not inhibited, contributing to increased toxicity
② *Clozapine:* Fluvoxamine markedly increases clozapine concentrations as a potent inhibitor of CYP1A2
③ *Cyclic antidepressants (clomipramine, desipramine, doxepin, imipramine, nortriptylline, trazadone):* Inhibition of metabolism (CYP1A2 and CYP3A4) leading to accumulation of cyclic antidepressants; dosage adjustments necessary
③ *Cyproheptadine:* Serotonin antagonist may partially reverse antidepressant and other effects
② *Dexfenfluramine:* Duplicate effects on inhibition of serotonin reuptake; inhibition of dexfenfluramine metabolism (CYP2D6) exaggerates effect; both mechanisms increase risk of serotonin syndrome
② *Fenfluramine:* Duplicate effects on inhibition of serotonin reuptake; inhibition of dexfenfluramine me-

tabolism (CYP2D6) exaggerates effect; both mechanisms increase risk of serotonin syndrome

❷ *HMG-CoA reductase inhibitors (atorvastatin, lovastatin, simvastatin):* Inhibition of statin metabolism (CYP3A4), by fluvoxamine, may lead to rhabdomyolysis

❸ *Lithium:* Neurotoxicity (tremor, confusion, ataxia, dizziness, dysarthria, and absence seizures) reported in patients receiving this combination; mechanism unknown

⚠ *MAOIs (isocarboxazid, phenelzine, tranylcypromine):* Increased CNS serotonergic effects have been associated with severe or fatal reactions with this combination

❸ *Mexiletine:* Reduced clearance of mexiletine, monitor serum mexiletine levels if co-administered

❸ *Methadone:* Significantly increased plasma methadone concentrations

❸ *Olanzapine:* May substantially increase olanzapine serum concentrations

❸ *Phenytoin:* Inhibition of metabolism and phenytoin toxicity

❸ *Quinidine:* Produces a modest increase in quinidine concentrations; increased quinidine effect or toxicity could result

❷ *Selegiline:* Sporadic cases of mania and hypertension

❸ *Sumatriptan:* Reports of weakness, hyperreflexia, and incoordination with SSRI and sumatriptan use, caution is advised

❷ *Tacrine:* Increased plasma tacrine concentrations, cholinergic side effects possible

❷ *Theophylline:* Theophylline toxicity increased via accumulation due to inhibition of metabolism (CYP1A2) by fluvoxamine

⚠ *Thioridazine:* Dose-related prolongation of the QTc interval, do not coadminister thioridazine and fluvoxamine

❷ *Tizanidine:* Increases tizanidine plasma concentrations

❷ *Tryptophan:* Additive serotonergic effects

❸ *Warfarin:* Increased hypothrombinemic response

SPECIAL CONSIDERATIONS

PATIENT/FAMILY EDUCATION

- May cause dizziness or drowsiness; use caution driving or performing tasks requiring alertness
- Maximum therapeutic response may require 4 wks or more to appear
- Do not discontinue the drug abruptly
- Take sips of tepid water and chew sugarless gum to relieve dry mouth

MONITORING PARAMETERS

- Assess appearance, behavior, level of interest, mood, and sleep pattern
- Assess pattern of daily bowel activity and stool consistency

folic acid/sodium folate (vitamin B_9)

(foe'-lik as'-id)

Rx: (folic acid) Folvite

Rx: (sodium folate) Folvite-parenteral

Chemical Class: Vitamin B complex

Therapeutic Class: Hematinic; vitamin

CLINICAL PHARMACOLOGY

Mechanism of Action: A coenzyme that stimulates production of platelets, RBCs, and WBCs. ***Therapeutic Effect:*** Essential for nucleoprotein synthesis and maintenance of normal erythropoiesis.

Pharmacokinetics

PO form almost completely absorbed from the GI tract (upper duodenum). Protein binding: high. Metabolized in the liver and plasma to active form. Excreted in urine. Removed by hemodialysis.

INDICATIONS AND DOSAGES

Vitamin B_9 deficiency

PO, IV, IM, Subcutaneous

Adults, Elderly, Children 12 yr and older. Initially, 1 mg/day. Maintenance: 0.5 mg/day.

Children 1-11 yr. Initially, 1 mg/day. Maintenance: 0.1-0.4 mg/day.

Infants. 50 mcg/day.

Dietary supplement

PO, IV, IM, Subcutaneous

Adults, Elderly, Children 4 yr and older. 0.4 mg/day.

Children 1-3 yr. 0.3 mg/day.

Children younger than 1 yr. 0.1 mg/day.

Pregnant women. 0.6 mg/day.

AVAILABLE FORMS

- *Tablets:* 0.4 mg, 0.8 mg, 1 mg.
- *Injection:* 5 mg/ml.

UNLABELED USES: To decrease the risk of colon cancer

CONTRAINDICATIONS: Anemias (aplastic, normocytic, pernicious, refractory)

PREGNANCY AND LACTATION: Pregnancy category A (C if used in doses above the recommended daily allowance); folic acid deficiency during pregnancy is a common problem in undernourished women and in women not receiving supplements; evidence has accumulated that folic acid deficiency, or abnormal folate metabolism, may be related to the occurrence of neural tube defects; actively excreted in human breast milk; compatible with breast-feeding; recommended daily allowance during lactation is 0.5 mg/day

SIDE EFFECTS

None known.

SERIOUS REACTIONS

- Allergic hypersensitivity occurs rarely with parenteral form. Oral folic acid is nontoxic.

INTERACTIONS

Drugs

[3] *Analgesics, carbamazepine, estrogens:* May increase folic acid requirements

[3] *Antacids, cholestyramine:* May decrease the absorption of folic acid

[3] *Methotrexate, triamterene, trimethoprim:* May antagonize the effects of folic acid

[3] *Phenytoin:* Decreased serum phenytoin concentrations; long-term phenytoin frequently leads to subnormal folate levels

❷ *Pyrimethamine:* Inhibition of antimicrobial effect of pyrimethamine

SPECIAL CONSIDERATIONS

- Recent evidence supports the premise that lowering elevated plasma homocysteine levels may reduce the risk of coronary heart disease

PATIENT/FAMILY EDUCATION

- Take only under medical supervision
- Eat foods rich in folic acid including fruits, vegetables, and organ meats

MONITORING PARAMETERS

- CBC; serum folate concentrations <0.005 mcg/ml indicate folic acid deficiency and concentrations <0.002 mcg/ml usually result in megaloblastic anemia
- Therapeutic improvement, including improved sense of well-being and relief from iron deficiency symptoms, such as fatigue, headache, pallor, dyspnea, and sore tongue

fomepizole

(foe-mep'-i-zoll)

Rx: Antizol

Chemical Class: Pyrazole derivative

Therapeutic Class: Antidote, ethylene glycol (antifreeze)

CLINICAL PHARMACOLOGY

Mechanism of Action: An alcohol dehydrogenase inhibitor that inhibits the enzyme that catalyzes the metabolism of ethanol, ethylene glycol, and methanol to their toxic metabolites. ***Therapeutic Effect:*** Inhibits conversion of ethylene glycol and methanol into toxic metabolites.

Pharmacokinetics

Protein binding: low. Rapidly distributes to total body water after IV infusion. Extensively metabolized by the liver. Minimal excretion in the urine. Removed by hemodialysis. ***Half-life:*** 5 hrs.

INDICATIONS AND DOSAGES

Ethylene glycol or methanol intoxication

IV infusion

Adults, Elderly. 15 mg/kg as loading dose, followed by 10 mg/kg q12h for 4 doses, then 15 mg/kg q12h until ethylene glycol or methanol concentrations are below 20 mg/dL. All doses should be administered as a slow IV infusion over 30 mins.

Dosage in renal impairment

During hemodialysis. 15 mg/kg as a loading dose, followed by 10 mg/kg q4h for 4 doses, then 15 mg/kg q4h until ethylene glycol or methanol concentrations are below 20 mg/dL.

After hemodialysis. If the time between the last dose and end of hemodialysis is less than 1 hr, do not give dose. If the time between is 1-3 hrs, give 50% of next scheduled dose. If time is greater than 3 hrs give next scheduled dose.

AVAILABLE FORMS

- *Solution for injection:* 1 g/ml (Antizol).

UNLABELED USES: Butoxyethanol intoxication, diethylene glycol intoxication, ethanol sensitivity

CONTRAINDICATIONS: Hypersensitivity to fomepizole or other pyrazoles

PREGNANCY AND LACTATION: Pregnancy category C

SIDE EFFECTS

Frequent

Hypertriglyceridemia, headache, nausea, dizziness

Occasional

Abnormal sense of smell, nystagmus, visual disturbances, ringing in ears, agitation, seizures, anorexia, heartburn, anxiety, vertigo, lightheadedness, altered sense of awareness

Rare

Anuria, disseminated intravascular coagulopathy

SERIOUS REACTIONS

- Mild allergic reactions including rash and eosinophilia occur rarely.
- Overdose may cause nausea, dizziness, and vertigo.

INTERACTIONS

Drugs

3 *Ethanol:* Reduced elimination rate of ethanol; reduced elimination rate of fomepizole

SPECIAL CONSIDERATIONS

PATIENT/FAMILY EDUCATION

- Common side effects are headache and nausea

MONITORING PARAMETERS

- Frequently monitor both ethylene glycol levels and acid-base balance, as determined by serum electrolyte (anion gap) or arterial blood gas analysis

• In patients with high ethylene glycol levels (≥50 mg/dL), significant metabolic acidosis or renal failure, consider hemodialysis to remove ethylene glycol and its toxic metabolites
• Treatment with fomepizole may be discontinued when ethylene glycol levels have been reduced to <20 mg/dL

fomivirsen sodium

(foh-mih-ver'-sen soe'-dee-um)
Rx: Vitravene
Chemical Class: Antisense oligonucleotide
Therapeutic Class: Antiviral

CLINICAL PHARMACOLOGY
Mechanism of Action: An antiviral that binds to messenger RNA, inhibiting the synthesis of viral proteins. ***Therapeutic Effect:*** Blocks replication of cytomegalovirus (CMV).
Pharmacokinetics
Minimal systemic absorption following intravitreal injection.
INDICATIONS AND DOSAGES
CMV retinitis
Intravitreal injection
Adults. 330 mcg (0.05 ml) every other week for 2 doses, then 330 mcg every 4 wks.
AVAILABLE FORMS
• *Intravitreal Injection:* 6.6 mg/ml.
CONTRAINDICATIONS: None known.
PREGNANCY AND LACTATION: Pregnancy category C; breast milk excretion unlikely
SIDE EFFECTS
Frequent (10%-5%)
Fever, headache, nausea, diarrhea, vomiting, abdominal pain, anemia, uveitis, abnormal vision
Occasional (5%-2%)
Chest pain, confusion, dizziness, depression, neuropathy, anorexia, weight loss, pancreatitis, dyspnea, cough
SERIOUS REACTIONS
• Thrombocytopenia may occur.
SPECIAL CONSIDERATIONS
PATIENT/FAMILY EDUCATION
• Does not treat systemic aspects of CMV infection
MONITORING PARAMETERS
• Ophthalmologic examination
• Monitor the patient for signs and symptoms of extraocular CMV infection, including pneumonitis and colitis. Also, assess for signs and symptoms of CMV infection in the untreated eye if only one eye is undergoing treatment

fondaparinux sodium

(fon-da-pa'-rin-ux)
Rx: Arixtra
Chemical Class: Pentasaccharide
Therapeutic Class: Anticoagulant

CLINICAL PHARMACOLOGY
Mechanism of Action: A factor Xa inhibitor and pentasaccharide that selectively binds to antithrombin, and increases its affinity for factor Xa, thereby inhibiting factor Xa and stopping the blood coagulation cascade. ***Therapeutic Effect:*** Indirectly prevents formation of thrombin and subsequently the fibrin clot.
Pharmacokinetics
Well absorbed after subcutaneous administration. Undergoes minimal, if any, metabolism. Highly bound to antithrombin III. Distributed mainly in blood and to a minor extent in extravascular fluid. Excreted unchanged in urine. Re-

moved by hemodialysis. ***Half-life:*** 17-21 hr (prolonged in patients with impaired renal function).

INDICATIONS AND DOSAGES

Prevention of venous thromboembolism

Subcutaneous

Adults. 2.5 mg once a day for 5-9 days after surgery. Initial dose should be given 6-8 hr after surgery. Dosage should be adjusted in the elderly and in those with renal impairment.

Treatment venous thromboembolism, pulmonary embolism

Subcutaneous

Adults, Elderly weighing greater than 100 kg. 10 mg once daily.

Adults, Elderly weighing 50-100 kg. 7.5 mg once daily.

Adults, Elderly weighing less than 50 kg. 5 mg once daily.

AVAILABLE FORMS

• *Injection:* 2.5 mg/0.5 ml prefilled syringe.

CONTRAINDICATIONS: Active major bleeding, bacterial endocarditis, body weight less than 50 kg, severe renal impairment (with creatinine clearance less than 30 ml/min), thrombocytopenia associated with antiplatelet antibody formation in the presence of fondaparinux

PREGNANCY AND LACTATION: Pregnancy category B; excreted in milk of lactating rats but human studies lacking; use caution in nursing mothers

SIDE EFFECTS

Occasional (14%)

Fever

Rare (4%-1%)

Injection site hematoma, nausea, peripheral edema

SERIOUS REACTIONS

• Accidental overdose may lead to bleeding complications ranging from local ecchymoses to major hemorrhage.

• Thrombocytopenia occurs rarely.

INTERACTIONS

Drugs

3 *Antithrombotic agents (aspirin, clopidogrel, ticlopidine, warfarin):* Increased risk of bleeding, close monitoring required

SPECIAL CONSIDERATIONS

• Slightly better at preventing DVT than enoxaparin; caused more bleeding than enoxaparin after knee replacement surgery; therapeutic niche not well defined

PATIENT/FAMILY EDUCATION

• The usual length of therapy is 5-9 days

• Do not take other medications, including OTC drugs (especially aspirin and NSAIDs), without physician approval

• Report severe or sudden headache, swelling in the feet or hands, unusual back pain, or unusual bleeding, bruising, or weakness

• Report bleeding from surgical site, chest pain, or dyspnea

• Use an electric razor and soft toothbrush to prevent bleeding during therapy

• The female patient should be aware that her menstrual flow may be heavier than usual

MONITORING PARAMETERS

• Periodic CBC, serum Cr, stool occult blood; there is no need for daily monitoring in patients with normal presurgical coagulation parameters

• Blood pressure, pulse—hypotension and tachycardia may indicate bleeding

• Assess for signs of bleeding, including bleeding at injection or surgical sites or from gums, blood in stool, ecchymosis, hematuria, and petechiae

formoterol fumarate

(for-moh'-te-role fyoo'-muh-rate)

Rx: Foradil Aerolizer

Chemical Class: Sympathomimetic amine; β_2-adrenergic agonist

Therapeutic Class: Antiasthmatic; bronchodilator

CLINICAL PHARMACOLOGY

Mechanism of Action: A long-acting bronchodilator that stimulates beta$_2$-adrenergic receptors in the lungs, resulting in relaxation of bronchial smooth muscle. Also inhibits release of mediators from various cells in the lungs, including mast cells, with little effect on heart rate. ***Therapeutic Effect:*** Relieves bronchospasm, reduces airway resistance. Improves bronchodilation, nighttime asthma control, and peak flow rates.

Pharmacokinetics

Route	*Onset*	*Peak*	*Duration*
Inhalation	1-3 mins	0.5-1 hrs	12 hrs

Absorbed from bronchi after inhalation. Metabolized in the liver. Primarily excreted in urine. Unknown if removed by hemodialysis. ***Half-life:*** 10 hr.

INDICATIONS AND DOSAGES

Asthma, chronic obstructive pulmonary disease (COPD)

Inhalation

Adults, Elderly, Children 5 yr and older. 12-mcg capsule q12h.

Exercise-induced bronchospasm

Inhalation

Adults, Elderly, Children 5 yr and older. 12-mcg capsule at least 15 min before exercise. Do not repeat for another 12 hrs.

AVAILABLE FORMS

• *Inhalation Powder in Capsules:* 12 mcg.

CONTRAINDICATIONS: None known.

PREGNANCY AND LACTATION: Pregnancy category C; β-agonists may potentially interfere with uterine contractility during labor; excretion into breast milk unknown; use caution in nursing mothers

SIDE EFFECTS

Occasional

Tremor, muscle cramps, tachycardia, insomnia, headache, irritability, irritation of mouth or throat

SERIOUS REACTIONS

• Excessive sympathomimetic stimulation may produce palpitations, extrasystole, and chest pain.

INTERACTIONS

Drugs

3 *Non-potassium sparing diuretics, xanthine derivatives, steroids:* Theoretical increase in the potential for hypokalemia

2 *β-blockers:* Decreased action of formoterol, cardioselective β-blockers preferable if concurrent use necessary (e.g., following myocardial infarction)

3 *Drugs that can prolong QT interval:* May potentiate cardiovascular effects

3 *MAO inhibitors, tricyclic antidepressants:* Theoretical increase in the potential for prolongation of QTc interval

SPECIAL CONSIDERATIONS

• Not indicated for patients whose asthma can be managed by occasional use of inhaled, short-acting, β_2-agonists

• Can be used concomitantly with short-acting β_2-agonists, inhaled or systemic corticosteroids, and theophylline

• Does not eliminate the need for treatment with an inhaled antiinflammatory agent

- Do not initiate therapy in patients with significantly worsening or acutely deteriorating asthma
- For use only with the Aerolizer Inhaler

PATIENT/FAMILY EDUCATION

- Should never be used more frequently than twice daily (morning and evening) at the recommended dose; do not use to treat acute symptoms
- Discontinue the regular use of short-acting β_2-agonists and use them only for symptomatic relief of acute asthma symptoms
- Seek medical advice immediately if a previously effective asthma medication regimen fails to provide the usual response
- For inhalation only, do not take orally
- Store in blister packaging, only remove immediately before use; handle capsules with dry hands
- Use the new Aerolizer Inhaler provided with each new prescription
- Drink plenty of fluids to decrease the thickness of lung secretions
- Avoid excessive use of caffeinated products, such as chocolate, cola, coffee, and tea

MONITORING PARAMETERS

- Pulmonary function tests
- Serum potassium
- Pulse rate and quality and respiratory rate, depth, rhythm, and type
- EKG

fosamprenavir calcium

(fos'-am-pren-a-veer kal'-see-um)

Rx: Lexiva

Chemical Class: HIV protease inhibitor

Therapeutic Class: Antiretroviral

F

CLINICAL PHARMACOLOGY

Mechanism of Action: An antiretroviral that is rapidly converted to amprenavir, which inhibits HIV-1 protease by binding to the enzyme's active site, thus preventing the processing of viral precursors and resulting in the formation of immature, noninfectious viral particles. ***Therapeutic Effect:*** Impairs HIV replication and proliferation.

Pharmacokinetics

Rapidly absorbed after PO administration. Protein binding: 90%. Metabolized in the liver. Excreted in urine and feces. ***Half-life:*** 7.7 hr.

INDICATIONS AND DOSAGES

HIV infection in patients who have not had previous protease inhibitor therapy

PO

Adults, Elderly. 1400 mg twice daily without ritonavir; or 1400 mg once daily plus ritonavir 200 mg once daily; or 700 mg twice daily plus ritonavir 100 mg twice daily.

HIV infection in patients who have had previous protease inhibitor therapy

PO

Adults, Elderly. 700 mg twice daily plus ritonavir 100 mg twice daily.

Concurrent therapy with efavirenz

PO

Adults, Elderly. In patients receiving fosamprenavir plus once-daily ritonavir in combination with efavirenz, an additional 100 mg/day ritonavir (300 mg total/day) should be given.

AVAILABLE FORMS

- *Tablets:* 700 mg (equivalent to 600 mg amprenavir).

CONTRAINDICATIONS: Concurrent use of amprenavir, dihydroergotamine, ergonovine, ergotamine, flecainide, methylergonovine, midazolam, pimozide, propafenone, ritonavir, triazolam

PREGNANCY AND LACTATION: Pregnancy category C, breast-feeding unsafe

SIDE EFFECTS

Frequent (39%-35%)

Nausea, rash, diarrhea

Occasional (19%-8%)

Headache, vomiting, fatigue, depression

Rare (7%-2%)

Pruritus, abdominal pain, perioral paresthesia

SERIOUS REACTIONS

- Severe and possibly life-threatening dermatologic reactions, including Stevens-Johnson syndrome, occur rarely.
- New onset or exacerbation of diabetes mellitus has been reported.

INTERACTIONS

Drugs

[3] *Abacavir:* Mild increase in fosamprenavir plasma level when given with abacavir

❷ *Alfuzosin:* Decreased clearance of alfuzosin

❷ *Alprazolam:* Decreased clearance of alprazolam

❷ *Amiodarone:* Decreased clearance of amiodarone

❷ *Amlodipine:* Decreased clearance of amlodipine

[3] *Antacids, didanosine:* May decrease the absorption of fosamprenavir

[3] *Atorvastatin:* Decreased clearance of atorvastatin

[3] *Barbiturates:* Increased clearance of fosamprenavir; reduced clearance of barbiturates

▲ *Bepredil:* Decreased clearance of bepredil

❷ *Carbamazepine:* Increased clearance of fosamprenavir; reduced clearance of carbamazepine

▲ *Cisapride:* Increased plasma levels of cisapride

[3] *Clozapine:* Increased blood concentrations of clozapine

[3] *Cyclosporine:* Decreased clearance of cyclosporine

[3] *Delavirdine:* Reduced clearance of fosamprenavir; fosamprenavir reduces clearance of erythromycin

❷ *Dexamethasone:* Decreased concentration of fosamprenavir

❷ *Efavirenz:* Efavirenz increases clearance of fosamprenavir

❷ *Eletriptan:* Decreased clearance of eletriptan; do not use within 72 hrs of fosamprenavir

▲ *Ergot alkaloids:* Increased plasma levels of ergot alkaloids

[3] *Erythromycin:* Reduced clearance of fosamprenavir; fosamprenavir reduces clearance of erythromycin

❷ *Felodipine:* Decreased clearance of felodipine

❷ *Garlic:* Decreased concentrations of fosamprenavir

❷ *Isradipine:* Decreased clearance of isradipine

❷ *Lidocaine:* Decreased clearance of lidocaine

▲ *Lovastatin:* Fosamprenavir reduces clearance of lovastatin

[3] *Methadone:* Decreased fosamprenavir concentrations

▲ *Midazolam:* Increased plasma levels of midazolam and prolonged effect

[3] *Nevirapine:* Reduces plasma fosamprenavir levels

[3] *Oral contraceptives:* Fosamprenavir may reduce efficacy

3 *Phenytoin:* Increased clearance of fosamprenavir; reduced clearance of phenytoin

❷ *Quinidine:* Decreased clearance of quinidine

❷ *Rifabutin:* Increased clearance of fosamprenavir; reduced clearance of rifabutin

⚠ *Rifampin:* Increased clearance of fosamprenavir

⚠ *Rifapentine:* Increased clearance of fosamprenavir

3 *Ritonavir:* Decreased clearance of fosamprenavir

3 *Saquinavir:* Decreased clearance of saquinavir; reduce dose of Fortovase (saquinavir soft gel capsule) to 800 mg tid

3 *Sildenafil:* Decreased clearance of sildenafil

⚠ *Simvastatin:* Decreased clearance of simvastatin

⚠ *St. John's wort:* Increased clearance of fosamprenavir

3 *Tacrolimus:* Decreased clearance of tacrolimus

❷ *Tadalafil:* Decreased clearance of tadalafil

⚠ *Triazolam:* Increased plasma levels of triazolam and prolonged effect

❷ *Tricyclic antidepressants:* Decreased clearance of tricyclic antidepressants

❷ *Vardenafil:* Decreased clearance of vardenafil

❷ *Verapamil:* Decreased clearance of verapamil

3 *Warfarin:* Increased blood concentrations of warfarin

SPECIAL CONSIDERATIONS

- Fosamprenavir is a prodrug for amprenavir, and allows fewer capsules to be administered per day, due to improved absorption

PATIENT/FAMILY EDUCATION

- Space doses evenly and continue taking fosamprenavir for the full course of treatment
- Consume small, frequent meals to help offset nausea and vomiting; consider taking OTC antidiarrheals if diarrhea occurs
- Fosamprenavir is not a cure for HIV infection, nor does it reduce the risk of transmitting HIV to others

MONITORING PARAMETERS

- HIV RNA level, CD4 count, CBC, metabolic panel, liver function tests, triglyceride and cholesterol levels
- Pattern of daily bowel activity and stool consistency
- Skin for rash

F

foscarnet sodium

(foss-car'-net soe'-dee-um)

Rx: Foscavir

Chemical Class: Pyrophosphate analog

Therapeutic Class: Antiviral

CLINICAL PHARMACOLOGY

Mechanism of Action: An antiviral that selectively inhibits binding sites on virus-specific DNA polymerase and reverse transcriptase. ***Therapeutic Effect:*** Inhibits replication of herpes virus.

Pharmacokinetics

Sequestered into bone and cartilage. Protein binding: 14%-17%. Primarily excreted unchanged in urine. Removed by hemodialysis. ***Half-life:*** 3.3-6.8 hrs (increased in impaired renal function).

INDICATIONS AND DOSAGES

Cytomegalovirus (CMV) retinitis

IV

Adults, Elderly. Initially, 60 mg/kg q8h or 100 mg/kg q12h for 2-3 wks. Maintenance: 90-120 mg/kg/day as a single IV infusion.

Herpes infection

IV

Adults. 40 mg/kg q8-12h for 2-3 wks or until healed.

Dosage in renal impairment

Dosages are individualized based on creatinine clearance. Refer to the dosing guide provided by the manufacturer.

AVAILABLE FORMS

• *Injection:* 24 mg/ml.

CONTRAINDICATIONS: None known.

PREGNANCY AND LACTATION: Pregnancy category C

SIDE EFFECTS

Frequent

Fever (65%); nausea (47%); vomiting, diarrhea (30%)

Occasional (5% or greater)

Anorexia, pain and inflammation at injection site, fever, rigors, malaise, headache, paresthesia, dizziness, rash, diaphoresis, abdominal pain

Rare (5%-1%)

Back or chest pain, edema, flushing, pruritus, constipation, dry mouth

SERIOUS REACTIONS

• Nephrotoxicity occurs to some extent in most patients.

• Seizures and serum mineral or electrolyte imbalances may be life-threatening.

INTERACTIONS

Drugs

3 *Nephrotoxic medications:* May increase the risk of nephrotoxicity

3 *Pentamidine (IV):* May cause reversible hypocalcemia, hypomagnesemia, and nephrotoxicity

3 *Quinolones:* Increased seizure risk (rare)

3 *Zidovudine (AZT):* May increase the risk of anemia

SPECIAL CONSIDERATIONS

• Hydration to establish diuresis both prior to and during administration is recommended to minimize renal toxicity; the standard 24 mg/ml sol may be used undiluted via a central venous catheter, dilute to 12 mg/ml with D_5W or NS when a peripheral vein catheter is used

PATIENT/FAMILY EDUCATION

• Foscarnet is not a cure for CMV retinitis

• Notify clinician of perioral tingling, numbness in the extremities, tremors, or paresthesias (could signify electrolyte imbalances)

MONITORING PARAMETERS

• Serum creatinine, calcium, phosphorus, potassium, magnesium at baseline and 2-3 times/wk during induction and at least every 1-2 wks during maintenance

• Hemoglobin

• Regular ophthalmologic examinations

• Signs and symptoms of serum electrolyte imbalances, especially hypocalcemia (numbness or tingling in the extremities or around the mouth) and hypokalemia (irritability, muscle cramps, numbness or tingling of the extremities, and weakness)

fosfomycin tromethamine

(fos-foe-mye′-sin troe-meth′-a-meen)

Rx: Monurol

Chemical Class: Phosphoric acid derivative

Therapeutic Class: Antibiotic

CLINICAL PHARMACOLOGY

Mechanism of Action: An antibiotic that prevents bacterial cell wall formation by inhibiting the synthesis of peptidoglycan. ***Therapeutic Effect:*** Bactericidal.

Pharmacokinetics

Rapidly absorbed following PO administration. Not bound to plasma proteins. Not metabolized. Partially excreted in urine; minimal elimination in feces. ***Half-life:*** 5.7 + 2.8 hr.

INDICATIONS AND DOSAGES

UTIs

PO (Uncomplicated)

Females. 3 g mixed in 4 oz water as a single dose.

PO (Complicated)

Males. 3 g/day q2-3days for 3 doses.

AVAILABLE FORMS

• *Powder for Oral Solution:* 3 g.

UNLABELED USES: Serious UTI in men

CONTRAINDICATIONS: None known.

PREGNANCY AND LACTATION: Pregnancy category B; excretion into breast milk unknown

SIDE EFFECTS

Occasional (9%-3%)

Diarrhea, nausea, headache, back pain

Rare (less than 2%)

Dysmenorrhea, pharyngitis, abdominal pain, rash

SERIOUS REACTIONS

• None known.

INTERACTIONS

Drugs

3 *Metoclopramide:* Decreased serum concentration and urinary excretion of fosfomycin

SPECIAL CONSIDERATIONS

• Inferior 5-11 day posttherapy microbiologic eradication rates compared to ciprofloxacin and co-trimoxazole for acute cystitis; eradication rates comparable to nitrofurantoin

• Reserve for women unable to tolerate or unlikely to comply with 3-day courses of co-trimoxazole or trimethoprim

PATIENT/FAMILY EDUCATION

• Always mix with water before ingesting

• Symptoms should improve 2-3 days after the initial dose of fosfomycin

fosinopril

(foe-sin'-oh-pril)

Rx: Monopril

Chemical Class: Angiotensin-converting enzyme (ACE) inhibitor, nonsulfhydryl

Therapeutic Class: Antihypertensive

F

CLINICAL PHARMACOLOGY

Mechanism of Action: An angiotensin-converting enzyme (ACE) inhibitor that suppresses the renin-angiotensin-aldosterone system and prevents conversion of angiotensin I to angiotensin II, a potent vasoconstrictor; may also inhibit angiotensin II at local vascular and renal sites. Decreases plasma angiotensin II, increases plasma renin activity, and decreases aldosterone secretion. ***Therapeutic Effect:*** Reduces peripheral arterial resistance, pulmonary capillary wedge pressure; improves cardiac output, and exercise tolerance.

Pharmacokinetics

Route	Onset	Peak	Duration
PO	1 hr	2-6 hrs	24 hrs

Slowly absorbed from the GI tract. Protein binding: 97%-98%. Metabolized in the liver and GI mucosa to active metabolite. Primarily excreted in urine. Minimal removal by hemodialysis. ***Half-life:*** 11.5 hrs.

INDICATIONS AND DOSAGES

Hypertension

PO

Adults, Elderly. Initially, 10 mg/day. Maintenance: 20-40 mg/day as a single or 2 divided doses. Maximum: 80 mg/day.

Children 6-16 yrs weighing more than 50 kg. Initially, 5-10 mg/day.

Heart failure
PO
Adults, Elderly. Initially, 10 mg/day. Maintenance: 20-40 mg/day. Maximum: 40 mg/day.

AVAILABLE FORMS

• *Tablets:* 10 mg, 20 mg, 40 mg.

UNLABELED USES: Treatment of diabetic and nondiabetic nephropathy, post-MI left ventricular dysfunction, renal crisis in scleroderma

CONTRAINDICATIONS: History of angioedema from previous treatment with ACE inhibitors, pregnancy

PREGNANCY AND LACTATION: Pregnancy category C (first trimester), category D (second and third trimesters); ACE inhibitors can cause fetal and neonatal morbidity and death when administered to pregnant women; when pregnancy is detected, discontinue ACE inhibitors as soon as possible; detectable in breast milk in trace amounts, a newborn would receive <0.1% of the mg/kg maternal dose; effect on nursing infant has not been determined; use with caution in nursing mothers

SIDE EFFECTS

Frequent (12%-9%)
Dizziness, cough

Occasional (4%-2%)
Hypotension, nausea, vomiting, upper respiratory tract infection

SERIOUS REACTIONS

• Excessive hypotension ("first-dose syncope") may occur in patients with CHF and in those who are severely salt and volume depleted.
• Angioedema (swelling of face and lips) and hyperkalemia occur rarely.
• Agranulocytosis and neutropenia may be noted in those with collagen vascular disease, including scleroderma and systemic lupus erythematosus, and impaired renal function.
• Nephrotic syndrome may be noted in those with history of renal disease.

INTERACTIONS

Drugs

3 *Alcohol:* May increase the effects of fosinopril

❷ *Allopurinol:* Combination may predispose to hypersensitivity reactions

3 *α-adrenergic blockers:* Exaggerated first-dose hypotensive response when added to fosinopril

3 *Aspirin:* May reduce hemodynamic effects of fosinopril; less likely at doses under 236 mg; less likely with nonacetylated salicylates

3 *Azathioprine:* Increased myelosuppression

3 *Cyclosporine:* Combination may cause renal insufficiency

3 *Insulin:* Fosinopril may enhance insulin sensitivity

3 *Iron:* Fosinopril may increase chance of systemic reaction to IV iron

3 *Lithium:* Reduced lithium clearance

3 *Loop diuretics:* Initiation of fosinopril may cause hypotension and renal insufficiency in patients taking loop diuretics

3 *NSAIDs:* May reduce hemodynamic effects of fosinopril

3 *Potassium-sparing diuretics:* Increased risk of hyperkalemia

3 *Trimethoprim:* Additive risk of hyperkalemia, especially in patient predisposed to renal insufficiency

Labs

• ACE inhibition can account for approximately 0.5 mEq/L rise in serum potassium

SPECIAL CONSIDERATIONS

PATIENT/FAMILY EDUCATION

• Caution with salt substitutes containing potassium chloride

• Rise slowly to sitting/standing position to minimize orthostatic hypotension
• Dizziness, fainting, lightheadedness may occur during first few days of therapy
• May cause altered taste perception or cough; persistent dry cough usually does not subside unless medication is stopped; notify clinician if these symptoms persist
• Report any signs or symptoms of infection, such as fever or sore throat
• Full therapeutic effect of fosinopril may take several weeks to appear
• Noncompliance with drug therapy or skipping fosinopril doses may cause severe, rebound hypertension

MONITORING PARAMETERS

• BUN, creatinine, potassium within 2 wk after initiation of therapy (increased levels may indicate acute renal failure)
• Blood pressure
• Intake and output
• In patients with CHF, assess for crackles and wheezes
• Urinalysis for proteinuria

frovatriptan succinate

(froe-va-trip'-tan suk'-si-nate)
Rx: Frova
Chemical Class: Serotonin derivative
Therapeutic Class: Antimigraine agent

CLINICAL PHARMACOLOGY

Mechanism of Action: A serotonin receptor agonist that binds selectively to vascular receptors, producing a vasoconstrictive effect on cranial blood vessels. ***Therapeutic Effect:*** Relieves migraine headache.

Pharmacokinetics

Well absorbed after PO administration. Metabolized by the liver to inactive metabolite. Eliminated in urine. ***Half-life:*** 26 hr (increased in hepatic impairment).

INDICATIONS AND DOSAGES

Acute migraine attack

PO

Adults, Elderly. Initially 2.5 mg. If headache improves but then returns, dose may be repeated after 2 hrs. Maximum: 7.5 mg/day.

AVAILABLE FORMS

• *Tablets:* 2.5 mg.

CONTRAINDICATIONS: Basilar or hemiplegic migraine, cerebrovascular or peripheral vascular disease, coronary artery disease, ischemic heart disease (including angina pectoris, history of MI, silent ischemia, and Prinzmetal's angina), severe hepatic impairment (Child-Pugh grade C), uncontrolled hypertension, use within 24 hrs of ergotamine-containing preparations or another serotonin receptor agonist, use within 14 days of MAOIs

PREGNANCY AND LACTATION: Pregnancy category C; excretion into breast milk unknown; use caution in nursing mothers

SIDE EFFECTS

Occasional (8%-4%)

Dizziness, paresthesia, fatigue, flushing

Rare (3%-2%)

Hot or cold sensation, dry mouth, dyspepsia

SERIOUS REACTIONS

• Cardiac reactions (including ischemia, coronary artery vasospasm, and MI), and noncardiac vasospasm-related reactions (such as cerebral hemorrhage and cerebrovascular accident [CVA]), occur rarely, particularly in patients with hypertension, diabetes, or a strong family history of coronary artery disease;

obese patients; smokers; males older than 40 yrs; and postmenopausal women.

INTERACTIONS

Drugs

▲ *Ergot-containing drugs:* Prolonged vasospastic reactions

3 *Oral contraceptives:* Decrease frovatriptan clearance and volume of distribution

3 *Propranolol:* May dramatically increase frovatriptan plasma concentration

2 *SSRIs:* Weakness, hyperreflexia, incoordination when coadministered

SPECIAL CONSIDERATIONS

- Triptans and dihydroergotamine are drugs of choice for moderate to severe migraine attacks; nasal sumatriptan is usually considered the triptan of choice due to its rapid onset; there are a number of oral triptans, including frovatriptan with more favorable biopharmaceutic profiles and high costs; comparisons not available
- There is no evidence that a second dose of frovatriptan is effective in patients who do not respond to a first dose of the drug for the same headache

PATIENT/FAMILY EDUCATION

- Useful medication for treatment of acute migraine attacks, not prevention; take a single dose of frovatriptan as soon as migraine symptoms appear
- Do not crush or chew film-coated tablets
- If the headache improves but then recurs, take a second dose at least 2 hrs after the first dose
- Avoid tasks that require mental alertness or motor skills until response to the drug has been established
- Notify the physician immediately if palpitations, pain or weakness in the extremities, pain or tightness in the chest or throat, or sudden or severe abdominal pain occurs
- The female patient of childbearing age should use contraceptives during therapy and inform the physician if she suspects she is pregnant
- Lie down in a dark, quiet room for additional benefit after taking frovatriptan

MONITORING PARAMETERS

- Headache response 1-4 hr after a dose (reduction from moderate or severe pain to minimal or no pain), functional disability, need for a second dose, headache recurrence, pulse, blood pressure

fulvestrant

(fool-ves′-trant)

Rx: Faslodex

Chemical Class: Estrogen derivative

Therapeutic Class: Antineoplastic

CLINICAL PHARMACOLOGY

Mechanism of Action: An estrogen antagonist that competes with endogenous estrogen at estrogen receptor binding sites. ***Therapeutic Effect:*** Inhibits tumor growth.

Pharmacokinetics

Extensively and rapidly distributed after IM administration. Protein binding: 99%. Metabolized in the liver. Eliminated by hepatobiliary route; excreted in feces. ***Half-life:*** 40 days in postmenopausal women. Peak serum levels occur in 7-9 days.

INDICATIONS AND DOSAGES

Breast cancer

IM

Adults, Elderly. 250 mg given once monthly.

AVAILABLE FORMS
• *Prefilled Syringe:* 50 mg/ml in 2.5-ml and 5-ml syringes.
UNLABELED USES: Endometriosis, uterine bleeding
CONTRAINDICATIONS: Known or suspected pregnancy
PREGNANCY AND LACTATION: Pregnancy category D; found in rat milk at levels significantly higher (approximately 12-fold) than plasma; excretion in human milk unknown; use with extreme caution in nursing mothers because of the potential for serious adverse reactions from fulvestrant in nursing infants
SIDE EFFECTS
Frequent (26%-13%)
Nausea, hot flashes, pharyngitis, asthenia, vomiting, vasodilatation, headache
Occasional (12%-5%)
Injection site pain, constipation, diarrhea, abdominal pain, anorexia, dizziness, insomnia, paresthesia, bone or back pain, depression, anxiety, peripheral edema, rash, diaphoresis, fever
Rare (2%-1%)
Vertigo, weight gain
SERIOUS REACTIONS
• UTIs, vaginitis, anemia, thromboembolic phenomena, and leukopenia occur rarely.

SPECIAL CONSIDERATIONS
• Store in refrigerator

PATIENT/FAMILY EDUCATION
• Notify the physician if weakness, hot flashes, or nausea become unmanageable

MONITORING PARAMETERS
• Blood chemistry and plasma lipid levels
• Evaluate the level of bone pain and ensure adequate pain relief if pain increases
• Assess for edema, especially in dependent areas
• Monitor for asthenia and dizziness and provide assistance with ambulation if these symptoms occur
• Assess for headache
• Offer an antiemetic, if ordered, to prevent or treat nausea and vomiting

furosemide
(fur-oh'-se-mide)
Rx: Lasix
Chemical Class: Anthranilic acid derivative
Therapeutic Class: Antihypertensive; diuretic, loop

CLINICAL PHARMACOLOGY
Mechanism of Action: A loop diuretic that enhances excretion of sodium, chloride, and potassium by direct action at the ascending limb of the loop of Henle. ***Therapeutic Effect:*** Produces diuresis and lower BP.
Pharmacokinetics

Route	Onset	Peak	Duration
PO	30-60 mins	1-2 hrs	6-8 hrs
IV	5 mins	20-60 mins	2 hrs
IM	30 mins	N/A	N/A

Well absorbed from the GI tract. Protein binding: 91%-97%. Partially metabolized in the liver. Primarily excreted in urine (nonrenal clearance increases in severe renal impairment). Not removed by hemodialysis. ***Half-life:*** 30-90 mins (increased in renal or hepatic impairment, and in neonates).
INDICATIONS AND DOSAGES
Edema, hypertension
PO
Adults, Elderly. Initially, 20-80 mg/dose; may increase by 20-40 mg/dose q6-8h. May titrate up to 600 mg/day in severe edematous states.

Children. 1-6 mg/kg/day in divided doses q6-12h.
Neonates. 1-4 mg/kg/dose 1-2 times a day.
IV, IM
Adults, Elderly. 20-40 mg/dose; may increase by 20 mg/dose q1-2h.
Children. 1-2 mg/kg/dose q6-12h.
Neonates. 1-2 mg/kg/dose q12-24h.
IV Infusion
Adults, Elderly. Bolus of 0.1 mg/kg, followed by infusion of 0.1 mg/kg/hr; may double q2h. Maximum: 0.4 mg/kg/hr.
Children. 0.05 mg/kg/hr; titrate to desired effect.

AVAILABLE FORMS
- *Oral Solution:* 10 mg/ml, 40 mg/5 ml.
- *Tablets:* 20 mg, 40 mg, 80 mg.
- *Injection:* 10 mg/ml.

UNLABELED USES: Hypercalcemia

CONTRAINDICATIONS: Anuria, hepatic coma, severe electrolyte depletion

PREGNANCY AND LACTATION: Pregnancy category C; (D if used in pregnancy-induced hypertension); cardiovascular disorders such as pulmonary edema, severe hypertension, or CHF are probably the only valid indications for this drug during pregnancy; furosemide has been used after the first trimester without causing fetal or newborn adverse effects; does not appear to significantly alter amniotic fluid volume; maternal use during pregnancy has not been associated with toxic or teratogenic effects, although metabolic complications have been observed (hyponatremia, hyperuricemia); reduces placental and/or maternal hepatic perfusion; excreted into breast milk; no reports of adverse effects in nursing infants

SIDE EFFECTS
Expected
Increased urinary frequency and urine volume
Frequent
Nausea, dyspepsia, abdominal cramps, diarrhea or constipation, electrolyte disturbances
Occasional
Dizziness, lightheadedness, headache, blurred vision, paresthesia, photosensitivity, rash, fatigue, bladder spasm, restlessness, diaphoresis
Rare
Flank pain

SERIOUS REACTIONS
- Vigorous diuresis may lead to profound water loss and electrolyte depletion, resulting in hypokalemia, hyponatremia, and dehydration.
- Sudden volume depletion may result in increased risk of thrombosis, circulatory collapse, and sudden death.
- Acute hypotensive episodes may occur, sometimes several days after beginning therapy.
- Ototoxicity—manifested as deafness, vertigo, or tinnitus—may occur, especially in patients with severe renal impairment.
- Furosemide use can exacerbate diabetes mellitus, systemic lupus erythematosus, gout, and pancreatitis.
- Blood dyscrasias have been reported.

INTERACTIONS
Drugs
❷ *Aminoglycosides (gentamicin, kanamycin, neomycin, streptomycin):* Additive ototoxicity (ethacrynic acid > furosemide, torsemide, bumetanide)
③ *Amphotericin B, nephrotoxic and ototoxic medications:* May in-

crease the risk of nephrotoxicity and ototoxicity

3 *Angiotensin-converting enzyme inhibitors:* Initiation of ACEI with intensive diuretic therapy may result in precipitous fall in blood pressure; ACEIs may induce renal insufficiency in the presence of diuretic-induced sodium depletion

3 *Anticoagulants, heparin:* May decrease the effects of these drugs

3 *Barbiturates (phenobarbital):* Reduced diuretic response

3 *Bile acid-binding resins (cholestyramine, colestipol):* Resins markedly reduce the bioavailability and diuretic response of furosemide

3 *Carbenoxolone:* Severe hypokalemia from coadministration

3 *Cephalosporins (cephaloridine, cephalothin):* Enhanced nephrotoxicity with coadministration

2 *Cisplatin:* Additive ototoxicity (ethacrynic acid > furosemide, torsemide, bumetanide)

3 *Clofibrate:* Enhanced effects of both drugs, especially in hypoalbuminemic patients

3 *Corticosteroids:* Concomitant loop diuretic and corticosteroid therapy can result in excessive potassium loss

3 *Digitalis glycosides (digoxin, digitoxin):* Diuretic-induced hypokalemia may increase risk of digitalis toxicity

2 *Lithium:* May increase the risk of lithium toxicity

3 *Nonsteroidal antiinflammatory drugs (flurbiprofen, ibuprofen, indomethacin, naproxen, piroxicam, aspirin, sulindac):* Reduced diuretic and antihypertensive effects

3 *Phenytoin:* Reduced diuretic response

3 *Probenecid:* May increase furosemide blood concentration

3 *Serotonin reuptake inhibitors (fluoxetine, paroxetine, sertraline):* Case reports of sudden death; enhanced hyponatremia proposed; causal relationships not established

3 *Terbutaline:* Additive hypokalemia

3 *Tubocurarine:* Prolonged neuromuscular blockade

Labs

- *Cortisol:* False increases
- *Glucose:* Falsely low urine tests with clinistix and diastix
- *Thyroxine:* Increased serum concentration
- *T_3 uptake:* Interference causes increased serum values

SPECIAL CONSIDERATIONS

PATIENT/FAMILY EDUCATION

- May cause GI upset, take with food or milk
- Take early in the day
- Avoid prolonged exposure to sunlight
- Expect an increase in the frequency and volume of urination
- Notify the physician if hearing abnormalities (ringing, roaring, or sense of fullness in the ears) or signs of an electrolyte imbalance (irregular heartbeat, muscle cramps or weakness, tremor) occur
- Eat foods high in potassium, including apricots, bananas, orange juice, potatoes, raisins, legumes, meat, and whole grains (such as cereals)

MONITORING PARAMETERS

- Urine volume, creatinine clearance, BUN electrolytes, reduction in edema, increased diuresis, decrease in body weight, reduction in blood pressure, glucose, uric acid, serum calcium (tetany), tinnitus, vertigo, hearing loss (especially in those at risk for ototoxicity—IV doses >120 mg; concomitant ototoxic drugs; renal disease)

gabapentin

(ga'-ba-pen-tin)

Rx: Neurontin

Chemical Class: Cyclohexanacetic acid derivative

Therapeutic Class: Anticonvulsant

CLINICAL PHARMACOLOGY

Mechanism of Action: An anticonvulsant and antineuralgic agent whose exact mechanism is unknown. May increase the synthesis or accumulation of gamma-aminobutyric acid by binding to as-yet-undefined receptor sites in brain tissue. ***Therapeutic Effect:*** Reduces seizure activity and neuropathic pain.

Pharmacokinetics

Well absorbed from the GI tract (not affected by food). Protein binding: less than 5%. Widely distributed. Crosses the blood-brain barrier. Primarily excreted unchanged in urine. Removed by hemodialysis. ***Half-life:*** 5-7 hr (increased in impaired renal function and the elderly).

INDICATIONS AND DOSAGES

Adjunctive therapy for seizure control

PO

Adults, Elderly, Children older than 12 yr. Initially, 300 mg 3 times a day. May titrate dosage. Range: 900-1800 mg/day in 3 divided doses. Maximum: 3600 mg/day.

Children 3-12 yr. Initially, 10-15 mg/kg/day in 3 divided doses. May titrate up to 25-35 mg/kg/day (for children 5-12 yr) and 40 mg/kg/day (for children 3-4 yr) Maximum: 50 mg/kg/day.

Adjunctive therapy for neuropathic pain

PO

Adults, Elderly. Initially, 100 mg 3 times a day; may increase by 300 mg/day at weekly intervals. Maximum: 3600 mg/day in 3 divided doses.

Children. Initially, 5 mg/kg/dose at bedtime, followed by 5 mg/kg/dose for 2 doses on day 2, then 5 mg/kg/dose for 3 doses on day 3. Range: 8-35 mg/kg/day in 3 divided doses.

Postherpetic neuralgia

PO

Adults, Elderly. 300 mg on day 1, 300 mg twice a day on day 2, and 300 mg 3 times a day on day 3. Titrate up to 1800 mg/day.

Dosage in renal impairment

Dosage and frequency are modified based on creatinine clearance:

Creatinine Clearance	*Dosage*
60 ml/min or higher	400 mg q8h
30-59 ml/min	300 mg q12h
16-29 ml/min	300 mg daily
less than 16 ml/min	300 mg every other day
Hemodialysis	200-300 mg after each 4-hr hemodialysis session

AVAILABLE FORMS

- *Capsules (Neurontin):* 100 mg, 300 mg, 400 mg.
- *Oral Solution (Neurontin):* 250 mg/5 ml.
- *Tablets (Neurontin):* 100 mg, 300 mg, 400 mg, 600 mg, 800 mg.

UNLABELED USES: Treatment of bipolar disorder, chronic pain, diabetic peripheral neuropathy, essential tremor, hot flashes, hyperhidrosis, migraines, psychiatric disorders (social phobia)

CONTRAINDICATIONS: None known.

PREGNANCY AND LACTATION: Pregnancy category C

SIDE EFFECTS

Frequent (19%-10%)

Fatigue, somnolence, dizziness, ataxia

Occasional (8%-3%)

Nystagmus, tremor, diplopia, rhinitis, weight gain

Rare (less than 2%)

Nervousness, dysarthria, memory loss, dyspepsia, pharyngitis, myalgia

SERIOUS REACTIONS

- Abrupt withdrawal may increase seizure frequency.
- Overdosage may result in diplopia, slurred speech, drowsiness, lethargy, and diarrhea.

INTERACTIONS

Drugs

3 *Antacids:* Reduce bioavailability of gabapentin by 20%

SPECIAL CONSIDERATIONS

PATIENT/FAMILY EDUCATION

- Do not stop abruptly; taper over 1 wk
- Take gabapentin only as prescribed
- Avoid tasks requiring mental alertness or motor skills until response to the drug is established
- Avoid alcohol while taking gabapentin
- Always carry an identification card or wear an identification bracelet that displays seizure disorder and anticonvulsant therapy

MONITORING PARAMETERS

- Drug level monitoring not necessary
- Weight, renal function, and behavior (in children)
- Seizure duration and frequency

galantamine hydrobromide

(ga-lan′-ta-meen hye-droe-broe′-mide)

Rx: Razadyne, Razadyne ER

Chemical Class: Benzazepine derivative; cholinesterase inhibitor

Therapeutic Class: Acetylcholinesterase inhibitor

CLINICAL PHARMACOLOGY

Mechanism of Action: A cholinesterase inhibitor that inhibits the enzyme acetylcholinesterase, thus increasing the concentration of acetylcholine at cholinergic synapses and enhancing cholinergic function in the CNS. ***Therapeutic Effect:*** Slows the progression of Alzheimer's disease.

Pharmacokinetics

Rapidly absorbed from the GI tract. Protein binding: 18%. Distributed to blood cells; binds to plasma proteins, mainly albumin. Metabolized in the liver. Excreted in urine. ***Half-life:*** 7 hr.

INDICATIONS AND DOSAGES

Alzheimer's disease

PO

Adults, Elderly. Initially, 4 mg twice a day (8 mg/day). After a minimum of 4 wk (if well tolerated), may increase to 8 mg twice a day (16 mg/day). After another 4 wk, may increase to 12 mg twice daily (24 mg/day). Range: 16-24 mg/day in 2 divided doses.

PO (Extended-Release)

Adults, Elderly. 8-24 mg/day as a single daily dose.

Dosage in renal impairment

For moderate impairment, maximum dosage is 16 mg/day. Drug is not recommended for patients with severe impairment.

AVAILABLE FORMS

• *Capsules (Extended-Release [Razadyne ER]):* 8 mg, 16 mg, 24 mg.
• *Oral Solution (Razadyne):* 4 mg/ml.
• *Tablets (Razadyne):* 4 mg, 8 mg, 12 mg.

CONTRAINDICATIONS: Severe hepatic or renal impairment

PREGNANCY AND LACTATION: Pregnancy category B; breast milk excretion information not known

SIDE EFFECTS

Frequent (17%-5%)

Nausea, vomiting, diarrhea, anorexia, weight loss

Occasional (9%-4%)

Abdominal pain, insomnia, depression, headache, dizziness, fatigue, rhinitis

Rare (less than 3%)

Tremors, constipation, confusion, cough, anxiety, urinary incontinence

SERIOUS REACTIONS

• Overdose may cause cholinergic crisis, characterized by increased salivation, lacrimation, severe nausea and vomiting, bradycardia, respiratory depression, hypotension, and increased muscle weakness. Treatment usually consists of supportive measures and an anticholinergic such as atropine.

INTERACTIONS

Drugs

3 *Anesthetics (inhaled):* Decreases neuromuscular blocking effects

3 *Anesthetics (local, esters):* Increases effects (possible toxicity) of local anesthetic (pseudocholinesterase competition)

3 *Anticholinergics:* Antagonistic effects; use to counteract undesirable muscarinic effects of cholinesterase inhibitors

2 *Bethanechol, pilocarpine, dexpanthanol, echothiophate:* Galantamine potentiates cholinergic agonists

3 *Cimetidine:* Increased bioavailability of galantamine (16%)

3 *Ketoconazole:* Strong inhibitor of CYP3A4; increases AUC of galantamine by 30%

3 *Erythromycin:* Moderate inhibitor of CYP3A4; increases AUC of galantamine by 10%

3 *Fluoxetine:* Inhibition of CYP2D6 may increase levels of galantamine

3 *Fluvoxamine:* Inhibition of CYP2D6 may increase levels of galantamine

3 *Paroxetine:* Strong inhibitor of CYP2D6; increases AUC of galantamine by 40%

2 *Succinylcholine:* Potentiates neuromuscular blockade

SPECIAL CONSIDERATIONS

• Extracted from the bulbs of the daffodil, *Narcissus pseudonarcissus*

PATIENT/FAMILY EDUCATION

• Patient and caregiver should be advised of high incidence of gastrointestinal effects and directions for resource and resolution
• Take galantamine with morning and evening meals to reduce the risk of nausea
• Avoid tasks that require mental alertness or motor skills until response to the drug has been established
• Notify the physician if excessive sweating, tearing, salivation, depression, dizziness, excessive fatigue, muscle weakness, insomnia, or persistent GI disturbances occurs
• Galantamine is not a cure for Alzheimer's disease but may slow the progression of its symptoms

MONITORING PARAMETERS

• Cognitive function (e.g., ADAS, Mini-Mental Status Exam [MMSE]), activities of daily living, global functioning, blood chemistry, complete blood counts, heart rate, blood pressure

• Periodically assess the 12-lead EKG and rhythm strips of patients with underlying arrhythmias

• Assess the patient for signs of GI distress, including nausea, vomiting, diarrhea, anorexia, and weight loss

ganciclovir sodium

(gan-sye'-kloe-veer soe'-dee-um)

Rx: Cytovene

Chemical Class: Acyclic purine nucleoside analog

Therapeutic Class: Antiviral

CLINICAL PHARMACOLOGY

Mechanism of Action: This synthetic nucleoside competes with viral DNA polymerase and is incorporated into growing viral DNA chains. ***Therapeutic Effect:*** Interferes with synthesis and replication of viral DNA.

Pharmacokinetics

Widely distributed. Protein binding: 1%-2%. Undergoes minimal metabolism. Excreted unchanged primarily in urine. Removed by hemodialysis. ***Half-life:*** 2.5-3.6 hr (increased in impaired renal function).

INDICATIONS AND DOSAGES

Cytomegalovirus (CMV) retinitis

IV

Adults, Children 3 mo and older. 10 mg/kg/day in divided doses q12h for 14-21 days, then 5 mg/kg/day as a single daily dose or 6 mg/kg 5 days a week.

Prevention of CMV disease in transplant patients

IV

Adults, Children. 10 mg/kg/day in divided doses q12h for 7-14 days, then 5 mg/kg/day as a single daily dose.

Other CMV infections

IV

Adults. Initially, 10 mg/kg/day in divided doses q12h for 14-21 days, then 5 mg/kg/day as a single daily dose. Maintenance: 1000 mg 3 times a day or 500 mg q3h (6 times a day).

Children. Initially, 10 mg/kg/day in divided doses q12h for 14-21 days, then 5 mg/kg/day as a single daily dose. Maintenance: 30 mg/kg/dose q8h.

Intravitreal implant

Adults. 1 implant q6-9mo plus oral ganciclovir.

Children 9 yr and older. 1 implant q6-9mo plus oral ganciclovir (30 mg/dose q8h).

Adult dosage in renal impairment

Dosage and frequency are modified based on creatinine clearance.

CrCl	*Induction Dosage*	*Maintenance Dosage*	*Oral*
50-69 ml/ min	2.5 mg/kg q12h	2.5 mg/kg q24h	1500 mg/ day
25-49 ml/ min	2.5 mg/kg q24h	1.25 mg/ kg q24h	1000 mg/ day
10-24 ml/ min	1.25 mg/kg q24h	0.625 mg/ kg q24h	500 mg/ day
less than 10 ml/ min	1.25 mg/kg 3 times/ wk	0.625 mg/kg 3 times/ wk	500 mg 3 times/ wk

AVAILABLE FORMS

• *Capsules (Cytovene):* 250 mg, 500 mg.

• *Powder for Injection (Cytovene):* 500 mg.

• *Implant (Vitrasert):* 4.5 mg.

UNLABELED USES: Treatment of other CMV infections, such as gastroenteritis, hepatitis, and pneumonitis

CONTRAINDICATIONS: Absolute neutrophil count less than 500/mm^3, platelet count less than 25,000/mm^3, hypersensitivity to acyclovir or ganciclovir, immunocompetent patients, patients with congenital or neonatal CMV disease

PREGNANCY AND LACTATION: Pregnancy category C; excretion into breast milk unknown; not recommended in nursing mothers due to potential for serious adverse reactions in the nursing infant; do not resume nursing for at least 72 hr after last dose of ganciclovir

SIDE EFFECTS

Frequent

Diarrhea (41%), fever (40%), nausea (25%), abdominal pain (17%), vomiting (13%)

Occasional (11%-6%)

Diaphoresis, infection, paresthesia, flatulence, pruritus

Rare (4%-2%)

Headache, stomatitis, dyspepsia, phlebitis

SERIOUS REACTIONS

- Hematologic toxicity occurs commonly: leukopenia in 41%-29% of patients and anemia in 25%-19%.
- Intra-ocular insertion occasionally results in visual acuity loss, vitreous hemorrhage, and retinal detachment.
- GI hemorrhage occurs rarely.

INTERACTIONS

Drugs

3 *Bone marrow depressants:* May increase bone marrow depression

3 *Didanosine:* Increased hematologic toxicity

3 *Imipenem, cilastin:* May increase the risk of seizures

▲ *Zidovudine (AZT):* Increased hematologic toxicity

SPECIAL CONSIDERATIONS

PATIENT/FAMILY EDUCATION

- Compliance with laboratory monitoring is essential
- Promptly report any new symptom to the physician
- Male patients should be aware that ganciclovir may temporarily or permanently inhibit sperm production
- Male patients should use barrier contraception during ganciclovir therapy and for 90 days afterward because of the drug's mutagenic potential
- Female patients should know that ganciclovir use may suppress fertility
- Female patients should use effective contraception during therapy
- Ganciclovir suppresses but does not cure CMV retinitis

MONITORING PARAMETERS

- CBC with differential and platelets q2days during induction and weekly thereafter
- Serum creatinine q2wk
- Intake and output
- Signs and symptoms of infiltration, phlebitis, pruritus, and rash
- Vision

gatifloxacin

(ga-ti-flocks'-a-sin)

Rx: Tequin, Tequin Teqpaq, Zymar

Chemical Class: Fluoroquinolone derivative

Therapeutic Class: Antibiotic

CLINICAL PHARMACOLOGY

Mechanism of Action: A fluoroquinolone that inhibits two enzymes, topoisomerase II and IV, in susceptible microorganisms. ***Therapeutic Effect:*** Interferes with bacterial DNA replication. Prevents or delays resistance emergence. Bactericidal.

Pharmacokinetics

Well absorbed from the GI tract after PO administration. Protein binding: 20%. Widely distributed. Metabolized in liver. Primarily excreted in urine. ***Half-life:*** 7-14 hr.

INDICATIONS AND DOSAGES

Chronic bronchitis, complicated urinary tract infections, pyelonephritis, skin infections

PO, IV

Adults, Elderly. 400 mg/day for 7-10 days (5 days for chronic bronchitis).

Sinusitis

PO, IV

Adults, Elderly. 400 mg/day for 10 days.

Pneumonia

PO, IV

Adults, Elderly. 400 mg/day for 7-14 days.

Cystitis

PO, IV

Adults, Elderly. 400 mg as a single dose or 200 mg/day for 3 days.

Urethral gonorrhea in men and women, endocervical and rectal gonorrhea in women

PO, IV

Adults, Elderly. 400 mg as a single dose.

Topical treatment of bacterial conjunctivitis due to susceptible strains of bacteria

Ophthalmic

Adults, Elderly, Children 1 yr and older. 1 drop q2h while awake for 2 days, then 1 drop up to 4 times/day for days 3-7.

Dosage in renal impairment

Creatinine Clearance	*Dosage*
40 ml/min	400 mg/day
less than 40 ml/min	Initially, 400 mg/day then 200 mg/day
Hemodialysis	Initially, 400 mg/day then 200 mg/day
Peritoneal dialysis	Initially, 400 mg/day then 200 mg/day

AVAILABLE FORMS

- *Tablets (Tequin, Tequin Teqpaq):* 200 mg, 400 mg.
- *Injection (Tequin):* 200-mg, 400-mg vials.
- *Ophthalmic Solution (Zymar):* 0.3%.

CONTRAINDICATIONS: Hypersensitivity to quinolones

PREGNANCY AND LACTATION: Pregnancy category C; breast milk excretion unknown

SIDE EFFECTS

Occasional (8%-3%)

Nausea, vaginitis, diarrhea, headache, dizziness

Ophthalmic: Conjunctival irritation, increased tearing, corneal inflammation

Rare (3%-0.1%)

Abdominal pain, constipation, dyspepsia, stomatitis, edema, insomnia, abnormal dreams, diaphoresis, altered taste, rash

Ophthalmic: Corneal swelling, dry eye, eye pain, eyelid swelling, headache, red eye, reduced visual acuity, altered taste

SERIOUS REACTIONS

- Pseudomembranous colitis, as evidenced by severe abdominal pain and cramps, severe watery diarrhea, and fever, may occur.
- Superinfection, manifested as genital or anal pruritus, ulceration or

changes in oral mucosa, and moderate to severe diarrhea, may occur.

INTERACTIONS

Drugs

3 *Aluminum:* Reduced absorption of gatifloxacin; do not take within 4 hr of dose

❷ *Amiodarone:* Additive cardiac toxicity

3 *Antacids (containing aluminum or magnesium):* Reduced absorption of gatifloxacin; do not take within 4 hr of dose

❷ *Antipsychotics:* Additive cardiac toxicity

3 *Didanosine (buffered formulation):* Markedly reduced absorption of gatifloxacin; take gatifloxacin 2 hr before didanosine

❷ *Erythromycin:* Coadministration may increase risk of cardiac toxicity due to gatifloxacin

3 *Foscarnet:* Coadministration increase seizure risk

3 *Iron:* Reduced absorption of gatifloxacin; do not take within 4 hr of dose

3 *Magnesium:* Reduced absorption of gatifloxacin; do not take within 4 hr of dose

3 *Probenecid:* Inhibits excretion of gatifloxacin

❷ *Procainamide:* Additive cardiac toxicity

❷ *Quinidine:* Additive cardiac toxicity

3 *Sodium bicarbonate:* Reduced absorption of gatifloxacin; do not take within 4 hr of dose

❷ *Sotalol:* Additive cardiac toxicity

3 *Sucralfate:* Reduced absorption of gatifloxacin; do not take within 4 hr of dose

❷ *Tricyclic antidepressants:* Additive cardiac toxicity

3 *Zinc:* Reduced absorption of gatifloxacin; do not take within 4 hr of dose

❷ *Ziprasidone:* Prolongs the QTc interval; theoretically, could increase the risk of ventricular arrhythmias

SPECIAL CONSIDERATIONS

PATIENT/FAMILY EDUCATION

- May be taken with or without meals
- Should be taken at least 4 hr before or 8 hr after multivitamins (containing iron or zinc), antacids (containing magnesium, calcium, or aluminum), sucralfate, or didanosine chewable/buffered tablets
- Discontinue treatment, rest and refrain from exercise, and inform prescriber if pain, inflammation, or rupture of a tendon occur
- Test reaction to this drug before operating an automobile or machinery or engaging in activities requiring mental alertness or coordination
- Drink plenty of fluids
- Avoid exposure to direct sunlight as this may cause a photosensitivity reaction
- Take for the full course of therapy

MONITORING PARAMETERS

- WBC count
- Signs of infection
- Pattern of daily bowel activity and stool consistency
- Evaluate for abdominal pain, altered sense of taste, dyspepsia (heartburn, indigestion), headache, and vomiting

gemfibrozil

(jem-fi′-broe-zil)

Rx: Lopid

Chemical Class: Fibric acid derivative

Therapeutic Class: Antilipemic

CLINICAL PHARMACOLOGY

Mechanism of Action: A fibric acid derivative that inhibits lipolysis of fat in adipose tissue; decreases liver uptake of free fatty acids and reduces hepatic triglyceride production. Inhibits synthesis of VLDL carrier apolipoprotein B. ***Therapeutic Effect:*** Lowers serum cholesterol and triglycerides (decreases VLDL, LDL; increases HDL).

Pharmacokinetics

Well absorbed from the GI tract. Protein binding: 99%. Metabolized in liver. Primarily excreted in urine. Not removed by hemodialysis. ***Half-life:*** 1.5 hr.

INDICATIONS AND DOSAGES

Hyperlipidemia

PO

Adults, Elderly. 1200 mg/day in 2 divided doses 30 min before breakfast and dinner.

AVAILABLE FORMS

• *Tablets:* 600 mg.

CONTRAINDICATIONS: Liver dysfunction (including primary biliary cirrhosis), preexisting gallbladder disease, severe renal dysfunction

PREGNANCY AND LACTATION: Pregnancy category C; excretion into breast milk unknown; use caution in nursing mothers

SIDE EFFECTS

Frequent (20%)

Dyspepsia

Occasional (10%-2%)

Abdominal pain, diarrhea, nausea, vomiting, fatigue

Rare (less than 2%)

Constipation, acute appendicitis, vertigo, headache, rash, pruritus, altered taste

SERIOUS REACTIONS

• Cholelithiasis, cholecystitis, acute appendicitis, pancreatitis, and malignancy occur rarely.

INTERACTIONS

Drugs

3 *Binding resins:* Reduced bioavailability of gemfibrozil, separate doses by >2 hr

3 *Glyburide:* Increased risk of hypoglycemia

2 *HMG CoA reductase inhibitors (atorvastatin, fluvastatin, lovastatin, pravastatin, simvastatin):* Increased likelihood of drug-induced myopathy

3 *Pioglitazone:* Increases pioglitazone plasma concentrations; enhanced hypoglycemic effect may occur

3 *Repaglinide:* Increases serum concentrations of repaglinide; enhanced hypoglycemic effects are likely to result

2 *Warfarin:* Increased hypoprothrombinemic, response to warfarin

SPECIAL CONSIDERATIONS

PATIENT/FAMILY EDUCATION

• May cause dizziness or blurred vision; use caution while driving or performing other tasks requiring alertness

• Notify clinician if GI side effects become pronounced

• Follow the prescribed diet

• Take gemfibrozil before meals

• Periodic laboratory tests are an essential part of therapy

MONITORING PARAMETERS

• Serum CK level in patients complaining of muscle pain, tenderness, or weakness

• Periodic CBC during first 12 mo of therapy

• Periodic LFTs; discontinue therapy if abnormalities persist
• Blood glucose
• Pattern of daily bowel activity and stool consistency
• Serum LDL, VLDL, triglyceride, and cholesterol levels for a therapeutic response
• Evaluate the patient for dizziness and headache
• Assess the patient for pain, especially in the right upper quadrant of the abdomen, because epigastric pain may indicate cholecystitis or cholelithiasis

gemifloxacin mesylate

(gem-ah-flox'-a-sin)

Rx: Factive

Chemical Class: Fluoroquinolone derivative

Therapeutic Class: Antibiotic

CLINICAL PHARMACOLOGY

Mechanism of Action: A fluoroquinolone that inhibits the enzyme DNA gyrase in susceptible microorganisms, interfering with bacterial cell replication and repair. ***Therapeutic Effect:*** Bactericidal.

Pharmacokinetics

Rapidly and well absorbed from the GI tract. Protein binding: 70%. Widely distributed. Penetrates well into lung tissue and fluid. Undergoes limited metabolism in the liver. Primarily excreted in feces; lesser amount eliminated in urine. Partially removed by hemodialysis. ***Half-life:*** 4-12 hr.

INDICATIONS AND DOSAGES

Acute bacterial exacerbation of chronic bronchitis

PO

Adults, Elderly. 320 mg once a day for 5 days.

Community-acquired pneumonia

PO

Adults, Elderly. 320 mg once a day for 7 days.

Dosage in renal impairment

Dosage and frequency are modified based on creatinine clearance.

Creatinine Clearance	Dosage
greater than 40 ml/min	320 mg once a day
40 ml/min or less	160 mg once a day

AVAILABLE FORMS

• *Tablets:* 320 mg.

CONTRAINDICATIONS: Concurrent use of amiodarone, quinidine, procainamide, or sotalol; history of prolonged QTc interval; hypersensitivity to fluoroquinolones; uncorrected electrolyte disorders (such as hypokalemia and hypomagnesemia)

PREGNANCY AND LACTATION: Pregnancy category C; breast milk excretion in humans unknown

SIDE EFFECTS

Occasional (4%-2%)

Diarrhea, rash, nausea

Rare (1% or less)

Headache, abdominal pain, dizziness

SERIOUS REACTIONS

• Antibiotic-associated colitis may result from altered bacterial balance.
• Hypersensitivity reactions, including photosensitivity (as evidenced by rash, pruritus, blisters, edema, and burning skin), have occurred.
• Tendonitis and rupture of the shoulder, hand, and Achilles tendons that required surgical repair or resulted in prolonged disability have been reported.

INTERACTIONS

Drugs

3 *Antacids containing aluminum, magnesium, or calcium:* Reduced

absorption of gemifloxacin; do not take within 3 hrs of dose of gemifloxacin

⚠ *Amiodarone:* Additive QT interval prolongation

3 *Cyclosporine:* Increases the risk of nephrotoxicity

3 *Didanosine, buffered form:* Markedly reduced absorption of gemifloxacin; do not take within 3 hrs of dose of gemifloxacin

⚠ *Erythromycin:* Additive QT interval prolongation

3 *Iron:* Reduced absorption of gemifloxacin; do not take within 3 hrs of dose of gemifloxacin

3 *Probenecid:* Increases gemifloxacin serum concentration

⚠ *Procainamide:* Additive QT interval prolongation

3 *Propranolol:* Inhibits metabolism of propranolol; increased plasma propranolol level

⚠ *Quinidine:* Additive QT interval prolongation

⚠ *Sotalol:* Additive QT interval prolongation

3 *Sucralfate:* Reduced absorption of gemifloxacin; do not take within 2 hrs of dose of gemifloxacin

3 *Zinc:* Reduced absorption of gemifloxacin; do not take within 3 hrs of dose of gemifloxacin

SPECIAL CONSIDERATIONS

- Use with caution in pneumonia due to *Klebsiella pneumoniae.* In clinical trials, 2 treatment failures occurred out of 13 cases

PATIENT/FAMILY EDUCATION

- May be taken with or without meals
- Do not chew pills
- Take for the full course of therapy
- Drink several glasses of water between meals
- Should not be taken within 3 hrs of multivitamins (containing iron or zinc), antacids (containing magnesium, calcium, or aluminum), sucralfate, or didanosine chewable/buffered tablets
- Discontinue treatment, rest and refrain from exercise, and inform prescriber if pain, inflammation, or rupture of a tendon occurs
- Test reaction to this drug before operating an automobile or machinery or engaging in activities requiring mental alertness or coordination

MONITORING PARAMETERS

- Liver function test results and WBC count
- Signs and symptoms of infection
- Pattern of daily bowel activity and stool consistency
- Skin for rash
- Be alert for signs and symptoms of superinfection, including genital pruritus and oral candidiasis
- Calculate the QT and QTc intervals to check for prolongation

gentamicin sulfate

(jen-ta-mye'-sin sul'-fate)

Rx: Garamycin, Garamycin Ophthalmic, Garamycin Topical, Genoptic, Gentacidin, Gentak, Gentacidin, Ocu-Mycin

Combinations

Rx: with prednisolone (Pred-G)

Chemical Class: Aminoglycoside

Therapeutic Class: Antibiotic

CLINICAL PHARMACOLOGY

Mechanism of Action: An aminoglycoside antibiotic that irreversibly binds to the protein of bacterial ribosomes. ***Therapeutic Effect:*** Interferes with protein synthesis of susceptible microorganisms. Bactericidal.

Pharmacokinetics

Rapid, complete absorption after IM administration. Protein binding: less than 30%. Widely distributed (does not cross the blood-brain barrier, low concentrations in CSF). Excreted unchanged in urine. Removed by hemodialysis. ***Half-life:*** 2-4 hr (increased in impaired renal function and neonates; decreased in cystic fibrosis and burn or febrile patients).

INDICATIONS AND DOSAGES

Acute pelvic, bone, intraabdominal, joint, respiratory tract, burn wound, postoperative, and skin or skin-structure infections; complicated UTIs; septicemia; meningitis

IV, IM

Adults, Elderly. Usual dosage, 3-6 mg/kg/day in divided doses q8h or 4-6.6 mg/kg once a day.

Children 5-12 yrs. Usual dosage, 2-2.5 mg/kg/dose q8h.

Children younger than 5 yrs. Usual dosage, 2.5 mg/kg/dose q8h.

Neonates. Usual dosage, 2.5-3.5 mg/kg/dose q8-12h.

Hemodialysis

IV, IM

Adults, Elderly. 0.5-0.7 mg/kg/dose after dialysis.

Children. 1.25-1.75 mg/kg/dose after dialysis.

Intrathecal

Adults. 4-8 mg/day.

Children 3 mo-12 yr. 1-2 mg/day.

Neonates. 1 mg/day.

Superficial eye infections

Ophthalmic Ointment

Adults, Elderly. Usual dosage, apply thin strip to conjunctiva 2-3 times a day.

Ophthalmic Solution

Adults, Elderly, Children. Usual dosage, 1-2 drops q2-4h up to 2 drops/hr.

Superficial skin infections

Topical

Adults, Elderly. Usual dosage, apply 3-4 times/day.

Dosage in renal impairment

Creatinine clearance greater than 41-60 ml/min. Dosage interval q12h.

Creatinine clearance 20-40 ml/min. Dosage interval q24h.

Creatinine clearance less than 20 ml/min. Monitor levels to determine dosage interval.

AVAILABLE FORMS

- *Injection:* 10 mg/ml, 40 mg/ml (Garamycin), 40 mg/50 ml-0.9%, 60 mg/50 ml-0.9%, 60 mg/100 ml-0.9%, 70 mg/50 ml-0.9%, 80 mg/50 ml-0.9%, 80 mg/100 ml-0.9%, 90 mg/100 ml-0.9%, 100 mg/50 ml-0.9%, 100 mg/100 ml-0.9%.
- *Ophthalmic Solution (Garamycin Ophthalmic, Gentacidin, Genoptic, Gentak, Ocu-Mycin):* 0.3%.
- *Ophthalmic Ointment (Gentak):* 0.3%.
- *Cream (Garamycin Topical):* 0.1%.
- *Ointment:* 0.1%.

UNLABELED USES: Topical: Prophylaxis of minor bacterial skin infections, treatment of dermal ulcer

CONTRAINDICATIONS: Hypersensitivity to other aminoglycosides (cross-sensitivity), or their components. Sulfite sensitivity may result in anaphylaxis, especially in asthmatic patients.

PREGNANCY AND LACTATION: Pregnancy category C; ototoxicity has not been reported as an effect of *in utero* exposure; 8th cranial nerve toxicity in the fetus is well known following exposure to other aminoglycosides and could potentially occur with gentamicin; potentiation of magnesium sulfate-induced neuromuscular weakness in neonates has been reported, use caution during the last 32 hr of pregnancy; data on excretion into breast milk are lacking

SIDE EFFECTS

Occasional

IM: Pain, induration

IV: Phlebitis, thrombophlebitis, hypersensitivity reactions (fever, pruritus, rash, urticaria)

Ophthalmic: Burning, tearing, itching, blurred vision

Topical: Redness, itching

Rare

Alopecia, hypertension, weakness

SERIOUS REACTIONS

• Nephrotoxicity (as evidenced by increased BUN and serum creatinine levels and decreased creatinine clearance) may be reversible if the drug is stopped at the first sign of symptoms.

• Irreversible ototoxicity (manifested as tinnitus, dizziness, ringing or roaring in the ears, and diminished hearing), and neurotoxicity (as evidenced by headache, dizziness, lethargy, tremor, and visual disturbances) occur occasionally. The risk of these effects increases with higher dosages or prolonged therapy and when the solution is applied directly to the mucosa.

• Superinfections, particularly with fungal infections, may result from bacterial imbalance no matter which administration route is used.

• Ophthalmic application may cause paresthesia of conjunctiva or mydriasis.

INTERACTIONS

Drugs

3 *Amphotericin B:* Synergistic nephrotoxicity

2 *Atracurium:* Gentamicin potentiates respiratory depression by atracurium

3 *Carbenicillin:* Potential for inactivation of gentamicin in patients with renal failure

3 *Carboplatin:* Additive nephrotoxicity or ototoxicity

3 *Cephalosporins:* Increased potential for nephrotoxicity in patients with preexisting renal disease

3 *Cisplatin:* Additive nephrotoxicity or ototoxicity

3 *Cyclosporine:* Additive nephrotoxicity

2 *Ethacrynic acid:* Additive ototoxicity

3 *Indomethacin:* Reduced renal clearance of gentamicin in premature infants

3 *Methoxyflurane:* Additive nephrotoxicity

2 *Nephrotoxic medications, other aminoglycosides, ototoxic medications:* May increase the risk of nephrotoxicity and ototoxicity

2 *Neuromuscular blocking agents:* Gentamicin potentiates respiratory depression by neuromuscular blocking agents

3 *NSAIDs:* May reduce renal clearance of gentamicin

3 *Penicillins (extended spectrum):* Potential for inactivation of gentamicin in patients with renal failure

3 *Piperacillin:* Potential for inactivation of gentamicin in patients with renal failure

2 *Succinylcholine:* Gentamicin potentiates respiratory depression by succinylcholine

3 *Ticarcillin:* Potential for inactivation of gentamicin in patients with renal failure

3 *Vancomycin:* Additive nephrotoxicity or ototoxicity

2 *Vecuronium:* Gentamicin potentiates respiratory depression by vecuronium

Labs

• *Amino acids:* Increase in urine amino acids
• *AST:* False elevations
• *Protein:* False urine elevations

SPECIAL CONSIDERATIONS

PATIENT/FAMILY EDUCATION

• Report headache, dizziness, loss of hearing, ringing, roaring in ears, or feeling of fullness in head
• Tilt head back, place medication in conjunctival sac, and close eyes
• Apply light finger pressure on lacrimal sac for 1 min following instillation (gtt)
• May cause temporary blurring of vision following administration (ophth)
• Notify clinician if stinging, burning, or itching becomes pronounced or if redness, irritation, swelling, decreasing vision, or pain persists or worsens (ophth)
• Do not touch tip of container to any surface (ophth)
• For external use only (ophth)
• Cleanse affected area of skin prior to application (top)
• Notify clinician if condition worsens or if rash or irritation develops (top)
• IM injection may cause discomfort

MONITORING PARAMETERS

• Urinalysis for proteinuria, cells, casts
• Urine output
• Serum peak, drawn at 30-60 min after IV INF or 60 min after IM inj, trough level drawn just before next dose; adjust dosage per levels (usual therapeutic plasma levels, peak 4-8 mcg/ml, trough ≤2 mcg/ml)
• Serum creatinine for CrCl calculation
• Serum calcium, magnesium, sodium
• Audiometric testing, assess hearing before, during, after treatment
• Evaluate the IV infusion site for signs and symptoms of phlebitis, such as heat, pain, and red streaking over the vein
• Skin for rash
• If giving ophthalmic gentamicin, monitor the patient's eye for burning, itching, redness, and tearing
• If giving topical gentamicin, monitor the patient for itching and redness
• Be alert for signs and symptoms of superinfection, particularly changes in the oral mucosa, diarrhea, and genital or anal pruritus
• In patients with neuromuscular disorders, assess the respiratory response carefully

glatiramer

(gla-teer'-a-mer)

Rx: Copaxone

Chemical Class: Polypeptide, synthetic

Therapeutic Class: Multiple sclerosis agent

CLINICAL PHARMACOLOGY

Mechanism of Action: An immunosuppressive whose exact mechanism is unknown. May act by modifying immune processes thought to be responsible for the pathogenesis of multiple sclerosis (MS). ***Therapeutic Effect:*** Slows progression of MS.

Pharmacokinetics

Substantial fraction of glatiramer is hydrolyzed locally. Some fraction of injected material enters lymphatic circulation, reaching regional lymph nodes; some may enter systemic circulation intact.

INDICATIONS AND DOSAGES

MS

Subcutaneous

Adults, Elderly. 20 mg once a day.

AVAILABLE FORMS

- *Injection:* 20 mg/ml in prefilled syringes.

CONTRAINDICATIONS: Hypersensitivity to mannitol

PREGNANCY AND LACTATION: Pregnancy category B; excretion into breast milk unknown; use caution in nursing mothers

SIDE EFFECTS

Expected (73%-40%)

Pain, erythema, inflammation, or pruritus at injection site; asthenia

Frequent (27%-18%)

Arthralgia, vasodilation, anxiety, hypertonia, nausea, transient chest pain, dyspnea, flu-like symptoms, rash, pruritus

Occasional (17%-10%)

Palpitations, back pain, diaphoresis, rhinitis, diarrhea, urinary urgency

Rare (8%-6%)

Anorexia, fever, neck pain, peripheral edema, ear pain, facial edema, vertigo, vomiting

SERIOUS REACTIONS

- Infection is a common effect.
- Lymphadenopathy occurs occasionally.

SPECIAL CONSIDERATIONS

- May be useful for relapsing-remitting multiple sclerosis in patients who are not benefiting from, or are intolerant of, interferon β-1 a/b; less effective in patients with advanced disease or chronic-progressive multiple sclerosis; not a cure for multiple sclerosis and benefits achieved are relatively modest
- Sites for injection include arms, abdomen, hips, and thighs

PATIENT/FAMILY EDUCATION

- Teach the patient and caregiver how to administer subcutaneous injections and properly dispose of needles
- Notify the physician if rash, weakness, difficulty breathing or swallowing, or itching or swelling of the legs occurs
- Avoid pregnancy during glatiramer therapy

MONITORING PARAMETERS

- Assess for injection site reactions
- Monitor the patient for fever, chills, and other evidence of infection

glimepiride

(glye'-meh-pye-ride)

Rx: Amaryl

Chemical Class: Sulfonylurea (2nd generation)

Therapeutic Class: Antidiabetic; hypoglycemic

CLINICAL PHARMACOLOGY

Mechanism of Action: A second-generation sulfonylurea that promotes release of insulin from beta cells of the pancreas and increases insulin sensitivity at peripheral sites. ***Therapeutic Effect:*** Lowers blood glucose concentration.

Pharmacokinetics

Route	Onset	Peak	Duration
PO	N/A	2-3 hrs	24 hrs

Completely absorbed from the GI tract. Protein binding: greater than 99%. Metabolized in the liver. Excreted in urine and eliminated in feces. ***Half-life:*** 5-9.2 hrs.

INDICATIONS AND DOSAGES

Diabetes mellitus

PO

Adults, Elderly. Initially, 1-2 mg once a day, with breakfast or first main meal. Maintenance: 1-4 mg once a day. After dose of 2 mg is reached, dosage should be increased in increments of up to 2 mg q1-2wk, based on blood glucose response. Maximum: 8 mg/day.

Dosage in renal impairment
PO
Adults. 1 mg once/day.

AVAILABLE FORMS

• *Tablets:* 1 mg, 2 mg, 4 mg.

CONTRAINDICATIONS: Diabetic complications, such as ketosis, acidosis, and diabetic coma; monotherapy for type 1 diabetes mellitus; severe hepatic or renal impairment; stress situations, including severe infection, trauma, and surgery

PREGNANCY AND LACTATION: Pregnancy category C; inappropriate for use during pregnancy due to inadequacy for blood glucose control, potential for prolonged neonatal hypoglycemia, and risk of congenital abnormalities; insulin is the drug of choice for control of blood sugars during pregnancy; breast milk secretion, unknown; the potential for neonatal hypoglycemia dictates caution in nursing mothers

SIDE EFFECTS

Frequent

Altered taste sensation, dizziness, somnolence, weight gain, constipation, diarrhea, heartburn, nausea, vomiting, stomach fullness, headache

Occasional

Increased sensitivity of skin to sunlight, peeling of skin, itching, rash

SERIOUS REACTIONS

• Overdose or insufficient food intake may produce hypoglycemia, especially with increased glucose demands.

• GI hemorrhage, cholestatic hepatic jaundice, leukopenia, thrombocytopenia, pancytopenia, agranulocytosis, and aplastic or hemolytic anemia occur rarely.

INTERACTIONS

Drugs

3 *Anabolic steroids:* Enhanced hypoglycemic response

3 *Angiotensin-converting enzyme inhibitors:* Increased risk of hypoglycemia

3 *Antacids:* Enhanced rate of absorption

3 *Aspirin:* Enhanced hypoglycemic effect

3 *β-Adrenergic blockers:* Altered response to hypoglycemia; prolonged recovery of normoglycemia, hypertension, blockade of tachycardia; may increase blood glucose concentration

3 *Clofibrate:* Enhanced effects of oral hypoglycemic drugs

3 *Corticosteroids:* Increased blood glucose in diabetic patients

3 *Cyclosporine:* Increased cyclosporine levels

⚠ *Ethanol:* Excessive intake may lead to altered glycemic control; Antabuse-like reaction may occur

3 *Gemfibrozil:* Increased risk of hypoglycemia

3 *H_2-receptor antagonists:* Enhanced rate of absorption

3 *MAOIs:* Excessive hypoglycemia may occur in patients with diabetes

3 *Oral anticoagulants:* May increase the effects of oral anticoagulants

2 *Phenylbutazole:* Increases serum concentrations of oral hypoglycemic drugs

3 *Proton pump blockers:* Enhanced rate of absorption

3 *Rifampin:* Reduced sulfonylurea concentrations

3 *Sulfonamides:* Enhanced hypoglycemic effects of sulfonylureas

3 *Thiazide diuretics:* Potential increased dosage requirement of antidiabetic drugs

SPECIAL CONSIDERATIONS

• No demonstrated advantage over existing second generation sulfonylureas

PATIENT/FAMILY EDUCATION

- Multiple drug interactions, including alcohol and salicylates
- Symptoms of hypoglycemia: tingling lips/tongue, nausea, confusion, fatigue, sweating, hunger, visual changes (spots)
- A prescribed diet is a principal part of treatment; do not skip or delay meals
- Carry candy, sugar packets, or other sugar supplements for immediate response to hypoglycemia and urge the patient to wear medical alert identification stating he or she has diabetes
- Consult the physician when glucose demands are altered, such as with fever, heavy physical activity, infection, stress, or trauma
- Wear sunscreen and protective eyewear to prevent the effects of light sensitivity

MONITORING PARAMETERS

- Self-monitored blood glucoses; glycosolated hemoglobin q3-6mo
- Assess for signs and symptoms of hypoglycemia (anxiety, cool wet skin, diplopia, dizziness, headache, hunger, numbness in mouth, tachycardia, tremors), or hyperglycemia (deep rapid breathing, dim vision, fatigue, nausea, polydipsia, polyphagia, polyuria, vomiting)
- Be alert to conditions that alter blood glucose requirements, such as fever, increased activity, stress, or a surgical procedure

glipizide

(glip'-i-zide)

Rx: Glucotrol, Glucotrol XL

Combinations

Rx: with metformin (Metaglip)

Chemical Class: Sulfonylurea (2nd generation)

Therapeutic Class: Antidiabetic; hypoglycemic

G

CLINICAL PHARMACOLOGY

Mechanism of Action: A second-generation sulfonylurea that promotes the release of insulin from beta cells of the pancreas and increases insulin sensitivity at peripheral sites. ***Therapeutic Effect:*** Lowers blood glucose concentration.

Pharmacokinetics

Route	*Onset*	*Peak*	*Duration*
PO	15-30 mins	2-3 hrs	12-24 hrs
Extended-release	2-3 hrs	6-12 hrs	24 hrs

Well absorbed from the GI tract. Protein binding: 99%. Metabolized in the liver. Excreted in urine. ***Half-life:*** 2-4 hrs.

INDICATIONS AND DOSAGES

Diabetes mellitus

PO

Adults. Initially, 5 mg/day or 2.5 mg in the elderly or those with hepatic disease. Adjust dosage in 2.5- to 5-mg increments at intervals of several days. Maximum single dose: 15 mg. Maximum dose/day: 40 mg. Maintenance (extended-release tablet): 20 mg/day.

Elderly. Initially, 2.5-5 mg/day. May increase by 2.5-5 mg/day q1-2wk.

AVAILABLE FORMS

- *Tablets (Glucotrol):* 5 mg, 10 mg.
- *Tablets (Extended-Release [Glucotrol XL]):* 2.5 mg, 5 mg, 10 mg.

CONTRAINDICATIONS: Diabetic ketoacidosis with or without coma, type 1 diabetes mellitus

PREGNANCY AND LACTATION: Pregnancy category C; inappropriate for use during pregnancy due to inadequate for blood glucose control, potential for prolonged neonatal hypoglycemia, and risk of congenital abnormalities; insulin is the drug of choice for control of blood sugars during pregnancy; breast milk secretion unknown; the potential for neonatal hypoglycemia dictates caution in nursing mothers

SIDE EFFECTS

Frequent

Altered taste sensation, dizziness, somnolence, weight gain, constipation, diarrhea, heartburn, nausea, vomiting, stomach fullness, headache

Occasional

Increased sensitivity of skin to sunlight, peeling of skin, itching, rash

SERIOUS REACTIONS

• Overdose or insufficient food intake may produce hypoglycemia, especially with increased glucose demands.

• GI hemorrhage, cholestatic hepatic jaundice, leukopenia, thrombocytopenia, pancytopenia, agranulocytosis, and aplastic or hemolytic anemia occurs rarely.

INTERACTIONS

Drugs

3 *Anabolic steroids:* Enhanced hypoglycemic response

3 *Angiotensin-converting enzyme inhibitor:* Increased risk of hypoglycemia

3 *Antacids:* Enhanced rate of absorption

3 *Aspirin:* Enhanced hypoglycemic effects

3 *β-Adrenergic blockers:* Altered response to hypoglycemia; prolonged recovery of normoglycemia, hypertension, blockade of tachycardia; may increase blood glucose concentration

3 *Clofibrate:* Enhanced effects of oral hypoglycemic drugs

3 *Corticosteroids:* Increased blood glucose in diabetic patients

▲ *Ethanol:* Excessive intake may lead to altered glycemic control; Antabuse-like reaction may occur

3 *Gemfibrozil:* Increased risk of hypoglycemia

3 *H_2-receptor antagonists (cimetidine, ranitidine, etc.):* Enhanced rate of absorption

3 *Lithium:* May decrease the effects of glipizide

3 *MAOIs:* Excessive hypoglycemia may occur in patient with diabetes

3 *Oral anticoagulants:* May increase the effects of oral anticoagulants

3 *Phenylbutazone:* Increases serum concentrations of oral hypoglycemics

3 *Quinidine, large doses of salicylates:* May increase the effects of glipizide

3 *Rifampin:* Reduced sulfonylurea concentrations

3 *Sulfonamides:* Enhanced hypoglycemic effects of sulfonylureas

3 *Thiazide diuretics:* Potential increased dosage requirement of antidiabetic drugs

SPECIAL CONSIDERATIONS

PATIENT/FAMILY EDUCATION

• Administer 30 min ac

• Notify clinician of fever, sore throat, rash, unusual bruising, or bleeding

• Multiple drug interactions, including alcohol and salicylates

• Symptoms of hypoglycemia: tingling lips/tongue, nausea, confusion, fatigue, sweating, hunger, visual changes (spots)

• Carry candy, sugar packets, or other sugar supplements for immediate response to hypoglycemia
• Notify clinician of fever, sore throat, rash, unusual bruising, or bleeding
• Diet is a principal part of treatment; do not skip or delay meals
• Wear sunscreen and protective eyewear to prevent the effects of light sensitivity

MONITORING PARAMETERS

• Self-monitored blood glucose; glycosylated hemoglobin q3-6 mo
• Assess the patient for signs and symptoms of hypoglycemia (anxiety, cool wet skin, diplopia, dizziness, headache, hunger, numbness in mouth, tachycardia, tremors), or hyperglycemia (deep rapid breathing, dim vision, fatigue, nausea, polydipsia, polyphagia, polyuria, vomiting)
• Be alert to conditions that alter blood glucose requirements, such as fever, increased activity, stress, or a surgical procedure

glucagon hydrochloride

(gloo'-ka-gon)

Rx: GlucaGen, GlucaGen Diagnostic Kit, Glucagon, Glucagon Diagnostic Kit, Glucagon Emergency Kit

Chemical Class: Polypeptide hormone

Therapeutic Class: Antihypoglycemic

CLINICAL PHARMACOLOGY

Mechanism of Action: A glucose elevating agent that promotes hepatic glycogenolysis, gluconeogenesis. Stimulates production of cyclic adenosine monophosphate (cAMP), which results in increased plasma glucose concentration, smooth muscle relaxation, and an inotropic myocardial effect. ***Therapeutic Effect:*** Increases plasma glucose level.

Pharmacokinetics

Onset of action occurs within 4-10 mins following IM administration. Recovery occurs within 12-32 mins. ***Half-life:*** 8-18 mins.

INDICATIONS AND DOSAGES

Hypoglycemia

IV, IM, Subcutaneous

Adults, Elderly, Children weighing more than 20 kg. 0.5-1 mg. May give 1 or 2 additional doses if response is delayed.

Children weighing 20 kg or less. 0.5 mg.

Diagnostic aid

IV, IM

Adults, Elderly. 0.25-2 mg 10 min prior to procedure.

AVAILABLE FORMS

• *Powder for Injection (GlucaGen, GlucaGen Diagnostic Kit, Glucagon, Glucagon Diagnostic Kit, Glucagon Emergency Kit):* 1 mg.

UNLABELED USES: Treatment of esophageal obstruction due to foreign bodies, toxicity associated with beta blockers or calcium channel blockers

CONTRAINDICATIONS: Hypersensitivity to glucagon or beef or pork proteins, known pheochromocytoma

PREGNANCY AND LACTATION: Pregnancy category B; excretion into breast milk unknown; use caution in nursing mothers

SIDE EFFECTS

Occasional

Nausea, vomiting

Rare

Allergic reaction, such as urticaria, respiratory distress, and hypotension

SERIOUS REACTIONS

• Overdose may produce persistent nausea and vomiting and hypokalemia, marked by severe weakness, decreased appetite, irregular heartbeat, and muscle cramps.

INTERACTIONS

Drugs

3 *Oral anticoagulants:* Enhanced hypoprothrombinemic response to warfarin and possibly other oral anticoagulants

SPECIAL CONSIDERATIONS

PATIENT/FAMILY EDUCATION

• Notify clinician when hypoglycemic reactions occur so that antidiabetic therapy can be adjusted

• Treat early signs of hypoglycemia with a simple sugar first, such as hard candy, honey, orange juice, sugar cubes, or table sugar dissolved in water or juice, followed by a protein source, such as cheese and crackers, half a sandwich, or a glass of milk

MONITORING PARAMETERS

• Blood sugar, level of consciousness

• Have IV dextrose readily available in case the patient does not awaken within 20 mins

• Assess the patient for evidence of an allergic reaction, including hypotension, respiratory difficulty, and urticaria

glyburide

(glye'-byoor-ide)

Rx: DiaBeta, Glycron, Glynase, Glynase Pres-Tab, Micronase

Combinations

Rx: with metformin (Glucovance)

Chemical Class: Sulfonylurea (2nd generation)

Therapeutic Class: Antidiabetic; hypoglycemic

CLINICAL PHARMACOLOGY

Mechanism of Action: A second-generation sulfonylurea that promotes release of insulin from beta cells of the pancreas and increases insulin sensitivity at peripheral sites. ***Therapeutic Effect:*** Lowers blood glucose concentration.

Pharmacokinetics

Route	*Onset*	*Peak*	*Duration*
PO	0.25-1 hr	1-2 hrs	12-24 hrs

Well absorbed from the GI tract. Protein binding: 99%. Metabolized in the liver to weakly active metabolite. Primarily excreted in urine. Not removed by hemodialysis. ***Half-life:*** 1.4-1.8 hr.

INDICATIONS AND DOSAGES

Diabetes mellitus

PO

Adults. Initially, 2.5-5 mg. May increase by 2.5 mg/day at weekly intervals. Maintenance: 1.25-20 mg/day. Maximum: 20 mg/day.

Elderly. Initially, 1.25-2.5 mg/day. May increase by 1.25-2.5 mg/day at 1- to 3-wk intervals.

PO (micronized tablets)

Adults, Elderly. Initially, 0.75-3 mg/day. May increase by 1.5 mg/day at weekly intervals. Maintenance: 0.75-12 mg/day as a single dose or in divided doses.

Dosage in renal impairment
Glyburide is not recommended in patients with creatinine clearance less than 50 ml/min.

AVAILABLE FORMS
- *Tablets (DiaBeta, Micronase):* 1.25 mg, 2.5 mg, 5 mg.
- *Tablets (Micronized [Glycron, Glynase]):* 1.5 mg, 3 mg, 4.5 mg, 6 mg.

CONTRAINDICATIONS: Diabetic ketoacidosis with or without coma, monotherapy for type 1 diabetes mellitus

PREGNANCY AND LACTATION: Pregnancy category C

SIDE EFFECTS
Frequent
Altered taste sensation, dizziness, somnolence, weight gain, constipation, diarrhea, heartburn, nausea, vomiting, stomach fullness, headache
Occasional
Increased sensitivity of skin to sunlight, peeling of skin, itching, rash

SERIOUS REACTIONS
- Overdose or insufficient food intake may produce hypoglycemia, especially in patients with increased glucose demands.
- Cholestatic jaundice, leukopenia, thrombocytopenia, pancytopenia, agranulocytosis, and aplastic or hemolytic anemia occur rarely.

INTERACTIONS
Drugs
3 *Anabolic steroids:* Enhanced hypoglycemic response
3 *Angiotensin-converting enzyme inhibitor:* Increased risk of hypoglycemia
3 *Antacids:* Enhanced rate of absorption
3 *Aspirin:* Enhanced hypoglycemic effects
3 *β-Adrenergic blockers:* Altered response to hypoglycemia; prolonged recovery of normoglycemia, hypertension, blockade of tachycardia; may increase blood glucose concentration
3 *Clofibrate:* Enhanced effects of oral hypoglycemic drugs
3 *Corticosteroids:* Increased blood glucose in diabetic patients
▲ *Ethanol:* Excessive intake may lead to altered glycemic control; Antabuse-like reaction may occur
3 *Gemfibrozil:* Increased risk of hypoglycemia
3 *H_2-receptor antagonists (cimetidine, ranitidine, etc.):* Enhanced rate of absorption
3 *MAOIs:* Excessive hypoglycemia may occur in patient with diabetes
3 *Phenylbutazone:* Increases serum concentrations of oral hypoglycemics
3 *Rifampin:* Reduced sulfonylurea concentrations
3 *Sulfonamides:* Enhanced hypoglycemic effects of sulfonylureas
3 *Thiazide diuretics:* Potential increased dosage requirement of antidiabetic drugs
3 *Warfarin:* Marked increase in warfarin response and bleeding
Labs
- *Protein:* False-urine increases with Ponceaus dye method

SPECIAL CONSIDERATIONS
- Micronized formulations do not provide bioequivalent serum concentrations to non-micronized formulations; retitrate patients when transferring from any hypoglycemic to micronized glyburide

PATIENT/FAMILY EDUCATION
- Multiple drug interactions including alcohol and salicylates
- Notify clinician of fever, sore throat, rash, unusual bruising, or bleeding
- Do not skip or delay meals
- Be aware of signs and symptoms of hypoglycemia and hyperglycemia

• Carry candy, sugar packets, or other sugar supplements for immediate response to hypoglycemia and wear medical alert identification stating that one has diabetes
• Consult the physician when glucose demands are altered, such as with fever, heavy physical activity, infection, stress, or trauma
• Wear sunscreen and protective eyewear to prevent the effects of light sensitivity

MONITORING PARAMETERS

• Self-monitored blood glucose; glycosylated Hgb q3-6mos
• Assess the patient for signs and symptoms of hypoglycemia (anxiety, cool wet skin, diplopia, dizziness, headache, hunger, perioral numbness, tachycardia, tremors), or hyperglycemia, (deep rapid breathing, dim vision, fatigue, nausea, polydipsia, polyphagia, polyuria, vomiting)
• Be alert to conditions that alter blood glucose requirements, such as fever, increased activity, stress, or a surgical procedure

glycerin

(gli'-ser-in)

Rx: Osmoglyn

OTC: Bausch & Lomb Computer Eye Drops, Fleet Bablylax, Fleet Liquid Glycerin Suppositories for Adults and Children, Fleet Maximum-Strength Glycerin Suppsitories, Fleet Glycerin Suppositories for Adults, Fleet Glycerin Suppositories for Children, Glyrol, Sani-Supp

Chemical Class: Trihydric alcohol

Therapeutic Class: Antiglaucoma agent; diuretic, osmotic; laxative

CLINICAL PHARMACOLOGY

Mechanism of Action: A osmotic dehydrating agent that increases osmotic pressure and draws fluid into colon and stimulates evacuation of inspissated feces. Lowers both intraocular and intracranial pressure by osmotic dehydrating effects. Increases blood flow to ischemic areas, decreases serum-free fatty acids, and increases synthesis of glycerides in the brain. ***Therapeutic Effect:*** Aids in fecal evacuation.

Pharmacokinetics

Well absorbed after PO administration but poorly absorbed after rectal administration. Widely distributed to extracellular space. Rapidly metabolized in liver. Primarily excreted in urine. ***Half-life:*** 30-45 min.

INDICATIONS AND DOSAGES

Constipation

Rectal

Adults, Elderly, Children 6 yrs and older. 3 g/day.

Children younger than 6 yrs. 1-1.5 g/day.

Ophthalmologic procedures

Ophthalmic

Adults, Elderly Children. 1 or 2 drops prior to examination q3-4h.

Reduction of intracranial pressure

PO

Adults, Elderly, Children. 1.5 g/kg/day q4h or 1 g/kg/dose q6h.

Reduction of intraocular pressure

PO

Adults, Elderly, Children. 1-1.8 g/kg 1-1.5 hrs preoperatively.

AVAILABLE FORMS

- *Ophthalmic Solution:* 1% (Bausch & Lomb Computer Eye Drops).
- *Oral Solution:* 50% (Osmoglyn).
- *Rectal Solution:* 2.3 g (Fleet Babylax), 5.6 g (Fleet Liquid Glycerin Suppositories).
- *Suppositories:* 1 g (Fleet Glycerin Suppositories for Children), 2 g (Fleet Glycerin Suppositories), 3 g (Fleet Maximum-Strength Glycerin Suppositories), 82.5% (Sani-Supp).

UNLABELED USES: Viral meningoencephalitis

CONTRAINDICATIONS: Hypersensitivity to any component in the preparation, well-established anuria, severe dehydration, frank or impending acute pulmonary edema, severe cardiac decompensation

PREGNANCY AND LACTATION: Pregnancy category C; data regarding use in breast-feeding are unavailable

SIDE EFFECTS

Frequent

Oral: Nausea, headache,vomiting

Rectal: Some degree of abdominal discomfort, nausea, mild cramps, headache,vomiting

Occasional

Oral: Diarrhea, dizziness, dry mouth or increased thirst

Ophthalmic: Pain and irritation may occur upon instillation

Rectal: Faintness, weakness, abdominal pain, bloating

SERIOUS REACTIONS

- Laxative abuse includes symptoms of abdominal pain, weakness, fatigue, thirst, vomiting, edema, bone pain, fluid and electrolyte imbalance, hypoalbuminemia, and syndromes that mimic colitis.

INTERACTIONS

Labs

- *Increase:* Amniotic fluid phosphatidylglycerol, serum triglycerides
- *Decrease:* Serum ionized calcium

SPECIAL CONSIDERATIONS

PATIENT/FAMILY EDUCATION

- Do not use laxative in the presence of abdominal pain, nausea, or vomiting
- Do not use longer than 1 wk
- Prolonged or frequent use may result in dependency or electrolyte imbalance
- Notify clinician if unrelieved constipation, rectal bleeding, muscle cramps, weakness, or dizziness occurs
- Institute measures to promote defecation such as increasing fluid intake, exercising, and eating a high-fiber diet

MONITORING PARAMETERS

- Blood glucose, intraocular pressure
- Daily bowel activity and stool consistency
- Hydration status
- Serum electrolytes
- Abdominal disturbances

glycopyrrolate

(glye-koe-pye'-roe-late)

Rx: Robinul, Robinul Forte

Chemical Class: Quaternary ammonium derivative

Therapeutic Class: Anticholinergic; antiulcer agent (adjunct); gastrointestinal

CLINICAL PHARMACOLOGY

Mechanism of Action: A quaternary anticholinergic that inhibits action of acetylcholine at postganglionic parasympathetic sites in smooth muscle, secretory glands, and CNS. ***Therapeutic Effect:*** Reduces salivation and excessive secretions of respiratory tract; reduces gastric secretions and acidity.

Pharmacokinetics

Poorly and irregularly absorbed from GI tract after oral administration. Metabolized in the liver. Primarily excreted in urine. ***Half-life:*** 1.7 hr.

INDICATIONS AND DOSAGES

Preoperative inhibition of salivation and excessive respiratory tract secretions

IM

Adults, Elderly. 4 mcg/kg 30-60 min before procedure.

Children 2 yr and older. 4 mcg/kg.

Children younger than 2 yr. 4-9 mcg/kg.

To block effects of anticholinesterase agents

IV

Adults, Elderly. 0.2 mg for each 1 mg neostigmine or 5 mg pyridostigmine.

Peptic ulcer disease, adjunct

IV, IM

Adults, Elderly. 0.1 mg IV or IM 3-4 times/day.

PO

Adults, Elderly. 1-2 mg 2-3 times/day. Maximum: 8 mg/day.

AVAILABLE FORMS

- *Injection (Robinul):* 0.2 mg/ml.
- *Tablets:* 1 mg (Robinul), 2 mg (Robinul Forte).

CONTRAINDICATIONS: Acute hemorrhage, myasthenia gravis, narrow-angle glaucoma, obstructive uropathy, paralytic ileus, tachycardia, ulcerative colitis

PREGNANCY AND LACTATION: Pregnancy category B; has been used prior to cesarean section to decrease gastric secretions; quaternary structure results in limited placental transfer; excretion into breast milk is unknown, but should be minimal due to quaternary structure

SIDE EFFECTS

Frequent

Dry mouth, decreased sweating, constipation

Occasional

Blurred vision, gastric bloating, urinary hesitancy, somnolence (with high dosage), headache, intolerance to light, loss of taste, nervousness, flushing, insomnia, impotence, mental confusion or excitement (particularly in the elderly and children), temporary lightheadedness (with parenteral form), local irritation (with parenteral form)

Rare

Dizziness, faintness

SERIOUS REACTIONS

- Overdose may produce temporary paralysis of ciliary muscle; pupillary dilation; tachycardia; palpitations; hot, dry, or flushed skin; absence of bowel sounds; hyperthermia; increased respiratory rate; EKG abnormalities; nausea; vomiting; rash over face or upper trunk; CNS stimulation; and psychosis (marked by agitation, restlessness, rambling speech, visual hallucinations, paranoid behavior, and delusions, followed by depression).

INTERACTIONS

Drugs

3 *IV anticholinergic agents:* Increased risk of developing ventricular arrhythmias

SPECIAL CONSIDERATIONS

PATIENT/FAMILY EDUCATION

- Glycopyrrolate may cause dry mouth
- Do not become overheated while exercising in hot weather because this may cause heat stroke
- Avoid hot baths and saunas
- Avoid tasks that require mental alertness or motor skills until response to the drug has been established

MONITORING PARAMETERS

- Blood pressure, body temperature, and heart rate
- Bowel sounds for peristalsis and mucous membranes and skin turgor for hydration status
- Palpate the patient's bladder for signs of urine retention, and monitor urine output

gonadorelin hydrochloride

(goe-nad-oh-rell'-in)

Rx: Gonadorelin acetate: Lutrepulse

Rx: Gonadorelin hydrochloride: Factrel

Chemical Class: Gonadotropin-releasing hormone, synthetic

Therapeutic Class: Diagnostic agent; ovulation stimulant

CLINICAL PHARMACOLOGY

Mechanism of Action: A synthetic luteinzing hormone that binds to specific transmembrane glycoprotein receptors on gonadotrophic cells of the anterior pituitary, which then stimulates synthesis and secretion of gonadotropins through mobilization of intracellular calcium, activation of protein kinase C, and gene transcription. ***Therapeutic Effect:*** Stimulates synthesis, release of luteinizing hormone (LH), follicle-stimulating hormone (FSH) from anterior pituitary. Stimulates release of gonadotropin-releasing hormone from hypothalamus.

Pharmacokinetics

Maximal LH release occurs within 20 mins. Metabolized in plasma. Excreted in urine as inactive metabolites. ***Half-life:*** 4 mins.

INDICATIONS AND DOSAGES

Primary hypothalamic amenorrhea

IV Pump

Adults. 5 mcg q90min (range 1-20 mcg); treatment interval 21 days. Refer to manufacturer's manual for proper dilutions/settings on pump. Response usually occurs 2-3 wk after initiation. Continue additional 2 wk after ovulation occurs (maintains corpus luteum).

Gonadotropin function evaluation

IV/Subcutaneous

Inhalation

Adults. 100 mcg. In females, perform test in early follicular phase of menstrual cycle.

AVAILABLE FORMS

- *Powder for Reconstitution, as Acetate:* 100 mcg (Lutrepulse).
- *Powder for Reconstitution, as Hydrochloride:* 100 mcg (Factrel).

UNLABELED USES: Hypothalmic anovulation, hypogonadotropic hypogonadism

CONTRAINDICATIONS: Any condition exacerbated by pregnancy, patients with ovarian cysts or causes of anovulation other than hypothalamic origin, the presence of a hormonally-dependent tumor, any conditions worsened by an increase of reproductive hormones, hypersensitivity to gonadorelin acetate or hydrochloride

PREGNANCY AND LACTATION: Pregnancy category B

SIDE EFFECTS

Occasional

Gonadorelin acetate: Multiple pregnancy, inflammation, infection, mild phlebitis, hematoma at catheter site

Gonadorelin hydrochloride: Swelling, pain, or itching at injection site with subcutanous administration, local or generalized skin rash with chronic subcutaneous administration

Rare

Gonadorelin acetate: Ovarian hyperstimulation

Gonadorelin hydrochloride: Headache, nausea, lightheadedness, abdominal discomfort, hypersensitivity reactions (bronchospasm, tachycardia, flushing, urticaria), induration at injection site

SERIOUS REACTIONS

- Anaphylactic reaction occurs rarely.

INTERACTIONS

Drugs

3 *Androgen, estrogen, glucocorticoid, progestin-containing preparations:* May reduce LH release from anterior pituitary

Labs

- Do not conduct diagnostic tests during administration of these agents

SPECIAL CONSIDERATIONS

PATIENT/FAMILY EDUCATION

- Notify the physician of any nausea, headache, or unusual vaginal discharge

MONITORING PARAMETERS

- Venous blood samples (for LH) drawn after administration at intervals of 15, 30, 45, 60, and 120 min

goserelin acetate

(goe'-se-rel-in)

Rx: Zoladex

Chemical Class: Gonadotropin-releasing hormone analog

Therapeutic Class: Antiendometriosis agent; antineoplastic

CLINICAL PHARMACOLOGY

Mechanism of Action: A gonadotropin-releasing hormone analog and antineoplastic agent that stimulates the release of luteinizing hormone (LH) and follicle-stimulating hormone (FSH) from the anterior pituitary gland. In males, increases testosterone concentrations initially, then suppresses secretion of LH and FSH, resulting in decreased testosterone levels. ***Therapeutic Effect:*** In females, causes a reduction in ovarian size and function, reduction in uterine and mammary gland size, and regression of sex-hormone-responsive tumors. In males, produces pharmacologic castration and decreases the growth of abnormal prostate tissue.

Pharmacokinetics

Protein binding: 27%. Metabolized in liver. Excreted in urine. ***Half-life:*** 4.2 hr (male); 2.3 hr (female).

INDICATIONS AND DOSAGES

Prostatic carcinoma

Implant

Adults older than 18 yr, Elderly. 3.6 mg every 28 days or 10.8 mg q12wk subcutaneously into upper abdominal wall.

Breast carcinoma, endometriosis
Implant
Adults. 3.6 mg every 28 days subcutaneously into upper abdominal wall.
Endometrial thinning
Implant
Adults. 3.6 mg subcutaneously into upper abdominal wall as a single dose or in 2 doses 4 wk apart.

AVAILABLE FORMS
- *Implant (Zoladex):* 3.6 mg, 10.8 mg.

CONTRAINDICATIONS: Pregnancy

PREGNANCY AND LACTATION: Pregnancy category D (advanced breast cancer), X (endometriosis, endometrial thinning); excretion into breast milk unknown; use caution in nursing mothers

SIDE EFFECTS
Frequent
Headache (60%), hot flashes (55%), depression (54%), diaphoresis (45%), sexual dysfunction (21%), decreased erection (18%), lower urinary tract symptoms (13%)
Occasional (10%-5%)
Pain, lethargy, dizziness, insomnia, anorexia, nausea, rash, upper respiratory tract infection, hirsutism, abdominal pain
Rare
Pruritus

SERIOUS REACTIONS
- Arrhythmias, CHF, and hypertension occur rarely.
- Ureteral obstruction and spinal cord compression have been observed. An immediate orchiectomy may be necessary if these conditions occur.

INTERACTIONS
- *Increase:* Alk phosphatase, estradiol, FSH, LH, testosterone levels (first week)
- *Decrease:* Testosterone levels (after first week), progesterone

SPECIAL CONSIDERATIONS
PATIENT/FAMILY EDUCATION
- Notify clinician if regular menstruation persists (females)
- An initial flare in bone pain may occur (prostate cancer therapy)
- The female patient should use nonhormonal contraceptive measures during goserelin therapy

MONITORING PARAMETERS
- Prostate-specific antigen, acid phosphatase, alk phosphatase
- Testosterone level (<25 ng/dl)
- Bone density if therapy prolonged

granisetron hydrochloride
(gra-ni'-se-tron hye-droe-klor'-ide)
Rx: Kytril
Chemical Class: Carbazole derivative
Therapeutic Class: Antiemetic

CLINICAL PHARMACOLOGY
Mechanism of Action: A 5-HT_3 receptor antagonist that acts centrally in the chemoreceptor trigger zone or peripherally at the vagal nerve terminals. ***Therapeutic Effect:*** Prevents nausea and vomiting.
Pharmacokinetics

Route	Onset	Peak	Duration
IV	1-3 mins	N/A	24 hrs

Rapidly and widely distributed to tissues. Protein binding: 65%. Metabolized in the liver to active metabolite. Eliminated in urine and feces. ***Half-life:*** 10-12 hrs (increased in the elderly).

INDICATIONS AND DOSAGES
Prevention of chemotherapy-induced nausea and vomiting
PO
Adults, Elderly. 2 mg 1 hr before chemotherapy or 1 mg 1 hr before and 12 hr after chemotherapy.

IV

Adults, Elderly, Children 2 yr and older. 10 mcg/kg/dose (or 1 mg/dose) within 30 min of chemotherapy.

Prevention of radiation-induced nausea and vomiting

PO

Adults, Elderly. 2 mg once a day, given 1 hr before radiation therapy.

Postoperative nausea or vomiting

PO

Adults, Elderly, Children 4 yr and older. 20-40 mcg/kg as a single postoperative dose.

IV

Adults, Elderly. 1 mg as a single postoperative dose.

Children older than 4 yr. 20-40 mcg/kg. Maximum: 1 mg.

AVAILABLE FORMS

- *Oral Solution:* 2 mg/10 ml.
- *Tablets:* 1 mg.
- *Injection:* 0.1 mg/ml, 1 mg/ml.

UNLABELED USES: PO: Prophylaxis of nausea or vomiting associated with radiation therapy

CONTRAINDICATIONS: None known.

PREGNANCY AND LACTATION: Pregnancy category B; breast milk excretion unknown

SIDE EFFECTS

Frequent (21%-14%)

Headache, constipation, asthenia

Occasional (8%-6%)

Diarrhea, abdominal pain

Rare (less than 2%)

Altered taste, hypersensitivity reaction

SERIOUS REACTIONS

- Hypertension, hypotension, arrhythmias such as sinus bradycardia, atrial fibrillation, varying degrees of AV block, ventricular ectopy including non-sustained tachycardia, and ECG abnormalities have been observed.
- Rare cases of hypersensitivity reactions, sometimes severe (e.g., anaphylaxis, shortness of breath, hypotension, urticaria) have been reported.

INTERACTIONS

Drugs

3 *Hepatic enzyme inducers:* May decrease the effects of granisetron

SPECIAL CONSIDERATIONS

PATIENT/FAMILY EDUCATION

- Granisetron is effective shortly after administration in preventing nausea and vomiting
- The drug may affect the sense of taste temporarily
- Use other methods of reducing nausea and vomiting, such as lying quietly and avoiding strong odors

MONITORING PARAMETERS

- Monitor for therapeutic effect
- Assess for headache
- Assess pattern of daily bowel activity and stool consistency

griseofulvin

(gri-see-oh-ful'-vin)

Rx: Fulvicin P/G, Fulvicin U/F, Grifulvin V, Grisactin 500, Griseofulicin, Gris-PEG

Chemical Class: Penicillium griseofulvum derivative

Therapeutic Class: Antifungal

CLINICAL PHARMACOLOGY

Mechanism of Action: An antifungal that inhibits fungal cell mitosis by disrupting mitotic spindle structure. ***Therapeutic Effect:*** Fungistatic.

Pharmacokinetics

Ultramicrosize is almost completely absorbed. Absorption is significantly enhanced after a fatty meal. Extensively metabolized in liver. Minimal excretion in urine. ***Half-life:*** 24 hr.

INDICATIONS AND DOSAGES

Tinea capitis, tinea corporis, tinea cruris, tinea pedis, tinea unguium

PO (Microsize Tablets, Oral Suspension)

Adults. Usual dosage, 500-1,000 mg as a single dose or in divided doses.

Children 2 yrs and older. Usual dosage, 10-20 mg/kg/day.

PO (Ultramicrosize Tablets)

Adults. Usual dosage, 330-750 mg/day as a single dose or in divided doses.

Children 2 yrs and older. 5-10 mg/kg/day.

AVAILABLE FORMS

- *Oral Suspension (Grifulvin V):* 125 mg/5 ml.
- *Tablets (Microsize [Fulvicin-U/F, Grisactin 500, Grifulvin V]):* 250 mg, 500 mg.
- *Tablets (Ultramicrosize):* 125 mg (Fulvicin P/G, Gris-PEG), 165 mg (Fulvicin P/G), 250 mg (Fulvicin P/G, Gris-PEG), 330 mg (Fulvicin P/G, Griseofulicin).

CONTRAINDICATIONS: Hepatocellular failure, porphyria

PREGNANCY AND LACTATION: Pregnancy category C; since the use of an antifungal is seldom essential during pregnancy, avoid use during this time; excretion into breast milk unknown; use caution in nursing mothers

SIDE EFFECTS

Occasional

Hypersensitivity reaction (including pruritus, rash, and urticaria), headache, nausea, diarrhea, excessive thirst, flatulence, oral thrush, dizziness, insomnia

Rare

Paresthesia of hands or feet, proteinuria, photosensitivity reaction

SERIOUS REACTIONS

- Granulocytopenia occurs rarely.

INTERACTIONS

Drugs

3 *Aspirin:* Reduces plasma salicylate level

3 *Cyclosporine:* Reduces plasma cyclosporine level

3 *Oral contraceptives:* Menstrual irregularities, increased risk of pregnancy possible

3 *Phenobarbital:* Reduces plasma griseofulvin level

3 *Tacrolimus:* Reduces plasma tacrolimus level

3 *Warfarin:* Reduces anticoagulant response

SPECIAL CONSIDERATIONS

- Prior to therapy, the type of fungus responsible for the infection should be identified

PATIENT/FAMILY EDUCATION

- Response to therapy may not be apparent for some time; complete entire course of therapy
- Avoid prolonged exposure to sunlight or sunlamps
- Notify clinician if sore throat or skin rash occurs
- Store oral suspensions at room temp in light-resistant container
- Avoid alcohol because flushing or tachycardia may occur
- Maintain good hygiene to help prevent superinfection
- Separate personal items that come in direct contact with affected areas
- Keep affected areas dry and wear light clothing for ventilation
- Take griseofulvin with foods high in fat, such as milk or ice cream, to reduce GI upset and assist in drug absorption

MONITORING PARAMETERS

- Periodic assessments of renal, hepatic, and hematopoietic function during prolonged therapy
- Skin for rash
- Therapeutic response to the drug
- Daily pattern of bowel activity and stool consistency

• Granulocyte count; if the patient develops granulocytopenia, notify the physician and expect to discontinue the drug
• In patients experiencing headache, establish and document the headache's location, onset, and type

guaifenesin

(gwye-fen'-e-sin)

Rx: Allfen, Amibid LA, Drituss G, Duratuss G, Fenesin, Ganidin NR, GG 200 NR, Guaibid-LA, Guaifenex G, Guaifenex LA, Gua-SR, Guiadrine G-1200, Guiatuss, Humavent LA, Humibid LA, Humibid Pediatric, Iofen, Iophen NR, Liquidbid, Liquidbid 1200, Liquidbid LA, Mucinex, Mucobid-L.A., Muco-Fen, Muco-Fen 1200, Muco-Fen 800, Organ-1 NR, Organidin NR, Pneumomist, Q-Bid LA, Respa-GF, Touro EX
OTC: Anti-Tuss, Breonesin, Genatuss, Glytuss, Guiatuss, Hytuss, Hytuss 2X, Mytussin, Naldecon Senior EX, Robitussin
Combinations
Rx: with codeine (Guiatussin AC); with dextromethorphan (Guaibid-DM); with hydrocodone (Hycotuss); with phenylpropanolamine (Entex LA)
Chemical Class: Glyceryl derivative
Therapeutic Class: Expectorant; mucolytic

CLINICAL PHARMACOLOGY
Mechanism of Action: An expectorant that stimulates respiratory tract secretions by decreasing adhesiveness and viscosity of phlegm. ***Therapeutic Effect:*** Promotes removal of viscous mucus.
Pharmacokinetics
Well absorbed from the GI tract. Metabolized in the liver. Excreted in urine. ***Half-life:*** 1 hr.

INDICATIONS AND DOSAGES
Expectorant
PO
Adults, Elderly, Children older than 12 yrs. 200-400 mg q4h.
Children 6-12 yrs. 100-200 mg q4h. Maximum: 1.2 g/day.
Children 2-5 yrs. 50-100 mg q4h. Maximum: 600 mg/day.
Children younger than 2 yrs. 12 mg/kg/day in 6 divided doses.
PO (Extended-Release)
Adults, Elderly, Children older than 12 yrs. 600-1200 mg q12h. Maximum: 2.4 g/day.
Children 6-12 yrs. 600 mg q12h. Maximum: 1.2 g/day.

AVAILABLE FORMS
• *Tablets (GG 200 NR, Iofen, Organ-1 NR, Organidin NR):* 200 mg.
• *Tablets (Extended-Release):* 300 mg (Humibid Pediatric), 575 mg (Touro EX), 600 mg (Amibid LA, Fenesin, Guaibid-LA, Guaifenex LA, Gua-SR, Humavent LA, Humibid LA, Liquidbid, Liquidbid LA, Mucinex, Mucobid-L.A., Pneumomist, A-Bid LA, Respa-GF), 800 mg (Muco-Fen 800), 1000 mg (Allfen, Muco-Fen), 1200 mg (Duratuss G, Guaifenex G, Guiadrine G-1200, Liquidbid 1200, Muco-Fen 1200).
• *Syrup (Ganidin NR, Guiatuss, Iophen NR, Robitussin, Tussin):* 100 mg/5 ml.

CONTRAINDICATIONS: None known.

PREGNANCY AND LACTATION: Pregnancy category C; excretion into breast milk unknown

SIDE EFFECTS
Rare
Dizziness, headache, rash, diarrhea, nausea, vomiting, abdominal pain
SERIOUS REACTIONS
• Overdose may produce nausea and vomiting.
INTERACTIONS
Labs
• *Interference:* Urine 5-HIAA, VMA

SPECIAL CONSIDERATIONS
PATIENT/FAMILY EDUCATION
• Drink a full glass of water with each dose to help further loosen mucus
• Notify clinician if cough persists after medication has been used for 7 days or cough is associated with headache, high fever, skin rash, or sore throat
• Do not take guaifenesin for chronic cough
• Avoid performing tasks that require mental alertness or motor skills until response to the drug has been established
MONITORING PARAMETERS
• Increase environmental humidity and fluid intake to lower the viscosity of the patient's lung secretions
• Assess the patient for clinical improvement, and record the onset of cough relief

guanabenz acetate
(gwan'-a-benz as'-eh-tayte)
Rx: Wytensin
Chemical Class: Dichlorobenzene derivative
Therapeutic Class: Antihypertensive; centrally acting sympathoplegic

CLINICAL PHARMACOLOGY
Mechanism of Action: An alpha-adrenergic agonist that stimulates alpha$_2$-adrenergic receptors. Inhibits sympathetic cardioaccelerator and vasoconstrictor center to heart, kidneys, peripheral vasculature. ***Therapeutic Effect:*** Decreases systolic, diastolic blood pressure (BP). Chronic use decreases peripheral vascular resistance.
Pharmacokinetics
Well absorbed from gastrointestinal (GI) tract. Widely distributed. Protein binding: 90%. Metabolized in liver. Excreted in urine and feces. Not removed by hemodialysis. ***Half-life:*** 6 hrs.
INDICATIONS AND DOSAGES
Hypertension
PO
Adults. Initially, 4 mg 2 times/day. Increase by 4-8 mg at 1-2-wk intervals.
Elderly. Initially, 4 mg/day. May increase q1-2 wks. Maintenance: 8-16 mg/day. Maximum: 32 mg/day.
AVAILABLE FORMS
• *Tablets:* 4 mg, 8 mg (Wytensin).
CONTRAINDICATIONS: History of hypersensitivity to guanabenz or any component of the formulation
PREGNANCY AND LACTATION: Pregnancy category C; excretion into breast milk unknown; use caution in nursing mothers

G

SIDE EFFECTS

Frequent

Drowsiness, dry mouth, dizziness

Occasional

Weakness, headache, nausea, decreased sexual ability

Rare

Ataxia, sleep disturbances, rash, itching, diarrhea, constipation, altered taste, muscle aches

SERIOUS REACTIONS

- Abrupt withdrawal may result in rebound hypertension manifested as nervousness, agitation, anxiety, insomnia, hand tingling, tremor, flushing, and sweating.
- Overdosage produces hypotension, somnolence, lethargy, irritability, bradycardia, and miosis (pupillary constriction).

INTERACTIONS

Drugs

3 *Alcohol, CNS depressants:* Increases sedation

3 *β-blockers:* Rebound hypertension from guanabenz withdrawal exacerbated by noncardioselective β-blockers

3 *Tricyclic antidepressants:* Inhibit the antihypertensive response

SPECIAL CONSIDERATIONS

PATIENT/FAMILY EDUCATION

- Avoid hazardous activities, since drug may cause drowsiness
- Do not discontinue drug abruptly, or withdrawal symptoms may occur (anxiety, increased BP, headache, insomnia, increased pulse, tremors, nausea, sweating)
- Do not use OTC (cough, cold, or allergy) products unless directed by clinician
- Rise slowly to sitting or standing position to minimize orthostatic hypotension, especially in elderly
- May cause dizziness, fainting, lightheadedness during first few days of therapy
- May cause dry mouth; use hard candy, saliva product, or frequent rinsing of mouth
- Avoid alcohol

MONITORING PARAMETERS

- Blood pressure (posturally), mental depression

guanfacine hydrochloride

(gwahn'-fa-seen hye-droe-klor'-ide)

Rx: Tenex

Chemical Class: Phenylacyl guanidine

Therapeutic Class: Antihypertensive, centrally acting sympathoplegic

CLINICAL PHARMACOLOGY

Mechanism of Action: An alpha-adrenergic agonist that stimulates alpha$_2$-adrenergic receptors and inhibits sympathetic cardioaccelerator and vasoconstrictor center to heart, kidneys, peripheral vasculature. ***Therapeutic Effect:*** Decreases systolic, diastolic blood pressure (BP). Chronic use decreases peripheral vascular resistance.

Pharmacokinetics

Well absorbed from gastrointestinal (GI) tract. Widely distributed. Protein binding: 71%. Metabolized in liver. Excreted in urine and feces. Not removed by hemodialysis. ***Half-life:*** 17 hrs.

INDICATIONS AND DOSAGES

Hypertension

PO

Adults, Elderly. Initially, 1 mg/day. Increase by 1 mg/day at intervals of 3-4 wks up to 3 mg/day in single or divided doses.

AVAILABLE FORMS

- *Tablets:* 1 mg, 2 mg (Tenex).

UNLABELED USES: Attention deficit hyperactivity disorder (ADHD), tic disorders

CONTRAINDICATIONS: History of hypersensitivity to guanfacine or any component of the formulation

PREGNANCY AND LACTATION: Pregnancy category B; excretion into human breast milk unknown

SIDE EFFECTS

Frequent

Dry mouth, somnolence

Occasional

Fatigue, headache, asthenia (loss of strength, energy), dizziness

SERIOUS REACTIONS

- Overdosage may produce difficult breathing, dizziness, faintness, severe drowsiness, bradycardia.

INTERACTIONS

Drugs

3 *β-blockers:* Rebound hypertension from guanfacine withdrawal exacerbated by noncardioselective β-blockers

3 *Cyclosporine, tacrolimus:* Increased immunosuppressant plasma levels

3 *Insulin, sulfonylureas hypoglycemics:* Diminished symptoms of hypoglycemia

3 *Neuroleptics, nitroprusside:* Severe hypotension possible

3 *Phenobarbital, phenytoin:* Reduces elimination half-life and plasma concentration

3 *Tricyclic antidepressants:* Inhibit the antihypertensive response

SPECIAL CONSIDERATIONS

PATIENT/FAMILY EDUCATION

- Avoid hazardous activities, since drug may cause drowsiness
- Do not discontinue oral drug abruptly, or withdrawal symptoms may occur after 3-4 days (anxiety, increased BP, headache, insomnia, increased pulse, tremors, nausea, sweating)
- Do not use OTC (cough, cold, or allergy) products unless directed by clinician
- Rise slowly to sitting or standing position to minimize orthostatic hypotension, especially in elderly
- Dizziness, fainting, lightheadedness may occur during first few days of therapy
- May cause dry mouth; use hard candy, saliva product, or frequent rinsing of mouth
- Avoid alcohol

MONITORING PARAMETERS

- Blood pressure (posturally), blood glucose in patients with diabetes mellitus; confusion, mental depression

---

halcinonide

(hal-sin'-o-nide)

Rx: Halog, Halog-E

Chemical Class: Corticosteroid, synthetic

Therapeutic Class: Corticosteroid, topical

CLINICAL PHARMACOLOGY

Mechanism of Action: A topical corticosteroid that has antiinflammatory, antipruritic, and vasoconstrictive properties. The exact mechanism of the antiinflammatory process is unclear. ***Therapeutic Effect:*** Reduces or prevents tissue response to the inflammatory process.

Pharmacokinetics

Well absorbed systemically. Large variation in absorption among sites. Protein binding: varies. Metabolized in liver. Primarily excreted in urine.

INDICATIONS AND DOSAGES

Dermatoses

Topical

Adults, Elderly. Apply sparingly 1-3 times/day.

AVAILABLE FORMS

- *Cream:* 0.1% (Halog).
- *Cream (emollient base):* 0.1% (Halog-E).
- *Ointment:* 0.1% (Halog).
- *Solution:* 0.1% (Halog).

CONTRAINDICATIONS: History of hypersensitivity to halcinonide or other corticosteroids

PREGNANCY AND LACTATION: Pregnancy category C; unknown whether top application could result in sufficient systemic absorption to produce detectable amounts in breast milk (systemic corticosteroids are secreted into breast milk in quantities not likely to have detrimental effects on infant)

SIDE EFFECTS

Occasional

Itching, redness, irritation, burning at site of application, dryness, folliculitis, acneiform eruptions, hypopigmentation

Rare

Allergic contact dermatitis, maceration of the skin, secondary infection, skin atrophy

SERIOUS REACTIONS

- The serious reactions of long-term therapy and the addition of occlusive dressings are reversible hypothalamic-pituitary-adrenal (HPA) axis suppression, manifestations of Cushing's syndrome, hyperglycemia, and glucosuria.

SPECIAL CONSIDERATIONS

PATIENT/FAMILY EDUCATION

- Apply sparingly only to affected area
- Avoid contact with the eyes
- Do not put bandages or dressings over treated area unless directed by clinician
- Do not use on weeping, denuded, or infected areas
- Discontinue drug, notify clinician if local irritation or fever develops
- Avoid exposure to sunlight

MONITORING PARAMETERS

- Skin for rash

halobetasol

(hal-oh-bay'-ta-sol)

Rx: Ultravate

Chemical Class: Corticosteroid, synthetic

Therapeutic Class: Corticosteroid, topical

CLINICAL PHARMACOLOGY

Mechanism of Action: A corticosteroid that inhibits accumulation of inflammatory cells at inflammation sites, phagocytosis, lysosomal enzyme release and synthesis or release of mediators of inflammation. ***Therapeutic Effect:*** Decreases or prevents tissue response to inflammatory process.

Pharmacokinetics

Variation in absorption among individuals and sites: scrotum 36%, forehead 7%, scalp 4%, forearm 1%.

INDICATIONS AND DOSAGES

Dermatoses, corticosteroid-unresponsive

Topical

Adults, Elderly, Children 12 yrs and older. Apply 1-2 times/day. Maximum: 50 g for 2 wks.

AVAILABLE FORMS

- *Cream:* 0.05% (Ultravate).
- *Ointment:* 0.05% (Ultravate).

CONTRAINDICATIONS: Hypersensitivity to halobetasol or other corticosteroids.

PREGNANCY AND LACTATION: Pregnancy category C; unknown whether top application could result in sufficient systemic absorption to produce detectable amounts in breast milk (systemic corticosteroids are secreted into breast milk in quantities not likely to have detrimental effects on infant)

SIDE EFFECTS

Frequent

Burning, stinging, pruritus

Rare

Cushing's syndrome, hyperglycemia, glucosuria, hypothalamic-pituitary-adrenal axis suppression

SERIOUS REACTIONS

- Overdosage can occur from topically applied halobetasol absorbed in sufficient amounts to produce systemic effects producing reversible adrenal suppression, manifestations of Cushing's syndrome, hyperglycemia, and glucosuria in some patients.

SPECIAL CONSIDERATIONS

PATIENT/FAMILY EDUCATION

- Apply sparingly only to affected area
- Avoid contact with the eyes
- Do not put bandages or dressings over treated area
- Do not use on weeping, denuded, or infected areas
- Discontinue drug, notify clinician if local irritation or fever develops
- Treatment should be limited to 2 wk, and amounts greater than 50 g/wk should not be used

MONITORING PARAMETERS

- Therapeutic response
- Sign of contact dermatitis or worsening of condition

haloperidol

(ha-loe-per'-idole)

Rx: Haldol, Haldol Decanoate

Chemical Class: Butyrophenone derivative

Therapeutic Class: Antipsychotic

CLINICAL PHARMACOLOGY

Mechanism of Action: An antipsychotic, antiemetic, and antidyskinetic agent that competitively blocks postsynaptic dopamine receptors, interrupts nerve impulse movement, and increases turnover of dopamine in the brain. Has strong extrapyramidal and antiemetic effects; weak anticholinergic and sedative effects. ***Therapeutic Effect:*** Produces tranquilizing effect.

Pharmacokinetics

Readily absorbed from the GI tract. Protein binding: 92%. Extensively metabolized in the liver. Primarily excreted in urine. Not removed by hemodialysis. ***Half-life:*** 12-37 hrs PO; 10-19 hr IV; 17-25 hr IM.

INDICATIONS AND DOSAGES

Acute psychosis, delirium

IV

Adults, Elderly. 0.5-50 mg at a rate of 5 mg/min. May repeat as needed.

Psychotic disorder

PO

Adults, Elderly. Initially, 0.5-5 mg 2-3 times a day. Maximum: 100 mg/day.

Severe behavioral problems

PO

Children 3-12 yrs, weighing 15-40 kg. 0.05-0.075 mg/kg/day. Initially, 0.5 mg/day. May increase by 0.5 mg/day q5-7days divided into 2-3 doses a day.

Tourette's disorder

PO

Adults, Elderly. 6-15 mg/day. May increase by 2-mg increments as needed. Maintenance: 9 mg/day.

Children 3-12 yr, weighing 15-40 kg. 0.05-0.075 mg/kg/day. Initially, 0.5 mg/day. May increase by 0.5 mg/day q5-7days divided into 2-3 doses a day.

AVAILABLE FORMS

- *Oral Concentrate:* 1 mg/ml, 2 mg/ml.
- *Tablets (Haldol):* 0.5 mg, 1 mg, 2 mg, 5 mg, 10 mg, 20 mg.
- *Injection (Lactate [Haldol]):* 5 mg/ml.
- *Injection (Decanoate [Haldol Decanoate]):* 50 mg/ml, 100 mg/ml.

UNLABELED USES: Treatment of Huntington's chorea, infantile autism, nausea or vomiting associated with cancer chemotherapy

CONTRAINDICATIONS: Angle-closure glaucoma, CNS depression, myelosuppression, Parkinson's disease, severe cardiac or hepatic disease

PREGNANCY AND LACTATION: Pregnancy category C; has been used for hyperemesis gravidarum, chorea gravidarum, and manic-depressive illness during pregnancy; excreted into breast milk; effect on nursing infant unknown, but may be of concern

SIDE EFFECTS

Frequent

Blurred vision, constipation, orthostatic hypotension, dry mouth, swelling or soreness of female breasts, peripheral edema

Occasional

Allergic reaction, difficulty urinating, decreased thirst, dizziness, decreased sexual function, drowsiness, nausea, vomiting, photosensitivity, lethargy

SERIOUS REACTIONS

- Extrapyramidal symptoms appear to be dose-related and typically occur in the first few days of therapy. Marked drowsiness and lethargy, excessive salivation, and fixed stare occur frequently. Less common reactions include severe akathisia (motor restlessness) and acute dystonias (such as torticollis, opisthotonos, and oculogyric crisis).
- Tardive dyskinesia (tongue protrusion, puffing of the cheeks, chewing or puckering of the mouth) may occur during long-term therapy or after discontinuing the drug and may be irreversible. Elderly female patients have a greater risk of developing this reaction.

INTERACTIONS

Drugs

3 *Alcohol, other CNS depressants:* May increase CNS depression

3 *Anticholinergics:* Inhibition of therapeutic effect of neuroleptics

3 *Barbiturates:* Potential reduction of serum neuroleptic concentrations

3 *Bromocriptine:* Inhibition of bromocriptine's ability to lower serum prolactin concentrations in patients with pituitary adenoma; theoretical inhibition of antipsychotic effects of neuroleptics

3 *Carbamazepine:* Decreased serum haloperidol concentrations

3 *Epinephrine:* May block alpha-adrenergic effects

3 *Extrapyramidal symptom-producing medications:* May increase extrapyramidal symptoms

3 *Guanethidine:* Inhibition of antihypertensive effect of guanethidine

3 *Indomethacin:* Increased incidence of adverse effects such as drowsiness, tiredness, and confusion

2 *Levodopa:* Inhibition of antiparkinsonian effects of levodopa

3 *Lithium:* Rare reports of severe neurotoxicity in patients receiving lithium and neuroleptics

3 *Quinidine:* Increases haldol concentrations; increased risk of toxicity

SPECIAL CONSIDERATIONS

PATIENT/FAMILY EDUCATION

- Do not mix liquid formulation with coffee or tea
- Use calibrated dropper
- Take with food or milk
- Arise slowly from reclining position
- Do not discontinue abruptly
- Use a sunscreen during sun exposure to prevent burns
- Take special precautions to stay cool in hot weather
- The drug's full therapeutic effect may take up to 6 wks to appear
- Drowsiness generally subsides with continued therapy
- Avoid tasks that require mental alertness or motor skills until response to the drug has been established
- Notify the physician if muscle stiffness occurs
- Take sips of tepid water or chew sugarless gum to help relieve dry mouth

MONITORING PARAMETERS

- Observe closely for signs of tardive dyskinesia
- Closely supervise suicidal patients during early therapy. As depression lessens, the patient's energy level improves, which increases the suicide potential
- Assess the patient for evidence of a therapeutic response, including improvement in self-care, increased interest in surroundings and ability to concentrate, and relaxed facial expression
- The therapeutic serum level for haloperidol is 0.2-1 mcg/ml, and the toxic serum level is greater than 1 mcg/ml

---

heparin sodium

(hep'-a-rin soe'-dee-um)

Rx: Hep-Lock, Hep-Pak CVC

Chemical Class: Glycosaminoglycan, sulfated

Therapeutic Class: Anticoagulant

CLINICAL PHARMACOLOGY

Mechanism of Action: A blood modifier that interferes with blood coagulation by blocking conversion of prothrombin to thrombin and fibrinogen to fibrin. ***Therapeutic Effect:*** Prevents further extension of existing thrombi or new clot formation. Has no effect on existing clots.

Pharmacokinetics

Well absorbed following subcutaneous administration. Protein binding: very high. Metabolized in the liver. Removed from the circulation via uptake by the reticuloendothelial system. Primarily excreted in urine. Not removed by hemodialysis. ***Half-life:*** 1-6 hr.

INDICATIONS AND DOSAGES

Line flushing

IV

Adults, Elderly, Children. 100 units q6-8h.

Infants weighing less than 10 kg. 10 units q6-8h.

Treatment of venous thrombosis, pulmonary embolism, peripheral arterial embolism, atrial fibrillation with embolism

Intermittent IV

Adults, Elderly. Initially, 10,000 units, then 50-70 units/kg (5000-10,000 units) q4-6h.

Children 1 yr and older. Initially, 50-100 units/kg, then 50-100 units q4h.
IV Infusion
Adults, Elderly. Loading dose: 80 units/kg, then 18 units/kg/hr, with adjustments based on aPTT. Range: 10-30 units/kg/hr.
Children 1 yr and older. Loading dose: 75 units/kg, then 20 units/kg/hr with adjustments based on aPTT.
Children younger than 1 yr. Loading dose: 75 units/kg, then 28 units/kg/hr.
Prevention of venous thrombosis, pulmonary embolism, peripheral arterial embolism, atrial fibrillation with embolism
Subcutaneous
Adult, Elderly. 5000 units q8-12h.

AVAILABLE FORMS

- *Injection:* 10 units/ml (Hep-Lock), 100 units/ml, 1000 units/ml, 2500 units/ml, 5000 units/ml, 7500 units/ml, 10,000 units/ml, 20,000 units/ml, 25,000 units/500 ml infusion.
- *Injectable Kit (Hep-Pak CVC):* 20 units/ml, 100 units/ml.

CONTRAINDICATIONS: Intracranial hemorrhage, severe hypotension, severe thrombocytopenia, subacute bacterial endocarditis, uncontrolled bleeding

PREGNANCY AND LACTATION: Pregnancy category C; does not cross the placenta, has major advantages over oral anticoagulants as the treatment of choice during pregnancy; is not excreted into breast milk due to its high molecular weight

SIDE EFFECTS

Occasional
Itching, burning (particularly on soles of feet) caused by vasospastic reaction

Rare
Pain, cyanosis of extremity 6-10 days after initial therapy lasting 4-6 hrs; hypersensitivity reaction, including chills, fever, pruritus, urticaria, asthma, rhinitis, lacrimation, and headache

SERIOUS REACTIONS

- Bleeding complications ranging from local ecchymoses to major hemorrhage occur more frequently in high-dose therapy, intermittent IV infusion, and in women 60 years of age and older.
- Antidote: Protamine sulfate 1-1.5 mg, IV, for every 100 units heparin subcutaneous within 30 mins of overdose, 0.5-0.75 mg for every 100 units heparin subcutaneous if within 30-60 mins of overdose, 0.25-0.375 mg for every 100 units heparin subcutaneous if 2 hrs have elapsed since overdose, 25-50 mg if heparin was given by IV infusion.

INTERACTIONS

Drugs

3 *Antithyroid medications, cefoperazone, cefotetan, valproic acid:* May cause hypoprothrombinemia

3 *Aspirin:* Increased risk of hemorrhage

3 *Feverfew, ginkgo biloba:* Increased risk of bleeding

3 *Probenecid:* May increase the effects of heparin

3 *Warfarin:* Warfarin may prolong the aPTT in patients receiving heparin; heparin may prolong the PT in patients receiving warfarin

SPECIAL CONSIDERATIONS

PATIENT/FAMILY EDUCATION

- Report any signs of bleeding: gums, under skin, urine, stools
- Use an electric razor and soft toothbrush, to prevent bleeding during heparin therapy

• Do not take other medications, including OTC drugs, without physician approval

• Inform the dentist and other physicians of heparin therapy

MONITORING PARAMETERS

• aPTT (usual goal is to prolong aPTT to a value that corresponds to a plasma heparin level of 0.2-0.4 U/ml by protamine titration or to an anti-factor Xa level of about 0.3-0.6 U/ml; this range must be determined for each individual laboratory), usually measure 6-8 hr after initiation of IV and 6-8 hr after INF rate changes; increase or decrease INF by 2-4 U/kg/hr dependent on aPTT

• For intermittent inj, measure aPTT 3.5-4 hr after IV inj; at midinterval after SC inj

• Platelet counts, signs of bleeding, Hgb, Hct, AST (SGOT) and ALT (SGPT) levels, and stool and urine cultures for occult blood

• Determine the amount of female patient's menstrual discharge and monitor for any increase

• Assess the patient's gums for erythema and gingival bleeding, skin for ecchymosis or petechiae, and urine for hematuria

• Evaluate the patient for abdominal or back pain, a decrease in blood pressure, an increase in pulse rate, and severe headache, which may be evidence of hemorrhage

• Check the patient's peripheral pulses for loss of peripheral circulation

• When converting to warfarin therapy, monitor the patient's PT results, as ordered. PT will be 10%-20% higher while heparin is being given concurrently

hydralazine hydrochloride

(hye-dral'-a-zeen hye-droe-klor'-ide)

Rx: Apresoline

Combinations

Rx: with hydrochlorothiazide (Apresazide); with hydrochlorothiazide, reserpine (Ser-Ap-Es)

Chemical Class: Phthalazine derivative

Therapeutic Class: Antihypertensive; direct vasodilator

H

CLINICAL PHARMACOLOGY

Mechanism of Action: An antihypertensive with direct vasodilating effects on arterioles. ***Therapeutic Effect:*** Decreases BP and systemic resistance.

Pharmacokinetics

Route	*Onset*	*Peak*	*Duration*
PO	20-30 mins	N/A	2-4 hrs
IV	5-20 mins	N/A	2-6 hrs

Well absorbed from the GI tract. Widely distributed. Protein binding: 85%-90%. Metabolized in the liver to active metabolite. Primarily excreted in urine. Not removed by hemodialysis. ***Half-life:*** 3-7 hr (increased with impaired renal function).

INDICATIONS AND DOSAGES

Moderate to severe hypertension

PO

Adults. Initially, 10 mg 4 times a day. May increase by 10-25 mg/dose q2-5 days. Maximum: 300 mg/day.

Elderly. Initially, 10 mg 2-3 times a day. May increase by 10-25 mg q2-3days.

Children. Initially, 0.75-1 mg/kg/day in 2-4 divided doses, not to exceed 25 mg/dose. May increase over 3-4 wk. Maximum: 7.5 mg/kg/day (5 mg/kg/day in infants). Maximum daily dose: 200 mg.

IV, IM

Adults, Elderly. Initially, 10-20 mg/dose q4-6h. May increase to 40 mg/ dose.

Children. Initially, 0.1-0.2 mg/kg/dose (maximum: 20 mg) q4-6h, as needed, up to 1.7-3.5 mg/kg/day in divided doses q4-6h.

Dosage in renal impairment

Dosage interval is based on creatinine clearance.

Creatinine Clearance	*Dosage Interval*
10-50 ml/min	q8h
less than 10 ml/min	q8-24h

AVAILABLE FORMS

- *Tablets:* 10 mg, 25 mg, 50 mg, 100 mg.
- *Injection:* 20 mg/ml.

UNLABELED USES: Treatment of CHF, hypertension secondary to eclampsia and preeclampsia, primary pulmonary hypertension.

CONTRAINDICATIONS: Coronary artery disease, lupus erythematosus, rheumatic heart disease

PREGNANCY AND LACTATION: Pregnancy category C; commonly used in pregnant women; excreted into breast milk; compatible with breast-feeding

SIDE EFFECTS

Frequent

Headache, palpitations, tachycardia (generally disappears in 7-10 days)

Occasional

GI disturbance (nausea, vomiting, diarrhea), paresthesia, fluid retention, peripheral edema, dizziness, flushed face, nasal congestion

SERIOUS REACTIONS

- High dosage may produce lupus erythematosus–like reaction, including fever, facial rash, muscle and joint aches, and splenomegaly.
- Severe orthostatic hypotension, skin flushing, severe headache, myocardial ischemia, and cardiac arrhythmias may develop.
- Profound shock may occur with severe overdosage.

INTERACTIONS

Drugs

3 *Diazoxide:* Severe hypotension

3 *Diuretics, other antihypertensives:* May increase the hypotensive effect

3 *NSAIDs:* Inhibited antihypertensive response to hydralazine

Labs

- *False increase:* Ca^{++} (slight); urine 17-ketogenic steroids; glucose, uric acid
- *False decrease:* Glucose, uric acid

SPECIAL CONSIDERATIONS

- Lupus-like syndrome more common in "slow acetylators" and following higher doses for prolonged periods

PATIENT/FAMILY EDUCATION

- Take with meals
- Notify clinician of any unexplained prolonged general tiredness or fever, muscle or joint aching, or chest pain
- Stools may turn black
- Rise slowly from a lying to a sitting position and permit legs to dangle from the bed momentarily before standing to reduce the hypotensive effect of hydralazine

MONITORING PARAMETERS

- CBC and ANA titer before and during prolonged therapy
- Pattern of daily bowel activity and stool consistency
- Monitor the patient for headache, palpitations, and tachycardia
- Assess for peripheral edema of the hands and feet

hydrochlorothiazide

(hye-droe-klor-oh-thye'-a-zide)

Rx: Aquazide H, Esidrix, HydroDIURIL, Microzide, Oretic

Combinations

Rx: with angiotensin-converting inhibitors: quinapril (Accuretic); captopril (Acediur, Capozide); lisinopril (Prinzide, Zestoretic); benazepril (Lotensin HCT); moexipril (Uniretic); enalapril (Vaseretic); with spironolactone (Aldactazide, Spirozide) with methyldopa (Aldoril), with hydralazine (Apresazide) with reserpine (Aqwesine, Hydropres, Hydroserpine, Hydrotensin, Mallopres, Marpres, Unipres) with angiotensin II receptor blockers: irbesartan (Avalide), valsartan (Diovan HCT), losartan (Hyzaar), with hydralazine and reserpine (Cam-ap-es, H.H.R., Hyserp, Lo-Ten, Ser-A-Gen, Seralazide, Ser-Ap-Es, Serpex, Uni-Serp), with triamterene: (Dyazide, Maxzide) with potassium (Esidrix-K) with guanethidine (Esimil), with β-blockers: propranolol: (Inderide); metoprolol: (Lopressor HCT); labetolol (Normazide, Trandate-HCT); timolol: (Timolide); bisoprolol (Ziac) with amiloride (Moduretic)

Chemical Class: Sulfonamide derivative

Therapeutic Class: Antihypertensive; diuretic, thiazide

CLINICAL PHARMACOLOGY

Mechanism of Action: A sulfonamide derivative that acts as a thiazide diuretic and antihypertensive. As a diuretic blocks reabsorption of water, sodium, and potassium at the cortical diluting segment of the distal tubule. As an antihypertensive reduces plasma, extracellular fluid volume, and peripheral vascular resistance by direct effect on blood vessels. ***Therapeutic Effect:*** Promotes diuresis; reduces BP.

Pharmacokinetics

Route	Onset	Peak	Duration
PO (diuretic)	2 hrs	4-6 hrs	6-12 hrs

Variably absorbed from the GI tract. Primarily excreted unchanged in urine. Not removed by hemodialysis. ***Half-life:*** 5.6-14.8 hrs.

INDICATIONS AND DOSAGES

Edema

PO

Adults, Elderly. 25-100 mg/day as a single or in divided doses.

Children 2-12 yrs. 1-2 mg/kg. Maximum: 100 mg/day.

Infants younger than 2 yrs. 1-2 mg/kg. Maximum: 37.5 mg/day.

Hypertension

PO

Adults, Elderly. Initially, 12.5-25 mg once daily. May increase up to 50-100 mg/day as a single or in divided doses.

Children 2-12 yrs. 1-2 mg/kg. Maximum: 100 mg/day.

Infants younger than 2 yrs. 1-2 mg/kg. Maximum: 37.5 mg/day.

AVAILABLE FORMS

- *Capsules (Microzide):* 12.5 mg.
- *Oral Solution:* 50 mg/5 ml.
- *Tablets (Aquazide, Oretic):* 25 mg, 50 mg, 100 mg.

UNLABELED USES: Treatment of diabetes insipidus, prevention of calcium-containing renal calculi

H

CONTRAINDICATIONS: Anuria, history of hypersensitivity to sulfonamides or thiazide diuretics, renal decompensation

PREGNANCY AND LACTATION: Pregnancy category B (D if used in pregnancy-induced hypertension); first trimester use may increase risk of congenital defects, use in later trimesters does not seem to carry this risk; therapy for preexisting hypertension can be continued throughout pregnancy with minimal risk; initiating for simple edema not recommended; few unequivocal indications for diuretic therapy in pregnancy except for pulmonary edema or congestive heart failure, excreted into breast milk in small amounts; considered compatible with breastfeeding

SIDE EFFECTS

Expected

Increase in urinary frequency and urine volume

Frequent

Potassium depletion

Occasional

Orthostatic hypotension, headache, GI disturbances, photosensitivity

SERIOUS REACTIONS

- Vigorous diuresis may lead to profound water and electrolyte depletion, resulting in hypokalemia, hyponatremia, and dehydration.
- Acute hypotensive episodes may occur.
- Hyperglycemia may occur during prolonged therapy.
- Pancreatitis, blood dyscrasias, pulmonary edema, allergic pneumonitis, and dermatologic reactions occur rarely.
- Overdose can lead to lethargy and coma without changes in electrolytes or hydration.

INTERACTIONS

Drugs

❷ *Angiotensin-converting enzyme inhibitors:* Risk of postural hypotension when added to ongoing diuretic therapy; more common with loop diuretics; first-dose hypotension possible in patients with sodium depletion or hypovolemia due to diuretics or sodium restriction; hypotensive response is usually transient; hold diuretic day of first dose

❸ *Calcium (high doses):* Risk of milk-alkali syndrome; monitor for hypercalcemia

❸ *Carbenoxolone:* Additive potassium wasting; severe hypokalemia

❸ *Cholestyramine/colestipol:* Reduced serum concentrations of thiazide diuretics

❸ *Corticosteroids:* Concomitant therapy may result in excessive potassium loss

❸ *Diazoxide:* Hyperglycemia

❸ *Digitalis glycosides:* Diuretic-induced hypokalemia may increase the risk of digitalis toxicity

❸ *Hypoglycemic agents:* Thiazide diuretics tend to increase blood glucose, may increase dosage requirements of antidiabetic drugs

❸ *Lithium:* Increased serum lithium concentrations, toxicity may occur

❸ *Methotrexate:* Increased bone marrow suppression

❸ *Nonsteroidal antiinflammatory drugs:* Concurrent use may reduce diuretic and antihypertensive effects

Labs

- *False decrease:* Urine estriol

SPECIAL CONSIDERATIONS

- May protect against osteoporotic hip fractures
- Loop diuretics or metolazone more effective if CrCl <40-50 ml/min

• Combinations with triamterene, lisinopril have potassium sparing effect

• Doses above 25 mg provide no further blood pressure reduction, but are more likely to induce metabolic disturbance (i.e., hypokalemia, hyperuricemia)

PATIENT/FAMILY EDUCATION

• Will increase urination temporarily (for about 3 wk); take early in the day

• May cause sensitivity to sunlight; avoid prolonged exposure to the sun and other ultraviolet light

• May cause gout attacks; notify clinician if sudden joint pain occurs

• Change positions slowly and let legs dangle momentarily before standing to reduce the drug's hypotensive effect

• Eat foods high in potassium, including apricots, bananas, raisins, orange juice, potatoes, legumes, meat, and whole grains (such as cereals)

MONITORING PARAMETERS

• Weight, urine output, serum electrolytes, BUN, creatinine, CBC, uric acid, glucose, lipids

Blood pressure

• Be especially alert for signs of potassium depletion, such as cardiac arrhythmias, in patients taking digoxin

• Assess the patient for constipation, which may occur with exercise diuresis

hydrocodone group

(hye-droe-koe'-done)

Rx: Hycodan

Combinations

Rx: Hydrocodone and acetaminophen, (Anexsia, Bancap HC, Ceta-Plus, Co-Gesic, Hydrocet, Hydrogesic, Lorcet 10/650, Lorcet-HD Lorcet Plus, Lortab, Margesic H, Maxidone, Norco, Stagesic, Vicodin, Vicodin ES, Vicodin HP, Zydone); Hydrocodone and aspirin (Damason-P); hydrocodone and chlorpheniramine (Tussionex), hydrocodone and guaifenesin (Codiclear DH, Hycosin, Hycotuss, Kwelcof, Pneumotussin, Vicoden Tuss, Vitussin); hydrocodone and homatropin (Hycodan and Hydromet, Hydropane, Tussigon); hydrocodone and ibuprofen, (Vicoprofen); hydrocodone and pseudoephedrine (Detussin, Histussin D, P-V Tussin); hydrocodone, chlorpheniramine, phenylephrine, acetaminophen, and caffeine (Hycomine Compound)

Chemical Class: Opiate derivative; phenanthrene derivative

Therapeutic Class: Antitussive; narcotic analgesic

DEA Class: Schedule III

CLINICAL PHARMACOLOGY

Mechanism of Action: Hydrocodone blocks pain perception in the cerebral cortex by binding to specific opiate receptors (mu and kappa) neuronal membranes of synapses. This binding results in a decreased synaptic chemical transmission throughout the CNS thus inhibiting the flow of pain sensations into the higher centers and cause analgesia. ***Therapeutic Effect:*** Alters perception of pain and produces analgesic effect.

Pharmacokinetics

Well absorbed. Metabolized in liver. Excreted in urine. ***Half-life:*** 3.3-3.4 hrs.

INDICATIONS AND DOSAGES

Hydrocodone & acetaminophen

Analgesia: PO

Adults, Children older than 13 yrs or more than 50 kg. 2.5-10 mg q4-6h. Maximum: 60 mg/day hydrocodone. Maximum dose of acetaminophen: 4 g/day.

Elderly. 2.5-5 mg hydrocodone q4-6h. Titrate dose to appropriate analgesic effect. Maximum: 4 g/day acetaminophen.

Children 2-13 yrs or less than 50 kg. 0.135 mg/kg/dose hydrocodone q4-6h. Maximum: 6 doses/day of hydrocodone or maximum recommended dose of acetaminophen.

Hydrocodone & aspirin

PO

Adults. 2.5-10 mg q4-6h. Maximum: 60 mg/day hydrocodone.

Elderly. 2.5-5 mg hydrocodone q4-6h. Titrate dose to appropriate analgesic effect.

Children 2-13 yrs or less than 50 kg. 0.135 mg/kg/dose hydrocodone q4-6h.

Hydrocodone & chlorpheniramine

PO

Adults, Elderly, Children 12 yrs and older. 5 ml q12h. Maximum: 10 ml/24h.

Children 6-12 yrs. 2.5 ml q12h. Maximum: 5 ml/24h.

Hydrocodone & guaifenesin

PO

Adults, Elderly, Children 12 yrs and older. 5 ml q4h. Maximum: 30 ml/24h.

Children 2-12 yrs. 2.5 ml q4h.

Children less than 2 yrs. 0.3 mg/kg/day (hydrocodone) in 4 divided doses.

Hydrocodone & homatropine

PO

Adults, Elderly. 10 mg (hydrocodone) q4-6h. A single dose should not exceed 15 mg and not more frequently than q4h.

Children. 0.6 mg/kg/day (hydrocodone) in 3-4 divided doses. Do not administer more frequently than q4h.

Hydrocodone & ibuprofen

PO

Adults. 7.5-15 mg (hydrocodone) q4-6h as needed for pain. Maximum: 5 tablets/day.

Hydrocodone & pseudoephedrine

PO

Adults, Elderly. 5 ml 4 times/day.

Hydrocodone, chlorpheniramine, phenylephrine, acetaminophen, & caffeine

PO

Adults, Elderly. 1 tablet q4h up to 4 times/day.

AVAILABLE FORMS

Hydrocodone & acetaminophen

- *Capsules:* Hydrocodone bitartrate 5 mg and acetaminophen 500 mg (Bancap HC, Ceta-Plus, Hydrocet, Hydrogesic, Lorcet-HD, Margesic H, Stagesic).
- *Elixir:* Hydrocodone bitartrate 7.5 mg and acetaminophen 500 mg/15 ml (Lortab).
- *Tablets:* Hydrocodone bitartrate 2.5 mg and acetaminophen 500 mg (Lortab), hydrocodone bitartrate 5 mg and acetaminophen 325 mg (Norco), hydrocodone bitartrate 5 mg and acetaminophen 400 mg (Zy-

done), hydrocodone bitartrate 5 mg and acetaminophen 500 mg (Anexsia, Co-Gesic, Lortab 5/500, Vicodin), hydrocodone bitartrate 7.5 mg and acetaminophen 325 mg (Norco), hydrocodone bitartrate 5 mg and acetaminophen 400 mg (Zydone), hydrocodone bitartrate 7.5 mg and acetaminophen 500 mg (Lortab 7.5/500), hydrocodone bitartrate 7.5 mg and acetaminophen 650 mg (Anexsia, Lorcet Plus), hydrocodone bitartrate 7.5 mg and acetaminophen 750 mg (Vicodin ES), hydrocodone bitartrate 10 mg and acetaminophen 325 mg (Norco), hydrocodone bitartrate 5 mg and acetaminophen 400 mg (Zydone), hydrocodone bitartrate 10 mg and acetaminophen 500 mg (Lortab 10/500), hydrocodone bitartrate 10 mg and acetaminophen 650 mg (Lorcet 10/650), hydrocodone bitartrate 10 mg and acetaminophen 660 mg (Vicodin HP), hydrocodone bitartrate 10 mg and acetaminophen 750 mg (Maxicodone).

Hydrocodone & aspirin

• *Tablets:* Hydrocodone bitartrate 5 mg and aspirin 500 mg (Damason-P).

Hydrocodone & chlorpheniramine

• *Syrup, Extended Release:* Hydrocodone polistirex 10 mg and chlorpheniramine polistirex 8 mg/5 ml (Tussionex).

Hydrocodone & guaifenesin

• *Liquid:* Hydrocodone bitartrate 2.5 mg and guaifenesin 200 mg/5 ml (Pneumotussin), hydrocodone bitartrate 5 mg and guaifenesin 100 mg/5 ml (Codiclear DH, Hycosin, Hycotuss, Kwelcof, Vicodin Tuss, Vitussin).

• *Tablets:* Hydrocodone bitartrate 2.5 mg and guaifenesin 300 mg (Pneumotussin).

Hydrocodone & homatropine

• *Syrup:* Hydrocodone bitartrate 5 mg and homatropine methylbromide 1.5 mg/5 ml (Hycodan, Hydromet, Hydropane).

• *Tablets:* Hydrocodone bitartrate 5 mg and homatropine methylbromide 1.5 mg (Hycodan, Tussigon).

Hydrocodone & ibuprofen

• *Tablets:* Hydrocodone bitartrate 7.5 mg and aspirin 200 mg (Vicoprofen).

Hydrocodone & pseudoephedrine

• *Liquid:* Hydrocodone bitartrate 5 mg and pseudoephedrine 60 mg/5 ml (Detussin, Histussin D).

• *Tablets:* Hydrocodone bitartrate 5 mg and pseudoephedrine 60 mg (P-V Tussin).

Hydrocodone, chlorpheniramine, phenylephrine, acetaminophen, & caffeine

• *Tablets:* Hydrocodone bitartrate 5 mg, chlorpheniramine maleate 2 mg, phenylephrine hydrochloride 10 mg, acetaminophen 250 mg, and caffeine 30 mg (Hycomine Compound).

CONTRAINDICATIONS: CNS depression, severe respiratory depression, hypersensitivity to hydrocodone, or any component of the formulation

PREGNANCY AND LACTATION: Pregnancy category B (category D if used for prolonged periods or in high doses at term); withdrawal could theoretically occur in infants exposed *in utero* to prolonged maternal ingestion; excretion into breast milk unknown; use caution in nursing mothers

Controlled Substance: Schedule III

SIDE EFFECTS

Frequent

Dizziness, sedation, drowsiness, bradycardia

Occasional
Anxiety, dysphoria, euphoria, fear, lethargy, lightheadedness, malaise, mental clouding, mental impairment, mood changes, physiologic dependence, sedation, somnolence, constipation, bradycardia, heartburn, nausea, vomiting
Rare
Hypersensitivity reaction, rash

SERIOUS REACTIONS

- Cardiac arrest, circulatory collapse, coma, hypotension, hypoglycemic coma, ureteral spasm, urinary retention, vesical sphincter spasm, agranulocytosis, bleeding time prolonged, hemolytic anemia, iron deficiency anemia, occult blood loss, thrombocytopenia, hepatic necrosis, hepatitis, skeletal muscle rigidity, renal toxicity, and renal tubular necrosis have been reported.
- Hearing impairment or loss have been reported with chronic overdose.
- Acute airway obstruction, apnea, dyspnea, and respiratory depression occur rarely and are usually dose related.

INTERACTIONS

Drugs

3 *Antihistamines, chloral hydrate, glutethimide, methocarbamol:* Enhanced depressant effects
3 *Barbiturates:* Additive respiratory and CNS depressant effects
3 *Cimetidine:* Increased respiratory and CNS depression
3 *Ethanol, other CNS depressants:* Additive CNS effects
2 *MAOIs:* May produce a severe, sometimes fatal reaction; plan to administer one-quarter of usual hydrocodone dose
3 *Protease inhibitors:* Enhanced CNS and respiratory depression

Labs

- False elevations of amylase and lipase

SPECIAL CONSIDERATIONS

PATIENT/FAMILY EDUCATION

- Report any symptoms of CNS changes, allergic reactions
- Physical dependency may result when used for extended periods
- Change position slowly, orthostatic hypotension may occur
- Avoid hazardous activities if drowsiness or dizziness occurs
- Avoid alcohol, other CNS depressants
- Minimize nausea by administering with food and remain lying down following dose
- Do not administer agonist/antagonist analgesics (i.e., pentazocine, nalbuphine, butorphanol, dezocine, buprenorphine) to patient who has received a prolonged course of hydrocodone (a pure agonist). In opioid-dependent patients, mixed agonist/antagonist analgesics may precipitate withdrawal symptoms

MONITORING PARAMETERS

- Clinical improvement of symptoms and record the onset of pain or cough relief
- Pattern of daily bowel activity and stool consistency

hydrocortisone

(hye-droe-kor'-ti-sone)

Rx: Acticort 100, Aeroseb-HC, A-HydroCort, Ala-Cort, Ala-Scalp HP, Anucort-HC, Anumed-HC, Anusol-HC, Anutone-HC, Caldecort, Cetacort, Colocort, Cortane, Cortaid, Cort-Dome High Potency, Cortef, Cortenema, Cortifoam, Cortizone-5, Cortizone-10, Cotacort, Emcort, Gly-Cort, Hemorrhoidal HC, Hemril-30, Hemril-HC Uniserts, Hydrocortone, Hydrocortone Phosphate, Hytone, Instacort 10, Lacticare-HC, Locoid, Locoid Lipocream, Nupercainal Hydrocortisone Cream, Nutracort, Orabase HCA, Pandel, Penecort, Preparation H Hydrocortisone, Protocort, Proctocream-HC, Procto-Kit 1%, Procto-Kit 2.5%, Proctosert HC, Proctosol-HC, Proctozone HC, Rectasol-HC, Rederm, Scalp-Aid, Solu-Cortef, Texacort, WestCort

OTC: Cortizone, Cortaid, Lanacort-5, Gynecort Female Creme, Dermolate, Tegrin-HC

Combinations

Rx: with choloramphenicol (Chloromycetin/HC suspension—ophthalmic); with neomycin and polymyxin B (Cortisporin Otic, Drotic, Otocort—otic); with neomycin, polymyxin B, and bacitracin (Cortisporin Ointment, Neotricin HC—ophthalmic); with oxytetracycline (Terra-Cortril—ophthalmic); with urea (Carmol HC)

Chemical Class: Glucocorticoid

Therapeutic Class: Corticosteroid, systemic; corticosteroid, topical

CLINICAL PHARMACOLOGY

Mechanism of Action: An adrenocortical steroid that inhibits accumulation of inflammatory cells at inflammation sites, phagocytosis, lysosomal enzyme release and synthesis and release of mediators of inflammation. ***Therapeutic Effect:*** Prevents or suppresses cell-mediated immune reactions. Decreases or prevents tissue response to inflammatory process.

Pharmacokinetics

Route	*Onset*	*Peak*	*Duration*
IV	N/A	4-6 hrs	8-12 hrs

Well absorbed after IM administration. Widely distributed. Metabolized in the liver. ***Half-life:*** Plasma, 1.5-2 hrs; biologic, 8-12 hrs.

INDICATIONS AND DOSAGES

Acute adrenal insufficiency

IV

Adults, Elderly. 100 mg IV bolus; then 300 mg/day in divided doses q8h.

Children. 1-2 mg/kg IV bolus; then 150-250 mg/day in divided doses q6-8h.

Infants. 1-2 mg/kg/dose IV bolus; then 25-150 mg/day in divided doses q6-8h.

Antiinflammation, immunosuppression

IV, IM

Adults, Elderly. 15-240 mg q12h.

Children. 1-5 mg/kg/day in divided doses q12h.

PO

Adults, Elderly. 15-240 mg q12h.

Children. 2.5-10 mg/kg/day.

Physiologic replacement

PO

Children. 0.5-0.75 mg/kg/day in divided doses q8h.

IM

Children. 0.25-0.35 mg/kg/day as a single dose.

Status asthmaticus

IV

Adults, Elderly. 100-500 mg q6h.

Children. 2 mg/kg/dose q6h.

Shock

IV

Adults, Elderly, Children 12 yr and older. 500 mg-2 g q2-6h.

Children younger than 12 yr. 50 mg/kg. May repeat in 4 hr, then q24h as needed.

Adjunctive treatment of ulcerative colitis

Rectal

Adults, Elderly. 100 mg at bedtime for 21 nights or until clinical and proctologic remission occurs (may require 2-3 mo of therapy).

Rectal (Cortifoam)

Adults, Elderly. 1 applicator 1-2 times a day for 2-3 wk, then every second day until therapy ends.

Topical

Adults, Elderly. Apply sparingly 2-4 times a day.

AVAILABLE FORMS

- *Tablets (Cortef):* 5 mg, 10 mg, 20 mg.
- *Oral Suspension, cypionate (Cortef):* 10 mg/5 ml
- *Cream (Rectal):* 1% (Nupercainal Hydrocortisone Cream, Cortizone-10, Preparation H Hydrocortisone, Proctocort, Procto-Kit 1%), 2.5% (Anusol-HC, Hemorrhoidal HC, Procto-Kit 2.5%, Proctosol-HC, Proctozone-HC).
- *Cream, butyrate (Topical [Locoid, Locoid Lipocream]):* 0.1%.
- *Cream, probutate (Topical [Pandel]):* 0.1%.
- *Cream, valerate (Topical [Westcort]):* 0.2%.
- *Cream (Topical):* 0.5% (Cortizone-5), 1% (Ala-Cort, Caldecort, Cortizone-10, Hycort, Hytone, Penecort), 2.5% (Hytone, Proctocream-HC).
- *Foam (Rectal [Cortifoam]):* 10%.
- *Gel (Topical [Instacort 10]):* 1%.
- *Lotion:* 0.5% (Cetacort), 1% (Ala-Cort, Cetacort, Cortone, Lacticare-HC, Nutracort), 2.5% (Hytone, Lacticare-HC, Nutracort).
- *Ointment, butyrate (Topical [Locoid]):* 0.1%.
- *Ointment, valerate (Topical [Westcort]):* 0.2%.
- *Ointment (Topical):* 0.5% (Cortizone-5), 1% (Anusol-HC, Cortaid, Cortizone-10, Hydrocortisone 1%, Hytone), 2.5% (Hytone).
- *Paste (Topical [Orabase HCA]):* 0.5%.
- *Solution (Topical):* 1% (Acticort 100, Gly-Cort, Penecort, Rederm, Scalp-Aid, Texacort), 2.5% (Texacort).
- *Solution, butyrate (Topical [Locoid]):* 0.1%.
- *Spray (Topical [Aeroseb-HC]):* 0.5%.
- *Suppositories:* 25 mg (Anucort-HC, Anumed-HC, Anusol-HC, Anutone-HC, Cort-Dome High Potency, Hemorrhoidal HC, Hemril-HC, Proctosol-HC, Rectasol-HC), 30 mg (Emcort, Hemril-30, Protocort, Proctosert HC).
- *Suppositories (Rectal [Colocort, Cortenema]):* 100 mg/60 ml.
- *Injection (A-hydro-Cort, Solu-Cortef):* 100 mg, 250 mg, 500 mg, 1 g.
- *Injectable Solution, sodium phosphate (Hydrocortone Phosphate):* 50 mg/ml.
- *Injectable Suspension, acetate:* 25 mg/ml, 50 mg/ml.

CONTRAINDICATIONS: Fungal, tuberculosis, or viral skin lesions; serious infections

PREGNANCY AND LACTATION: Pregnancy category C (D if used in first trimester); excreted in breast milk; could interfere with infant's growth and endogenous corticosteroid production

SIDE EFFECTS

Frequent

Insomnia, heartburn, nervousness, abdominal distention, diaphoresis, acne, mood swings, increased appetite, facial flushing, delayed wound healing, increased susceptibility to infection, diarrhea or constipation

Occasional

Headache, edema, change in skin color, frequent urination

Topical: Itching, redness, irritation

Rare

Tachycardia, allergic reaction (such as rash and hives), psychologic changes, hallucinations, depression

Topical: Allergic contact dermatitis, purpura

Systemic: Absorption more likely with use of occlusive dressings or extensive application in young children

SERIOUS REACTIONS

• Long-term therapy may cause hypocalcemia, hypokalemia, muscle wasting (especially in arms and legs), osteoporosis, spontaneous fractures, amenorrhea, cataracts, glaucoma, peptic ulcer disease, and CHF.

• Abruptly withdrawing the drug after long-term therapy may cause anorexia, nausea, fever, headache, sudden severe joint pain, rebound inflammation, fatigue, weakness, lethargy, dizziness, and orthostatic hypotension.

INTERACTIONS

Drugs

3 *Aminoglutethamide:* Enhanced elimination of hydrocortisone; reduction in corticosteroid response

3 *Amphotericin:* Increases the risk of hypokalemia

3 *Antidiabetics:* Increased blood glucose in patients with diabetes

3 *Barbiturates:* Reduction in the serum concentrations of corticosteroids

3 *Cholestyramine, colestipol:* Possible reduced absorption of corticosteroids

3 *Cyclosporine:* Increased levels of both drugs increases the risk of seizures

3 *Digoxin:* May increase the risk of digoxin toxicity caused by hypokalemia

3 *Diuretics, potassium supplements:* May decrease the effects of these drugs

3 *Estrogens:* Enhanced effects of corticosteroids

3 *Hepatic enzyme inducers:* May decrease the effects of hydrocortisone

3 *Isoniazid (INH):* Reduced INH levels, enhanced corticosteroid effect

3 *IUDs:* Inhibition of inflammation may decrease contraceptive effect

3 *Live-virus vaccines:* May decrease the patient's antibody response to vaccine, increase vaccine side effects, and potentiate virus replication

3 *NSAIDs:* Increased risk GI ulceration

3 *Phenytoin:* Reduced therapeutic effect of corticosteroids

3 *Rifampin:* Reduced therapeutic effect of corticosteroids

3 *Salicylates:* Enhanced elimination of salicylates; subtherapeutic salicylate concentrations possible

Labs

• *False negative:* Skin allergy tests

SPECIAL CONSIDERATIONS

PATIENT/FAMILY EDUCATION

• May cause GI upset; take with meals or snacks

• Take single daily doses in a.m.

• Increased dose of rapidly acting corticosteroids may be necessary in patients subjected to unusual stress

• Signs of adrenal insufficiency include fatigue, anorexia, nausea, vomiting, diarrhea, weight loss, weakness, dizziness, and low blood sugar

• Avoid abrupt withdrawal of therapy following high-dose or long-term therapy

• May mask infections

• Do not give live-virus vaccines to patients on prolonged therapy

• Patients on chronic steroid therapy should wear medical alert bracelet

• Avoid alcohol and limit caffeine intake during hydrocortisone therapy

• Notify the dentist and other physicians that he or she is taking hydrocortisone or has taken it within the past 12 mos

• Avoid contact with eyes

• Apply topical hydrocortisone valerate after a bath or shower for best absorption. Do not cover the affected area with plastic pants, tight diapers, or other types of coverings unless the physician instructs otherwise

• Steroids often cause mood swings, ranging from euphoria to depression

MONITORING PARAMETERS

• Serum K and glucose

• Edema, blood pressure, CHF, mental status, weight

• Growth in children on prolonged therapy

• Electrolytes

• Pattern of daily bowel activity and stool consistency

• Monitor the patient for signs and symptoms of hypocalcemia (such as cramps and muscle twitching), or hypokalemia (such as EKG changes, irritability, nausea and vomiting, numbness or tingling of lower extremities, and weakness)

hydroflumethiazide

(hye-droe-floo-meth-eye'-a-zide)

Rx: Diucardin, Saluron

Combinations

Rx: reserpine (Salutensin, Salutensin-Demi)

Chemical Class: Sulfonamide derivative

Therapeutic Class: Antihypertensive; diuretic, thiazide

CLINICAL PHARMACOLOGY

Mechanism of Action: A diuretic that blocks reabsorption of water, the electrolytes sodium and potassium at cortical diluting segment of distal tubule. As an antihypertensive it reduces plasma and extracellular fluid volume and decreases peripheral vascular resistance (PVR) by direct effect on blood vessels. ***Therapeutic Effect:*** Promotes diuresis, reduces blood pressure (BP).

Pharmacokinetics

Rapidly but incompletely absorbed from the gastrointestinal (GI) tract. Metabolized to metabolite that is extensively bound to red blood cells and has a longer half-life than parent compound. Primarily excreted in urine. Not removed by hemodialysis. ***Half-life:*** 2-17 hrs.

INDICATIONS AND DOSAGES

Edema

PO

Adults, Elderly. Initially, 50 mg 2 times/day. Maintenance: 25-200 mg/day.

Hypertension

Initially, 50 mg 2 times/day. Maintenance: 50-100 mg/day.

Adults, Elderly, Children. 1 mg/kg/day.

AVAILABLE FORMS

• *Tablets:* 50 mg (Diucardin, Saluron).

UNLABELED USES: Treatment of diabetes insipidus

CONTRAINDICATIONS: Anuria, history of hypersensitivity to sulfonamides or thiazide diuretics, renal decompensation, pregnancy

PREGNANCY AND LACTATION: Pregnancy category C; therapy for preexisting hypertension can be continued throughout pregnancy with minimal risk; initiating for simple edema not recommended; few unequivocal indications for diuretic therapy in pregnancy except for pulmonary edema or congestive heart failure; excreted into breast milk in small amounts; considered compatible with breast-feeding

SIDE EFFECTS

Expected

Increase in urine frequency and volume

Frequent

Potassium depletion

Occasional

Postural hypotension, headache, GI disturbances, photosensitivity reaction

SERIOUS REACTIONS

• Vigorous diuresis may lead to profound water loss and electrolyte depletion, resulting in hypokalemia, hyponatremia, and dehydration.

• Acute hypotensive episodes may occur.

• Hyperglycemia may be noted during prolonged therapy.

• GI upset, pancreatitis, dizziness, paresthesias, headache, blood dyscrasias, pulmonary edema, allergic pneumonitis, and dermatologic reactions occur rarely.

• Overdosage can lead to lethargy and coma without changes in electrolytes or hydration.

INTERACTIONS

Drugs

❷ *Angiotensin-converting enzyme inhibitors:* Risk of postural hypotension when added to ongoing diuretic therapy; more common with loop diuretics; first-dose hypotension possible in patients with sodium depletion or hypovolemia due to diuretics or sodium restriction; hypotensive response is usually transient; hold diuretic day of first dose

❸ *Calcium (high dose):* Risk of milk-alkali syndrome. Monitor for hypoglycemia

❸ *Cholestyramine, colestipol:* Reduced serum concentrations of thiazide diuretics

❸ *Corticosteroids:* Concomitant therapy may result in excessive potassium loss

❸ *Diazoxide:* Hyperglycemia

❸ *Digitalis glycosides:* Diuretic-induced hypokalemia may increase the risk of digitalis toxicity

❸ *Hypoglycemic agents:* Thiazide diuretics tend to increase blood glucose; may increase dosage requirements of hypoglycemic agents

❸ *Lithium:* Increased serum lithium concentrations, toxicity may occur

❸ *Methotrexate:* Increased bone marrow suppression

❸ *Nonsteroidal antiinflammatory drugs:* Concurrent may reduce diuretic and antihypertensive effects

Labs

• *False decrease:* Urine estriol

SPECIAL CONSIDERATIONS

• May protect against osteoporotic hip fractures
• Loop diuretics or metolazone more effective if CrCl <40-50 ml/min

PATIENT/FAMILY EDUCATION

• Will increase urination temporarily (approximately 3 wk); take early in the day to prevent sleep disturbance
• May cause sensitivity to sunlight; avoid prolonged exposure to the sun and other ultraviolet light
• May cause gout attacks; notify clinician if sudden joint pain occurs
• Change positions slowly and let legs dangle momentarily before standing to reduce the drug's hypotensive effect
• Eat foods high in potassium, including apricots, bananas, raisins, orange juice, potatoes, legumes, meat, and whole grains (such as cereals)

MONITORING PARAMETERS

• Weight, urine output, serum electrolytes, BUN, creatinine, CBC, uric acid, glucose, lipids
• Blood pressure
• Be especially alert for signs of potassium depletion, such as cardiac arrhythmias, in patients taking digoxin
• Assess the patient for constipation, which may occur with exercise diuresis

hydromorphone hydrochloride

(hye-droe-mor'-fone hye-droe-klor'-ide)

Rx: Dilaudid, Dilaudid-5, Dilaudid HP, Hydromorph, Hydrostat IR

Chemical Class: Opiate derivative; phenanthrene derivative

Therapeutic Class: Antitussive; narcotic analgesic

DEA Class: Schedule II

CLINICAL PHARMACOLOGY

Mechanism of Action: An opioid agonist that binds to opioid receptors in the CNS, reducing the intensity of pain stimuli from sensory nerve endings. ***Therapeutic Effect:*** Alters the perception of and emotional response to pain; suppresses cough reflex.

Pharmacokinetics

Route	*Onset*	*Peak*	*Duration*
PO	30 mins	90-120 mins	4 hrs
IV	10-15 mins	15-30 mins	2-3 hrs
IM	15 mins	30-60 mins	4-5 hrs
Subcutaneous	15 mins	30-90 mins	4 hrs
Rectal	15-30 mins	N/A	N/A

Well absorbed from the GI tract after IM administration. Widely distributed. Metabolized in the liver. Excreted in urine. ***Half-life:*** 1-3 hrs.

INDICATIONS AND DOSAGES

Analgesia

PO

Adults, Elderly, Children weighing 50 kg and more. 2-4 mg q3-4h. Range: 2-8 mg/dose.

Children older than 6 mos and weighing less than 50 kg. 0.03-0.08 mg/kg/dose q3-4h.

IV

Adults, Elderly, Children weighing more than 50 kg. 0.2-0.6 mg q2-3h.

Children weighing 50 kg or less. 0.015 mg/kg/dose q3-6h as needed.

Rectal

Adults, Elderly. 3 mg q4-8h.

Patient-controlled analgesia (PCA)

IV

Adults, Elderly. 0.05-0.5 mg at 5-15-min lockout. Maximum (4-hr): 4-6 mg.

Epidural

Adults, Elderly. Bolus dose of 1-1.5 mg at rate of 0.04-0.4 mg/hr. Demand dose of 0.15 mg at 30-min lockout.

Cough

PO

Adults, Elderly, Children older than 12 yrs. 1 mg q3-4h.

Children 6-12 yrs. 0.5 mg q3-4h.

AVAILABLE FORMS

- *Liquid:* 1 mg/ml (Dilaudid-5), 5 mg/5 ml (Dilaudid).
- *Tablets:* 2 mg (Dilaudid, Hydrostat IR), 3 mg (Dilaudid, Hydrostat IR), 4 mg (Dilaudid), 8 mg (Dilaudid).
- *Injection:* 1 mg/ml (Dilaudid), 2 mg/ml (Dilaudid), 4 mg/ml (Dilaudid), 10 mg/ml (Dilaudid HP).
- *Suppository (Dilaudid):* 3 mg.

CONTRAINDICATIONS: Obstetric analgesia, respiratory depression in the absence of resuscitative equipment, status asthmaticus

PREGNANCY AND LACTATION: Pregnancy category B (category D if used for prolonged periods or in high doses at term); use during labor produces neonatal respiratory depression; excretion into breast milk unknown; use caution in nursing mothers

SIDE EFFECTS

Frequent

Somnolence, dizziness, hypotension (including orthostatic hypotension), decreased appetite

Occasional

Confusion, diaphoresis, facial flushing, urine retention, constipation, dry mouth, nausea, vomiting, headache, pain at injection site

Rare

Allergic reaction, depression

SERIOUS REACTIONS

- Overdose results in respiratory depression, skeletal muscle flaccidity, cold or clammy skin, cyanosis, and extreme somnolence progressing to seizures, stupor, and coma.
- The patient who uses hydromorphone repeatedly may develop a tolerance to the drug's analgesic effect as well as physical dependence.
- This drug may have a prolonged duration of action and cumulative effect in patients with hepatic or renal impairment.

INTERACTIONS

Drugs

3 *Antihistamines, chloral hydrate, glutethimide, methocarbamol:* Enhanced depressant effects

3 *Barbiturates:* Additive respiratory and CNS depressant effects

3 *Cimetidine:* Increased respiratory and CNS depression

3 *Ethanol, other CNS depressants:* Additive CNS effects

3 *MAOIs:* May produce a severe, fatal reaction; plan to administer one-quarter of usual hydromorphone dose

Labs

- *False increase:* Amylase and lipase

SPECIAL CONSIDERATIONS

- Do not administer agonist/antagonist analgesics (i.e., pentazocine, nalbuphine, butorphanol, dezocine, buprenorphine) to patient who has received a prolonged course of hydromorphone (a pure agonist). In opioid-dependent patients, mixed agonist/antagonist analgesics may precipitate withdrawal symptoms.

PATIENT/FAMILY EDUCATION

- Physical dependency may result when used for extended periods
- Avoid hazardous activities if drowsiness or dizziness occurs
- Avoid alcohol, other CNS depressants unless directed by clinician
- Minimize nausea by administering with food and remain lying down following dose
- Be alert to the onset of pain because the drug is less effective if a full pain response recurs before the next dose
- Change positions slowly to avoid orthostatic hypotension

MONITORING PARAMETERS

- Vital signs
- Pattern of daily bowel activity and stool consistency, especially with long-term use
- Keep in mind that the drug's effect is reduced if the full pain response recurs before the next dose
- For patients being treated for a cough, auscultate the lungs for adventitious breath sounds and increase fluid intake and environmental humidity to decrease the viscosity of lung secretions
- Initiate deep-breathing and coughing exercises, particularly in patients with impaired respiratory function
- Clinical improvement and record the onset of pain or cough relief

hydroquinone

(hye-droe-kwin'-one)

Rx: Alphaquin HP, Alustra, Claripel, Eldopaque, Eldopaque Forte, Eldoquin, EpiQuin Micro, Esoterica Regular, Glyquin, Lustra, Lustra-AF, Melanex, Melpaque HP, Melquin-3, Melquin HP, NeoStrata AHA, Nuquin HP, Neostrata HQ, Palmer's Skin Success Fade Cream, Solaquin, Solaquin Forte

Combinations

Rx: with fluocinolone/tretinoin (Tri-Luma)

Chemical Class: Monobenzone derivative

Therapeutic Class: Depigmenting agent

CLINICAL PHARMACOLOGY

Mechanism of Action: A depigmenting agent that suppresses melanocyte metabolic processes of the skin. Inhibits the enzymatic oxidation of tyrosine to DOPA (3, 4-dihydroxyphenylalanine). Sun exposure reverses this effect and causes repigmentation. ***Therapeutic Effect:*** Lighten hyperpigmented areas.

Pharmacokinetics

Onset and duration of depigmentation vary among individuals. About 35% is absorbed.

INDICATIONS AND DOSAGES

Hyperpigmentation, melanin

Topical

Adults, Elderly, Children 12 yrs and older. Apply twice daily.

AVAILABLE FORMS

- *Cream:* 2% (Eldopaque, Esoterica Regular, Palmer's Skin Success Fade Cream) 4% (Alphaquin HP, Alustra, EpiQuin Micro, Lustra, Melquin HP, Nuquin HP).

• *Cream, with sunscreen:* 2% (Solaquin), 4% (Claripel, Glyquin, Solaquin, Solaquin Forte, Lustra-AF, Melpaque HP).
• *Gel:* 2% (NeoStrata AHA).
• *Gel, with sunscreen:* 4% (Nuqiun HP, Solaquin Forte.

UNLABELED USES: None known.

CONTRAINDICATIONS: Hypersensitivity to hydroquinone, sulfites, or any other component of its formulation

PREGNANCY AND LACTATION: Pregnancy category C; degree of systemic absorption unknown; excretion into breast milk unknown

SIDE EFFECTS

Occasional

Burning, itching, stinging, erythema such as localized contact dermatitis

Rare

Conjunctival changes, fingernail staining

SERIOUS REACTIONS

• Gradual blue-black darkening of skin has been reported.
• Occasional cutaneous hypersensitivity (localized contact dermatitis) may occur.

INTERACTIONS

Labs

• *False decrease:* Urine glucose

SPECIAL CONSIDERATIONS

PATIENT/FAMILY EDUCATION

• Apply small amount to an unbroken patch of skin and check in 24 hr; if vesicle formation, itching, or excessive inflammation occurs, further treatment not advised
• Positive response may require 3 wks-6 mos
• Protect the treated area from UV light by using a sunscreen, sun block, or protective clothing
• Avoid application to lips or near eyes

MONITORING PARAMETERS

• Skin for any irritation or rash

hydroxocobalamin (vitamin B_{12})

(hye-drox'-oh-co-bal'-a-min)

Rx: Alphamin, Hydrobexan, Hydro-Cobex, Hydro-Crysti-12, Hydroxy-Cobal, LA-12, Vibal LA

Chemical Class: Vitamin B complex

Therapeutic Class: Antidote, nitroprusside; hematinic; vitamin

H

CLINICAL PHARMACOLOGY

Mechanism of Action: A coenzyme for metabolic functions, including fat and carbohydrate metabolism and protein synthesis. ***Therapeutic Effect:*** Necessary for growth, cell replication, hematopoiesis, and myelin synthesis.

Pharmacokinetics

Rapidly absorbed after IM administration. Protein binding: high. Primarily excreted in urine. Metabolized in liver. ***Half-life:*** 6 days.

INDICATIONS AND DOSAGES

Vitamin B_{12} deficiency

IM

Adults, Elderly. 30 mcg/day for 5-10 days then 100-200 mcg monthly.
Children. 1-5 mg in single doses of 100 mcg over 2 or more wks then 30-50 mcg monthly.

AVAILABLE FORMS

• *Injection:* 100 mcg/ml (Alphamin), 1000 mcg/ml (Alphamin, Hydrobexan, Hydro-Cobex, Hydro-Crysti-12, Hydroxy-Cobal, LA-12, Vibal LA).

CONTRAINDICATIONS: Folate-deficient anemia, hereditary optic nerve atrophy, hypersensitivity to cobalt, hypersensitivity to hydroxocobalamin or any component of the formulation

PREGNANCY AND LACTATION: Pregnancy category A (C if dose exceeds recommended daily allowance); vitamin B_{12} is an essential vitamin and needs are increased during pregnancy; excreted into breast milk; 2.6 mcg/day should be consumed during pregnancy and lactation

SIDE EFFECTS

Occasional

Diarrhea, itching, pain at injection site

SERIOUS REACTIONS

- Rare allergic reaction, generally due to impurities in preparation, may occur.
- May produce peripheral vascular thrombosis, pulmonary edema, hypokalemia, and congestive heart failure (CHF).

INTERACTIONS

Labs

- *False positive:* Intrinsic factor
- *Interference:* Methotrexate, pyrimethamine and most antibiotics interfere with vitamin B_{12} assay

SPECIAL CONSIDERATIONS

PATIENT/FAMILY EDUCATION

- Therapy may require life-long monthly injections
- Notify the physician if symptoms of an infection occur

MONITORING PARAMETERS

- Serum potassium for first 48 hr during treatment of severe megaloblastic anemia
- Reticulocyte counts, Hct, vitamin B_{12}, iron, and folic acid plasma levels prior to treatment, between days 5 and 7 of treatment, then frequently until Hct is normal

hydroxychloroquine sulfate

(hye-drox-ee-klor'-oh-kwin sul'-fate)

Rx: Plaquenil

Chemical Class: 4-aminoquinoline derivative

Therapeutic Class: Antimalarial; disease-modifying antirheumatic drug (DMARD)

CLINICAL PHARMACOLOGY

Mechanism of Action: An antimalarial and antirheumatic that concentrates in parasite acid vesicles, increasing the pH of the vesicles and interfering with parasite protein synthesis. Antirheumatic action may involve suppressing formation of antigens responsible for hypersensitivity reactions. ***Therapeutic Effect:*** Inhibits parasite growth.

Pharmacokinetics

Variable rate of absorption. Widely distributed in body tissues (eyes, kidneys, liver, lungs). Protein binding: 45%. Partially metabolized in liver. Partially excreted in urine. ***Half-life:*** 32 days (in plasma); 50 days (in blood).

INDICATIONS AND DOSAGES

Treatment of acute attack of malaria (dosage in mg base)

PO

Dose	Times	Adults	Children
Initial	Day 1	620 mg	10 mg/kg
Second	6 hr later	310 mg	5 mg/kg
Third	Day 2	310 mg	5 mg/kg
Fourth	Day 3	310 mg	5 mg/kg

Suppression of malaria

PO

Adults. 310 mg base weekly on same day each week, beginning 2 wks before entering an endemic area and continuing for 4-6 wks after leaving the area.

Children. 5 mg base/kg/wk, beginning 2 wk before entering an endemic area and continuing for 4-6 wk after leaving the area. If therapy is not begun before exposure, administer a loading dose of 10 mg base/kg in 2 equally divided doses 6 hr apart, followed by the usual dosage regimen.

Rheumatoid arthritis

PO

Adults. Initially, 400-600 mg (310-465 mg base) daily for 5-10 days, gradually increased to optimum response level. Maintenance (usually within 4-12 wk): Dosage decreased by 50% and then continued at maintenance dose of 200-400 mg/day. Maximum effect may not be seen for several months.

Lupus erythematosus

PO

Adults. Initially, 400 mg once or twice a day for several weeks or months. Maintenance: 200-400 mg/day.

AVAILABLE FORMS

• *Tablets:* 200 mg (155 mg base).

UNLABELED USES: Treatment of juvenile arthritis, sarcoid-associated hypercalcemia

CONTRAINDICATIONS: Long-term therapy for children, porphyria, psoriasis, retinal or visual field changes

PREGNANCY AND LACTATION: Pregnancy category C; excreted in breast milk; safe use during nursing has not been established

SIDE EFFECTS

Frequent

Mild, transient headache; anorexia; nausea; vomiting

Occasional

Visual disturbances, nervousness, fatigue, pruritus (especially of palms, soles, and scalp), irritability, personality changes, diarrhea

Rare

Stomatitis, dermatitis, impaired hearing

SERIOUS REACTIONS

• Ocular toxicity, especially retinopathy, may occur and may progress even after drug is discontinued.

• Prolonged therapy may result in peripheral neuritis, neuromyopathy, hypotension, EKG changes, agranulocytosis, aplastic anemia, thrombocytopenia, seizures, and psychosis.

• Overdosage may result in headache, vomiting, visual disturbances, drowsiness, seizures, and hypokalemia followed by cardiovascular collapse and death.

INTERACTIONS

Drugs

3 *Digitalis glycosides:* Increased serum digoxin concentrations

3 *Methotrexate:* Increases the plasma concentration of methotrexate; an increase in both methotrexate efficacy and toxicity may occur

3 *Penicillamine:* May increase blood penicillamine concentration and the risk of hematologic, renal, or severe skin reactions

3 *Praziquantel:* Reduced praziquantel concentration

SPECIAL CONSIDERATIONS

PATIENT/FAMILY EDUCATION

• Report any muscle weakness, visual disturbances, difficulty hearing, or ringing in ears to clinician

• Continue taking hydroxychloroquine for the full course of treatment

• Therapeutic response may not be evident for up to 6 mos

MONITORING PARAMETERS

• Baseline and periodic ophthalmologic examinations (visual acuity, slit lamp, funduscopic, and visual field tests); periodic tests of knee and ankle reflexes to detect muscular weakness

• Periodic CBCs during prolonged therapy

- Liver function test
- Assess the patient's buccal mucosa and skin, and check for pruritus
- Evaluate the patient for GI distress

hydroxyprogesterone

Rx: Gestrol LA

Chemical Class: Progestin derivative

Therapeutic Class: Antineoplastic; progestin

CLINICAL PHARMACOLOGY

Mechanism of Action: A hormone that influences proliferative endometrium and transforms into secretory endometrium. Secretion of pituitary gonadotropins is inhibited, which prevents follicular maturation and ovulation. ***Therapeutic Effect:*** Facilitates ureteral dilatation associated with hydronephrosis of pregnancy.

INDICATIONS AND DOSAGES

Amenorrhea

IM

Adults. 375 mg given at any point in the menstrual cycle.

Endogenous estrogen production

IM

Adults. 125-250 mg beginning on the tenth day of cycle and repeated every 7 days until suppression is no longer desired.

Endometrial carcinoma

IM

Adults. 1000 mg 1 or more times weekly.

Abnormal uterine bleeding

IM

Adults. 5-10 mg for 6 days. When estrogen is given concomitantly, begin progesterone after 2 wks of estrogen therapy; discontinue when menstrual flow begins.

Prevention of endometrial hyperplasia

IM

Adults. 200 mg in evening for 12 days per 28-day cycle in combination with daily conjugated estrogen.

Premature labor

IM

Adults. 250-500 mg once weekly.

AVAILABLE FORMS

- *Injection:* 250 mg/ml (Gestrol LA).

UNLABELED USES: Alopecia, stress incontinence, menopausal symptoms, preterm delivery, treatment of prostatic hyperplasia, seborrhea, ureteral stones

CONTRAINDICATIONS: Breast cancer, cerebral apoplexy or history of these conditions, missed abortion, severe liver dysfunction, thromboembolic disorders, thrombophlebitis, undiagnosed vaginal bleeding, genital malignancy, use as a diagnostic test for pregnancy

PREGNANCY AND LACTATION: Pregnancy category D; an increased risk of hypospadias in the male fetus and mild virilization of the female fetus have been reported with progestin use; progestins compatible with breast-feeding

SIDE EFFECTS

Frequent

Breakthrough bleeding or spotting at beginning of therapy, amenorrhea, change in menstrual flow, breast tenderness

Occasional

Edema, weight gain or loss, rash, pruritus, photosensitivity, skin pigmentation

Rare

Pain or swelling at injection site, acne, mental depression, alopecia, hirsutism

SERIOUS REACTIONS

• Thrombophlebitis, cerebrovascular disorders, retinal thrombosis, and pulmonary embolism rarely occur.

INTERACTIONS

Drugs

3 *Aminoglutethimide:* Decreases progestin concentration

3 *Bromocriptine:* May interfere with the effects of bromocriptine

SPECIAL CONSIDERATIONS

PATIENT/FAMILY EDUCATION

• Take protective measures against exposure to UV light or sunlight
• Notify the physician of abnormal vaginal bleeding or other symptoms
• The female patient should contact the physician, and stop taking the drug, as prescribed, if she suspects she is pregnant
• Do not smoke tobacco

MONITORING PARAMETERS

• Weight
• Blood pressure
• Skin for rash and urticaria

hydroxyzine

(hye-drox'-i-zeen)

Rx: Atarax, Hyzine, Vistaject-50, Vistaril, Vistaril IM

Chemical Class: Piperidine derivative

Therapeutic Class: Antiemetic (parenteral); antihistamine; anxiolytic; sedative/hypnotic

CLINICAL PHARMACOLOGY

Mechanism of Action: A piperazine derivative that competes with histamine for receptor sites in the GI tract, blood vessels, and respiratory tract. May exert CNS depressant activity in subcortical areas. Diminishes vestibular stimulation and depresses labyrinthine function. ***Therapeutic Effect:*** Produces anxiolytic, anticholinergic, antihistaminic, and analgesic effects; relaxes skeletal muscle; controls nausea and vomiting.

Pharmacokinetics

Route	*Onset*	*Peak*	*Duration*
PO	15-30 mins	N/A	4-6 hrs

Well absorbed from the GI tract and after parenteral administration. Metabolized in the liver. Primarily excreted in urine. Not removed by hemodialysis. ***Half-life:*** 20-25 hr (increased in the elderly).

INDICATIONS AND DOSAGES

Anxiety

PO

Adults, Elderly. 25-100 mg 4 times a day. Maximum: 600 mg/day.

Nausea and vomiting

IM

Adults, Elderly. 25-100 mg/dose q4-6h.

Pruritus

PO

Adults, Elderly. 25 mg 3-4 times a day.

Preoperative sedation

PO

Adults, Elderly. 50-100 mg.

IM

Adults, Elderly. 25-100 mg.

Usual pediatric dosage

PO

Children. 2 mg/kg/day in divided doses q6-8h.

IM

Children. 0.5-1 mg/kg/dose q4-6h.

AVAILABLE FORMS

• *Capsules (Vistaril):* 25 mg, 50 mg, 100 mg.
• *Oral Suspension (Vistaril):* 25 mg/5 ml.
• *Syrup (Atarax):* 10 mg/5 ml.
• *Tablets (Atarax):* 10 mg, 25 mg, 50 mg, 100 mg.

• *Injection (Hyzine, Vistacot, Vistaject-50, Vistaril IM):* 25 mg/ml, 50 mg/ml.

CONTRAINDICATIONS: None known.

PREGNANCY AND LACTATION: Pregnancy category C (but no excess in birth defects documented); safe during labor for relief of anxiety; no data on breast-feeding

SIDE EFFECTS

Side effects are generally mild and transient.

Frequent

Somnolence, dry mouth, marked discomfort with IM injection

Occasional

Dizziness, ataxia, asthenia, slurred speech, headache, agitation, increased anxiety

Rare

Paradoxical CNS reactions, such as hyperactivity or nervousness in children and excitement or restlessness in elderly or debilitated patients (generally noted during first 2 wks of therapy, particularly in presence of uncontrolled pain)

SERIOUS REACTIONS

• A hypersensitivity reaction, including wheezing, dyspnea, and chest tightness, may occur.

INTERACTIONS

Drugs

3 *Alcohol, other CNS depressants:* May increase CNS depressant effects

3 *MAOIs:* May increase anticholinergic and CNS depressant effects

Labs

• *False increase:* Urine 17-hydroxycorticosteroids and 17-ketogenic steroids

SPECIAL CONSIDERATIONS

PATIENT/FAMILY EDUCATION

• The IM injection may cause marked discomfort

• Drowsiness usually diminishes with continued therapy

• Avoid tasks that require mental alertness and motor skills until response to the drug has been established

• Take sips of tepid water and chew sugarless gum to help relieve dry mouth

MONITORING PARAMETERS

• CBC and blood chemistry tests periodically for patients on long-term therapy

• Breath sounds for signs of a hypersensitivity reaction, such as wheezing

• Electrolytes

• Assess the patient for paradoxical CNS reactions, particularly early in therapy

hyoscyamine sulfate

(hye-oh-sye'-a-meen sul'-fate)

Rx: A-Spas S/L, Anaspaz, Cystospaz, Cystospaz-M, Donnamar, Hyosine, IV-Stat, Levbid, Levsin, Levsin S/L, Levsinex, Neosol, NuLev, Spasdel, Symax SL, Symax SR

Combinations

Rx: with phenobarbital (Levsin PB)

Chemical Class: Belladonna alkaloid

Therapeutic Class: Anticholinergic; gastrointestinal

CLINICAL PHARMACOLOGY

Mechanism of Action: A GI antispasmodic and anticholinergic agent that inhibits the action of acetylcholine at postganglionic (muscarinic) receptor sites. ***Therapeutic Effect:*** Decreases secretions (bronchial, salivary, sweat gland) and gastric juices and reduces motility of GI and urinary tract.

Pharmacokinetics

Completely absorbed following PO administration. Partially hydrolyzed. Majority of hyoscyamine dose is excreted unchanged in urine. Removed by hemodialysis. ***Half-life:*** 3.5 hr (immediate-release); 7 hr (sustained-release).

INDICATIONS AND DOSAGES

GI tract disorders

PO

Adults, Elderly, Children 12 yr and older. 0.125-0.25 mg q4h as needed. Extended-release: 0.375-0.75 mg q12h. Maximum: 1.5 mg/day.

Children 2-11 yr. 0.0625-0.125 mg q4h as needed. Extended-release: 0.375 mg q12h. Maximum: 0.75 mg/day.

IV, IM

Adults, Elderly, Children 12 yr and older. 0.25-0.5 mg q4h for 1-4 doses.

Hypermotility of lower urinary tract

PO, Sublingual

Adults, Elderly. 0.15-0.3 mg 4 times a day; or extended-release 0.375 mg q12h.

Infant colic

PO

Infants. Individualized drops dosed q4h as needed.

AVAILABLE FORMS

- *Tablets (Anaspaz, Cystospaz, Levsin, Spacol):* 0.125 mg.
- *Tablets (Oral-Disintegrating [NuLev]):* 0.125 mg.
- *Tablets (Sublingual [Levsin S/L, Symax SL]):* 0.125 mg.
- *Tablets (Extended-Release [Levbid, Spacol T/S, Symax SR]):* 0.375 mg.
- *Capsules (Extended-Release [Cystospaz-M, Levsinex]):* 0.375 mg.
- *Liquid (Hyosine, Spacol):* 0.125 mg/5 ml.
- *Oral Drops (Hyosine, Levsin):* 0.125 mg/ml.
- *Oral Solution (Hyosine, Levsin):* 0.125 mg/5 ml.

CONTRAINDICATIONS: GI or GU obstruction, myasthenia gravis, narrow-angle glaucoma, paralytic ileus, severe ulcerative colitis

PREGNANCY AND LACTATION: Pregnancy category C; excreted in breast milk; infants sensitive to anticholinergics

SIDE EFFECTS

Frequent

Dry mouth (sometimes severe), decreased sweating, constipation

Occasional

Blurred vision; bloated feeling; urinary hesitancy; somnolence (with high dosage); headache; intolerance to light; loss of taste; nervousness; flushing; insomnia; impotence; mental confusion or excitement (particularly in the elderly and children); temporary lightheadedness (with parenteral form); local irritation (with parenteral form)

Rare

Dizziness, faintness

SERIOUS REACTIONS

- Overdose may produce temporary paralysis of ciliary muscle; pupillary dilation; tachycardia; palpitations; hot, dry, or flushed skin; absence of bowel sounds; hyperthermia; increased respiratory rate; EKG abnormalities; nausea; vomiting; rash over face or upper trunk; CNS stimulation; and psychosis (marked by agitation, restlessness, rambling speech, visual hallucinations, paranoid behavior, and delusions, followed by depression).

INTERACTIONS

Drugs

3 *Antacids, antidiarrheals:* May decrease the absorption of hyoscyamine

3 *Ketoconazole:* May decrease the absorption of this drug

3 *Other anticholinergics:* May increase the effects of hyoscyamine

3 *Potassium chloride:* May increase the severity of GI lesions with the matrix formulation of potassium chloride

SPECIAL CONSIDERATIONS

PATIENT/FAMILY EDUCATION

• Dry mouth may occur during hyoscyamine therapy; maintain good oral hygiene because the lack of saliva may increase the risk of cavities
• Notify the physician if constipation, difficulty urinating, eye pain, or rash occurs
• Avoid hot baths and saunas
• Avoid tasks that require mental alertness or motor skills until response to the drug has been established

MONITORING PARAMETERS

• Pattern of daily bowel activity and stool consistency
• Blood pressure, body temperature

ibandronate sodium

(i-ban'-droh-nate soe'-dee-um)

Rx: Boniva

Chemical Class: Pyrophosphate analog

Therapeutic Class: Antiosteoporotic; bisphosphonate

CLINICAL PHARMACOLOGY

Mechanism of Action: A bisphosphonate that binds to bone hydroxyapatite (part of the mineral matrix of bone) and inhibits osteoclast activity. ***Therapeutic Effect:*** Reduces rate of bone turnover and bone resorption, resulting in a net gain in bone mass.

Pharmacokinetics

Absorbed in the upper GI tract. Extent of absorption impaired by food or beverages (other than plain water). Rapidly binds to bone. Unabsorbed portion is eliminated in urine. Protein binding: 90%. ***Half-life:*** 10-60 hr.

INDICATIONS AND DOSAGES

Osteoporosis

PO

Adults, Elderly. 2.5 mg daily. Alternatively, 150 mg once monthly.

AVAILABLE FORMS

• *Tablets:* 2.5 mg, 150 mg.

CONTRAINDICATIONS: Hypersensitivity to other bisphosphonates, including alendronate, etidronate, pamidronate, risedronate, and tiludronate; inability to stand or sit upright for at least 60 mins; severe renal impairment with creatinine clearance less than 30 ml/min; uncorrected hypocalcemia

PREGNANCY AND LACTATION: Pregnancy category C; breast milk excretion unknown

SIDE EFFECTS

Frequent (13%-6%)

Back pain; dyspepsia, including epigastric distress and heartburn; peripheral discomfort; diarrhea; headache; myalgia

Occasional (4%-3%)

Dizziness, arthralgia, asthenia

Rare (2% or less)

Vomiting, hypersensitivity reaction

SERIOUS REACTIONS

• Upper respiratory tract infection occurs occasionally.
• Overdose causes hypocalcemia, hypophosphatemia, and significant GI disturbances.

INTERACTIONS

Drugs

3 *Antacids: calcium and other multivalent cations (aluminum, magnesium, iron):* Reduced absorption

3 *Food (including coffee and juice):* Decreases bioavailability drastically (see Pharmacokinetics)

3 *Aspirin, nonsteroidal antiinflammatory drugs:* Theoretical increased risk of gastropathy

Labs

• Decreases in alkaline phosphatase levels

• Bisphosphonate class effect—interference with the use of bone-imaging agents

SPECIAL CONSIDERATIONS

• Clinicians should remain alert to signs or symptoms signaling possible esophageal irritation reaction (dysphagia, retrosternal pain, or heartburn)

PATIENT/FAMILY EDUCATION

• To maximize absorption and clinical benefit, patients should be instructed to take drug at least 60 mins before first food or drink of the day or other oral medications (particularly calcium, antacids, or vitamins)

• To reduce potential for esophageal irritation, patients should be instructed to swallow tablets intact (not chew or suck) with a full glass of plain water (not mineral water) while remaining in the standing or sitting upright position for 60 mins

• Patients should receive supplemental calcium and vitamin D if dietary intake is inadequate

• Consider beginning weight-bearing exercises and modifying behavioral factors, such as reducing alcohol consumption and stopping cigarette smoking

MONITORING PARAMETERS

• Bone mass density (T-score, hip, spine), N-telopeptide; serum calcium (adjusted for hypoalbuminemia), phosphorus, magnesium, renal function, liver function, serum electrolytes, signs and symptoms of toxicity (i.e., esophageal irritation)

ibuprofen

(eye-byoo'-proe-fen)

Rx: Advil, Advil Pediatric, Children's Advil, Ibu, Ibu-4, Ibu-6, Ibu-8, Ibu-Tab, Motrin

OTC: Advil, Arthritis Foundation Pain Reliever, Children's Motrin, Ibuprin, Junior Advil, Junior Strength Motrin, Motrin IB, Nuprin, Pediacare Fever

Combinations

Rx: with Hydrocodone (Vicoprofen); with oxycodone (Combunox)

OTC: With pseudoephedrine (Sine-Aid IB, Motrin IB Sinus)

Chemical Class: Propionic acid derivative

Therapeutic Class: NSAID; antipyretic; nonnarcotic analgesic

CLINICAL PHARMACOLOGY

Mechanism of Action: An NSAID that inhibits prostaglandin synthesis. Also produces vasodilation by acting centrally on the heat-regulating center of the hypothalamus.

Therapeutic Effect: Produces analgesic and antiinflammatory effects and decreases fever.

Pharmacokinetics

Route	*Onset*	*Peak*	*Duration*
PO (analgesic)	0.5 hrs	N/A	4-6 hrs
PO (antirheumatic)	2 days	1-2 wks	N/A

Rapidly absorbed from the GI tract. Protein binding: greater than 90%. Metabolized in the liver. Primarily excreted in urine. Not removed by hemodialysis. ***Half-life:*** 2-4 hr.

INDICATIONS AND DOSAGES

Acute or chronic rheumatoid arthritis, osteoarthritis, migraine pain, gouty arthritis

PO

Adults, Elderly. 400-800 mg 3-4 times a day. Maximum: 3.2 g/day.

Mild to moderate pain, primary dysmenorrhea

PO

Adults, Elderly. 200-400 mg q4-6h as needed. Maximum: 1.6 g/day.

Fever, minor aches or pain

PO

Adults, Elderly. 200-400 mg q4-6h. Maximum: 1.6 g/day.

Children. 5-10 mg/kg/dose q6-8h. Maximum: 40 mg/kg/day. OTC: 7.5 mg/kg/dose q6-8h. Maximum: 30 mg/kg/day.

Juvenile arthritis

PO

Children. 30-70 mg/kg/day in 3-4 divided doses. Maximum: 400 mg/day in children weighing less than 20 kg, 600 mg/day in children weighing 20-30 kg, 800 mg/day in children weighing greater than 30-40 kg.

AVAILABLE FORMS

- *Caplets (Advil, Menadol, Motrin):* 200 mg.
- *Capsules (Advil, Advil Migraine):* 200 mg.
- *Gelcaps (Advil, Motrin IB):* 200 mg.
- *Tablets:* 200 mg (Advil, Motrin IB), 400 mg (Ibu, Ibu-4, Ibu-6, Ibu-8, Ibu-Tab, Motrin), 600 mg (Ibu, Ibu-4, Ibu-6, Ibu-8, Ibu-Tab, Motrin), 800 mg (Ibu, Ibu-4, Ibu-6, Ibu-8, Ibu-Tab, Motrin).
- *Tablets (Chewable):* 50 mg (Children's Advil, Children's Motrin), 100 mg (Junior Advil, Junior Strength Motrin).
- *Oral Suspension (Advil, Children's Advil, Children's Motrin):* 100 mg/5 ml.
- *Oral Drops (Advil Pediatric, Infant Advil, Infant Motrin, Children's Motrin, Pediacare Fever):* 40 mg/ml.

UNLABELED USES: Treatment of psoriatic arthritis, vascular headaches

CONTRAINDICATIONS: Active peptic ulcer, chronic inflammation of GI tract, GI bleeding disorders or ulceration, history of hypersensitivity to aspirin or NSAIDs

PREGNANCY AND LACTATION: Pregnancy category B (D if used in third trimester or near delivery); reduces amniotic fluid volume, constriction of the ductus arteriosus in third trimester; compatible with breast-feeding

SIDE EFFECTS

Occasional (9%-3%)

Nausea with or without vomiting, dyspepsia, dizziness, rash

Rare (less than 3%)

Diarrhea or constipation, flatulence, abdominal cramps or pain, pruritus

SERIOUS REACTIONS

- Acute overdose may result in metabolic acidosis.
- Rare reactions with long-term use include peptic ulcer disease, GI bleeding, gastritis, a severe hepatic reaction (cholestasis, jaundice), nephrotoxicity (dysuria, hematuria, proteinuria, nephrotic syndrome), and a severe hypersensitivity reaction (particularly in patients with systemic lupus erythematosus or other collagen diseases).

INTERACTIONS

Drugs

3 *Aminoglycosides:* Reduced clearance with elevated aminoglycoside levels and potential for toxicity (especially indomethacin in premature infants; other NSAIDs probably)

3 *Anticoagulants:* Excessive hypoprothrombinemia, decreased platelet aggregation with increased risk of GI bleeding

3 *Antihypertensives (α-blockers, angiotensin-converting enzyme inhibitors, angiotensin II receptor blockers, β-blockers, diuretics):* Inhibition of antihypertensive and other favorable hemodynamic effects

3 *Aspirin, other salicylates:* May increase the risk of GI side effects such as bleeding

3 *Bone marrow depressants:* May increase the risk of hematologic reactions

3 *Corticosteroids:* Increased risk of GI ulceration

3 *Cyclosporine:* Increased nephrotoxicity risk

3 *Lithium:* Decreased clearance of lithium (mediated via prostaglandins) resulting in elevated serum lithium levels and risk of toxicity

3 *Methotrexate:* Decreased renal secretion of methotrexate resulting in elevated methotrexate levels and risk of toxicity

3 *Phenylpropanolamine:* Possible acute hypertensive reaction

3 *Probenecid:* May increase the ibuprofen blood concentration

3 *Potassium-sparing diuretics:* Additive hyperkalemia potential

3 *Triamterene:* Acute renal failure reported with addition of indomethacin; caution with other NSAIDs

Labs

- *False decrease:* ALT, AST

SPECIAL CONSIDERATIONS

- Administer with food or antacids if GI symptoms occur

PATIENT/FAMILY EDUCATION

- Do not chew or crush enteric-coated ibuprofen tablets
- Ibuprofen may cause dizziness
- Avoid alcohol and aspirin during ibuprofen therapy because these substances increase the risk of GI bleeding
- Avoid performing tasks that require mental alertness or motor skills until response to the drug has been established

MONITORING PARAMETERS

- Initial hemogram and fecal occult blood test within 3 mos of starting regular chronic therapy; repeat every 6-12 mos (more frequently in high-risk patients: >65 years, peptic ulcer disease, concurrent steroids or anticoagulants); electrolytes, creatinine, and BUN within 3 mo of starting regular chronic therapy; repeat every 6-12 mos
- Body temperature for fever
- CBC, platelet count, serum alkaline phosphatase, bilirubin, AST (SGOT) and ALT (SGPT) levels
- Pattern of daily bowel activity and stool consistency
- Therapeutic response, such as improved grip strength, increased joint mobility, and decreased pain, tenderness, stiffness, and swelling

ibutilide fumarate

(eye-byoo′-ti-lide)

Rx: Corvert

Chemical Class: Methanesulfonamide derivative

Therapeutic Class: Antiarrhythmic, class III

CLINICAL PHARMACOLOGY

Mechanism of Action: An antiarrhythmic that prolongs both atrial and ventricular action potential duration and increases the atrial and ventricular refractory period. Activates slow, inward current (mostly of sodium), produces mild slowing of sinus node rate and AV conduction, and causes dose-related prolongation of QT interval. ***Therapeutic Effect:*** Converts arrhythmias to sinus rhythm.

Pharmacokinetics

After IV administration, highly distributed, rapidly cleared. Protein binding: 40%. Primarily excreted in urine as metabolite. ***Half-life:*** 2-12 hr (average: 6 hr).

INDICATIONS AND DOSAGES

Rapid conversion of atrial fibrillation or flutter of recent onset to normal sinus rhythm

IV Infusion

Adults, Elderly weighing 60 kg and more. One vial (1 mg) given over 10 min. If arrhythmia does not stop within 10 min after end of initial infusion, a second 1 mg/10-min infusion may be given.

Adults, Elderly weighing less than 60 kg. 0.01 mg/kg given over 10 min. If arrhythmia does not stop within 10 min after end of initial infusion, a second 0.01 mg/kg, 10-min infusion may be given.

AVAILABLE FORMS

• *Injection:* 0.1 mg/ml solution.

CONTRAINDICATIONS: None known.

PREGNANCY AND LACTATION: Pregnancy category C; excretion into breast milk unknown; breastfeeding not recommended

SIDE EFFECTS

Ibutilide is generally well tolerated.

Occasional

Ventricular extrasystoles (5.1%), ventricular tachycardia (4.9%), headache (3.6%), hypotension, orthostatic hypotension (2%)

Rare

Bundle-branch block, AV block, bradycardia, hypertension

SERIOUS REACTIONS

• Sustained polymorphic ventricular tachycardia, occasionally with QT prolongation (torsades de pointes) occurs rarely.

• Overdose results in CNS toxicity, including CNS depression, rapid gasping breathing, and seizures.

• Expect that prolongation of repolarization may be exaggerated.

• Existing arrhythmias may worsen or new arrhythmias may develop.

INTERACTIONS

Drugs

3 *Disopyramide, quninidine, procainamide, amiodarone, sotalol:* Potential to prolong refractoriness

❷ *Phenothiazines, tricyclic antidepressants, terfenadine, astemizole:* Increased potential for prodysrhythmia due to prolongation of QT interval

SPECIAL CONSIDERATIONS

PATIENT/FAMILY EDUCATION

• Blood pressure and EKG will be continuously monitored during therapy

• Immediately report palpitations or other adverse reactions

MONITORING PARAMETERS

• Continuous ECG monitoring for at least 4 hr following infusion or until QTc returns to baseline (longer

monitoring if dysrhythmic activity noted). Defibrillator must be available
- Blood pressure

imatinib mesylate

(im'-a-tin-ib mes'-sil-ate)

Rx: Gleevec

Chemical Class: Phenylaminopyrimidine derivative

Therapeutic Class: Antineoplastic

CLINICAL PHARMACOLOGY

Mechanism of Action: Inhibits Bcr-Abl tyrosine kinase, an enzyme created by the Philadelphia chromosome abnormality found in patients with chronic myeloid leukemia (CML). ***Therapeutic Effect:*** Suppresses tumor growth during the three stages of CML: blast crisis, accelerated phase, and chronic phase.

Pharmacokinetics

Well absorbed after PO administration. Binds to plasma proteins, particularly albumin. Metabolized in the liver. Eliminated mainly in the feces as metabolites. ***Half-life:*** 18 hr.

INDICATIONS AND DOSAGES

CML

PO

Adults, Elderly. 400 mg/day for patients in chronic-phase CML; 600 mg/day for patients in accelerated phase or blast crisis. May increase dosage from 400 to 600 mg/day for patients in chronic phase or from 600 to 800 mg (given as 300-400 mg twice a day) for patients in accelerated phase or blast crisis in the absence of a severe drug reaction or severe neutropenia or thrombocytopenia in the following circumstances: progression of the disease, failure to achieve a satisfactory hematologic response after 3 mos or more of treatment, or loss of a previously achieved hematologic response.

Children. 260 mg/m^2 a day as a single daily dose or in 2 divided doses.

GI stromal tumors

PO

Adults, Elderly. 400 or 600 mg once daily

AVAILABLE FORMS

- *Tablets:* 100 mg, 400 mg.
- *Capsules:* 100 mg.

CONTRAINDICATIONS: Pregnancy

PREGNANCY AND LACTATION: Pregnancy category D; breast-feeding not recommended

SIDE EFFECTS

Frequent (68%-24%)

Nausea, diarrhea, vomiting, headache, fluid retention (periorbital, lower extremities), rash, musculoskeletal pain, muscle cramps, arthralgia

Occasional (23%-10%)

Abdominal pain, cough, myalgia, fatigue, fever, anorexia, dyspepsia, constipation, night sweats, pruritus

Rare (less than 10%)

Nasopharyngitis, petechiae, asthenia, epistaxis

SERIOUS REACTIONS

- Severe fluid retention (manifested as pleural effusion, pericardial effusion, pulmonary edema, and ascites) and hepatotoxicity occur rarely.
- Neutropenia and thrombocytopenia are expected responses to the drug.
- Respiratory toxicity, manifested as dyspnea and pneumonia, may occur.

INTERACTIONS

Drugs

3 *Ketoconazole, itraconazole, erythromycin, clarithromycin (CYP3A4 inhibitors):* Increased imatinib concentrations

3 *Virus vaccines:* May potentiate viral replication, increase vaccine side effects, and decrease the patient's antibody response to the vaccine

3 *Simvastatin, cyclosporin, dihydropyridine calcium channel blockers, triazolo-benzodiazepines, pimozide (inhibition of CYP3A4 by imatinib):* Increased concentrations of these drugs

3 *Phenytoin, dexamethasone, carbamezepine, rifampicin, phenobarbital, St. John's wort (CYP3A4 inducers):* Decreased imatinib concentrations

2 *Warfarin:* Altered metabolism of warfarin, use standard or low molecular weight heparin

2 *Acetaminophen:* Possible increased hepatotoxicity (single report of patient death)

SPECIAL CONSIDERATIONS

- Median time to hematologic response 1 mo
- Manage fluid retention with interruption of therapy, diuretics, dose reduction
- If bilirubin increases >3 × upper limits normal (ULN) or transaminases >5 × ULN, withhold until bilirubin <1.5 × ULN and transaminases <2.5 × ULN; reduce dose and continue treatment
- If in chronic phase and ANC <1 × 10^9/L and/or platelets <50 × 10^9/L, stop therapy until ANC = 1.5 × 10^9/L and platelets = 75 × 10^9/L, resume at reduced dose; if patient in accelerated phase or blast crisis, check if cytopenia related to leukemia
- There are no controlled trials in pediatric patients demonstrating a clinical benefit, such as improvement in disease-related symptoms or increased survival

PATIENT/FAMILY EDUCATION

- Take with food and large glass of water to minimize GI side effects
- Avoid acetaminophen (hepatotoxicity)
- Numerous drugs may interact with imatinib, discuss with prescriber
- Avoid receiving vaccinations and coming in contact with crowds, people with known infections, and anyone who has recently received a live-virus vaccine

MONITORING PARAMETERS

- Follow weights and monitor for fluid retention
- LFTs before treatment and every month, CBC, serum chemistry, bone marrow assessment (including cytogenic analysis)
- Pattern of daily bowel activity and stool consistency

imipenem-cilastatin sodium

(i-mi-pen'-em sye-la-stat'-in soe'-dee-um)

Rx: Primaxin IM, Primaxin IV

Chemical Class: Carbapenem; renal dipeptidase inhibitor (cilistatin); thienamycin derivative

Therapeutic Class: Antibiotic

CLINICAL PHARMACOLOGY

Mechanism of Action: A fixed-combination carbapenem. Imipenem penetrates the bacterial cell membrane and binds to penicillin-binding proteins, inhibiting cell wall synthesis. Cilastatin competitively inhibits the enzyme dehydropeptidase, preventing renal metabolism of imipenem. ***Therapeutic Effect:*** Produces bacterial cell death.

Pharmacokinetics

Readily absorbed after IM administration. Protein binding: 13%-21%. Widely distributed. Metabolized in the kidneys. Primarily excreted in urine. Removed by hemodialysis. ***Half-life:*** 1 hr (increased in impaired renal function).

INDICATIONS AND DOSAGES

Serious respiratory tract, skin and skin-structure, gynecologic, bone, joint, intraabdominal, nosocomial, and polymicrobic infections; UTIs; endocarditis; septicemia

IV

Adults, Elderly. 2-4 g/day in divided doses q6h.

Mild to moderate respiratory tract, skin and skin-structure, gynecologic, bone, joint, intraabdominal, and polymicrobic infections; UTIs; endocarditis; septicemia

IV

Adults, Elderly. 1-2 g/day in divided doses q6-8h.

Children older than 3 mo-12 yr. 60-100 mg/kg/day in divided doses q6h. Maximum: 4 g/day.

Children 1-3 mo. 100 mg/kg/day in divided doses q6h.

Children younger than 1 mo. 20-25 mg/kg/dose q8-24h.

IM

Adults, Elderly. 500-750 mg q12h.

Dosage in renal impairment

Dosage and frequency are modified based on creatinine clearance and the severity of the infection.

Creatinine Clearance	*Dosage (IV)*
31-70 ml/mins	500 mg q8h
21-30 ml/mins	500 mg q12h
5-20 ml/mins	250 mg q12h

AVAILABLE FORMS

• *IV Injection (Primaxin IV):* 250 mg, 500 mg.

• *IM Injection (Primaxin IM):* 500 mg, 750 mg.

CONTRAINDICATIONS: *IM:* Severe shock or heart block, hypersensitivity to local anesthetics of the amide type. *IV:* Patients with meningitis.

PREGNANCY AND LACTATION: Pregnancy category C; unknown if excreted in breast milk

SIDE EFFECTS

Occasional (3%-2%)

Diarrhea, nausea, vomiting

Rare (2%-1%)

Rash

SERIOUS REACTIONS

• Antibiotic-associated colitis and other superinfections may occur.

• Anaphylactic reactions have been reported.

INTERACTIONS

Drugs

3 *Cyclosporine, tacrolimus:* Risk of CNS toxicity

2 *Ganciclovir:* Generalized seizures have been reported when these drugs have been used concomitantly

3 *Theophylline:* Increased seizure risk without elevated theophylline levels

Labs

• *Interference:* Clindamycin, erythromycin, metronidazole, polymyxin, tetracycline, trimethoprim colistin levels

SPECIAL CONSIDERATIONS

PATIENT/FAMILY EDUCATION

• Notify the physician if severe diarrhea occurs

MONITORING PARAMETERS

• Daily bowel activity and stool consistency

• Liver and renal function

imipramine hydrochloride

(im-ip′-ra-meen hye-droe-klor′-ide)

Rx: Tofranil, Tofranil PM

Chemical Class: Dibenzazepine derivative; tertiary amine

Therapeutic Class: Antidepressant, tricyclic; antiincontinence agent

CLINICAL PHARMACOLOGY

Mechanism of Action: A tricyclic antidepressant, antibulimic, anticataplectic, antinarcoleptic, antineuralgic, antineuritic, and antipanic agent that blocks the reuptake of neurotransmitters, such as norepinephrine and serotonin, at presynaptic membranes, increasing their concentration at postsynaptic receptor sites. ***Therapeutic Effect:*** Relieves depression and controls nocturnal enuresis.

Pharmacokinetics

Rapidly, well absorbed following PO administration. Protein binding: more than 90%. Metabolized in liver, with first-pass effect. Excreted in urine as metabolites. ***Half-life:*** 6-18 hr.

INDICATIONS AND DOSAGES

Depression

PO

Adults. Initially, 75-100 mg/day. May gradually increase to 300 mg/day then reduce dosage to effective maintenance level, 50-150 mg/day.

Elderly. Initially, 10-25 mg/day at bedtime. May increase by 10-25 mg every 3-7 days. Range: 50-150 mg/day.

Children. 1.5 mg/kg/day. May increase by 1 mg/kg every 3-4 days. Maximum: 5 mg/kg/day.

Enuresis

PO

Children older than 6 yr. Initially, 10-25 mg at bedtime. May increase by 25 mg/day. Maximum: 50 mg for children older than 12 yr.

AVAILABLE FORMS

- *Tablets (Tofranil):* 10 mg, 25 mg, 50 mg.
- *Capsules (Tofranil-PM):* 75 mg, 100 mg, 125 mg, 150 mg.

UNLABELED USES: Treatment of attention-deficit hyperactivity disorder, cataplexy associated with narcolepsy, neurogenic pain, panic disorder

CONTRAINDICATIONS: Acute recovery period after MI, use within 14 days of MAOIs

PREGNANCY AND LACTATION: Pregnancy category D

SIDE EFFECTS

Frequent

Somnolence, fatigue, dry mouth, blurred vision, constipation, delayed micturition, orthostatic hypotension, diaphoresis, impaired concentration, increased appetite, urine retention, photosensitivity

Occasional

GI disturbances (nausea, metallic taste)

Rare

Paradoxical reactions, (agitation, restlessness, nightmares, insomnia), extrapyramidal symptoms (particularly fine hand tremor)

SERIOUS REACTIONS

- Overdose may produce seizures; cardiovascular effects, such as severe orthostatic hypotension, dizziness, tachycardia, palpitations, and arrhythmias; and altered temperature regulation, including hyperpyrexia or hypothermia.
- Abrupt discontinuation after prolonged therapy may produce headache, malaise, nausea, vomiting, and vivid dreams.

INTERACTIONS

Drugs

3 *Altretamine:* Orthostatic hypotension

3 *Amphetamines:* Theoretical increase in amphetamine effect

3 *Antidiabetics:* Possible enhanced hypoglycemic effects

3 *Antithyroid agents:* May increase the risk of agranulocytosis

❷ *Bethanidine, clonidine:* Inhibition of antihypertensive effect, possible hypertensive crisis

3 *Carbamazepine, cholestyramine, colestipol, barbiturates:* Reduces imipramine levels

❷ *Epinephrine, norepinephrine:* Hypertension and dysrhythmias

3 *Ethanol:* Enhanced motor skill impairment

3 *Ginkgo biloba:* May decrease the seizure threshold

3 *Guanethidine, guanfacine:* Inhibition of antihypertensive effect

3 *Isoproterenol and possibly other β-agonists:* Increased risk of arrhythmias

3 *Lithium:* Possible increased CNS toxicity, especially in elderly

▲ *MAOIs:* Serotonin syndrome, some fatal

❷ *Moclobemide:* Risk serotonin syndrome

3 *Phenothiazines, cimetidine (not with other H_2 blockers), calcium channel blockers, selective serotonin reuptake inhibitors, quinidine, ritonavir, indinavir:* Increased imipramine levels

3 *Phenylephrine:* Enhanced pressor response

3 *Phenytoin:* May decrease imipramine blood concentration

3 *Propantheline:* Excessive anticholinergic effects

3 *St. John's Wort:* May increase imipramine's pharmacologic effects and risk of toxicity

3 *Venlafaxine:* Increases imipramine serum concentrations

Labs

- *False increase:* Carbamazepine levels
- *False decrease:* Urine 5-HIAA, VMA

SPECIAL CONSIDERATIONS

PATIENT/FAMILY EDUCATION

- Withdrawal symptoms (headache, nausea, vomiting, muscle pain, weakness) may occur if drug discontinued abruptly
- At doses of 20 mg/kg ventricular arrhythmias occur
- Improvement may occur 2-5 days after starting therapy but the full therapeutic effect will likely occur within 2-3 wks
- Change positions slowly to help prevent dizziness
- The patient will develop tolerance to the drug's anticholinergic, hypotensive, and sedative effects during early therapy
- Avoid tasks that require mental alertness or motor skills until response to the drug has been established
- Take sips of tepid water and chew sugarless gum to relieve dry mouth

MONITORING PARAMETERS

- Closely monitor suicidal patients during early therapy. As depression lessens, the patient's energy level generally improves, increasing the likelihood of suicide attempts
- Assess the patient's appearance, behavior, level of interest, mood, and sleep pattern before and during therapy
- Pattern of daily bowel activity and stool consistency
- Blood pressure, pulse rate
- Evidence of urine retention
- The therapeutic serum level for imipramine is 225-300 ng/ml; the toxic serum level is greater than 500 ng/ml

imiquimod

(i-mi-kwi′-mod)

Rx: Aldara

Chemical Class: Imidazoquinoline amine

Therapeutic Class: Antiviral

CLINICAL PHARMACOLOGY

Mechanism of Action: An immune response modifier whose mechanism of action is uknown. ***Therapeutic Effect:*** Reduces genital and perianal warts.

Pharmacokinetics

Minimal absorption after topical administration. Minimal excretion in urine and feces.

INDICATIONS AND DOSAGES

Warts/condyloma acuminata

Topical

Adults, Elderly, Children 12 yrs and older. Apply 3 times/wk before normal sleeping hours; leave on skin 6-10 hrs. Remove following treatment period. Continue therapy for maximum of 16 wks.

AVAILABLE FORMS

- *Cream:* 5% (Aldara).

CONTRAINDICATIONS: History of hypersensitivity to imiquimod

PREGNANCY AND LACTATION: Pregnancy category C; excretion into breast milk unknown but would be expected to be small given minimal systemic absorption

SIDE EFFECTS

Frequent

Local skin reactions: erythema, itching, burning, erosion, excoriation/flaking, fungal infections (women)

Occasional

Pain, induration, ulceration, scabbing, soreness, headache, flu-like symptoms

SERIOUS REACTIONS

- None reported.

SPECIAL CONSIDERATIONS

- New option for treatment of genital and perianal warts, which can be applied by patient at home and appears to have low toxicity compared to podofilox
- Response rates approximately 50% and relapses are common

PATIENT/FAMILY EDUCATION

- Apply thin layer to wart(s) and rub in until cream is no longer visible
- Do not occlude application site
- Should severe local reaction occur, remove cream by washing with soap and water; treatment may be resumed once skin reaction has subsided
- Wash hands before and after application

MONITORING PARAMETERS

- Skin for local reaction

inamrinone lactate

(in-am′-ri-nohn lack′-tate)

Rx: Inamrinone

Chemical Class: Bipyridine derivative

Therapeutic Class: Cardiac inotropic agent

CLINICAL PHARMACOLOGY

Mechanism of Action: A positive inotropic agent that inhibits myocardial myocardial cyclic adenosine monophosphate (cAMP) phosphodiesterase activity and directly stimulates cardiac contractility. Peripheral vasodilation reduces both preload and afterload. ***Therapeutic Effect:*** Reduces preload and afterload; increases cardiac output.

Pharmacokinetics

After IV administration, rapidly absorbed from the gastrointestinal (GI) tract. Protein binding: 10%-49%. Partially metabolized in liver. Excreted in urine as both inamrinone and its metabolites. ***Half-life:*** 3-6 hr (half-life increased with congestive heart failure).

INDICATIONS AND DOSAGES

Short-term management of intractable heart failure

IV infusion (continuous)

Adults. Initially, 0.75 mg/kg loading dose over 2-3 mins followed by a maintenance infusion of 5 and 10 mcg/kg/min. A bolus dose of 0.75 mg/kg may be given 30 mins after the initiation of therapy. Use within 24 hr and do not dilute with solutions that contain dextrose. Maximum: 10 mg/kg/day.

AVAILABLE FORMS

- *Injection:* 5mg/ml (Inamrinone).

CONTRAINDICATIONS: Severe aortic or pulmonic valvular disease; hypersensitivity to inamrinone or bisulfites.

PREGNANCY AND LACTATION: Pregnancy category C

SIDE EFFECTS

Occasional

Arrhythmia, nausea, hypotension, thrombocytopenia

Rare

Fever, vomiting, abdominal pain, anorexia, chest pain, decreased tear production, hepatotoxicity and burning at the site of injection, hypersensitivity to inamrinone

SERIOUS REACTIONS

- Overdose may cause severe hypotension.

INTERACTIONS

Drugs

3 *Digoxin:* May increase inotropic effects

3 *Furosemide:* Precipitates when furosemide is injected into an IV line infusing inamrinone

Labs

- *Increase:* Serum digoxin (Abbott TdX method)

SPECIAL CONSIDERATIONS

PATIENT/FAMILY EDUCATION

- Report dizziness or trouble swallowing

MONITORING PARAMETERS

- BP and pulse q5min during infusion; if BP drops 30 mm Hg, stop infusion
- Cardiac output and pulmonary capillary wedge pressure
- Monitor platelet count and serum K, Na, Cl, Ca, BUN, creatinine, ALT, AST, and bilirubin daily

indapamide

(in-dap'-a-mide)

Rx: Lozol

Chemical Class: Indoline derivative

Therapeutic Class: Antihypertensive; diuretic, thiazide-like

CLINICAL PHARMACOLOGY

Mechanism of Action: A thiazide-like diuretic that blocks reabsorption of water, sodium, and potassium at the cortical diluting segment of the distal tubule; also reduces plasma and extracellular fluid volume and peripheral vascular resistance by direct effect on blood vessels. ***Therapeutic Effect:*** Promotes diuresis and reduces BP.

Pharmacokinetics

Almost completely absorbed following PO administration. Protein binding: 71%-79%. Extensively metabolized in liver. Excreted in urine. ***Half-life:*** 14-15 hr.

INDICATIONS AND DOSAGES

Edema

PO

Adults. Initially, 2.5 mg/day, may increase to 5 mg/day after 1 wk.

Hypertension
PO
Adults, Elderly. Initially, 1.25 mg, may increase to 2.5 mg/day after 4 wk or 5 mg/day after additional 4 wk.

AVAILABLE FORMS
• *Tablets:* 1.25 mg, 2.5 mg.

CONTRAINDICATIONS: Anuria, hypersensitivity to sulfonamides

PREGNANCY AND LACTATION: Pregnancy category B (D if used in pregnancy-induced hypertension); therapy for preexisting hypertension can be continued throughout pregnancy with minimal risk; initiating for edema not recommended; few unequivocal indications for diuretic therapy in pregnancy except for pulmonary edema or congestive heart failure; not known if excreted in breast milk

SIDE EFFECTS
Frequent (5% and greater)
Fatigue, numbness of extremities, tension, irritability, agitation, headache, dizziness, lightheadedness, insomnia, muscle cramps
Occasional (less than 5%)
Tingling of extremities, urinary frequency, urticaria, rhinorrhea, flushing, weight loss, orthostatic hypotension, depression, blurred vision, nausea, vomiting, diarrhea or constipation, dry mouth, impotence, rash, pruritus

SERIOUS REACTIONS
• Vigorous diuresis may lead to profound water and electrolyte depletion, resulting in hypokalemia, hyponatremia, and dehydration.
• Acute hypotensive episodes may occur.
• Hyperglycemia may occur during prolonged therapy.
• Pancreatitis, blood dyscrasias, pulmonary edema, allergic pneumonitis, and dermatologic reactions occur rarely.
• Overdose can lead to lethargy and coma without changes in electrolytes or hydration.

INTERACTIONS
Drugs
❷ *Angiotensin-converting enzyme inhibitors:* Risk of postural hypotension when added to ongoing diuretic therapy; more common with loop diuretics; first-dose hypotension possible in patients with sodium depletion or hypovolemia due to diuretics or sodium restriction; hypotensive response is usually transient; hold diuretic day of first dose
❸ *Corticosteroids:* Concomitant therapy may result in excessive potassium loss
❸ *Diazoxide:* Blunt insulin secretion; results in hyperglycemia
❷ *Digoxin:* May increase the risk of digoxin toxicity associated with indapamide-induced hypokalemia
❸ *Lithium:* Concurrent use may result in elevated serum levels of lithium; monitor carefully
❸ *Nonsteroidal antiinflammatory drugs:* Concurrent use may reduce diuretic and antihypertensive effects

SPECIAL CONSIDERATIONS

PATIENT/FAMILY EDUCATION
• May cause sensitivity to sunlight; avoid prolonged exposure to the sun and other ultraviolet light
• May cause gout attacks; notify clinician if sudden joint pain occurs
• May worsen control or increase requirements of hypoglycemic agents
• Take indapamide early in the day to avoid urination at night
• Change positions slowly and let legs dangle momentarily before standing to reduce the drug's hypotensive effect

• Eat foods high in potassium, such as apricots, bananas, raisins, orange juice, potatoes, legumes, meat, and whole grains (such as cereals)

MONITORING PARAMETERS

• Weight, urine output, serum electrolytes, BUN, creatinine, CBC, uric acid, glucose, lipids
• Blood pressure

indinavir

(in-din′-a-veer)

Rx: Crixivan

Chemical Class: Protease inhibitor, HIV

Therapeutic Class: Antiretroviral

CLINICAL PHARMACOLOGY

Mechanism of Action: A protease inhibitor that suppresses HIV protease, an enzyme necessary for splitting viral polyprotein precursors into mature and infectious viral particles. ***Therapeutic Effect:*** Interrupts HIV replication, slowing the progression of HIV infection.

Pharmacokinetics

Rapidly absorbed after PO administration. Protein binding: 60%. Metabolized in the liver. Primarily excreted in urine. Unknown if removed by hemodialysis. ***Half-life:*** 1.8 hr (increased in impaired hepatic function).

INDICATIONS AND DOSAGES

HIV infection (in combination with other antiretrovirals)

PO

Adults. 800 mg (two 400-mg capsules) q8h.

Dosage adjustments when given concomitantly

Delavirdine, itraconazole, ketoconazole: Reduce dose to 600 mg q8h.

Efavirenz: Increase dose to 1000 mg q8h.

Lopinavir/ritonavir: Reduce dose to 600 mg twice a day.

Nevirapine: Increase dose to 1000 mg q8h.

Rifabutin: Reduce rifabutin by ½ and increase indinavir to 1000 mg q8h.

Ritonavir: 100-200 mg twice a day and indinavir 800 mg twice a day or ritonavir 400 mg twice a day and indinavir 400 mg twice a day.

HIV infection in patients with hepatic insufficiency

PO

Adults. 600 mg q8h.

AVAILABLE FORMS

• *Capsules:* 100 mg, 200 mg, 333 mg, 400 mg.

UNLABELED USES: Prophylaxis following occupational exposure to HIV

CONTRAINDICATIONS: Concurrent use with terfenadine, cisapride, astemizole, triazolam, midazolam, pimozide, ergot derivatives; nephrolithiasis

PREGNANCY AND LACTATION: Pregnancy category C; not recommended for breast-feeding mothers

SIDE EFFECTS

Frequent

Nausea (12%), abdominal pain (9%), headache (6%), diarrhea (5%)

Occasional

Vomiting, asthenia, fatigue (4%); insomnia; accumulation of fat in waist, abdomen, or back of neck

Rare

Abnormal taste sensation, heartburn, symptomatic urinary tract disease, transient renal dysfunction

SERIOUS REACTIONS

• Nephrolithiasis (flank pain with or without hematuria) occurs in 4% of patients.

INTERACTIONS

Drugs

3 *Barbiturates:* Increased clearance of indinavir; reduced clearance of barbiturates

❷ *Carbamazepine:* Increased clearance of indinavir; reduced clearance of carbamazepine

▲ *Cisapride:* Increased plasma levels of cisapride

3 *Clarithromycin:* Indinavir reduces clearance of clarithromycin

3 *Delavirdine:* Decreased clearance of indinavir; reduce dose of indinavir to 600 mg q8h

❷ *Efavirenz:* Reduced indinavir level; increase indinavir dose to 1000 mg q8h

▲ *Ergot alkaloids:* Increased plasma levels of ergot alkaloids

3 *Erythromycin:* Reduced clearance of indinavir; indinavir reduces clearance of erythromycin

3 *Grapefruit, grapefruit juice:* May decrease indinavir blood concentration and effect

3 *High-fat, high-calorie, high-protein meals:* May decrease indinavir blood concentration

3 *Ketoconazole:* Decreased clearance of indinavir; decrease indinavir dose to 600 mg tid

▲ *Lovastatin:* Indinavir reduces clearance of lovastatin

▲ *Midazolam:* Increased plasma levels of midazolam and prolonged effect

3 *Nelfinavir:* Decreased clearance of indinavir; reduce dose of indinavir to 1200 mg bid

3 *Nevirapine:* Reduces plasma indinavir levels; no dose adjustment needed

3 *Omeprazole:* Reduces the absorption of indinavir; loss of antiviral efficacy may result

3 *Oral contraceptives:* Indinavir may reduce efficacy

3 *Phenytoin:* Increased clearance of indinavir; reduced clearance of phenytoin

❷ *Rifabutin:* Increased clearance of indinavir; reduced clearance of rifabutin—reduce rifabutin dose to 150 mg qd and increase indinavir dose to 1000 mg tid

▲ *Rifampin:* Increased clearance of indinavir

3 *Ritonavir:* Decreased clearance of indinavir; decrease indinavir dose to 400 mg bid

3 *Saquinavir:* Decreased clearance of saquinavir; reduce dose of Fortovase (saquinavir soft gel capsule) to 800 mg tid

3 *Sildenafil:* Increases sildenafil plasma concentrations; increased toxic effects may occur

▲ *Simvastatin:* Indinavir reduces clearance of simvastatin

3 *St. John's Wort:* Reduces plasma concentration of indinavir

▲ *Terfenadine:* Increased plasma levels of terfenadine

▲ *Triazolam:* Increased plasma levels of triazolam and prolonged effect

3 *Troleandomycin:* Reduced clearance of indinavir; indinavir reduces clearance of troleandomycin

SPECIAL CONSIDERATIONS

- Antiretroviral activity of indinavir may be increased when used in combination with reverse transcriptase inhibitors

PATIENT/FAMILY EDUCATION

- Drink plenty of water, at least 48 oz/day
- Take with water or light, low-fat meals (dry toast, apple juice, corn flakes, skim milk). High-fat meals and grapefruit juice reduce absorption
- Capsules sensitive to moisture. Keep dessicant in bottle
- If dose is missed take next dose on schedule; do not double this dose

• Separate dosing with didanosine by 1 hr
• Take 1 hr before or 2 hrs after meals; may take with skim milk or low-fat meal

MONITORING PARAMETERS
• Serum amylase, bilirubin, cholesterol, lipase, and triglyceride levels; blood glucose level; CBC; CD4+ cell count; and liver function test results
• Monitor for signs and symptoms of nephrolithiasis (flank pain and hematuria), and notify the physician if symptoms occur; if nephrolithiasis occurs, expect therapy to be interrupted for 1-3 days
• Pattern of daily bowel activity and stool consistency

indomethacin

(in-doe-meth'-a-sin)

Rx: Indocin, Indocin IV, Indocin SR, Indo-Lemmon

Chemical Class: Indole acetic acid derivative

Therapeutic Class: NSAID; antipyretic; nonnarcotic analgesic

CLINICAL PHARMACOLOGY

Mechanism of Action: An NSAID that produces analgesic and antiinflammatory effects by inhibiting prostaglandin synthesis. Also increases the sensitivity of the premature ductus to the dilating effects of prostaglandins. ***Therapeutic Effect:*** Reduces the inflammatory response and intensity of pain. Closure of the patent ductus arteriosus.

Pharmacokinetics

Rectal absorption more rapid than oral administration. Protein binding: 99%. Metabolized in liver. Excreted in urine. ***Half-life:*** 4.5 hr.

INDICATIONS AND DOSAGES

Moderate to severe rheumatoid arthritis, osteoarthritis, ankylosing spondylitis

PO

Adults, Elderly. Initially, 25 mg 2-3 times a day; increased by 25-50 mg/wk up to 150-200 mg/day. Or 75 mg/day (extended-release) up to 75 mg twice a day.

Children. 1-2 mg/kg/day. Maximum: 150-200 mg/day.

Acute gouty arthritis

PO

Adults, Elderly. Initially, 100 mg, then 50 mg 3 times a day.

Acute shoulder pain

PO

Adults, Elderly. 75-150 mg/day in 3-4 divided doses.

Usual rectal dosage

Adults, Elderly. 50 mg 4 times a day.

Children. Initially, 1.5-2.5 mg/kg/day, increased up to 4 mg/kg/day. Maximum: 150-200 mg/day.

Patent ductus arteriosus

IV

Neonates. Initially, 0.2 mg/kg. Subsequent doses are based on age, as follows:

Neonates older than 7 days. 0.25 mg/kg for second and third doses.

Neonates 2-7 days. 0.2 mg/kg for second and third doses.

Neonates less than 48 hr. 0.1 mg/kg for second and third doses.

AVAILABLE FORMS
• *Capsules (Indocin):* 25 mg, 50 mg.
• *Capsules (Sustained-Release [Indocin SR]):* 75 mg.
• *Oral Suspension (Indocin):* 25 mg/5 ml.
• *Powder for Injection (Indocin IV):* 1 mg.
• *Suppositories:* 50 mg.

UNLABELED USES: Treatment of fever due to malignancy, pericarditis, psoriatic arthritis, rheumatic complications associated with Paget's disease of bone, vascular headache

CONTRAINDICATIONS: Active GI bleeding or ulcerations; hypersensitivity to aspirin, indomethacin, or other NSAIDs; renal impairment, thrombocytopenia

PREGNANCY AND LACTATION: Pregnancy category B; crosses placenta; excreted in breast milk

SIDE EFFECTS

Frequent (11%-3%)

Headache, nausea, vomiting, dyspepsia, dizziness

Occasional (less than 3%)

Depression, tinnitus, diaphoresis, somnolence, constipation, diarrhea, bleeding disturbances in patent ductus arteriosus

Rare

Hypertension, confusion, urticaria, pruritus, rash, blurred vision

SERIOUS REACTIONS

- Paralytic ileus and ulceration of the esophagus, stomach, duodenum, or small intestine may occur.
- Patients with impaired renal function may develop hyperkalemia and worsening of renal impairment.
- Indomethacin use may aggravate epilepsy, parkinsonism, and depression or other psychiatric disturbances.
- Nephrotoxicity, including dysuria, hematuria, proteinuria, and nephrotic syndrome, occurs rarely.
- Metabolic acidosis or alkalosis, apnea, and bradycardia occur rarely in patients with patent ductus arteriosus.

INTERACTIONS

Drugs

3 *Aminoglycosides:* Reduced clearance with elevated aminoglycoside levels and potential for toxicity (especially indomethacin in premature infants; other NSAIDs probably)

3 *Anticoagulants:* Excessive hypoprothrombinemia, decreased platelet aggregation with increased risk of GI bleeding

3 *Antihypertensives (α-blockers, angiotensin-converting enzyme,inhibitors, angiotensin II receptor blockers, β-blockers, diuretics:* Inhibition of antihypertensive and other favorable hemodynamic effects

3 *Aspirin, other salicylates:* May increase the risk of GI side effects such as bleeding

3 *Bone marrow depressants:* May increase the risk of hematologic reactions

3 *Corticosteroids:* Increased risk of GI ulceration

3 *Cyclosporine:* Increased nephrotoxicity risk

3 *Feverfew:* May decrease the effects of feverfew

3 *Ginkgo biloba:* May increase the risk of bleeding

3 *Lithium:* Decreased clearance of lithium (mediated via prostaglandins) resulting in elevated serum lithium levels and risk of toxicity

3 *Methotrexate:* Decreased renal secretion of methotrexate resulting in elevated methotrexate levels and risk of toxicity

3 *Phenylpropanolamine:* Possible acute hypertensive reaction

3 *Potassium-sparing diuretics:* Additive hyperkalemia potential

3 *Probenecid:* May increase the indomethacin blood concentration

3 *Triamterene:* Acute renal failure reported with addition of indomethacin; caution with other NSAIDs

3 *Vancomycin:* May increase the concentration of vancomycin in neonates; vancomycin toxicity may result

SPECIAL CONSIDERATIONS

PATIENT/FAMILY EDUCATION

- Take with food
- No significant advantage over other oral NSAIDs; cost and clinical situation should govern use
- Swallow capsules whole and do not chew, open, or crush them
- Avoid tasks that require mental alertness or motor skills until response to the drug has been established
- Avoid alcohol and aspirin during indomethacin therapy because these substances increase the risk of GI bleeding

MONITORING PARAMETERS

- Renal and hepatic function with prolonged use: check after 3 mos, then q6-12mos
- Initial CBC and fecal occult blood test within 3 mos of starting regular chronic therapy; repeat q6-12mos (more frequently in high-risk patients)
- Blood pressure, EKG, heart rate, platelet count, serum sodium and blood glucose levels, and urine output

infliximab

(in-flix'-i-mab)

Rx: Remicade

Chemical Class: Monoclonal antibody

Therapeutic Class: Tumor necrosis factor α (TNF-α) antibody

CLINICAL PHARMACOLOGY

Mechanism of Action: A monoclonal antibody that binds to tumor necrosis factor (TNF), inhibiting functional activity of TNF. Reduces infiltration of inflammatory cells. ***Therapeutic Effect:*** Decreases inflamed areas of the intestine.

Pharmacokinetics

Route	Onset	Peak	Duration
IV (Crohn's disease)	1-2 wks	N/A	8-48 wks
IV (Rheumatoid arthritis [RA])	3-7 days	N/A	6-12 wks

Absorbed into the GI tissue; primarily distributed in the vascular compartment. ***Half-life:*** 9.5 days.

INDICATIONS AND DOSAGES

Crohn's disease, moderate to severe, ulcerative colitis, psoriatic arthritis

IV Infusion

Adults, Elderly. Initially, 5 mg/kg at weeks 0, 2, and 6. Maintenance: 5 mg/kg q8wk thereafter.

Ankylosing spondylitis

IV Infusion

Adults, Elderly. Initially, 5 mg/kg at weeks 0, 2, and 6. Maintenance: 5 mg/kg q6wk thereafter.

Fistulizing Crohn's disease

IV Infusion

Adults, Elderly. Initially, 5 mg/kg followed by additional 5-mg/kg doses at 2 and 6 wk after first infusion.

Rheumatoid arthritis (RA)

IV Infusion

Adults, Elderly. 3 mg/kg; followed by additional doses at 2 and 6 wk after first infusion, then q8wk.

AVAILABLE FORMS

- *Powder for Injection:* 100 mg.

UNLABELED USES: CHF, juvenile arthritis, psoriasis, reactive arthritis, sciatica

CONTRAINDICATIONS: Sensitivity to murine proteins, sepsis, serious active infection

PREGNANCY AND LACTATION: Pregnancy category B; breast milk excretion unknown; nursing not recommended

SIDE EFFECTS

Frequent (22%-10%)

Headache, nausea, fatigue, fever

Occasional (9%-5%)

Fever or chills during infusion, pharyngitis, vomiting, pain, dizziness, bronchitis, rash, rhinitis, cough, pruritus, sinusitis, myalgia, back pain

Rare (4%-1%)

Hypotension or hypertension, paresthesia, anxiety, depression, insomnia, diarrhea, urinary tract infection

SERIOUS REACTIONS

- Serious infections, including sepsis, occur rarely.
- Hypersensitivity reaction, lupus-like syndrome, and severe hepatic reactions may occur.

INTERACTIONS

Drugs

3 *Immunosuppressants:* May reduce frequency of infusion reactions and antibodies to infliximab

- *Live virus vaccines:* No information on vaccine response or secondary transmission of infection

SPECIAL CONSIDERATIONS

- Evaluate for risk of TB (TB skin test) prior to initiating therapy

PATIENT/FAMILY EDUCATION

- More susceptible to infections; avoid crowds, people with URI, flu, etc.
- Expect follow-up tests, such as ESR, C-reactive protein measurement, and urinalysis
- Report signs of infection, such as fever
- The patient with rheumatoid arthritis should report increase in pain, stiffness, or swelling of joints
- The patient with Crohn's disease should report changes in stool color, consistency, or elimination pattern

MONITORING PARAMETERS

- Decreased levels of serum IL-6, C-reactive protein, ESR, rheumatoid factor, signs and symptoms of disease, urinalysis, blood chemistry, human anti-cA2 titers, blood pressure (during and after infusion), temperature, body weight, signs and symptoms of infection (including TB)

insulin group

(in′-su-lin)

Rx: *Rapid-Acting:* Insulin Lispro (Humalog), Insulin Aspart (Novolog, NovoMix 30[AUS], Novorapid[AUS])

Rx: *Regular Short-Acting:* Actrapid(AUS), Humulin R, Novolin R, Regular Iletin II

Rx: *Intermediate-Acting:* NPH (Humulin N, Novolin N, NPH Iletin II)

Rx: *Lente:* Humulin L, Lente Iletin II, Monotard(AUS), Novolin L

Rx: *Long-Acting:* Insulin Glargine (Lantus Ultralente), Insulin Detemir (Levemir)

Rx: *Intermediate- and Short-Acting Mixtures:* Humulin 50/50, Humulin 70/30, Humalog Mix 75/25, Humalog Mix 50/50, Novolin 70/30, Novolog Mix 70/30

Chemical Class: Exogenous insulin

Therapeutic Class: Antidiabetic; hypoglycemic

CLINICAL PHARMACOLOGY

Mechanism of Action: An exogenous insulin that facilitates passage of glucose, potassium, and magnesium across the cellular membranes of skeletal and cardiac muscle and adipose tissue. Controls storage and metabolism of carbohydrates, protein, and fats. Promotes conversion of glucose to glycogen in the liver. ***Therapeutic Effect:*** Controls glucose levels in diabetic patients.

Pharmacokinetics

Drug Form	*Onset (hr)*	*Peak (hr)*	*Duration (hr)*
Lispro	0.25	0.5-1.5	4-5
Insulin aspart	1/6	1-3	3-5
Regular	0.5-1	2-4	5-7
NPH	1-2	6-14	24+
Lente	1-3	6-14	24+
Insulin glargine	N/A	N/A	24

INDICATIONS AND DOSAGES

Treatment of insulin-dependent type 1 diabetes mellitus and non-insulin-dependent type 2 diabetes mellitus when diet or weight control has failed to maintain satisfactory blood glucose levels or in event of fever, infection, pregnancy, surgery, or trauma, or severe endocrine, hepatic or renal dysfunction; emergency treatment of ketoacidosis (regular insulin); to promote passage of glucose across cell membrane in hyperalimentation (regular insulin); to facilitate intracellular shift of potassium in hyperkalemia (regular insulin)

Subcutaneous

Adults, Elderly, Children. 0.5-1 unit/kg/day.

Adolescents (during growth spurt). 0.8-1.2 unit/kg/day.

AVAILABLE FORMS

• All insulins are available as 100 units/ml concentrations.

• *Rapid-Acting:* Humulin R, Novolin R, Novolog, Humalog, Regular Iletin II.

• *Intermediate-Acting:* Humulin L, Novolin L, Lente Iletin II, Humulin N, Novolin N, NPH Illetin II.

• *Long-Acting:* Lantus Ultralente, Levemir.

• *Intermediate- and Short-Acting Mixtures:* Humulin 50/50, Humulin 70/30, Humalog Mix 75/25, Humalog Mix 50/50, Novolin 70/30, Novolog Mix 70/30.

CONTRAINDICATIONS: Hypersensitivity or insulin resistance may require change of type or species source of insulin

PREGNANCY AND LACTATION: Pregnancy category B; insulin requirements of pregnant diabetic patients often decreased in first half and increased in the latter half of pregnancy; elevated blood glucose levels associated with congenital abnormalities; does not pass into breast milk

SIDE EFFECTS

Occasional

Localized redness, swelling, and itching caused by improper injection technique or allergy to cleansing solution or insulin

Infrequent

Somogyi effect, including rebound hyperglycemia with chronically excessive insulin dosages: systemic allergic reaction, marked by rash, angioedema, and anaphylaxis; lipodystrophy or depression at injection site due to breakdown of adipose tissue; lipohypertrophy or accumulation of subcutaneous tissue at injection site due to inadequate site rotation

Rare

Insulin resistance

SERIOUS REACTIONS

• Severe hypoglycemia caused by hyperinsulinism may occur with insulin overdose, decrease or delay of food intake, or excessive exercise and in those with brittle diabetes.

• Diabetic ketoacidosis may result from stress, illness, omission of insulin dose, or long-term poor insulin control.

INTERACTIONS

Drugs

3 *β-blockers:* Increased glucose levels, hypoglycemia symptoms masked (except sweating)

3 *Cigarette smoking, marijuana, corticosteroids, thiazides:* Increased glucose levels

3 *Clonidine, guanfacine, guanabenz:* Hypoglycemia symptoms masked

⚠ *Ethanol (excessive):* Hypoglycemia

3 *Salicylates, ACE inhibitors, anabolic steroids, MAO inhibitors:* Enhanced hypoglycemic response

SPECIAL CONSIDERATIONS

PATIENT/FAMILY EDUCATION

• Symptoms of hypoglycemia include fatigue, weakness, confusion, headache, convulsions, hunger, nausea, pallor, sweating, rapid breathing

• For hypoglycemia, give 1 mg glucagon, glucose 25 g IV (via dextrose 50% sol, 50 ml) or oral glucose if tolerated

• When mixing insulins, draw up short-acting first

• Dosage adjustment may be necessary when changing insulin products

• Human insulin considered insulin of choice secondary to antigenicity of animal insulins

• The regimen of exercise, good hygiene (including foot care), prescribed diet, and weight control is an integral part of treatment

• Carry candy, sugar packets, or other sugar supplements for immediate response to hypoglycemia

MONITORING PARAMETERS

• Assess the patient for signs and symptoms of hypoglycemia (anxiety, cool wet skin, diplopia, dizziness, headache, hunger, numbness in mouth, tachycardia, tremors), or hyperglycemia, (deep rapid breathing [Kussmaul's respirations], dim vision, fatigue, nausea, polydipsia, polyphagia, polyuria, vomiting)

• Be alert to conditions that alter blood glucose requirements, such as fever, increased activity, stress, or a surgical procedure

• Monitor the sleeping patient for diaphoresis and restlessness

interferon alfa-2a/2b

(in-ter-feer'-on)

Rx: Roferon-A (alfa-2a), Intron-A (alfa-2b)

Combinations

Rx: Interferon alfa-2b with ribavirin (Rebetron Combination Therapy)

Chemical Class: Recombinant interferon

Therapeutic Class: Antineoplastic; antiviral

CLINICAL PHARMACOLOGY

Mechanism of Action: A biologic response modifier that inhibits viral replication in virus-infected cells. ***Therapeutic Effect:*** Suppresses cell proliferation; increases phagocytic action of macrophages; augments specific lymphocytic cell toxicity.

Pharmacokinetics

Interferon alfa-2a: Well absorbed after IM, subcutaneous administration. Undergoes proteolytic degradation during reabsorption in kidney. ***Half-life:*** IM: 2 hrs; Subcutaneous: 3 hrs.

Interferon alfa-2b: Well absorbed after IM, subcutaneous administration. Undergoes proteolytic degradation during reabsorption in kidney. ***Half-life:*** 2-3 hrs.

UNLABELED USES: Treatment of acquired immunodeficiency syndrome (AIDS), AIDS-related Kaposi's sarcoma, malignant melanoma, renal cell carcinoma

CONTRAINDICATIONS: Hypersensitivity to albumin, interferon

PREGNANCY AND LACTATION: Pregnancy category C; possible abortifacient; not known if excreted into breast milk; avoid in nursing mothers

SIDE EFFECTS

Frequent

Interferon beta-1a: Headache (67%), flu-like symptoms (61%), myalgia (34%), upper respiratory infection (31%), pain (24%), asthenia, chills (21%), sinusitis (18%), infection (11%)

Interferon beta-1a: Injection site reaction (85%), headache (84%), flu-like symptoms (76%), fever (59%), pain (52%), asthenia (49%), myalgia (44%), sinusitis (36%), diarrhea, dizziness (35%), mental status changes (29%), constipation (24%), diaphoresis (23%), vomiting (21%)

Occasional

Interferon beta-1a: Abdominal pain, arthralgia (9%), chest pain, dyspnea (6%), malaise, syncope (4%)

Interferon beta-1b: Malaise (15%), somnolence (6%), alopecia (4%)

Rare

Interferon beta-1a: Injection site reaction, hypersensitivity reaction (3%)

SERIOUS REACTIONS

- Anemia occurs in 8% of patients taking interferon beta-1a.
- Seizures occur rarely in patients taking interferon beta-1b.

INTERACTIONS

Drugs

3 *Zidovudine, theophylline:* Increased levels of these drugs

SPECIAL CONSIDERATIONS

PATIENT/FAMILY EDUCATION

- Use acetaminophen for relief of flu-like symptoms
- Avoid prolonged sun exposure (photosensitivity)
- Benefit in chronic progressive multiple sclerosis has not been evaluated
- Patients treated × 2 yr had significantly longer time to progression of disability compared with placebo group
- Do not change drug dosage or administration schedule without consulting the physician
- Document the type and severity of injection site reaction; these reactions will not require discontinuation of therapy, but should be reported immediately

MONITORING PARAMETERS

- CBC, platelets, liver function tests, and blood chemistries q3mo
- DC for ANC <750/m^3, ALT/AST >10 × upper normal limits; when labs return to these levels, restart at 50% of dose
- Assess for flu-like symptoms, headache, and myalgia
- Evaluate for depression and suicidal ideation

interferon gamma-1b

(in-ter-feer'-on)

Rx: Actimmune

Chemical Class: Recombinant interferon

Therapeutic Class: Biologic response modifier

CLINICAL PHARMACOLOGY

Mechanism of Action: A biologic response modifier that induces activation of macrophages in blood monocytes to phagocytes, which is necessary in the body's cellular immune response to intracellular and extracellular pathogens. Enhances phagocytic function and antimicrobial activity of monocytes. ***Therapeutic Effect:*** Decreases signs and symptoms of serious infections in chronic granulomatous disease.

Pharmacokinetics

Slowly absorbed after subcutaneous administration. ***Half-life:*** 0.5-1 hr.

INDICATIONS AND DOSAGES

Chronic granulomatous disease; severe, malignant osteopetrosis

Subcutaneous

Adults, Children older than 1 yr. 50 mcg/m^2 (1.5 million units/m^2) in patients with body surface area (BSA) greater than 0.5 m^2; 1.5 mcg/kg/dose in patients with BSA 0.5 m^2 or less. Give 3 times a week.

AVAILABLE FORMS

- *Injection:* 100 mcg (2 million units).

CONTRAINDICATIONS: Hypersensitivity to *Escherichia coli*–derived products

PREGNANCY AND LACTATION: Pregnancy category C; possible abortifacient; not known if excreted in breast milk; not recommended in breast-feeding

SIDE EFFECTS

Frequent

Fever (52%); headache (33%); rash (17%); chills, fatigue, diarrhea (14%)

Occasional (13%-10%)

Vomiting, nausea

Rare (6%-3%)

Weight loss, myalgia, anorexia

SERIOUS REACTIONS

- Interferon gamma-1b may exacerbate preexisting CNS disturbances, including decreased mental status, gait disturbance, and dizziness, as well as cardiac disorders.

INTERACTIONS

Drugs

3 *Bone marrow depressants:* May increase myelosuppression

3 *Theophylline, zidovudine:* Increased levels of these drugs

SPECIAL CONSIDERATIONS

- Optimal sites for inj are the right and left deltoid and anterior thigh

PATIENT/FAMILY EDUCATION

- Use acetaminophen to relieve fever, headache
- Store vials in the refrigerator
- Teach the patient how to properly administer the drug and dispose of needles and syringes
- Flu-like symptoms may be alleviated or minimized by taking doses at bedtime and tend to diminish with continued therapy
- Avoid performing tasks that require mental alertness or motor skills until response to the drug has been established

MONITORING PARAMETERS

- Monitor the patient for flu-like symptoms, including chills, fatigue, fever, and myalgia
- Skin for rash

iodine; potassium iodide

Rx: Pima, SSKI

Chemical Class: Iodine product

Therapeutic Class: Antithyroid agent; expectorant

CLINICAL PHARMACOLOGY

Mechanism of Action: An agent that reduces viscosity of mucus by increasing respiratory tract secretions. Inhibits secretion of thyroid hormone, fosters colloid accumulation in thyroid follicles. ***Therapeutic Effect:*** Blocks thyroid radioiodine uptake.

Pharmacokinetics

Oral onset 24-48 hrs, peak 10-15 days, duration 6 wks. Primarily excreted in the urine.

INDICATIONS AND DOSAGES

Expectorant

PO

Adults, Elderly, Children 3 yrs and older. 325-650 mg q8h (Pima); 300-600 mg 3-4 times/day (SSKI).

Children less than 3 yrs. 162 mg q8h.

Preoperative thyroidectomy

PO

Adults, Elderly, Children. 0.1-0.3 ml (3-5 drops of Lugol's solution) q8h or 50-250 mg (1-5 drops of SSKI) q8h. Administer 10 days before surgery.

Radiation protectant to radioactive isotopes of iodine

PO

Adults, Elderly. 195 mg/day (Pima) for 10 days. Start 24 hrs prior to exposure.

Children more than 1 yr. 130 mg/day for 10 days. Start 24 hrs prior to exposure.

Children less than 1 yr. 65 mg/day for 10 days. Start 24 hrs prior to exposure.

Reduce risk of thyroid cancer following nuclear accident

PO

Adults, Elderly, Children more than 68 kg. 130 mg/day.

Children 3-18 yrs. 65 mg/day.

Children 1 mo-3 yrs. 32 mg/day.

Children 1 mo and younger. 16 mg/day.

Sporotrichosis

PO

Adults, Elderly. Initally, 5 drops (SSKI) q8h and increase to 40-50 drops q8h as tolerated for 3-6 mos.

Thyrotoxic crisis

PO

Adults, Elderly. 300-500 mg (6-19 drops SSKI) q8h or 1 ml (Lugol's solution) q8h.

AVAILABLE FORMS

- *Solution:* 1 mg/ml (SSKI), 100 mg/ml (Lugol's solution).
- *Syrup:* 325/5 ml (Pima).
- *Tablets:* 130 mg (Iosat).

CONTRAINDICATIONS: Hypersensitivity to potassium, iodine compounds, or any of its component, pulmonary edema, hyperkalemia, impaired renal function, hyperthyroidism, iodine-induced goiter, pregnancy

PREGNANCY AND LACTATION: Pregnancy category D; use of iodides as expectorants during pregnancy is contraindicated; concentrated in breast milk; may affect infant's thyroid activity but considered compatible with breast-feeding

SIDE EFFECTS

Occasional

Irregular heartbeat, confusion, drowsiness, fever, rash, diarrhea, GI bleeding, metallic taste, nausea, stomach pain, vomiting, numbness, tingling, weakness

Rare

Goiter, salivary gland swelling and tenderness, thyroid adenoma, swelling of the throat and neck, myxedema, lymph node swelling

SERIOUS REACTIONS

- Hypersensitivity symptoms include angioedema, muscle weakness, paralysis, peaked T-waves, flattened P-waves, prolongation of QRS complex, ventricular arrhythmias.

INTERACTIONS

Drugs

3 *Lithium:* Increased likelihood of hypothyroidism

SPECIAL CONSIDERATIONS

PATIENT/FAMILY EDUCATION

- Dilute sol with water or fruit juice to improve taste, drink sol through straw
- Administer with food or milk
- May experience a metallic taste while taking potassium iodide
- Notify the physician if they experiences any stomach pain, nausea, vomiting, black or tarry stools, or unresolved weakness

MONITORING PARAMETERS

- Thyroid function tests if used for thyroid-related conditions

iodoquinol

(eye-oh-do-kwin′-ole)

Rx: Yodoxin

Chemical Class: Hydroxyquinoline derivative

Therapeutic Class: Amebicide

CLINICAL PHARMACOLOGY

Mechanism of Action: An antibacterial, antifungal, and antitrichomonal agent that works in the intestinal lumen by an unknown mechanism. ***Therapeutic Effect:*** Amebicidal.

Pharmacokinetics

Partially and irregularly absorbed from the gastrointestinal (GI) tract. Metabolized in liver. Primarily excreted in feces.

INDICATIONS AND DOSAGES

Intestinal amebiasis

PO

Adults, Elderly. 630-650 mg 3 times a day for 20 days.

Children. 40 mg/kg in 3 divided doses for up to 20 days. Maximum: 650 mg/day.

AVAILABLE FORMS

- *Tablets:* 210 mg, 650 mg (Yodoxin).
- *Powder:* 25 g, 100 g (Yodoxin).

CONTRAINDICATIONS: Hepatic impairment, renal impairment, chronic diarrhea (especially in children), hypersensitivity to iodine and 8-hydroxyquinolones

PREGNANCY AND LACTATION: Pregnancy category C; excretion into breast milk unknown

SIDE EFFECTS

Occasional

Fever, chills, headache, nausea, vomiting, diarrhea, cramps, urticaria, pruritus

SERIOUS REACTIONS

- Optic neuritis, atrophy, and peripheral neuropathy have been reported with high dosages and long-term use.

SPECIAL CONSIDERATIONS

PATIENT/FAMILY EDUCATION

- Take full course of therapy
- Nausea, diarrhea, or GI upset may occur
- Skin, hair, and clothing may be temporarily stained yellow-brown following iodoquinol use

MONITORING PARAMETERS

- Therapeutic response to therapy

ipecac syrup

(ip′-e-kak)

OTC: Ipecac

Chemical Class: Cephaelis ipecacuanha derivative

Therapeutic Class: Emetic

CLINICAL PHARMACOLOGY

Mechanism of Action: An antidote that acts centrally by stimulating medullary chemoreceptor trigger zone and locally by irritating gastric mucosa. ***Therapeutic Effect:*** Produces emesis.

Pharmacokinetics

Onset of action occurs within 20-30 mins. Eliminated very slowly in urine.

INDICATIONS AND DOSAGES
Poisoning, acute
PO
Adults, Elderly, Children 12 yrs and older. 15-30 ml followed by 200-300 ml of water.
Children 6-12 yrs. 5-10 ml followed by 10-20 ml/kg.
Children 1-12 yrs. 15 ml followed by 10-20 ml/kg.
Children 6 mos-1 yr. 5-10 ml, followed by 10-20 ml/kg.
AVAILABLE FORMS
• *Syrup:* 70 mg/ml.
CONTRAINDICATIONS: Ingestion of petroleum distillate, ingestion of strong acids or bases, ingestion of strychnine, unconsciousness or absence of gag reflex, hypersensitivity to ipecac or any component of the formulation
PREGNANCY AND LACTATION: Pregnancy category C; not known if excreted in breast milk
SIDE EFFECTS
Expected response
Nausea, vomiting, drowsiness and mild CNS depression after vomiting
Occasional
Diarrhea, lethargy, muscle aching, stomach cramps
SERIOUS REACTIONS
• Cardiotoxicity may occur if ipecac syrup is not vomited (noted as hypotension, tachycardia, precordial chest pain, pulmonary congestion, dyspnea, ventricular tachycardia and fibrillation, cardiac arrest).
• Overdose may produce diarrhea, fast/irregular heartbeat, nausea continuing >30 min, stomach pain, respiratory difficulty, unusually tired, and aching/stiff muscles.
INTERACTIONS
Drugs
3 *Activated charcoal:* Decreased effect of ipecac; if both drugs used, give activated charcoal after emesis induced

ipratropium bromide

(eye-pra-troep′-ee-um broe′-mide)
Rx: Atrovent, Atrovent Nasal
Combinations
Rx: with albuterol (Combivent)
Chemical Class: Quaternary ammonium compound
Therapeutic Class: COPD agent; bronchodilator

CLINICAL PHARMACOLOGY
Mechanism of Action: An anticholinergic that blocks the action of acetylcholine at parasympathetic sites in bronchial smooth muscle. ***Therapeutic Effect:*** Causes bronchodilation and inhibits nasal secretions.
Pharmacokinetics

Route	Onset	Peak	Duration
Inhalation	1-3 mins	1-2 hrs	4-6 hrs

Minimal systemic absorption after inhalation. Metabolized in the liver (systemic absorption). Primarily eliminated in feces. ***Half-life:*** 1.5-4 hr.
INDICATIONS AND DOSAGES
Bronchospasm
Inhalation
Adults, Elderly. 2 inhalations 4 times a day. Maximum: 12 inhalations/day.
Children 3-14 yrs. 1-2 inhalations 3 times a day. Maximum: 6 inhalations/day.
Nebulization
Adults, Elderly. 500 mcg 3-4 times a day.
Children. 125-250 mcg 3 times a day.
Rhinorrhea (perennial allergic and non-allergic rhinitis)
Intranasal (0.03%)

Adults, Elderly, Children 6 yr and older. 2 sprays per nostril 2-3 times a day.

Rhinorrhea (common cold)

Intranasal (0.06%)

Adults, Elderly. 2 sprays per nostril 3-4 times a day for up to 4 days.

Children 5 yr and older. 2 sprays per nostril 3 times a day for up to 4 days.

Rhinorrhea (seasonal allergy)

Intranasal (0.06%)

Adults, Elderly, Children 5 yr and older. 2 sprays per nostril 4 times a day for up to 3 wk.

AVAILABLE FORMS

- *Oral Inhalation:* 18 mcg/actuation.
- *Aerosol Solution for Inhalation:* 0.02%.
- *Nasal Spray:* 0.03%, 0.06%.

CONTRAINDICATIONS: History of hypersensitivity to atropine, soya lecithin, or related food products such as soybean and peanut

PREGNANCY AND LACTATION: Pregnancy category B; not known if excreted in breast milk, but little systemic absorption when administered by INH

SIDE EFFECTS

Frequent

Inhalation (6%-3%): Cough, dry mouth, headache, nausea

Nasal: Dry nose and mouth, headache, nasal irritation

Occasional

Inhalation (2%): Dizziness, transient increased bronchospasm

Rare (less than 1%)

Inhalation: Hypotension, insomnia, metallic or unpleasant taste, palpitations, urine retention

Nasal: Diarrhea or constipation, dry throat, abdominal pain, stuffy nose

SERIOUS REACTIONS

- Worsening of angle-closure glaucoma, acute eye pain, and hypotension occur rarely.

INTERACTIONS

Drugs

3 *Cromolyn inhalation solution:* Avoid mixing these drugs because they form a precipitate

SPECIAL CONSIDERATIONS

- Bronchodilator of choice for COPD

PATIENT/FAMILY EDUCATION

- Do not take more than 2 inhalations at a time because excessive use decreases the drug's effectiveness and may cause paradoxical bronchoconstriction
- Rinse mouth with water immediately after inhalation to prevent mouth and throat dryness
- Drink plenty of fluids to decrease the thickness of lung secretions
- Avoid excessive use of caffeinated products, such as chocolate, cocoa, cola, coffee, and tea

MONITORING PARAMETERS

- Pulse rate and quality and respiratory rate, depth, rate, rhythm, and type
- Breath sounds for crackles, rhonchi, and wheezing
- ABG levels
- Examine the patient's lips and fingernails for a blue or gray color in light-skinned patients and a gray color in dark-skinned patients, which are signs of hypoxemia
- Observe the patient for clavicular, intercostal, and sternal retractions and a hand tremor
- Evaluate the patient for evidence of clinical improvement, such as cessation of retractions, quieter and slower respirations, and a relaxed facial expression

irbesartan

(ir-be-sar'-tan)

Rx: Avapro

Combinations

Rx: with hydrochlorothiazide (Avalide)

Chemical Class: Angiotensin II receptor antagonist

Therapeutic Class: Antihypertensive

CLINICAL PHARMACOLOGY

Mechanism of Action: An angiotensin II receptor, type AT_1, antagonist that blocks the vasoconstrictor and aldosterone-secreting effects of angiotensin II, inhibiting the binding of angiotensin II to the AT_1 receptors. ***Therapeutic Effect:*** Causes vasodilation, decreases peripheral resistance, and decreases BP.

Pharmacokinetics

Rapidly and completely absorbed after PO administration. Protein binding: 90%. Undergoes hepatic metabolism to inactive metabolite. Recovered primarily in feces and, to a lesser extent, in urine. Not removed by hemodialysis. ***Half-life:*** 11-15 hr.

INDICATIONS AND DOSAGES

Hypertension alone or in combination with other antihypertensives

PO

Adults, Elderly, Children 13 yr and older. Initially, 75-150 mg/day. May increase to 300 mg/day.

Children 6-12 yr. Initially, 75 mg/day. May increase to 150 mg/day.

Nephropathy

PO

Adults, Elderly. Target dose of 300 mg/day.

AVAILABLE FORMS

• *Tablets:* 75 mg, 150 mg, 300 mg.

UNLABELED USES: Treatment of atrial fibrillation, CHF

CONTRAINDICATIONS: Bilateral renal artery stenosis, biliary cirrhosis or obstruction, primary hyperaldosteronism, severe hepatic insufficiency

PREGNANCY AND LACTATION: Pregnancy category C (first trimester—category D, second and third trimesters); drugs acting directly on the renin-angiotensin-aldosterone system are documented to cause fetal harm (hypotension, oligohydramnios, neonatal anemia, hyperkalemia, neonatal skull hypoplasia, anuria, and renal failure; neonatal limb contractures, craniofacial deformities, and hypoplastic lung development; breast milk excretion unknown

SIDE EFFECTS

Occasional (9%-3%)

Upper respiratory tract infection, fatigue, diarrhea, cough

Rare (2%-1%)

Heartburn, dizziness, headache, nausea, rash

SERIOUS REACTIONS

• Overdosage may manifest as hypotension and tachycardia. Bradycardia occurs less often.

INTERACTIONS

3 *Hydrochlorothiazide:* Further reduces blood pressure

SPECIAL CONSIDERATIONS

• Potentially as or more effective than angiotensin-converting enzyme inhibitors, without cough; no evidence for reduction in morbidity and mortality as first-line agents in hypertension, yet; whether they provide the same cardiac and renal protection also still tentative; like ACE inhibitors, less effective in black patients

PATIENT/FAMILY EDUCATION

• Call your clinician immediately if note following side effects: wheezing; lip, throat, or face swelling; hives or rash

• Female patients should be aware of the consequences of second- and third-trimester exposure to irbesartan

• Avoid tasks that require mental alertness or motor skills until response to the drug has been established

• Report signs and symptoms of infection, including fever and sore throat

• Avoid outdoor exercise during hot weather to avoid the risks of dehydration and hypotension

MONITORING PARAMETERS

• Baseline electrolytes, urinalysis, blood urea nitrogen and creatinine with recheck at 2-4 wks after initiation (sooner in volume-depleted patients); monitor sitting blood pressure; watch for symptomatic hypotension, particularly in volume-depleted patients

iron dextran

(iron dex′-tran)

Rx: InFeD, Dexferrum

Chemical Class: Ferric hydroxide complexed with dextran

Therapeutic Class: Hematinic

CLINICAL PHARMACOLOGY

Mechanism of Action: A trace element and essential component in the formation of Hgb. Necessary for effective erythropoiesis and transport and utilization of oxygen. Serves as cofactor of several essential enzymes. ***Therapeutic Effect:*** Replenishes Hgb and depleted iron stores.

Pharmacokinetics

Readily absorbed after IM administration. Most absorption occurs within 72 hr; remainder within 3-4 wk. Bound to protein to form hemosiderin, ferritin, or transferrin. No physiologic system of elimination. Small amounts lost daily in shedding of skin, hair, and nails and in feces, urine, and perspiration. ***Half-life:*** 5-20 hr.

INDICATIONS AND DOSAGES

Iron deficiency anemia (no blood loss)

Dosage is expressed in terms of milligrams of elemental iron, degree of anemia, patient weight, and presence of any bleeding. Expect to use periodic hematologic determinations as guide to therapy.

IV, IM

Adults, Elderly. Mg iron = 0.66 × weight (kg) × (100 − Hgb [g/dl]/14.8

Iron replacement secondary to blood loss

IV, IM

Adults, Elderly. Replacement iron (mg) = blood loss (ml) times Hct.

Maximum daily dosages

Adults weighing more than 50 kg. 100 mg.

Children weighing 10-50 kg. 100 mg.

Children weighing 5-less than 10 kg. 50 mg.

Infants weighing less than 5 kg. 25 mg.

AVAILABLE FORMS

• *Injection (DexFerrum, Infed):* 50 mg/ml.

CONTRAINDICATIONS: All anemias except iron deficiency anemia, including pernicious, aplastic, normocytic, and refractory

PREGNANCY AND LACTATION: Pregnancy category C; excreted in breast milk

SIDE EFFECTS

Frequent

Allergic reaction (such as rash and itching), backache, myalgia, chills, dizziness, headache, fever, nausea, vomiting, flushed skin, pain or redness at injection site, brown discoloration of skin, metallic taste

SERIOUS REACTIONS

- Anaphylaxis has occurred during the first few minutes after injection, causing death rarely.
- Leukocytosis and lymphadenopathy occur rarely.

INTERACTIONS

Drugs

3 *Enalapril:* Three patients on enalapril receiving IV iron developed systemic reactions (GI symptoms, hypotension); causality not established

3 *Vitamin E:* Decreased reticulocyte response in anemic children

Labs

- *False increase:* Serum calcium, serum glucose, serum iron
- *False positive:* Stool guaiac

SPECIAL CONSIDERATIONS

- Discontinue oral iron before giving
- Delayed reaction (fever, myalgias, arthralgias, nausea) may occur 1-2 days after administration
- When giving IM, give only in gluteal muscle

PATIENT/FAMILY EDUCATION

- Pain and brown staining of the skin may occur at the injection site
- Do not take oral iron while receiving iron injections
- Stools may become black during iron therapy; this side effect is harmless unless accompanied by abdominal cramping or pain and red streaking or sticky consistency of stool
- Report abdominal cramping or pain, back pain, fever, headache, or red streaking or a sticky consistency of stool
- Chew gum, suck on hard candy, and maintain good oral hygiene to prevent or reduce the metallic taste

isocarboxazid

(eye-soe-kar-box'-a-zid)

Rx: Marplan

Chemical Class: Hydrazine derivative

Therapeutic Class: Antidepressant, monoamine oxidase inhibitor (MAOI)

CLINICAL PHARMACOLOGY

Mechanism of Action: An antidepressant that inhibits the MAO enzyme system at central nervous system (CNS) storage sites. The reduced MAO activity causes an increased concentration in epinephrine, norepinephrine, serotonin, and dopamine at neuron receptor sites. ***Therapeutic Effect:*** Produces antidepressant effect.

INDICATIONS AND DOSAGES

Depression refractory to other antidepressants or electroconvulsive therapy

PO

Adults, Elderly. Initially, 10 mg 3 times/day. May increase to 60 mg/day.

AVAILABLE FORMS

- *Tablets:* 10 mg (Marplan).

UNLABELED USES: Treatment of panic disorder, vascular or tension headaches

CONTRAINDICATIONS: Cardiovascular disease (CVD), cerebrovascular disease, liver impairment, pheochromocytoma, liver impairment

PREGNANCY AND LACTATION: Pregnancy category C; breast-feeding data not available

SIDE EFFECTS

Frequent (more than 10%)

Postural hypotension, drowsiness, decreased sexual ability, weakness, trembling, visual disturbances

Occasional (10%-1%)

Tachycardia, peripheral edema, nervousness, chills, diarrhea, anorexia, constipation, xerostomia

Rare (less than 1%)

Hepatitis, leukopenia, parkinsonian syndrome

SERIOUS REACTIONS

• Hypertensive crisis, marked by severe hypertension, occipital headache radiating frontally, neck stiffness or soreness, nausea, vomiting, sweating, fever or chilliness, clammy skin, dilated pupils, palpitations, tachycardia or bradycardia, and constricting chest pain.

INTERACTIONS

Drugs

3 *Barbiturates:* Prolonged action of barbiturate

▲ *Dextromethorphan:* Agitation, seizure, increased BP, hyperpyrexia

▲ *Ephedrine, amphetamines, phenylephrine, phenylpropanolamine, pseudoephedrine:* Hypertension, severe

▲ *Ethanol:* Alcoholic beverages containing tyramine may cause severe hypertensive reaction

3 *Guanethidine:* Decreased antihypertensive response to guanethidine

3 *Levodopa:* Hypertension, severe

❷ *Lithium:* Hyperpyrexia possible

▲ *Meperidine:* Sweating, rigidity, hypertension

▲ *Methotrimeprazine:* Case report of fatality in patient taking these drugs, causality not established

3 *Norepinephrine:* Increased pressor response to norepinephrine

▲ *Reserpine:* Potential for hypertensive reaction, clinical evidence lacking

▲ *Sertraline, fluoxetine, fluvoxamine, paroxetine, venlafaxine:* Increased CNS effects (serotonergic)

▲ *Tricyclic antidepressants:* Excessive sympathetic response, mania, hyperpyrexia

SPECIAL CONSIDERATIONS

• Phentolamine for severe hypertension

PATIENT/FAMILY EDUCATION

• Avoid high-tyramine foods: cheese (aged), sour cream, beer, wine, pickled products, liver, raisins, bananas, figs, avocados, meat tenderizers, chocolate, yogurt; soy sauce, caffeine

• Do not discontinue medication quickly after long-term use

• Notify the physician if headache or neck soreness or stiffness occurs

• Avoid using OTC preparations for colds, hayfever, and weight reduction

MONITORING PARAMETERS

• Blood pressure, heart rate, weight

• Diet

• Mood

• Monitor the patient for occipital headache radiating frontally and neck stiffness or soreness, which may be the first sign of impending hypertensive crisis

isoetharine hydrochloride/ isoetharine mesylate

(eye-soe-eth'-a-reen hye-droe-klor'-ide/eye-soe-eth'-a-reen mes'-sil-ate)

Rx: Beta-2, Bronkosol, Dey-Lute

Rx: Bronkometer

Chemical Class: Sympathomimetic amine; β_2-adrenergic agonist

Therapeutic Class: Antiasthmatic; bronchodilator

CLINICAL PHARMACOLOGY

Mechanism of Action: A sympathomimetic (adrenergic agonist) that stimulates beta$_2$-adrenergic receptors in the lungs, resulting in relaxation of bronchial smooth muscle. ***Therapeutic Effect:*** Relieves bronchospasm, reduces airway resistance.

Pharmacokinetics

Rapidly, well absorbed from the gastrointestinal (GI) tract. Extensive metabolism in GI tract. Unknown extent metabolized in liver and lungs. Excreted in urine. ***Half-life:*** 4 hrs.

INDICATIONS AND DOSAGES

Bronchospasm

Hand-Bulb Nebulizer

Adults, Elderly. 4 inhalations (range: 3-7 inhalations) undiluted. May be repeated up to 5 times/day.

Metered Dose Inhalation

Adults, Elderly. 1-2 inhalations q4h. Wait 1 min before administering second inhalation.

IPPB, Oxygen Aerolization

Adults, Elderly. 0.5-1 ml of a 0.5% or 0.5 ml of a 1% solution diluted 1:3.

AVAILABLE FORMS

- *Metered Spray:* 0.61% (Brokometer).
- *Solution for Inhalation:* 0.08% (Dey-Lute), 0.1% (Dey-Lute), 0.17% (Dey-Lute), 1% (Beta-2, Brokosol).

CONTRAINDICATIONS: History of hypersensitivity to sympathomimetics

PREGNANCY AND LACTATION: Pregnancy category C; no breast-feeding data available

SIDE EFFECTS

Occasional

Tremor, nausea, nervousness, palpitations, tachycardia, peripheral vasodilation, dryness of mouth, throat, dizziness, vomiting, headache, increased BP, insomnia.

SERIOUS REACTIONS

- Excessive sympathomimetic stimulation may produce palpitations, extrasystoles, tachycardia, chest pain, slight increase in BP followed by a substantial decrease, chills, sweating, and blanching of skin.
- Too-frequent or excessive use may lead to loss of bronchodilating effectiveness and severe and paradoxical bronchoconstriction.

INTERACTIONS

Drugs

❷ *β-blockers:* Decreased action of isoetharine, cardioselective β-blockers preferable if concurrent use necessary

❸ *Furosemide:* Potential for additive hypokalemia

SPECIAL CONSIDERATIONS

- Inhalation technique critical
- Re-educate routinely

PATIENT/FAMILY EDUCATION

- Increase fluid intake to decrease the viscosity of pulmonary secretions

- Rinse mouth with water immediately after inhalation
- Avoid excessive use of caffeine derivatives, such as chocolate, cocoa, coffee, cola, and tea

MONITORING PARAMETERS

- Lung sounds for rhonchi, wheezing, and rales
- Clinical improvement (quieter, slower respirations, relaxed facial expression, cessation of clavicular retractions)

isoniazid

(eye-soe-nye'-a-zid)

Rx: *INH:* Nydrazid

Combinations

Rx: with rifampin (Rifamate); with rifampin, pyrazinamide (Rifater)

Chemical Class: Isonicotinic acid derivative

Therapeutic Class: Antituberculosis agent

CLINICAL PHARMACOLOGY

Mechanism of Action: An isonicotinic acid derivative that inhibits mycolic acid synthesis and causes disruption of the bacterial cell wall and loss of acid-fast properties in susceptible mycobacteria. Active only during bacterial cell division. ***Therapeutic Effect:*** Bactericidal against actively growing intracelleluar and extracellular susceptible mycobacteria.

Pharmacokinetics

Readily absorbed from the GI tract. Protein binding: 10%-15%. Widely distributed (including to CSF). Metabolized in the liver. Primarily excreted in urine. Removed by hemodialysis. ***Half-life:*** 0.5-5 hrs.

INDICATIONS AND DOSAGES

Tuberculosis (in combination with one or more antituberculars)

PO, IM

Adults, Elderly. 5 mg/kg/day as a single dose. Maximum 300 mg/day.

Children. 10-15 mg/kg/day as a single dose. Maximum 300 mg/day.

Prevention of tuberculosis

PO, IM

Adults, Elderly. 300 mg/day as a single dose.

Children. 10 mg/kg/day as a single dose. Maximum 300 mg/day.

AVAILABLE FORMS

- *Tablets:* 100 mg, 300 mg.
- *Syrup:* 50 mg/5 ml.
- *Injection (Nydrazid):* 100 mg/ml.

CONTRAINDICATIONS: Acute hepatic disease, history of hypersensitivity reactions or hepatic injury with previous isoniazid therapy

PREGNANCY AND LACTATION: Pregnancy category C; the American Thoracic Society recommends use of isoniazid for tuberculosis during pregnancy; excreted in breast milk; women can safely breast-feed their infants while taking isoniazid if the infant is periodically examined for signs and symptoms of peripheral neuritis or hepatitis

SIDE EFFECTS

Frequent

Nausea, vomiting, diarrhea, abdominal pain

Rare

Pain at injection site, hypersensitivity reaction

SERIOUS REACTIONS

- Rare reactions include neurotoxicity (as evidenced by ataxia and paraesthesia), optic neuritis, and hepatotoxicity.

INTERACTIONS

Drugs

3 *Acetaminophen:* Increased acetaminophen concentrations, potential for hepatotoxicity

3 *Antacids:* Reduced plasma isoniazid concentrations
3 *Carbamazepine:* Increased serum carbamazepine concentrations, toxicity may occur
3 *Corticosteroids:* Reduced plasma concentrations of isoniazid
3 *Cycloserine:* Increased potential for CNS toxicity
3 *Diazepam, triazolam:* Increased concentrations of these drugs
2 *Disulfiram:* Adverse mental changes and coordination problems
3 *Ethanol:* Higher incidence of isoniazid-induced hepatitis in alcoholics
3 *Hepatotoxic medications:* May increase the risk of hepatotoxicity
3 *Ketoconazole:* May decrease ketoconazole blood concentration
3 *Phenytoin:* Predictable increases in serum phenytoin concentrations, toxicity possible
3 *Rifampin:* Increased hepatotoxicity of isoniazid in some patients; more common with slow acetylators of isoniazid, and/or preexisting liver disease
3 *Theophylline:* Increased theophylline concentrations, toxicity possible
3 *Valproic acid:* Increased valproic acid concentration possible
3 *Warfarin:* Potential for enhanced hypoprothrombinemic response to warfarin

Labs

- *False increase:* Serum AST, serum uric acid
- *False decrease:* Serum glucose
- *False positive:* Urine sugar

SPECIAL CONSIDERATIONS

PATIENT/FAMILY EDUCATION

- Take on empty stomach if possible; however, may be taken with food to decrease GI upset
- Minimize daily alcohol consumption to lessen the risk of hepatitis
- Notify clinician of weakness, fatigue, loss of appetite, nausea and vomiting, yellowing of skin or eyes, darkening of urine, numbness or tingling of hands and feet
- Do not skip doses and continue taking isoniazid for the full course of therapy (6-24 mos)
- Avoid foods containing tyramine, including aged cheeses, sauerkraut, smoked fish, and tuna, because these foods may cause headache, a hot or clammy feeling, lightheadedness, pounding heartbeat, and red or itching skin

MONITORING PARAMETERS

- Periodic ophthalmologic examinations even when visual symptoms do not occur
- Periodic liver function tests
- Assess the patient for burning, numbness, and tingling of the extremities. Be aware that patients at risk for neuropathy, such as alcoholics, those with chronic hepatic disease, diabetics, the elderly, and malnourished individuals, may receive pyridoxine prophylactically
- Be alert for signs and symptoms of a hypersensitivity reaction, including fever and skin eruptions

isoproterenol hydrochloride

(eye-soe-proe-ter'-e-nole hye-droe-klor'-ide)

Rx: Isuprel

Combinations

Rx: with phenylephrine (Duo-Medihaler)

Chemical Class: Catecholamine, synthetic

Therapeutic Class: Antiasthmatic; bronchodilator; sympathomimetic; vasopressor; ß-adrenergic agonist

CLINICAL PHARMACOLOGY

Mechanism of Action: A sympathomimetic (adrenergic agonist) that stimulates $beta_1$-adrenergic receptors. ***Therapeutic Effect:*** Increases myocardial contractility, stroke volume, cardiac output.

Pharmacokinetics

Readily absorbed. Metabolized in liver. Primarily excreted in urine. ***Half-life:*** 2.5-5 min.

INDICATIONS AND DOSAGES

Arrhythmias

IV Bolus

Adults, Elderly. Initially, 0.02-0.06 mg (1-3 ml of diluted solution). Subsequent dose range: 0.01-0.2 mg (0.5-10 ml of diluted solution).

IV Infusion

Adults, Elderly. Initially, 5 mcg/min (1.25 ml/min of diluted solution). Subsequent dose range: 2-20 mcg/min.

Children. 2.5 mcg/min or 0.1 mcg/kg per min.

Complete heart block following closure of ventricular septal defects

IV

Adults, Elderly. 0.04-0.06 mg (2-3 ml of diluted solution).

Infants. 0.01-0.03 (0.5-1.5 ml of diluted solution).

Shock

IV Infusion

Adults, Elderly. Rate of 0.5-5 mcg/min (0.25-2.5 ml of 1:500,000 dilution); rate of infusion based on clinical response (heart rate, central venous pressure, systemic BP, urine flow measurements).

AVAILABLE FORMS

- *Injection:* 0.02 mg/ml (Isuprel).

CONTRAINDICATIONS: Tachycardia due to digitalis toxicity, preexisting arrhythmias, angina, precordial distress, hypersensitivity to isoproterenol or any component of the formulation

PREGNANCY AND LACTATION: Pregnancy category C; no reports linking isoproterenol with congenital defects have been located; excretion into breast milk unknown; use caution in nursing mothers

SIDE EFFECTS

Frequent

Palpitations, tachycardia, restlessness, nervousness, tremor, insomnia, anxiety

Occasional

Increased sweating, headache, nausea, flushed skin, dizziness, coughing

SERIOUS REACTIONS

- Excessive sympathomimetic stimulation may cause palpitations, extrasystoles, tachycardia, chest pain, slight increase in BP followed by a substantial decrease, chills, sweating, and blanching of skin.
- Ventricular arrhythmias may occur if heart rate is above 130 beats/min.
- Parotid gland swelling may occur with prolonged use.

INTERACTIONS

Drugs

3 *Amitriptyline:* Combined use may result in predisposition to cardiac arrhythmias

3 *β-blockers:* Reduced effectiveness of isoproterenol in the treatment of asthma

3 *Epinephrine:* May induce serious arrhythmias

3 *MAOIs, tricyclic antidepressants:* May increase cardiovascular effects

Labs

• *False increase:* Serum AST, serum bilirubin, serum glucose

SPECIAL CONSIDERATIONS

PATIENT/FAMILY EDUCATION

• Notify the physician of chest pain, palpitations, or pain or burning at the injection site

MONITORING PARAMETERS

• Blood pressure, pulse, urine output, EKG

isosorbide dinitrate/isosorbide mononitrate

(eye-soe-sore'-bide)

Rx: (isosorbide dinitrate) Dilatrate, Dilatrate-SR, ISDN, Isochron, Isordil, Isordil Tembids, Isordil Titradose, Sorbitrate

Rx: (isosorbide mononitrate) Imdur, ISMO, Monoket

Chemical Class: Nitrate, organic

Therapeutic Class: Antianginal

CLINICAL PHARMACOLOGY

Mechanism of Action: A nitrate that stimulates intracellular cyclic guanosine monophosphate. ***Therapeutic Effect:*** Relaxes vascular smooth muscle of both arterial and venous vasculature. Decreases preload and afterload.

Pharmacokinetics

Route	*Onset*	*Peak*	*Duration*
Dinitrate			
Sublingual	2-5 mins	N/A	1-2 hrs
Oral (Chewable)	2-5 mins	N/A	1-2 hrs
Oral	15-40 mins	N/A	4-6 hrs
Oral (Sustained-Release)	30 mins	N/A	12 hrs
Mononitrate			
Oral (Extended-Release)	60 mins	N/A	N/A

Dinitrate poorly absorbed and metabolized in the liver to its activate metabolite isosorbide mononitrate. Mononitrate well absorbed after PO administration. Excreted in urine and feces. ***Half-life:*** Dinitrate, 1-4 hrs; mononitrate, 4 hrs.

INDICATIONS AND DOSAGES

Angina

PO (isosorbide dinitrate)

Adults, Elderly. 5-40 mg 4 times a day. Sustained-release: 40 mg q8-12h.

PO (isosorbide mononitrate)

Adults, Elderly. 5-10 mg twice a day given 7 hrs apart. Sustained-release: Initially, 30-60 mg/day in morning as a single dose. May increase dose at 3-day intervals. Maximum: 240 mg/day.

AVAILABLE FORMS

• *Capsules (Sustained-Release [Dilatrate, Isordil Tembids]):* 40 mg.

• *Tablets:* 5 mg (ISDN, Isordil, Isordil Titradose), 10 mg (ISDN, ISMO, Isordil, Isordil Titradose, Monoket), 20 mg (ISDN, ISMO, Isordil, Isordil Titradose, Monoket), 30 mg (ISDN,

Isordil, Isordil Titradose), 40 mg (ISDN, Isordil, Isordil Titradose).

- *Tablets (Chewable [Sorbitrate]):* 5 mg, 10 mg.
- *Tablets (Extended-Release [Imdur]):* 30 mg, 60 mg, 120 mg.
- *Tablets (Sublingual [Isordil]):* 2.5 mg, 5 mg, 10 mg.

UNLABELED USES: CHF, dysphagia, pain relief, relief of esophageal spasm with gastroesophageal reflux

CONTRAINDICATIONS: Closed-angle glaucoma, GI hypermotility or malabsorption (extended-release tablets), head trauma, hypersensitivity to nitrates, increased intracranial pressure, orthostatic hypotension, severe anemia (extended-release tablets)

PREGNANCY AND LACTATION: Pregnancy category C; excretion into breast milk unknown; use caution in nursing mothers

SIDE EFFECTS

Frequent

Burning and tingling at oral point of dissolution (sublingual), headache (possibly severe) occurs mostly in early therapy, diminishes rapidly in intensity, and usually disappears during continued treatment, transient flushing of face and neck, dizziness (especially if patient is standing immobile or is in a warm environment), weakness, orthostatic hypotension, nausea, vomiting, restlessness

Occasional

GI upset, blurred vision, dry mouth

SERIOUS REACTIONS

- Blurred vision or dry mouth may occur (drug should be discontinued).
- Isosorbide administration may cause severe orthostatic hypotension manifested by fainting, pulselessness, cold or clammy skin, and diaphoresis.
- Tolerance may occur with repeated, prolonged therapy, but may not occur with the extended-release form. Minor tolerance may be seen with intermittent use of sublingual tablets.
- High dosage tends to produce severe headache.

INTERACTIONS

Drugs

3 *Alcohol:* Exaggerated hypotension and cardiac collapse

3 *Calcium channel blockers:* Exaggerated symptomatic orthostatic hypotension

3 *Dihydroergotamine:* Increases the bioavailability of dihydroergotamine with resultant increase in mean standing systolic blood pressure; functional antagonism, decreasing effects

3 *Sildenafil:* Excessive hypotensive effects

SPECIAL CONSIDERATIONS

PATIENT/FAMILY EDUCATION

- Headache may be a marker for drug activity; do not try to avoid by altering treatment schedule; contact clinician if severe or persistent; aspirin or acetaminophen may be used for relief
- Dissolve SL tablets under tongue; do not crush, chew, or swallow
- Do not crush chewable tablets before administering
- Avoid alcohol
- Make changes in position slowly to prevent fainting

MONITORING PARAMETERS

- Monitor and document the number of anginal episodes and orthostatic blood pressure
- Assess for dizziness or lightheadedness and facial or neck flushing

isotretinoin

(eye-soe-tret′-i-noyn)

Rx: Accutane

Chemical Class: Retinoid; vitamin A derivative

Therapeutic Class: Antiacne agent

CLINICAL PHARMACOLOGY

Mechanism of Action: Reduces the size of sebaceous glands and inhibits their activity. ***Therapeutic Effect:*** Decreases sebum production; produces antikeratinizing and antiinflammatory effects.

Pharmacokinetics

Metabolized in the liver; major metabolite active. Eliminated in urine and feces. ***Half-life:*** 21 hr; metabolite, 21-24 hr.

INDICATIONS AND DOSAGES

Recalcitrant cystic acne that is unresponsive to conventional acne therapies

PO

Adults. Initially, 0.5-2 mg/kg/day divided into 2 doses for 15-20 wk. May repeat after at least 2 mo off therapy.

Treatment of gram-negative folliculitis, severe keratinization disorders, severe rosacea

AVAILABLE FORMS

- *Capsules:* 10 mg, 20 mg, 40 mg.

CONTRAINDICATIONS: Hypersensitivity to isotretinoin or parabens (component of capsules)

PREGNANCY AND LACTATION: Pregnancy category X; isotretinoin is a potent human teratogen; excretion into breast milk unknown, but based on the close relationship to vitamin A, the presence of isotretinoin in breast milk should be expected; avoid use in nursing mothers

SIDE EFFECTS

Frequent (90%-20%)

Cheilitis (inflammation of lips), dry skin and mucous membranes, skin fragility, pruritus, epistaxis, dry nose and mouth, conjunctivitis, hypertriglyceridemia, nausea, vomiting, abdominal pain

Occasional (16%-5%)

Musculoskeletal symptoms (including bone pain, arthralgia, generalized myalgia), photosensitivity

Rare

Decreased night vision, depression

SERIOUS REACTIONS

- Inflammatory bowel disease and pseudotumor cerebri (benign intracranial hypertension) have been associated with isotretinoin therapy.

INTERACTIONS

Drugs

3 *Carbamazepine:* Decreased concentrations of carbamazepine in one patient

3 *Vitamin A supplements:* Possible additive toxic effects

3 *Oral contraceptives:* May decrease the effectiveness of oral contraceptives; two forms of contraception should be used simultaneously during isotretinoin therapy

2 *Tetracyclines:* Concomitant use of isotretinoin and tetracyclines associated with pseudotumor cerebri

SPECIAL CONSIDERATIONS

- Have patient complete consent form included with package insert prior to initiating therapy

PATIENT/FAMILY EDUCATION

- Administer with meals
- Avoid alcohol
- Do not take vitamin supplements containing vitamin A
- **Women of childbearing potential should practice contraception during therapy and for 1 mo before and after therapy**
- Notify clinician immediately if pregnancy is suspected

- A transient exacerbation of acne may occur during the initiation of therapy
- Avoid prolonged exposure to sunlight or sunlamps
- Do not donate blood during and for 30 days after stopping therapy
- Use caution driving or operating any vehicle at night
- Discontinue drug if visual difficulties occur and have an ophthalmologic exam

MONITORING PARAMETERS

- Pregnancy test initially, during first 5 days of menstrual period then monthly
- CBC with differential, platelet count, baseline sedimentation rate, serum triglycerides (baseline and biweekly for 4 wk), liver enzymes
- Skin and mucous membranes for excessive dryness

isradipine

(is-rad′-i-peen)

Rx: DynaCirc, DynaCirc CR

Chemical Class: Dihydropyridine

Therapeutic Class: Antianginal; antihypertensive; calcium channel blocker

CLINICAL PHARMACOLOGY

Mechanism of Action: An antihypertensive that inhibits calcium movement across cardiac and vascular smooth-muscle cell membranes. Potent peripheral vasodilator that does not depress SA or AV nodes. ***Therapeutic Effect:*** Produces relaxation of coronary vascular smooth muscle and coronary vasodilation. Increases myocardial oxygen delivery to those with vasospastic angina.

Pharmacokinetics

Route	*Onset*	*Peak*	*Duration*
PO	2-3 hrs	2-4 wks (with multiple doses) 8-16 hrs (with single dose)	N/A
PO (Controlled-release)	2 hrs	8-10 hrs	N/A

Well absorbed from the GI tract. Protein binding: 95%. Metabolized in the liver (undergoes first-pass effect). Primarily excreted in urine. Not removed by hemodialysis. ***Half-life:*** 8 hr.

INDICATIONS AND DOSAGES

Hypertension

PO

Adults, Elderly. Initially, 2.5 mg twice a day. May increase by 2.5 mg at 2- to 4-wk intervals. Range: 5-20 mg/day

AVAILABLE FORMS

- *Capsules (Dynacirc):* 2.5 mg, 5 mg.
- *Capsules (Controlled-Release [Dynacirc-CR]):* 5 mg, 10 mg.

UNLABELED USES: Treatment of chronic angina pectoris, Raynaud's phenomenon

CONTRAINDICATIONS: Cardiogenic shock, CHF, heart block, hypotension, sinus bradycardia, ventricular tachycardia

PREGNANCY AND LACTATION: Pregnancy category C; excretion into breast milk unknown; use caution in nursing mothers

SIDE EFFECTS

Frequent (7%-4%)

Peripheral edema, palpitations (higher frequency in females)

Occasional (3%)

Facial flushing, cough

Rare (2%-1%)

Angina, tachycardia, rash, pruritus

SERIOUS REACTIONS

• Overdose produces nausea, drowsiness, confusion, and slurred speech.
• CHF occurs rarely.

INTERACTIONS

Drugs

3 *β-blockers:* May have an additive effect

3 *Cimetidine:* Increased blood levels of isradipine with cimetidine

3 *Digitalis glycosides:* Increased digitalis levels; increased risk of toxicity

3 *Fentanyl:* Severe hypotension or increased fluid volume requirements

3 *Grapefruit, grapefruit juice:* May increase the absorption of isradipine

3 *Lovastatin:* Decreased lovastatin concentrations

SPECIAL CONSIDERATIONS

PATIENT/FAMILY EDUCATION

• Do not abruptly discontinuing isradipine
• Compliance with the treatment regimen is essential to control hypertension
• Rise slowly from a lying to a sitting position and wait momentarily before standing to avoid isradipine's hypotensive effect
• Notify the physician if an irregular heartbeat, nausea, pronounced dizziness, or shortness of breath occurs
• Avoid grapefruit and grapefruit juice because these foods may increase the absorption of isradipine

MONITORING PARAMETERS

• Blood pressure for hypotension and pulse for bradycardia
• Assess for peripheral edema behind the medial malleolus in ambulatory patients or in the sacral area in bedridden patients
• Observe the patient for signs and symptoms of CHF and examine the patient's skin for flushing

itraconazole

(it-ra-con'-a-zol)

Rx: Sporanox

Chemical Class: Triazole derivative

Therapeutic Class: Antifungal

CLINICAL PHARMACOLOGY

Mechanism of Action: A fungistatic antifungal that inhibits the synthesis of ergosterol, a vital component of fungal cell formation. ***Therapeutic Effect:*** Damages the fungal cell membrane, altering its function.

Pharmacokinetics

Moderately absorbed from the GI tract. Absorption is increased if the drug is taken with food. Protein binding: 99%. Widely distributed, primarily in the fatty tissue, liver, and kidneys. Metabolized in the liver to active metabolite. Primarily excreted in urine. Not removed by hemodialysis. ***Half-life:*** 21 hr; metabolite, 12 hr.

INDICATIONS AND DOSAGES

Blastomycosis, histoplasmosis

PO

Adults, Elderly. Initially, 200 mg once a day. Maximum: 400 mg/day in 2 divided doses.

IV

Adults, Elderly. 200 mg twice a day for 4 doses, then 200 mg once a day.

Aspergillosis

PO

Adults, Elderly. 600 mg/day in 3 divided doses for 3-4 days, then 200-400 mg/day in 2 divided doses.

IV

Adults, Elderly. 200 mg twice a day for 4 doses, then 200 mg once a day.

Esophageal candidiasis

PO

Adults, Elderly. Swish 100-200 mg (10-20 ml) in mouth for several seconds, then swallow. Maximum: 200 mg/day.

Oropharyngeal candidiasis

PO

Adults, Elderly. 200 mg (10 ml) oral solution, swish and swallow once a day for 7-14 days.

Febrile neutropenia

IV

Adults, Elderly. 200 mg twice a day for 4 doses, then 200 mg for up to 14 days. Then give PO 200 mg twice a day until neutropenia resolves.

Onychomycosis (fingernail)

PO

Adults, Elderly. 200 mg twice a day for 7 days, off for 21 days, repeat 200 mg twice a day for 7 days.

Onychomycosis (toenail)

PO

Adults, Elderly. 200 mg once daily for 12 wk.

AVAILABLE FORMS

- *Capsules:* 100 mg.
- *Oral Solution:* 10 mg/ml.
- *Injection:* 10 mg/ml (25-ml ampule).

UNLABELED USES: Suppression of histoplasmosis; treatment of disseminated sporotrichosis, fungal pneumonia and septicemia, or ringworm of the hand

CONTRAINDICATIONS: Hypersensitivity to fluconazole, ketoconazole, or miconazole

PREGNANCY AND LACTATION: Pregnancy category C; excreted into breast milk; do not administer to nursing mothers

SIDE EFFECTS

Frequent (11%-9%)

Nausea, rash

Occasional (5%-3%)

Vomiting, headache, diarrhea, hypertension, peripheral edema, fatigue, fever

Rare (2% or less)

Abdominal pain, dizziness, anorexia, pruritus

SERIOUS REACTIONS

- Hepatitis (as evidenced by anorexia, abdominal pain, unusual fatigue or weakness, jaundice skin or sclera, and dark urine) occurs rarely.

INTERACTIONS

Drugs

3 *Alprazolam:* Increased plasma alprazolam concentration

3 *Aluminum:* Reduced itraconazole absorption

3 *Amprenavir:* Increased plasma amprenavir concentration

3 *Antacids:* Reduced itraconazole absorption

▲ *Astemizole:* QT prolongation and life-threatening dysrhythmia

3 *Atevirdine:* Increased plasma atevirdine concentration

3 *Atorvastatin:* Increased plasma atorvastatin concentration with risk of rhabdomyolysis

3 *Buspirone:* Increased plasma buspirone concentration

3 *Calcium:* Reduced itraconazole absorption

3 *Cerivastatin:* Increased plasma cerivastatin concentration with risk of rhabdomyolysis

3 *Chlordiazepoxide:* Increased plasma chlordiazepoxide concentration

3 *Cimetidine:* Reduced itraconazole absorption

▲ *Cisapride:* QT prolongation and life-threatening dysrhythmia

3 *Clarithromycin:* Increased plasma itraconazole concentration

3 *Cyclosporine:* Increased plasma cyclosporine concentration

3 *Diazepam:* Increased plasma diazepam concentration

3 *Digoxin:* Increased plasma digoxin concentration

3 *Didanosine:* Reduced itraconazole absorption

3 *Erythromycin:* Increased plasma itraconazole concentration

3 *Ethanol:* Disulfiram-like reaction possible
3 *Famotidine:* Reduced itraconazole absorption
3 *Felodipine:* Increased plasma felodipine concentration
3 *Fluvastatin:* Increased plasma fluvastatin concentration with risk of rhabdomyolysis
3 *Food:* Increased intraconazole absorption
3 *Grapefruit, grapefruit juice:* May alter itraconazole absorption
3 *Haloperidol:* Increases the plasma concentrations of haloperidol
3 *Indinavir:* Increased plasma indinavir concentration
3 *Lansoprazole:* Reduced itraconazole absorption
2 *Lovastatin:* Increased plasma lovastatin concentration with risk of rhabdomyolysis
3 *Magnesium:* Reduced itraconazole absorption
3 *Methadone:* Increased plasma methadone concentration
3 *Methylprednisolone:* Increased plasma methylprednisolone concentration
3 *Midazolam:* Increased plasma midazolam concentration
3 *Nelfinavir:* Increased plasma nelfinavir concentration
3 *Nifedipine:* Increases nifedipine concentrations and enhances the hypotensive effects
3 *Nizatidine:* Reduced itraconazole absorption
3 *Omeprazole:* Reduced itraconazole absorption
3 *Oral anticoagulants:* Increased hypoprothrombinemic response
2 *Phenytoin:* Markedly reduced plasma itraconazole concentration
1 *Pimozide:* Increased plasma pimozide concentration, QT prolongation and life-threatening dysrhythmia
3 *Pravastatin:* Increased plasma pravastatin concentration with risk of rhabdomyolysis
1 *Quinidine:* Increased plasma quinidine concentration, QT prolongation and life-threatening dysrhythmia
3 *Repaglinide:* Increases serum concentration of repaglinide; enhances hypoglycemic effect
3 *Rifampin:* Decreased plasma itraconazole concentration; decreased plasma rifampin concentration
3 *Ritonavir:* Increased plasma ritonavir concentration
3 *Saquinavir:* Increased plasma saquinavir concentration
2 *Simvastatin:* Increased plasma simvastatin concentration with risk of rhabdomyolysis
3 *Sodium bicarbonate:* Reduced itraconazole absorption
3 *Sucralfate:* Reduced itraconazole absorption
3 *Tacrolimus:* Increased plasma tacrolimus concentration
1 *Terfenadine:* QT prolongation and life-threatening dysrhythmia
3 *Tolbutamide:* Increased plasma tolbutamide concentration
2 *Triazolam:* Increased plasma triazolam concentration
3 *Warfarin:* Increased hypoprothrombinemic response

SPECIAL CONSIDERATIONS

PATIENT/FAMILY EDUCATION

- Take with food to ensure maximal absorption
- Avoid antacids within 2 hr of itraconazole administration
- Report decreased appetite, dark urine, nausea, vomiting, pale stools, unusual fatigue, or yellow skin to the physician
- Avoid grapefruit and grapefruit juice because they may alter itraconazole absorption

MONITORING PARAMETERS
- Liver function tests in patients with preexisting abnormalities

---

ivermectin
(eye-ver-mek′-tin)
Rx: Stromectol
Chemical Class: Avermectin derivative
Therapeutic Class: Antihelmintic

CLINICAL PHARMACOLOGY
Mechanism of Action: Selectively binds to chloride ion channels in invertebrate nerve/muscle cells, increasing permeability to chloride ions. In general the following organisms are susceptible to ivermectin: *Onchocerca volvulus, Pediculosis capitis, Strongyloides stercoralis, Sarcoptes scabiei,* and *Wuchereria bancrofti.* ***Therapeutic effects:*** Causes paralysis/death of parasites.
Pharmacokinetics
Does not readily cross the blood-brain barrier. Metabolized in the liver. Excreted in the feces. ***Half-life:*** 4 hrs. Well absorbed with plasma concentrations proportional to the dose.
INDICATIONS AND DOSAGES
Strongyloidiasis
PO
Adults, Elderly, Children >33 lbs: 200 mcg/kg as a single dose.
Onchoceriasis
PO
Adults, Elderly, Children >33 lbs: 150 mcg/kg as a single dose at 3-12-month intervals.
Scabies
PO
Adults. 200 mcg/kg as a single dose and repeat 2 wks later.
Norwegian scabies (crusted scabies infection), superinfected scabies, or resistant scabies
PO
Adults. 200 mcg/kg with repeated treatments or combined with a topical scabicide.
Pediculosis
PO
Adults. A regimen of 2 doses of 200 mcg/kg with each dose separated by 10 days.
Bancroft's filariasis
PO
Adults, Children >15 kg. 150 mcg/kg as a single dose. May repeat 1 or 2 more times (each dose a week apart) if larva continues to migrate 1 wk after the previous dose.
AVAILABLE FORMS
- ***Tablets:*** 3 mg, 6 mg.

UNLABELED USES: Cutaneous larva migrans, filariasis, pediculosis, scabies, *Wuchereria bancrofti*
CONTRAINDICATIONS: Hypersensitivity to ivermectin or to any one of its components. Should not be used in women who are pregnant or infants.
PREGNANCY AND LACTATION: Pregnancy category C; excreted in breast milk in low concentrations
SIDE EFFECTS
Occasional
Abdominal pain, anorexia, arthralgia, constipation, diarrhea, dizziness, drowsiness, edema, fatigue, fever, lymphadenopathy, maculopapular or unspecified rash, nausea, vomiting, orthostatic hypotension, pruritis, Stevens-Johnson syndrome, toxic epidermal necrolysis, tremor, urticaria, vertigo, visual impairment, weakness
INTERACTIONS
Drugs
3 *Carbamazepine:* May decrease concentrations

SPECIAL CONSIDERATIONS

PATIENT/FAMILY EDUCATION

- Rapid killing of microfilariae may induce systemic or ocular inflammatory response (Mazzotti reaction, manifest by pruritus, rash, lymphadenopathy, and fever)
- Complete full course of therapy
- Keep hands away from mouth

MONITORING PARAMETERS

- Stool for parasites; blood for microfilaria and eosinophils

kanamycin sulfate

(kan-a-mye'-sin sul'-fate)

Rx: Kantrex

Chemical Class: Aminoglycoside

Therapeutic Class: Antibiotic

CLINICAL PHARMACOLOGY

Mechanism of Action: An aminoglycoside antibiotic that irreversibly binds to protein on bacterial ribosomes. ***Therapeutic Effect:*** Interferes with protein synthesis of susceptible microorganisms.

Pharmacokinetics

Negligible amounts are absorbed through intact intestinal mucosa. Protein binding: 0%-3%. Minimally metabolized in liver. Partially excreted in feces; small amounts eliminated in urine. Removed by hemodialysis. ***Half-life:*** approximately 2 hr.

INDICATIONS AND DOSAGES

Short-term treatment of serious infections

IV

Adults. 15 mg/kg/day.

IM

Adults, Children. 15 mg/kg/day in 2 divided dosages administered at equally divided intervals (75 mg/kg q12h). If continuously high blood levels are desired, the daily dose of 15 mg/kg may be given in equally divided doses q6-8h.

Dosage in renal impairment

Dosage and frequency are modified based on the degree of renal impairment and serum drug concentration.

AVAILABLE FORMS

- *Injection:* 1 g/3 ml.

CONTRAINDICATIONS: Hypersensitivity to other aminoglycosides (cross-sensitivity), or their components, long-term therapy

PREGNANCY AND LACTATION: Pregnancy category: unavailable for irrigating solution.; 8th cranial nerve toxicity in the fetus has been reported; excreted into breast milk in low concentrations; poor oral availability reduces potential for ototoxicity for the infant; compatible with breast-feeding

SIDE EFFECTS

Occasional

Hypersensitivity reactions (fever, pruritus, rash, urticaria)

Rare

Headache

SERIOUS REACTIONS

- Serious reactions may include nephrotoxicity (as evidenced by increased thirst, decreased appetite, nausea, vomiting, increased BUN and serum creatinine levels, and decreased creatinine clearance), neurotoxicity (manifested as muscle twitching, visual disturbances, seizures, and tingling), and ototoxicity (as evidenced by tinnitus, dizziness, and loss of hearing).

INTERACTIONS

Drugs

3 *Amphotericin B:* Synergistic nephrotoxicity

2 *Atracurium:* Kanamycin potentiates respiratory depression by atracurium

3 *Carbenicillin:* Potential for inactivation of kanamycin in patients with renal failure
3 *Carboplatin:* Additive nephrotoxicity or ototoxicity
3 *Cephalosporins:* Increased potential for nephrotoxicity in patients with preexisting renal disease
3 *Cisplatin:* Additive nephrotoxicity or ototoxicity
3 *Cyclosporine:* Additive nephrotoxicity
2 *Ethacrynic acid:* Additive ototoxicity
3 *Indomethacin:* Reduced renal clearance of kanamycin in premature infants
3 *Methoxyflurane:* Additive nephrotoxicity
2 *Neuromuscular blocking agents:* Kanamycin potentiates respiratory depression by neuromuscular blocking agents
3 *NSAIDs:* May reduce renal clearance of kanamycin
3 *Penicillins(extended-spectrum):* Potential for inactivation of kanamycin in patients with renal failure
3 *Piperacillin:* Potential for inactivation of kanamycin in patients with renal failure
2 *Succinylcholine:* Kanamycin potentiates respiratory depression by succinylcholine
3 *Ticarcillin:* Potential for inactivation of kanamycin in patients with renal failure
3 *Vancomycin:* Additive nephrotoxicity or ototoxicity
2 *Vecuronium:* Kanamycin potentiates respiratory depression by vecuronium

Labs

- *False increase:* Urine amino acids

SPECIAL CONSIDERATIONS

PATIENT/FAMILY EDUCATION

- Report headache, dizziness, loss of hearing, ringing, roaring in ears, or feeling of fullness in head

MONITORING PARAMETERS

- Urinalysis
- Urine output
- Serum peak drawn at 30-60 min after IV INF or 60 min after IM inj, trough level drawn just before next dose; adjust dosage per levels, especially in renal function impairment (usual therapeutic plasma levels; peak 15-30 mg/L, trough $\leq$10 mg/L)
- Serum creatinine for CrCl calculation
- Serum calcium, magnesium, sodium
- Audiometric testing; assess hearing before, during, after treatment
- RBCs, WBCs

kaolin; pectin

(kay'-oh-lin; pek'-tin)

OTC: Kao-Spen, Kapectolin

Combinations

OTC: with bismuth subcarbonate (K-C); with bismuth subsalicylate (Kaodene non-narcotic)

Chemical Class: Kaolin: hydrous magnesium aluminum silicate; pectin: purified carbohydrate product

Therapeutic Class: Antidiarrheal

CLINICAL PHARMACOLOGY

Mechanism of Action: An antidiarrheal agent that acts as an adsorbent and protectant. ***Therapeutic Effect:*** Absorbs bacteria, toxins, and reduces water loss.

Pharmacokinetics

Not absorbed orally. Up to 90% of pectin decomposed in gastrointestinal (GI) tract.

INDICATIONS AND DOSAGES
Antidiarrheal
PO
Adults, Elderly. 60-120 ml after each loose bowel movement (LBM).
Children 12 yrs and older. 60 ml after each LBM.
Children 6-12 yrs. 30-60 ml after each LBM.
Children 3-6 yrs. 15-30 ml after each LBM.

AVAILABLE FORMS
- *Suspension:* 5.2 g kaolin and 260 mg pectin /30 ml (Kao-Spen), 5.85 g kaolin and 130 mg pectin/30 ml (Kaopectolin).

CONTRAINDICATIONS: Diarrhea secondary to pseudomembranous enterocolitis or toxigenic bacteria, hypersensitivity to kaolin/pectin products

PREGNANCY AND LACTATION: Pregnancy category C; neither agent is systemically absorbed; should have no effect on lactation or nursing infant

SIDE EFFECTS
Rare
Constipation

SERIOUS REACTIONS
- Dehydration may occur.

INTERACTIONS
Drugs
❷ *Clindamycin, lincomycin:* Reduced antibacterial efficacy of these drugs
❸ *Digoxin:* Reduced bioavailability of digoxin tablets, capsules not affected
❸ *Lovastatin:* Pectin inhibits cholesterol lowering effects of lovastatin
❸ *Quinidine:* Reduced plasma quinidine concentrations

SPECIAL CONSIDERATIONS

PATIENT/FAMILY EDUCATION
- Do not self-medicate diarrhea for >48 hr without consulting a provider

MONITORING PARAMETERS
- Pattern of daily bowel activity and stool consistency

ketoconazole
(kee-toe-kon′-na-zole)
Rx: Nizoral, Nizoral Topical
OTC: Nizoral AD
Chemical Class: Imidazole derivative
Therapeutic Class: Antifungal

CLINICAL PHARMACOLOGY
Mechanism of Action: A fungistatic antifungal that inhibits the synthesis of ergosterol, a vital component of fungal cell formation. ***Therapeutic Effect:*** Damages the fungal cell membrane, altering its function.
Pharmacokinetics
Well absorbed from GI tract following PO administration. Protein binding: 91%-99%. Metabolized in liver. Primarily excreted in bile with minimal elimination in urine. Negligible systemic absorption following topical absorption. Ketoconazole is not detected in plasma after shampooing or topical administration. ***Half-life:*** 2-12 hr.

INDICATIONS AND DOSAGES
Histoplasmosis, blastomycosis, systemic candidiasis, chronic mucocutaneous candidiasis, coccidioidomycosis, paracoccidioidomycosis, chromomycosis, seborrheic dermatitis, tinea corporis, tinea capitis, tinea manus, tinea cruris, tinea pedis, tinea unguium (onychomycosis), oral thrush, candiduria
PO
Adults, Elderly. 200-400 mg/day.
Children. 3.3-6.6 mg/kg/day. Maximum: 800 mg/day in 2 divided doses.

K

Topical
Adults, Elderly. Apply to affected area 1-2 times a day for 2-4 wk.
Shampoo
Adults, Elderly. Use twice weekly for 4 wk, allowing at least 3 days between shampooing. Use intermittently to maintain control.

AVAILABLE FORMS

- *Tablets (Nizoral):* 200 mg.
- *Cream (Nizoral Topical):* 2%.
- *Shampoo (Nizoral AD):* 1%.

UNLABELED USES: *Systemic:* Treatment of fungal pneumonia, prostate cancer, septicemia

CONTRAINDICATIONS: None known.

PREGNANCY AND LACTATION: Pregnancy category C; has been used, apparently without harm, for the treatment of vaginal candidiasis during pregnancy; not detected in plasma with chronic shampoo use; unknown if cream absorbed; oral ketoconazole probably excreted in breast milk; use in breast-feeding not recommended

SIDE EFFECTS

Occasional (10%-3%)
Nausea, vomiting
Rare (less than 2%)
Abdominal pain, diarrhea, headache, dizziness, photophobia, pruritus
Topical: itching, burning, irritation

SERIOUS REACTIONS

- Hematologic toxicity (as evidenced by thrombocytopenia, hemolytic anemia, and leukopenia) occurs occasionally.
- Hepatotoxicity may occur within 1 week to several months after starting therapy.
- Anaphylaxis occurs rarely.

INTERACTIONS

Drugs

3 *Alprazolam:* Increased plasma alprazolam concentration
3 *Aluminum:* Reduced ketoconazole absorption
3 *Amprenavir:* Increased plasma amprenavir concentration
3 *Antacids:* Reduced ketoconazole absorption
▲ *Astemizole:* QT prolongation and life-threatening dysrhythmia
3 *Atevirdine:* Increased plasma atevirdine concentration
3 *Atorvastatin:* Increased plasma atorvastatin concentration with risk of rhabdomyolysis
3 *Buspirone:* Increased plasma buspirone concentration
3 *Calcium:* Reduced ketoconazole absorption
3 *Chlordiazepoxide:* Increased plasma chlordiazepoxide concentration
3 *Cimetidine:* Reduced ketoconazole absorption
❷ *Cisapride:* QT prolongation and dysrhythmia
3 *Cyclosporine:* Increased plasma cyclosporine concentration
3 *Diazepam:* Increased plasma diazepam concentration
3 *Didanosine:* Reduced ketoconazole absorption
3 *Ethanol:* Disulfiram-like reaction possible
3 *Famotidine:* Reduced ketoconazole absorption
3 *Felodipine:* Increased plasma felodipine concentration
3 *Fluvastatin:* Increased plasma fluvastatin concentration with risk of rhabdomyolysis
3 *Indinavir:* Increased plasma indinavir concentration
3 *Lansoprazole:* Reduced ketoconazole absorption
3 *Loratadine:* Increases loratadine plasma concentrations
❷ *Lovastatin:* Increased plasma lovastatin concentration with risk of rhabdomyolysis

3 *Magnesium:* Reduced ketoconazole absorption
3 *Methadone:* Increased plasma methadone concentration
3 *Methylprednisolone:* Increased plasma methylprednisolone concentration
3 *Midazolam:* Increased plasma midazolam concentration
3 *Nelfinavir:* Increased plasma nelfinavir concentration
3 *Nisoldipine:* Increases nisoldipine concentrations; increased hypotensive effects may occur
3 *Nizatidine:* Reduced ketoconazole absorption
3 *Omeprazole:* Reduced ketoconazole absorption
3 *Oral anticoagulants:* Increased hypoprothrombinemic response
❷ *Pimozide:* Elevated pimozide concentrations and cardiac arrhythmias may occur
3 *Pravastatin:* Increased plasma pravastatin concentration with risk of rhabdomyolysis
3 *Quetiapine:* Increases quetiapine plasma concentrations; expect side effects in some patients
3 *Quinidine:* Increased plasma quinidine concentration
3 *Ranitidine:* Reduces the plasma concentrations of ketoconazole, potentially resulting in loss of antifungal effect
3 *Rifampin:* Decreased plasma ketoconazole concentration; decreased plasma rifampin concentration
3 *Ritonavir:* Increased plasma ritonavir concentration
3 *Rosiglitazone:* Increases rosiglitazone concentrations and may increase the hypoglycemic effect of rosiglitazone
3 *Sirolimus:* Marked increase in the plasma concentration of sirolimus; sirolimus-induced toxicity may result
3 *Saquinavir:* Increased plasma saquinavir concentration
❷ *Simvastatin:* Increased plasma simvastatin concentration with risk of rhabdomyolysis
3 *Sodium bicarbonate:* Reduced ketoconazole absorption
3 *Sucralfate:* Reduced ketoconazole absorption
3 *Tacrolimus:* Increased plasma tacrolimus concentration
⚠ *Terfenadine:* QT prolongation and life-threatening dysrhythmia
3 *Tolbutamide:* Increased plasma tolbutamide concentration
3 *Tolterodine:* Moderately increased tolterodine serum concentrations
3 *Triazolam:* Increased plasma triazolam concentration
3 *Warfarin:* Increased hypoprothrombinemic response
3 *Ziprasidone:* Modest increase in ziprasidone plasma concentrations; some increase in side effects might occur
3 *Zolpidem:* Increases zolpidem concentrations; increased sedation may occur

SPECIAL CONSIDERATIONS

PATIENT/FAMILY EDUCATION

- For shampoo, moisten hair and scalp, apply shampoo, and gently massage over entire scalp for 1 min; rinse with warm water; repeat, leaving shampoo on scalp for additional 3 min
- Do not take tab with antacids or H_2-receptor antagonists; separate doses by at least 2 hr
- Take tablets with food
- Prolonged therapy over weeks or months is usually necessary
- Do not miss a dose and continue therapy for as long as directed
- Avoid alcohol to minimize the risk of liver damage

• Avoid tasks that require mental alertness or motor skills until response to the drug is established
• Notify the physician if dark urine, pale stools, yellow skin or eyes, increased irritation (with topical use), or other new symptoms occurs
• The patient using topical ketoconazole should avoid drug contact with the eyes, keep the skin clean and dry, rub the drug well into affected areas, and wear light clothing for ventilation
• Separate personal items that come in direct contact with the affected area

MONITORING PARAMETERS
• Liver function tests at baseline and periodically during treatment
• CBC for evidence of hematologic toxicity
• Pattern of daily bowel activity and stool consistency
• Skin for rash, pruritus, urticaria, burning, or irritation

ketoprofen

(kee-toe-proe'-fen)
Rx: Oruvail
OTC: Actron, Orudis KT
Chemical Class: Propionic acid derivative
Therapeutic Class: NSAID; antipyretic; nonnarcotic analgesic

CLINICAL PHARMACOLOGY
Mechanism of Action: An NSAID that produces analgesic and antiinflammatory effects by inhibiting prostaglandin synthesis. ***Therapeutic Effect:*** Reduces the inflammatory response and intensity of pain.
Pharmacokinetics
Immediate-release capsules are rapidly and well absorbed following PO administration; extended-release capsules are also well absorbed. Protein binding: 99%. Metabolized in liver. Excreted in urine; less than 10% excreted as unchanged (unconjugated) drug. ***Half-life:*** 2.4 hr.

INDICATIONS AND DOSAGES
Acute or chronic rheumatoid arthritis and osteoarthritis
PO
Adults. Initially, 75 mg 3 times a day or 50 mg 4 times a day.
Elderly. Initially, 25-50 mg 3-4 times a day. Maintenance: 150-300 mg/day in 3-4 divided doses.
PO (Extended-Release)
Adults, Elderly. 100-200 mg once a day.
Mild to moderate pain, dysmenorrhea
PO
Adults, Elderly. 25-50 mg q6-8h. Maximum: 300 mg/day.
Over-the-counter (OTC) dosage
PO
Adults, Elderly. 12.5 mg q4-6h. Maximum: 6 tabs/day.
Dosage in renal impairment
Mild. 150 mg/day maximum.
Severe. 100 mg/day maximum.

AVAILABLE FORMS
• *Capsules:* 25 mg, 50 mg, 75 mg.
• *Capsules (Extended-Release [Oruvail]):* 100 mg, 150 mg, 200 mg.
• *Tablets (Orudis KT):* 12.5 mg (OTC).

UNLABELED USES: Treatment of acute gouty arthritis, psoriatic arthritis, ankylosing spondylitis, vascular headache

CONTRAINDICATIONS: Active peptic ulcer disease, chronic inflammation of the GI tract, GI bleeding or ulceration, history of hypersensitivity to aspirin or NSAIDs

PREGNANCY AND LACTATION: Pregnancy category B (category D if used in third trimester); could cause constriction of the ductus arteriosus *in utero;* persistent pulmonary hypertension of the newborn or prolonged labor; unknown if excreted into human breast milk

SIDE EFFECTS

Frequent (11%)

Dyspepsia

Occasional (more than 3%)

Nausea, diarrhea or constipation, flatulence, abdominal cramps, headache

Rare (less than 2%)

Anorexia, vomiting, visual disturbances, fluid retention

SERIOUS REACTIONS

• Rare reactions with long-term use include peptic ulcer disease, GI bleeding, gastritis, and severe hepatic reactions (cholestasis, jaundice), nephrotoxicity (dysuria, hematuria, proteinuria, nephrotic syndrome), and severe hypersensitivity reaction (bronchospasm, angioedema).

INTERACTIONS

Drugs

3 *Aminoglycosides:* Reduced clearance with elevated aminoglycoside levels and potential for toxicity (especially indomethacin in premature infants; other NSAIDs probably)

3 *Anticoagulants:* Excessive hypoprothrombinemia, decreased platelet aggregation with increased risk of GI bleeding

3 *Antihypertensives (α-blockers, angiotensin-converting enzyme inhibitors, angiotensin II receptor blockers, β-blockers, diuretics):* Inhibition of antihypertensive and other favorable hemodynamic effects

3 *Aspirin, other salicylates:* May increase the risk of GI side effects such as bleeding

3 *Bone marrow depressants:* May increase the risk of hematologic reactions

3 *Corticosteroids:* Increased risk of GI ulceration

3 *Cyclosporine:* Increased nephrotoxicity risk

3 *Lithium:* Decreased clearance of lithium (mediated via prostaglandins) resulting in elevated serum lithium levels and risk of toxicity

3 *Methotrexate:* Decreased renal secretion of methotrexate resulting in elevated methotrexate levels and risk of toxicity

3 *Phenylpropanolamine:* Possible acute hypertensive reaction

3 *Potassium-sparing diuretics:* Additive hyperkalemia potential

3 *Probenecid:* May increase ketoprofen blood concentration

3 *Triamterene:* Acute renal failure reported with addition of indomethacin; caution with other NSAIDs

Labs

• *False decrease:* Serum ALT, AST; serum lactate dehydrogenase

SPECIAL CONSIDERATIONS

• No significant advantage over other NSAIDs; cost should govern use

PATIENT/FAMILY EDUCATION

• Avoid aspirin and alcoholic beverages

• Take with food, milk, or antacids to decrease GI upset

• Swallow capsules whole and do not chew or crush them

• Inform the physician if the female patient plans to become pregnant

MONITORING PARAMETERS

• Initial hemogram and fecal occult blood test within 3 mo of starting regular chronic therapy; repeat every 6-12 mo (more frequently in high-risk patients [>65 years, peptic ulcer disease, concurrent steroids or anticoagulants]); electrolytes, creatinine, and BUN within 3 mo of starting regular chronic therapy; repeat every 6-12 mo

- Therapeutic response, such as improved grip strength, increased mobility, improved range of motion, and decreased pain, tenderness, stiffness, and swelling

ketorolac tromethamine

(kee-toe-role'-ak troe-meth'-a-meen)

Rx: Acular, Acular LS, Acular PF, Toradol, Toradol IM, Toradol IV/IM

Chemical Class: Acetic acid derivative

Therapeutic Class: NSAID; antipyretic; nonnarcotic analgesic

CLINICAL PHARMACOLOGY

Mechanism of Action: An NSAID that inhibits prostaglandin synthesis and reduces prostaglandin levels in the aqueous humor. ***Therapeutic Effect:*** Relieves pain stimulus and reduces intraocular inflammation.

Pharmacokinetics

Route	Onset	Peak	Duration
PO	30-60 mins	1.5-4 hrs	4-6 hrs
IV/IM	30 mins	1-2 hrs	4-6 hrs

Readily absorbed from the GI tract, after IM administration. Protein binding: 99%. Largely metabolized in the liver. Primarily excreted in urine. Not removed by hemodialysis. ***Half-life:*** 3.8-6.3 hrs (increased with impaired renal function and in the elderly).

INDICATIONS AND DOSAGES

Short-term relief of mild to moderate pain (multiple doses)

PO

Adults, Elderly. 10 mg q4-6h. Maximum: 40 mg/24 hr.

IV, IM

Adults younger than 65 yrs. 30 mg q6h. Maximum: 120 mg/24 hrs.

Adults 65 yrs and older, those with renal impairment, those weighing less than 50 kg. 15 mg q6h. Maximum: 60 mg/24 hrs.

Children 2-16 yrs. 0.5 mg/kg q6h.

Short-term relief of mild to moderate pain (single dose)

IV

Adults younger than 65 yrs, Children 17 yr and older weighing more than 50 kg. 30 mg.

Adults 65 yrs and older, with renal impairment, weighing less than 50 kg. 15 mg.

Children 2-16 yrs. 0.5 mg/kg. Maximum: 15 mg.

IM

Adults younger than 65 yrs, Children 17 yrs and older, weighing more than 50 kg. 60 mg.

Adults 65 yrs and older, with renal impairment, weighing less than 50 kg. 30 mg.

Children 2-16 yrs. 1 mg/kg. Maximum: 15 kg.

Allergic conjunctivitis

Ophthalmic

Adults, Elderly, Children 3 yrs and older. 1 drop 4 times a day.

Cataract extraction

Ophthalmic

Adults, Elderly. 1 drop 4 times a day. Begin 24 hr after surgery and continue for 2 wks.

Refractive surgery

Ophthalmic

Adults, Elderly. 1 drop 4 times a day for 3 days.

AVAILABLE FORMS

- *Tablets (Toradol):* 10 mg.

• *Injection (Toradol, Toradol IM, Toradol IV/IM):* 15 mg/ml, 30 mg/ml.
• *Ophthalmic Solution:* 0.4% (Acular LS), 0.5% (Acular, Acular PF).

UNLABELED USES: Prevention or treatment of ocular inflammation (ophthalmic form)

CONTRAINDICATIONS: Active peptic ulcer disease, chronic inflammation of GI tract, GI bleeding or ulceration, history of hypersensitivity to aspirin or NSAIDs

PREGNANCY AND LACTATION: Pregnancy category C (D if used in third trimester); excreted into breast milk; not recommended in lactation

SIDE EFFECTS

Frequent (17%-12%)

Headache, nausea, abdominal cramps or pain, dyspepsia

Occasional (9%-3%)

Diarrhea

Ophthalmic: Transient stinging and burning

Rare (3%-1%)

Constipation, vomiting, flatulence, stomatitis, dizziness

Ophthalmic: Ocular irritation, allergic reactions, superficial ocular infection, keratitis

SERIOUS REACTIONS

• Rare reactions with long-term use include peptic ulcer disease, GI bleeding, gastritis, severe hepatic reactions (cholestasis, jaundice), nephrotoxicity (glomerular nephritis, interstitial nephritis, nephrotic syndrome), and an acute hypersensitivity reaction (including fever, chills, and joint pain).

INTERACTIONS

Drugs

3 *Aminoglycosides:* Reduced clearance with elevated aminoglycoside levels and potential for toxicity (especially indomethacin in premature infants; other NSAIDs probably)

3 *Anticoagulants:* Excessive hypoprothrombinemia, decreased platelet aggregation with increased risk of GI bleeding

3 *Antihypertensives (α-blockers, angiotensin-converting enzyme inhibitors, angiotensin II receptor blockers, β-blockers, diuretics):* Inhibition of antihypertensive and other favorable hemodynamic effects

3 *Aspirin, other salicylates:* May increase the risk of GI side effects such as bleeding

3 *Bone marrow depressants:* May increase the risk of hematologic reactions

3 *Corticosteroids:* Increased risk of GI ulceration

3 *Cyclosporine:* Increased nephrotoxicity risk

3 *Lithium:* Decreased clearance of lithium (mediated via prostaglandins) resulting in elevated serum lithium levels and risk of toxicity

3 *Methotrexate:* Decreased renal secretion of methotrexate resulting in elevated methotrexate levels and risk of toxicity

3 *Phenylpropanolamine:* Possible acute hypertensive reaction

3 *Potassium-sparing diuretics:* Additive hyperkalemia potential

3 *Probenecid:* May increase ketorolac blood concentration

3 *Triamterene:* Acute renal failure reported with addition of indomethacin; caution with other NSAIDs

SPECIAL CONSIDERATIONS

PATIENT/FAMILY EDUCATION

• Not for chronic use
• No significant advantage over other oral NSAIDs; cost and clinical situation should govern use; no reason to continue parenteral course of therapy with oral ketorolac (more expensive, more toxic)

• Combined use of ketorolac parenteral and oral should not exceed 5 days
• Take ketorolac with food or milk if GI upset occurs
• Do not administer ketorolac ophthalmic solution while wearing soft contact lenses; transient burning and stinging may occur after instillation
• Avoid tasks that require mental alertness or motor skills until response to the drug has been established
• Inform the physician if the female patient plans to become pregnant

MONITORING PARAMETERS

• CBC, liver and renal function test results, urine output, BUN level, and serum alkaline phosphatase, bilirubin, and creatinine levels
• Be alert for signs of bleeding, which may also occur with ophthalmic use if systemic absorption occurs
• Therapeutic response, such as improved grip strength, increased joint mobility, and decreased pain, tenderness, stiffness, and swelling

labetalol hydrochloride

(la-bet'-a-lole hye-droe-klor'-ide)

Rx: Normodyne, Trandate

Combinations

Rx: with hydrochlorothiazide (Normozide, Trandate HCT)

Chemical Class: α-adrenergic blocker, peripheral; β-adrenergic blocker, nonselective

Therapeutic Class: Antihypertensive

CLINICAL PHARMACOLOGY

Mechanism of Action: An antihypertensive that blocks alpha$_1$-, beta$_1$-, and beta$_2$-(large doses) adrenergic receptor sites. Large doses increase airway resistance. ***Therapeutic Effect:*** Slows sinus heart rate; decreases peripheral vascular resistance, cardiac output, and BP.

Pharmacokinetics

Route	Onset	Peak	Duration
PO	0.5-2 hrs	2-4 hrs	8-12 hrs
IV	2-5 mins	5-15 mins	2-4 hrs

Completely absorbed from the GI tract. Protein binding: 50%. Undergoes first-pass metabolism. Metabolized in the liver. Primarily excreted in urine. Not removed by hemodialysis. ***Half-life:*** PO, 6-8 hrs; IV, 5.5 hrs.

INDICATIONS AND DOSAGES

Hypertension

PO

Adults. Initially, 100 mg twice a day adjusted in increments of 100 mg twice a day q2-3 days. Maintenance: 200-400 mg twice a day. Maximum: 2.4 g/day.

Elderly. Initially, 100 mg 1-2 times a day. May increase as needed.

Severe hypertension, hypertensive emergency

IV

Adults. Initially, 20 mg. Additional doses of 20-80 mg may be given at 10-min intervals, up to total dose of 300 mg.

IV Infusion

Adults. Initially, 2 mg/min up to total dose of 300 mg.

PO (after IV therapy)

Adults. Initially, 200 mg; then, 200-400 mg in 6-12 hr. Increase dose at 1-day intervals to desired level.

AVAILABLE FORMS

• *Tablets (Normodyne, Trandate):* 100 mg, 200 mg, 300 mg.
• *Injection (Trandate):* 5 mg/ml.

UNLABELED USES: Control of hypotension during surgery, treatment of chronic angina pectoris

CONTRAINDICATIONS: Bronchial asthma, cardiogenic shock, overt cardiac failure, second- or third-degree heart block, severe bradycardia, uncontrolled CHF, other conditions associated with severe and prolonged hypotension

PREGNANCY AND LACTATION: Pregnancy category C (D if used in second or third trimester); similar drug, atenolol, frequently used in the third trimester for treatment of hypertension (many studies of efficacy and safety of atenolol in pregnancy-induced hypertension); long-term use has been associated with intrauterine growth retardation; only a small amount of drug appears in milk (0.004% of dose); unlikely to be therapeutically significant

SIDE EFFECTS

Frequent

Drowsiness, difficulty sleeping, unusual fatigue or weakness, diminished sexual ability, transient scalp tingling

Occasional

Dizziness, dyspnea, peripheral edema, depression, anxiety, constipation, diarrhea, nasal congestion, nausea, vomiting, abdominal discomfort

Rare

Altered taste, dry eyes, increased urination, paresthesia

SERIOUS REACTIONS

• Labetalol administration may precipitate or aggravate CHF because of decreased myocardial stimulation.

• Abrupt withdrawal may precipitate ischemic heart disease, producing sweating, palpitations, headache, and tremor.

• May mask signs and symptoms of acute hypoglycemia (tachycardia, BP changes) in patients with diabetes.

INTERACTIONS

Drugs

3 *α_1-adrenergic blockers:* Potential enhanced first-dose response (marked initial drop in blood pressure, particularly on standing)

3 *Amiodarone:* Symptomatic bradycardia and sinus arrest, especially patients with bradycardia, sick sinus syndrome, or partial AV node block

3 *Cimetidine:* Increased plasma labetolol concentrations

3 *Clonidine:* Withdrawal of clonidine abruptly may exaggerate the hypertension due to unopposed alpha stimulation; safer than other β-blockers, however

3 *Digoxin:* Additive prolongation of AV conduction time

3 *Dihydropyridine calcium channel blockers:* Severe hypotension or impaired cardiac performance; most prevalent with impaired left ventricular function, cardiac arrhythmias, or aortic stenosis

3 *Diltiazem:* Potentiates β-adrenergic effects; hypotension, left ventricular failure, and AV conduction disturbances problematic in elderly, patients with left ventricular dysfunction, aortic stenosis, or with large doses of either drug

3 *Diuretics:* May increase hypotensive effect

3 *Epinephrine:* Increased diastolic pressure and bradycardia during epinephrine infusions

3 *Hypoglycemic agents:* Masked hypoglycemia, hyperglycemia

3 *MAOIs:* May produce hypertension

3 *NSAIDs:* Reduced hypotensive effects of β-blockers

3 *Sympathomimetics, xanthines:* May mutually inhibit effects
❷ *Theophylline:* Antagonistic pharmacodynamic effects
3 *Verapamil:* Potentiates β-adrenergic effects; hypotension, left ventricular failure, and AV conduction disturbances problematic in elderly, patients with ventricular dysfunction, aortic stenosis, or with large doses of either drug

Labs

• *False positive:* Urine amphetamine
• *False increase:* Urinary catecholamines, plasma epinephrine

SPECIAL CONSIDERATIONS

PATIENT/FAMILY EDUCATION

• Do not discontinue abruptly; may require taper; rapid withdrawal may produce rebound hypertension or angina
• Transient scalp tingling may occur, especially when treatment is initiated
• May mask the symptoms of hypoglycemia, except for sweating, in diabetic patients
• Maintain compliance
• Avoid tasks that require mental alertness or motor skills until response to the drug has been established
• Notify the physician if excessive fatigue, headache, prolonged dizziness, shortness of breath, or weight gain occurs
• Do not take nasal decongestants and OTC cold preparations, especially those containing stimulants, without physician approval

MONITORING PARAMETERS

• Angina: Reduction in nitroglycerin usage; frequency, severity, onset, and duration of angina pain; heart rate
• Arrhythmias: Heart rate
• Congestive heart failure: Functional status, cough, dyspnea on exertion, paroxysmal nocturnal dyspnea, exercise tolerance, and ventricular function
• Hypertension: Blood pressure
• Postmyocardial infarction: Left ventricular function, lower resting heart rate
• Toxicity: Blood glucose, bronchospasm, hypotension, bradycardia, depression, confusion, hallucination, sexual dysfunction

lactulose

(lak'-tyoo-lose)

Rx: Cholac, Constilac, Constulose, Enulose, Generlac, Kristalose

Chemical Class: Disaccharide lactose analog

Therapeutic Class: Ammonia detoxicant; laxative

CLINICAL PHARMACOLOGY

Mechanism of Action: A lactose derivative that retains ammonia in colon and decreases serum ammonia concentration, producing osmotic effect. ***Therapeutic Effect:*** Promotes increased peristalsis and bowel evacuation, which expels ammonia from the colon.

Pharmacokinetics

Route	*Onset*	*Peak*	*Duration*
PO	24-48 hrs	N/A	N/A
Rectal	30-60 mins	N/A	N/A

Poorly absorbed from the GI tract. Acts in the colon. Primarily excreted in feces.

INDICATIONS AND DOSAGES

Constipation

PO

Adults, Elderly. 15-30 ml (10-20 g)/day, up to 60 ml(40 g)/day.
Children. 7.5 ml(5 g)/day after breakfast.

Portal-systemic encephalopathy
PO
Adults, Elderly. Initially, 30-45 ml every hr. Then, 30-45 ml (20-30 g) 3-4 times a day. Adjust dose q1-2 days to produce 2-3 soft stools a day.
Children. 40-90 ml/day in divided doses.
Infants. 2.5-10 ml/day in divided doses.
Rectal (as retention enema)
Adults, Elderly. 300 ml with 700 ml water or saline solution; patient should retain 30-60 min. Repeat q4-6h. If evacuation occurs too promptly, repeat immediately.

AVAILABLE FORMS
- *Syrup:* 10 g/15 ml.
- *Packets:* 10 g, 20 g.

CONTRAINDICATIONS: Abdominal pain, appendicitis, nausea, patients on a galactose-free diet, vomiting

PREGNANCY AND LACTATION: Pregnancy category B

SIDE EFFECTS
Occasional
Abdominal cramping, flatulence, increased thirst, abdominal discomfort
Rare
Nausea, vomiting

SERIOUS REACTIONS
- Diarrhea indicates overdose.
- Long-term use may result in laxative dependence, chronic constipation, and loss of normal bowel function.

INTERACTIONS
Drugs
3 *Oral medications:* May decrease transit time of concurrently administered oral medications, decreasing lactulose absorption
Labs
- *False increase:* Serum creatinine

SPECIAL CONSIDERATIONS
PATIENT/FAMILY EDUCATION
- May be mixed with fruit juice, water, or milk to increase palatability
- Do not take other laxatives while on lactulose therapy
- When receiving lactulose rectally, retain the liquid until cramping is felt; evacuation occurs in 24-48 hrs of the initial drug dose
- Institute measures to promote defecation, such as increasing fluid intake, exercising, and eating a high-fiber diet

MONITORING PARAMETERS
- Serum electrolytes, carbon dioxide periodically during chronic treatment
- Daily bowel activity and stool consistency, record time of evacuation
- Serum ammonia levels, looking for a reduction
- Mental status, and watch for signs of reduced ammonia level, such as lessening of asterixis

lamivudine
(la-mi'-vyoo-deen)
Rx: Epivir, Epivir-HBV
Combinations
Rx: with abacavir (Epzicom); with zidovudine: (Combivir)
Chemical Class: Nucleoside analog
Therapeutic Class: Antiretroviral

CLINICAL PHARMACOLOGY
Mechanism of Action: An antiviral that inhibits HIV reverse transcriptase by viral DNA chain termination. Also inhibits RNA- and DNA-dependent DNA polymerase, an enzyme necessary for HIV repli-

cation. ***Therapeutic Effect:*** Interrupts HIV replication, slowing the progression of HIV infection.

Pharmacokinetics

Rapidly and completely absorbed from the GI tract. Protein binding: less than 36%. Widely distributed (crosses the blood-brain barrier). Primarily excreted unchanged in urine. Not removed by hemodialysis or peritoneal dialysis. ***Half-life:*** 11-15 hr (intracellular), 2-11 hr (serum, adults), 1.7-2 hr (serum, children) (increased in impaired renal function).

INDICATIONS AND DOSAGES

HIV infection (in combination with other antiretrovirals)

PO

Adults, Children 12-16 yr, weighing 50 kg (100 lb) or more. 150 mg twice a day or 300 mg once a day.

Adults weighing less than 50 kg. 2 mg/kg twice a day.

Children 3 mo-11 yr. 4 mg/kg twice a day (up to 150 mg/dose).

Chronic hepatitis B

PO

Adults, Children 17 yr and older. 100 mg/day.

Children younger than 17 yr. 3 mg/kg/day. Maximum: 100 mg/day.

Dosage in renal impairment

Dosage and frequency are modified based on creatinine clearance.

Creatinine Clearance (ml/min)	*Dosage*
50 ml/min or higher	150 mg twice a day
30-49 ml/min	150 mg once a day
15-29 ml/min	150 mg first dose, then 100 mg once a day
5-14 ml/min	150 mg first dose, then 50 mg once a day
less than 5 ml/min	50 mg first dose, then 25 mg once a day

AVAILABLE FORMS

• *Oral Solution:* 5 mg/ml (Epivir-HBV), 10 mg/ml (Epivir).

• *Tablets:* 100 mg (Epivir-HBV), 150 mg (Epivir), 300 mg (Epivir).

UNLABELED USES: Prophylaxis in health care workers at risk of acquiring HIV after occupational exposure

CONTRAINDICATIONS: None known.

PREGNANCY AND LACTATION: Pregnancy category C; not recommended in nursing mothers

SIDE EFFECTS

Frequent

Headache (35%), nausea (33%), malaise and fatigue (27%), nasal disturbances (20%), diarrhea, cough (18%), musculoskeletal pain, neuropathy (12%), insomnia (11%), anorexia, dizziness, fever or chills (10%)

Occasional

Depression (9%); myalgia (8%); abdominal cramps (6%); dyspepsia, arthralgia (5%)

SERIOUS REACTIONS

• Lactic acidosis and severe hepatomegaly with steatosis, including fatal cases, have been reported.

• Pancreatitis occurs in 13% of pediatric patients.

• Anemia, neutropenia, and thrombocytopenia occur rarely.

INTERACTIONS

Drugs

3 *Co-trimoxazole:* Increases lamivudine blood concentration

3 *St. John's Wort:* May decrease lamivudine blood concentration and effect

SPECIAL CONSIDERATIONS

PATIENT/FAMILY EDUCATION

• Space lamivudine doses evenly around the clock and continue taking the drug for the full course of treatment

• Advise the parents of a pediatric patient to closely monitor the child for symptoms of pancreatitis, such as clammy skin, hypotension, nausea, severe and steady abdominal pain that often radiates to the back, and vomiting accompanyied by abdominal pain
• Avoid performing tasks that require mental alertness or motor skills until response to the drug has been established
• Lamivudine is not a cure for HIV, nor does it reduce the risk of transmitting HIV to others

MONITORING PARAMETERS

• Serum amylase, BUN, and serum creatinine levels
• Pattern of daily bowel activity and stool consistency
• Evaluate for altered sleep patterns, cough, dizziness, headache, and nausea
• If pancreatitis occurs in a pediatric patient, help the patient to sit up or flex at the waist to relieve abdominal pain aggravated by movement

---

lamotrigine

(la-moe-trih'-jeen)

Rx: Lamictal, Lamictal CD

Chemical Class: Phenyltriazine derivative

Therapeutic Class: Anticonvulsant

CLINICAL PHARMACOLOGY

Mechanism of Action: An anticonvulsant whose exact mechanism is unknown. May block voltage-sensitive sodium channels, thus stabilizing neuronal membranes and regulating presynaptic transmitter release of excitatory amino acids. ***Therapeutic Effect:*** Reduces seizure activity.

Pharmacokinetics

Rapidly absorbed from the GI tract. Protein binding: 55%. Metabolized primarily by glucuronic acid conjugation. Excreted in the urine. ***Half-life:*** 13-30 hr.

INDICATIONS AND DOSAGES

Seizure control in patients receiving enzyme-inducing antiepileptic drugs (EIAEDs), but not valproic acid

PO

Adults, Elderly, Children older than 12 yr. Recommended as add-on therapy: 50 mg once a day for 2 wk, followed by 100 mg/day in 2 divided doses for 2 wk. Maintenance: Dosage may be increased by 100 mg/day every week, up to 300-500 mg/day in 2 divided doses.

Children 2-12 yr. 0.6 mg/kg/day in 2 divided doses for 2 wk, then 1.2 mg/kg/day in 2 divided doses for wk 3 and 4. Maintenance: 5-15 mg/kg/day. Maximum: 400 mg/day.

Seizure control in patients receiving combination therapy of EIAEDs and valproic acid

PO

Adults, Elderly, Children older than 12 yr. 25 mg every other day for 2 wk, followed by 25 mg once a day for 2 wk. Maintenance: Dosage may be increased by 25-50 mg/day q1-2wk, up to 150 mg/day in 2 divided doses.

Children 2-12 yr. 0.15 mg/kg/day in 2 divided doses for 2 wk, then 0.3 mg/kg/day in 2 divided doses for wk 3 and 4. Maintenance: 1-5 mg/kg/day in 2 divided doses. Maximum: 200 mg/day.

Conversion to monotherapy for patients receiving EIAEDs

PO

Adults, Elderly, Children 16 yr and older. 500 mg/day in 2 divided doses. Titrate to desired dose while maintaining EIAED at fixed level, then withdraw EIAED by 20% each wk over a 4-wk period.

Conversion to monotherapy for patients receiving valproic acid

PO

Adults, Elderly, Children 16 yr and older. Titrate lamotrigine to 200 mg/day, maintaining valproic acid dose. Maintain lamotrigine dose and decrease valproic acid to 500 mg/day, no greater than 500 mg/day/wk, then maintain 500 mg/day for 1 wk. Increase lamotrigine to 300 mg/day and decrease valproic acid to 250 mg/day. Maintain for 1 wk, then discontinue valproic acid and increase lamotrigine by 100 mg/day each wk until maintenance dose of 500 mg/day reached.

Bipolar disorder in patients receiving EIAEDs

PO

Adults, Elderly. 50 mg/day for 2 wk, then 100 mg/day for 2 wk, then 200 mg/day for 1 wk, then 300 mg/day for 1 wk, then up to usual maintenance dose 400 mg/day in divided doses.

Bipolar disorder in patients receiving valproic acid

PO

Adults, Elderly. 25 mg/day every other day for 2 wk, then 25 mg/day for 2 wk, then 50 mg/day for 1 wk, then 100 mg/day. Usual maintenance dose with valproic acid: 100 mg/day.

Discontinuation therapy

Adults, Children older than 12 yr. A dosage reduction of approximately 50% per week over at least 2 wk is recommended.

AVAILABLE FORMS

- *Tablets:* 25 mg, 100 mg, 150 mg, 200 mg.
- *Tablets (Chewable):* 2 mg, 5 mg, 25 mg.

CONTRAINDICATIONS: None known.

PREGNANCY AND LACTATION: Pregnancy category C; passes into breast milk; effects on infants exposed by this route are unknown

SIDE EFFECTS

Frequent

Dizziness (38%), diplopia (28%), headache (29%), ataxia (22%), nausea (19%), blurred vision (16%), somnolence, rhinitis (14%)

Occasional (10%-5%)

Rash, pharyngitis, vomiting, cough, flu-like symptoms, diarrhea, dysmenorrhea, fever, insomnia, dyspepsia

Rare

Constipation, tremor, anxiety, pruritus, vaginitis, hypersensitivity reaction

SERIOUS REACTIONS

- Abrupt withdrawal may increase seizure frequency.
- Serious rashes, including Stevens-Johnson syndrome, requiring hospitalization and discontinuation of treatment have been reported.

INTERACTIONS

Drugs

3 *Carbamazepine:* Increased carbamazepine epoxide levels; decreased lamotrigine levels

3 *Phenobarbital, primidone, phenytoin:* Decreased lamotrigine concentrations

3 *Valproic acid:* Increased lamotrigine concentration; decreased valproic acid concentration

SPECIAL CONSIDERATIONS

PATIENT/FAMILY EDUCATION

- Notify clinician immediately if a skin rash develops
- Avoid prolonged exposure to direct sunlight

• Do not discontinue the drug abruptly after long-term therapy; strict maintenance of drug therapy is essential for seizure control
• Avoid alcohol and tasks that require mental alertness or motor skills until response to the drug is established

MONITORING PARAMETERS
• Notify the physician promptly if rash occurs, and expect to discontinue the drug
• Assess for signs of clinical improvement, including a decrease in the frequency and intensity of seizures
• Assess the patient for headache and visual abnormalities

lansoprazole

(lan-soe-pra'-zole)

Rx: Prevacid, Prevacid IV, Prevacid Solu-Tab

Combinations

Rx: with naproxen (Napra-PAC)

Chemical Class: Benzimidazole derivative

Therapeutic Class: Antiulcer agent; gastrointestinal antisecretory agent

CLINICAL PHARMACOLOGY

Mechanism of Action: A proton pump inhibitor that selectively inhibits the parietal cell membrane enzyme system (hydrogen-potassium adenosine triphosphatase) or proton pump. ***Therapeutic Effect:*** Suppresses gastric acid secretion.

Pharmacokinetics

Route	Onset	Peak	Duration
PO (15 mg)	2-3 hrs	N/A	24 hrs
PO (30 mg)	1-2 hrs	N/A	longer than 24 hrs

Rapid and complete absorption (food may decrease absorption) once drug has left stomach. Protein binding: 97%. Distributed primarily to gastric parietal cells and converted to two active metabolites. Extensively metabolized in the liver. Eliminated in bile and urine. Not removed by hemodialysis. ***Half-life:*** 1.5 hr (increased in the elderly and in those with hepatic impairment).

INDICATIONS AND DOSAGES

Duodenal ulcer

PO

Adults, Elderly. 15 mg/day, before eating, preferably in the morning, for up to 4 wk. Maintenance: 15 mg/day.

Erosive esophagitis

PO

Adults, Elderly. 30 mg/day, before eating, for up to 8 wks. If healing does not occur within 8 wks (in 5%-10% of cases), may give for additional 8 wk. Maintenance: 15 mg/day.

IV

Adults, Elderly. 30 mg once a day for up to 7 days. Switch to oral lansoprazole therapy as soon as patient can tolerate oral route.

Gastric ulcer

PO

Adults. 30 mg/day for up to 8 wk.

NSAID gastric ulcer

PO

Adults, Elderly. (Healing): 30 mg/day for up to 8 wk. (Prevention): 15 mg/day for up to 12 wk.

Healed duodenal ulcer, gastroesophageal reflux disease

PO

Adults. 15 mg/day.

Usual pediatric dosage

Children 3 mos-14 yrs, weighing more than 20 kg. 30 mg once daily.

Children 3 mos-14 yrs, weighing 10-20 kg. 15 mg once daily.

Children 3 mos-14 yrs, weighing less than 10 kg. 7.5 mg once daily.

H. pylori infection

PO

Adults, Elderly. (triple drug therapy) 30 mg q12h for 10-14 days. (dual drug therapy) 30 mg q8h for 14 days.

Pathologic hypersecretory conditions (including Zollinger-Ellison syndrome)

PO

Adults, Elderly. 60 mg/day. Individualize dosage according to patient needs and for as long as clinically indicated. Administer up to 120 mg/day in divided doses.

AVAILABLE FORMS

• *Capsules (Delayed-Release [Prevacid]):* 15 mg, 30 mg.

• *Granules for Oral Suspension (Prevacid):* 15 mg/pack; 30 mg/pack.

• *Injection Powder for Reconstitution (Prevacid IV):* 30 mg.

• *Orally Disintegrating Tablets (Prevacid Solu-Tab):* 15 mg, 30 mg.

CONTRAINDICATIONS: None known.

PREGNANCY AND LACTATION: Pregnancy category B; excretion into breast milk unknown

SIDE EFFECTS

Occasional (3%-2%)

Diarrhea, abdominal pain, rash, pruritus, altered appetite

Rare (1%)

Nausea, headache

SERIOUS REACTIONS

• Bilirubinemia, eosinophilia, and hyperlipemia occur rarely.

INTERACTIONS

Drugs

3 *Ampicillin, iron salts:* May interfere with the absorption of these agents

3 *Cefpodoxime, cefuroxime, ketoconazole, enoxacin:* Reduced concentrations of these drugs

3 *Digoxin, nifedipine:* Increased serum concentrations of these drugs

3 *Food:* 50% decrease in absorption if given 30 min after food compared to the fasting condition

3 *Glipizide, glyburide, tolbutamide:* Increased concentrations of these drugs, potential for hypoglycemia

3 *Sucralfate:* Delayed absorption of lansoprazole and reduced bioavailability, administer lansoprazole at least 30 min prior to sucralfate

SPECIAL CONSIDERATIONS

• For patients with a nasogastric tube, capsules may be opened and the intact granules mixed with 40 ml of apple juice and injected through tube into stomach

• For patients unable to swallow capsules, capsule can be opened and the intact granules sprinkled on 1 tablespoon of applesauce and swallowed immediately; do not crush or chew granules

• For oral suspension, empty contents of packet into 30 ml of water only, do not use other liquids, do not crush or chew granules; if material remains add more water, stir, and drink immediately

MONITORING PARAMETERS

• Monitor the patient's ongoing laboratory results

• Assess for abdominal pain, diarrhea, and nausea and watch for therapeutic response (relief of GI symptoms)

lanthanum carbonate

(lan-thah'-num car-bo'-nate)

Rx: Fosrenol

Chemical Class: Naturally occurring rare earth element

Therapeutic Class: Phosphate adsorbent

CLINICAL PHARMACOLOGY

Mechanism of Action: A phosphate regulator that dissociates in the acidic environment of the upper GI tract to lanthanum ions, which bind to dietary phosphate released from food during digestion, forming highly insoluble lanthanum phosphate complexes. ***Therapeutic Effect:*** Reduces phosphate absorption.

Pharmacokinetics

Very low absorption following oral administration. Protein binding: greater than 99%. Not metabolized. Phosphate complexes are eliminated in urine. ***Half-life:*** 53 hr (in plasma); 2-3.6 yrs. (from bone).

INDICATIONS AND DOSAGES

Reduce serum phosphate in end-stage renal disease

PO

Adults, Elderly. 750 mg-1500 mg in divided doses, taken with or immediately after a meal. Dosage may be titrated in 750-mg increments q2-3wk based on serum phosphate levels.

AVAILABLE FORMS

• *Tablets (Chewable):* 250 mg, 500 mg.

CONTRAINDICATIONS: None known.

PREGNANCY AND LACTATION: Pregnancy category C; as the effect of lanthanum on the absorption of vitamins and other nutrients has not been studied, use during pregnancy is not recommended; excretion into human breast milk unknown, use caution in nursing mothers

SIDE EFFECTS

Frequent

Nausea (11%), vomiting (9%), dialysis graft occlusion (8%), abdominal pain (5%)

SERIOUS REACTIONS

• Dialysis graft occlusion has been reported.

INTERACTIONS

Drugs

3 : Products known to interact with antacids should not be taken within 2 hrs of lanthanum

SPECIAL CONSIDERATIONS

• A calcium and aluminum free phosphate binding agent; can be used as an alternative to aluminum- and calcium-containing agents, especially in patients who are at risk for calcium or aluminum toxicity

• Enables separation of control of calcium from phosphate

• Has not been compared directly to sevelemer, which also has low systemic absorption and is calcium and aluminum free

PATIENT/FAMILY EDUCATION

• Take with or immediately after meals

• Chew completely before swallowing, do not swallow intact tablets

MONITORING PARAMETERS

• Serum phosphate concentrations during titration, then at regular intervals thereafter

leflunomide

(leh-floo'-no-mide)

Rx: Arava

Chemical Class: Isoxazole derivative

Therapeutic Class: Disease-modifying antirheumatic drug (DMARD); immunomodulatory agent

CLINICAL PHARMACOLOGY

Mechanism of Action: An immunomodulatory agent that inhibits dihydroorotate dehydrogenase, the enzyme involved in autoimmune process that leads to rheumatoid arthritis. ***Therapeutic Effect:*** Reduces signs and symptoms of rheumatoid arthritis and slows structural damage.

Pharmacokinetics

Well absorbed after PO administration. Protein binding: greater than 99%. Metabolized to active metabolite in the GI wall and liver. Excreted through both renal and biliary systems. Not removed by hemodialysis. ***Half-life:*** 16 days.

INDICATIONS AND DOSAGES

Rheumatoid arthritis

PO

Adults, Elderly. Initially, 100 mg/day for 3 days, then 10-20 mg/day.

AVAILABLE FORMS

• *Tablets:* 10 mg, 20 mg.

CONTRAINDICATIONS: Pregnancy or plans to become pregnant

PREGNANCY AND LACTATION: Pregnancy category X; amount of excretion into breast milk unknown; use of leflunomide by nursing mothers is not recommended since the potential risk to nursing infants is considered serious

SIDE EFFECTS

Frequent (20%-10%)

Diarrhea, respiratory tract infection, alopecia, rash, nausea

SERIOUS REACTIONS

• Transient thrombocytopenia and leukopenia occur rarely.

• Rare cases of severe hepatic injury, including cases with fatal outcome, have been reported during treatment.

INTERACTIONS

Drugs

3 *Cholestyramine, charcoal:* Coadministration results in rapid and significant decrease in active metabolite

3 *Nonsteroidal antiinflammatory drugs:* Inhibition of CYP2C9, decreases the metabolism of many NSAIDS

3 *Rifampin:* Leflunomide levels increased 40%

SPECIAL CONSIDERATIONS

• Discuss potential risks of pregnancy and recommend appropriate contraception

MONITORING PARAMETERS

• *Efficacy:* ESR, C-reactive protein, platelet count, hemoglobin, improvement of RA; *toxicity:* LFTs (baseline, then monthly until stable)

lepirudin

(leh-peer'-yoo-din)

Rx: Refludan

Chemical Class: Hirudin derivative; thrombin inhibitor

Therapeutic Class: Anticoagulant

CLINICAL PHARMACOLOGY

Mechanism of Action: An anticoagulant that inhibits thrombogenic action of thrombin (independent of antithrombin II and not inhibited by platelet factor 4). One molecule of lepirudin binds to one molecule of thrombin. ***Therapeutic Effect:*** Produces dose-dependent increases in aPTT.

Pharmacokinetics

Distributed primarily in extracellular fluid. Primarily eliminated by the kidneys. ***Half-life:*** 1.3 hr (increased in impaired renal function).

INDICATIONS AND DOSAGES

Heparin-induced thrombocytopenia and associated thromboembolic disease to prevent further thromboembolic complications

IV, IV Infusion

Adults, Elderly. 0.2-0.4 mg/kg, IV slowly over 15-20 sec, followed by IV infusion of 0.1-0.15 mg/kg/hr for 2-10 days or longer.

Dosage in renal impairment

Initial dose is decreased to 0.2 mg/kg, with infusion rate adjusted based on creatinine clearance.

Creatinine Clearance (ml/min)	*% of standard infusion rate*	*Infusion rate (mg/kg/hr)*
45-60	50	0.075
30-44	30	0.045
15-29	15	0.0225

AVAILABLE FORMS

• *Powder for Injection:* 50 mg.

CONTRAINDICATIONS: None known.

PREGNANCY AND LACTATION: Pregnancy category B; use caution in nursing mothers

SIDE EFFECTS

Frequent (14%-5%)

Bleeding from gums, puncture sites, or wounds, hematuria, fever, GI and rectal bleeding

Occasional (3%-1%)

Epistaxis; allergic reaction, such as rash and pruritus; vaginal bleeding

SERIOUS REACTIONS

• Overdose is characterized by excessively high aPTT.

• Intracranial bleeding occurs rarely.

• Abnormal hepatic function occurs in 6% of patients.

INTERACTIONS

Drugs

3 *Thrombolytics:* Increased risk of bleeding complications; enhanced effect of lepirudin on aPTT prolongation

3 *Antithrombotic agents (warfarin, aspirin, ticlopidine, clopidogrel, dipyridamole):* Increased risk of bleeding

SPECIAL CONSIDERATIONS

• Untreated, HIT can lead to thrombosis, venous thromboembolism, acute MI, peripheral artery occlusion, and stroke; mortality rate approaches 20%-30%

• All sources of heparin must be discontinued as soon as HIT is detected

• In clinical trials the cumulative risk of death 35 days after starting treatment was 9% in the lepirudin-treated patients, compared with 18% in historic controls; cumulative risk of new thromboembolic complications was 6% with lepirudin and 22% in historic controls

PATIENT/FAMILY EDUCATION

• Report bleeding, breathing difficulty, bruising, dizziness, edema, fever, itching, lightheadedness, or rash

• Use an electric razor and soft toothbrush to prevent bleeding during lepirudin therapy

• Do not take other medications, including OTC drugs (especially aspirin), without physician approval

• Menstrual flow may be heavier than usual

MONITORING PARAMETERS

• aPTT ratio (patient aPTT over median of laboratory normal range for aPTT); target range 1.5-2.5; do not start in patients with baseline aPTT

ratio ≥2.5; determine aPTT ratio 4 hr following start of INF and at least daily thereafter
• CBC with platelet count (to detect bleeding complications and monitor recovery of platelets)
• Hct; renal function studies; BUN, serum creatinine, AST, and ALT levels; and stool and urine specimen for occult blood
• Assess for abdominal or back pain, a decrease in BP, an increase in pulse rate, and severe headache, which may be evidence of hemorrhage
• Determine the amount of female patient's menstrual discharge and monitor for any increase

letrozole
(let'-roe-zole)
Rx: Femara
Chemical Class: Benzhydryltriazole derivative
Therapeutic Class: Antineoplastic

CLINICAL PHARMACOLOGY
Mechanism of Action: Decreases the level of circulating estrogen by inhibiting aromatase, an enzyme that catalyzes the final step in estrogen production. ***Therapeutic Effect:*** Inhibits the growth of breast cancers that are stimulated by estrogens.
Pharmacokinetics
Rapidly and completely absorbed. Metabolized in the liver. Primarily eliminated by the kidneys. Unknown if removed by hemodialysis. ***Half-life:*** Approximately 2 days.

INDICATIONS AND DOSAGES
Breast cancer
PO
Adults, Elderly. 2.5 mg/day. Continue until tumor progression is evident.

AVAILABLE FORMS
• *Tablets:* 2.5 mg.

CONTRAINDICATIONS: None known.

PREGNANCY AND LACTATION: Pregnancy category D; excretion into breast milk unknown; use caution in nursing mothers

SIDE EFFECTS
Frequent (21%-9%)
Musculoskeletal pain (back, arm, leg), nausea, headache
Occasional (8%-5%)
Constipation, arthralgia, fatigue, vomiting, hot flashes, diarrhea, abdominal pain, cough, rash, anorexia, hypertension, peripheral edema
Rare (4%-1%)
Asthenia, somnolence, dyspepsia, weight gain, pruritus

SERIOUS REACTIONS
• Pleural effusion, pulmonary embolism, bone fracture, thromboembolic disorder, and MI have been reported.

INTERACTIONS
Drugs
3 *Tamoxifen:* Decreases letrozole concentrations by 38%

SPECIAL CONSIDERATIONS
PATIENT/FAMILY EDUCATION
• May take without regard to meals
• Notify the physician if weakness, hot flashes, or nausea becomes unmanageable

MONITORING PARAMETERS
• Consider CBC, TFTs, electrolytes, serum transaminases, creatinine until more toxicity information available
• Monitor for asthenia and dizziness
• Assess the patient for headache
• Administer an antiemetic, if ordered, to prevent or treat nausea and vomiting
• Evaluate for evidence of musculoskeletal pain, and provide analgesics, if ordered

leucovorin calcium (folinic acid, citrovorum factor)

(loo-koe-vor'-in kal'-see-um)

Rx: Wellcovorin

Chemical Class: Folic acid derivative

Therapeutic Class: Antidote, dihydrofolate reductase inhibitor; hematinic

CLINICAL PHARMACOLOGY

Mechanism of Action: An antidote to folic acid antagonists that may limit methotrexate action on normal cells by competing with methotrexate for the same transport processes into the cells. ***Therapeutic Effect:*** Reverses toxic effects of folic acid antagonists. Reverses folic acid deficiency.

Pharmacokinetics

Readily absorbed from the GI tract. Widely distributed. Primarily concentrated in the liver. Metabolized in the liver and intestinal mucosa to active metabolite. Primarily excreted in urine. ***Half-life:*** 15 min; metabolite, 30-35 min.

INDICATIONS AND DOSAGES

Conventional rescue dosage in high-dose methotrexate therapy

PO, IV, IM

Adults, Elderly, Children. 10 mg/m^2 IM or IV one time, then PO q6h until serum methotrexate level is less than 10^{-8} M. If 24-hr serum creatinine level increases by 50% or greater over baseline or methotrexate level exceeds 5×10^{-6} M or 48-hr level exceeds 9×10^{-7} M, increase to 100 mg/m^2 IV q3h until methotrexate level is less than 10^{-8} M.

Folic acid antagonist overdose

PO

Adults, Elderly, Children. 2-15 mg/day for 3 days or 5 mg every 3 days.

Megaloblastic anemia secondary to folate deficiency

IM

Adults, Elderly, Children. 1 mg/day.

Colon cancer

IV

Adults, Elderly. 200 mg/m^2 followed by 370 mg/m^2 fluorouracil daily for 5 days. Repeat course at 4-wk intervals for 2 courses, then 4-5-wks intervals or 20 mg/m^2 followed by 425 mg/m^2 fluorouracil daily for 5 days. Repeat course at 4-wk intervals for 2 courses, then 4-5-wks intervals.

AVAILABLE FORMS

- *Tablets:* 5 mg, 10 mg, 15 mg, 25 mg.
- *Powder for Injection:* 50 mg, 100 mg, 200 mg, 350 mg, 500 mg.

UNLABELED USES: Treatment of Ewing's sarcoma, gestational trophoblastic neoplasms, or non-Hodgkin's lymphoma; treatment adjunct for head and neck carcinoma

CONTRAINDICATIONS: Pernicious anemia, other megaloblastic anemias secondary to vitamin B_{12} deficiency

PREGNANCY AND LACTATION: Pregnancy category C; has been used in the treatment of megaloblastic anemia during pregnancy; compatible with breast-feeding

SIDE EFFECTS

Frequent

When combined with chemotherapeutic agents: Diarrhea, stomatitis, nausea, vomiting, lethargy or malaise or fatigue, alopecia, anorexia

Occasional

Urticaria, dermatitis

INTERACTIONS

Drugs

3 *Anticonvulsants:* May decrease the effects of anticonvulsants

3 *Chemotherapeutic agents:* May increase the effects and toxicity of these drugs when taken in combination

SPECIAL CONSIDERATIONS

- Administer as soon as possible following overdoses of dihydrofolate reductase inhibitors

PATIENT/FAMILY EDUCATION

- Encourage the patient with folic acid deficiency to eat foods high in folic acid, including dried beans, meat proteins, and green leafy vegetables
- Notify the physician if an allergic reaction or vomiting occurs

MONITORING PARAMETERS

- CBC with differential and platelets, electrolytes, and liver function tests prior to each treatment with leucovorin/5-fluorouracil combination
- Plasma methotrexate concentrations as a therapeutic guide to high-dose methotrexate therapy with leucovorin rescue; continue leucovorin until plasma methotrexate concentrations are $<5 \times 10^{-8}$M (see dosage)
- Serum creatinine
- Monitor the patient for vomiting, which may require a change from oral to parenteral therapy

leuprolide acetate

(loo′-proe-lide)

Rx: Eligard, Lupron, Lupron Depot, Lupron Depot-Gyn, Lupron Depot-Ped, Viadur

Chemical Class: Gonadotropin-releasing hormone analog

Therapeutic Class: Antiendometriosis agent; antineoplastic

CLINICAL PHARMACOLOGY

Mechanism of Action: A gonadotropin-releasing hormone analog and antineoplastic agent that stimulates the release of luteinizing hormone (LH) and follicle-stimulating hormone (FSH) from the anterior pituitary gland. ***Therapeutic Effect:*** Produces pharmacologic castration and decreases the growth of abnormal prostate tissue in males; causes endometrial tissue to become inactive and atrophic in females; and decreases the rate of pubertal development in children with central precocious puberty.

Pharmacokinetics

Rapidly and well absorbed after subcutaneous administration. Absorbed slowly after IM administration. Protein binding: 43%-49%. ***Half-life:*** 3-4 hr.

INDICATIONS AND DOSAGES

Advanced prostatic carcinoma

IM (Lupron Depot)

Adults, Elderly. 7.5 mg every month or 22.5 mg q3mo or 30 mg q4mo.

Subcutaneous (Eligard)

Adults, Elderly. 7.5 mg every month or 22.5 mg q3mo or 30 mg q4mo.

Subcutaneous (Lupron)

Adults, Elderly. 1 mg/day.

Subcutaneous (Viadur)

Adults, Elderly. 65 mg implanted q12mo.

Endometriosis

IM (Lupron Depot)

Adults, Elderly. 3.75 mg/mo for up to 6 mos or 11.25 mg q3mo for up to 2 doses.

Uterine leiomyomata

IM (with iron [Lupron Depot])

Adults, Elderly. 3.75 mg/mo for up to 3 mos or 11.25 mg as a single injection.

Precocious puberty

IM (Lupron Depot)

Children. 0.3 mg/kg/dose every 28 days. Minimum: 7.5 mg. If down regulation is not achieved, titrate upward in 3.75-mg increments q4wk.

Subcutaneous (Lupron)

Children. 20-45 mcg/kg/day. Titrate upward by 10 mcg/kg/day if down regulation is not achieved.

AVAILABLE FORMS

- *Implant (Viadur):* 65 mg.
- *Injection Depot Formulation:* 3.75 (Lupron Depot), 7.5 mg (Eligard, Lupron Depot, Lupron Depot-Ped), 11.25 (Lupron Depot, Lupron Depot-Ped, Lupron Depot-Gyn), 15 mg (Lupron Depot-Ped), 22.5 mg (Eligard, Lupron Depot), 30 mg (Lupron Depot).
- *Injection Solution (Lupron):* 5 mg/ml.

CONTRAINDICATIONS: Lactation, pernicious anemia, pregnancy, undiagnosed vaginal bleeding; Eligard 7.5 mg is contraindicated in patients with hypersensitivity to GnRH, GnRH agonist analogs or any of the components, 30 mg Lupron Depot contraindicated in women, the implant form is contraindicated in women and children

PREGNANCY AND LACTATION: Pregnancy category X; spontaneous abortions or intrauterine growth retardation are possible; not recommended during lactation

SIDE EFFECTS

Frequent

Hot flashes (ranging from mild flushing to diaphoresis)

Females: Amenorrhea, spotting

Occasional

Arrhythmias; palpitations; blurred vision; dizziness; edema; headache; burning, itching, or swelling at injection site; nausea; insomnia; weight gain

Females: Deepening voice, hirsutism, decreased libido, increased breast tenderness, vaginitis, altered mood

Males: Constipation, decreased testicle size, gynecomastia, impotence, decreased appetite, angina

Rare

Males: Thrombophlebitis

SERIOUS REACTIONS

- Signs and symptoms of metastatic prostatic carcinoma (such as bone pain, dysuria or hematuria, and weakness or paresthesia of the lower extremities) occasionally worsen 1-2 wks after the initial dose but then subside with continued therapy.
- Pulmonary embolism and MI occur rarely.

SPECIAL CONSIDERATIONS

PATIENT/FAMILY EDUCATION

- May cause increase in bone pain and difficulty urinating during first few weeks of treatment for prostate cancer, may also cause hot flashes
- Gonadotropin and sex steroids rise above baseline initially; side effects greatest in first weeks
- Continuous therapy vital for treatment of central precocious puberty
- Females may experience menses or spotting during first 2 mos of therapy for central precocious puberty; notify provider if continues into second treatment month; nonhormonal contraception should be used
- To the patient with prostate cancer, signs and symptoms of the disease may worsen temporarily during the first few weeks of leuprolide therapy
- Avoid performing tasks that require mental alertness or motor skills until response to the drug has been established

MONITORING PARAMETERS

- Monitor response to therapy for prostate cancer by measuring prostate specific antigen (PSA) levels
- GnRH stimulation test and sex steroid levels 1-2 mo after starting therapy for central precocious puberty,

measurement of bone age for advancement q6-12mo
• Monitor the patient for arrhythmias and palpitations
• Assess the patient for peripheral edema
• Evaluate the patient's sleep pattern
• Monitor the patient for visual difficulties

levetiracetam

(lev-a-tear-as′-e-tam)

Rx: Keppra

Chemical Class: Pyrrolidone derivative

Therapeutic Class: Anticonvulsant

CLINICAL PHARMACOLOGY

Mechanism of Action: An anticonvulsant that inhibits burst firing without affecting normal neuronal excitability. ***Therapeutic Effect:*** Prevents seizure activity.

Pharmacokinetics

Rapidly and almost completely absorbed through the GI tract. Protein binding: less than 10%. Insignificant amount metabolized in liver. Excreted in urine. Removed by hemodialysis. ***Half-life:*** 7 hr.

INDICATIONS AND DOSAGES

Partial-onset seizures

PO

Adults, Elderly. Initially, 500 mg q12h. May increase by 1000 mg/day q2wk. Maximum: 3000 mg/day.

Children 4-16 yr. 10-20 mg/kg/day in 2 divided doses. May increase at weekly intervals by 10-20 mg/kg. Maximum: 60 mg/kg.

Dosage in renal impairment

Dosage is modified based on creatinine clearance.

Creatinine Clearance (ml/min)	*Dosage*
Higher than 80 ml/min	500-1500 mg q12h
50-80 ml/min	500-1000 mg q12h
30-50 ml/min	250-750 mg q12h
less than 30 ml/min	250-500 mg q12h
End stage renal disease using dialysis	500-1000 mg q12h, after dialysis, a 250- to 500-mg supplemental dose is recommended.

AVAILABLE FORMS

• *Oral solution:* 100 mg/ml.
• *Tablets:* 250 mg, 500 mg, 750 mg.

CONTRAINDICATIONS: None known.

PREGNANCY AND LACTATION: Pregnancy category C; developmental toxicity in animals; excretion into breast milk unknown

SIDE EFFECTS

Frequent (15%-10%)

Somnolence, asthenia, headache, infection

Occasional (9%-3%)

Dizziness, pharyngitis, pain, depression, nervousness, vertigo, rhinitis, anorexia

Rare (less than 3%)

Amnesia, anxiety, emotional lability, cough, sinusitis, anorexia, diplopia

SERIOUS REACTIONS

• Acute psychosis and seizures have been reported. Sudden discontinuance increases the risk of seizure activity.

INTERACTIONS

Drugs

3 *Ginkgo biloba:* May decrease the anticonvulsant effectiveness

SPECIAL CONSIDERATIONS

• Reserve as an alternative treatment for patients with partial onset seizures not responding to first-line agents

PATIENT/FAMILY EDUCATION

- Notify clinician if female patients intend to or become pregnant
- Caution about common adverse effects, i.e., dizziness and somnolence; these side effects usually diminish with continued therapy
- Avoid tasks that require mental alertness or motor skills until response to the drug is established
- Do not discontinue levetiracetam therapy abruptly because this may precipitate seizures; strict maintenance of drug therapy is essential for seizure control

MONITORING PARAMETERS

- Therapeutic plasma concentrations not established; base dosing on therapeutic response (reduction in severity and frequency of seizures)
- Renal function tests

levocabastine

(lee-voe-kab′-as-teen)

Rx: Livostin

Chemical Class: Phenylisonipecotic acid derivative

Therapeutic Class: Ophthalmic antihistamine

CLINICAL PHARMACOLOGY

Mechanism of Action: An antiallergic agent that selectively antagonizes H_1 receptor. ***Therapeutic Effect:*** Blocks histamine-associated symptoms of seasonal allergic conjunctivitis.

Pharmacokinetics

Duration of action is about 2 hrs. Minimal systemic absorption.

INDICATIONS AND DOSAGES

Allergic conjunctivitis

Ophthalmic

Adults, Elderly, Children 12 yrs or older. 1 drop 4 times/day, for up to 2 wks.

AVAILABLE FORMS

- *Ophthalmic Suspension:* 0.05% (Livostin).

CONTRAINDICATIONS: Wearing of soft contact lenses (product contains benzalkonium chloride), hypersensitivity to levocabastine or any component of the formulation

PREGNANCY AND LACTATION: Pregnancy category C; excreted in human breast milk at very low concentrations due to minimal systemic absorption following ocular administration

SIDE EFFECTS

Frequent

Transient stinging, burning, discomfort, headache

Occasional

Dry mouth, fatigue, eye dryness, lacrimation/discharge, eyelid edema

Rare

Rash, erythema, nausea, dyspnea

SERIOUS REACTIONS

- None reported.

SPECIAL CONSIDERATIONS

- Shake well before using
- Do not wear soft contact lenses during therapy
- Mild burning or stinging may occur upon instillation

MONITORING PARAMETERS

- Therapeutic response to medication

levodopa

(lee-voe-doe'-pa)

Rx: Dopar, Larodopa

Combinations

Rx: with Carbidopa (Sinemet, Sinemet CR)

Chemical Class: Catecholamine precursor

Therapeutic Class: Anti-Parkinson's agent; antidyskinetic

CLINICAL PHARMACOLOGY

Mechanism of Action: A dopamine prodrug that is converted to dopamine in basal ganglia. Increases dopamine concentrations in the brain, inhibiting hyperactive cholinergic activity. ***Therapeutic Effect:*** Decreases signs and symptoms of Parkinson's disease.

Pharmacokinetics

About 30% absorbed. May be reduced with high-protein meal. Protein binding: minimal. Crosses blood-brain barrier. Converted to dopamine. Eliminated primarily in urine and to a lesser amount in feces and expired air. Not removed by hemodialysis. ***Half-life:*** 0.75-1.5 hrs.

INDICATIONS AND DOSAGES

Parkinsonism

PO

Adults, Elderly. Initially, 0.5-1 g 2-4 times/day. May increase in increments not exceeding 0.75 g every 3-7 days, up to a maximum of 8 g/day.

AVAILABLE FORMS

- *Capsules:* 100 mg, 250 mg, 500 mg (Dopar).
- *Tablets:* 100 mg, 250 mg, 500 mg (Larodopa).

CONTRAINDICATIONS: Nonselective MAOI therapy, hypersensitivity to levodopa or any component of its formulation.

PREGNANCY AND LACTATION: Pregnancy category C; do not use in nursing mothers

SIDE EFFECTS

Frequent

Uncontrolled body movements of the face, tongue, arms and upper body, nausea and vomiting, anorexia

Occasional

Depression, anxiety, confusion, nervousness, difficulty urinating, irregular heartbeats, hiccoughs, dizziness, lightheadedness, decreased appetite, blurred vision, constipation, dry mouth, flushed skin, headache, insomnia, diarrhea, unusual tiredness, darkening of urine, discolored sweat

Rare

Hypertension, ulcer, hemolytic anemia, marked by tiredness or weakness.

SERIOUS REACTIONS

- High incidence of involuntary dystonic and dyskinetic movements may be noted in patients on long-term therapy.
- Mental changes, such as paranoid ideation, psychotic episodes, and depression, may be noted.
- Numerous mild to severe central nervous system (CNS) psychiatric disturbances may include reduced attention span, anxiety, nightmares, daytime somnolence, euphoria, fatigue, paranoia, and hallucinations.

INTERACTIONS

Drugs

3 *Benzodiazepines:* Diazepam and chlordiazepoxide have exacerbated parkinsonism in a few patients receiving levodopa, effect of other benzodiazepines not clinically established

3 *Food:* High-protein diets may inhibit the efficacy of levodopa

3 *Iron:* Reduced levodopa bioavailability possible

3 *Methionine, phenytoin, pyridoxine, spiramycin, tacrine:* Inhibited clinical response to levodopa
3 *Moclobemide:* Increased risk of adverse effects from levodopa
3 *MAOIs:* Hypertensive response
2 *Neuroleptics:* Inhibited clinical response to levodopa

Labs

- *False positive:* Urine ferric chloride test, urine ketones, urine glucose, Coombs test
- *False negative:* Urine glucose (glucose oxidase), urine guaiacols spot test
- *False increase:* Serum acid phosphatase, urine amino acids, serum AST, serum bilirubin, plasma catecholamines, serum cholinesterase, serum creatinine, urine creatinine, creatinine clearance, serum glucose, urine hydroxy-methoxymandelic acid, urine ketones, serum lithium, urine protein, urine sugar, serum uric acid, urine uric acid
- *False decrease:* Serum bilirubin (conjugated and unconjugated), serum glucose, urine glucose, serum triglycerides, serum urea nitrogen, serum uric acid, VMA

SPECIAL CONSIDERATIONS

- Combination with carbidopa is preferred preparation

PATIENT/FAMILY EDUCATION

- Full benefit may require up to 6 mo
- Take with food to minimize GI upset
- Avoid sudden changes in posture
- May cause darkening of the urine or sweat
- Avoid tasks that require mental alertness or motor skills until response to the drug is established
- Avoid alcohol
- Take sips of tepid water or chew sugarless gum to relieve dry mouth
- Avoid meals that are high in protein because it may delay the effects of levodopa

MONITORING PARAMETERS

- CBC, renal function, liver function, ECG, intraocular pressure
- Be alert to neurologic effects including agitation, headache, lethargy, and mental confusion
- Monitor the patient for dyskinesia, characterized by difficulty with movement
- Assess the patient for clinical reversal of symptoms, such as improvement of masklike facial expression, muscular rigidity, shuffling gait, and resting tremors of hands and head

levofloxacin

(lee-voe-flox'-a-sin)

Rx: Iquix, Levaquin, Levaquin Leva-Pak, Quixin

Chemical Class: Fluoroquinolone derivative

Therapeutic Class: Antibiotic

CLINICAL PHARMACOLOGY

Mechanism of Action: A fluoroquinolone that inhibits the DNA enzyme gyrase in susceptible microorganisms, interfering with bacterial cell replication and repair. ***Therapeutic Effect:*** Bactericidal.

Pharmacokinetics

Well absorbed after both PO and IV administration. Protein binding: 24%-8%. Penetrates rapidly and extensively into leukocytes, epithelial cells, and macrophages. Lung concentrations are 2-5 times higher than those of plasma. Eliminated unchanged in the urine. Partially removed by hemodialysis. ***Half-life:*** 8 hr.

INDICATIONS AND DOSAGES

Bacterial sinusitis

PO

Adults, Elderly. 500 mg once daily for 10 days or 750 mg once daily for 5 days.

Bronchitis

PO, IV

Adults, Elderly. 500 mg q24h for 7 days.

Community-acquired pneumonia

PO

Adults, Elderly. 750 mg/day for 5 days or 500 mg for 7-14 days.

Pneumonia, nosocomial

PO, IV

Adults, Elderly. 750 mg q24h for 7-14 days.

Acute maxillary sinusitis

PO, IV

Adults, Elderly. 500 mg q24h for 10-14 days.

Skin and skin-structure infections

PO, IV

Adults, Elderly. (Uncomplicated) 500 mg q24h for 7-10 days. (Complicated) 750 mg q24h for 7-14 days.

Prostatitis

IV, PO

Adults, Elderly. 500 mg q24h for 28 days.

Uncomplicated UTI

IV, PO

Adults, Elderly. 250 mg q24h for 3 days.

UTIs, acute pyelonephritis

PO, IV

Adults, Elderly. 250 mg q24h for 10 days.

Bacterial conjunctivitis

Ophthalmic

Adults, Elderly, Children 1 yr and older. 1-2 drops q2h for 2 days (up to 8 times a day), then 1-2 drops q4h for 5 days.

Corneal ulcer

Ophthalmic

Adults, Elderly, Children older than 5 yr. Days 1-3: Instill 1-2 drops q30min to 2 hrs while awake and 4-6 hrs after retiring. Days 4 through completion: 1-2 drops q1-4h while awake.

Dosage in renal impairment

For bronchitis, pneumonia, sinusitis, and skin and skin-structure infections, dosage and frequency are modified based on creatinine clearance.

Creatinine Clearance	*Dosage*
50-80 ml/min	No change
20-49 ml/min	500 mg initially, then 250 mg q24h
10-19 ml/min	500 mg initially, then 250 mg q48h

Dialysis 500 mg initially, then 250 mg q48h

For UTIs and pyelonephritis, dosage and frequency are modified based on creatinine clearance.

Creatinine Clearance	*Dosage*
20 ml/min	No change
10-19 ml/min	250 mg initially, then 250 mg q48h

AVAILABLE FORMS

- *Oral Solution:* 25 mg/ml.
- *Tablets (Levaquin, Levaquin Leva-Pak):* 250 mg, 500 mg, 750 mg.
- *Injection (Levaquin):* 500-mg/20-ml vials.
- *Premixed Solution (Levaquin):* 25 mg/ml, 250 mg/50 ml, 500 mg/100 ml, 750 mg/150 ml.
- *Ophthalmic Solution:* 0.5% (Iquix), 1.5% (Quixin).

UNLABELED USES: Anthrax, gonorrhea, pelvic inflammatory disease (PID)

CONTRAINDICATIONS: Hypersensitivity to other fluoroquinolones or nalidixic acid

PREGNANCY AND LACTATION: Pregnancy category C; excretion into breast milk unknown; due to the potential for arthropathy and osteochondrosis, use extreme caution in nursing mothers

SIDE EFFECTS

Occasional (3%-1%)

Diarrhea, nausea, abdominal pain, dizziness, drowsiness, headache, lightheadedness

Ophthalmic: Local burning or discomfort, margin crusting, crystals or scales, foreign body sensation, ocular itching, altered taste

Rare (less than 1%)

Flatulence; altered taste; pain; inflammation or swelling in calves, hands, or shoulder; chest pain; difficulty breathing; palpitations; edema; tendon pain

Ophthalmic: Corneal staining, keratitis, allergic reaction, eyelid swelling, tearing, reduced visual acuity

SERIOUS REACTIONS

• Antibiotic-associated colitis and other superinfections may occur from altered bacterial balance. Hypersensitivity reactions, including photosensitivity (as evidenced by rash, pruritus, blisters, edema, and burning skin), have occurred in patients receiving fluoroquinolones.

INTERACTIONS

Drugs

3 *Aluminum:* Reduced absorption of levofloxacin; do not take within 4 hr of dose

3 *Antacids:* Reduced absorption of levofloxacin; do not take within 4 hr of dose

3 *Calcium:* Reduced absorption of levofloxacin; do not take within 4 hr of dose

3 *Cimetidine:* Reduced absorption of levofloxacin

3 *Didanosine:* Markedly reduced absorption of levofloxacin; take levofloxacin 2 hr before didanosine

3 *Famotidine:* Reduced absorption of levofloxacin

3 *Iron:* Reduced absorption of levofloxacin; do not take within 4 hr of dose

3 *Lansoprazole:* Reduced absorption of levofloxacin

3 *Magnesium:* Reduced absorption of levofloxacin; do not take within 4 hr of dose

3 *Nizatidine:* Reduced absorption of levofloxacin

3 *NSAIDs:* May increase the risk of CNS stimulation or seizures

3 *Omeprazole:* Reduced absorption of levofloxacin

3 *Ranitidine:* Reduced absorption of levofloxacin

3 *Sodium bicarbonate:* Reduced absorption of levofloxacin; do not take within 4 hr of dose

3 *Sucralfate:* Reduced absorption of levofloxacin; do not take within 4 hr of dose

3 *Warfarin:* May increase hypoprothrombinemic response to warfarin

3 *Zinc:* Reduced absorption of levofloxacin; do not take within 4 hr of dose

SPECIAL CONSIDERATIONS

• L-isomer of the racemate, ofloxacin (a commercially available quinolone antibiotic)

PATIENT/FAMILY EDUCATION

• Avoid direct exposure to sunlight (even when using sunscreen)

• Drink fluids liberally

• Avoid tasks that require mental alertness or motor skills until response to the drug is established

• Notify the physician if chest pain, difficulty breathing, palpitations, persistent diarrhea, edema, or tendon pain occurs

L

MONITORING PARAMETERS

- Blood glucose levels and liver and renal function tests
- Assess for any hypersensitivity reactions, including photosensitivity, pruritus, skin rash, and urticaria
- Be alert for signs and symptoms of superinfection, such as anal or genital pruritus, moderate to severe diarrhea, new or increased fever, and ulceration or changes in the oral mucosa
- Evaluate food tolerance and change in taste sensation

levonorgestrel

(lee-voe-nor-jes'-trel)

Rx: Norplant, Plan B

Combinations

Rx: Transdermal with estradiol (Climara Pro); See oral contraceptives monograph for combined oral contraceptives containing levonorgestrel

Chemical Class: 19-nortestosterone derivative; progestin derivative

Therapeutic Class: Contraceptive; progestin

CLINICAL PHARMACOLOGY

Mechanism of Action: A contraceptive hormone that causes thickening of cervical mucus, inhibition of ovulation, and inhibition of implantation. ***Therapeutic Effect:*** Prevents ovulation or fertilization.

Pharmacokinetics

Levonorgestrel is rapidly and completely absorbed after oral administration. Maximum serum concentrations of approximately 15 ng/ml occur at an average of 2 hrs. Does not appear to be extensively metabolized by the liver. Protein binding: 97.5%. Primarily excreted in the urine, with smaller amounts recovered in the feces.

INDICATIONS AND DOSAGES

Long-term prevention of pregnancy

Intrauterine

Adults, Elderly: Insert 1 system into uterine cavity within 7 days of onset of menstruation or immediately after first trimester abortion. Releases 20 mcg levonorgestrol daily over 5 yrs.

Emergency contraception

PO

Adults, Elderly: One 0.75-mg tablet as soon as possible within 72 hrs of unprotected sexual intercourse. A second 0.75-mg tablet 12 hrs after the first dose.

AVAILABLE FORMS

- *Tablet:* 0.75 mg.
- *Intrauterine:* 20 mcg/day.

CONTRAINDICATIONS: Active thrombophlebitis or thromboembolic disorders, undiagnosed abnormal genital bleeding, known or suspected pregnancy, acute liver disease, benign or malignant liver tumors, known or suspected carcinoma of the breast, history of idiopathic intracranial hypertension, hypersensitivity to levonorgestrel or any of the components of the levonorgestrel implants

PREGNANCY AND LACTATION: Pregnancy category X; compatible with breast-feeding

SIDE EFFECTS

Occasional

Hypertension, headache, depression, nervousness, breast pain, dysmenorrhea, decreased libido, abdominal pain, nausea, weight gain, leukorrhea, vaginitis

Rare

Alopecia, anemia, cervicitis, dyspareunia, eczema, failed insertion, migraine, sepsis, vomiting

SERIOUS REACTIONS

• None known.

INTERACTIONS

Drugs

3 *Carbamazepine, phenobarbital, phenytoin, rifampin:* Decreased efficacy of levonorgestrel, pregnancy has occurred

SPECIAL CONSIDERATIONS

PATIENT/FAMILY EDUCATION

• Most women can expect some variation in menstrual bleeding; these irregularities should diminish with continued use

• Capsules can be removed at any time for any reason or at the end of 5 yr. Removal is more difficult than insertion

• Failure rate 0.2%-1.0%, increases to 5% in patients ≥70 kg (Norplant)

• Efficacy of emergency contraception is better as soon as possible after unprotected intercourse. Causes less nausea and vomiting than other products for emergency contraception. Decreases risk of pregnancy from 8% to 19%

• Based on WHO study, levonorgesterel (norgestrel)-only pills preferred emergency contraception; equal efficacy and 50% less nausea, vomiting compared to combined regimen

• About 80% of women wishing to become pregnant conceived within 12 mo after removal of intrauterine device

• Avoid smoking

• Pain, redness, swelling, or warmth in the calf, chest pain, migraine headache, peripheral paresthesia, sudden decrease in vision, and sudden shortness of breath should be reported immediately

MONITORING PARAMETERS

• Blood glucose, blood pressure, hepatic enzymes, weight

• Pregnancy

levorphanol

(lee-vor′-fa-nole)

Rx: Levo-Dromoran

Chemical Class: Opiate derivative; phenanthrene derivative

Therapeutic Class: Narcotic analgesic

DEA Class: Schedule II

CLINICAL PHARMACOLOGY

Mechanism of Action: An opioid agonist that binds at opiate receptor sites in central nervous system (CNS). ***Therapeutic Effect:*** Reduced intensity of pain stimuli incoming from sensory nerve endings, altering pain perception and emotional response to pain.

Pharmacokinetics

Rapidly absorbed. Protein binding: 40%-50%. Extensively distributed. Metabolized in liver. Excreted in urine. ***Half-life:*** 11 hrs.

INDICATIONS AND DOSAGES

Pain

PO

Adults, Elderly. 2 mg. May be increased to 3 mg, if needed.

IM/Subcutaneous

Adults, Elderly: 1-2 mg as a single dose. May repeat in 6-8 hrs as needed. Maximum: 3-8 mg/day.

IV

Adults. Up to 1 mg injection in divided doses. May repeat in 3-6 hrs as needed. Maximum: 4-8 mg/day.

Preoperative

IM/Subcutaneous

Adults, Elderly. 1-2 mg as a single dose 60-90 min before surgery.

AVAILABLE FORMS

• *Tablets:* 2 mg (Lev-Dromoran).

• *Injection:* 2 mg/ml (Levo-Dromoran).

CONTRAINDICATIONS: Hypersensitivity to levorphanol or any component of the formulation

PREGNANCY AND LACTATION: Pregnancy category C (category D if used for prolonged periods or in high doses at term); use during labor produces neonatal depression

Controlled Substance: Schedule II

SIDE EFFECTS

Effects are dependent on dosage amount, route of administration. Ambulatory patients and those not in severe pain may experience dizziness, nausea, vomiting, hypotension more frequently than those in supine position or having severe pain

Frequent

Dizziness, drowsiness, hypotension, nausea, vomiting

Occasional

Shortness of breath, confusion, decreased urination, stomach cramps, altered vision, constipation, dry mouth, headache, difficult or painful urination

Rare

Allergic reaction (rash, itching), histamine reaction (decreased BP, increased sweating, flushed face, wheezing)

SERIOUS REACTIONS

- Overdosage results in respiratory depression, skeletal muscle flaccidity, cold clammy skin, cyanosis, extreme somnolence progressing to convulsions, stupor, coma.
- Tolerance to analgesic effect, physical dependence may occur with repeated use.
- Paralytic ileus may occur with prolonged use.

INTERACTIONS

Drugs

3 *Antihistamines, chloral hydrate, glutethimide, methocarbamol:* Enhanced depressant effects

3 *Barbiturates:* Additive respiratory and CNS depressant effects

3 *Cimetidine:* Increased respiratory and CNS depression

3 *Ethanol:* Additive CNS effects

Labs

- *False increase:* Amylase and lipase

levothyroxine sodium

(lee-voe-thye-rox'-een soe'-dee-um)

Rx: Levo-T, Levothroid, Levoxyl, Synthroid, Unithroid

Combinations

Rx: with liothyronine (Euthroid, Thyrolar)

Chemical Class: Synthetic levo isomer of thyroxine (T_4)

Therapeutic Class: Thyroid hormone

CLINICAL PHARMACOLOGY

Mechanism of Action: A synthetic isomer of thyroxine involved in normal metabolism, growth, and development, especially of the CNS in infants. Possesses catabolic and anabolic effects. ***Therapeutic Effect:*** Increases basal metabolic rate, enhances gluconeogenesis, and stimulates protein synthesis.

Pharmacokinetics

Variable, incomplete absorption from the GI tract. Protein binding: greater than 99%. Widely distributed. Deiodinated in peripheral tissues, minimal metabolism in the liver. Eliminated by biliary excretion. ***Half-life:*** 6-7 days.

INDICATIONS AND DOSAGES

Hypothyroidism

PO

Adults, Elderly, Children older than 12 yrs, growth and puberty complete. 1.7 mcg/kg/day as single daily dose. Usual maintenance: 100-200 mcg/day.

Children older than 12 yrs, growth and puberty incomplete. 2-3 mcg/kg/day.

Children 6-12 yrs. 4-5 mcg/kg/day.
Children 1-5 yrs. 5-6 mcg/kg/day.
Children 6-12 mos. 6-8 mcg/kg/day.
Children 3-6 mos. 8-10 mcg/kg/day.
Children younger than 3 mos. 10-15 mcg/kg/day.

Myxedema coma

IV

Adults, Elderly. Initially, 300-500 mcg. Maintenance: 75-100 mcg/day.

Pituitary TSH suppression

PO

Adults, Elderly. Doses greater than 2 mcg/kg/day usually required to suppress TSH below 0.1 milliunits/liter.

AVAILABLE FORMS

• *Tablets (Levo-T, Levothroid, Levoxyl, Synthroid, Unithroid):* 0.025 mg, 0.05 mg, 0.075 mg, 0.088 mg, 0.1 mg, 0.112 mg, 0.125 mg, 0.137 mg, 0.15 mg, 0.175 mg, 0.2 mg, 0.3 mg.
• *Injection (Synthroid):* 200 mcg, 500 mcg.

CONTRAINDICATIONS: Hypersensitivity to tablet components, such as tartrazine; allergy to aspirin; lactose intolerance; MI and thyrotoxicosis uncomplicated by hypothyroidism; treatment of obesity

PREGNANCY AND LACTATION: Pregnancy category A; little or no transplacental passage at physiologic serum concentrations; excreted into breast milk in low concentrations (inadequate to protect a hypothyroid infant; too low to interfere with neonatal thyroid screening programs)

SIDE EFFECTS

Occasional

Reversible hair loss at the start of therapy (in children)

Rare

Dry skin, GI intolerance, rash, hives, pseudotumor cerebri or severe headache in children

SERIOUS REACTIONS

• Excessive dosage produces signs and symptoms of hyperthyroidism, including weight loss, palpitations, increased appetite, tremors, nervousness, tachycardia, hypertension, headache, insomnia, and menstrual irregularities.
• Cardiac arrhythmias occur rarely.

INTERACTIONS

Drugs

3 *Aluminum and magnesium antacids, bile acid sequestrants, calcium carbonate, ferrous sulfate, kayexalate, simethicone, sucralfate:* Reduced serum thyroid concentrations through binding and delaying or preventing absorption of levothyroxine, administer these agents at least 4 hr apart

3 *Antidepressants (tricyclics, tetracyclics, selective serotonin reuptake inhibitors):* Potential increase in therapeutic and toxic effects of levothyroxine and tri/tetracyclics; increased levothyroxine requirements with sertraline

3 *Carbamazepine, phenobarbital, phenytoin, rifampin:* Increased elimination of thyroid hormones; possible increased requirement for thyroid hormones in hypothyroid patients

3 *Digoxin:* Levothyroxin may reduce therapeutic effects of digitalis glycosides

❷ *Ketamine:* Concurrent use with thyroid hormones may cause hypertension and tachycardia

3 *Oral anticoagulants:* Thyroid hormones increase catabolism of vitamin K–dependent clotting factors; an increase or decrease in clinical thyroid status will increase or decrease the hypoprothrombinemic response to oral anticoagulants

3 *Sympathomimetics:* Concurrent use may increase the effects of thyroid hormones or sympathomimetics

3 *Theophylline:* Reduced serum theophylline concentrations with initiation of thyroid therapy

Labs

- *False increase:* Serum triiodothyronine

SPECIAL CONSIDERATIONS

- Bioequivalence problems have been documented in the past for products marketed by different manufacturers; however, studies in patients have shown comparable clinical efficacy between brands based on the results of thyroid function tests; brand interchange should be limited to products with demonstrated therapeutic equivalence

PATIENT/FAMILY EDUCATION

- Transient, partial hair loss may be experienced by children in the first few months of therapy
- Take as a single daily dose, preferably before breakfast
- Do not abruptly discontinue the drug
- Maintain follow-up office visits; thyroid function tests are essential
- Report chest pain, insomnia, nervousness, tremors, or weight loss
- Full therapeutic effect of the drug may take 1-3 wks to appear

MONITORING PARAMETERS

- TSH
- Pulse for rate and rhythm; report a marked increase in pulse rate or one that exceeds 100 beats/minute
- Evaluate the patient's appetite and sleep pattern

lidocaine

(lye'-doe-kane)

Rx: Lidoderm, Xylocaine

OTC: DermaFlex, Solarcaine, Zilactin-L

Combinations

Rx: with epinephrine (LidoSite, Xylocaine with Epinephrine); Prilocaine (EMLA)

Chemical Class: Amide derivative

Therapeutic Class: Anesthetic, local

CLINICAL PHARMACOLOGY

Mechanism of Action: An amide anesthetic that inhibits conduction of nerve impulses. ***Therapeutic Effect:*** Causes temporary loss of feeling and sensation. Also an antiarrhythmic that decreases depolarization, automaticity, excitability of the ventricle during diastole by direct action. ***Therapeutic Effect:*** Inhibits ventricular arrhythmias.

Pharmacokinetics

Route	Onset	Peak	Duration
IV	30-90 sec	N/A	10-20 min
Local anesthetic	2.5 min	N/A	30-60 min

Completely absorbed after IM administration. Protein binding: 60%-80%. Widely distributed. Metabolized in the liver. Primarily excreted in urine. Minimally removed by hemodialysis. ***Half-life:*** 1-2 hr.

INDICATIONS AND DOSAGES

Rapid control of acute ventricular arrhythmias after an MI, cardiac catheterization, cardiac surgery, or digitalis-induced ventricular arrhythmias

IM

Adults, Elderly. 300 mg (or 4.3 mg/kg). May repeat in 60-90 min.

IV
Adults, Elderly. Initially, 50-100 mg (1 mg/kg) IV bolus at rate of 25-50 mg/min. May repeat in 5 min. Give no more than 200-300 mg in 1 hr. Maintenance: 20-50 mcg/kg/min (1-4 mg/min) as IV infusion.
Children, Infants. Initially, 0.5-1 mg/kg IV bolus; may repeat but total dose not to exceed 3-5 mg/kg. Maintenance: 10-50 mcg/kg/min as IV infusion.

Dental or surgical procedures, childbirth
Infiltration or nerve block
Adults. Local anesthetic dosage varies with procedure, degree of anesthesia, vascularity, duration. Maximum dose: 4.5 mg/kg. Do not repeat within 2 hrs.

Local skin disorders (minor burns, insect bites, prickly heat, skin manifestations of chickenpox, abrasions), and mucous membrane disorders (local anesthesia of oral, nasal, and laryngeal mucous membranes; local anesthesia of respiratory, urinary tract; relief of discomfort of pruritus ani, hemorrhoids, pruritus vulvae)
Topical
Adults, Elderly. Apply to affected areas as needed.

Treatment of shingles-related skin pain
Topical (Dermal patch)
Adults, Elderly. Apply to intact skin over most painful area (up to 3 applications once for up to 12 hrs in a 24-hr period).

AVAILABLE FORMS
- *IM Injection:* 300 mg/3 ml.
- *Direct IV Injection:* 10 mg/ml, 20 mg/ml.
- *IV Admixture Injection:* 40 mg/ml, 100 mg/ml, 200 mg/ml.
- *IV Infusion:* 2 mg/ml, 4 mg/ml, 8 mg/ml.
- *Injection (anesthesia):* 0.5%, 1%, 1.5%, 2%, 4%.
- *Liquid:* 2.5%, 5%.
- *Ointment:* 2.5%, 5%.
- *Cream:* 0.5%.
- *Gel:* 0.5%, 2.5%.
- *Topical Spray:* 0.5%.
- *Topical Solution:* 2%, 4%.
- *Topical Jelly:* 2%.
- *Dermal Patch:* 5%.

CONTRAINDICATIONS: Adams-Stokes syndrome, hypersensitivity to amide-type local anesthetics, septicemia (spinal anesthesia), supraventricular arrhythmias, Wolff-Parkinson-White syndrome

PREGNANCY AND LACTATION: Pregnancy category B; has been used as a local anesthetic during labor and delivery; may produce CNS depression and bradycardia in the newborn with high serum levels; compatible with breast-feeding

SIDE EFFECTS
CNS effects are generally dose related and of short duration.
Occasional
IM: Pain at injection site
Topical: Burning, stinging, tenderness at application site
Rare
Generally with high dose: Drowsiness; dizziness; disorientation; light-headedness; tremors; apprehension; euphoria; sensation of heat, cold, or numbness; blurred or double vision; ringing or roaring in ears (tinnitus); nausea

SERIOUS REACTIONS
- Although serious adverse reactions to lidocaine are uncommon, high dosage by any route may produce cardiovascular depression, bradycardia, hypotension, arrhythmias, heart block, cardiovascular collapse, and cardiac arrest.
- Potential for malignant hyperthermia.

• CNS toxicity may occur, especially with regional anesthesia use, progressing rapidly from mild side effects to tremors, somnolence, seizures, vomiting, and respiratory depression.

• Methemoglobinemia (evidenced by cyanosis) has occurred following topical application of lidocaine for teething discomfort and laryngeal anesthetic spray.

INTERACTIONS

Drugs

3 *Anticonvulsants:* May increase cardiac depressant effects

3 *Disopyramide:* Induction of dysrhythmia or heart failure in predisposed patients

3 *Metoprolol, nadolol, propranolol, cimetidine:* Increased serum lidocaine concentrations

3 *Morphine:* Respiratory depression and loss of consciousness have been reported

3 *Other antiarrhythmics:* May increase cardiac effects

Labs

• *False increase:* Serum creatinine, CSF protein

lindane (gamma benzene hexachloride)

(lin'-dane)

Rx: Lindane

Chemical Class: Cyclic chlorinated hydrocarbon

Therapeutic Class: Pediculicide; scabicide

CLINICAL PHARMACOLOGY

Mechanism of Action: A scabicidal agent that is directly absorbed by parasites and ova through the exoskeleton. ***Therapeutic Effect:*** Stimulates the nervous system, resulting in seizures and death of parasitic arthropods.

Pharmacokinetics

May be absorbed systemically. Metabolized in liver. Excreted in the urine and feces. ***Half-life:*** 17-22 hrs.

INDICATIONS AND DOSAGES

Treatment of scabies

Topical

Adults, Elderly, Children. Apply thin layer. Massage on skin from neck to the toes. Bathe and remove drug after 8-12 hrs.

Head lice, crab lice

Topical

Adults, Elderly, Children. Apply about 30 ml of shampoo to dry hair and massage into hair for 4 min. Add small amounts of water to hair until lather forms, then rinse hair thoroughly and comb with a fine tooth comb to remove nits. Maximum: 60 ml of shampoo.

AVAILABLE FORMS

• *Lotion:* 1% (Lindane).
• *Shampoo:* 1% (Lindane).

CONTRAINDICATIONS: Hypersensitivity to lindane or any component of the formulation, uncontrolled seizure disorders, crusted (Norwegian) scabies, acutely inflamed skin or raw, weeping surfaces, or other skin conditions that may increase systemic absorption

PREGNANCY AND LACTATION: Pregnancy category B; use no more than twice during a pregnancy; amounts excreted in breast milk probably clinically insignificant

SIDE EFFECTS

Rare (less than 1%)

Burning, stinging, cardiac arrhythmia, ataxia, dizziness, headache, restlessness, seizures, pain, alopecia, contact dermatitis, skin and adipose tissue may act as repositories, eczematous eruptions, pruritus, urticaria, nausea, vomiting, aplastic anemia, hepatitis, paresthesias, hematuria, pulmonary edema

SERIOUS REACTIONS

• Seizures rarely occur.

SPECIAL CONSIDERATIONS

PATIENT/FAMILY EDUCATION

• Do not exceed prescribed dosage
• Do not apply to face
• Avoid getting in eyes
• Wear rubber gloves for application
• Do not use oil-based hair products (e.g., conditioners) after using product
• Treat sexual and household contacts concurrently

MONITORING PARAMETERS

• Skin for local burning, itching, and irritation

linezolid

(li-ne'-zoh-lid)

Rx: Zyvox

Chemical Class: Oxazolidinone derivative

Therapeutic Class: Antibiotic

CLINICAL PHARMACOLOGY

Mechanism of Action: An oxalodinone antiinfective that binds to a site on bacterial 23S ribosomal RNA, preventing the formation of a complex that is essential for bacterial translation. ***Therapeutic Effect:*** Bacteriostatic against enterococci and staphylococci; bactericidal against streptococci.

Pharmacokinetics

Rapidly and extensively absorbed after PO administration. Protein binding: 31%. Metabolized in the liver by oxidation. Excreted in urine. ***Half-life:*** 4-5.4 hr.

INDICATIONS AND DOSAGES

Vancomycin-resistant infections (VRE)

PO, IV

Adults, Elderly, Children older than 11 yrs. 600 mg q12h for 14-28 days.

Children 11 yrs and younger. 10 mg/kg q8-12h for 14-28 days.

Pneumonia, complicated skin and skin structure infections

PO, IV

Adults, Elderly, Children older than 11 yrs. 600 mg q12h for 10-14 days.

Children 11 yrs and younger. 10 mg/kg q8h for 10-14 days.

Uncomplicated skin and skin structure infections

PO

Adults, Elderly. 400 mg q12h for 10-14 days.

Children older than 11 yrs. 600 mg q12h for 10-14 days.

Children 5-11 yrs. 10 mg/kg/dose q12h for 10-14 days.

Children younger than 5 yrs. 10 mg/kg q8h for 10-14 days.

Usual neonate dosage

PO, IV

Neonates. 10 mg/kg/dose q8-12h.

AVAILABLE FORMS

• *Powder for Oral Suspension:* 100 mg/5 ml.
• *Tablets:* 400 mg, 600 mg.
• *Injection:* 2 mg/ml in 100-ml, 200-ml, 300-ml bags.

CONTRAINDICATIONS: None known.

PREGNANCY AND LACTATION: Pregnancy category C; breast milk excretion unknown

SIDE EFFECTS

Occasional (5%-2%)

Diarrhea, nausea, headache

Rare (less than 2%)

Altered taste, vaginal candidiasis, fungal infection, dizziness, tongue discoloration

SERIOUS REACTIONS

• Thrombocytopenia and myelosuppression occur rarely.

• Antibiotic-associated colitis and other superinfections may result from altered bacterial balance.

INTERACTIONS

Drugs

❷ *Amphetamines, alcoholic beverages containing tyramine, metaraminol, phenylephrine, phenylpropanolamine, pseudoephedrine, tyramine:* Severe hypertensive reaction

❷ *Antidepressants, cyclic:* Excessive sympathetic response

❷ *Dextromethorphan:* Severe hypertensive reaction

❷ *Dopamine:* Severe hypertensive reaction

❷ *Epinephrine:* Severe hypertensive reaction

❸ *Levodopa:* Hypertension

❸ *MAOIs:* Decreases the effects of MAOIs

❷ *Meperidine:* Severe hypertensive reaction

❷ *Selective serotonin reuptake inhibitors (SSRIs):* Serotonin syndrome (hyperpyrexia, cognitive dysfunction)

❷ *Sibutramine:* Serotonin syndrome (hyperpyrexia, cognitive dysfunction)

❷ *Trazodone:* Serotonin syndrome (hyperpyrexia, cognitive dysfunction)

❷ *Venlafaxine:* Serotonin syndrome (hyperpyrexia, cognitive dysfunction)

SPECIAL CONSIDERATIONS

• Most appropriate use is when vancomycin-resistant *Enterococcus faecium* infection is documented or strongly suspected, or for oral therapy of methicillin-resistant *Staphylococcus aureus* infection

PATIENT/FAMILY EDUCATION

• Avoid high-tyramine foods (consume less than 100 mg per meal)

• Space drug doses evenly around the clock and continue linezolid therapy for the full course of treatment

• Take with food or milk if GI upset occurs

MONITORING PARAMETERS

• CBC weekly if treatment longer than 2 wks, ALT, AST, renal function

• Pattern of daily bowel activity and stool consistency; mild GI effects may be tolerable, but severe symptoms may indicate the onset of antibiotic-associated colitis

• Be alert for signs and symptoms of superinfection, such as abdominal pain, moderate to severe diarrhea, severe anal or genital pruritus, and severe mouth soreness

---

liothyronine (T_3)

(lye-oh-thye′-roe-neen)

Rx: Cytomel, Triostat

Combinations

Rx: with levothyroxine (Euthroid, Thyrolar)

Chemical Class: Synthetic triiodothyronine (T_3)

Therapeutic Class: Thyroid hormone

CLINICAL PHARMACOLOGY

Mechanism of Action: A synthetic form of triiodothyronine (T_3), a thyroid hormone involved in normal metabolism, growth, and development, especially of the CNS in infants. Possesses catabolic and anabolic effects. ***Therapeutic Effect:*** Increases basal metabolic rate, enhances gluconeogenesis, and stimulates protein synthesis.

Pharmacokinetics

Almost completely absorbed following PO administration. Absorption is reduced to 43% in congestive heart failure (CHF) patients. Not firmly bound to serum protein. Excreted in urine. ***Half-life:*** 25 hr.

INDICATIONS AND DOSAGES

Hypothyroidism

PO

Adults, Elderly. Initially, 25 mcg/day. May increase in increments of 12.5-25 mcg/day q1-2wk. Maximum: 100 mcg/day.

Children. Initially, 5 mcg/day. May increase by 5 mcg/day q3-4wk. Maintenance: 100 mcg/day (children older than 3 yr); 50 mcg/day (children 1-3 yr); 20 mcg/day (infants).

Myxedema

PO

Adults, Elderly. Initially, 5 mcg/day. Increase by 5-10 mcg q1-2wk (after 25 mcg/day has been reached, may increase in 12.5-mcg increments). Maintenance: 50-100 mcg/day.

Nontoxic goiter

PO

Adults, Elderly. Initially, 5 mcg/day. Increase by 5-10 mcg/day q1-2wk. When 25 mcg/day has been reached, may increase by 12.5-25 mcg/day q1-2wk. Maintenance: 75 mcg/day.

Children. 5 mcg/day. May increase by 5 mcg q1-2wk. Maintenance: 15-20 mcg/day.

Congenital hypothyroidism

PO

Children. Initially, 5 mcg/day. Increase by 5 mcg/day q3-4 days. Maintenance: Full adult dosage (children older than 3 yrs); 50 mcg/day (children 1-3 yrs); 20 mcg/day (infants).

T_3 suppression test

PO

Adults, Elderly. 75-100 mcg/day for 7 days; then repeat I^{131} thyroid uptake test.

Myxedema coma, precoma

IV

Adults, Elderly. Initially, 25-50 mcg (10-20 mcg in patients with cardiovascular disease). Total dose at least 65 mcg/day.

AVAILABLE FORMS

- *Tablets (Cytomel):* 5 mcg, 25 mcg, 50 mcg.
- *Injection (Triostat):* 10 mcg/ml.

CONTRAINDICATIONS: MI and thyrotoxicosis uncomplicated by hypothyroidism; obesity; uncorrected adrenal cortical insufficiency

PREGNANCY AND LACTATION: Pregnancy category A; little or no transplacental passage at physiologic serum concentrations; excreted into breast milk in low concentrations (inadequate to protect a hypothyroid infant; too low to interfere with neonatal screening programs)

SIDE EFFECTS

Occasional

Reversible hair loss at start of therapy (in children)

Rare

Dry skin, GI intolerance, rash, hives, pseudotumor cerebri or severe headache in children

SERIOUS REACTIONS

- Excessive dosage produces signs and symptoms of hyperthyroidism, including weight loss, palpitations, increased appetite, tremors, nervousness, tachycardia, hypertension, headache, insomnia, and menstrual irregularities.
- Cardiac arrhythmias occur rarely.

INTERACTIONS

Drugs

3 *Bile acid sequestrants:* Reduced serum thyroid hormone concentrations

3 *Carbamazepine, phenytoin, rifampin:* Increased elimination of thyroid hormones; possible increased requirement for thyroid hormones in hypothyroid patients

3 *Oral anticoagulants:* Thyroid hormones increase catabolism of vitamin K–dependent clotting factors; an increase or decrease in clinical thyroid status will increase or decrease the hypoprothrombinemic response to oral anticoagulants

3 *Sympathommimetics:* May increase the risk of coronary insufficiency and the effects of liothyronine

3 *Theophylline:* Reduced serum theophylline concentrations with initiation of thyroid therapy

SPECIAL CONSIDERATIONS

PATIENT/FAMILY EDUCATION

- Transient, partial hair loss may be experienced by children in the first few months of therapy
- Other thyroid products have longer half-lives. Take this into consideration when switching from them to liothyronine
- Take as single daily dose, preferably before breakfast
- Do not discontinue this drug
- Do not change brands of the drug
- Promptly report chest pain, insomnia, nervousness, tremors, or weight loss

MONITORING PARAMETERS

- TSH
- Pulse for rate and rhythm
- Appetite and sleep pattern

lisinopril

(ly-sin'-oh-pril)

Rx: Prinivil, Zestril

Combinations

Rx: with hydrochlorothiazide (Prinzide, Zestoretic)

Chemical Class: Angiotensin-converting enzyme (ACE) inhibitor, nonsulfhydryl

Therapeutic Class: Antihypertensive

CLINICAL PHARMACOLOGY

Mechanism of Action: This angiotensin-converting enzyme (ACE) inhibitor suppresses the renin-angiotensin-aldosterone system and prevents conversion of angiotensin I to angiotensin II, a potent vasoconstrictor; may also inhibit angiotensin II at local vascular and renal sites. Decreases plasma angiotensin II, increases plasma renin activity, and decreases aldosterone secretion.

Therapeutic Effect: Reduces peripheral arterial resistance, BP, afterload, pulmonary capillary wedge pressure (preload), and pulmonary vascular resistance. In those with heart failure, also decreases heart size, increases cardiac output, and exercise tolerance time.

Pharmacokinetics

Route	*Onset*	*Peak*	*Duration*
PO	1 hr	6 hr	24 hr

Incompletely absorbed from the GI tract. Protein binding: 25%. Primarily excreted unchanged in urine. Removed by hemodialysis. ***Half-life:*** 12 hr (half-life is prolonged in those with impaired renal function).

INDICATIONS AND DOSAGES

Hypertension (used alone)

PO

Adults. Initially, 10 mg/day. May increase by 5-10 mcg/day at 1-2 wk intervals. Maximum: 40 mg/day.

Elderly. Initially, 2.5-5 mg/day. May increase by 2.5-5 mg/day at 1-2-wk intervals. Maximum: 40 mg/day.

Hypertension (used in combination with other antihypertensives)

PO

Adults. Initially, 2.5-5 mg/day titrated to patient's needs.

Adjunctive therapy for management of heart failure

PO

Adults, Elderly. Initially, 2.5-5 mg/day. May increase by no more than 10 mg/day at intervals of at least 2 wk. Maintenance: 5-40 mg/day.

Improve survival in patients after a myocardial infarction (MI)

PO

Adults, Elderly. Initially, 5 mg, then 5 mg after 24 hr, 10 mg after 48 hr, then 10 mg/day for 6 wk. For patients with low systolic BP, give 2.5 mg/day for 3 days, then 2.5-5 mg/day.

Dosage in renal impairment

Titrate to patient's needs after giving the following initial dose:

Creatinine Clearance	*% Normal Dose*
10-50 ml/min	50-75
less than 10 ml/min	25-50

AVAILABLE FORMS

• *Tablets (Prinivil, Zestril):* 2.5 mg, 5 mg, 10 mg, 20 mg, 30 mg, 40 mg.

UNLABELED USES: Treatment of hypertension or renal crises with scleroderma

CONTRAINDICATIONS: History of angioedema from previous treatment with ACE inhibitors

PREGNANCY AND LACTATION: Pregnancy category C (first trimester), category D (second and third trimesters); ACE inhibitors can cause fetal and neonatal morbidity and death when administered to pregnant women; when pregnancy is detected, discontinue ACE inhibitors as soon as possible; detectable in breast milk in trace amounts; a newborn would receive <0.1% of the mg/kg maternal dose; effect on nursing infant has not been determined

SIDE EFFECTS

Frequent (12%-5%)

Headache, dizziness, postural hypotension

Occasional (4%-2%)

Chest discomfort, fatigue, rash, abdominal pain, nausea, diarrhea, upper respiratory infection

Rare (1% or less)

Palpitations, tachycardia, peripheral edema, insomnia, paresthesia, confusion, constipation, dry mouth, muscle cramps

SERIOUS REACTIONS

• Excessive hypotension ("first-dose syncope") may occur in patients with CHF and severe salt and volume depletion.

• Angioedema (swelling of face and lips) and hyperkalemia occurs rarely.

• Agranulocytosis and neutropenia may be noted in patients with collagen vascular disease, including scleroderma and systemic lupus erythematosus, and impaired renal function.

• Nephrotic syndrome may be noted in patients with history of renal disease.

INTERACTIONS

Drugs

❷ *Allopurinol:* Predisposition to hypersensitivity reactions to ACE inhibitors

③ *Aspirin, NSAIDs:* Inhibition of the antihypertensive response to ACE inhibitors

③ *Azathioprine:* Increased myelosuppression

3 *Insulin:* Enhanced insulin sensitivity
3 *Lithium:* Increased risk of serious lithium toxicity
3 *Loop diuretics:* Initiation of ACE inhibitor therapy in the presence of intensive diuretic therapy results in a precipitous fall in blood pressure in some patients; ACE inhibitors may induce renal insufficiency in the presence of diuretic-induced sodium depletion
3 *Potassium-sparing diuretics:* Increased risk for hyperkalemia
3 *Prazosin, terazosin, doxazosin:* Exaggerated first-dose hypotensive response to α-blockers
3 *Trimethoprim:* Additive risk of hyperkalemia, especially in patient predisposed to renal insufficiency
3 *Rofecoxib:* Inhibits the antihypertensive effect of lisinopril
3 *Tizanidine:* Isolated cases of acute hypotension have occurred

Labs

- ACE inhibition can account for approximately 0.5 mEq/L rise in serum potassium

SPECIAL CONSIDERATIONS

PATIENT/FAMILY EDUCATION

- Caution with salt substitutes containing potassium chloride
- Rise slowly to sitting/standing position to minimize orthostatic hypotension
- Dizziness, fainting, lightheadedness may occur during first few days of therapy
- May cause altered taste perception or cough; persistent dry cough usually does not subside unless medication is stopped; notify clinician if these symptoms persist
- Do not skip doses or discontinue the drug
- Avoid taking OTC cold preparations or nasal decongestants

MONITORING PARAMETERS

- BUN, creatinine, potassium within 2 wk after initiation of therapy (increased levels may indicate acute renal failure)
- Intake and output
- Daily weights
- Assess for edema
- Pattern of daily bowel activity and stool consistency

---

lithium carbonate/lithium citrate

(lith'-ee-um)

Rx: (lithium carbonate) Eskalith, Lithobid

Rx: (lithium citrate) Cibalith-S

Chemical Class: Monovalent cation

Therapeutic Class: Antimanic; psychotherapeutic agent

CLINICAL PHARMACOLOGY

Mechanism of Action: A psychotherapeutic agent that affects the storage, release, and reuptake of neurotransmitters. Antimanic effect may result from increased norepinephrine reuptake and serotonin receptor sensitivity. ***Therapeutic Effect:*** Produces antimanic and antidepressant effects.

Pharmacokinetics

Rapidly and completely absorbed from the GI tract. Primarily excreted unchanged in urine. Removed by hemodialysis. ***Half-life:*** 18-24 hr (increased in elderly).

INDICATIONS AND DOSAGES:

Alert: During acute phase, a therapeutic serum lithium concentration of 1-1.4 mEq/L is required. For long-term control, the desired level is 0.5-1.3 mEq/L. Monitor serum drug concentration and clinical response to determine proper dosage.

Prevention or treatment of acute mania, manic phase of bipolar disorder (manic-depressive illness)
PO
Adults. 300 mg 3-4 times a day or 450-900 mg slow-release form twice a day. Maximum: 2.4 g/day.
Elderly. 900-1200 mg/day. Maintenance: 300 mg twice a day. May increase by 300 mg/day q1wk.
Children 12 yr and older. 600-1800 mg/day in 3-4 divided doses (2 doses/day for slow-release).
Children younger than 12 yr. 15-60 mg/kg/day in 3-4 divided doses, not to exceed usual adult dose.

AVAILABLE FORMS

- *Capsules:* 150 mg, 300 mg, 600 mg.
- *Syrup:* 300 mg/ml.
- *Tablets:* 300 mg.
- *Tablets (Controlled-Release):* 450 mg.
- *Tablets (Slow-Release):* 300 mg.

UNLABELED USES: Prevention of vascular headache; treatment of depression, neutropenia

CONTRAINDICATIONS: Debilitated patients, severe cardiovascular disease, severe dehydration, severe renal disease, severe sodium depletion

PREGNANCY AND LACTATION: Pregnancy category D; avoid use in pregnancy if possible, especially during the first trimester; excreted in breast milk; contraindicated in nursing mothers

SIDE EFFECTS

Alert: Side effects are dose related and seldom occur at lithium serum levels less than 1.5 mEq/L.

Occasional
Fine hand tremor, polydipsia, polyuria, mild nausea

Rare
Weight gain, bradycardia or tachycardia, acne, rash, muscle twitching, cold and cyanotic extremities, pseudotumor cerebri (eye pain, headache, tinnitus, vision disturbances)

SERIOUS REACTIONS

- A lithium serum concentration of 1.5-2.0 mEq/L may produce vomiting, diarrhea, drowsiness, confusion, incoordination, coarse hand tremor, muscle twitching, and T-wave depression on EKG.
- A lithium serum concentration of 2.0-2.5 mEq/L may result in ataxia, giddiness, tinnitus, blurred vision, clonic movements, and severe hypotension.
- Acute toxicity may be characterized by seizures, oliguria, circulatory failure, coma, and death.

INTERACTIONS

Drugs

3 *ACE inhibitors, methyldopa:* Increased risk of lithium toxicity

3 *Acetazolamide, sodium bicarbonate, urea:* Increased lithium renal clearance, decreased lithium efficacy

3 *Aminophylline, caffeine, dyphylline, oxtriphylline, theophylline:* Increased lithium renal clearance, decreased lithium efficacy

3 *Diltiazem, verapamil, amitriptyline, carbamazepine, fluoxetine, fluvoxamine:* Neurotoxicity, including seizures

3 *Haloperidol:* May increase extrapyramidal symptoms and the risk of neurologic toxicity

2 *MAOIs:* Malignant hyperpyrexia

3 *Mefenamic acid:* Isolated cases of lithium toxicity have been associated with mefenamic acid therapy

3 *Metronidazole:* Increased risk of lithium toxicity

3 *Molindone:* May increase the risk of neurotoxicity

3 *Neuroleptics:* Reduced neuroleptic response; severe neurotoxicity possible in acute manic patients receiving lithium and neuroleptics

3 *Neuromuscular blocking agents:* Prolonged effect of neuromuscular blocking agents possible

3 *NSAIDs (including COX-2 inhibitors):* Increased lithium concentrations

3 *Phenothiazines:* May decrease the absorption of phenothiazines, increase the intracellular concentration and renal excretion of lithium, and increase delirium and extrapyramidal symptoms. Antiemetic effect of some phenothiazines may mask early signs of lithium toxicity

3 *Phenytoin:* Development of lithium toxicity has been reported

3 *Potassium iodide:* Increased risk for hypothyroidism

3 *Sodium bicarbonate:* Decreased plasma lithium concentrations

3 *Sodium chloride:* High sodium intake may reduce serum lithium concentrations; sodium restriction may increase serum lithium

3 *Theophylline:* Increased lithium renal clearance, decreased lithium efficacy

3 *Thiazide diuretics:* Decreased lithium renal clearance, increased lithium concentrations

Labs

- *False increase:* Serum creatinine

SPECIAL CONSIDERATIONS

PATIENT/FAMILY EDUCATION

- Take with meals to avoid stomach upset
- Discontinue medication and contact clinician for diarrhea, vomiting, unsteady walking, coarse hand tremor, severe drowsiness, muscle weakness
- Lithium may cause excessive thirst and increased urination
- Drink 8-12 glasses of water or other liquid every day
- Do not restrict sodium in diet
- Regular monitoring of lithium blood levels is necessary to determine proper dosage
- Limit consumption of alcohol and caffeine
- Avoid tasks that require mental alertness or motor skills until response to the drug has been established

MONITORING PARAMETERS

- Serum lithium concentrations drawn immediately prior to next dose (8-12 hr after previous dose), monitor biweekly until stable then q2-3mo; therapeutic range 0.8-1.2 mEq/L (acute), 0.5-1.0 mEq/L (maintenance)
- Serum creatinine, CBC, urinalysis, serum electrolytes, fasting glucose, ECG, TSH
- Assess for increased urine output and persistent thirst
- Therapeutic response to the drug, as characterized by increased ability to concentrate, improvement in self-care, interest in surroundings, and a relaxed facial expression

Iodoxamide tromethamine

(loe-dox'-a-mide)

Rx: Alomide

Chemical Class: Dioxamic acid derivative; mast cell stabilizer

Therapeutic Class: Ophthalmic antiinflammatory

CLINICAL PHARMACOLOGY

Mechanism of Action: A mast cell stabilizer that prevents increase in cutaneous vascular permeability, antigen-stimulated histamine release, and may prevent calcium influx into mast cells. ***Therapeutic Effect:*** Inhibits sensitivity reaction.

Pharmacokinetics
Non-detectable absorption. ***Half-life:*** 8.5 hrs.
INDICATIONS AND DOSAGES
Treatment of vernal keratoconjunctivitis, conjunctivitis, and keratitis
Ophthalmic
Adults, Elderly, Children 2 yrs or older. 1-2 drops 4 times/day, for up to 3 mos.
AVAILABLE FORMS
• *Ophthalmic Solution:* 0.1% (Alomide).
CONTRAINDICATIONS: Wearing soft contact lenses (product contains benzalkonium chloride), hypersensitivity to lodoxamide tromethamine or any component of the formulation
PREGNANCY AND LACTATION: Pregnancy category B; excretion into breast milk unknown but would be expected to be almost nothing since plasma levels are not measurable following ocular administration of therapeutic doses
SIDE EFFECTS
Frequent
Transient stinging, burning, instillation discomfort
Occasional
Ocular itching, blurred vision, dry eye, tearing/discharge/foreign body sensation, headache
Rare
Scales on lid/lash, ocular swelling, sticky sensation, dizziness, somnolence, nausea, sneezing, dry nose, rash
SERIOUS REACTIONS
• None reported.
SPECIAL CONSIDERATIONS
PATIENT/FAMILY EDUCATION
• Do not wear soft contact lenses during therapy
• Mild burning and stinging may occur upon instillation
MONITORING PARAMETERS
• Therapeutic response to medication

lomefloxacin hydrochloride
(loe-me-flox'-a-sin hy-droe-klor'-ide)
Rx: Maxaquin
Chemical Class: Fluoroquinolone derivative
Therapeutic Class: Antibiotic

CLINICAL PHARMACOLOGY
Mechanism of Action: A quinolone that inhibits the enzyme DNA gyrase in susceptible microorganisms, interfering with bacterial cell replication and repair. ***Therapeutic Effect:*** Bactericidal.
Pharmacokinetics
Well absorbed from the GI tract. Protein binding: 10%. Widely distributed. Metabolized in the liver. Primarily excreted in urine. Not removed by hemodialysis. ***Half-life:*** 4-6 hr (increased with impaired renal function and in the elderly).
INDICATIONS AND DOSAGES
Complicated UTIs
PO
Adults, Elderly. 400 mg/day for 10-14 days.
Uncomplicated UTIs
PO
Adults (females). 400 mg/day for 3 days.
Lower respiratory tract infections
PO
Adults, Elderly. 400 mg/day for 10 days.
Surgical prophylaxis
PO
Adults, Elderly. 400 mg 2-6 hr before surgery.

Dosage in renal impairment

Dosage and frequency are modified based on creatinine clearance.

Creatinine Clearance	*Dosage*
41 ml/min and higher	No change
10-40 ml/min	400 mg initially, then 200 mg/day for 10-14 days

AVAILABLE FORMS

• *Tablets:* 400 mg.

CONTRAINDICATIONS: Hypersensitivity to quinolones

PREGNANCY AND LACTATION: Pregnancy category C; excretion into breast milk unknown; due to the potential for arthropathy and osteochondrosis, use extreme caution in nursing mothers

SIDE EFFECTS

Occasional (3%-2%)

Nausea, headache, photosensitivity, dizziness

Rare (1%)

Diarrhea

SERIOUS REACTIONS

• Antibiotic-associated colitis and other superinfections may result from altered bacterial balance.

• Hypersensitivity reactions, including photosensitivity (as evidenced by rash, pruritus, blisters, edema, and burning skin), have occurred in patients receiving fluoroquinolones.

• Arthropathy may occur if the drug is given to children younger than 18 yrs.

INTERACTIONS

Drugs

3 *Antacids (aluminum and magnesium containing):* Reduced absorption of lomefloxacin; take lomefloxacin 2 hr before or 4 hr after antacids

3 *Caffeine:* May increase the effects of these drugs

3 *Calcium, iron, zinc:* Reduced absorption of lomefloxacin; do not take lomefloxacin 2 hr before or after

3 *Cimetidine:* Interference with the elimination of other quinolones

3 *Cyclosporine:* Increased plasma cyclosporine concentrations with other quinolones

3 *Didanosine (buffered formulations):* Markedly reduced absorption of lomefloxacin; take lomefloxacin 2 hr before or 4 hr after didanosine

3 *Probenecid:* Probenecid slows the renal elimination of lomefloxacin, possibly resulting in increased plasma lomefloxacin concentrations

3 *Sodium bicarbonate:* Reduced absorption of lomefloxacin; do not take within 4 hr of dose

3 *Sucralfate:* Reduced absorption of lomefloxacin; take lomefloxacin 2 hr before or 4 hr after sucralfate

3 *Theophylline:* Decreases clearance and may increase blood concentration and risk of toxicity of theophylline

3 *Warfarin:* May increase hypoprothrombinemic response to warfarin

SPECIAL CONSIDERATIONS

PATIENT/FAMILY EDUCATION

• Avoid direct and indirect exposure to sunlight (even when using sunscreen), discontinue at first signs of phototoxicity, avoid re-exposure to sunlight until completely recovered from reaction

• Take dose in the evening to reduce risk of phototoxicity

• Take without regard to meals

• Drink fluids liberally

• Do not take antacids containing magnesium or aluminum or products containing iron or zinc within 4 hr before or 2 hr after dosing

• Do not skip drug doses and continue taking lomefloxacin for the full course of therapy

MONITORING PARAMETERS

• WBC count
• Mental status
• Monitor for dizziness, headache, and signs and symptoms of infection
• Be alert for signs and symptoms of superinfection, such as anal or genital pruritus, fever, oral candidiasis, and vaginitis

loperamide hydrochloride

(loe-per′-a-mide hye-droe-klor′-ide)

Rx: Imodium

OTC: Imodium A-D, Maalox Anti-Diarrheal

Combinations

OTC: with simethicone (Imodium Advanced)

Chemical Class: Piperidine derivative

Therapeutic Class: Antidiarrheal

CLINICAL PHARMACOLOGY

Mechanism of Action: An antidiarrheal that directly affects the intestinal wall muscles. ***Therapeutic Effect:*** Slows intestinal motility and prolongs transit time of intestinal contents by reducing fecal volume, diminishing loss of fluid and electrolytes, and increasing viscosity and bulk of stool.

Pharmacokinetics

Poorly absorbed from the GI tract. Protein binding: 97%. Metabolized in the liver. Eliminated in feces and excreted in urine. Not removed by hemodialysis. ***Half-life:*** 9.1-14.4 hr.

INDICATIONS AND DOSAGES

Acute diarrhea

PO (capsules)

Adults, Elderly. Initially, 4 mg; then 2 mg after each unformed stool. Maximum: 16 mg/day.

Children 9-12 yrs, weighing more than 30 kg. Initially, 2 mg 3 times a day for 24 hr.

Children 6-8 yrs, weighing 20-30 kg. Initially, 2 mg twice a day for 24 hr.

Children 2-5 yrs, weighing 13-20 kg. Initially, 1 mg 3 times a day for 24 hr. Maintenance: 1 mg/10 kg only after loose stool.

Chronic diarrhea

PO

Adults, Elderly. Initially, 4 mg; then 2 mg after each unformed stool until diarrhea is controlled.

Children. 0.08-0.24 mg/kg/day in 2-3 divided doses. Maximum: 2 mg/dose.

Traveler's diarrhea

PO

Adults, Elderly. Initially, 4 mg; then 2 mg after each loose bowel movement (LBM). Maximum: 8 mg/day for 2 days.

Children 9-11 yrs. Initially, 2 mg; then 1 mg after each LBM. Maximum: 6 mg/day for 2 days.

Children 6-8 yrs. Initially, 1 mg; then 1 mg after each LBM. Maximum: 4 mg/day for 2 days.

AVAILABLE FORMS

• *Capsules:* 2 mg.
• *Liquid:* 1 mg/5 ml.
• *Tablets:* 2 mg.

CONTRAINDICATIONS: Acute ulcerative colitis (may produce toxic megacolon), diarrhea associated with pseudomembranous enterocolitis due to broad-spectrum antibiotics or to organisms that invade intestinal mucosa (such as *Escherichia coli,* shigella, and salmonella), patients who must avoid constipation

PREGNANCY AND LACTATION: Pregnancy category B; unknown if excreted in breast milk; compatible with breast-feeding

SIDE EFFECTS

Rare

Dry mouth, somnolence, abdominal discomfort, allergic reaction (such as rash and itching)

SERIOUS REACTIONS

- Toxicity results in constipation, GI irritation, including nausea and vomiting, and CNS depression. Activated charcoal is used to treat loperamide toxicity.

INTERACTIONS

Drugs

3 *Opioid (narcotic) analgesics:* May increase the risk of constipation

SPECIAL CONSIDERATIONS

PATIENT/FAMILY EDUCATION

- Do not self-medicate diarrhea for >48 hr without consulting provider
- Notify the physician if abdominal distention and pain, diarrhea that does not stop within 3 days, or fever occurs
- Loperamide may cause dry mouth
- Avoid alcohol during loperamide therapy
- Avoid tasks that require mental alertness or motor skills until response to the drug has been established

MONITORING PARAMETERS

- Bowel sounds for peristalsis
- Pattern of daily bowel activity and stool consistency

lopinavir; ritonavir

(low-pin′-a-veer; ri-toe′-na-veer)

Rx: Kaletra

Chemical Class: Protease inhibitor, HIV

Therapeutic Class: Antiviral

CLINICAL PHARMACOLOGY

Mechanism of Action: A protease inhibitor combination drug in which lopinavir inhibits the activity of the enzyme protease late in the HIV replication process and ritonavir increases plasma levels of lopinavir. ***Therapeutic Effect:*** Formation of immature, noninfectious viral particles.

Pharmacokinetics

Readily absorbed after PO administration (absorption increased when taken with food). Protein binding: 98%-99%. Metabolized in the liver. Eliminated primarily in feces. Not removed by hemodialysis. ***Half-life:*** 5-6 hr.

INDICATIONS AND DOSAGES

HIV infection

PO

Adults. 3 capsules (400 mg lopinavir/100 mg ritonavir) or 5 ml twice a day. Increase to 4 capsules (533 mg lopinavir/133 mg ritonavir) or 6.5 ml when taken with efavirenz or nevirapine.

Children weighing 15-40 kg who are not taking efavirenz or nevirapine. 10 mg/kg twice a day.

Children weighing 7-14 kg who are not taking alprenavir, efavirenz, nelfinavir, nevirapine. 12 mg/kg twice a day.

Children weighing 15-40 kg who are taking efavirenz or nevirapine. 11 mg/kg twice a day.

Children weighing 7-14 kg who are taking efavirenz or nevirapine. 13 mg/kg twice a day.

PO (Once Daily)

Alert: Once daily dosing is not recommended in therapy-experienced patients and has not been evaluated in children.

Adults. 6 capsules (800 mg lopinavir/200 mg ritonavir) or 10 ml once daily. Increase to 8 capsules (1066 mg lopinavir/266 mg ritonavir) or 13 ml when taken with efavirenz or nevirapine.

AVAILABLE FORMS

- *Capsules:* 133.3 mg lopinavir/ 33.3 mg ritonavir.
- *Oral Solution:* 80 mg/ml lopinavir/20 mg/ml ritonavir.

CONTRAINDICATIONS: Concomitant use of ergot derivatives (causes peripheral ischemia of extremities and vasospasm), flecainide, midazolam, pimozide, propafenone (increases the risk of serious cardiac arrhythmias), or triazolam (increases sedation or respiratory depression); hypersensitivity to lopinavir or ritonavir

PREGNANCY AND LACTATION: Pregnancy category C; breast milk excretion unknown; the CDC recommends that HIV-infected mothers not breast-feed their infants to avoid risking postnatal transmission of HIV

SIDE EFFECTS

Frequent (14%)

Mild to moderate diarrhea

Occasional (6%-2%)

Nausea, asthenia, abdominal pain, headache, vomiting

Rare (less than 2%)

Insomnia, rash

SERIOUS REACTIONS

- Anemia, leukopenia, lymphadenopathy, deep vein thrombosis, Cushing's syndrome, pancreatitis, and hemorrhagic colitis occur rarely.

INTERACTIONS

Drugs

❷ *Amiodarone:* Increased plasma levels of amiodarone

[3] *Amprenavir:* Increased plasma level of amprenavir; consider dose adjustment of amprenavir to 750 mg bid

▲1 *Astemizole:* Increased plasma levels of astemizole

[3] *Atorvastatin:* Increased plasma level of atorvastatin

[3] *Atovaquone:* Decreased level of atovaquone

[3] *Barbiturates:* Increased clearance of lopinavir/ritonavir; reduced clearance of barbiturates

❷ *Bepredil:* Increased plasma levels of bepredil

❷ *Carbamazepine:* Increased clearance of lopinavir/ritonavir; reduced clearance of carbamazepine

[3] *Cerivastatin:* Increased plasma level of cerivastatin

▲1 *Cisapride:* Increased plasma levels of cisapride

❷ *Clarithromycin:* Reduced clearance of lopinavir/ritonavir; lopinavir/ritonavir reduces clearance of clarithromycin; reduce clarithromycin dose for renal insufficiency if coadministered

[3] *Cyclosporine:* Increased plasma level of cyclosporine

[3] *Dexamethasone:* Decreased plasma level of lopinavir/ritonavir

[3] *Didanosine (buffered formulation):* Reduces absorption of lopinavir/ritonavir, take didanosine 1 hr before or 2 hr after dose of lopinavir/ ritonavir

[3] *Dihydropyridine calcium channel blockers (amlodipine, felodipine, nifedipine, nicardipine):* Increased plasma level of these drugs

[3] *Efavirenz:* Increased clearance of lopinavir/ritonavir, increase dose to 533/133 mg bid

❷ *Encainide:* Increased plasma levels of encainide

▲ *Ergot alkaloids:* Increased plasma levels of ergot alkaloids

[3] *Erythromycin:* Reduced clearance of lopinavir/ritonavir; lopinavir/ritonavir reduces clearance of erythromycin

▲ *Flecainide:* Increased plasma levels of flecainide

▲ *Flurazepam:* Increased plasma levels of flurazepam

[3] *Indinavir:* Increased plasma level of indinavir; consider dose reduction to 600 mg bid

[3] *Itraconazole:* Lopinavir/ritonavir reduces clearance of itraconazole; reduce itraconazole dose

[3] *Ketoconazole:* Lopinavir/ritonavir reduces clearance of ketoconazole; reduce ketoconazole dose

❷ *Lidocaine:* Increased plasma levels of lidocaine

❷ *Lovastatin:* Lopinavir/ritonavir reduces clearance of lovastatin

❷ *Meperidine:* Increased plasma levels of meperidine

[3] *Methadone:* Lopinavir/ritonavir reduces methadone plasma concentration by 50%

▲ *Midazolam:* Increased plasma levels of midazolam and prolonged effect

[3] *Nevirapine:* Increased clearance of lopinavir/ritonavir, increase dose to 533/133 mg bid

[3] *Oral contraceptives:* Lopinavir/ritonavir may reduce efficacy

[3] *Phenytoin:* Increased clearance of lopinavir/ritonavir; reduced clearance of phenytoin

▲ *Pimozide:* Increased plasma levels of pimozide

▲ *Propafenone:* Increased plasma levels of propafenone

❷ *Propoxyphene:* Increased plasma levels of propoxyphene

❷ *Quinidine:* Increased plasma levels of quinidine

[3] *Rapamycin:* Increased plasma level of rapamycin

❷ *Rifabutin:* Increased clearance of lopinavir/ritonavir; reduced clearance of rifabutin; reduce rifabutin dose to 150 mg qod

❷ *Rifampin:* Increased clearance of lopinavir/ritonavir

[3] *Saquinavir:* Decreased clearance of saquinavir; reduce dose of Fortovase (saquinavir soft gel capsule) to 800 mg bid

❷ *Sildenafil:* Increased plasma level of sildenafil, reduce dose to 25 mg q48h

❷ *Simvastatin:* Lopinavir/ritonavir reduces clearance of simvastatin

❷ *St. John's Wort (hypericum perforatum):* Increased clearance of lopinavir/ritonavir

[3] *Tacrolimus:* Increased plasma level of tacrolimus

❷ *Tadalafil, vardenafil:* Increases the adverse effects of these drugs

▲ *Terfenadine:* Increased plasma levels of terfenadine

[3] *Tenofovir:* Lopinavir/ritonavir increases tenofovir AUC by 34%; tenofovir decreases AUC of lopinavir/ritonavir by 24% (when co-administered with lopinavir/ritonavir, tenofovir should be administered 2 hours before or one hour after administration of lopinavir/ritonavir)

▲ *Triazolam:* Increased plasma levels of triazolam and prolonged effect

[3] *Troleandomycin:* Reduced clearance of lopinavir/ritonavir; lopinavir/ritonavir reduces clearance of troleandomycin

[3] *Warfarin:* May reduce warfarin effect

❷ *Zolpidem:* Increased plasma levels of zolpidem

SPECIAL CONSIDERATIONS

PATIENT/FAMILY EDUCATION

- Take with food to improve bioavailability
- Be aware of many potential drug interactions
- This drug is not a cure for HIV infection, nor does it reduce the risk of transmitting HIV to others

MONITORING PARAMETERS

- Plasma glucose, lipid levels, hepatic function tests
- CBC with differential, CD4+ cell count, HIV RNA level (viral load), serum electrolytes
- Weight
- Pattern of daily bowel activity and stool consistency
- Assess for signs and symptoms of opportunistic infections, such as fever, oral mucosa changes, and a cough or other respiratory symptoms

loracarbef

(lor-a-kar'-bef)

Rx: Lorabid, Lorabid Pulvules

Chemical Class: Carbacephem derivative

Therapeutic Class: Antibiotic

CLINICAL PHARMACOLOGY

Mechanism of Action: A second-generation cephalosporin that binds to bacterial cell membranes and inhibits cell wall synthesis. ***Therapeutic Effect:*** Bactericidal.

Pharmacokinetics

Well absorbed from GI tract. Protein binding: 25%. Widely distributed. Primarily excreted unchanged in urine. Moderately removed by hemodialysis. ***Half-life:*** 1 hr (increased in impaired renal function).

INDICATIONS AND DOSAGES

Bronchitis

PO

Adults, Elderly, Children 12 yrs and older. 200-400 mg q12h for 7 days.

Pharyngitis

PO

Adults, Elderly, Children 12 yrs and older. 200 mg q12h for 10 days.

Children 6 mos-11 yrs. 7.5 mg/kg q12h for 10 days.

Pneumonia

PO

Adults, Elderly, Children 12 yrs and older. 400 mg q12h for 14 days.

Sinusitis

PO

Adults, Elderly, Children 12 yrs and older. 400 mg q12h for 10 days.

Children 6 mos-11 yrs. 15 mg/kg q12h for 10 days.

Skin and soft-tissue infections

PO

Adults, Elderly, Children 12 yrs and older. 200 mg q12h for 7 days.

Children 6 mos-11 yrs. 7.5 mg/kg q12h for 7 days.

UTIs

PO

Adults, Elderly, Children 6 mos-12 yrs. 200-400 mg q12h for 7-14 days.

Otitis media

PO

Children 6 mos-12 yrs. 15 mg/kg q12h for 10 days.

AVAILABLE FORMS

- *Capsules (Lorabid Pulvules):* 200 mg, 400 mg.
- *Powder for Oral Suspension (Lorabid):* 100 mg/5 ml, 200 mg/5 ml.

CONTRAINDICATIONS: History of anaphylactic reaction to penicillins or hypersensitivity to cephalosporins

PREGNANCY AND LACTATION: Pregnancy category B; unknown if excreted into breast milk

L

SIDE EFFECTS

Frequent

Abdominal pain, anorexia, nausea, vomiting, diarrhea

Occasional

Rash, pruritus

Rare

Dizziness, headache, vaginitis

SERIOUS REACTIONS

- Antibiotic-associated colitis and other superinfections may result from altered bacterial balance.
- Hypersensitivity reactions (ranging from rash, urticaria, and fever to anaphylaxis) occur in fewer than 5% of patients, most commonly in patients with a history of drug allergies, especially to penicillins.

INTERACTIONS

Drugs

3 *Probenecid:* Increases serum concentration of loracarbef

SPECIAL CONSIDERATIONS

- Essentially same spectrum and utility as cefaclor
- Take 1 hr before eating or 2 hr after eating

MONITORING PARAMETERS

- Pattern of daily bowel activity and stool consistency
- Skin for a rash, especially in the diaper area in infants and toddlers
- Intake and output, renal function reports, and urinalysis results for signs of nephrotoxicity
- Assess for nausea or vomiting
- Be alert for signs and symptoms of superinfection, including abdominal pain or cramping, anal or genital pruritus or discharge, moderate to severe diarrhea, and severe mouth or tongue soreness

loratadine

(lor-at'-a-deen)

OTC: Claritin, Claritin Reditabs

Combinations

OTC: with pseudoephedrine (Claritin-D)

Chemical Class: Piperidine derivative

Therapeutic Class: Antihistamine

CLINICAL PHARMACOLOGY

Mechanism of Action: A long-acting antihistamine that competes with histamine for H_1 receptor sites on effector cells. ***Therapeutic Effect:*** Prevents allergic responses mediated by histamine, such as rhinitis, urticaria, and pruritus.

Pharmacokinetics

Route	Onset	Peak	Duration
PO	1-3 hr	8-12 hr	longer than 24 hr

Rapidly and almost completely absorbed from the GI tract. Protein binding: 97%; metabolite, 73%-77%. Distributed mainly to the liver, lungs, GI tract, and bile. Metabolized in the liver to active metabolite; undergoes extensive first-pass metabolism. Eliminated in urine and feces. Not removed by hemodialysis. ***Half-life:*** 8.4 hr; metabolite, 28 hr (increased in elderly and hepatic impairment).

INDICATIONS AND DOSAGES

Allergic rhinitis, urticaria

PO

Adults, Elderly, Children 6 yrs and older. 10 mg once a day.

Children 2-5 yrs. 5 mg once a day.

Dosage in renal and hepatic impairment

PO

Adults, Elderly, Children 6 yr and older. 10 mg every other day.

Children 2-5 yr. 5 mg every other day.

AVAILABLE FORMS

- *Syrup (Claritin):* 10 mg/10 ml.
- *Tablets (Alavert, Claritin, Tavist ND):* 10 mg.
- *Tablets (Rapidly Disintegrating [Alavert, Claritin RediTab]):* 10 mg.

UNLABELED USES: Adjunct treatment of bronchial asthma

CONTRAINDICATIONS: Hypersensitivity to loratadine or its ingredients

PREGNANCY AND LACTATION: Pregnancy category B; excreted into breast milk at levels equivalent to serum levels

SIDE EFFECTS

Frequent (12%-8%)

Headache, fatigue, somnolence

Occasional (3%)

Dry mouth, nose, or throat

Rare

Photosensitivity

SERIOUS REACTIONS

- Abnormal hepatic function, including jaundice, hepatitis, and hepatic necrosis; alopecia; anaphylaxis; breast enlargement; erythema multiforme; peripheral edema; and seizures have been reported.

INTERACTIONS

Drugs

3 *Itraconazole, ketoconazole, miconazole, clarithromycin, erythromycin:* Increased loratadine levels but no increase in toxicity reported

3 *Food:* Delays the absorption of loratadine

SPECIAL CONSIDERATIONS

- Effective, but expensive nonsedating antihistamine; reserve for patients unable to tolerate sedating antihistamines like chlorpheniramine

PATIENT/FAMILY EDUCATION

- May cause drowsiness
- Avoid tasks requiring mental alertness or motor skills until response to the drug has been established
- Drink plenty of water to help prevent dry mouth
- Avoid direct exposure to sunlight and wear sunscreen outdoors to prevent a photosensitivity reaction
- Avoid alcohol during loratadine therapy

MONITORING PARAMETERS

- Increase fluid intake in patients with upper respiratory allergies to decrease the viscosity of secretions, offset thirst, and replace fluids lost from diaphoresis
- Monitor for relief of symptoms, including rhinorrhea, sneezing, and itching, red, watery eyes

L

lorazepam

(lor-a'-ze-pam)

Rx: Ativan, Lorazepam Intensol

Chemical Class: Benzodiazepine

Therapeutic Class: Anticonvulsant; anxiolytic; sedative/hypnotic

DEA Class: Schedule IV

CLINICAL PHARMACOLOGY

Mechanism of Action: A benzodiazepine that enhances the action of the inhibitory neurotransmitter gamma-aminobutyric acid in the CNS, affecting memory, as well as motor, sensory, and cognitive function. ***Therapeutic Effect:*** Produces anxiolytic, anticonvulsant, sedative, muscle relaxant, and antiemetic effects.

Pharmacokinetics

Route	Onset	Peak	Duration
PO	60 min	N/A	8-12 hr
IV	15-30 min	N/A	8-12 hr
IM	30-60 min	N/A	8-12 hr

Well absorbed after PO and IM administration. Protein binding: 85%. Widely distributed. Metabolized in the liver. Primarily excreted in urine. Not removed by hemodialysis. ***Half-life:*** 10-20 hr.

INDICATIONS AND DOSAGES

Anxiety

PO

Adults. 1-10 mg/day in 2-3 divided doses. Average: 2-6 mg/day.

Elderly. Initially, 0.5-1 mg/day. May increase gradually. Range: 0.5-4 mg.

IV

Adults, Elderly. 0.02-0.06 mg/kg q2-6h.

IV Infusion

Adults, Elderly. 0.01-0.1 mg/kg/h.

PO, IV

Children. 0.05 mg/kg/dose q4-8h. Range: 0.02-0.1 mg/kg. Maximum: 2 mg/dose.

Insomnia due to anxiety

PO

Adults. 2-4 mg at bedtime.

Elderly. 0.5-1 mg at bedtime.

Preoperative sedation

IV

Adults, Elderly. 0.044 mg/kg 15-20 min before surgery. Maximum total dose: 2 mg.

IM

Adults, Elderly. 0.05 mg/kg 2 hr before procedure. Maximum total dose: 4 mg.

Status epilepticus

IV

Adults, Elderly. 4 mg over 2-5 min. May repeat in 10-15 min. Maximum: 8 mg in 12-hr period.

Children. 0.1 mg/kg over 2-5 min. May give second dose of 0.05 mg/kg in 15-20 min. Maximum: 4 mg.

Neonates. 0.05 mg/kg. May repeat in 10-15 min.

AVAILABLE FORMS

- *Tablets (Ativan):* 0.5 mg, 1 mg, 2 mg.
- *Injection (Ativan):* 2 mg/ml, 4 mg/ml.
- *Oral Solution (Lorazepam Intensol):* 2 mg/ml.

UNLABELED USES: Treatment of alcohol withdrawal, panic disorders, skeletal muscle spasms, chemotherapy-induced nausea or vomiting, tension headache, tremors; adjunctive treatment before endoscopic procedures (diminishes patient recall)

CONTRAINDICATIONS: Angle-closure glaucoma, preexisting CNS depression, severe hypotension, severe uncontrolled pain

PREGNANCY AND LACTATION: Pregnancy category D (other benzodiazepines associated with cleft lip, cleft palate, microcephaly, pyloric stenosis); neonatal withdrawal, hypotonia; excreted into breast milk in low quantities; effect on infant unknown

Controlled Substance: Schedule IV

SIDE EFFECTS

Frequent

Somnolence (initially in the morning), ataxia, confusion

Occasional

Blurred vision, slurred speech, hypotension, headache

Rare

Paradoxical CNS restlessness or excitement in elderly or debilitated

SERIOUS REACTIONS

• Abrupt or too-rapid withdrawal may result in pronounced restlessness, irritability, insomnia, hand tremor, abdominal or muscle cramps, diaphoresis, vomiting, and seizures.

• Overdose results in somnolence, confusion, diminished reflexes, and coma.

INTERACTIONS

Drugs

3 *Ethanol, other CNS depressants:* Increased adverse psychomotor effects of lorazepam

2 *Fluconazole:* Potential for increased lorazepam concentrations

3 *Itraconazole:* Potential for increased lorazepam concentrations

3 *Kava kava, valerian:* May increase CNS depression

3 *Loxapine:* Isolated cases of respiratory depression, stupor, and hypotension have been observed in patients receiving loxapine and lorazepam

3 *Smoking:* Reduces the effectiveness of lorazepam

SPECIAL CONSIDERATIONS

• A good choice for elderly or patients with liver dysfunction who need benzodiazepines due to phase II metabolism to inactive metabolites (less likely to accumulate)

PATIENT/FAMILY EDUCATION

• Do not discontinue abruptly after long-term use, withdrawal syndrome (seizures, anxiety, insomnia, nausea, vomiting, flu-like illness, confusion, hallucinations, memory impairment) can occur

• Drowsiness usually disappears with continued therapy

• Avoid tasks that require mental alertness or motor skills until response to the drug has been established

• Avoid smoking, drinking alcoholic beverages, and taking other CNS depressants; smoking reduces the effectiveness of lorazepam, and alcohol and CNS depressants increase sedation

• The female patient on long-term therapy should use effective contraception during therapy and should notify the physician immediately if she becomes or may be pregnant

MONITORING PARAMETERS

• Blood pressure, heart rate, respiratory rate, CBC with differential, and hepatic function. For those on long-term therapy, expect blood chemistry studies and hepatic and renal function tests to be performed periodically

• Therapeutic response, such as a calm facial expression and decreased restlessness and insomnia

• The therapeutic serum level for lorazepam is 50-240 ng/ml; the toxic serum level is unknown

losartan potassium

(lo-sar'-tan poe-tass'-ee-um)

Rx: Cozaar

Combinations

Rx: with hydrochlorothiazide (Hyzaar)

Chemical Class: Angiotensin II receptor antagonist

Therapeutic Class: Antihypertensive

CLINICAL PHARMACOLOGY

Mechanism of Action: An angiotensin II receptor, type AT_1, antagonist that blocks vasoconstrictor and aldosterone-secreting effects of angiotensin II, inhibiting the binding of angiotensin II to the AT_1 receptors. ***Therapeutic Effect:*** Causes vasodilation, decreases peripheral resistance, and decreases BP.

Pharmacokinetics

Route	Onset	Peak	Duration
PO	N/A	6 hr	24 hr

Well absorbed after PO administration. Protein binding: 98%. Undergoes first-pass metabolism in the liver to active metabolites. Excreted in urine and via the biliary system. Not removed by hemodialysis. ***Half-life:*** 2 hrs, metabolite: 6-9 hr.

INDICATIONS AND DOSAGES

Hypertension

PO

Adults, Elderly. Initially, 50 mg once a day. Maximum: May be given once or twice a day, with total daily doses ranging from 25-100 mg.

Nephropathy

PO

Adults, Elderly. Initially, 50 mg/day. May increase to 100 mg/day based on BP response.

Stroke reduction

PO

Adults, Elderly. 50 mg/day. Maximum: 100 mg/day.

Hypertension in patients with impaired hepatic function

PO

Adults, Elderly. Initially, 25 mg/day.

AVAILABLE FORMS

• *Tablets:* 25 mg, 50 mg, 100 mg.

UNLABELED USES: CHF, erythrocytosis

CONTRAINDICATIONS: None known.

PREGNANCY AND LACTATION: Pregnancy category C (D if used in second or third trimesters)

SIDE EFFECTS

Frequent (8%)

Upper respiratory tract infection

Occasional (4%-2%)

Dizziness, diarrhea, cough

Rare (1% or less)

Insomnia, dyspepsia, heartburn, back and leg pain, muscle cramps, myalgia, nasal congestion, sinusitis

SERIOUS REACTIONS

• Overdosage may manifest as hypotension and tachycardia. Bradycardia occurs less often.

INTERACTIONS

Drugs

3 *Cimetidine:* May increase the effects of losartan

3 *Fluconazole:* Decreased conversion to active metabolite (CYP2C9 inhibition), loss of antihypertensive effects

2 *Lithium:* Increased renal lithium reabsorption at the proximal tubular site due to the natriuresis associated with the inhibition of aldosterone secretion; increased risk of lithium toxicity

3 *NSAIDs:* May reduce hemodynamic effects of losartan

3 *Phenobarbital:* May decrease the effects of losartan

3 *Potassium-sparing diuretics:* Increased risk of hyperkalemia

3 *Rifampin:* Induced metabolism of losartan and metabolite, resulting in a decrease in the area under the concentration-time curve (AUC) and half-life of both compounds and reduced losartan efficacy

SPECIAL CONSIDERATIONS

• Potentially as or more effective than angiotensin-converting enzyme inhibitors, without cough; no evidence for reduction in morbidity and mortality as first-line agents in hypertension, yet; whether they provide the same cardiac and renal protection also still tentative; like ACE inhibitors, less effective in black patients

PATIENT/FAMILY EDUCATION

• Call your clinician immediately if note following side effects: wheezing; lip, throat or face swelling; hives or rash

• Advise female patients of the consequences of second- and third-trimester exposure to losartan
• Stress to the female patient that she should immediately notify the physician if she becomes pregnant
• Avoid tasks that require mental alertness or motor skills until response to the drug has been established
• Avoid cold preparations or nasal decongestants while on losartan therapy
• Do not abruptly discontinue the drug

MONITORING PARAMETERS

• Baseline electrolytes, urinalysis, blood urea nitrogen, and creatinine with recheck at 2-4 wks after initiation (sooner in volume-depleted patients); monitor sitting blood pressure; pulse rate; watch for symptomatic hypotension, particularly in volume-depleted patients
• Pattern of daily bowel activity and stool consistency

lovastatin

(loe'-va-sta-tin)

Rx: Altocor, Mevacor

Combinations

Rx: With niacin, extended-release (Advicor)

Chemical Class: Substituted hexahydronaphthalene

Therapeutic Class: HMG-CoA reductase inhibitor; antilipemic

CLINICAL PHARMACOLOGY

Mechanism of Action: An antihyperlipidemic that inhibits HMG-CoA reductase, the enzyme that catalyzes the early step in cholesterol synthesis. ***Therapeutic Effect:*** Decreases LDL cholesterol, VLDL cholesterol, plasma triglycerides; increases HDL cholesterol.

Pharmacokinetics

Route	*Onset*	*Peak*	*Duration*
PO	3 days	4-6 wk	N/A

Incompletely absorbed from the GI tract (increased on empty stomach). Protein binding: 95%. Hydrolyzed in the liver to active metabolite. Primarily eliminated in feces. Not removed by hemodialysis. ***Half-life:*** 1.1-1.7 hrs.

INDICATIONS AND DOSAGES

Atherosclerosis, coronary artery disease

PO

Adults, Elderly. Initially, 20 mg/day. Maintenance: 10-80 mg once daily or in 2 divided doses. Maximum: 80 mg/day.

Hypercholesterolemia

PO

Adults, Elderly. Initially, 20 mg/day. Maintenance: 10-80 mg once daily or in 2 divided doses. Maximum: 80 mg/day.

PO (Extended-Release)

Adults, Elderly. Initially, 20-60 mg once daily at bedtime. Maintenance: 10-60 mg once daily at bedtime.

Heterozygous familial hypercholesterolemia

PO

Children 10-17 yr. Initially, 10 mg/day. May increase to 20 mg/day after 8 wk and 40 mg/day after 16 wk if needed.

AVAILABLE FORMS

• *Tablets (Mevacor):* 10 mg, 20 mg, 40 mg.
• *Tablets (Extended-Release [Altocor]):* 20 mg, 40 mg, 60 mg.

CONTRAINDICATIONS: Active liver disease, pregnancy, unexplained elevated liver function tests

PREGNANCY AND LACTATION: Pregnancy category X (may produce skeletal malformations); excretion into breast milk unknown, contraindicated in nursing mothers

L

SIDE EFFECTS

Generally well tolerated. Side effects usually mild and transient.

Frequent (9%-5%)

Headache, flatulence, diarrhea, abdominal pain or cramps, rash and pruritus

Occasional (4%-3%)

Nausea, vomiting, constipation, dyspepsia

Rare (2%-1%)

Dizziness, heartburn, myalgia, blurred vision, eye irritation

SERIOUS REACTIONS

- There is a potential for cataract development.
- Lovastatin occasionally produces myopathy manifested as muscle pain, tenderness, or weakness with elevated creatine kinase. Myopathy may take the form of rhabdomyolysis fatalities.

INTERACTIONS

Drugs

3 *Cholestyramine, colestipol:* Decreased bioavailability of lovastatin possible, potentially reduced benefit overcome by additive lipid-lowering effects of concurrent therapy

2 *Clarithromycin, danazol, erythromycin, nefazodone:* Severe myopathy or rhabdomyolysis

2 *Clofibrate, fenofibrate, gemfibrozil:* Severe myopathy or rhabdomyolysis with combination possible, especially at high doses; if used concomitantly lovastatin dose should not exceed 20 mg/day

3 *Cyclosporine:* Concomitant administration increases risk of severe myopathy or rhabdomyolysis; if used concomitantly lovastatin dose should not exceed 20 mg/day

3 *Diltiazem, verapamil:* Increased risk of myopathy

2 *Fluconazole, itraconazole, ketoconazole:* Large increases in lovastatin concentration, myopathy, or rhabdomyolysis possible

3 *Grapefruit juice:* Increased risk of myopathy or rhabdomyolysis with large quantities of grapefruit juice (>1 quart/day)

3 *Imatinib:* Increased risk of myopathy or rhabdomyolysis with combination

3 *Isradipine:* Reduction in lovastatin concentration

3 *Niacin:* Concomitant administration increases risk of severe myopathy or rhabdomyolysis; if used concomitantly lovastatin dose should not exceed 20 mg/day

3 *Pectin:* Reduced cholesterol-lowering effect of lovastatin

2 *Protease inhibitors:* Severe myopathy or rhabdomyolysis with combination possible

2 *Telithromycin:* Causes a large increase in lovastatin concentrations

3 *Warfarin:* Increased prothrombin times and bleeding reported with concomitant use

SPECIAL CONSIDERATIONS

- Less effective in homozygous familial hypercholesterolemia (lack of functional LDL receptors); these patients also more likely to have adverse reaction of elevated transaminases
- Statin selection based on lipid-lowering prowess, cost, and availability

PATIENT/FAMILY EDUCATION

- Report symptoms of myalgia, muscle tenderness, or weakness
- Take daily doses in the evening for increased effect
- Take with meals
- A prescribed diet and periodic laboratory tests are essential parts of therapy
- Avoid consuming grapefruit juice

MONITORING PARAMETERS

- Cholesterol (max therapeutic response 4-6 wk)

• LFTs (AST, ALT) at baseline and at 12 wk of therapy; if no change, no further monitoring necessary (discontinue if elevations persist >3 × upper limit of normal)
• CPK in patients complaining of diffuse myalgia, muscle tenderness, or weakness
• Daily pattern of bowel activity
• Assess the patient for pruritus and rash

loxapine succinate

(lox'-a-peen suk'-si-nate)
Rx: Loxitane
Chemical Class: Dibenzoxazepine derivative; tertiary amine
Therapeutic Class: Antipsychotic

CLINICAL PHARMACOLOGY
Mechanism of Action: A dibenzodiazepine derivative that interferes with the binding of dopamine at postysnaptic receptor sites in brain. Strong anticholinergic effects. ***Therapeutic Effect:*** Suppresses locomotor activity, produces tranquilization.
Pharmacokinetics
Onset of action occurs within 1 hr. Metabolized to active metabolites 8-hydroxyloxapine, 7-hydroxyloxapine, and 8-hydroxyamoxapine. Excreted in urine. ***Half-life:*** 4 hrs.
INDICATIONS AND DOSAGES
Psychotic disorders
PO
Adults. 10 mg 2 times/day. Increase dosage rapidly during first week to 50 mg, if needed. Usual therapeutic, maintenance range: 60-100 mg daily in 2-4 divided doses. Maximum: 250 mg/day.

AVAILABLE FORMS
• *Capsules:* 5 mg, 10 mg, 25 mg, 50 mg (Loxitane).
CONTRAINDICATIONS: Severe central nervous system (CNS) depression, comatose states, hypersensivitiy to loxapine or any component of the formulation
PREGNANCY AND LACTATION: Pregnancy category C; no data in lactating women
SIDE EFFECTS
Frequent
Blurred vision, confusion, drowsiness, dry mouth, dizziness, lightheadedness
Occasional
Allergic reaction (rash, itching), decreased urination, constipation, decreased sexual ability, enlarged breasts, headache, photosensitivity, nausea, vomiting, insomnia, weight gain
SERIOUS REACTIONS
• Extrapyramidal symptoms frequently noted are akathisia (motor restlessness, anxiety). Less frequently noted are akinesia (rigidity, tremor, salivation, masklike facial expression, reduced voluntary movements). Infrequently noted dystonias: torticollis (neck muscle spasm), opisthotonos (rigidity of back muscles), and oculogyric crisis (rolling back of eyes). Tardive dyskinesia (protrusion of tongue, puffing of cheeks, chewing/puckering of mouth) occurs rarely but may be irreversible. Risk is greater in female elderly patients.
INTERACTIONS
Drugs
3 *Anticholinergics:* Decreased neuroleptic effect
3 *Bromocriptine:* Decreased lowering of prolactin by bromocriptine in patients with pituitary adenoma

❷ *Epinephrine:* Inhibition of vasopressor effect of epinephrine
❸ *Lithium:* Increased neurotoxicity
❸ *Lorazepam:* Isolated cases of respiratory depression, stupor, and hypotension have been observed

SPECIAL CONSIDERATIONS

PATIENT/FAMILY EDUCATION

- Avoid alcohol; caution with activities requiring mental alertness
- Mix oral concentrate in orange or grapefruit juice
- Full therapeutic effect may take up to 6 wks
- Report any visual disturbances
- Chew sugarless gum or take sips of tepid water to relieve dry mouth
- Do not abruptly discontinue loxapine
- Avoid tasks that require mental alertness or motor skills until response to the drug is established

MONITORING PARAMETERS

- Therapeutic response including increased ability to concentrate, improvement in self-care, interest in surroundings, and relaxed facial expression

---

mafenide

(ma′-fe-nide)
Rx: Sulfamylon
Chemical Class: Sulfonamide derivative
Therapeutic Class: Antibiotic, topical

CLINICAL PHARMACOLOGY

Mechanism of Action: A topical antiinfective that decreases number of bacteria avascular tissue of second- and third-degree burns. ***Therapeutic Effect:*** Bacteriostatic. Promotes spontaneous healing of deep partial-thickness burns.

Pharmacokinetics

Absorbed through devascularzied areas into systemic circulation following topical administration. Excreted in the form of its metabolite rho-carboxybenzenesulfonamide.

INDICATIONS AND DOSAGES

Burns

Topical

Adults, Elderly, Children. Apply 1-2 times/day.

AVAILABLE FORMS

- *Cream:* 85 mg base/g (Sulfamylon).

CONTRAINDICATIONS: Hypersensitivity to mafenide or sulfite or any other component of the formulation

PREGNANCY AND LACTATION: Pregnancy category C; compatible with breast-feeding except in G-6-PD deficiency and ill, jaundiced, or premature infants

SIDE EFFECTS

Difficult to distinguish side effects and effects of severe burn

Frequent

Pain, burning upon application

Occasional

Allergic reaction (usually 10-14 days after initiation): itching, rash, facial edema, swelling; unexplained syndrome of marked hyperventilation with respiratory alkalosis

Rare

Delay in eschar separation, excoriation of new skin

SERIOUS REACTIONS

- Hemolytic anemia, porphyria, bone marrow depression, superinfections (especially with fungi), metabolic acidosis occurs rarely.

INTERACTIONS

Labs

- *False increase:* Urine amino acids

SPECIAL CONSIDERATIONS

PATIENT/FAMILY EDUCATION

- Topical application may cause temporary pain or bruising

• Do not interrupt therapy
• Bathe burn area daily

MONITORING PARAMETERS

• Assess burn area and surrounding skin

magaldrate

OTC: Riopan, Iosopan Plus, Lowsium Plus

Combinations

OTC: with simethicone (Riopan Plus)

Chemical Class: Aluminum and magnesium hydroxide and sulfate mixture

Therapeutic Class: Antacid

CLINICAL PHARMACOLOGY

Mechanism of Action: An antacid that causes less hydrogen ion available for diffusion through the gastrointestinal (GI) mucosa. ***Therapeutic Effect:*** Reduces and neutralizes gastric acid.

INDICATIONS AND DOSAGES

Hyperacidity and gas

PO

Adults, Elderly. 540-1080 mg between meals and at bedtime.

AVAILABLE FORMS

• *Suspension:* Magaldrate 540 mg and simethicone 20 mg/5 ml, magaldrate 540 mg and simethicone 40 mg/5 ml, magaldrate 1080 mg and simethicone 40 mg/5 ml.
• *Tablets (chewable):* Magaldrate 540 mg and simethicone 20 mg, magaldrate 1080 mg and simethicone 20 mg.

CONTRAINDICATIONS: Hypersensitivity to magaldrate, colostomy or ileostomy, appendicitis, ulcerative colitis, diverticulits

PREGNANCY AND LACTATION: Pregnancy category C

SIDE EFFECTS

Rare

Constipation, diarrhea, fluid retention, dizziness or lightheadedness, continuing discomfort, irregular heartbeat, loss of appetite, mood or mental changes, muscle weakness, unusual tiredness or weakness, weight loss, chalky taste

SERIOUS REACTIONS

• None known.

INTERACTIONS

Drugs

3 *Allopurinol, cefpodoxime, ciprofloxacin, isoniazid, ketoconazole, quinolones, tetracyclines, digoxin, iron salts, indomethacin:* Decreased GI absorption of these drugs

3 *Pseudoephedrine, enteric-coated aspirin, diazepam:* Increased GI absorption of these drugs

3 *Quinidine:* Increased quinidine levels

3 *Salicylates:* Increased urinary excretion of salicylates

SPECIAL CONSIDERATIONS

PATIENT/FAMILY EDUCATION

• Take other medications at least 2 hrs before or after dosing with magaldrate
• Drink several glasses of water a day to help reduce possible constipation
• Notify the physician if diarrhea occurs

MONITORING PARAMETERS

• Pattern of daily bowel activity and stool consistency

magnesium chloride/ magnesium citrate/ magnesium hydroxide/ magnesium oxide/magnesium protein complex/ magnesium sulfate

(mag-nee'-zhum)

OTC: (magnesium chloride) Mag-Delay SR, Slow-Mag

OTC: (magnesium citrate) Citrate of Magnesia

OTC: (magnesium hydroxide) Phillips Milk of Magnesia

OTC: (magnesium oxide) Mag-Ox 400, Uro-Mag

OTC: (magnesium protein complex) Mg-PLUS

OTC: (magnesium sulfate) Epsom salt, magnesium sulfate injection, Sulfamag

Chemical Class: Divalent cation

Therapeutic Class: Antacid; antiarrhythmic; electrolyte supplement; laxative; uterine relaxant

CLINICAL PHARMACOLOGY

Mechanism of Action: An antacid, laxative, electrolyte, and anticonvulsant. As an antacid acts in the stomach to neutralize gastric acid. ***Therapeutic Effect:*** Increases pH. As a laxative has an osmotic effect, primarily in the small intestine, and draws water into the intestinal lumen. ***Therapeutic Effect:*** Produces distention and promotes peristalsis and bowel evacuation. As a systemic dietary supplement and electrolyte replacement, is found primarily in intracellular fluids and is essential for enzyme activity, nerve conduction, and muscle contraction. As an anticonvulsant, blocks neuromuscular transmission and the amount of acetylcholine released at the motor end plate. ***Therapeutic Effect:*** Controls seizure. Maintains and restores magnesium levels.

Pharmacokinetics

Antacid, laxative: Minimal absorption through the intestine. Absorbed dose primarily excreted in urine. Systemic: Widely distributed. Primarily excreted in urine.

INDICATIONS AND DOSAGES

Hypomagnesemia

PO (magnesium sulfate)

Adults, Elderly. 3 g q6h for 4 doses as needed.

IV, IM

Adults, Elderly. 1-12 g/day in divided doses.

Children. 25-50 mg/kg/dose q4-6h for 3-4 doses. Maintenance: 30-60 mg/kg/day.

Hypertension, seizures

IV, IM (magnesium sulfate)

Children. 20-100 mg/kg/dose q4-6h as needed.

IV

Adults. Initially, 4 g then 1-4 g/hr by continuous infusion.

Arrhythmias

IV (magnesium sulfate)

Adults, Elderly. Initially, 1-2 g then infusion of 1-2 g/hr.

Constipation

PO (magnesium sulfate)

Adults, Elderly, Children 12 yrs and older. 10-30 g/day in divided doses.

Children 6-11 yrs. 5-10 g/day in divided doses.

Children 2-5 yrs. 2.5-5 g/kg/day in divided doses.

PO (magnesium hydroxide)

Adults, Elderly, Children 12 yrs and older. 6-8 tablets or 30-60 ml/day.

Children 6-11 yrs. 3-4 tablets or 7.5-15 ml/day.

Children 2-5 yrs. 1-2 tablets or 2.5-7.5 ml/day.

INDICATIONS AND DOSAGES

Arthritis, inflammation, musculoskeletal disorders (backache)

PO

Adults, Elderly. 650 mg times/day or 1090 mg 3 times/day. May increase to 3.6-4.8 g/day in 3-4 divided doses.

AVAILABLE FORMS

• *Tablets:* 467 mg (Backache Pain Relief Extra Strength, Momentum), 325 mg (Doan's Original), 500 mg (Extra Strength Doan's), 650 mg (Keygesic-10), 600 mg (Mobidin).

CONTRAINDICATIONS: Severe renal impairment, hypersensitivity to magnesium salicylate or any component of the formulation

PREGNANCY AND LACTATION: Pregnancy category C; excreted into breast milk; use caution in nursing mothers due to potential adverse effects in nursing infant

SIDE EFFECTS

Occasional

Gastric mucosal irritation, bleeding

SERIOUS REACTIONS

• Overdosage may cause tinnitus.

• Toxic levels may be reached quickly in dehydrated, febrile children. Marked toxicity is manifested as hyperthermia, restlessness, abnormal breathing patterns, convulsions, respiratory failure, and coma.

INTERACTIONS

Drugs

3 *Oral anticoagulants:* May increase the risk of bleeding

3 *Probenecid:* May increase magnesium salicylate blood concentration

3 *Spironolactone:* Inhibits the diuretic action of spironolactone

3 *Sulfonylureas, methotrexate, barbiturates, diphenylhydantoin:* May displace these agents from plasma protein binding sites, resulting in enhanced action of these agents

Labs

• *False increase:* Serum bicarbonate, CSF protein, serum theophylline

• *False decrease:* Urine cocaine, urine estrogen, serum glucose, urine 17-hydroxycorticosteroids, urine opiates

• *False positive:* Urine ferric chloride test

SPECIAL CONSIDERATIONS

• Consider for patients with GI intolerance to aspirin or patients in whom interference with normal platelet function by aspirin or other NSAIDs is undesirable

PATIENT/FAMILY EDUCATION

• Report ringing in ears or persistent GI pain

MONITORING PARAMETERS

• AST, ALT, bilirubin, creatinine, CBC, if patient is on long-term therapy

mannitol

(man'-i-tall)

Rx: Osmitrol, Resectisol

Chemical Class: Hexahydric alcohol

Therapeutic Class: Antiglaucoma agent; diuretic, osmotic; genitourinary irrigant

CLINICAL PHARMACOLOGY

Mechanism of Action: An osmotic diuretic, antiglaucoma, and antihemolytic agent that elevates osmotic pressure of the glomerular filtrate, inhibiting tubular reabsorption of water and electrolytes, resulting in increased flow of water into interstitial fluid and plasma. ***Therapeutic Effect:*** Produces diuresis; reduces IOP; reduces ICP and cerebral edema.

Pharmacokinetics

Route	Onset	Peak	Duration
IV (diuresis)	15-30 min	N/A	2-8 hr
IV (Reduced ICP)	15-30 min	N/A	3-8 hr
IV (Reduced IOP)	N/A	30-60 min	4-8 hr

Remains in extracellular fluid. Primarily excreted in urine. Removed by hemodialysis. ***Half-life:*** 100 min.

INDICATIONS AND DOSAGES

Intracranial pressure

IV

Adults, Elderly. 0.25-1 g/kg q6-8h. Maximum: 6 g/24 hr.

Children. 0.25-1 g/kg as needed. Maximum: 2 g/kg/dose.

Intraocular pressure (IOP)

IV

Adults, Elderly. 1.5-2 g/kg as a 15%-20% solution. Maximum: 6 g/24 hr.

Children. 1-2 g/kg. Maximum: 2 g/kg/dose.

Renal impairment, oliguria

IV

Adults, Elderly. Use test dose. 300-400 mg/kg or up to 100 g given as a single dose.

Children. 0.25-2 g/kg. Maximum: 6 g/kg/24 hr.

Toxicity, poisoning

IV

Adults, Elderly. Continuous infusion as a 5%-20% solution.

Children. Up to 2 g/kg as 5%-10% solution.

AVAILABLE FORMS

- *Injection (Osmitrol):* 5%, 10%, 15%, 20%, 25%.
- *Irrigation Solution (Resectisol):* 5%.

CONTRAINDICATIONS: Dehydration, intracranial bleeding, severe pulmonary edema and congestion; several renal disease (anuria), increasing oliguria and azotemia

PREGNANCY AND LACTATION: Pregnancy category C

SIDE EFFECTS

Frequent

Dry mouth, thirst

Occasional

Blurred vision, increased urinary frequency and urine volume, headache, arm pain, backache, nausea, vomiting, urticaria, dizziness, hypotension or hypertension, tachycardia, fever, angina-like chest pain

SERIOUS REACTIONS

- Fluid and electrolyte imbalance may occur from rapid administration of large doses or inadequate urine output resulting in overexpansion of extracellular fluid.
- Circulatory overload may produce pulmonary edema and CHF.
- Excessive diuresis may produce hypokalemia and hyponatremia.
- Fluid loss in excess of electrolyte excretion may produce hypernatremia and hyperkalemia.

INTERACTIONS

Drugs

3 *Digoxin:* Increases the risk of digoxin toxicity associated with mannitol-induced hypokalemia

Labs

- *False increase:* Serum osmolality, serum phosphate, CSF protein
- *False decrease:* Serum phosphate

SPECIAL CONSIDERATIONS

PATIENT/FAMILY EDUCATION

- Expect an increase in the frequency and volume of urination
- Mannitol may cause dry mouth
- Weigh him- or herself daily

MONITORING PARAMETERS

- Serum electrolytes, urine output
- BUN and liver function tests
- Weight

maprotiline hydrochloride

(mah-pro-'-tih-leen)

Rx: Ludiomil

Chemical Class: Dibenzo-bicyclo-octadiene derivative

Therapeutic Class: Antidepressant, tetracyclic

CLINICAL PHARMACOLOGY

Mechanism of Action: A tetracyclic compound that blocks reuptake norepinephrine by CNS presynaptic neuronal membranes, increasing availability at postsynaptic neuronal receptor sites, and enhances synaptic activity. ***Therapeutic Effect:*** Produces antidepressant effect, with prominent sedative effects and low anticholinergic activity.

Pharmacokinetics

Slowly and completely absorbed after PO administration. Protein binding: 88%. Metabolized in liver by hydroxylation and oxidative modification. Excreted in urine. Unknown if removed by hemodialysis. ***Half-life:*** 27-58 hrs.

INDICATIONS AND DOSAGES

Mild to moderate depression

PO

Adults. 75 mg/day to start, in 1-4 divided doses. Elderly: 50-75 mg/day. In 2 wks, increase dosage gradually in 25 mg increments until therapeutic response is achieved. Reduce to lowest effective maintenance level.

Severe depression

PO

Adults. 100-150 mg/day in 1-4 divided doses. May increase gradually to maximum 225 mg/day.

Usual elderly dosage

PO

Initially, 25 mg at bedtime. May increase by 25 mg q3-7 days. Maintenance: 50-75 mg/day.

AVAILABLE FORMS

- *Tablets:* 25 mg, 50 mg, 75 mg (Ludiomil).

CONTRAINDICATIONS: Acute recovery period following myocardial infarction (MI) within 14 days of MAOI ingestion, known or suspected seizure disorder, hypersensitivity to maprotiline or any component of the formulation

PREGNANCY AND LACTATION: Pregnancy category B; excreted into breast milk; milk:plasma ratios of 1:5 and 1:3 have been reported; significance to the nursing infant unknown

SIDE EFFECTS

Frequent

Drowsiness, fatigue, dry mouth, blurred vision, constipation, delayed micturition, postural hypotension, excessive sweating, disturbed concentration, increased appetite, urinary retention

Occasional

GI disturbances (nausea, GI distress, metallic taste sensation), photosensitivity

Rare

Paradoxical reaction (agitation, restlessness, nightmares, insomnia), extrapyramidal symptoms (particularly fine hand tremor)

SERIOUS REACTIONS

- Higher incidence of seizures than with tricyclic antidepressants, especially in those with no previous history of seizures.
- High dosage may produce cardiovascular effects, such as severe postural hypotension, dizziness, tachycardia, palpitations, and arrhythmias.
- May also result in altered temperature regulation (hyperpyrexia or hypothermia).

• Abrupt withdrawal from prolonged therapy may produce headache, malaise, nausea, vomiting, and vivid dreams.

INTERACTIONS

Drugs

3 *Barbiturates:* Reduced serum concentrations of cyclic antidepressants

❷ *Bethanidine:* Reduced antihypertensive effect of bethanidine

3 *Carbamazepine:* Reduced cyclic antidepressant serum concentrations

3 *Cimetidine:* Increased maprotiline concentrations

❷ *Clonidine:* Reduced antihypertensive response to clonidine; enhanced hypertensive response with abrupt clonidine withdrawal

3 *Debrisoquin:* Inhibited antihypertensive response of debrisoquin

❷ *Epinephrine:* Markedly enhanced pressor response to IV epinephrine

3 *Ethanol:* Additive impairment of motor skills; abstinent alcoholics may eliminate cyclic antidepressants more rapidly than non-alcoholics

3 *Fluoxetine, fluvoxamine:* Marked increases in cyclic antidepressant plasma concentrations

3 *Grapefruit juice:* Marked increase in cyclic antidepressant plasma concentrations

3 *Guanethidine:* Inhibited antihypertensive response to guanethidine

❷ *Moclobemide:* Potential association with fatal or non-fatal serotonin syndrome

▲ *MAOIs:* Excessive sympathetic response, mania, or hyperpyrexia possible

3 *Neuroleptics:* Increased therapeutic and toxic effects of both drugs

❷ *Norepinephrine:* Markedly enhanced pressor response to norepinephrine

❷ *Phenylephrine:* Enhanced pressor response to IV phenylephrine

3 *Propantheline:* Excessive anticholinergic effects

3 *Propoxyphene:* Enhanced effect of cyclic antidepressants

3 *Quinidine:* Increased cyclic antidepressant serum concentrations

3 *Tolazemide:* Enhanced hypoglycemic effects of tolazemide

Labs

• *False negative:* Serum tricyclic antidepressants screen

SPECIAL CONSIDERATIONS

• Not first-line agent due to risk of seizures

PATIENT/FAMILY EDUCATION

• Use caution in driving or other activities requiring alertness

• Do not discontinue abruptly after long-term use

• Wear protective clothing and use sunscreen to protect skin for ultraviolet light or sunlight

• Report visual disturbances

• Take sips of tepid water or chew sugarless gum to relieve dry mouth

MONITORING PARAMETERS

• CBC

• Weight

• *Mental status:* mood, sensorium, affect, suicidal tendencies

• Determination of maprotiline plasma concentrations is not routinely recommended, but may be useful in identifying toxicity, drug interactions, or noncompliance (adjustments in dosage should be made according to clinical response not plasma concentrations); therapeutic plasma levels 200-300 ng/ml (including active metabolite)

• Blood pressure, pulse

mazindol

(may'-zin-doll)

Rx: Sanorex

Chemical Class: Imidazoline derivative

Therapeutic Class: Anorexiant

DEA Class: Schedule IV

CLINICAL PHARMACOLOGY

Mechanism of Action: An isoindole that stimulates the central nervous system and primarily exerting its effect on the limbic system. ***Therapeutic Effect:*** Stimulates the hypothalamus to reduce appetite.

Pharmacokinetics

Slow but complete absorption. Protein binding: greater than 99%. Metabolized in liver to metabolites. Primarily excreted in urine as well as feces. Unknown if removed by hemodialysis. ***Half-life:*** 30-50 hrs.

INDICATIONS AND DOSAGES

Obesity

PO

Adults. 1 mg/day. Maximum: 3 mg/day.

AVAILABLE FORMS

• *Tablets:* 1 mg, 2 mg (Sanorex).

UNLABELED USES: Narcolepsy

CONTRAINDICATIONS: Agitated states, glaucoma, history of drug abuse, symptomatic cardiovascular disease (arrhythmias), coadministration with or within 14 days of MAOI therapy, hypersensitivity to mazindol

PREGNANCY AND LACTATION: Pregnancy category C

SIDE EFFECTS

Occasional

Insomnia, headache, tachycardia, palpitations, tremors, nervousness, restlessness, dry mouth, constipation

Rare

Blurred vision, impotence, insulin sensitivity, rash, sweating, weakness

SERIOUS REACTIONS

• Overdosage includes symptoms of irritability, agitation, hyperactivity, tachycardia, arrhythmia, tachypnea.

INTERACTIONS

Drugs

3 *Furazolidone:* Hypertensive crisis

3 *Guanethidine:* Decreased antihypertensive effects

2 *MAOIs:* Hypertensive crisis

3 *Pressor amines:* Potentiates the pressor effect of these agents

2 *Sympathomimetics:* May increase the risk of hypertension and tachycardia

3 *Tricyclic antidepressants:* Decreased anorexiant effects

Labs

• *False positive:* Chlordiazepoxide, flurazepam, methadone, methapyrilene, methylphenidate, phendimetrazine

SPECIAL CONSIDERATIONS

PATIENT/FAMILY EDUCATION

• May cause insomnia; avoid taking late in the day

• Use caution while driving or performing other tasks requiring alertness; may cause dizziness or blurred vision

• Take with food if stomach upset occurs

• Do not discontinue abruptly

• Mazindol is not for long-term use

MONITORING PARAMETERS

• Blood glucose

• Weight

mebendazole

(me-ben′-da-zole)

Rx: Vermox

Chemical Class: Benzimidazole derivative

Therapeutic Class: Antihelmintic

CLINICAL PHARMACOLOGY

Mechanism of Action: A synthetic benzimidazole derivative that degrades parasite cytoplasmic microtubules and irreversibly blocks glucose uptake in helminths and larvae. Vermicidal. ***Therapeutic Effect:*** Depletes glycogen, decreases ATP, causes helminth death.

Pharmacokinetics

Poorly absorbed from GI tract (absorption increases with food). Metabolized in liver. Primarily eliminated in feces. ***Half-life:*** 2.5-9 hrs (half-life increased with impaired renal function).

INDICATIONS AND DOSAGES

Trichuriasis, ascariasis, hookworm

PO

Adults, Elderly, Children older than 2 yrs. 1 tablet in morning and at bedtime for 3 days.

Enterobiasis

PO

Adults, Elderly, Children older than 2 yrs: 1 tablet one time.

AVAILABLE FORMS

• *Tablets, chewable:* 100 mg (Vermox).

UNLABELED USES: Ancylostoma duodenale or Necator americanus

CONTRAINDICATIONS: Hypersensitivity to mebendazole or any component of the formulation

PREGNANCY AND LACTATION: Pregnancy category C; consider treatment if the parasite is causing clinical disease or may cause public health problems; it is doubtful that enough mebendazole is absorbed to be excreted into breast milk in significant quantities

SIDE EFFECTS

Occasional

Nausea, vomiting, headache, dizziness, transient abdominal pain, diarrhea with massive infection and expulsion of helminths

Rare

Fever

SERIOUS REACTIONS

• High dosage may produce reversible myelosuppression (granulocytopenia, leukopenia, neutropenia).

INTERACTIONS

Drugs

3 *Carbamazepine:* Decreased mebendazole concentrations and effect via induction of metabolism

2 *Phenytoin:* Decreased mebendazole concentrations; possible impairment of therapeutic effect

SPECIAL CONSIDERATIONS

PATIENT/FAMILY EDUCATION

• Chew or crush tablets and administer with food

• Parasite death and removal from digestive tract may take up to 3 days after treatment

• Consult clinician if not cured in 3 wk

• For pinworms, all household contacts of patient should be treated

• Strict hygiene essential to prevent reinfection; disinfect toilet facilities, change and launder undergarments, bed linens, towels, and nightclothes

MONITORING PARAMETERS

• Collect stool or perianal specimens, as required

• CBC with high dosage

mecamylamine hydrochloride

(mek-a-mill'-a-meen hye-droe-klor-ide)

Rx: Inversine

Chemical Class: Ganglionic blocker

Therapeutic Class: Antihypertensive; ganglionic blocker

CLINICAL PHARMACOLOGY

Mechanism of Action: A ganglionic blocker that inhibits acetylcholine at the autonomic ganglia. Blocks central nicotinic cholinergic receptors, which inhibits effects of nicotine. ***Therapeutic Effect:*** Reduces blood pressure; decreases desire to smoke.

Pharmacokinetics

Completely absorbed following PO administration. Widely distributed. Excreted in urine. ***Half-life:*** 24 hrs.

INDICATIONS AND DOSAGES

Hypertension

PO

Adults. Initially, 2.5 mg q12h for 2 days, then increase by 2.5-mg increments at more than 2-day intervals until desired blood pressure is achieved. The average daily dose is 25 mg in 3 divided doses.

Smoking cessation

PO

Adults. Initially, 2.5 mg q12h for 2 days, then increase by 2.5-mg increments during the first week of therapy. Range: 10-20 mg in divided doses.

AVAILABLE FORMS

• *Tablets:* 2.5 mg (Inversine).

UNLABELED USES: Tourette's syndrome, hyperreflexia

CONTRAINDICATIONS: Coronary insufficiency, pyloric stenosis, glaucoma, uremia, recent myocardial infarction, unreliable patients

PREGNANCY AND LACTATION: Pregnancy category C; not recommended in nursing mothers

SIDE EFFECTS

Occasional

Nausea, diarrhea, orthostatic hypotension, tachycardia, drowsiness, urinary retention, blurred vision, dilated pupils, confusion, mental depression, decreased sexual ability, loss of appetite

Rare

Pulmonary edema, pulmonary fibrosis, paresthesias

SERIOUS REACTIONS

• Overdosage includes symptoms such as hypotension, nausea, vomiting, urinary retention and constipation.

INTERACTIONS

Drugs

3 *Alcohol, anesthesia, thiazide diuretics:* May increase the action of these agents

SPECIAL CONSIDERATIONS

PATIENT/FAMILY EDUCATION

• Take after meals

• Arise slowly from reclining position

• Orthostatic changes are exacerbated by alcohol, exercise, hot weather

• Notify the physician if loose bowel movements occur

MONITORING PARAMETERS

• Maintenance doses should be limited to dose that causes slight faintness or dizziness in the standing position

• Blood pressure

• Intake and output, urinary frequency

meclizine hydrochloride

(mek'-li-zeen hye-droe-klor'-ide)

Rx: Antivert, Meclicot, Meni-D

OTC: Bonine

Chemical Class: Piperazine derivative

Therapeutic Class: Antihistamine; antivertigo agent

CLINICAL PHARMACOLOGY

Mechanism of Action: An anticholinergic that reduces labyrinthine excitability and diminishes vestibular stimulation of the labyrinth, affecting the chemoreceptor trigger zone. ***Therapeutic Effect:*** Reduces nausea, vomiting, and vertigo.

Pharmacokinetics

Route	*Onset*	*Peak*	*Duration*
PO	30-60 min	N/A	12-24 hr

Well absorbed from the GI tract. Widely distributed. Metabolized in the liver. Primarily excreted in urine. ***Half-life:*** 6 hr.

INDICATIONS AND DOSAGES

Motion sickness

PO

Adults, Elderly, Children 12 yrs and older. 12.5-25 mg 1 hr before travel. May repeat q12-24h. May require a dose of 50 mg.

Vertigo

PO

Adults, Elderly, Children 12 yrs and older. 25-100 mg/day in divided doses, as needed.

AVAILABLE FORMS

- *Tablets (Antivert, Meclicot, Meni-D):* 12.5 mg, 25 mg, 50 mg.
- *Tablets (Chewable [Bonine]):* 25 mg.

CONTRAINDICATIONS: None known.

PREGNANCY AND LACTATION: Pregnancy category B; used for treatment of nausea and vomiting during pregnancy; excretion into breast milk unknown

SIDE EFFECTS

Frequent

Drowsiness

Occasional

Blurred vision; dry mouth, nose, or throat

SERIOUS REACTIONS

- A hypersensitivity reaction, marked by eczema, pruritus, rash, cardiac disturbances, and photosensitivity, may occur.
- Overdose may produce CNS depression (manifested as sedation, apnea, cardiovascular collapse, or death) or severe paradoxical reactions (such as hallucinations, tremor, and seizures).
- Children may experience paradoxical reactions, including restlessness, insomnia, euphoria, nervousness, and tremors.
- Overdose in children may result in hallucinations, seizures, and death.

INTERACTIONS

Drugs

3 *Alcohol, CNS depressants:* May increase CNS depressant effect

SPECIAL CONSIDERATIONS

PATIENT/FAMILY EDUCATION

- Meclizine commonly causes dizziness, drowsiness, and dry mouth
- Avoid tasks that require mental alertness or motor skills until response to the drug has been established
- Avoid alcohol during meclizine therapy
- Take sips of tepid water and chew sugarless gum to help relieve dry mouth

MONITORING PARAMETERS

- Blood pressure, especially in elderly patients, who are at increased risk for hypotension

- Electrolytes
- Hydration status

meclofenamate sodium

(me-kloe-fen'-a-mate soe'-dee-um)

Chemical Class: Anthranilic acid derivative

Therapeutic Class: NSAID; antipyretic; nonnarcotic analgesic

CLINICAL PHARMACOLOGY

Mechanism of Action: A nonsteroidal antiinflammatory drug that inhibits prostaglandin synthesis by decreasing activity of the enzyme, cyclooxygenase, which results in decreased formation of prostaglandin precursors. ***Therapeutic Effect:*** Reduces inflammatory response and intensity of pain stimulus reaching sensory nerve endings.

Pharmacokinetics

PO route, onset 15 mins, peak 0.5-1.5 hrs, duration 2-4 hrs. Completely absorbed from the gastrointestinal (GI) tract. Widely distributed. Protein binding: greater than 99%. Metabolized in liver. Primarily excreted in urine and feces as metabolites. Not removed by hemodialysis. ***Half-life:*** 2-3.3 hrs.

INDICATIONS AND DOSAGES

Mild to moderate pain

PO

Adults, Elderly. 50 mg q4-6h as needed.

Excessive menstrual blood loss and primary dysmenorrhea

PO

Adults, Elderly. 100 mg 3 times/day for 6 days, starting at the onset of menstrual flow.

Rheumatoid arthritis, osteoarthritis

PO

Adults, Elderly. 200-400 mg 3-4 times/day.

AVAILABLE FORMS

- *Capsules:* 50 mg, 100 mg.

CONTRAINDICATIONS: Active peptic ulcer disease, chronic inflammation of GI tract, GI bleeding disorders, GI ulceration, history of hypersensitivity to aspirin or NSAIDs

PREGNANCY AND LACTATION: Pregnancy category B (category D if used in third trimester); may inhibit labor and prolong pregnancy, cause constriction of the ductus arteriosus *in utero,* or cause persistent pulmonary hypertension of the newborn

SIDE EFFECTS

Frequent (33%-10%)

Diarrhea, nausea, abdominal cramping/pain, dyspepsia (heartburn, indigestion, epigastric pain)

Occasional (9%-1%)

Flatulence, rash, dizziness

Rare (less than 1%)

Constipation, anorexia, stomatitis, headache, ringing in the ears, rash

SERIOUS REACTIONS

- Overdosage may result in headache, seizure, vomiting, and cerebral edema.
- Peptic ulcer disease, GI bleeding, gastritis, severe hepatic reactions, such as jaundice, nephrotoxicity, marked by hematuria, dysuria, proteinuria, and severe hypersensitivity reaction, including bronchospasm, and facial edema occur rarely.

INTERACTIONS

Drugs

3 *Aminoglycosides:* Reduced clearance with elevated aminoglycoside levels and potential for toxicity (especially indomethacin in premature infants; other NSAIDs probably)

M

3 *Anticoagulants:* Excessive hypoprothrombinemia, decreased platelet aggregation with increased risk of GI bleeding

3 *Antihypertensives (α-blockers, angiotensin-converting enzyme inhibitors, angiotensin II receptor blockers, β-blockers, diuretics):* Inhibition of antihypertensive and other favorable hemodynamic effects

3 *Aspirin:* May lower meclofenamate sodium plasma levels

3 *Corticosteroids:* Increased risk of GI ulceration

3 *Cyclosporine:* Increased nephrotoxicity risk

3 *Lithium:* Decreased clearance of lithium (mediated via prostaglandins) resulting in elevated serum lithium levels and risk of toxicity

3 *Methotrexate:* Decreased renal secretion of methotrexate resulting in elevated methotrexate levels and risk of toxicity

3 *Phenylpropanolamine:* Possible acute hypertensive reaction

3 *Potassium-sparing diuretics:* Additive hyperkalemia potential

3 *Triamterene:* Acute renal failure reported with addition of indomethacin; caution with other NSAIDs

SPECIAL CONSIDERATIONS

- No significant advantage over other NSAIDs; cost should govern use

PATIENT/FAMILY EDUCATION

- Swallow capsules whole and do not open, chew, or crush capsules
- Avoid alcohol and aspirin during meclofenamate therapy
- Notify the physician if edema, GI distress, headache, rash, signs of bleeding, or visual disturbances occurs
- The female patient should notify the physician if she suspects pregnancy or if she plans to become pregnant

MONITORING PARAMETERS

- Initial hemogram and fecal occult blood test within 3 mo of starting regular chronic therapy; repeat every 6-12 mo (more frequently in high-risk patients [>65 years, peptic ulcer disease, concurrent steroids or anticoagulants]); electrolytes, creatinine, and BUN within 3 mo of starting regular chronic therapy; repeat every 6-12 mo

---

medroxyprogesterone acetate

(me-drox'-ee-proe-jes'-te-rone as'-eh-tayte)

Rx: Depo-Provera, Depo-Provera Contraceptive, Depo-SubQ-Provera 104, Provera

Combinations

Rx: with estradiol (Lunelle)

Chemical Class: 17α-hydroxyprogesterone derivative

Therapeutic Class: Antineoplastic; contraceptive; progestin

CLINICAL PHARMACOLOGY

Mechanism of Action: A hormone that transforms endometrium from proliferative to secretory in an estrogen-primed endometrium. Inhibits secretion of pituitary gonadotropins. ***Therapeutic Effect:*** Prevents follicular maturation and ovulation. Stimulates growth of mammary alveolar tissue and relaxes uterine smooth muscle. Corrects hormonal imbalance.

Pharmacokinetics

Slowly absorbed after IM administration. Protein binding: 90%. Metabolized in the liver. Primarily excreted in urine. ***Half-life:*** 30 days.

INDICATIONS AND DOSAGES

Hormone replacement therapy

PO

Adults. 5-10 mg for 12-14 consecutive days a month, beginning on day 1 or 16 of cycle given as part of regimen with conjugated estrogens.

Endometrial hyperplasia

PO

Adults. 2.5-10 mg/day for 14 days.

Secondary amenorrhea

PO

Adults. 5-10 mg/day for 5-10 days, beginning at any time during menstrual cycle or 2.5 mg/day.

Abnormal uterine bleeding

PO

Adults. 5-10 mg/day for 5-10 days, beginning on calculated day 16 or day 21 of menstrual cycle.

Endometrial, renal carcinoma

IM

Adults, Elderly. Initially, 400-1000 mg; repeat at 1-wk intervals. If improvement occurs and disease is stabilized, begin maintenance with as little as 400 mg/mo.

Pregnancy prevention

IM (Depo-Provera)

Adults. 150 mg q3mo.

Subcutaneous (Depo-SubQ-Provera 104)

Adults. 104 mg q3mo (q12-14wk).

AVAILABLE FORMS

- *Tablets (Provera):* 2.5 mg, 5 mg, 10 mg.
- *Injection:* 104 mg/0.65 ml prefilled syringe (Depo-SubQ-Provera 104), 150 mg/ml (Depo-Provera Contraceptive), 400 mg/ml (Depo-Provera).

UNLABELED USES: Hormone replacement therapy in estrogen-treated menopausal women, treatment of endometriosis

CONTRAINDICATIONS: Carcinoma of breast; estrogen-dependent neoplasm; history of or active thrombotic disorders, such as cerebral apoplexy, thrombophlebitis, or thromboembolic disorders; hypersensitivity to progestins; known or suspected pregnancy; missed abortion; severe hepatic dysfunction; undiagnosed abnormal genital bleeding; use as pregnancy test

PREGNANCY AND LACTATION: Pregnancy category X; compatible with breast-feeding

SIDE EFFECTS

Frequent

Transient menstrual abnormalities (including spotting, change in menstrual flow or cervical secretions, and amenorrhea) at initiation of therapy

Occasional

Edema, weight change, breast tenderness, nervousness, insomnia, fatigue, dizziness

Rare

Alopecia, depression, dermatologic changes, headache, fever, nausea

SERIOUS REACTIONS

- Thrombophlebitis, pulmonary or cerebral embolism, and retinal thrombosis occur rarely.
- Women who use medroxyprogesterone injection may lose significant bone mineral density.

INTERACTIONS

Drugs

3 *Aminoglutethimide:* Reduced plasma medroxyprogesterone concentrations

3 *Bromocriptine:* May interfere with the effects of bromocriptine

Labs

- *Feces:* Green color

SPECIAL CONSIDERATIONS

PATIENT/FAMILY EDUCATION

- Take protective measures against exposure to ultraviolet light
- Diabetic patients must monitor blood glucose carefully during therapy

- Take with food if GI upset occurs
- When used as contraceptive, menstrual cycle may be disrupted and irregular and unpredictable bleeding or spotting results; usually decreases to the point of amenorrhea as treatment continues (55% at 1 yr)
- After stopping injections, 50% of women who become pregnant will do so in about 10 mo after the last injection, 93% within 18 mo; not related to length of time drug used; women with lower body weights conceive sooner
- Failure rate 0.3% in first year of constant use
- Immediately report chest pain, migraine headache, numbness of an arm or leg, sudden decrease in vision, sudden shortness of breath, and pain, redness, swelling, or warmth in the calf

MONITORING PARAMETERS
- Blood pressure
- Skin for rash
- Weight

mefenamic acid

(me-fe-nam′-ik as′-id)

Rx: Ponstel

Chemical Class: Anthranilic acid derivative

Therapeutic Class: NSAID; antipyretic; nonnarcotic analgesic

CLINICAL PHARMACOLOGY

Mechanism of Action: A nonsteroidal antiinflammatory drug that produces analgesic and antiinflammatory effect by inhibiting prostaglandin synthesis. ***Therapeutic Effect:*** Reduces inflammatory response and intensity of pain stimulus reaching sensory nerve endings.

Pharmacokinetics

Rapidly absorbed from the gastrointestinal (GI) tract. Protein binding: high. Metabolized in liver. Partially excreted in urine and partially in the feces. Not removed by hemodialysis. ***Half-life:*** 3.5 hrs.

INDICATIONS AND DOSAGES

Mild to moderate pain, lower back pain, dysmenorrhea

PO

Adults, Elderly, Children 14 yrs and older. Initially, 500 mg to start, then 250 mg q4h as needed. Maximum: 1 wk of therapy.

AVAILABLE FORMS
- *Capsules:* 250 mg (Ponstel).

UNLABELED USES: Cataract prevention, menorrhagia, osteoarthritis, premenstrual syndrome, rheumatoid arthritis

CONTRAINDICATIONS: History of hypersensitivity to aspirin or NSAIDs, pregnancy

PREGNANCY AND LACTATION: Pregnancy category C (category D if used in third trimester)

SIDE EFFECTS

Occasional (10%-1%)

Dyspepsia, including heartburn, indigestion, flatulence, abdominal cramping, constipation, nausea, diarrhea, epigastric pain, vomiting, headache, nervousness, dizziness, bleeding, elevated liver function tests, tinnitus

Rare (less than 1%)

Fluid retention, arrhythmias, tachycardia, confusion, drowsiness, rash, dry eyes, blurred vision, hot flashes

SERIOUS REACTIONS
- Peptic ulcer, GI bleeding, gastritis, and severe hepatic reaction, such as cholestasis and jaundice, occur rarely.
- Nephrotoxicity, including dysuria, hematuria, proteinuria, and nephrotic syndrome and severe hy-

persensitivity reaction, marked by bronchospasm, and angioedema occur rarely.

INTERACTIONS

Drugs

3 *Aminoglycosides:* Reduced clearance with elevated aminoglycoside levels and potential for toxicity (especially indomethacin in premature infants; other NSAIDs probably)

3 *Anticoagulants:* Excessive hypoprothrombinemia, decreased platelet aggregation with increased risk of GI bleeding

3 *Antihypertensives (α-blockers, angiotensin-converting enzyme inhibitors, angiotensin II receptor blockers, β-blockers, diuretics):* Inhibition of antihypertensive and other favorable hemodynamic effects

3 *Corticosteroids:* Increased risk of GI ulceration

3 *Cyclosporine:* Increased nephrotoxicity risk

3 *Lithium:* Decreased clearance of lithium (mediated via prostaglandins) resulting in elevated serum lithium levels and risk of toxicity

2 *Methotrexate:* Decreased renal secretion of methotrexate resulting in elevated methotrexate levels and risk of toxicity

3 *Phenylpropanolamine:* Possible acute hypertensive reaction

3 *Potassium-sparing diuretics:* Additive hyperkalemia potential

3 *Triamterene:* Acute renal failure reported with addition of indomethacin; caution with other NSAIDs

SPECIAL CONSIDERATIONS

- No significant advantage over other NSAIDs; cost should govern use
- Use beyond 1 wk is not recommended

PATIENT/FAMILY EDUCATION

- Avoid alcohol and aspirin during mefenamic acid therapy
- Swallow capsules whole
- Take the drug with food if GI upset occurs
- The female patient should inform the physician if she suspects pregnancy or plans to become pregnant

MONITORING PARAMETERS

- Initial hemogram and fecal occult blood test within 3 mo of starting regular chronic therapy; repeat 6-12 mo (more frequently in high-risk patients [>65 years, peptic ulcer disease, concurrent steroids or anticoagulants]); electrolytes, creatinine, and BUN within 3 mo of starting regular chronic therapy; repeat every 6-12 mo

mefloquine hydrochloride

(me′-floe-kwin hye-droe-klor′-ide)

Rx: Lariam

Chemical Class: Quinolinemethanol derivative

Therapeutic Class: Antimalarial

CLINICAL PHARMACOLOGY

Mechanism of Action: A quinolone-methanol compound structurally similar to quinine that destroys the asexual blood forms of malarial pathogens, *Plasmodium falciparum, P. vivax, P. malariae, P. ovale*. ***Therapeutic Effect:*** Inhibits parasite growth.

Pharmacokinetics

Well absorbed from the gastrointestinal (GI) tract. Protein binding: 98%. Widely distributed, including cerebrospinal fluid (CSF). Metabolized in liver. Primarily excreted in urine. ***Half-life:*** 21-22 days.

INDICATIONS AND DOSAGES

Suppression of malaria

PO

Adults. 250 mg base weekly starting 1 wk before travel, continuing weekly during travel and for 4 wks after leaving endemic area.

Children more than 45 kg. 250 mg weekly starting 1 wk before travel, continuing weekly during travel and for 4 wks after leaving endemic area.

Children 45-31 kg. 187.5 mg (¾ tablet) weekly starting 1 wk before travel, continuing weekly during travel and for 4 wks after leaving endemic area.

Children 30-20 kg. 125 mg (½ tablet) weekly starting 1 wk before travel, continuing weekly during travel and for 4 wks after leaving endemic area.

Children 19-15 kg. 62.5 mg (¼ tablet) weekly starting 1 wk before travel, continuing weekly during travel and for 4 wks after leaving endemic area.

Treatment of malaria

PO

Adults. 1250 mg as a single dose.

Children. 15-25 mg/kg in a single dose. Maximum: 1250 mg.

AVAILABLE FORMS

- *Tablets:* 250 mg.

CONTRAINDICATIONS: Cardiac abnormalities, severe psychiatric disorders, epilepsy, history of hypersensitivity to mefloquine

PREGNANCY AND LACTATION: Pregnancy category C; use caution during the first 12-14 wks of pregnancy; excreted in breast milk in amounts not thought to be harmful to the nursing infant and insufficient to provide adequate protection against malaria

SIDE EFFECTS

Occasional

Mild transient headache, difficulty concentrating, insomnia, lightheadedness, vertigo, diarrhea, nausea, vomiting, visual disturbances, tinnitus

Rare

Aggressive behavior, anxiety, bradycardia, depression, hallucinations, hypotension, panic attacks, paranoia, psychosis, syncope, tremor

SERIOUS REACTIONS

- Prolonged therapy may result in peripheral neuritis, neuromyopathy, hypotension, electrocardiogram (EKG) changes, agranulocytosis, aplastic anemia, thrombocytopenia, seizures, and psychosis.
- Overdosage may result in headache, vomiting, visual disturbance, drowsiness, and seizures.

INTERACTIONS

Drugs

3 *β-blockers:* Increased risk of bradycardia

SPECIAL CONSIDERATIONS

PATIENT/FAMILY EDUCATION

- Do not take on an empty stomach
- Take medication with at least 8 oz water
- Caution, initially, when driving, operating machinery, where concentration necessary
- Promptly report any visual disturbances

MONITORING PARAMETERS

- Liver function tests and ophthalmic examinations during prolonged therapy

megestrol acetate

(me-jess'-trole as'-eh-tayte)

Rx: Megace, Megace ES

Chemical Class: Progestin derivative

Therapeutic Class: Antineoplastic; appetite stimulant

CLINICAL PHARMACOLOGY

Mechanism of Action: A hormone and antineoplastic agent that suppresses the release of luteinizing hormone from the anterior pituitary gland by inhibiting pituitary function. ***Therapeutic Effect:*** Shrinks tumors. Also increases appetite by an unknown mechanism.

Pharmacokinetics

Well absorbed from the GI tract. Metabolized in the liver; excreted in urine. ***Half-life:*** 13-105 hr (mean 34 hr).

INDICATIONS AND DOSAGES

Palliative treatment of advanced breast cancer

PO

Adults, Elderly. 160 mg/day in 4 equally divided doses.

Palliative treatment of advanced endometrial carcinoma

PO

Adults, Elderly. 40-320 mg/day in divided doses. Maximum: 800 mg/day in 1-4 divided doses.

Anorexia, cachexia, weight loss

PO

Adults, Elderly. 800 mg (20 ml)/day.

PO (Megace ES)

Adults, Elderly. 625 mg/day.

AVAILABLE FORMS

- *Tablets (Megace):* 20 mg, 40 mg.
- *Suspension:* 40 mg/ml (Megace), 625 mg/5 ml (equivalent to 800 mg/20 ml) (Megace ES).

UNLABELED USES: Appetite stimulant, treatment of hormone-dependent or advanced prostate carcinoma, treatment of uterine bleeding

CONTRAINDICATIONS: Suspension: Known or suspected pregnancy

PREGNANCY AND LACTATION: Pregnancy category X; not recommended during the first 4 mos of pregnancy

SIDE EFFECTS

Frequent

Weight gain secondary to increased appetite

Occasional

Nausea, breakthrough bleeding, backache, headache, breast tenderness, carpal tunnel syndrome

Rare

Feeling of coldness

SERIOUS REACTIONS

- Thrombophlebitis and pulmonary embolism occur rarely.

SPECIAL CONSIDERATIONS

- Average weight gain in AIDS patients 11 lbs in 12 wk. Begin therapy only after treatable causes of weight loss are sought and addressed
- Contraception is imperative during megestrol therapy
- Notify the physician if calf pain, difficulty breathing, or vaginal bleeding occurs
- Megestrol may cause backache, breast tenderness, headache, nausea, and vomiting

MONITORING PARAMETERS

- Signs and symptoms of a therapeutic response to the drug

meloxicam

(mel-ox'-i-kam)

Rx: Mobic

Chemical Class: Oxicam derivative

Therapeutic Class: NSAID; antipyretic; nonnarcotic analgesic

CLINICAL PHARMACOLOGY

Mechanism of Action: An NSAID that produces analgesic and antiinflammatory effects by inhibiting prostaglandin synthesis. ***Therapeutic Effect:*** Reduces the inflammatory response and intensity of pain.

Pharmacokinetics

Route	*Onset*	*Peak*	*Duration*
PO (analgesic)	30 min	4-5 hr	N/A

Well absorbed after PO administration. Protein binding: 99%. Metabolized in the liver. Eliminated in urine and feces. Not removed by hemodialysis. ***Half-life:*** 15-20 hrs.

INDICATIONS AND DOSAGES

Osteoarthritis, rheumatoid arthritis

PO

Adults. Initially, 7.5 mg/day. Maximum: 15 mg/day.

AVAILABLE FORMS

- *Tablets:* 7.5 mg, 15 mg.
- *Oral Suspension:* 7.5 mg/5 ml.

UNLABELED USES: Ankylosing spondylitis

CONTRAINDICATIONS: Aspirin-induced nasal polyps associated with bronchospasm

PREGNANCY AND LACTATION: Pregnancy category C (D if used in third trimester or near delivery); animal studies document both teratogenic and nonteratongenic (premature PDA closure) in animals; no studies in humans; no human studies on breast milk excretion; in rats, milk concentrations are twice that of plasma

SIDE EFFECTS

Frequent (9%-7%)

Dyspepsia, headache, diarrhea, nausea

Occasional (4%-3%)

Dizziness, insomnia, rash, pruritus, flatulence, constipation, vomiting

Rare (less than 2%)

Somnolence, urticaria, photosensitivity, tinnitus

SERIOUS REACTIONS

- Rare reactions with long-term use include peptic ulcer disease, GI bleeding, gastritis, severe hepatic reaction (jaundice), nephrotoxicity (hematuria, dysuria, proteinuria), and a severe hypersensitivity reaction (bronchospasm, angioedema).

INTERACTIONS

Drugs

❷ *Anticoagulants (heparin, low-molecular-weight heparin, warfarin, etc.):* Increased risk of hematoma and major and minor bleeding

❷ *Aspirin:* Increased risk of GI ulceration, especially with high dose aspirin; potential negation of protective cardiac effects

3 *ACE inhibitors, angiotensin II receptor blockers:* Diminished antihypertensive effect

3 *β-blockers:* Diminished antihypertensive effect

3 *Cholestyramine:* Increases clearance of meloxicam (50%), with reduction in $t_{1/2}$ and AUC

3 *Corticosteroids:* Additive effects; increased risk of GI bleeding, sodium/water retention

3 *Cyclosporine:* Additive nephrotoxicity

3 *Diuretics:* Reduced natriuretic effects

3 *Ginkgo biloba:* May increase the risk of bleeding

❷ *Lithium:* Addition of meloxicam may result in increased lithium blood levels (21%)

❷ *Warfarin:* Additive effects on coagulation; prothrombin times as INR have increased with the addition of meloxicam

Labs

• *Guaiac (Hemoccult) assay:* False positives

SPECIAL CONSIDERATIONS

• Partial, not pure, COX-2 selective inhibitor; most studies have compared it with non-selective agents, making final assessment of place in therapy difficult

PATIENT/FAMILY EDUCATION

• Take with food or milk; report gastrointestinal adverse effects

• The female patient should inform the physician if she suspects pregnancy or plans to become pregnant

• Avoid tasks that require mental alertness or motor skills until response to the drug has been established

MONITORING PARAMETERS

• Acute phase reactants for efficacy in rheumatoid arthritis; pain, stiffness, number of swollen joints, range of motion, functional capacity, structural damage, fecal occult blood, hemogram, renal and hepatic function

memantine hydrochloride

(mem'-an-teen hye-droe-klor'-ide)

Rx: Namenda

Chemical Class: Adamantane derivative; tricyclic amine

Therapeutic Class: Antidementia agent

CLINICAL PHARMACOLOGY

Mechanism of Action: A neurotransmitter inhibitor that decreases the effects of glutamate, the principle excitatory neurotransmitter in the brain. Persistent CNS excitation by glutamate is thought to cause the symptoms of Alzheimer's disease. ***Therapeutic Effect:*** May reduce clinical deterioration in moderate to severe Alzheimer's disease.

Pharmacokinetics

Rapidly and completely absorbed after PO administration. Protein binding: 45%. Undergoes little metabolism; most of the dose is excreted unchanged in urine. ***Half-life:*** 60-80 hr.

INDICATIONS AND DOSAGES

Alzheimer's disease

PO

Adults, Elderly. Initially, 5 mg once a day. May increase dosage at intervals of at least 1 wk in 5-mg increments to 10 mg/day (5 mg twice a day), then 15 mg/day (5 mg and 10 mg as separate doses), and finally 20 mg/day (10 mg twice a day). Target dose: 20 mg/day.

AVAILABLE FORMS

• *Tablets:* 5 mg, 10 mg.

• *Oral Solution:* 2 mg/ml.

CONTRAINDICATIONS: Severe renal impairment

PREGNANCY AND LACTATION: Pregnancy category B; breast milk excretion unknown

M

SIDE EFFECTS

Occasional (7%-4%)

Dizziness, headache, confusion, constipation, hypertension, cough

Rare (3%-2%)

Back pain, nausea, fatigue, anxiety, peripheral edema, arthralgia, insomnia

SERIOUS REACTIONS

• None known.

INTERACTIONS

Drugs

3 *Carbonic anhydrase inhibitors (acetazolamide, dichlorphenamide, methazolamide):* Memantine renal clearance reduced by 80% under alkaline urine conditions (pH 8)

3 *Cimetidine, hydrochlorothiazide, nicotine, quinidine, ranitidine:* May alter plasma levels of both drugs

SPECIAL CONSIDERATIONS

• Combination memantine-donepezil more likely to show a smaller decline or an improvement

PATIENT/FAMILY EDUCATION

• Twice daily for doses above 5 mg and minimum interval, 1 wk dose escalation

• Do not abruptly discontinue memantine or adjust the drug dosage

• If therapy is interrupted for several days, restart the drug at the lowest dose and increase the dosage at intervals of at least 1 wk to the most recent dose, as prescribed

• Maintain adequate fluid intake

MONITORING PARAMETERS

• *Efficacy:* Improvement or maintenance of mental status and functional quality of life scales

• *Toxicity:* Pharmacotoxic psychosis (hallucinations, nervousness, changes in behavior, tremor, akathisia, restlessness, increased motor activity, insomnia, depression)

• Renal function, urine pH because alkaline urine may lead to an accumulation of the drug and a possible increase in side effects

menotropins

(men-oh-troe'-pins)

Rx: Humegon, Pergonal, Repronex

Chemical Class: Human pituitary gonadotropins, purified

Therapeutic Class: Ovulation stimulant

CLINICAL PHARMACOLOGY

Mechanism of Action: A mixture of equal activity of follicle stimulating hormone (FSH) and luteinizing hormone (LH) that are isolated from the urine of postmenopausal women and are necessary for the development, maturation, and release of ova from ovaries and for spermatogenesis in the testes. ***Therapeutic Effect:*** Promotes ovulation and pregnancy in infertile women.

Pharmacokinetics

Not absorbed from the gastrointestinal (GI) tract. Cleared from circulation by glomular filtration. Degraded in proximal tubule or excreted unchanged in urine. ***Half-life:*** 2.2-2.9 hr.

INDICATIONS AND DOSAGES

Follicle maturation, ovulation and pregnancy induction

IM

Adults. Initially, 75 International Units (IU) daily for 7-12 days followed by hCG, 5000-10,000 units one day after the last dose of menotropins. Treat until indices of estrogen activity are equivalent to or greater than those of the normal individual. If signs of ovulation are present but pregnancy does not occur, repeat this dosage regimen for at least 2 more courses before increasing the dose of menotropins.

Follicle maturation, ovulation and pregnancy induction

IM

Adults. After 3 course failures at 75 IU, increase dose to 150 IU daily for 7-12 days followed by 5000-10,000 units of hCG 1 day after the last dose of menotropins. If signs of ovulation are present but pregnancy does not develop, repeat the same dose for 2 more courses.

Stimulation of spermatogenesis

IM

Adults. Pretreatment with 5000 units hCG 3 times weekly is required prior to initiating concomitant therapy with menotropins. Continue pretreatment until serum testosterone levels are in the normal range and masculinization is reached (may require 4-6 mos); then initiate therapy with menotropins 75 IU 3 times weekly and 2000 units hCG twice weekly for a minimum of 4 mos. If the patient has not responded after 4 mos, continue treatment with 75 IU menotropins 3 times weekly or increase dose to 150 IU 3 times weekly, keeping the dose for hCG the same.

AVAILABLE FORMS

• *Injection:* 75 units FSH activity and 150 units LH activity/2 ml ampule (Humegon, Pergonal, Repronex), 150 units FSH activity and 150 units LH activity/2 ml ampule (Humegon, Pergonal, Repronex).

CONTRAINDICATIONS: Prior hypersensitivity to menotropins

Women: Known or suspected pregnancy, high FSH level indicating primary ovarian failure, abnormal bleeding of undetermined origin, an organic intracranial lesion such as a pituitary tumor, elevated gonadotropin levels indicating primary testicular failure, presence of any cause of infertility other than anovulation, unless they are candidates for in vitro fertilization, ovarian cysts or enlargement not due to polycystic ovary syndrome, uncontrolled thyroid and adrenal dysfunction

Men: Infertility disorders other than hypogonadotropic hypogonadism, normal gonadotropin levels indicating normal pituitary function

PREGNANCY AND LACTATION: Pregnancy category X

SIDE EFFECTS

Occasional

Women: Abdominal pain, bloating, diarrhea, nausea, vomiting, body rash, dizziness, dyspnea, tachypnea, ovarian cysts, ovarian enlargement, pain, rash, swelling at injection site, tachycardia

Men: Gynecomastia

SERIOUS REACTIONS

• Acute respiratory distress syndrome, atelectasis, pulmonary embolism, pulmonary infarction, arterial occlusion, cerebral vascular occlusion, venous thrombophlebitis, congenital abnormalities, ectopic pregnancy, and ovarian hyperstimulation syndrome have been reported.

SPECIAL CONSIDERATIONS

PATIENT/FAMILY EDUCATION

• Multiple births occur in approximately 20% of women treated with menotropins and HCG

• Couple should engage in intercourse daily, beginning on the day prior to HCG administration, until ovulation occurs

• Ovarian enlargement regresses without treatment in 2-3 wk

MONITORING PARAMETERS

• Urinary estrogen; do not administer HCG if >150 mcg/24 hr (increased risk of hyperstimulation of ovaries syndrome)

• Sonographic visualization of ovaries; estradiol levels

meperidine hydrochloride

(me-per'-i-deen hye-droe-klor'-ide)

Rx: Demerol

Combinations

Rx: with promethazine (Mepergan)

Chemical Class: Opiate derivative; phenylpiperidine derivative

Therapeutic Class: Narcotic analgesic

DEA Class: Schedule II

CLINICAL PHARMACOLOGY

Mechanism of Action: An opioid agonist that binds to opioid receptors in the CNS. ***Therapeutic Effect:*** Alters the perception of and emotional response to pain.

Pharmacokinetics

Route	Onset	Peak	Duration
PO	15 min	60 min	2-4 hr
IV	less than 5 min	5-7 min	2-3 hr
IM	10-15 min	30-50 min	2-4 hr
Subcutaneous	10-15 min	30-50 min	2-4 hr

Variably absorbed from the GI tract; well absorbed after IM administration. Protein binding: 60%-80%. Widely distributed. Metabolized in the liver to active metabolite. Primarily excreted in urine. Not removed by hemodialysis. ***Half-life:*** 2.4-4 hr; metabolite 8-16 hr (increased in hepatic impairment and disease).

INDICATIONS AND DOSAGES

Analgesia

PO, IM, Subcutaneous

Adults, Elderly. 50-150 mg q3-4h.

Children. 1.1-1.5 mg/kg q3-4h. Do not exceed single dose of 100 mg.

Patient-controlled analgesia (PCA)

IV

Adults. Loading dose: 50-100 mg. Intermittent bolus: 5-30 mg. Lockout interval: 10-20 min. Continuous infusion: 5-40 mg/hr. Maximum (4-hr): 200-300 mg.

Dosage in renal impairment

Dosage is based on creatinine clearance.

Creatinine Clearance	Dosage
10-50 ml/min	75% of usual dose
less than 10 ml/min	50% of usual dose

AVAILABLE FORMS

- *Syrup:* 50 mg/5 ml.
- *Tablets:* 50 mg, 100 mg.
- *Injection:* 10 mg/ml, 25 mg/ml, 50 mg/ml, 75 mg/ml, 100 mg/ml.

CONTRAINDICATIONS: Delivery of premature infant, diarrhea due to poisoning, use within 14 days of MAOIs

PREGNANCY AND LACTATION: Pregnancy category B (category D if used for prolonged periods or in high doses at term); use during labor may produce neonatal respiratory depression; compatible with breast-feeding

Controlled Substance: Schedule II

SIDE EFFECTS

Frequent

Sedation, hypotension (including orthostatic hypotension), diaphoresis, facial flushing, dizziness, nausea, vomiting, constipation

Occasional

Confusion, arrhythmias, tremors, urine retention, abdominal pain, dry mouth, headache, irritation at injection site, euphoria, dysphoria

Rare

Allergic reaction (rash, pruritus), insomnia

SERIOUS REACTIONS

• Overdose results in respiratory depression, skeletal muscle flaccidity, cold or clammy skin, cyanosis, and extreme somnolence progressing to seizures, stupor, and coma. The antidote is 0.4 mg naloxone.

• The patient who uses meperidine repeatedly may develop a tolerance to the drug's analgesic effect and physical dependence.

INTERACTIONS

Drugs

3 *Antihistamines, chloral hydrate, glutethimide, methocarbamol:* Enhanced depressant effects

3 *Barbiturates:* Additive respiratory and CNS depressant effects

3 *Cimetidine:* Increased respiratory and CNS depression

3 *Ethanol:* Additive CNS effects

▲ *MAOIs:* Accumulation of CNS serotonin leading to agitation, blood pressure changes, hyperpyrexia, seizures

3 *Neuroleptics:* Hypotension, excessive CNS depression

3 *Phenytoin:* Enhanced metabolism; reduced meperidine concentrations

❷ *Selegiline:* Though primarily MAO-B inhibitor, residual MAO-A activity; see MAOI description

❷ *Sibutramine:* Increases risk of serotonin syndrome

Labs

• *False increase:* Amylase and lipase

SPECIAL CONSIDERATIONS

PATIENT/FAMILY EDUCATION

• Physical dependency may result when used for extended periods

• Do not administer agonist/antagonist analgesics (i.e., pentazocine, nalbuphine, butorphanol, dezocine, buprenorphine) to patient who has received a prolonged course of meperidine (a pure agonist). In opioid-dependent patients, mixed agonist/antagonist analgesics may precipitate withdrawal symptoms.

• Change position slowly; orthostatic hypotension may occur

• Avoid hazardous activities if drowsiness or dizziness occurs

• Avoid alcohol, other CNS depressants unless directed by clinician

• Minimize nausea by administering with food and remain lying down following dose

• The injection may cause discomfort

• Increase fluid intake and consumption of high-fiber foods to prevent constipation

MONITORING PARAMETERS

• Monitor the patient's vital signs for 15-30 mins after an IM or subcutaneous dose and for 5-10 mins after an IV dose. Be alert for decreased blood pressure, as well as a change in quality and rate of pulse

• Level of pain and sedation

• Pattern of daily bowel activity and stool consistency

• Therapeutic serum drug level is 100-550 ng/ml; toxic serum drug level is greater than 1000 ng/ml

mephobarbital

(me'-foe-bar'-bi-tal)

Rx: Mebaral

Chemical Class: Barbituric acid derivative

Therapeutic Class: Anticonvulsant; sedative/hypnotic

DEA Class: Schedule IV

CLINICAL PHARMACOLOGY

Mechanism of Action: A barbiturate that increases seizure threshold in the motor cortex. ***Therapeutic Effect:*** Depresses monosynaptic and polysynaptic transmission in the central nervous system (CNS).

Pharmacokinetics

PO route onset 20-60 mins, peak N/A, duration 6-8 hrs. Well absorbed after PO administration. Widely distributed. Metabolized in liver to active metabolite, a form of phenobarbital. Minimally excreted in urine. Removed by hemodialysis.

Half-life: 34 hrs.

INDICATIONS AND DOSAGES

Epilepsy

PO

Adults, Elderly. 400-600 mg/day in divided doses or at bedtime.

Children more than 5 yrs. 32-64 mg 3 or 4 times/day.

Children less than 5 yrs. 16 -32 mg 3 or 4 times/day.

Sedation

PO

Adults, Elderly. 32-100 mg/day in 3-4 divided doses.

Children. 16-32 mg in 3-4 divided doses.

AVAILABLE FORMS

- *Tablets:* 32 mg, 50 mg, 100 mg (Mebaral).

CONTRAINDICATIONS: Porphyria, history of hypersensitivity to mephobarbital or other barbituates

PREGNANCY AND LACTATION: Pregnancy category D; has caused major adverse effects in some nursing infants; should be given with caution to nursing women

SIDE EFFECTS

Frequent

Dizziness, lightheadedness, somnolence

Occasional

Confusion, headache, insomnia, mental depression, nervousness, nightmares, unusual excitement

Rare

Rash, paradoxical CNS hyperactivity or nervousness in children, excitement or restlessness in elderly, generally noted during first 2 wks of therapy, particularly noted in presence of uncontrolled pain

SERIOUS REACTIONS

- Abrupt withdrawal after prolonged therapy may produce effects including markedly increased dreaming, nightmares or insomnia, tremor, sweating, vomiting, to hallucinations, delirium, seizures, and status epilepticus.
- Skin eruptions appear as hypersensitivity reaction.
- Blood dyscrasias, liver disease, and hypocalcemia occur rarely.
- Overdosage produces cold or clammy skin, hypothermia, severe CNS depression, cyanosis, rapid pulse, and Cheyne-Stokes respirations.
- Toxicity may result in severe renal impairment.

INTERACTIONS

Drugs

3 *Acetaminophen:* Enhanced hepatotoxic potential of acetaminophen overdoses

3 *Antidepressants:* Reduced serum concentration of cyclic antidepressants

3 *β-adrenergic blockers:* Reduced serum concentrations of β-blockers, which are extensively metabolized

3 *Calcium channel blockers:* Reduced serum concentrations of verapamil and dihydropyridines

3 *Chloramphenicol:* Increased barbiturate concentrations; reduced serum chloramphenicol concentrations

3 *Corticosteroids:* Reduced serum concentrations of corticosteroids; may impair therapeutic effect

3 *Cyclosporine:* Reduced serum concentration of cyclosporine

3 *Digitoxin:* Reduced serum concentration of digitoxin

3 *Disopyramide:* Reduced serum concentration of disopyramide

3 *Doxycycline:* Reduced serum doxycycline concentrations
3 *Estrogen:* Reduced serum concentration of estrogen
3 *Ethanol:* Excessive CNS depression
3 *Griseofulvin:* Reduced griseofulvin absorption
3 *Methoxyflurane:* Enhanced nephrotoxic effect
3 *MAOIs:* Prolonged effect of barbiturates
3 *Narcotic analgesics:* Increased toxicity of meperidine; reduced effect of methadone; additive CNS depression
3 *Neuroleptics:* Reduced effect of either drug
2 *Oral anticoagulants:* Decrease hypoprothrombinemic response to oral anticoagulants
3 *Oral contraceptives:* Reduced efficacy of oral contraceptives
3 *Phenytoin:* Unpredictable effect on serum phenytoin levels
3 *Propafenone:* Reduced serum concentration of propafenone
3 *Quinidine:* Reduced quinidine plasma concentrations
3 *Tacrolimus:* Reduced serum concentration of tacrolimus
3 *Theophylline:* Reduced serum theophylline concentrations
3 *Valproic acid:* Increased serum concentrations of amobarbital
2 *Warfarin:* See oral anticoagulants

Labs

- *Phenobarbital:* Falsely increased result

SPECIAL CONSIDERATIONS

PATIENT/FAMILY EDUCATION

- Avoid driving or other activities requiring alertness
- Avoid alcohol ingestion or CNS depressants
- Do not discontinue medication abruptly after long-term use
- Notify clinician of fever, sore throat, mouth sores, easy bruising or bleeding, broken blood vessels under skin
- Mephobarbital may be habit-forming

MONITORING PARAMETERS

- Periodic CBC, liver and renal function tests, serum folate, vitamin D during prolonged therapy
- Blood pressure, heart rate, respiratory rate
- CNS status

meprobamate

(me-proe'-ba-mate)

Rx: Miltown

Chemical Class: Carbamate derivative

Therapeutic Class: Anxiolytic; sedative/hypnotic

DEA Class: Schedule IV

CLINICAL PHARMACOLOGY

Mechanism of Action: A carbamate derivative that affects the thalamus and limbic system. Appears to inhibit multi-neuronal spinal reflexes. ***Therapeutic Effect:*** Relieves pain or muscle spasms.

Pharmacokinetics

Slowly absorbed from the gastrointestinal (GI) tract. Protein binding: 0%-30%. Metabolized in liver. Excreted in urine and feces. Moderately dialyzable. ***Half-life:*** 10 hrs.

INDICATIONS AND DOSAGES

Anxiety disorders

PO

Adults, Children 12 yrs and older. 400 mg 3-4 times. Maximum: 2400 mg/day.

Children 6-12 yrs. 100-200 mg 2-3 times/day.

Elderly. Use lowest effective dose. 200 mg 2-3 times/day.

Dosage in renal impairment

Creatinine Clearance	*Dosage Interval*
10-50 ml/min	every 9-12 hrs
less than 10 ml/min	every 12-18 hrs

AVAILABLE FORMS

• *Tablets:* 200 mg, 400 mg, 600 mg (Miltown).

UNLABELED USES: Muscle contraction, headache, premenstrual tension, external sphincter spasticity, muscle rigidity, opisthotonos-associated with tetanus

CONTRAINDICATIONS: Acute intermittent porphyria, hypersensitivity to meprobamate or related compounds

PREGNANCY AND LACTATION: Pregnancy category D; excreted into breast milk in concentrations 2-4 times that of maternal plasma; effect on nursing infant unknown

SIDE EFFECTS

Frequent

Drowsiness, dizziness

Occasional

Tachycardia, palpitations, headache, lightheadedness, dermatitis, diarrhea, nausea, vomiting, dyspnea, rash, weakness, blurred vision, wheezing

SERIOUS REACTIONS

• Agranulocytosis, aplastic anemia, leucopenia, anaphylaxis, cardiac arrhythmias, hypotensive crisis, syncope, Stevens-Johnson syndrome, and bullous dermatitis have been reported.

• Overdose may cause CNS depression, ataxia, coma, shock, hypotension, and death.

INTERACTIONS

Drugs

3 *Ethanol:* Enhanced CNS depression

Labs

• *17-Hydroxycorticosteroids:* Urine, increased

• *17-Ketogenic steroids:* Urine, increased

SPECIAL CONSIDERATIONS

PATIENT/FAMILY EDUCATION

• Avoid alcohol

• Do not discontinue abruptly following long-term use

• This drug may cause dizziness or drowsiness

MONITORING PARAMETERS

• Periodic CBC with differential and platelets during prolonged therapy

• Renal function tests, BUN, serum creatinine, liver function tests

• Therapeutic levels range between 6-12 ng/ml

meropenem

(mer-oh-pen′-em)

Rx: Merrem

Chemical Class: Carbapenem

Therapeutic Class: Antibiotic

CLINICAL PHARMACOLOGY

Mechanism of Action: A carbapenem that binds to penicillin-binding proteins and inhibits bacterial cell wall synthesis. ***Therapeutic Effect:*** Produces bacterial cell death.

Pharmacokinetics

After IV administration, widely distributed into tissues and body fluids, including CSF. Protein binding: 2%. Primarily excreted unchanged in urine. Removed by hemodialysis. ***Half-life:*** 1 hr.

INDICATIONS AND DOSAGES

Intraabdominal infections

IV

Adults, Elderly, Children weighing more than 50 kg. 1 g q8h.

Children 3 mo and older, weighing 50 kg and less. 20 mg/kg q8h. Maximum: 1 g q8h.

Meningitis
IV
Adults, Elderly, Children weighing 50 kg or more. 2 g q8h.
Children 3 mo and older weighing less than 50 kg. 40 mg/kg q8h. Maximum: 2 g/dose.

Dosage in renal impairment
Dosage and frequency are modified based on creatinine clearance.

Creatinine Clearance	*Dosage*	*Interval*
26-49 ml/min	Recommended dose (1000 mg)	q12h
10-25 ml/min	½ of recommended dose	q12h
less than 10 ml/min	½ of recommended dose	q24h

AVAILABLE FORMS
- *Powder for Injection:* 500 mg, 1 g.

UNLABELED USES: Lower respiratory tract infections, febrile neutropenia, gynecologic and obstetric infections, sepsis

CONTRAINDICATIONS: History of seizures or CNS abnormality, hypersensitivity to penicillins

PREGNANCY AND LACTATION: Pregnancy category B; unknown if excreted into human milk

SIDE EFFECTS
Frequent (5%-3%)
Diarrhea, nausea, vomiting, headache, inflammation at injection site
Occasional (2%)
Oral candidiasis, rash, pruritus
Rare (less than 2%)
Constipation, glossitis

SERIOUS REACTIONS
- Antibiotic-associated colitis and other superinfections may occur.
- Anaphylactic reactions have been reported.
- Seizures may occur in those with CNS disorders (including brain lesions and a history of seizures), bacterial meningitis, or impaired renal function.

INTERACTIONS
Drugs
3 *Probenecid:* Inhibits renal excretion of meropenem
3 *Valproic acid:* Two reports of decreased valproate concentrations

SPECIAL CONSIDERATIONS
- Less likely to induce seizures than imipenem-cilastin

PATIENT/FAMILY EDUCATION
- Immediately notify the physician if severe diarrhea occurs and avoid taking antidiarrheals until directed to do so
- Notify the physician of troublesome or serious adverse reactions, including infusion site pain, redness, or swelling; nausea or vomiting; or a rash or itching

MONITORING PARAMETERS
- Renal, hepatic, and hematopoietic function during prolonged therapy
- Pattern of daily bowel activity and stool consistency
- Hydration status, and check for nausea and vomiting
- Check the IV injection site for inflammation
- Check skin for a rash
- Electrolyte levels (especially potassium), intake and output, and renal function test results
- Observe the patient's mental status, and be alert for seizures or tremors
- Blood pressure and body temperature at least twice a day

mesalamine/5 aminosalicylic acid/5-ASA)

(mez-al'-a-meen)

Rx: Asacol, Pentasa, Rowasa

Chemical Class: 5-amino derivative of salicylic acid

Therapeutic Class: Gastrointestinal antiinflammatory

CLINICAL PHARMACOLOGY

Mechanism of Action: A salicylic acid derivative that locally inhibits arachidonic acid metabolite production, which is increased in patients with chronic inflammatory bowel disease. ***Therapeutic Effect:*** Blocks prostaglandin production and diminishes inflammation in the colon.

Pharmacokinetics

Poorly absorbed from the colon. Moderately absorbed from the GI tract. Metabolized in the liver to active metabolite. Unabsorbed portion eliminated in feces; absorbed portion excreted in urine. Unknown if removed by hemodialysis. ***Half-life:*** 0.5-1.5 hr; metabolite, 5-10 hr.

INDICATIONS AND DOSAGES

Treatment of ulcerative colitis

PO (capsule)

Adults, Elderly. 1 g 4 times a day.

Children. 50 mg/kg/day divided q6-12h.

PO (tablet)

Adults, Elderly. 800 mg 3 times a day.

Children. 50 mg/kg/day divided q8-12h.

Maintenance of remission in ulcerative colitis

PO (capsule)

Adults, Elderly. 1 g 4 times a day.

PO (tablet)

Adults, Elderly. 1.6 g/day in divided doses.

Distal ulcerative colitis, proctosigmoiditis, proctitis

Rectal (retention enema)

Adults, Elderly. 60 ml (4 g) at bedtime; retained overnight for approximately 8 hrs for 3-6 wks.

Rectal (500-mg suppository)

Adults, Elderly. Twice a day. May increase to 3 times a day.

Rectal (1000-mg suppository)

Adults, Elderly. Once daily at bedtime. Continue therapy for 3-6 wks.

AVAILABLE FORMS

- *Tablets (Delayed-Release [Asacol]):* 400 mg.
- *Capsules (Controlled-Release [Pentasa]):* 250 mg.
- *Rectal Suspension (Rowasa):* 4 g/60 ml.
- *Suppositories (Canasa):* 500 mg, 1 g.

CONTRAINDICATIONS: None known.

PREGNANCY AND LACTATION: Pregnancy category B; has produced adverse effects in a nursing infant and should be used with caution during breast-feeding; observe nursing infant closely for changes in stool consistency

SIDE EFFECTS

Mesalamine is generally well tolerated, with only mild and transient effects.

Frequent (greater than 6%)

PO: Abdominal cramps or pain, diarrhea, dizziness, headache, nausea, vomiting, rhinitis, unusual fatigue

Rectal: Abdominal or stomach cramps, flatulence, headache, nausea

Occasional (6%-2%)

PO: Hair loss, decreased appetite, back or joint pain, flatulence, acne

Rectal: Hair loss

Rare (less than 2%)

Rectal: Anal irritation

SERIOUS REACTIONS

• Sulfite sensitivity may occur in susceptible patients, manifested by cramping, headache, diarrhea, fever, rash, hives, itching, and wheezing. Discontinue drug immediately.

• Hepatitis, pancreatitis, and pericarditis occur rarely with oral forms.

INTERACTIONS

Drugs

3 *Warfarin:* Inhibits warfarin effect

SPECIAL CONSIDERATIONS

PATIENT/FAMILY EDUCATION

• Swallow tabs whole, do not break the outer coating

• Intact or partially intact tabs may be found in stool; notify clinician if this occurs repeatedly

• Avoid excess handling of suppositories

• Lie on left side during enema administration (to facilitate migration into the sigmoid colon)

• Avoid tasks that require mental alertness or motor skills until response to the drug has been established

• Mesalamine may discolor urine yellow-brown

MONITORING PARAMETERS

• Pattern of daily bowel activity and stool consistency and record time of evacuation

• Skin for rash and urticaria

mesna

(mes´-na)

Rx: Mesnex

Chemical Class: Thiol derivative

Therapeutic Class: Antidote, ifosfamide

CLINICAL PHARMACOLOGY

Mechanism of Action: An antineoplastic adjunct and cytoprotective agent that binds with and detoxifies urotoxic metabolites of ifosfamide and cyclophosphamide. ***Therapeutic Effect:*** Inhibits ifosfamide- and cyclophosphamide-induced hemorrhagic cystitis.

Pharmacokinetics

Rapidly metabolized after IV administration to mesna disulfide, which is reduced to mesna in kidney. Excreted in urine. ***Half-life:*** 24 min.

INDICATIONS AND DOSAGES

Prevention of hemorrhagic cystitis in patients receiving ifosfamide

IV

Adults, Elderly. 20% of ifosfamide dose at time of ifosfamide administration and 4 and 8 hr after each dose of ifosfamide. Total dose: 60% of ifosfamide dosage. Range: 60%-160% of the daily ifosfamide dose.

Hemorrhagic cystitis (chronic low-dose cyclophosphamide)

PO

Adults, Elderly. 20 mg/kg q3-4h.

Hemorrhagic cystitis (high-dose cyclophosphamide)

IV

Adults, Elderly. 40% of cyclophosphamide dose at 0, 3, 6, 9 hr and IV fluids.

AVAILABLE FORMS

• *Tablets:* 400 mg.

• *Injection:* 100 mg/ml.

M

CONTRAINDICATIONS: None known.

PREGNANCY AND LACTATION: Pregnancy category B; use caution in nursing mothers

SIDE EFFECTS

Frequent (more than 17%)

Bad taste, soft stools

Large doses: Diarrhea, myalgia, headache, fatigue, nausea, hypotension, allergic reaction

SERIOUS REACTIONS

• Hematuria occurs rarely.

INTERACTIONS

Labs

• *False positive:* Urinary ketones, β-hydroxybutyrate

SPECIAL CONSIDERATIONS

PATIENT/FAMILY EDUCATION

• Notify the physician or nurse if headache, myalgia, or nausea occurs

MONITORING PARAMETERS

• Urinalysis each day prior to ifosfamide administration

• Reduction or discontinuation of ifosfamide may be initiated in patients developing hematuria (>50 RBC/hpf)

• Pattern of daily bowel activity and stool consistency; record the time of evacuation

• Blood pressure for hypotension

---

mesoridazine besylate

(mez-oh-rid'-a-zeen bess'-il-late)

Rx: Serentil

Chemical Class: Piperidine phenothiazine derivative

Therapeutic Class: Antipsychotic

CLINICAL PHARMACOLOGY

Mechanism of Action: A phenothiazine that blocks dopamine at postsynaptic receptor sites in the brain. ***Therapeutic Effect:*** Diminishes schizophrenic behavior. Also has anticholinergic and sedative effects.

Pharmacokinetics

Absorption may be erratic. Protein binding: 75%-91%. Undergoes first-pass metabolism. Small portions are metabolized in liver. Excreted in urine and feces. ***Half-life:*** Unknown.

INDICATIONS AND DOSAGES

Schizophrenia

PO

Adults, Elderly. 25-50 mg 3 times a day. Maximum: 400 mg/day.

IM

Adults, Elderly. Initially, 25 mg. May repeat in 30-60 min. Range: 25-200 mg.

Severe behavioral problems (combativeness or explosive, hyperexcitable behavior) associated with neurologic diseases

PO

Elderly. Initially, 10 mg once or twice a day. May increase at 4-7-day intervals. Maximum: 250 mg.

IM

Adults, Elderly. Initially, 25 mg. May repeat in 30-60 min. Range: 25-200 mg.

AVAILABLE FORMS

• *Oral Solution:* 25 mg/ml.

• *Tablets:* 10 mg, 25 mg, 50 mg, 100 mg.

• *Injection:* 25 mg/ml.

CONTRAINDICATIONS: Coma, concurrent administration of drugs that cause QTc-interval prolongation, myelosuppression, severe cardiovascular disease, severe CNS depression, subcortical brain damage

PREGNANCY AND LACTATION: Pregnancy category C; bulk of evidence indicates that phenothiazines are safe for mother and fetus; effect on nursing infant is unknown, but may be of concern

SIDE EFFECTS

Frequent

Orthostatic hypotension, dizziness, syncope (occur frequently after first injection, occasionally after subsequent injections, and rarely with oral form)

Occasional

Somnolence (during early therapy), dry mouth, blurred vision, lethargy, constipation or diarrhea, nasal congestion, peripheral edema, urine retention

Rare

Ocular changes, altered skin pigmentation (in those taking high doses for prolonged periods), darkening of urine

SERIOUS REACTIONS

- Abrupt withdrawal after long-term therapy may precipitate nausea, vomiting, gastritis, dizziness, and tremors.
- Blood dyscrasias, particularly agranulocytosis and mild leukopenia, may occur.
- Mesoridazine use may lower the seizure threshold.

INTERACTIONS

Drugs

3 *Alcohol, other CNS depressants:* May increase CNS and respiratory depression and the hypotensive effects of mesoridazine

3 *Anticholinergics:* Inhibited therapeutic response to antipsychotic; enhanced anticholinergic side effects

3 *Antidepressants:* Increased serum concentrations of some cyclic antidepressants

3 *Antimalarials:* Mesoridazine serum levels increased

3 *Antithyroid agents:* May increase the risk of agranulocytosis

3 *Attapulgite:* Reduced mesoridazine via decreased absorption

3 *Barbiturates:* Reduced effect of antipsychotic

3 *β-blockers:* Enhanced effects of both drugs

3 *Bromocriptine, lithium:* Reduced effects of both drugs

3 *Clonidine:* Hypotension

3 *Epinephrine:* Reversed pressor response to epinephrine

3 *Extrapyramidal symptom–producing medications:* May increase extrapyramidal symptoms

3 *Guanadrel:* Mesoridazine inhibits antihypertensive response

3 *Guanethidine:* Inhibited antihypertensive response to guanethidine

2 *Levodopa:* Inhibited effect of levodopa on Parkinson's disease

3 *Narcotic analgesics:* Excessive CNS depression, hypotension, respiratory depression

3 *Orphenadrine:* Reduced serum neuroleptic concentrations; excessive anticholinergic effects

3 *Phenylpropanolamine:* Case report of patient death on combination of these two drugs

SPECIAL CONSIDERATIONS

PATIENT/FAMILY EDUCATION

- Do not discontinue abruptly
- Concentrate may be diluted just prior to administration with distilled water, acidified tap water, orange or grape juice
- Full therapeutic effect may take up to 6 wks to appear
- Drowsiness generally subsides with continued therapy
- The drug may darken the urine

MONITORING PARAMETERS

- Observe closely for signs of tardive dyskinesia
- Periodic CBC with platelets during prolonged therapy
- Pattern of daily bowel activity and stool consistency
- Closely supervise suicidal patients during early therapy. As depression lessens, the patient's energy level improves, which increases the suicide potential

metaproterenol sulfate

(met-a-proe-ter′-e-nole sul′-fate)

Rx: Alupent

Chemical Class: Sympathomimetic amine; β_2-adrenergic agonist

Therapeutic Class: Antiasthmatic; bronchodilator

CLINICAL PHARMACOLOGY

Mechanism of Action: A sympathomimetic that stimulates beta$_2$-adrenergic receptors, resulting in relaxation of bronchial smooth muscle. ***Therapeutic Effect:*** Relieves bronchospasm and reduces airway resistance.

Pharmacokinetics

Systemic absorption is rapid following aerosol administration; however, serum concentrations at recommended doses are very low. Metabolized in liver. Excreted in urine primarily as glucoside metabolite. ***Half-life:*** Unknown.

INDICATIONS AND DOSAGES

Treatment of bronchospasm

PO

Adults, Children 10 yrs and older. 20 mg 3-4 times a day.

Elderly. 10 mg 3-4 times a day. May increase to 20 mg/dose.

Children 6-9 yrs. 10 mg 3-4 times a day.

Children 2-5 yrs. 1.3-2.6 mg/kg/day in 3-4 divided doses.

Children younger than 2 yrs. 0.4 mg/kg 3-4 times a day.

Inhalation

Adults, Elderly, Children 12 yrs and older. 2-3 inhalations q3-4h. Maximum: 12 inhalations/24 hr.

Nebulization

Adults, Elderly, Children 12 yrs and older. 10-15 mg (0.2-0.3 ml) of 5% q4-6h.

Children younger than 12 yr, Infants. 0.5-1 mg/kg (0.01-0.02 ml/kg) of 5% q4-6h.

AVAILABLE FORMS

- *Syrup:* 10 mg/5 ml.
- *Tablets:* 10 mg, 20 mg.
- *Aerosol Oral Inhalation:* 0.65 mg/inhalation.
- *Solution for Oral Inhalation:* 0.4%, 0.6%, 5%.

CONTRAINDICATIONS: Angle-closure glaucoma, preexisting arrhythmias associated with tachycardia

PREGNANCY AND LACTATION: Pregnancy category C; has been used to prevent premature labor; long-term evaluation of infants exposed *in utero* to β-agonists has been reported, but not specifically for metaproterenol, no harmful effects were observed

SIDE EFFECTS

Frequent (over 10%)

Rigors, tremors, anxiety, nausea, dry mouth

Occasional (9%-1%)

Dizziness, vertigo, asthenia, headache, GI distress, vomiting, cough, dry throat

Rare (less than 1%)

Somnolence, diarrhea, altered taste

SERIOUS REACTIONS

- Excessive sympathomimetic stimulation may cause palpitations, extrasystoles, tachycardia, chest pain, a slight increase in BP followed by a substantial decrease, chills, diaphoresis, and blanching of skin.
- Too-frequent or excessive use may lead decreased drug effectiveness and severe, paradoxical bronchoconstriction.

INTERACTIONS

Drugs

3 *Furosemide:* Potential for additive hypokalemia

❷ *β-blockers:* Decreased action of metaproterenol, cardio selective β-blockers preferable if concurrent use necessary

❸ *Digoxin, other sympathomimetics:* May increase the risk of arrhythmias

❷ *MAOIs:* May increase the risk of hypertensive crisis

❸ *Tricyclic antidepressants:* May increase cardiovascular effects

Labs

• *Glucose:* Urine, increase via Benedict's reagent

SPECIAL CONSIDERATIONS

PATIENT/FAMILY EDUCATION

• Proper inhalation technique is vital for MDIs

• Excessive use may lead to adverse effects

• Notify clinician if no response to usual doses

• Drink plenty of fluids to decrease the thickness of lung secretions

• Notify the physician if chest pain, difficulty breathing, dizziness, flushing, headache, palpitations, tachycardia, or tremors occurs

• Avoid use of caffeine derivatives such as chocolate, cocoa, cola, coffee, and tea

MONITORING PARAMETERS

• Pulse rate and quality and respiratory rate depth, rhythm, and type

• ABG levels and pulmonary function test results

• Evidence of cyanosis, a blue or a dusky color in light-skinned patients and a gray color in dark-skinned patients

• Evaluate the patient for signs of clinical improvement, such as cessation of retractions, quieter and slower respirations, and a relaxed facial expression

metaraminol bitartrate

(met-ar-am′-e-nol bye-tar′-trate)

Rx: Aramine

Chemical Class: Catecholamine, synthetic

Therapeutic Class: Vasopressor; α-adrenergic sympathomimetic amine

CLINICAL PHARMACOLOGY

Mechanism of Action: An alpha-adrenergic receptor agonist that causes vasoconstriction, reflex bradycardia, inhibits GI smooth muscle and vascular smooth muscle supplying skeletal muscle, and increases heart rate and force of heart muscle contraction. ***Therapeutic Effect:*** Increases both systolic and diastolic pressure.

Pharmacokinetics

Route	*Onset*	*Peak*	*Duration*
IM (pressor effect)	10 min	N/A	20-60 min
IV	1-2 min	N/A	
SC	5-20 min	N/A	

Metabolized in the liver. Excreted in the urine and the bile.

INDICATIONS AND DOSAGES

Prevention of hypotension

IM/SC

Adults, Elderly. 2-10 mg as a single dose.

Children. 0.01 mg/kg as a single dose.

Adjunctive treatment of hypotension

IV

Adults, Elderly. 15-100 mg IV infusion, administered at a rate to maintain the desired blood pressure.

M

Severe shock
IV
Adults, Elderly. 0.5-5 mg direct IV injection followed by 15-100 mg IV infusion in 250-500 ml fluid for control of blood pressure.

AVAILABLE FORMS
• *Injection:* 10 mg/ml (Aramine).

CONTRAINDICATIONS: Cyclopropane or halothane anesthesia, use of MAOIs, pregnancy, hypersensitivity to metaraminol

PREGNANCY AND LACTATION: Pregnancy category D; use could cause reduced uterine blood flow and fetal hypoxia

SIDE EFFECTS
Occasional
Tachycardia, hypertension, cardiac arrhythmias, flushing, palpitations, hypotension, angina, tremors, nervousness, headache, dizziness, weakness, sloughing of skin, nausea, abscess formation, diaphoresis

SERIOUS REACTIONS
• Overdosage produces hypertension, cerebral hemorrhage, cardiac arrest, and seizures.

INTERACTIONS
Drugs
③ *Guanethidine:* Reversed antihypertensive effects
② *Halogenated hydrocarbon anesthetics:* Sensitized myocardium to the effects of catecholamines, arrhythmias possible
⚠ *MAOIs:* Severe hypertensive response
③ *Oxytocic drugs:* Concomitant use may cause severe persistent hypertension
③ *Tricyclic antidepressants:* Vasopressor response decreased; higher sympathomimetic may be necessary

SPECIAL CONSIDERATIONS

PATIENT/FAMILY EDUCATION
• Notify the physician immediately if increased heart rate or palpitations occurs

MONITORING PARAMETERS
• Maximum effect is not immediately apparent; allow at least 10 min to elapse before increasing the dose
• BP and pulse

---

metaxalone
(me-tax'-a-lone)
Rx: Skelaxin
Chemical Class: Oxazolidinedione derivative
Therapeutic Class: Skeletal muscle relaxant

CLINICAL PHARMACOLOGY
Mechanism of Action: A central depressant whose exact mechanism is unknown. Many effects due to its central depressant actions. ***Therapeutic Effect:*** Relieves pain or muscle spasms.
Pharmacokinetics
PO route onset 1 hr, peak 3 hrs, duration 4-6 hrs. Well absorbed from the gastrointestinal (GI) tract. Metabolized in liver. Primarily excreted in urine. ***Half-life:*** 9 hrs.

INDICATIONS AND DOSAGES
Muscle relaxant
PO
Adults, Elderly, Children older than 12 yrs. 800 mg 3-4 times/day.

AVAILABLE FORMS
• *Tablets:* 400 mg, 800 mg (Skelaxin).

CONTRAINDICATIONS: Impaired renal or hepatic function, history of drug-induced hemolytic anemias or other anemias, history of hypersensitivity to metaxalone

PREGNANCY AND LACTATION: Pregnancy category C

SIDE EFFECTS
Occasional
Drowsiness, headache, lightheadedness, dermatitis, nausea, vomiting, stomach cramps, dyspnea

SERIOUS REACTIONS

• Overdose may cause CNS depression, coma, shock, and respiratory depression.

INTERACTIONS

Drugs

3 *Alcohol, barbiturates, other CNS depressants:* May enhance the effects of these agents

Labs

• *False positive:* Glucose, urine via Benedict's reagent

SPECIAL CONSIDERATIONS

PATIENT/FAMILY EDUCATION

• Drowsiness usually diminishes with continued therapy
• Avoid tasks that require mental alertness or motor skills until response to the drug is established
• Avoid alcohol or other depressants while taking metaxalone
• Avoid sudden changes in posture to help avoid hypotensive effects

MONITORING PARAMETERS

• Therapeutic response; decreased intensity of skeletal muscle pain, stiffness, and tenderness, improved mobility

metformin hydrochloride

(met-for'-min hye-droe-klor'-ide)

Rx: Fortamet, Glucophage, Glucophage XL, Glumetza, Riomet

Combinations

Rx: with rosiglitazone (Avandamet); with glyburide (Glucovance)

Chemical Class: Biguanide

Therapeutic Class: Antidiabetic; hypoglycemic

CLINICAL PHARMACOLOGY

Mechanism of Action: An antihyperglycemic that decreases hepatic production of glucose. Decreases absorption of glucose and improves insulin sensitivity. ***Therapeutic Effect:*** Improves glycemic control, stabilizes or decreases body weight, and improves lipid profile.

Pharmacokinetics

Slowly, incompletely absorbed after oral administration. Food delays or decreases the extent of absorption. Protein binding: negligible. Primarily distributed to intestinal mucosa and salivary glands. Primarily excreted unchanged in urine. Removed by hemodialysis. ***Half-life:*** 3-6 hr.

INDICATIONS AND DOSAGES

Diabetes mellitus

PO (Immediate-Release Tablets, Solution)

Adults, Elderly. Initially, 500 mg twice a day or 850 mg once daily. Maintenance: 1-2.55 g/day in 2-3 divided doses. Maximum: 2500 mg/day.

Children 10-16 yr. Initially, 500 mg twice a day. Maintenance: Titrate in 500-mg increments weekly. Maximum: 2000 mg/day.

PO (Extended-Release Tablets [Glucophage XL])

Adults, Elderly. Initially, 500 mg once daily. Maintenance: 1-2 g daily. Maximum: 2000 mg/day.

PO (Extended-Release Tablets [Fortamet, Glumetza])

Adults, Elderly. 500 mg-1 g once daily. Maintenance: 1-2.5 g once daily. Maximum: 2500 mg/day.

AVAILABLE FORMS

• *Oral Solution (Riomet):* 100 mg/ml.
• *Tablets (Glucophage):* 500 mg, 850 mg, 1000 mg.
• *Tablets (Extended-Release):* 500 mg (Fortamet, Glucophage XL, Glumetza), 750 mg (Glucophage

XL), 1000 mg (Fortamet, Glumetza).

UNLABELED USES: Treatment of HIV liopodystrophy syndrome, metabolic complications of AIDS, polycystic ovary syndrome, prediabetes, weight reduction

CONTRAINDICATIONS: Acute CHF, MI, cardiovascular collapse, renal disease or dysfunction, respiratory failure, septicemia

PREGNANCY AND LACTATION: Pregnancy category B; breast milk excretion unknown

SIDE EFFECTS

Occasional (greater than 3%)

GI disturbances (including diarrhea, nausea, vomiting, abdominal bloating, flatulence, and anorexia) that are transient and resolve spontaneously during therapy.

Rare (3%-1%)

Unpleasant or metallic taste that resolves spontaneously during therapy

SERIOUS REACTIONS

• Lactic acidosis occurs rarely but is a fatal complication in 50% of cases. Lactic acidosis is characterized by an increase in blood lactate levels (greater than 5 mmol/L), a decrease in blood pH, and electrolyte disturbances. Signs and symptoms of lactic acidosis include unexplained hyperventilation, myalgia, malaise, and somnolence, which may advance to cardiovascular collapse (shock), acute CHF, acute MI, and prerenal azotemia.

INTERACTIONS

Drugs

3 *Alcohol, amiloride, digoxin, furosemide, morphine, nifedipine, procainamide, quinidine, quinine, ranitidine, triamterene, trimethoprim, vancomycin:* Increase metformin blood concentration

3 *Cimetidine:* Increased metformin AUC 50%, peak concentrations 81%, and decreased renal clearance 27%, increasing the risk of lactic acidosis

3 *Iodinated contrast studies:* May cause acute renal failure and increased risk of lactic acidosis

3 *Monoamine oxidase (MAO) inhibitors:* Stimulate insulin secretion via β-adrenergic stimulation; excessive and prolonged hypoglycemia may occur in some individuals

SPECIAL CONSIDERATIONS

• May also lower triglycerides

• May decrease insulin requirement in insulin-requiring diabetics

PATIENT/FAMILY EDUCATION

• Administer with food

• Avoid excessive alcohol

• Notify clinician of diarrhea, severe muscle pain or cramping, shallow and fast breathing, unusual tiredness and weakness, unusual sleepiness (signs of lactic acidosis)

MONITORING PARAMETERS

• Glycosylated hemoglobin q3-6 mo (<7.0%); self-monitored preprandial blood sugars <150 mg/dL; absence of hyperglycemia (e.g., polyuria, polyphagia, polydipsia, blurred vision)

• Renal and hepatic function tests before and annually during therapy

• Serum vitamin B_{12} annually during chronic therapy

• Assess the patient concurrently taking oral sulfonylureas for signs and symptoms of hypoglycemia, including anxiety, cool wet skin, diplopia, dizziness, headache, hunger, numbness in mouth, tachycardia, and tremors

• Be alert to conditions that alter blood glucose requirements, such as fever, increased activity, stress, or a surgical procedure

methacholine chloride

(meth-a-ko'-leen klor'-ide)

Rx: Provocholine

Chemical Class: Choline ester

Therapeutic Class: Diagnostic agent

CLINICAL PHARMACOLOGY

Mechanism of Action: A cholinergic, parasympathomimetic, synthetic analog of acetylcholine that stimulates muscarinic, postganglionic parasympathetic receptors. ***Therapeutic Effect:*** Results in smooth muscle contraction of the airways and increased tracheobronchial secretions.

Pharmacokinetics

PO route onset rapid, peak 1-4 mins, duration 15-75 mins or 5 mins if methacholine challenge is followed with a beta-agonist agent. Undergoes rapid hydrolysis in the plasma by acetylcholinesterase.

INDICATIONS AND DOSAGES

Asthma diagnosis

Inhalation

Challenge test: Before inhalation challenge, perform baseline pulmonary function tests; the patient must have an FEV_1 of at least 70% of the predicted value. The following is a suggested schedule for administration of methacholine challenge. Calculate cumulative units by multiplying number of breaths by concentration given. Total cumulative units are the sum of cumulative units for each concentration given.

Vial E

- Serial concentration: 0.025 mg/ml
- No. of breaths: 5
- Cumulative units per concentration: 0.125
- Total cumulative units: 0.125

Vial D

- Serial concentration: 0.25 mg/ml
- No. of breaths: 5
- Cumulative units per concentration: 1.25
- Total cumulative units: 1.375

Vial C

- Serial concentration: 2.5 mg/ml
- No. of breaths: 5
- Cumulative units per concentration: 12.5
- Total cumulative units: 13.88

Vial B

- Serial concentration: 10 mg/ml
- No. of breaths: 5
- Cumulative units per concentration: 50
- Total cumulative units: 63.88

Vial A

- Serial concentration: 25 mg/ml
- No. of breaths: 5
- Cumulative units per concentration: 125
- Total cumulative units: 188.88

Determine FEV_1 within 5 mins of challenge; a positive challenge is a 20% reduction in FEV_1.

AVAILABLE FORMS

- *Powder for oral inhalation:* 100 mg/5 ml (Provocholine).

UNLABELED USES: Adie syndrome diagnosis, familial dysautonomia diagnosis, peripheral ischemia, parotitis

CONTRAINDICATIONS: Asthma, wheezing, or very low baseline pulmonary function tests, concomitant use of beta-blockers, hypersensitivity to the drug; because of the potential for severe bronchoconstriction

PREGNANCY AND LACTATION: Pregnancy category C

SIDE EFFECTS

Occasional

Headache, lightheadedness, itching, throat irritation, wheezing

M

SERIOUS REACTIONS

• Severe bronchoconstriction and reduction in respiratory function can result. Patients with severe hyperreactivity of the airways can experience bronchoconstriction at a dosage as low as 0.025 mg/ml (0.125 cumulative units). If severe bronchoconstriction occurs, reverse immediately by administration of a rapid-acting inhaled bronchodilator (beta-agonist).

INTERACTIONS

Drugs

3 *β-blockers:* Exaggerated response to methacholine challenge, prolonged recovery, poor response to treatment

SPECIAL CONSIDERATIONS

PATIENT/FAMILY EDUCATION

• Notify the physician immediately of difficulty breathing

MONITORING PARAMETERS

• FEV_1 3-5 min after administration of each serial concentration; procedure is complete when there is a ≥20% reduction in FEV_1 compared to baseline (positive response) or when 5 inhalations have been administered at each concentration and FEV_1 has been reduced by ≤14% (negative response)

methadone hydrochloride

(meth'-a-done hye-droe-klor'-ide)

Rx: Dolophine, Methadone Intensol, Methadose

Chemical Class: Diphenylheptane derivative; opiate derivative

Therapeutic Class: Narcotic analgesic

DEA Class: Schedule II

CLINICAL PHARMACOLOGY

Mechanism of Action: An opioid agonist that binds with opioid receptors in the CNS. ***Therapeutic Effect:*** Alters the perception of and emotional response to pain; reduces withdrawal symptoms from other opioid drugs.

Pharmacokinetics

Route	*Onset*	*Peak*	*Duration*
Oral	0.5-1 hr	1.5-2 hrs	6-8 hrs
IM	10-20 mins	1-2 hrs	4-5 hrs
IV	N/A	15-30 mins	3-4 hrs

Well absorbed after IM injection. Protein binding: 80%-85%. Metabolized in the liver. Primarily excreted in urine. Not removed by hemodialysis. ***Half-life:*** 15-25 hrs.

INDICATIONS AND DOSAGES

Analgesia

PO

Adults, Elderly. Initially, 5-10 mg q3-4h.

Children. 0.1-0.2 mg/kg q6h as needed. Maximum: 10 mg/dose.

IV, IM, Subcutaneous

Adults, Elderly. Initially, 2.5-10 mg q3-4h.

Narcotic addiction

IM, PO

Adults, Elderly. 15-40 mg once daily or as needed. Reduce dose at 1-2 day-

intervals based on patient response.
Maintenance: Individualized.

AVAILABLE FORMS

- *Oral Concentrate (Methadone Intensol, Methadose):* 10 mg/ml.
- *Oral Solution:* 5 mg/5 ml, 10 mg/ 5 ml.
- *Tablets (Dolophine, Methadose):* 5 mg, 10 mg.
- *Tablets (Dispersible [Methadose]):* 40 mg.
- *Injection (Dolophine):* 10 mg/ml.

CONTRAINDICATIONS: Delivery of premature infant, diarrhea due to poisoning, hypersensitivity to narcotics, labor

PREGNANCY AND LACTATION: Pregnancy category B (category D if used for prolonged periods or in high doses at term); compatible with breast-feeding if mother consumes ≤20 mg/24 hr

Controlled Substance: Schedule II

SIDE EFFECTS

Frequent

Sedation, decreased BP (including orthostatic hypotension), diaphoresis, facial flushing, constipation, dizziness, nausea, vomiting

Occasional

Confusion, urine retention, palpitations, abdominal cramps, visual changes, dry mouth, headache, decreased appetite, anxiety, insomnia

Rare

Allergic reaction (rash, pruritus)

SERIOUS REACTIONS

- Overdose results in respiratory depression, skeletal muscle flaccidity, cold or clammy skin, cyanosis, and extreme somnolence progressing to seizures, stupor, and coma. The antidote is 0.4 mg naloxone.
- The patient who uses methadone long-term may develop a tolerance to the drug's analgesic effect and physical dependence.

INTERACTIONS

Drugs

3 *Anticoagulants:* Potentiation of warfarin's anticoagulant effect

3 *Antihistamines, chloral hydrate, glutethimide, methocarbamol:* Enhanced depressant effects

3 *Barbiturates:* Additive respiratory and CNS depressant effects

3 *Carbamazepine, phenobarbital, primidone, rifampin:* Reduced serum methadone concentrations; increased symptoms associated with narcotic withdrawal

3 *Cimetidine:* Increased effect of narcotic analgesics

3 *Ethanol:* Additive CNS effects

3 *Neuroleptics:* Hypotension and excessive CNS depression

3 *Nevirapine:* Reduces methadone concentrations, methadone withdrawal symptoms may occur

2 *Phenytoin:* As with carbamazepine above

3 *Protease inhibitors:* Increased respiratory and CNS depression

3 *Somatostatin:* Inhibited the analgesic effect of methadone

3 *St. John's Wort:* Reduces methadone plasma concentrations and may lead to symptoms of methadone withdrawal

Labs

- *Morphine:* Urine, increased
- *Pregnancy tests:* Urine, false positive (Gravindex)
- *False increase:* Amylase and lipase

SPECIAL CONSIDERATIONS

- When used for the treatment of narcotic addiction in detoxification or maintenance programs, can only be dispensed by approved hospital pharmacies, approved community pharmacies, and maintenance programs approved by the Food and Drug Administration and the designated state authority

• Do not administer agonist/antagonist analgesics (i.e., pentazocine, nalbuphine, butorphanol, dezocine, buprenorphine) to patient who has received a prolonged course of methadone (a pure agonist). In opioid-dependent patients, mixed agonist/antagonist analgesics may precipitate withdrawal symptoms.

PATIENT/FAMILY EDUCATION

• Change position slowly; orthostatic hypotension may occur
• Minimize nausea by administering with food and remain lying down following dose
• Avoid tasks that require mental alertness or motor skills until response to the drug has been established

MONITORING PARAMETERS

• Vital signs
• Assess for adequate voiding
• Clinical improvement and onset of relief of pain

---

methamphetamine hydrochloride

(meth-am-fet'-a-meen hye-droe-klor'-ide)

Rx: Desoxyn, Gradumet
Chemical Class: Amphetamine derivative
Therapeutic Class: Anorexiant; central nervous system stimulant
DEA Class: Schedule II

CLINICAL PHARMACOLOGY

Mechanism of Action: A sympathomimetic amine related to amphetamine and ephedrine that enhances CNS stimulant activity. Peripheral actions include elevation of systolic and diastolic blood pressure and weak bronchodilator and respiratory stimulant action. ***Therapeutic Effect:*** Increases motor activity, mental alertness; decreases drowsiness, fatigue.

Pharmacokinetics

Rapidly absorbed from the gastrointestinal (GI) tract. Metabolized in liver. Primarily excreted in the urine. Unknown if removed by hemodialysis. *Half-life:* 4-5 hrs.

INDICATIONS AND DOSAGES

Attention deficit/hyperactivity disorder (ADHD)

PO

Adults, Children 6 yrs and older. Initially, 2.5-5 mg 1-2 times/day. Increase by 5 mg/day at weekly intervals until therapeutic response achieved.

Appetite suppressant

PO

Adults, Children 12 yrs and older. 5 mg daily, given 30 min before meals. Extended-release 10-15 mg in the morning.

AVAILABLE FORMS

• *Tablets:* 5 mg.
• *Tablets (Extended-Release):* 5 mg, 10 mg, 15 mg (Desoxyn, Gradumet).

UNLABELED USES: Narcolepsy

CONTRAINDICATIONS: Advanced arteriosclerosis, agitated states, glaucoma, history of drug abuse, history of hypersensitivity to sympathomimetic amines, hyperthyroidism, moderate to severe hypertension, symptomatic cardiovascular disease, within 14 days following discontinuation of an MAOI

PREGNANCY AND LACTATION: Pregnancy category C; use of amphetamine for medical indications does not pose a significant risk to the fetus for congenital anomalies; mild withdrawal symptoms may be observed in the newborn; illicit maternal use presents significant risks to the fetus and newborn including intrauterine growth retardation, premature delivery, and the potential for increased maternal, fetal, and neonatal morbidity; concentrated in breast milk; contraindicated during breast-feeding

Controlled Substance: Schedule II

SIDE EFFECTS

Frequent

Irregular pulse, increased motor activity, talkativeness, nervousness, mild euphoria, insomnia

Occasional

Headache, chills, dry mouth, gastrointestinal (GI) distress, worsening depression in patients who are clinically depressed, tachycardia, palpitations, chest pain

SERIOUS REACTIONS

- Overdose may produce skin pallor, flushing, arrhythmias, and psychosis.
- Abrupt withdrawal following prolonged administration of high dosage may produce lethargy, which may last for weeks.
- Prolonged administration to children with ADHD may produce a temporary suppression of normal weight and height patterns.

INTERACTIONS

Drugs

3 *Acetazolamide:* Increased serum amphetamine concentrations and prolonged amphetamine effects

3 *Antidepressants:* Increased effect of amphetamines, clinical evidence lacking

3 *Furazolidone:* Hypertensive reactions

3 *Guanadrel, guanethidine:* Inhibition of the antihypertensive response

3 *Insulin:* Requirements in diabetes mellitus may be altered in association with the use of methamphetamine

⚠ *MAOIs:* Severe hypertensive reactions possible

3 *Phenothiazines:* Antagonizes the CNS stimulant action of methamphetamine

3 *Selegiline:* Potential for enhanced pressor effect if used in combination

3 *Sodium bicarbonate:* Large doses of sodium bicarbonate inhibit the elimination and increase the effect of amphetamines

Labs

- *Amino acids:* Urine, increased
- *Amphetamine:* Urine, positive at 1.0 mcg/ml

SPECIAL CONSIDERATIONS

PATIENT/FAMILY EDUCATION

- Take early in the day
- Do not discontinue abruptly
- Avoid hazardous activities until stabilized on medication
- Avoid OTC preparations unless approved by clinician

methazolamide

(meth-a-zoe'-la-mide)

Rx: Glauctabs, Neptazane

Chemical Class: Carbonic anhydrase inhibitor; sulfonamide derivative

Therapeutic Class: Antiglaucoma agent

CLINICAL PHARMACOLOGY

Mechanism of Action: A noncompetitive inhibitor of carbonic anhydrase that inhibits the enzyme at the luminal border of cells of the proximal tubule. Increases urine volume and changes to an alkaline pH with subsequent decreases in the excretion of titratable acid and ammonia. ***Therapeutic Effect:*** Produces a diuretic and antiglaucoma effect.

Pharmacokinetics

PO route onset 2-4 hrs, peak 6-8 hrs, duration 10-18 hrs. Well absorbed slowly from the gastrointestinal (GI) tract. Protein binding: 55%. Distributed into the tissues (including CSF). Metabolized slowly from the GI tract. Partially excreted in urine. Not removed by hemodialysis. ***Half-life:*** 14 hrs.

INDICATIONS AND DOSAGES

Glaucoma

PO

Adults, Elderly. 50-100 mg/day 2-3 times/day.

AVAILABLE FORMS

• *Tablets:* 25 mg, 50 mg.

UNLABELED USES: Motion sickness, essential tremor

CONTRAINDICATIONS: Kidney or liver dysfunction, severe pulmonary obstruction, hypersensitivity to methazolamide or any component of the formulation

PREGNANCY AND LACTATION: Pregnancy category C

SIDE EFFECTS

Occasional

Paresthesias, hearing dysfunction or tinnitus, fatigue, malaise, loss of appetite, taste alteration, nausea, vomiting, diarrhea, polyuria, drowsiness, confusion, hypokalemia

Rare

Metabolic acidosis, electrolyte imbalance, transient myopia, urticaria, melena, hematuria, glycosuria, hepatic insufficiency, flaccid paralysis, photosensitivity, convulsions, and rarely, crystalluria, renal calculi

SERIOUS REACTIONS

• Malaise and complaints of tiredness and myalgia are signs of excessive dosing and acidosis in the elderly.

• Stevens-Johnson syndrome, toxic epidermal necrolysis, fulminant hepatic necrosis, agranulocytosis, aplastic anemia, and other blood dyscrasias have been reported and have caused fatalities.

INTERACTIONS

Drugs

3 *Amphetamines:* Increased amphetamine serum concentrations and prolonged effects

3 *Antiarrhythmics (flecainide, mexiletine):* Alkalinization of urine increases concentrations of these drugs

3 *Cyclosporine:* Increased trough cyclosporine levels with potential for neurotoxicity and nephropathy

3 *Ephedrine:* Increased ephedrine concentrations

3 *Methenamine compounds:* Interference with antibacterial activity

3 *Phenytoin:* Increased risk of osteomalacia with prolonged use of both agents

3 *Quinidine:* Alkalinization of urine increases quinidine concentrations

2 *Salicylates:* Increased concentrations of methazolamide leading to CNS toxicity; also see furosemide for other general diuretic interactions

3 *Steroids:* Potential for developing hypokalemia

Labs

• *Increase:* Blood glucose levels, bilirubin, blood ammonia, calcium, chloride

• *Decrease:* Urine citrate, serum potassium

• *False positive:* Urinary protein

SPECIAL CONSIDERATIONS

PATIENT/FAMILY EDUCATION

• Take with food if GI upset occurs

• Methazolamide may cause drowsiness and impair judgment or coordination

• Methazolamide may cause altered taste

MONITORING PARAMETERS

• Intraocular pressure, reduction in AMS symptoms, serum electrolytes, creatinine, CO_2

methenamine

(meth-en′-a-meen)

Rx: Hiprex, Mandelamine, Urex

Chemical Class: Formaldehyde precursors

Therapeutic Class: Urinary antiinfective

CLINICAL PHARMACOLOGY

Mechanism of Action: A hippuric acid salt that hydrolyzes to formaldehyde and ammonia in acidic urine. ***Therapeutic Effect:*** Formaldehyde has antibacterial action. Bacteriocidal.

Pharmacokinetics

Readily absorbed from the gastrointestinal (GI) tract. Partially metabolized by hydrolysis (unless protected by enteric coating) and partially by the liver. Primarily excreted in urine. ***Half-life:*** 3-6 hrs.

INDICATIONS AND DOSAGES

Urinary tract infection (UTI)

PO

Adults, Elderly. 1 g 2 times/day (as hippurate). 1 g 4 times/day (as mandelate).

Children 6-12 yrs. 25-50 mg/kg/day q12h (as hippurate). 50-75 mg/kg/day q6h (as mandelate).

AVAILABLE FORMS

- *Oral Suspension, as mandelate:* 0.5 g/5 ml.
- *Tablets, as hippurate:* 1 g (Urex, Hiprex).
- *Tablets, enteric coated, as mandelate:* 500 mg, 1 g (Mandelamine).

UNLABELED USES: Hyperhidrosis

CONTRAINDICATIONS: Moderate to severe renal impairment, hepatic impairment (hippurate salt), tartrazine sensitivity (Hiprex contains tartrazine), hypersensitivity to methenamine or any of its components

PREGNANCY AND LACTATION: Pregnancy category C; excreted into breast milk; no adverse effects on nursing infants have been reported

SIDE EFFECTS

Occasional

Rash, nausea, dyspepsia, difficulty urinating

Rare

Bladder irritation, increased liver enzymes

SERIOUS REACTIONS

- Crystalluria can occur when methenamine is given in large doses.

INTERACTIONS

Drugs

3 *Acetazolamide:* Acetazolamide interferes with the urinary antibacterial activity of methenamine

3 *Antacids (magnesium, aluminum, sodium bicarbonate):* Interfere with urinary antibacterial activity of methenamine

3 *Sulfadiazine (sulfamethizole, sulfathiazole):* Combination may yield crystalluria

Labs

- *Catecholamines:* Plasma, increased
- *Estriol:* Urine, decreased
- *Estrogens:* Urine, decreased
- *PSP Excretion:* Urine, increased
- *Sugar:* Urine, increased via Benedict's reagent
- *Urobilinogen:* Urine, increased

SPECIAL CONSIDERATIONS

PATIENT/FAMILY EDUCATION

- Keep urine acidic (pH <5.5) by eating food that acidifies urine (meats, eggs, fish, gelatin products, prunes, plums, cranberries); may need to add ascorbic acid
- Fluids must be increased to 3 L/day to avoid crystallization in kidneys
- Take at evenly spaced intervals around clock for best results
- Take with food to reduce GI upset

MONITORING PARAMETERS
- Periodic liver function tests (hippurate); urine pH
- Renal function
- Skin for rash

methimazole

(meth-im'-a-zole)

Rx: Tapazole

Chemical Class: Thioimidazole derivative

Therapeutic Class: Antithyroid agent

CLINICAL PHARMACOLOGY

Mechanism of Action: A thiomidazole derivative that inhibits synthesis of thyroid hormone by interfering with the incorporation of iodine into tyrosyl residues. ***Therapeutic Effect:*** Effectively treats hyperthyroidism by decreasing thyroid hormone levels.

Pharmacokinetics

Rapid absorption following PO administration. Protein binding: Not significant. Widely distributed throughout the body. Metabolized in liver. Excreted in urine. ***Half-life:*** 5-6 hr.

INDICATIONS AND DOSAGES

Hyperthyroidism

PO

Adults, Elderly. Initially, 15-60 mg/day in 3 divided doses. Maintenance: 5-15 mg/day.

Children. Initially, 0.4 mg/kg/day in 3 divided doses. Maintenance: One-half the initial dose.

AVAILABLE FORMS
- *Tablets:* 5 mg, 10 mg, 20 mg.

CONTRAINDICATIONS: None known.

PREGNANCY AND LACTATION: Pregnancy category D; use smallest possible dose to control maternal disease (propylthiouracil preferable, less likely to cross the placenta); excreted into breast milk

SIDE EFFECTS

Frequent (5%-4%)

Fever, rash, pruritus

Occasional (3%-1%)

Dizziness, loss of taste, nausea, vomiting, stomach pain, peripheral neuropathy or numbness in fingers, toes, face

Rare (less than 1%)

Swollen lymph nodes or salivary glands

SERIOUS REACTIONS
- Agranulocytosis as long as 4 mos after therapy, pancytopenia, and hepatitis have occurred.

INTERACTIONS

Drugs

3 *Amiodarone, iodinated glycerol, iodine, potassium iodide:* May decrease response to methimazole

3 *Digoxin:* May increase the blood concentration of digoxin as patient becomes euthyroid

3 *I^{131}:* May decrease thyroid uptake of I^{131}

3 *Oral anticoagulants:* Reduced hypoprothrombinemic response to oral anticoagulants

3 *Theophylline:* Physiologic response to antithyroid drug will increase theophylline concentrations via decreased clearance

Labs
- *False increase:* Glucose

SPECIAL CONSIDERATIONS
- Methimazole is the thioamide of choice based on improved patient adherence and outcomes

PATIENT/FAMILY EDUCATION
- Notify clinician of fever, sore throat, unusual bleeding or bruising, rash, yellowing of skin, vomiting

• Do not exceed the prescribed dosage
• Space do[illegible]venly around the clo[illegible] consumption of iodine products and seafood

[illegible]NITORING PARAMETERS

• [illegible]BC periodically during therapy [illegible]pecially during initial 3 mo), [illegible]SH
• Prothrombin time
• Serum hepatic enzymes
• Pulse
• Weight
• Skin for rash

---

methocarbamol

(meth-oh-kar'-ba-mole)

Rx: Carbacot, Robaxin

Combinations

Rx: with aspirin (Robaxisal)

Chemical Class: Carbamate derivative

Therapeutic Class: Skeletal muscle relaxant

CLINICAL PHARMACOLOGY

Mechanism of Action: A carbamate derivative of guaifenesin that causes skeletal muscle relaxation by general CNS depression. ***Therapeutic Effect:*** Relieves muscle spasticity.

Pharmacokinetics

Rapidly and almost completely absorbed from the gastrointestinal (GI) tract. Protein binding: 46%-50%. Metabolized in liver by dealkylation and hydroxylation. Primarily excreted in urine as metabolites. ***Half-life:*** 1-2 hrs.

INDICATIONS AND DOSAGES

Musculoskeletal spasm

IM/IV

Adults, Children 16 yrs and older. 1 g q8h for no more than 3 consecutive days. May repeat course of therapy after a drug-free interval of 48 hrs.

PO

Adults, Children 16 yrs and older. 1.5 g 4 times/day for 2-3 days (up to 8 g/day may be given in severe conditions). Decrease to 4-4.5 g/day in 3-6 divided doses.

Elderly. Initially, 500 mg 4 times a day. May gradually increase dosage.

Tetanus spasm

IV

Adults. 1-3 g q6h until oral dosing is possible. Injection should be used no more than 3 consecutive days.

Children. 15 mg/kg/dose or 500 mg/m^2/dose q6h as needed. Maximum: 1.8 g/m^2/day for 3 days only.

AVAILABLE FORMS

• *Injection:* 100 mg/ml (Robaxin).
• *Tablets:* 325 mg, 500 mg (Carbacot, Robaxin), 750 mg (Carbacot).

CONTRAINDICATIONS: Hypersensitivity to methocarbamol or any component of the formulation, renal impairment (injection formulation)

PREGNANCY AND LACTATION: Pregnancy category C; compatible with breast-feeding

SIDE EFFECTS

Frequent

Transient drowsiness, weakness, dizziness, lightheadedness, nausea, vomiting

Occasional

Headache, constipation, anorexia, hypotension, confusion, blurred vision, vertigo, facial flushing, rash

Rare

Paradoxical CNS excitement and restlessness, slurred speech, tremor, dry mouth, diarrhea, nocturia, impotence, bradycardia, hypotension, syncope

SERIOUS REACTIONS

• Anaphylactoid reactions, leukopenia, and seizures (intravenous form) have been reported.
• Methocarbamol overdosage results in cardiac arrhythmias, nausea, vomiting, drowsiness, and coma.

INTERACTIONS

Drugs

3 *Pyridostigmine bromide:* May inhibit the effect of pyridostigmine bromide

Labs

- *Color:* Urine brown, green, blue, or black on standing
- *5-hydroxyindole acetic acid:* Urine, increased
- *Vanillylmandelic acid (VMA):* Urine, increased

SPECIAL CONSIDERATIONS

PATIENT/FAMILY EDUCATION

- Drowsiness usually diminishes with continued therapy
- Avoid tasks that require mental alertness or motor skills until response to the drug is established
- Do not abruptly discontinue methocarbamol after long-term therapy

MONITORING PARAMETERS

- Therapeutic response, such as decreased intensity of skeletal muscle pain

---

methotrexate sodium

(meth-oh-trex'-ate soe'-dee-um)

Rx: Rheumatrex, Trexall

Chemical Class: Dihydrofolate reductase inhibitor

Therapeutic Class: Antineoplastic; antipsoriatic; disease-modifying antirheumatic drug (DMARD)

CLINICAL PHARMACOLOGY

Mechanism of Action: An antimetabolite that competes with enzymes necessary to reduce folic acid to tetrahydrofolic acid, a component essential to DNA, RNA, and protein synthesis. This action inhibits DNA, RNA, and protein synthesis. ***Therapeutic Effect:*** Causes death of cancer cells.

Pharmacokinetics

Variably absorbed from the GI tract. Completely absorb[illegible] IM administration. Protein binding[illegible] 60%. Widely distributed. Metabo[illegible]lized intracellularly in the li[illegible]. Primarily excreted in urine. Re[illegible]moved by hemodialysis but not by peritoneal dialysis. ***Half-life:*** 8-12 hr (large doses, 8-15 hr).

INDICATIONS AND DOSAGES

Trophoblastic neoplasms

PO, IM

Adults, Elderly. 15-30 mg/day for 5 days; repeat in 7 days for 3-5 courses.

Head and neck cancer

PO, IV, IM

Adults, Elderly. 25-50 mg/m^2 once weekly.

Choriocarcinoma, chorioadenoma destruens, hydatidiform mole

PO, IM

Adults, Elderly. 15-30 mg/day for 5 days; repeat 3-5 times with 1-2 wk between courses.

Breast cancer

IV

Adults, Elderly. 30-60 mg/m^2 days 1 and 8 q3-4wk.

Acute lymphocytic leukemia

PO, IV, IM

Adults, Elderly. Induction: 3.3 mg/m^2/day in combination with other chemotherapeutic agents. Maintenance: 30 mg/m^2/wk PO or IM in divided doses or 2.5 mg/kg IV every 14 days.

Burkitt's lymphoma

PO

Adults. 10-25 mg/day for 4-8 days; repeat with 7- to 10-day rest between courses.

Lymphosarcoma

PO

Adults, Elderly. 0.625-2.5 mg/kg/day.

ment along with intensified monitoring during early therapy is recommended—CBCs at 1, 2, and 4 wk of treatment; if stable dose may be increased and subsequent CBCs should be performed at monthly intervals
- BUN, serum uric acid, urine ClCr, electrolytes before, during therapy
- Liver function tests before and during therapy

methoxsalen

(meth-ox'-a-len)

Rx: 8-MOP, Oxsoralen, Oxsoralen-Ultra, Uvadex

Chemical Class: Psoralen derivative

Therapeutic Class: Antipsoriatic; pigmenting agent

CLINICAL PHARMACOLOGY

Mechanism of Action: A member of the family of psoralens that induces an augmented sunburn reaction followed by hyperpigmentation in the presence of long-wave ultraviolet radiation. Bonds covalently to pyrimidine bases in DNA, inhibits the synthesis of DNA, and suppresses cell division. The augmented sunburn reaction involves excitation of the methoxsalen molecule by radiation in the long-wave ultraviolet light (UVA), resulting in transference of energy to the methoxsalen molecule producing an excited state or "triplet electronic state". The molecule, in this "triplet state", then reacts with cutaneous DNA. ***Therapeutic Effect:*** Results in symptomatic control of severe, recalcitrant disabling psoriasis, repigmentation of idiopathic vitiligo, palliative treatment of skin manifestations of cutaneous T-cell lymphoma (CTCL), repigmentation of idiopathic vitiligo, and palliative treatment of skin manifestations of CTCL.

Pharmacokinetics

Absorption varies. Food increases peak serum levels. Reversibly bound to albumin. Metabolized in the liver. Excreted in the urine. ***Half-life:*** 2 hrs.

INDICATIONS AND DOSAGES

Psoriasis

PO

Adults, Elderly. 10-70 mg 1.5 -2 hrs before exposure to UVA light, repeated 2-3 times/week. Give at least 48 hrs apart. Dosage is based upon patient's body weight and skin type:

Less than 30 kg: 10 mg.
30-50 kg: 20 mg.
51-65 kg: 30 mg.
66-80 kg: 40 mg.
81-90 kg: 50 mg.
91-115 kg: 60 mg.
more than 115 kg: 70 mg.

Vitiligo

PO

Adults, Elderly, Children older than 12 yrs. 20 mg 2-4 hrs before exposure to UVA light. Give at least 48 hrs apart.

Topical

Adults, Elderly, Children older than 12 yrs. Apply 1-2 hrs. before exposure to UVA light, no more than once weekly.

CTCL

Extracorporeal

Adults, Elderly. Inject 200 mcg into the photoactivation bag during collection cycle using the UVAR photopheresis system, 2 consecutive days every 4 wks for a minimum of 7 treatment cycles.

AVAILABLE FORMS

- *Capsule:* 10 mg (8-MOP).
- *Gelcap:* 10 mg (Oxsoralen-Ultra).
- *Lotion:* 1% (Oxsoralen).
- *Solution:* 20 mcg/ml (Uvadex).

UNLABELED USES: Dermographism, eczema, hypereosinophilic syndrome, hypopigmented sarcoidosis, ichthyosis linearis circumflexa, lymphomatoid papulosis, mycosis fungoides, palmoplantar pustulosis, pruritus, scleromyxedema, systemic sclerosis

CONTRAINDICATIONS: Cataract, invasive squamous cell cancer, aphakia, melanoma, pregnancy (Uvadex), diseases associated with photosensitivity, hypersensitivity to methoxsalen (psoralens) or any component of the formulation

PREGNANCY AND LACTATION: Pregnancy category C; excretion into breast milk unknown

SIDE EFFECTS

Occasional

Nausea, pruritus, edema, hypotension, nervousness, vertigo, depression, dizziness, headache, malaise, painful blistering, burning, rash, urticaria, loss of muscle coordination, leg cramps

SERIOUS REACTIONS

• Hypersensitivity reaction, such as nausea and severe burns, may occur.

SPECIAL CONSIDERATIONS

• Hard and soft caps are not equivalent

PATIENT/FAMILY EDUCATION

• Do not sunbathe during 24 hr prior to methoxsalen ingestion and UVA exposure

• Wear UVA-absorbing sunglasses for 24 hr following treatment to prevent cataract

• Avoid sun exposure for at least 8 hr after methoxsalen ingestion

• Avoid concurrent photosensitizing drugs

• Avoid furocoumarin-containing foods (e.g., limes, figs, parsley, parsnips, mustard, carrots, celery)

• Repigmentation of vitiligo may require 6-9 mo

MONITORING PARAMETERS

• Weight

• UVA exposure

methscopolamine bromide

(meth-scoe-pol-a-meen broe'-mide)

Rx: Carbacot, Pamine, Robaxin

Chemical Class: Quaternary ammonium derivative

Therapeutic Class: Antiulcer agent (adjunct)

CLINICAL PHARMACOLOGY

Mechanism of Action: A carbamate derivative of guaifenesin that causes skeletal muscle relaxation by general CNS depression. ***Therapeutic Effect:*** Relieves muscle spasticity.

Pharmacokinetics

Rapidly and almost completely absorbed from the gastrointestinal (GI) tract. Protein binding: 46%-50%. Metabolized in liver by dealkylation and hydroxylation. Primarily excreted in urine as metabolites. ***Half-life:*** 1-2 hrs.

INDICATIONS AND DOSAGES

Musculoskeletal spasm

IM/IV

Adults, Children 16 yrs and older. 1 g q8h for no more than 3 consecutive days. May repeat course of therapy after a drug-free interval of 48 hrs.

PO

Adults, Children 16 yrs and older. 1.5 g 4 times/day for 2-3 days (up to 8 g/day may be given in severe conditions). Decrease to 4-4.5 g/day in 3-6 divided doses.

Elderly. Initially, 500 mg 4 times a day. May gradually increase dosage.

Tetanus spasm

IV

Adults. 1-3 g q6h until oral dosing is possible. Injection should be used no more than 3 consecutive days.

Children. 15 mg/kg/dose or 500 mg/m^2/dose q6h as needed. Maximum: 1.8 g/m^2/day for 3 days only.

AVAILABLE FORMS

- *Injection:* 100 mg/ml (Robaxin).
- *Tablets:* 325 mg, 500 mg (Carbacot, Robaxin), 750 mg (Carbacot).

CONTRAINDICATIONS: Hypersensitivity to methocarbamol or any component of the formulation, renal impairment (injection formulation)

PREGNANCY AND LACTATION: Pregnancy category C; excretion into breast milk unknown, although would be expected to be minimal due to quaternary structure (see also atropine)

SIDE EFFECTS

Frequent

Transient drowsiness, weakness, dizziness, lightheadedness, nausea, vomiting

Occasional

Headache, constipation, anorexia, hypotension, confusion, blurred vision, vertigo, facial flushing, rash

Rare

Paradoxical CNS excitement and restlessness, slurred speech, tremor, dry mouth, diarrhea, nocturia, impotence, bradycardia, hypotension, syncope

SERIOUS REACTIONS

- Anaphylactoid reactions, leukopenia, and seizures (intravenous form) have been reported.
- Methocarbamol overdosage results in cardiac arrhythmias, nausea, vomiting, drowsiness, and coma.

INTERACTIONS

Drugs

3 *Amantadine, rimantadine:* Methscopolamine potentiates the CNS side effects of antivirals; antivirals potentiate the anticholinergic side effects of other anticholinergics

3 *Antacids:* May interfere with the absorption of methscopolamine

3 *Antidepressants (amitriptyline, doxepin, imipramine, maprotiline, nortriptyline, protriptyline, trimipramine):* Excessive anticholinergic effects

3 *Neuroleptics (chlorpromazine, haloperidol):* Methscopolamine may inhibit the therapeutic response to neuroleptics; excessive anticholinergic effects with combination

3 *Tacrine:* Tacrine may inhibit the therapeutic effects of anticholinergic agents; centrally acting anticholinergics may inhibit the therapeutic effects of tacrine

SPECIAL CONSIDERATIONS

- Has not been shown to be effective in contributing to the healing of peptic ulcer, decreasing the rate of recurrence, or preventing complications

PATIENT/FAMILY EDUCATION

- Avoid performing tasks that require mental alertness or motor skills until response to the drug is established
- Notify the physician if blood in stool occurs

MONITORING PARAMETERS

- Upper gastrointestinal contrast radiology or endoscopy to ensure healing
- Stool tests for occult blood and blood hemoglobin or hematocrit values to rule out bleeding from ulcer

methsuximide

(meth-sux'-i-mide)

Rx: Celontin

Chemical Class: Succinimide derivative

Therapeutic Class: Anticonvulsant

CLINICAL PHARMACOLOGY

Mechanism of Action: An anticonvulsant agent that increases the seizure threshold, suppresses paroxysmal spike-and-wave pattern in absence seizures, and depresses nerve transmission in the motor cortex. ***Therapeutic Effect:*** Controls absence (petit mal) seizures.

Pharmacokinetics

Rapidly metabolized in liver to active metabolite, *N*-desmethylmethsuximide. Primarily excreted in urine. Unknown if removed by hemodialysis. ***Half-life:*** 1.4 hr.

INDICATIONS AND DOSAGES

Absence seizures

PO

Adults, Elderly. Initially, 300 mg/day for the first week. Increase dosage by 300 mg/day at weekly intervals until response is attained. Maintenance: 1200 mg/day at 2-4 times/day. Do not exceed 1000 mg/day in children 12-15 yrs, 1200 mg/day in patients older than 15 yr.

Children. Initially, 10-15 mg/kg/day 3-4 times/day. Increase at weekly intervals. Maximum: 30 mg/kg/day.

AVAILABLE FORMS

• *Capsules:* 150 mg, 300 mg (Celontin).

UNLABELED USES: Partial complex (psychomotor) seizures

CONTRAINDICATIONS: Hypersensitivity to succinimides or any component of the formulation

PREGNANCY AND LACTATION: Pregnancy category C

SIDE EFFECTS

Frequent

Drowsiness, dizziness, nausea, vomiting

Occasional

Visual abnormalities, such as spots before eyes, difficulty focusing, blurred vision, dry mouth or pharynx, tongue irritation, nervousness, insomnia, headache, constipation or diarrhea, rash, weight loss, proteinuria, edema

SERIOUS REACTIONS

• Toxic reactions appear as blood dyscrasias, including aplastic anemia, agranulocytosis, thrombocytopenia, leukopenia, leukocytosis, eosinophilia, cardiovascular disturbances, such as congestive heart failure (CHF), hypotension or hypertension, thrombophlebitis, arrhythmias, and dermatologic effects, such as rash, urticaria, pruritus, photosensitivity.

• Abrupt withdrawal may precipitate status epilepticus.

INTERACTIONS

Drugs

3 *Other antiepileptic agents:* May increase plasma concentrations of these drugs

Labs

• *Ethosuximide:* False positive metabolite cross-reacts

SPECIAL CONSIDERATIONS

PATIENT/FAMILY EDUCATION

• Take with food or milk

• Do not discontinue abruptly

• Drowsiness usually subsides with continued therapy

• Avoid tasks that require mental alertness and motor skills until response to the drug is established

• Notify the physician of visual disturbances, rash, or unusual bleeding

MONITORING PARAMETERS

• CBC with differential; liver enzymes

• Serum *N*-desmethylmethsuximide concentrations at trough for efficacy (range 10-40 mcg/ml) and 3 hr post-dose for toxicity (>40 mcg/ml)
• Clinical improvement

methyclothiazide

(meth-i-kloe-thye'-ah-zide)

Rx: Aquatensen, Enduron

Combinations

Rx: with reserpine (Diutensen-R)

Chemical Class: Sulfonamide derivative

Therapeutic Class: Antihypertensive; diuretic, thiazide

CLINICAL PHARMACOLOGY

Mechanism of Action: A sulfonamide derivative that acts as a thiazide diuretic and antihypertensive. As a diuretic it blocks the reabsorption of water, sodium, and potassium at cortical diluting segment of distal tubule. As an antihypertensive it reduces plasma and extracellular fluid volume and decreases peripheral vascular resistance (PVR) by direct effect on blood vessels. ***Therapeutic Effect:*** Promotes diuresis, reduces blood pressure (BP).

Pharmacokinetics

Variably absorbed from the gastrointestinal (GI) tract. Primarily excreted unchanged in urine. Not removed by hemodialysis. ***Half-life:*** 24 hrs.

INDICATIONS AND DOSAGES

Edema

PO

Adults. 2.5-10 mg/day.

Hypertension

PO

Adults. 2.5-5 mg/day.

AVAILABLE FORMS

• *Tablets:* 2.5 mg, 5 mg (Aquatensen, Enduron).

UNLABELED USES: Treatment of diabetes insipidus, prevention of calcium-containing renal stones

CONTRAINDICATIONS: Anuria, history of hypersensitivity to sulfonamides or thiazide diuretics, renal decompensation

PREGNANCY AND LACTATION: Pregnancy category B; therapy for preexisting hypertension can be continued throughout pregnancy with minimal risk; initiating for simple edema not recommended; few unequivocal indications for diuretic therapy in pregnancy except for pulmonary edema or congestive heart failure; excreted into breast milk in small amounts; considered compatible with breast-feeding

SIDE EFFECTS

Expected

Increase in urinary frequency and volume

Frequent

Potassium depletion

Occasional

Postural hypotension, headache, GI disturbances, photosensitivity reaction, anorexia

SERIOUS REACTIONS

• Vigorous diuresis may lead to profound water loss and electrolyte depletion leading to hypokalemia, hyponatremia, and dehydration.
• Acute hypotensive episodes may occur.
• Hyperglycemia may be noted during prolonged therapy.
• GI upset, pancreatitis, dizziness, paresthesias, headache, blood dyscrasias, pulmonary edema, allergic pneumonitis, and dermatologic reactions occur rarely.
• Overdosage can lead to lethargy and coma without changes in electrolytes or hydration.

INTERACTIONS

Drugs

3 *Alcohol, barbiturates, narcotics:* Potentiation of orthostatic hypotension may occur

2 *Angiotensin-converting enzyme inhibitors:* Risk of postural hypotension when added to ongoing diuretic therapy; more common with loop diuretics; first-dose hypotension possible in patients with sodium depletion or hypovolemia due to diuretics or sodium restriction; hypotensive response is usually transient; hold diuretic day of first dose

3 *Calcium:* Large doses can lead to milk-alkali syndrome

3 *Carbenoxolone:* Severe hypokalemia

3 *Binding resins (cholestyramine, colestipol):* Reduces thiazide serum levels and lessened diuretic effects

3 *Corticosteroids:* Concomitant therapy may result in excessive potassium loss

3 *Diazoxide:* Hyperglycemia

3 *Digitalis glycosides:* Diuretic-induced hypokalemia may potentiate the risk of digitalis toxicity

3 *Hypoglycemic agents:* Thiazide diuretics tend to increase blood glucose; may increase dosage requirements of hypoglycemic agents.

3 *Insulin:* Increased blood glucose, increased dosage requirement of antidiabetic drugs

3 *Lithium:* Increased lithium concentrations

3 *Methotrexate:* Increased methotrexate effects; potentiates bone marrow toxicity

3 *Nonsteroidal antiinflammatory drugs:* Concurrent use may reduce diuretic and antihypertensive effects.

3 *Pressor amines (e.g., norepinephrine):* Possible decreased response to pressor amines

SPECIAL CONSIDERATIONS

- Doses above 2.5 mg provide no further blood pressure reduction, but are more likely to induce metabolic disturbance (i.e., hypokalemia, hyperuricemia)
- May protect against osteoporotic hip fractures
- Loop diuretics or metolazone more effective if CrCl <40-50 ml/min

PATIENT/FAMILY EDUCATION

- Will increase urination temporarily (approx. 3 wks); take early in the day to prevent sleep disturbance
- May cause sensitivity to sunlight; avoid prolonged exposure to the sun and other ultraviolet light
- May cause gout attacks; notify clinician if sudden joint pain occurs
- Rise slowly from lying to sitting position and permit legs to dangle momentarily before standing to reduce the drug's hypotensive effect

MONITORING PARAMETERS

- Weight, urine output, serum electrolytes, BUN, creatinine, CBC, uric acid, glucose, lipids

methylcellulose

(meth-ill-sell'-you-lose)

OTC: Citrucel, Cologel

Chemical Class: Hydrophilic semisynthetic cellulose derivative

Therapeutic Class: Laxative

CLINICAL PHARMACOLOGY

Mechanism of Action: A bulk-forming laxative that dissolves and expands in water. ***Therapeutic Effect:*** Provides increased bulk and moisture content in stool, increasing peristalsis and bowel motility.

Pharmacokinetics

Route	Onset	Peak	Duration
PO	12-24 hr	N/A	N/A

Acts in small and large intestines. Full effect may not be evident for 2-3 days.

INDICATIONS AND DOSAGES

Constipation

PO

Adults, Elderly. 1 tbsp (15 ml) in 8 oz water 1-3 times a day.

Children 6-12 yr. 1 tsp (5 ml) in 4 oz water 3-4 times a day.

AVAILABLE FORMS

• *Powder (Citrucel, Cologel).*

CONTRAINDICATIONS: Abdominal pain, dysphagia, nausea, partial bowel obstruction, symptoms of appendicitis, vomiting

PREGNANCY AND LACTATION: Pregnancy category C; bulk-forming laxatives are the laxative of choice during pregnancy; compatible with breast-feeding

SIDE EFFECTS

Rare

Some degree of abdominal discomfort, nausea, mild cramps, griping, faintness

SERIOUS REACTIONS

• Esophageal or bowel obstruction may occur if administered with less than 250 ml or 1 full glass of liquid.

INTERACTIONS

Drugs

3 *Digoxin, oral anticoagulants, salicylates:* May decrease the effects of digoxin, oral anticoagulants, and salicylates by decreasing absorption of these drugs

3 *Potassium-sparing diuretics, potassium supplements:* May interfere with the effects of potassium-sparing diuretics and potassium supplements

SPECIAL CONSIDERATIONS

PATIENT/FAMILY EDUCATION

• Notify clinician of unrelieved constipation, rectal bleeding

• Ensure adequate fluids, proper dietary fiber intake, and regular exercise

• Take each dose with a full glass of water; taking methylcellulose with an inadequate amount of fluid may cause choking or swelling in the throat

MONITORING PARAMETERS

• Pattern of daily bowel activity and stool consistency, time of evacuation

• Electrolytes

---

methyldopa

(meth-ill-doe′-pa)

Rx: Aldomet, Methyldopate

Combinations

Rx: with HCTZ (Aldoril); with chlorothiazide (Aldoclor)

Chemical Class: Catecholamine, synthetic

Therapeutic Class: Antihypertensive; centrally acting sympathoplegic

---

CLINICAL PHARMACOLOGY

Mechanism of Action: An antihypertensive agent that stimulates central inhibitory alpha-adrenergic receptors, lowers arterial pressure, and reduces plasma renin activity. ***Therapeutic Effect:*** Reduces BP.

Pharmacokinetics

Absorption from GI tract is variable. Protein binding: negligible. Metabolized in liver. Excreted in urine. Removed by hemodialysis. ***Half-life:*** 1.7 hr.

M

INDICATIONS AND DOSAGES
Hypertension
IV
Adults, Elderly. 250-500 mg q6h. Maximum: 1 g q6h.
Children. 5-10 mg/kg/dose q6-8h. Maximum: 65 mg/kg/day or 3g/24 hr.
PO
Adults, Elderly. Initially, 250 mg 2-3 times a day. May increase at 2-day intervals up to 3 g/day. Range: 250-1000 mg/day in 2 divided doses.
Children. Initially, 10 mg/kg/day in 2-4 divided doses. May increase at 2-day intervals up to 65 mg/kg/day. Maximum: 3 g/day.

AVAILABLE FORMS
- *Tablets (Aldomet):* 125 mg, 250 mg, 500 mg.
- *Oral Suspension (Methyldopate):* 250 mg/5 ml.
- *Injection:* 50 mg/ml.

CONTRAINDICATIONS: Hepatic disease, hepatic disorders previously associated with methyldopa therapy, MAOIs, pheochromocytoma

PREGNANCY AND LACTATION: Pregnancy category B (oral); C (IV); no adverse reactions have been reported despite rather wide use during pregnancy; compatible with breast-feeding

SIDE EFFECTS
Frequent
Peripheral edema, somnolence, headache, dry mouth
Occasional
Mental changes (such as anxiety, depression), decreased sexual function or libido, diarrhea, swelling of breasts, nausea, vomiting, lightheadedness, paresthesia, rhinitis

SERIOUS REACTIONS
- Hepatotoxicity (abnormal liver function test results, jaundice, hepatitis), hemolytic anemia, unexplained fever and flu-like symptoms may occur. If these conditions appear, discontinue the medication and contact the physician.

INTERACTIONS
Drugs
3 *β-blockers:* Rebound hypertension from methyldopa withdrawal exacerbated by noncardioselective β-blockers
3 *Hypotensive-producing medications:* May increase the effects of methyldopa
3 *Iron:* Inhibited antihypertensive response to methyldopa
3 *Lithium:* Lithium toxicity not necessarily associated with excessive lithium concentrations
3 *MAOIs:* May cause hyperexcitability
3 *Norepinephrine:* May prolong the pressor response to norepinephrine
3 *NSAIDs:* May decrease the effects of methyldopa
3 *Tricyclic antidepressants:* Inhibit the antihypertensive response
Labs
- *Interference:* Plasma and urine catecholamines, serum creatinine, glucose, serum, urine uric acid, and acetaminophen, AST
- *False increase:* Urine amino acids, serum bilirubin, urine ferric chloride test, urine ketones, metanephrines, VMA
- *False decrease:* Serum cholesterol, triglycerides
- *False positive:* Guaiacols spot test, urine melanogen, urine Thormahlen test

SPECIAL CONSIDERATIONS
- Perform both direct and indirect Coombs test if blood transfusion needed. If indirect Coombs test positive, interference may occur with cross match. Positive direct Coombs test will not interfere

PATIENT/FAMILY EDUCATION

- Urine exposed to air after voiding may darken
- Do not discontinue abruptly
- Initial sedation usually improves
- Avoid tasks requiring mental alertness and motor skills until response to the drug has been established

MONITORING PARAMETERS

- CBC, liver function tests periodically during therapy
- Direct Coombs test before therapy and after 6-12 mo. If positive rule out hemolytic anemia
- Blood pressure, pulse
- Weight

methylene blue

(meth'-i-leen bloo)

Rx: Urolene Blue

Chemical Class: Thiazine dye

Therapeutic Class: Antidote, cyanide; antidote, drug-induced methemoglobinemia; diagnostic agent

CLINICAL PHARMACOLOGY

Mechanism of Action: A weak germicide that hastens the conversion of methemoglobin to hemoglobin in low concentrations. At high concentrations, it has the opposite effect by converting ferrous ion of reduced hemoglobin to ferric iron to form methemoglobin. In cyanide toxicity, it combines with cyanide to form cyanmethemoglobin, preventing interference of cyanide with the cytochrome system. ***Therapeutic Effect:*** Antidote for drug-induced methemoglobinemia.

Pharmacokinetics

Erratic absorption. Protein binding: unknown. Metabolized in tissues to leucomethylene blue. Excreted unchanged in urine and feces. Unknown if removed by hemodialysis. ***Half-life:*** Unknown.

INDICATIONS AND DOSAGES

Methemoglobinemia, drug-induced

IV

Adults, Elderly, Children. 1-2 mg/kg (0.1-0.2 ml/kg of 1% solution) injected very slowly over several minutes.

NADPH-methemoglobin reductase deficiency

PO

Children. 1-1.5 mg/kg/day. Maximum: 300 mg/day.

Genitourniary antiseptic

PO

Adults. 65-130 mg 3 times/day. Maximum: 390 mg/day.

Dosage in renal impairment

Specific guidelines are unavailable although dosage adjustment should be considered.

AVAILABLE FORMS

- *Injection:* 10 mg/ml.
- *Tablets:* 65 mg (Urolene Blue).

CONTRAINDICATIONS: Hypersensitivity to methylene blue or any component of its formulation, glucose-6-phosphate dehydrogenase (G6PD) deficiency, intraspinal injection, severe renal insufficiency, treatment of methemoglobinemia in cyanide poisoning

PREGNANCY AND LACTATION: Pregnancy category C (category D if inj intra-amniotically); deep blue staining of the newborn, hemolytic anemia, hyperbilirubinemia, and methemoglobinemia in the newborn may occur after inj into the amniotic fluid

SIDE EFFECTS

Occasional

Dizziness, headache, mental confusion, abdominal pain, diarrhea, nausea, vomiting, hypertension, hypotension, sweating

M

Rare
Arrhythmias, hemolytic anemia, methemoglobinemia

SERIOUS REACTIONS

- Hemolytic anemia and methemoglobinemia occur rarely.

SPECIAL CONSIDERATIONS

PATIENT/FAMILY EDUCATION

- Photosensitivity may occur
- Methylene blue may discolor urine and feces blue-green
- Take after meals with a full glass of water
- Remove any stains from methylene blue using hypochlorite solution

MONITORING PARAMETERS

- Hct
- Blood pressure
- CBC

methylergonovine maleate

(meth-ill-er-goe-noe'-veen)

Rx: Methergine

Chemical Class: Ergot alkaloid

Therapeutic Class: Oxytocic

CLINICAL PHARMACOLOGY

Mechanism of Action: An ergot alkaloid that stimulates alpha-adrenergic and serotonin receptors, producing arterial vasoconstriction. Causes vasospasm of coronary arteries and directly stimulates uterine muscle. ***Therapeutic Effect:*** Increases strength and frequency of uterine contractions. Decreases uterine bleeding.

Pharmacokinetics

Route	*Onset*	*Peak*	*Duration*
PO	5-10 mins	N/A	N/A
IV	Immediate	N/A	3 hr
IM	2-5 mins	N/A	N/A

Rapidly absorbed from the GI tract after IM administration. Distributed rapidly to plasma, extracellular fluid, and tissues. Metabolized in the liver and undergoes first-pass effect. Primarily excreted in urine. ***Half-life:*** IV (alpha phase), 2-3 min or less; IV (beta phase), 20-30 min or longer.

INDICATIONS AND DOSAGES

Prevention and treatment of postpartum and post-abortion hemorrhage due to atony or involution

PO

Adults. 0.2 mg 3-4 times a day. Continue for up to 7 days.

IV, IM

Adults. Initially, 0.2 mg. May repeat q2-4h for no more than a total of 5 doses.

AVAILABLE FORMS

- *Tablets:* 0.2 mg.
- *Injection:* 0.2 mg/ml.

UNLABELED USES: Treatment of incomplete abortion

CONTRAINDICATIONS: Hypertension, pregnancy, toxemia, untreated hypocalcemia

PREGNANCY AND LACTATION: Pregnancy category C; small quantity appears in breast milk; adverse effects have not been described

SIDE EFFECTS

Frequent
Nausea, uterine cramping, vomiting

Occasional
Abdominal pain, diarrhea, dizziness, diaphoresis, tinnitus, bradycardia, chest pain

Rare
Allergic reaction, such as rash and itching; dyspnea; severe or sudden hypertension

SERIOUS REACTIONS

- Severe hypertensive episodes may result in cerebrovascular accident (CVA), serious arrhythmias, and seizures. Hypertensive effects are more frequent with patient susceptibility, rapid IV administration, and concurrent use of regional anesthesia or vasoconstrictors.

• Peripheral ischemia may lead to gangrene.

INTERACTIONS

Drugs

3 *Vasoconstrictors, vasopressors:* May increase the effects of methylergonovine

SPECIAL CONSIDERATIONS

PATIENT/FAMILY EDUCATION

• Report increased blood loss, severe abdominal cramps, increased temperature, or foul-smelling lochia.

• Symptoms of ergotism occur with overdosage (nausea, vomiting, diarrhea, seizure, hallucinations, delirium, numb/gangrenous extremities)

• Avoid smoking because of added effects of vasoconstriction

MONITORING PARAMETERS

• Blood pressure, pulse, and uterine response

---

methylphenidate hydrochloride

(meth-ill-fen′-i-date)

Rx: Concerta, Metadate CD, Metadate ER, Methylin, Methylin ER, Ritalin, Ritalin-LA, Ritalin-SR

Chemical Class: Piperidine derivative of amphetamine

Therapeutic Class: Cerebral stimulant

DEA Class: Schedule II

CLINICAL PHARMACOLOGY

Mechanism of Action: A CNS stimulant that blocks the reuptake of norepinephrine and dopamine into presynaptic neurons. ***Therapeutic Effect:*** Decreases motor restlessness and fatigue; increases motor activity, attention span, and mental alertness; produces mild euphoria.

Pharmacokinetics

Onset	Peak	Duration
Immediate-release	2 hrs	3-5 hrs
Sustained-release	4-7 hrs	3-8 hrs
Extended-release	N/A	8-12 hrs

Slowly and incompletely absorbed from the GI tract. Protein binding: 15%. Metabolized in the liver. Eliminated in urine and in feces by biliary system. Unknown if removed by hemodialysis. ***Half-life:*** 2-4 hrs.

INDICATIONS AND DOSAGES

Attention deficit hyperactivity disorder (ADHD)

PO

Children 6 yr and older. Immediate release: Initially, 2.5-5 mg before breakfast and lunch. May increase by 5-10 mg/day at weekly intervals. Maximum: 60 mg/day.

PO (Concerta)

Children 6 yr and older. Initially, 18 mg once a day; may increase by 18 mg/day at weekly intervals. Maximum: 72 mg/day.

PO (Metadate CD)

Children 6 yr and older. Initially, 20 mg/day. May increase by 20 mg/day at weekly intervals. Maximum: 60 mg/day.

PO (Ritalin LA)

Children 6 yr and older. Initially, 20 mg/day. May increase by 10 mg/day at weekly intervals. Maximum: 60 mg/day.

PO (Metadate ER, Methylin ER, Ritalin SR)

Children 6 yr and older. May replace regular tablets after daily dose is titrated and 8-hr dosage corresponds to sustained-release or extended-release tablet size.

M

Narcolepsy
PO
Adults, Elderly. 10 mg 2-3 times a day. Range: 10-60 mg/day.

AVAILABLE FORMS
- *Capsules (Extended-Release [Metadate CD]):* 10 mg, 20 mg, 30 mg.
- *Capsules (Extended-Release [Ritalin LA]):* 10 mg, 20 mg, 30 mg, 40 mg.
- *Tablets (Ritalin):* 5 mg, 10 mg, 20 mg.
- *Tablets (Extended-Release [Mentadate ER, Mehtylin ER]):* 10 mg, 20 mg.
- *Tablets (Extended-Release [Concerta]):* 18 mg, 27 mg, 36 mg, 54 mg, 72 mg.
- *Tablets (Sustained-Release [Ritalin SR]):* 20 mg.
- *Tablets (Chewable [Methylin]):* 2.5 mg, 5 mg, 10 mg.
- *Oral Solution (Methylin):* 5 mg/5 ml, 10 mg/5 ml.

UNLABELED USES: Treatment of disease-related fatigue, secondary mental depression,

CONTRAINDICATIONS: Use within 14 days of MAOIs

PREGNANCY AND LACTATION: Pregnancy category C
Controlled Substance: Schedule II

SIDE EFFECTS
Frequent
Anxiety, insomnia, anorexia
Occasional
Dizziness, drowsiness, headache, nausea, abdominal pain, fever, rash, arthralgia, vomiting
Rare
Blurred vision, Tourette syndrome (marked by uncontrolled vocal outbursts, repetitive body movements, and tics), palpitations

SERIOUS REACTIONS
- Prolonged administration to children with ADHD may delay growth.
- Overdose may produce tachycardia, palpitations, arrhythmias, chest pain, psychotic episode, seizures, and coma.
- Hypersensitivity reactions and blood dyscrasias occur rarely.

INTERACTIONS
Drugs
③ *CNS stimulants:* May have an additive effect
③ *Guanethidine:* Inhibition of guanethidine antihypertensive effect
② *MAOIs:* Hypertensive reactions
③ *Ma huang:* May increase CNS stimulation
③ *Phenytoin:* Increased phenytoin levels with risk of toxicity
③ *Tricyclic antidepressants:* Increased serum concentrations of tricyclic antidepressants
Labs
- *False positive:* Urine amphetamine

SPECIAL CONSIDERATIONS
- Overdosage may cause vomiting, agitation, tremor, muscle twitching, seizures, confusion, tachycardia, hypertension, arrhythmias

PATIENT/FAMILY EDUCATION
- Take last daily dose prior to 6 p.m. to avoid insomnia
- Do not discontinue abruptly
- Avoid OTC preparations unless approved by clinician
- Do not crush or chew sustained-release formulation
- Avoid performing tasks that require mental alertness or motor skills until response to the drug is established
- Dry mouth may be relieved by sugarless gum and sips of tepid water
- Report nervousness, palpitations, fever, vomiting, or skin rash

MONITORING PARAMETERS
- Periodic CBC with differential and platelet count

methylprednisolone/ methylprednisolone acetate/ methylprednisolone sodium succinate

(meth-ill-pred-niss'-oh-lone)

Rx: Adlone-40, Adlone-80, A-Methapred, Depmedalone, Dep Medalone 80, Depoject-80, Depo-Medrol, Depopred, Med-Jec-40, Medralone 80, Medrol, Medrol Dosepak, Methacort 40, Methacort 80, Methylcotol, Methylcotolone, Methylpred DP, Solu-Medrol

Chemical Class: Glucocorticoid, synthetic

Therapeutic Class: Corticosteroid, systemic

CLINICAL PHARMACOLOGY

Mechanism of Action: An adrenocortical steroid that suppresses migration of polymorphonuclear leukocytes and reverses increased capillary permeability. ***Therapeutic Effect:*** Decreases inflammation.

Pharmacokinetics

Route	Onset	Peak	Duration
PO	N/A	1-2 hrs	30-36 hrs
IM	N/A	4-8 days	1-4 wks

Well absorbed from the GI tract after IM administration. Widely distributed. Metabolized in the liver. Excreted in urine. Removed by hemodialysis. ***Half-life:*** 3.5 hrs.

INDICATIONS AND DOSAGES

Antiinflammatory, immunosuppressive

IV

Adults, Elderly. 10-40 mg. May repeat as needed.

Children. 0.5-1.7 mg/kg/day or 5-25 mg/m^2/day in 2-4 divided doses.

PO

Adults, Elderly. 2-60 mg/day in 1-4 divided doses.

Children. 0.5-1.7 mg/kg/day or 5-25 mg/m^2/day in 2-4 divided doses.

Status asthmaticus

IV

Adults, Elderly, Children. Initially, 2 mg/kg/dose, then 0.5-1 mg/kg/dose q6h for up to 5 days.

Spinal cord injury

IV Bolus

Adults, Elderly. 30 mg/kg over 15 min. Maintenance dose: 5.4 mg/kg/h over 23 hr, to be given within 45 min of bolus dose.

IM (methylprednisolone acetate)

Adults, Elderly. 10-80 mg/day.

Children. 0.5-1.7 mg/kg/day or 5-25 mg/m^2/day in 2-4 divided doses.

Intraarticular, Intralesional

Adults, Elderly. 4-40 mg, up to 80 mg q1-5wk.

AVAILABLE FORMS

- *Tablets (Medrol, Medrol Dosepak, Methylpred DP):* 2 mg, 4 mg, 8 mg, 16 mg, 32 mg.
- *Injection Powder for Reconstitution (A-Methapred, Solu-Medrol):* 40 mg, 125 mg, 500 mg, 1 g.
- *Injection Suspension:* 20 mg/ml (Depo-Medrol), 40 mg/ml (Adlone-40, Depo-Medrol, Depopred, Depmedalone, Med-Jec-40, Methylcotol), 80 mg/ml (Adlone-80, Depmedalone, Dep Medalone 80, Depoject-80, Depopred, Depo-Medrol, Medralone 80, Methacort 80, Methylcotolone).

CONTRAINDICATIONS: Administration of live virus vaccines, systemic fungal infection

PREGNANCY AND LACTATION: Pregnancy category C; excreted in breast milk; could suppress infant's growth and interfere with endogenous corticosteroid production

SIDE EFFECTS

Frequent

Insomnia, heartburn, anxiety, abdominal distention, diaphoresis, acne, mood swings, increased appetite, facial flushing, GI distress, delayed wound healing, increased susceptibility to infection, diarrhea or constipation

Occasional

Headache, edema, tachycardia, change in skin color, frequent urination, depression

Rare

Psychosis, increased blood coagulability, hallucinations

SERIOUS REACTIONS

- Long-term therapy may cause hypocalcemia, hypokalemia, muscle wasting (especially in arms and legs), osteoporosis, spontaneous fractures, amenorrhea, cataracts, glaucoma, peptic ulcer disease, and CHF.
- Abruptly withdrawing the drug after long-term therapy may cause anorexia, nausea, fever, headache, sudden severe myalgia, rebound inflammation, fatigue, weakness, lethargy, dizziness, and orthostatic hypotension.

INTERACTIONS

Drugs

3 *Aminoglutethamide:* Enhanced elimination of corticosteroids; marked reduction in corticosteroid response; increased clearance of methylprednisolone; doubling of dose may be necessary

3 *Amphotericin:* May increase hypokalemia

3 *Antidiabetics:* Increased blood glucose

3 *Barbiturates, carbamazepine:* Reduced serum concentrations of corticosteroids; increased clearance of methylprednisolone

3 *Cholestyramine, colestipol:* Possible reduced absorption of corticosteroids

3 *Cyclosporine:* Possible increased concentration of both drugs, seizures

3 *Digoxin:* May increase the risk of digoxin toxicity caused by hypokalemia

3 *Diuretics, potassium supplements:* May decrease the effects of these drugs

3 *Erythromycin, troleandomycin, clarithromycin, ketoconazole:* Possible enhanced steroid effect

3 *Estrogens, oral contraceptives:* Enhanced effects of corticosteroids

3 *Isoniazid:* Reduced plasma concentrations of isoniazid

3 *IUDs:* Inhibition of inflammation may decrease contraceptive effect

3 *Live-virus vaccines:* May decrease the patient's antibody response to vaccine, increase vaccine side effects, and potentiate virus replication

3 *NSAIDs:* Increased risk GI ulceration

3 *Rifampin:* Reduced therapeutic effect of corticosteroids; may reduce hepatic clearance of methylprednisolone

3 *Salicylates:* Subtherapeutic salicylate concentrations possible

Labs

- *False increase:* Cortisol, digoxin, theophylline level
- *False decrease:* Urine glucose (Clinistix, Diastix only, Testape no effect)
- *False negative:* Skin allergy tests

SPECIAL CONSIDERATIONS

PATIENT/FAMILY EDUCATION

- Take single daily doses in a.m.
- May mask infections

• Increased dose of rapidly acting corticosteroids may be necessary in patients subjected to unusual stresses
• Signs of adrenal insufficiency include fatigue, anorexia, nausea, vomiting, diarrhea, weight loss, weakness, dizziness, and low blood sugar
• Avoid abrupt withdrawal of therapy following high dose or long-term therapy. Relative insufficiency may exist for up to 1 yr after discontinuation
• Patients on chronic steroid therapy should wear Medic Alert bracelet
• Do not give live-virus vaccines to patients on prolonged therapy
• Take oral methylprednisolone with food or milk

MONITORING PARAMETERS

• Serum K and glucose
• Growth of children on prolonged therapy
• Intake and output
• Weight
• Pattern of daily bowel activity
• Vital signs
• Signs and symptoms of hypocalcemia (such as cramps and muscle twitching), or hypokalemia (such as EKG changes, irritability, nausea and vomiting, numbness or tingling of lower extremities, and weakness)

methyltestosterone

(meth-il-tes-tos'-te-rone)

Rx: Android, Android-10, Android-25, Oreton Methyl, Testred, Virilon

Chemical Class: Androgen; testosterone derivative

Therapeutic Class: Androgen; antineoplastic

DEA Class: Schedule III

CLINICAL PHARMACOLOGY

Mechanism of Action: A synthetic testosterone derivative with androgen activity that promotes growth and development of male sex organs and maintains secondary sex characteristics in androgen-deficient males. ***Therapeutic Effect:*** Treats hypogonadism and delayed puberty in males.

Pharmacokinetics

Well absorbed from the gastrointestinal (GI) tract. Protein binding: 98%. Metabolized in liver. Primarily excreted in urine. Unknown if removed by hemodialysis. ***Half-life:*** 10-100 min.

INDICATIONS AND DOSAGES

Breast cancer

PO

Adults, Elderly. 50-200 mg/day.

Delayed puberty

PO

Adults. 10-50 mg/day.

Adults, Elderly. 50-200 mg/day.

Hypogonadism

PO

Adults. 10-50 mg/day.

AVAILABLE FORMS

• *Capsules:* 10 mg (Android, Testred, Virilon).
• *Tablets:* 10 mg (Android-10, Oreton Methyl), 25 mg (Android-25).

UNLABELED USES: Hereditary angiodema

M

CONTRAINDICATIONS: Pregnancy, prostatic or breast cancer in males, hypersensitivity to methyltestosterone or any other component of its formulation

PREGNANCY AND LACTATION: Pregnancy category X; causes virilization of female fetuses; excretion into breast milk unknown; use extreme caution in nursing mothers

Controlled Substance: Schedule III

SIDE EFFECTS

Frequent

Gynecomastia, acne, amenorrhea or other menstrual irregularities

Females: Hirsutism, deepening of voice, clitoral enlargement that may not be reversible when drug is discontinued

Occasional

Edema, nausea, insomnia, oligospermia, priapism, male pattern of baldness, bladder irritability, hypercalcemia in immobilized patients or those with breast cancer, hypercholesterolemia

Rare

Polycythemia

SERIOUS REACTIONS

- Cholestatic jaundice, hepatocellular neoplasms, peliosis hepatitis, edema with or without congestive heart failure and suppression of clotting factors II, V, VII, and X have been reported.

INTERACTIONS

Drugs

❷ *Bupropion:* May increase the risk of seizures by decreasing seizure threshold

❸ *Cyclosporine:* Increased cyclosporine concentrations

❸ *Liver toxic medications:* May increase liver toxicity

❷ *Warfarin:* Enhanced hypoprothrombinemic response to oral anticoagulants

SPECIAL CONSIDERATIONS

PATIENT/FAMILY EDUCATION

- Do not swallow buccal tablets, allow to dissolve between cheek and gum
- Avoid eating, drinking, or smoking while buccal tablet in place

MONITORING PARAMETERS

- LFTs, lipids, Hct, Hgb
- Growth rate in children (X-rays for bone age q6mo)
- Report weight gains of 5 lbs or more
- Weight
- Blood pressure

metoclopramide hydrochloride

(met'-oh-kloe-pra'-mide hye-droe-klor'-ide)

Rx: Reglan

Chemical Class: Para-aminobenzoic acid derivative

Therapeutic Class: Antiemetic; gastrointestinal prokinetic agent

CLINICAL PHARMACOLOGY

Mechanism of Action: A dopamine receptor antagonist that stimulates motility of the upper GI tract and decreases reflux into the esophagus. Also raises the threshold of activity in the chemoreceptor trigger zone. ***Therapeutic Effect:*** Accelerates intestinal transit and gastric emptying; relieves nausea and vomiting.

Pharmacokinetics

Route	Onset	Peak	Duration
PO	30-60 min	N/A	N/A
IV	1-3 min	N/A	N/A
IM	10-15 min	N/A	N/A

Well absorbed from the GI tract. Metabolized in the liver. Protein binding: 30%. Primarily excreted in urine. Not removed by hemodialysis. ***Half-life:*** 4-6 hr.

INDICATIONS AND DOSAGES

Prevention of chemotherapy-induced nausea and vomiting

IV

Adults, Elderly, Children. 1-2 mg/kg 30 min before chemotherapy; repeat q2h for 2 doses, then q3h as needed for total of 5 doses/day.

Postoperative nausea, vomiting

IV

Adults, Elderly. 10-20 mg q4-6h as needed.

Children. 0.25 mg/kg/dose q6-8h as needed.

Diabetic gastroparesis

PO, IV

Adults. 10 mg 30 min before meals and at bedtime for 2-8 wk.

PO

Elderly. Initially, 5 mg 30 min before meals and at bedtime. May increase to 10 mg.

IV

Elderly. 5 mg over 1-2 min. May increase to 10 mg.

Symptomatic gastroesophageal reflux

PO

Adults. 10-15 mg up to 4 times a day, or single doses up to 20 mg as needed.

Elderly. Initially, 5 mg 4 times a day. May increase to 10 mg.

Children. 0.4-0.8 mg/kg/day in 4 divided doses.

To facilitate small bowel intubation (single dose)

IV

Adults, Elderly. 10 mg as a single dose.

Children 6-14 yr. 2.5-5 mg as a single dose.

Children younger than 6 yr. 0.1 mg/kg as a single dose.

Dosage in renal impairment

Dosage is modified based on creatinine clearance.

Creatinine Clearance	*% of normal dose*
40-50 ml/min	75%
10-40 ml/min	50%
less than 10 ml/min	25%-50%

AVAILABLE FORMS

- *Syrup:* 5 mg/5 ml.
- *Tablets:* 5 mg, 10 mg.
- *Injection:* 5 mg/ml.

UNLABELED USES: Prevention of aspiration pneumonia; treatment of drug-related postoperative nausea and vomiting, gastric stasis in preterm infants, persistent hiccups, slow gastric emptying, vascular headaches

CONTRAINDICATIONS: Concurrent use of medications likely to produce extrapyramidal reactions, GI hemorrhage, GI obstruction or perforation, history of seizure disorders, pheochromocytoma

PREGNANCY AND LACTATION: Pregnancy category B; has been used during pregnancy as an antiemetic and to decrease gastric emptying time; excreted into milk; use during lactation a concern because of the potent CNS effects the drug is capable of producing

SIDE EFFECTS

Frequent (10%)

Somnolence, restlessness, fatigue, lethargy

Occasional (3%)

Dizziness, anxiety, headache, insomnia, breast tenderness, altered menstruation, constipation, rash, dry mouth, galactorrhea, gynecomastia

Rare (less than 3%)

Hypotension or hypertension, tachycardia

SERIOUS REACTIONS

• Extrapyramidal reactions occur most commonly in children and young adults (18-30 yrs) receiving large doses (2 mg/kg) during chemotherapy and are usually limited to akathisia (involuntary limb movement and facial grimacing).

INTERACTIONS

Drugs

3 *Alcohol, other CNS depressants:* May increase CNS depressant effect

3 *Cyclosporine:* Increased bioavailability and serum concentrations of cyclosporine

3 *Digitalis glycosides:* Reduced serum digoxin concentration when coadministered with generic formulations

3 *Ethanol:* Increased sedative effects of ethanol

3 *MAOIs:* Metoclopramide releases catecholamines, use cautiously with MAOIs

3 *Insulin:* Dosage and timing of insulin may need to be adjusted

SPECIAL CONSIDERATIONS

• Dystonic reactions can be managed with 50 mg diphenhydramine or 1-2 mg benztropine IM

PATIENT/FAMILY EDUCATION

• Use caution while diving or during other activities requiring alertness; may cause drowsiness

• Notify the physician if involuntary eye, facial, or limb movement occurs

• Avoid alcohol during metoclopramide therapy

MONITORING PARAMETERS

• Blood pressure, heart rate, BUN and serum creatinine levels to assess renal function

metolazone

(me-tole'-a-zone)

Rx: Mykrox (rapid acting), Zaroxolyn (slow acting)

Chemical Class: Quinazoline derivative

Therapeutic Class: Antihypertensive; diuretic, thiazide-like

CLINICAL PHARMACOLOGY

Mechanism of Action: A thiazide-like diuretic and antihypertensive. As a diuretic, blocks reabsorption of sodium, potassium, and chloride at the distal convoluted tubule, increasing renal excretion of sodium and water. As an antihypertensive, reduces plasma and extracellular fluid volume and peripheral vascular resistance. ***Therapeutic Effect:*** Promotes diuresis and reduces BP.

Pharmacokinetics

Route	*Onset*	*Peak*	*Duration*
PO (diuretic)	1 hr	2 hrs	12-24 hrs

Incompletely absorbed from the GI tract. Protein binding: 95%. Primarily excreted unchanged in urine. Not removed by hemodialysis. ***Half-life:*** 14 hrs.

INDICATIONS AND DOSAGES

Edema

PO (Zaroxolyn)

Adults, Elderly. 5-10 mg/day. May increase to 20 mg/day in edema associated with renal disease or heart failure.

Children. 0.2-0.4 mg/kg/day in 1-2 divided doses.

Hypertension

PO (Zaroxolyn)

Adults, Elderly. 2.5-5 mg/day.

PO (Mykrox)

Adults, Elderly. Initially, 0.5 mg/day. May increase up to 1 mg/day.

AVAILABLE FORMS

• *Tablets (Prompt-Release [Mykrox]):* 0.5 mg.

• *Tablets (Extended-Release [Zaroxolyn]):* 2.5 mg, 5 mg, 10 mg.

CONTRAINDICATIONS: Anuria, hepatic coma or precoma, history of hypersensitivity to sulfonamides or thiazide diuretics, renal decompensation

PREGNANCY AND LACTATION: Pregnancy category B (D if used in pregnancy-induced hypertension); therapy for preexisting hypertension can be continued throughout pregnancy with minimal risk; initiating for simple edema not recommended; few unequivocal indications for diuretic therapy in pregnancy except for pulmonary edema or congestive heart failure; excreted into breast milk in small amounts; considered compatible with breastfeeding

SIDE EFFECTS

Expected

Increase in urinary frequency and urine volume

Frequent (10%-9%)

Dizziness, lightheadedness, headache

Occasional (6%-4%)

Muscle cramps and spasm, fatigue, lethargy

Rare (less than 2%)

Asthenia, palpitations, depression, nausea, vomiting, abdominal bloating, constipation, diarrhea, urticaria

SERIOUS REACTIONS

• Vigorous diuresis may lead to profound water and electrolyte depletion, resulting in hypokalemia, hyponatremia, and dehydration.

• Acute hypotensive episodes may occur.

• Hyperglycemia may occur during prolonged therapy.

• Pancreatitis, paresthesia, blood dyscrasias, pulmonary edema, allergic pneumonitis, and dermatologic reactions occur rarely.

• Overdose can lead to lethargy and coma without changes in electrolytes or hydration.

INTERACTIONS

Drugs

❷ *Angiotensin-converting enzyme inhibitors:* Risk of postural hypotension when added to ongoing diuretic therapy; more common with loop diuretics; first-dose hypotension possible in patients with sodium depletion or hypovolemia due to diuretics or sodium restriction; hypotensive response is usually transient; hold diuretic day of first dose

3 *Calcium:* Milk-alkali syndrome

3 *Carbenoxolone:* Enhanced hypokalemia

3 *Cholestyramine, colestipol:* Reduced serum concentrations of metolazone

3 *Corticosteroids:* Concomitant therapy may result in excessive potassium loss

3 *Diazoxide:* Hyperglycemia

3 *Digitalis glycosides:* Diuretic-induced hypokalemia may increase the risk of digitalis toxicity

3 *Hypoglycemic agents:* Metolazone increases blood glucose

3 *Lithium:* Increased serum lithium concentrations, toxicity may occur

3 *Methotrexate:* Enhanced bone marrow suppression

3 *Nonsteroidal antiinflammatory drugs:* Concurrent use may reduce diuretic and antihypertensive effects

SPECIAL CONSIDERATIONS

• More effective than other thiazide-type diuretics in patients with impaired renal function

• Metolazone formulations are not bioequivalent or therapeutically equivalent at the same doses. Mykrox is more rapidly and completely bioavailable; do not interchange brands.

PATIENT/FAMILY EDUCATION

• Will increase urination; take early in the day to prevent sleep disturbance
• May cause sensitivity to sunlight; avoid prolonged exposure to the sun and other ultraviolet light
• May cause gout attacks; notify clinician if sudden joint pain occurs
• Change position slowly and let legs dangle momentarily before standing to reduce the drug's hypotensive effect
• Eat foods high in potassium such as apricots, bananas, raisins, orange juice, potatoes, legumes, meat, and whole grains (such as cereals)

MONITORING PARAMETERS

• Weight, urine output, serum electrolytes, BUN, creatinine, CBC, uric acid, glucose, lipids

metoprolol tartrate

(me-toe-proe'-lole)

Rx: Lopressor, Toprol XL

Combinations

Rx: with hydrochlorothiazide (Lopressor Hct)

Chemical Class: β_1-adrenergic blocker, cardioselective

Therapeutic Class: Antianginal; antihypertensive

CLINICAL PHARMACOLOGY

Mechanism of Action: An antianginal, antihypertensive, and MI adjunct that selectively blocks $beta_1$-adrenergic receptors; high dosages may block $beta_2$-adrenergic receptors. Decreases oxygen requirements. Large doses increase airway resistance. ***Therapeutic Effect:*** Slows sinus node heart rate, decreases cardiac output, and reduces BP. Also decreases myocardial ischemia severity.

Pharmacokinetics

Route	Onset	Peak	Duration
PO	10-15 mins	N/A	6 hrs
PO (extended release)	N/A	6-12 hrs	24 hrs
IV	Immediate	20 mins	5-8 hrs

Well absorbed from the GI tract. Protein binding: 12%. Widely distributed. Metabolized in the liver (undergoes significant first-pass metabolism). Primarily excreted in urine. Removed by hemodialysis. ***Half-life:*** 3-7 hrs.

INDICATIONS AND DOSAGES

Mild to moderate hypertension

PO

Adults. Initially, 100 mg/day as single or divided dose. Increase at weekly (or longer) intervals. Maintenance: 100-450 mg/day.

Elderly. Initially, 25 mg/day. Range: 25-300 mg/day.

PO (Extended-Release)

Adults. 50-100 mg/day as single dose. May increase at least at weekly intervals until optimum BP attained. Maximum: 200 mg/day.

Elderly. Initially, 25-50 mg/day as a single dose. May increase at 1-2-week intervals.

Chronic, stable angina pectoris

PO

Adults. Initially, 100 mg/day as single or divided dose. Increase at weekly (or longer) intervals. Maintenance: 100-450 mg/day.

PO (Extended-Release)
Adults. Initially, 100 mg/day as single dose. May increase at least at weekly intervals until optimum clinical response achieved. Maximum: 200 mg/day.

Congestive heart failure
PO (Extended-Release)
Adults. Initially, 25 mg/day. May double dose q2wk. Maximum: 200 mg/day.

Early treatment of MI
IV
Adults. 5 mg q2min for 3 doses, followed by 50 mg orally q6h for 48 hr. Begin oral dose 15 min after last IV dose. Or, in patients who do not tolerate full IV dose, give 25-50 mg orally q6h, 15 min after last IV dose.

Late treatment and maintenance after an MI
PO
Adults. 100 mg twice a day for at least 3 mo.

AVAILABLE FORMS
- *Tablets (Lopressor):* 25 mg, 50 mg, 100 mg.
- *Tablets (Extended-Release [Toprol XL]):* 25 mg, 50 mg, 100 mg, 200 mg.
- *Injection (Lopressor):* 1 mg/ml.

UNLABELED USES: To increase survival rate in diabetic patients with coronary artery disease (CAD); treatment or prevention of anxiety; cardiac arrhythmias; hypertrophic cardiomyopathy; mitral valve prolapse syndrome; pheochromocytoma; tremors; thyrotoxicosis; vascular headache

CONTRAINDICATIONS: Cardiogenic shock, MI with a heart rate less than 45 beats/min or systolic BP less than 100 mm Hg, overt heart failure, second- or third-degree heart block, sinus bradycardia

PREGNANCY AND LACTATION: Pregnancy category C; (D if used in second or third trimester); similar drug, atenolol, frequently used in the third trimester for treatment of hypertension (many studies of efficacy and safety of atenolol in pregnancy-induced hypertension); long-term use has been associated with intrauterine growth retardation; excreted into breast milk in insignificant concentrations; prudent to monitor infant for signs of β-blockade

SIDE EFFECTS
Metoprolol is generally well tolerated, with transient and mild side effects.

Frequent
Diminished sexual function, drowsiness, insomnia, unusual fatigue or weakness

Occasional
Anxiety, nervousness, diarrhea, constipation, nausea, vomiting, nasal congestion, abdominal discomfort, dizziness, difficulty breathing, cold hands or feet

Rare
Altered taste, dry eyes, nightmares, paraesthesia, allergic reaction (rash, pruritus)

SERIOUS REACTIONS
- Overdose may produce profound bradycardia, hypotension, and bronchospasm.
- Abrupt withdrawal of metoprolol may result in diaphoresis, palpitations, headache, tremulousness, exacerbation of angina, MI, and ventricular arrhythmias.
- Metoprolol administration may precipitate CHF and MI in patients with heart disease; thyroid storm in those with thyrotoxicosis; and peripheral ischemia in those with existing peripheral vascular disease.
- Hypoglycemia may occur in patients with previously controlled diabetes mellitus.

INTERACTIONS

Drugs

3 *α-adrenergic blockers:* Potential enhanced first-dose response (marked initial drop in blood pressure), particularly on standing (especially prazosin)

3 *Amiodarone:* Bradycardia, cardiac arrest, or ventricular dysrhythmia

3 *Antidiabetics:* Altered response to hypoglycemia, prolonged recovery of normoglycemia, hypertension, blockade of tachycardia; may increase blood glucose and impair peripheral circulation

3 *Antipyrine:* Increased antipyrine concentrations

3 *Barbiturates:* Reduced β-blocker concentrations

2 *β-agonists:* Antagonism of bronchodilating effect

3 *Bromazepam, diazepam, oxazepam:* Increased benzodiazepine effect (lorazepam and alprazolam unaffected)

3 *Cimetidine, etintidine, propafenone, propoxyphene, quinidine:* Increased plasma metoprolol concentration

3 *Clonidine:* Abrupt withdrawal of clonidine while on a β-blocker may exaggerate the rebound hypertension due to unopposed alpha stimulation

3 *Digoxin:* Additive prolongation of atrioventricular (AV) conduction time

3 *Dihydropyridines (nicardipine, nifedipine, felodipine, isradipine, nisoldipine):* Increased β-blocker effects

3 *Diltiazem:* Potentiates β-adrenergic effects; hypotension, left ventricular failure, and AV conduction disturbances problematic in elderly, patients with left ventricular dysfunction, aortic stenosis, or with large doses of either drug

3 *Dipyridamole, tacrine:* Bradycardia

3 *Fluoxetine:* Enhanced effect of β-blocker

3 *Isoproterenol:* Potential reduction in effectiveness of isoproterenol in the treatment of asthma; less likely with cardioselective agents like metoprolol

3 *Local anesthetics:* Use of local anesthetics containing epinephrine may result in hypertensive reactions in patients taking β-blockers

3 *NSAIDs:* Reduced hypotensive effects of β-blockers

3 *Phenylephrine:* Enhanced pressor response to phenylephrine, particularly when it is administered IV

3 *Prazosin:* First-dose response to prazosin may be enhanced by β-blockade

3 *Quinolones:* Inhibition of β-blocker metabolism, increased β-blocker effects

3 *Rifampin:* Reduced plasma metoprolol concentration

3 *Theophylline:* Antagonistic pharmacodynamic effects

3 *Verapamil:* Potentiates β-adrenergic effects; hypotension, left ventricular failure, and AV conduction disturbances problematic in elderly, patients with left ventricular dysfunction, aortic stenosis, or with large doses of either drug

SPECIAL CONSIDERATIONS

PATIENT/FAMILY EDUCATION

- Do not discontinue abruptly; may require taper; rapid withdrawal may produce rebound hypertension or angina
- Avoid driving or other activities requiring alertness until response to therapy is determined
- Take with or immediately following meals

• Extended-release tablets are scored and can be divided; whole or half tablet should be swallowed whole and not chewed or crushed

MONITORING PARAMETERS

• Angina: Reduction in nitroglycerin usage; frequency, severity, onset, and duration of angina pain; heart rate
• Arrhythmias: heart rate
• Congestive heart failure: Functional status, cough, dyspnea on exertion, paroxysmal nocturnal dyspnea, exercise tolerance, and ventricular function
• Hypertension: Blood pressure
• Migraine headache: Reduction in the frequency, severity, and duration of attacks
• Postmyocardial infarction: Left ventricular function, lower resting heart rate
• Toxicity: Blood glucose, bronchospasm, hypotension, bradycardia, depression, confusion, hallucination, sexual dysfunction

---

metronidazole

(me-troe-ni′-da-zole)

Rx: Flagyl, Flagyl 375, Flagyl ER, Flagyl I.V. RTU, MetroCream, MetroGel, MetroGel-Vaginal, Metro I.V., MetroLotion, Metronidazole Benzoate, Noritate, Protostat, Rozex

Chemical Class: Nitroimidazole derivative

Therapeutic Class: Antibiotic; antihelmintic; antiprotozoal

CLINICAL PHARMACOLOGY

Mechanism of Action: A nitroimidazole derivative that disrupts bacterial and protozoal DNA, inhibiting nucleic acid synthesis. ***Therapeutic Effect:*** Produces bactericidal, antiprotozoal, amebicidal, and trichomonacidal effects. Produces antiinflammatory and immunosuppressive effects when applied topically.

Pharmacokinetics

Well absorbed from the GI tract; minimally absorbed after topical application. Protein binding: less than 20%. Widely distributed; crosses blood-brain barrier. Metabolized in the liver to active metabolite. Primarily excreted in urine; partially eliminated in feces. Removed by hemodialysis. ***Half-life:*** 8 hr (increased in alcoholic hepatic disease and in neonates).

INDICATIONS AND DOSAGES

Anaerobic infections

PO, IV

Adults, Elderly, Children. Initially, 15 mg/kg once, then 7.5 mg/kg/dose q6h. Maximum: 4 g/day.

Amebic dysentery

PO

Adults, Elderly. 750 mg 3 times a day for 5-10 days.

Children. 35-50 mg/kg/day in 3 divided doses for 10 days. Maximum: 750 mg/dose.

Amebic liver abscess

PO

Adults, Elderly. 500-750 mg 3 times a day for 5-10 days.

Children. 50 mg/kg/day in 3 divided doses. Maximum: 750 mg/dose.

Giardiasis

PO

Adults, Elderly. 250 mg 3 times a day for 5 days.

Children. 15 mg/kg/day in 3 divided doses for 7-10 days. Maximum: 250 mg/dose.

Pseudomembranous colitis

PO

Adults, Elderly. 500-750 mg 3 times a day or 250-500 mg 4 times a day.

Children. 7.5 mg/kg q6h for 7-10 days.

Trichomoniasis

PO

Adults, Elderly. 250 mg 3 times a day or 375 mg twice a day or 500 mg twice a day or 2 g as a single dose.

Children. 15 mg/kg/day in 3 divided doses for 7 days.

Bacterial vaginosis

PO

Adults. (non-pregnant): 500 mg twice a day for 7 days or 750 mg (extended-release) once daily for 7 days or 2 g as a single dose. (pregnant): 250 mg 3 times a day for 7 days.

Intravaginal

Adults. (Pregnant, non-pregnant): (0.75%) Apply twice a day for 5 days. Center for Disease Control (CDC) does not recommend the use of topical agents during pregnancy.

Rosacea

Topical

Adults, Elderly. (1%): Apply to affected area once daily. (0.75%): Apply to affected area twice a day.

AVAILABLE FORMS

- *Capsules (Flagyl 375):* 375 mg.
- *Tablets (Flagyl, Protostat):* 250 mg, 500 mg.
- *Tablets (Extended-Release [Flagyl ER]):* 750 mg.
- *Injection (Infusion [Flagyl I.V. RTU]):* 500 mg/100 ml.
- *Topical Cream:* 0.75% (MetroCream, Rozex), 1% (Noritate).
- *Topical Gel (MetroGel):* 0.75%, 1%.
- *Topical Lotion (MetroLotion):* 0.75%.
- *Vaginal Gel (MetroGel-Vaginal):* 0.75%.

UNLABELED USES: Treatment of bacterial vaginosis, grade III-IV decubitus ulcers with anaerobic infection, *H. pylori*–associated gastritis and duodenal ulcer, inflammatory bowel disease; topical treatment of acne rosacea

CONTRAINDICATIONS: Hypersensitivity to other nitroimidazole derivatives (also parabens with topical application)

PREGNANCY AND LACTATION: Pregnancy category B; use in pregnancy controversial; use in first trimester and single-dose therapy often avoided; use with caution during breast-feeding; if single-dose therapy is used, discontinue breast-feeding for 12-24 hr to allow excretion of the drug

SIDE EFFECTS

Frequent

Systemic: Anorexia, nausea, dry mouth, metallic taste

Vaginal: Symptomatic cervicitis and vaginitis, abdominal cramps, uterine pain

Occasional

Systemic: Diarrhea or constipation, vomiting, dizziness, erythematous rash, urticaria, reddish brown urine

Topical: Transient erythema, mild dryness, burning, irritation, stinging, tearing when applied too close to eyes

Vaginal: Vaginal, perineal, or vulvar itching; vulvar swelling

Rare

Mild, transient leukopenia; thrombophlebitis with IV therapy

SERIOUS REACTIONS

- Oral therapy may result in furry tongue, glossitis, cystitis, dysuria, pancreatitis, and flattening of T waves on EKG readings.
- Peripheral neuropathy, manifested as numbness and tingling in hands or feet, is usually reversible if treatment is stopped immediately after neurologic symptoms appear.
- Seizures occur occasionally.

INTERACTIONS

Drugs

3 *Carbamazepine:* Increased carbamazepine levels

3 *Cholestyramine, colestipol:* Reduced metronidazole absorption
3 *Disulfiram:* CNS toxicity
3 *Ethanol:* Disulfiram-like reaction
2 *Fluorouracil:* Enhanced toxicity of fluorouracil
3 *IV phenytoin, phenobarbital, diazepam, nitroglycerine, trimethoprim-sulfamethoxazole:* Disulfiram-like reaction due to ethanol in IV preparations
2 *Oral anticoagulants:* Increased hypoprothrombinemic response to warfarin
3 *Phenytoin:* Increased phenytoin levels

Labs

• *Interference:* Glucose
• *False decrease:* AST, zidovudine level
• *False positive increase:* Clindamycin, erythromycin, polymyxin, tetracycline, and trimethoprim assays

SPECIAL CONSIDERATIONS

• Treat sexual partner(s) for trichomoniasis

PATIENT/FAMILY EDUCATION

• Drug may cause GI upset; take with food
• Avoid alcoholic beverages during therapy and for at least 24 hr following last dose (disulfiram-like reaction possible)
• Drug may cause darkening of urine
• May cause an unpleasant metallic taste
• H_2 blocker must be prescribed with Helidac kit
• Avoid tasks requiring mental alertness or motor skills until response to the drug is established
• The patient taking metronidazole for trichomoniasis should refrain from sexual intercourse until the full treatment is completed
• The patient using topical metronidazole should avoid drug contact with eyes

MONITORING PARAMETERS

• CBC
• Pattern of daily bowel activity and stool consistency
• Intake and output and assess for urinary problems
• Skin for rash and urticaria
• Be alert for signs and symptoms of superinfection, such as anal or genital pruritus, furry tongue, ulceration or change of oral mucosa, and vaginal discharge

metyrosine

(me-tye'-roe-seen)

Rx: Demser

Chemical Class: α-methyl-L-tyrosine

Therapeutic Class: Pheochromocytoma agent

CLINICAL PHARMACOLOGY

Mechanism of Action: A tyrosine hydroxylase inhibitor that blocks conversion of tyrosine to dihydroxyphenylalanine, the rate limiting step in the biosynthetic pathway of catecholamines. ***Therapeutic Effect:*** Reduces levels of endogenous catecholamines.

Pharmacokinetics

Well absorbed from the gastrointestinal (GI) tract. Metabolized in the liver. Excreted primarily in the urine. ***Half-life:*** 7.2 hrs.

INDICATIONS AND DOSAGES

Pheochromocytoma (preoperative)

PO

Adults, Elderly. Initially, 250 mg 4 times/day. Increase by 250-500 mg/day up to 4 g/day. Maintenance: 2-4 g/day in 4 divided doses for 5-7 days.

M

AVAILABLE FORMS
• *Capsule:* 250 mg (Demser).
UNLABELED USES: Tourette syndrome
CONTRAINDICATIONS: Hypertension of unknown etiology, hypersensitivity to metyrosine or any component of the formulation
PREGNANCY AND LACTATION: Pregnancy category C
SIDE EFFECTS
Frequent
Drowsiness, extrapyramidal symptoms, diarrhea
Occasional
Galactorrhea, edema of the breasts, nausea, vomiting, dry mouth, impotence, nasal congestion
Rare
Lower extremity edema, urinary problems, urticaria, anemia, depression, disorientation
SERIOUS REACTIONS
• Serious or life-threatening allergic reaction characterized hallucinations, hematuria, hyperstimulation after withdrawal, severe lower extremity edema, and parkinsonism.
INTERACTIONS
Drugs
3 *Alcohol:* May increase CNS depression
3 *Phenothiazines, haloperidol:* Potentiation of EPS
Labs
• *False increase:* Urinary catecholamines (due to presence of metyrosine metabolites)

SPECIAL CONSIDERATIONS

PATIENT/FAMILY EDUCATION
• Maintain a daily liberal fluid intake
• Avoid alcohol or CNS depressants
• Avoid tasks that require mental alertness or motor skills until response to the drug is established
MONITORING PARAMETERS
• Blood pressure, ECG

mexiletine hydrochloride

(mex′-i-le-teen hye-droe-klor′-ide)
Rx: Mexitil
Chemical Class: Lidocaine derivative
Therapeutic Class: Antiarrhythmic, class IB

CLINICAL PHARMACOLOGY
Mechanism of Action: An antiarrhythmic that shortens duration of action potential and decreases effective refractory period in the His-Purkinje system of the myocardium by blocking sodium transport across myocardial cell membranes. ***Therapeutic Effect:*** Suppresses ventricular arrhythmias.
Pharmacokinetics
Well absorbed from the GI tract. Protein binding: 50%-60%. Metabolized in liver. Approximately 10% is excreted unchanged in urine. ***Half-life:*** 10-12 hr.
INDICATIONS AND DOSAGES
Arrhythmia
PO
Adults, Elderly. Initially, 200 mg q8h. Adjust dosage by 50-100 mg at 2- to 3-day intervals. *Maximum:* 1200 mg/day.
AVAILABLE FORMS
• *Capsules:* 150 mg, 200 mg, 250 mg.
UNLABELED USES: Treatment of diabetic neuropathy
CONTRAINDICATIONS: Cardiogenic shock, preexisting second- or third-degree AV block, right bundle-branch block without presence of pacemaker
PREGNANCY AND LACTATION: Pregnancy category C; limited data do not suggest significant risk to the

fetus; compatible with breast-feeding

SIDE EFFECTS

Frequent (greater than 10%)

GI distress, including nausea, vomiting, and heartburn; dizziness; lightheadedness; tremor

Occasional (10%-1%)

Nervousness, change in sleep habits, headache, visual disturbances, paresthesia, diarrhea or constipation, palpitations, chest pain, rash, respiratory difficulty, edema

SERIOUS REACTIONS

• Mexiletine has the ability to worsen existing arrhythmias or produce new ones.

• CHF may occur and existing CHF may worsen.

• Abnormal liver function tests have been reported, some in the first few weeks of therapy with mexiletine.

INTERACTIONS

Drugs

3 *Acetazolamide, sodium bicarbonate:* Alkalinization of urine retards mexiletine elimination

3 *Antacids:* May reduce mexiletine absorption

3 *Cimetidine:* May increase mexiletine blood concentration

3 *Metoclopramide:* May increase mexiletine absorption

3 *Phenytoin, rifampin, phenobarbital:* Reduced mexiletine concentrations

3 *Quinidine:* Elevated mexiletine concentrations

2 *Theophylline:* Elevated theophylline serum concentrations and toxicity

SPECIAL CONSIDERATIONS

• Because of proarrhythmic effects, not recommended for non–life-threatening arrhythmias

• Antiarrhythmic drugs have not been shown to increase survival of patients with ventricular arrhythmias

• Initiate therapy in facilities capable of providing continuous ECG monitoring and managing life-threatening dysrhythmias

PATIENT/FAMILY EDUCATION

• Take with food or antacid

• Notify the physician if dark urine, cough, generalized fatigue, nausea, pale stools, severe or persistent abdominal pain, shortness of breath, unexplained sore throat or fever, vomiting, or yellowing of the eyes or skin occurs

• Do not use nasal decongestants and OTC cold preparations without physician approval

MONITORING PARAMETERS

• Therapeutic mexiletine concentrations 0.5-2 mcg/ml

• EKG and vital signs for cardiac side effects

• Pulse for rate and quality and irregularity

• Pattern of bowel activity and stool consistency

• Signs and symptoms of CHF

miconazole

(mye-con'-a-zole)

Rx: Femizol-M, Micatin, Monistat-3, Monistat-7, Monistat-Derm

Chemical Class: Imidazole derivative

Therapeutic Class: Antifungal

CLINICAL PHARMACOLOGY

Mechanism of Action: An imidazole derivative that inhibits synthesis of ergosterol (vital component of fungal cell formation), damaging cell membraine. ***Therapeutic Effect:*** Fungistatic; may be fungicidal, depending on concentration.

Pharmacokinetics

Parenteral: Widely distributed in tissues. Metabolized in liver. Primarily excreted in urine. ***Half-life:*** 24 hrs. Topical: No systemic absorption following application to intact skin. Intravaginally: Small amount absorbed systemically.

INDICATIONS AND DOSAGES

Coccidioidomycosis

IV

Adults, Elderly. 1.8-3.6 g/day for 3-20 wks or longer.

Cryptococcosis

IV

Adults, Elderly. 1.2-2.4 g/day for 3-12 wks or longer.

Petriellidiosis

IV

Adults, Elderly. 0.6-3.0 g/day for 5-20 wks or longer.

Candidiasis

IV

Adults, Elderly. 0.6-1.8 g/day for 1-20 wks or longer.

Paracoccidioidomycosis

IV

Adults, Elderly. 0.2-1.2 g/day for 2-16 wks or longer.

Children. Usual dosage for children

IV

20-40 mg/kg/day in 3 divided doses. (Do not exceed 15 mg/kg for any 1 infusion).

Vulvovaginal candidiasis

Intravaginally

Adults, Elderly. One 200-mg suppository at bedtime for 3 days; one 100-mg suppository or one applicatorful at bedtime for 7 days.

Topical fungal infections, cutaneous candidiasis

Topical

Adults, Elderly, Children 2 yrs and older. Apply liberally 2 times/day, morning and evening.

AVAILABLE FORMS

- *Injection:* 10 mg/ml.
- *Vaginal Suppository:* 100 mg (Monistat-7), 200 mg (Monistat-3).
- *Topical Cream:* 2% (Micatin, Monistat-Derm).
- *Vaginal Cream:* 2% (Femizol-M).
- *Topical Powder:* 2% (Micatin).
- *Topical Spray:* 2% (Lotrimin-AF).

CONTRAINDICATIONS: Children younger than 1 yr old, hypersensitivity to miconazole or any component of the formulation

Topically: Children younger than 2 yrs old

PREGNANCY AND LACTATION: Pregnancy category C (Top category B); unknown if excreted into breast milk

SIDE EFFECTS

Frequent

Phlebitis, fever, chills, rash, itching, nausea, vomiting

Occasional

Dizziness, drowsiness, headache, flushed face, abdominal pain, constipation, diarrhea, decreased appetite

Topical: Itching, burning, stinging, erythema, urticaria

Vaginal: Vulvovaginal burning, itching, irritation, headache, skin rash

SERIOUS REACTIONS

- Anemia, thrombocytopenia, and liver toxicity occur rarely.

INTERACTIONS

Drugs

3 *Aminoglycosides:* Decreased antibiotic peak levels

❷ *Cisapride:* Increased cisapride concentrations, toxicity and arrhythmias

3 *Cyclosporine:* Possible increased cyclosporine levels

3 *Felodipine:* Enhanced vasodilation, hypotension

❷ *HMG CoA reductase inhibitors (e.g., lovastatin):* Increased toxicity, rhabdomyolysis

❸ *Loratadine:* Increased loratadine concentrations

❸ *Midazolam:* Reduced midazolam metabolism

❸ *Quinidine:* Increased quinidine concentrations

❸ *Tacrolimus:* Possible increased tacrolimus levels

❸ *Tolbutamide:* Inhibition of tolbutamide metabolism

❸ *Triazolam:* Reduced triazolam metabolism

❸ *Warfarin:* Enhanced anticoagulant effect

Labs

• The base in suppository products may interfere with latex; do not use these with contraceptive diaphragms, condoms

SPECIAL CONSIDERATIONS

PATIENT/FAMILY EDUCATION

• Avoid getting into eyes

• Continue for the full length of treatment

MONITORING PARAMETERS

• Assess for vaginal burning and itching

• Pattern of daily bowel activity and stool consistency

midazolam hydrochloride

(mid′-ay-zoe-lam hye-droe-klor′-ide)

Rx: Versed

Chemical Class: Benzodiazepine

Therapeutic Class: Sedative/hypnotic

DEA Class: Schedule IV

CLINICAL PHARMACOLOGY

Mechanism of Action: A benzodiazepine that enhances the action of gamma-aminobutyric acid, one of the major inhibitory neurotransmitters in the brain. ***Therapeutic Effect:*** Produces anxiolytic, hypnotic, anticonvulsant, muscle relaxant, and amnestic effects.

Pharmacokinetics

Route	*Onset*	*Peak*	*Duration*
PO	10-20 mins	N/A	N/A
IV	1-5 mins	5-7 mins	20-30 mins
IM	5-15 mins	15-60 mins	2-6 hrs

Well absorbed after IM administration. Protein binding: 97%. Metabolized in the liver to active metabolite. Primarily excreted in urine. Not removed by hemodialysis. ***Half-life:*** 1-5 hrs.

INDICATIONS AND DOSAGES

Preoperative sedation

PO

Children. 0.25-0.5 mg/kg. Maximum: 20 mg.

IV

Adults, Elderly. 0.02-0.04 mg/kg.

Children 6-12 yr. 0.025-0.05 mg/kg.

Children 6 mo-5 yr. 0.05-0.1 mg/kg.

IM

Adults, Elderly. 0.07-0.08 mg/kg 30-60 min before surgery.

Children. 0.1-0.15 mg/kg 30-60 min before surgery. Maximum: 10 mg.

Conscious sedation for diagnostic, therapeutic, and endoscopic procedures

IV

Adults, Elderly. 1-2.5 mg over 2 min. Titrate as needed. Maximum total dose: 2.5-5 mg.

Children 6-12 yr. 0.025-0.05 mg/kg. Total dose of 0.4 mg/kg may be necessary. Maximum total dose: 10 mg.

Children 6 mo-5 yr. 0.05-0.1 mg/kg. Total dose of 0.6 mg/kg may be necessary. Maximum total dose: 6 mg.

Conscious sedation during mechanical ventilation

IV

Adults, Elderly. Initially, 0.02-0.08 mg/kg. May repeat at 5-15-mins intervals or continuous infusion rate of 0.04-0.2 mg/kg/hr and titrated to desired effect.

Children. Initially, 0.05-0.2 mg/kg followed by a continuous infusion of 0.06-0.12 mg/kg/hr (1-2 mcg/kg/minute) titrated to desired effect.

Status epilepticus

IV

Children older than 2 mo. Loading dose of 0.15 mg/kg followed by continuous infusion of 1 mcg/kg/min. Titrate as needed. Range: 1-18 mcg/kg/min.

AVAILABLE FORMS

- *Syrup:* 2 mg/ml.
- *Injection:* 1 mg/ml, 5 mg/ml.
- *Injection (Preservative-Free):* 1 mg/ml, 5 mg/ml.

UNLABELED USES: Anxiety, status epilepticus

CONTRAINDICATIONS: Acute alcohol intoxication, acute angle-closure glaucoma, allergies to cherries, coma, shock

PREGNANCY AND LACTATION: Pregnancy category D; excreted in breast milk, use with caution in nursing mothers

Controlled Substance: Schedule IV

SIDE EFFECTS

Frequent (10%-4%)

Decreased respiratory rate, tenderness at IM or IV injection site, pain during injection, oxygen desaturation, hiccups

Occasional (3%-2%)

Hypotension, paradoxical CNS reaction

Rare (less than 2%)

Nausea, vomiting, headache, coughing

SERIOUS REACTIONS

- Inadequate or excessive dosage or improper administration may result in cerebral hypoxia, agitation, involuntary movements, hyperactivity, and combativeness.
- A too-rapid IV rate, excessive doses, or a single large dose increases the risk of respiratory depression or arrest.
- Respiratory depression or apnea may produce hypoxia and cardiac arrest.

INTERACTIONS

Drugs

3 *Calcium channel blockers, erythromycin, ketoconazole, itraconazole:* Increased midazolam levels; increased sedation; respiratory depression

3 *CNS depressants, alcohol:* Additive effects with other CNS depressants

3 *Grapefruit, grapefruit juice:* Increases the oral absorption and systemic availability of midazolam

3 *Kava kava, valerian:* May increase CNS depression

3 *Phenytoin:* Reduces the effect of oral midazolam, but parenteral midazolam is less likely to be affected

3 *Rifampin:* Reduces midazolam plasma concentrations; loss of efficacy is likely to occur

3 *Saquinavir:* Increases midazolam concentrations, particularly following oral midazolam; increased midazolam-induced sedation is likely to result

SPECIAL CONSIDERATIONS

PATIENT/FAMILY EDUCATION

- Midazolam produces an amnesic effect
- The female patient on long-term therapy should use effective contraception during therapy and notify the physician immediately if she becomes or may be pregnant

MONITORING PARAMETERS

- Monitor the patient's respiratory rate and oxygen saturation continuously during parenteral administration to detect apnea and respiratory depression
- Monitor the patient's level of sedation every 3-5 mins, and assess vital signs during the recovery period

midodrine hydrochloride

(mye'-doe-drene hye-droe-klor'-ide)

Rx: ProAmatine

Chemical Class: Catecholamine, synthetic

Therapeutic Class: Vasopressor; α-adrenergic sympathomimetic amine

CLINICAL PHARMACOLOGY

Mechanism of Action: A vasopressor that forms the active metabolite desglymidodrine, an $alpha_1$-agonist, activating alpha receptors of the arteriolar and venous vasculature. ***Therapeutic Effect:*** Increases vascular tone and BP.

Pharmacokinetics

Rapid absorption from the GI tract following PO administration. Protein binding: low. Undergoes enzymatic hydrolysis (deglycination) in the systemic circulation. Excreted in urine. ***Half-life:*** 0.5 hr.

INDICATIONS AND DOSAGES

Orthostatic hypotension

PO

Adults, Elderly. 10 mg 3 times a day. Give during the day when patient is upright, such as upon arising, midday, and late afternoon. Do not give later than 6 p.m.

Dosage in renal impairment

For adults and elderly patients, give 2.5 mg 3 times a day; increase gradually, as tolerated.

AVAILABLE FORMS

- *Tablets:* 2.5 mg, 5 mg, 10 mg.

UNLABELED USES: Infection-related hypotension, intradialytic hypotension, psychotropic agent–induced hypotension, urinary incontinence

CONTRAINDICATIONS: Acute renal function impairment, persistent hypertension, pheochromocytoma, severe cardiac disease, thyrotoxicosis, urine retention

PREGNANCY AND LACTATION: Pregnancy category C; unknown if excreted in breast milk

SIDE EFFECTS

Frequent (20%-7%)

Paresthesia, piloerection, pruritus, dysuria, supine hypertension

Occasional (less than 7%-1%)

Pain, rash, chills, headache, facial flushing, confusion, dry mouth, anxiety

SERIOUS REACTIONS

- Increased systolic arterial pressure has been reported.

INTERACTIONS

Drugs

2 *α-adrenergic agonists:* Enhanced pressor response

M

3 *α-adrenergic antagonists:* Antagonism of midodrine's effects

3 *Cardiac glycosides, β-blockers:* Increased risk of bradycardia, AV block, arrhythmia

3 *Sodium-retaining steroids (such as fludrocortisone):* May increase sodium retention

3 *Vasoconstrictors:* May have an additive vasocontricting effect

SPECIAL CONSIDERATIONS

- Advantages include rapid and nearly complete absorption, a long elimination $t_{1/2}$, lack of central nervous system (CNS) penetration, and minimal to no cardiac effects
- Supine hypertension has been a therapy-limiting complication

PATIENT/FAMILY EDUCATION

- To minimize supine hypertension, avoid taking drug after the evening meal
- Use OTC medications, such as cough, cold, and diet preparations, cautiously because they may affect blood pressure

MONITORING PARAMETERS

- Blood pressure, liver and renal function

---

mifepristone

(mi-fe'-pri-stone)

Rx: Mifeprex

Chemical Class: Antiprogestational agent; progestin derivative

Therapeutic Class: Abortifacient

CLINICAL PHARMACOLOGY

Mechanism of Action: An abortifacient that has antiprogestational activity resulting from competitive interaction with progesterone. Inhibits the activity of endogenous or exogenous progesterone. Also has antiglucocorticoid and weak antiandrogenic activity. ***Therapeutic Effect:*** Terminates pregnancy.

Pharmacokinetics

Protein binding: 98%. Metabolized in liver. Primarily eliminated in feces; minimal excretion in urine. ***Half-life:*** 20-54 hrs.

INDICATIONS AND DOSAGES

Termination of pregnancy

PO

Adults. Day 1: 600 mg as single dose. Day 3: 400 mcg misoprostol. Day 14: Post-treatment examination.

AVAILABLE FORMS

- *Tablets:* 200 mg.

UNLABELED USES: Breast or ovarian cancer, Cushing's syndrome, endometriosis, intrauterine fetal death or nonviable early pregnancy, postcoital contraception or contragestation, unresectable meningioma

CONTRAINDICATIONS: Chronic adrenal failure, concurrent long-term steroid or anticoagulant therapy, confirmed or suspected ectopic pregnancy, intrauterine device (IUD) in place, hemorrhagic disorders or concurrent anticoagulant therapy, inherited porphyria, hypersensitivity to misoprostol or other prostaglandins

PREGNANCY AND LACTATION: Pregnancy category X; excretion in human milk unknown but likely

SIDE EFFECTS

Frequent (greater than 10%)

Headache, dizziness, abdominal pain, nausea, vomiting, diarrhea, fatigue

Occasional (10%-3%)

Uterine hemorrhage, insomnia, vaginitis, dyspepsia, back pain, fever, viral infections, rigors

Rare (2%-1%)

Anxiety, syncope, anemia, asthenia, leg pain, sinusitis, leukorrhea

SERIOUS REACTIONS

• None known.

INTERACTIONS

Drugs

3 *Ketoconazole, itraconazole, erythromycin, grapefruit juice:* May inhibit mifepristone metabolism, raising serum levels

3 *Rifampin, dexamethasone, St. John's Wort, phenytoin, phenobarbital, carbamazepine:* May induce mifepristone metabolism, lowering serum levels

3 *St. John's Wort:* May increase the metabolism of mifepristone

SPECIAL CONSIDERATIONS

• Provided only to licensed physicians who sign and return a Prescriber's Agreement. Not available through pharmacies

• Patients should be given the Medication Guide and sign the Patient Agreement (Danco Laboratories, 1-877-432-7596)

• Provide medication for cramping and GI symptoms, instructions on what to do if significant bleeding or other adverse reactions occur

• Advise patient bleeding/spotting occur for average of 9-16 days; 8% have some bleeding for >30 days

• Expulsion occurs within the first 48 hrs in 6%, in 63%-72% within 24 hrs of misoprostol administration (most of these within 4 hrs), surgical intervention in 4.5%-8%

• Quantitative hCG levels not decisive until ≥10 days following mifepristone administration. Confirm continuing pregnancy by ultrasound scan. Uterine debris does not necessarily require surgical removal

• Report adverse events (blood transfusion, hospitalization, ongoing pregnancy) in writing to Medical Director, Danco Laboratories LLC, PO Box 4816, New York, NY 10185

• For 24 hr/day consultation, contact Danco Laboratories at 1-877-432-7596

PATIENT/FAMILY EDUCATION

• Completing treatment schedule is important, including the 48-hr visit for misoprostol and the post-treatment follow-up visit at 14 days

• Vaginal bleeding and uterine cramping will occur, but are not proof of complete expulsion

• There is a risk of fetal malformation if treatment fails

• Treatment failure is managed by surgical termination

• Contraception should be initiated as soon as pregnancy termination has been confirmed

MONITORING PARAMETERS

• Hgb and Hct

---

milrinone lactate

(mill'-re-none)

Rx: Primacor, Primacor I.V.

Chemical Class: Bipyridine derivative

Therapeutic Class: Cardiac inotropic agent

CLINICAL PHARMACOLOGY

Mechanism of Action: A cardiac inotropic agent that inhibits phosphodiesterase, which increases cyclic adenosine monophosphate and potentiates the delivery of calcium to myocardial contractile systems. ***Therapeutic Effect:*** Relaxes vascular muscle, causing vasodilation. Increases cardiac output; decreases pulmonary capillary wedge pressure and vascular resistance.

Pharmacokinetics

Route	Onset	Peak	Duration
IV	5-15 mins	N/A	N/A

Protein binding: 70%. Primarily excreted unchanged in urine. ***Half-life:*** 2.4 hr.

INDICATIONS AND DOSAGES

Short-term management of CHF

IV

Adults. Initially, 50 mcg/kg over 10 min. Continue with maintenance infusion rate of 0.375-0.75 mcg/kg/min based on hemodynamic and clinical response. Total daily dosage: 0.59-1.13 mg/kg.

Dosage in renal impairment

For patients with severe renal impairment, reduce dosage to 0.2-0.43 mcg/kg/min.

AVAILABLE FORMS

• *Injection (Primacor, Primacor I.V.):* 1 mg/ml, 10-ml single-dose vial, 20-ml single-dose vial, 50-ml single-dose vial, 5-ml sterile cartridge unit.

• *Injection (Premix [Primacor]):* 200 mcg/ml.

CONTRAINDICATIONS: None known.

PREGNANCY AND LACTATION: Pregnancy category C; caution with breast-feeding until more known about excretion in breast milk

SIDE EFFECTS

Occasional (3%-1%)

Headache, hypotension

Rare (less than 1%)

Angina, chest pain

SERIOUS REACTIONS

• Supraventricular and ventricular arrhythmias (12%), nonsustained ventricular tachycardia (2%), and sustained ventricular tachycardia (1%) may occur.

INTERACTIONS

Drugs

3 *Other cardiac glycosides:* Produces additive inotropic effects

SPECIAL CONSIDERATIONS

PATIENT/FAMILY EDUCATION

• Immediately report palpitations or chest pain

• Milrinone is not a cure for CHF but will help relieve symptoms

MONITORING PARAMETERS

• Fluid and electrolyte changes, renal function

• Improvement in cardiac output may increase diuresis, and K^+ loss

• Blood pressure, EKG, heart rate, serum potassium levels

• Signs and symptoms of CHF

minocycline hydrochloride

(mi-noe-sye'-kleen hye-droe-klor'-ide)

Rx: Arestin, Dynacin, Minocin, Myrac, Vectrin

Chemical Class: Tetracycline derivative

Therapeutic Class: Antibiotic

CLINICAL PHARMACOLOGY

Mechanism of Action: A tetracycline antibiotic that inhibits bacterial protein synthesis by binding to ribosomes. ***Therapeutic Effect:*** Bacteriostatic.

Pharmacokinetics

Protein binding: 76%. Partial elimination in feces; minimal excretion in urine. Not removed by hemodialysis. ***Half-life:*** 11-12 hr (oral capsule).

INDICATIONS AND DOSAGES

Mild, moderate, or severe prostate, urinary tract, and CNS infections (excluding meningitis); uncomplicated gonorrhea; inflammatory acne; brucellosis; skin granulomas; cholera; trachoma; nocardiasis; yaws; and syphilis when penicillins are contraindicated

PO

Adults, Elderly. Initially, 100-200 mg, then 100 mg q12h or 50 mg q6h.

IV

Adults, Elderly. Initially, 200 mg, then 100 mg q12h up to 400 mg/day.

PO, IV

Children older than 8 yr. Initially, 4 mg/kg, then 2 mg/kg q12h.

AVAILABLE FORMS

• *Capsules (Dynacin, Minocin, Vectrin):* 50 mg, 75 mg, 100 mg.

• *Capsules (Pellet-Filled [Minocin]):* 50 mg, 100 mg.

• *Tablets (Minocin, Myrac):* 50 mg, 75 mg, 100 mg.

• *Powder for Injection (Minocin, Myrac):* 100 mg.

UNLABELED USES: Treatment of atypical mycobacterial infections, rheumatoid arthritis, scleroderma

CONTRAINDICATIONS: Children younger than 8 yrs, hypersensitivity to tetracyclines, last half of pregnancy

PREGNANCY AND LACTATION: Pregnancy category D; not recommended in last half of pregnancy secondary to adverse effects on fetal teeth; not recommended in breast-feeding

SIDE EFFECTS

Frequent

Dizziness, light-headedness, diarrhea, nausea, vomiting, abdominal cramps, possibly severe photosensitivity, drowsiness, vertigo

Occasional

Altered pigmentation of skin or mucous membranes, rectal or genital pruritus, stomatitis

SERIOUS REACTIONS

• Superinfection (especially fungal), anaphylaxis, and benign intracranial hypertension may occur.

• Bulging fontanelles occur rarely in infants.

INTERACTIONS

Drugs

3 *Antacids:* Decreased effect of minocycline

3 *Barbiturates:* Decreased effect of minocycline

2 *Bismuth:* Inhibited antibiotic absorption

3 *Carbamazepine:* Decreased effect of minocycline

3 *Colestipol, cholestyramine:* Inhibited antibiotic absorption

3 *Digoxin:* Increased digoxin levels in 10% of patients

3 *Iron:* Decreased minocycline absorption

2 *Methoxyflurane:* Renal toxicity

3 *Oral contraceptives:* Decreased contraceptive efficacy

3 *Penicillins:* Antagonizes antibacterial effect of penicillins

3 *St. John's Wort:* May increase the risk of photosensitivity

3 *Warfarin:* Possible increase in hypoprothrombinemic response

SPECIAL CONSIDERATIONS

PATIENT/FAMILY EDUCATION

• May take with food

• Avoid sun exposure

• Drink a full glass of water

• Space doses evenly around the clock and continue taking minocycline for the full course of treatment

• Avoid tasks that require mental alertness or motor skills until response to the drug is established

• Notify the physician if diarrhea, rash, or other new symptoms occur

MONITORING PARAMETERS

• Pattern of daily bowel activity and stool consistency

• Skin for rash

• Blood pressure

• Be alert for signs and symptoms of superinfection, such as anal or genital pruritus, diarrhea, and stomatitis

minoxidil

(min-nox'-i-dill)

Rx: Loniten

OTC: Rogaine

Chemical Class: Piperidinopyrimidine derivative

Therapeutic Class: Antihypertensive; direct vasodilator; hair growth stimulant (topical use)

CLINICAL PHARMACOLOGY

Mechanism of Action: An antihypertensive and hair growth stimulant that has direct action on vascular smooth muscle, producing vasodilation of arterioles. ***Therapeutic Effect:*** Decreases peripheral vascular resistance and BP; increases cutaneous blood flow; stimulates hair follicle epithelium and hair follicle growth.

Pharmacokinetics

Route	Onset	Peak	Duration
PO	0.5 hrs	2-8 hrs	2-5 days

Well absorbed from the GI tract; minimal absorption after topical application. Protein binding: none. Widely distributed. Metabolized in the liver to active metabolite. Primarily excreted in urine. Removed by hemodialysis. ***Half-life:*** 4.2 hrs.

INDICATIONS AND DOSAGES

Severe symptomatic hypertension, hypertension associated with organ damage, hypertension that has failed to respond to maximal therapeutic dosages of a diuretic or two other antihypertensives

PO

Adults, Children 12 yr and older. Initially, 5 mg/day. Increase with at least 3-day intervals to 10 mg, then 20 mg, then up to 40 mg/day in 1-2 doses.

Elderly. Initially, 2.5 mg/day. May increase gradually. Maintenance: 10-40 mg/day. Maximum: 100 mg/day.

Children younger than 12 yr. Initially, 0.1-0.2 mg/kg (5 mg maximum) daily. Gradually increase at a minimum of 3-day intervals. Maintenance: 0.25-1 mg/kg/day in 1-2 doses. Maximum: 50 mg/day.

Hair regrowth

Topical

Adults. 1 ml to affected areas of scalp 2 times a day. Total daily dose not to exceed 2 ml.

AVAILABLE FORMS

- *Tablets (Loniten):* 2.5 mg, 10 mg.
- *Topical Solution:* 2% (20 mg/ml) (Rogaine), 5% (50 mg/ml) (Rogaine ExtraStrength).

CONTRAINDICATIONS: Pheochromocytoma

PREGNANCY AND LACTATION: Pregnancy category C; compatible with breast-feeding

SIDE EFFECTS

Frequent

PO: Edema with concurrent weight gain, hypertrichosis (elongation, thickening, increased pigmentation of fine body hair; develops in 80% of patients within 3-6 wks after beginning therapy)

Occasional

PO: T-wave changes (usually revert to pretreatment state with continued therapy or drug withdrawal)

Topical: Pruritus, rash, dry or flaking skin, erythema

Rare

PO: Breast tenderness, headache, photosensitivity reaction

Topical: Allergic reaction, alopecia, burning sensation at scalp, soreness at hair root, headache, visual disturbances

SERIOUS REACTIONS

• Tachycardia and angina pectoris may occur because of increased oxygen demands associated with increased heart rate and cardiac output.

• Fluid and electrolyte imbalance and CHF may occur, especially if a diuretic is not given concurrently with minoxidil.

• Too-rapid reduction in BP may result in syncope, cerebrovascular accident (CVA), MI, and ocular or vestibular ischemia.

• Pericardial effusion and tamponade may be seen in patients with impaired renal function who are not on dialysis.

INTERACTIONS

Drugs

❷ *Guanethidine:* Orthostatic hypotension, may be severe

③ *NSAIDs:* May decrease the hypotensive effects of minoxidil

③ *Parenteral antihypertensives:* May increase hypotensive effect

Labs

• No known interactions with top sol

SPECIAL CONSIDERATIONS

• Must be used in conjunction with diuretic (except dialysis patients) and β-blocker or other sympathetic nervous system depressant (to prevent reflex tachycardia)

PATIENT/FAMILY EDUCATION

• At least 4 mo of bid application necessary before evidence of hair growth with topical solution

• Continued treatment necessary to maintain or increase hair growth with topical solution

• Maximum blood pressure response occurs 3-7 days after initiation of minoxidil therapy

• Avoid exposure to sunlight and artificial light sources

mirtazapine

(mir-taz'-a-peen)

Rx: Remeron, Remeron Soltab

Chemical Class: Tetracyclic piperazino-azepine derivative

Therapeutic Class: Antidepressant

CLINICAL PHARMACOLOGY

Mechanism of Action: A tetracyclic compound that acts as an antagonist at presynaptic alpha$_2$-adrenergic receptors, increasing both norepinephrine and serotonin neurotransmission. Has low anticholinergic activity. ***Therapeutic Effect:*** Relieves depression and produces sedative effects.

Pharmacokinetics

Rapidly and completely absorbed after PO administration; absorption not affected by food. Protein binding: 85%. Metabolized in the liver. Primarily excreted in urine. Unknown if removed by hemodialysis. ***Half-life:*** 20-40 hr (longer in males [37 hr] than females [26 hr]).

INDICATIONS AND DOSAGES

Depression

PO

Adults. Initially, 15 mg at bedtime. May increase by 15 mg/day q1-2wk. Maximum: 45 mg/day.

Elderly. Initially, 7.5 mg at bedtime. May increase by 7.5-15 mg/day q1-2wk. Maximum: 45 mg/day.

AVAILABLE FORMS

• *Tablets:* 7.5 mg, 15 mg, 30 mg, 45 mg.

• *Tablets (Disintegrating):* 15 mg, 30 mg, 45 mg.

CONTRAINDICATIONS: Use within 14 days of MAOIs

PREGNANCY AND LACTATION: Pregnancy category C

SIDE EFFECTS

Frequent

Somnolence (54%), dry mouth (25%), increased appetite (17%), constipation (13%), weight gain (12%)

Occasional

Asthenia (8%), dizziness (7%), flu-like symptoms (5%), abnormal dreams (4%)

Rare

Abdominal discomfort, vasodilation, paresthesia, acne, dry skin, thirst, arthralgia

SERIOUS REACTIONS

- Mirtazapine poses a higher risk of seizures than tricyclic antidepressants, especially in those with no previous history of seizures.
- Overdose may produce cardiovascular effects, such as severe orthostatic hypotension, dizziness, tachycardia, palpitations, and arrhythmias.
- Abrupt discontinuation after prolonged therapy may produce headache, malaise, nausea, vomiting, and vivid dreams.
- Agranulocytosis occurs rarely.

INTERACTIONS

Drugs

3 *Alcohol, diazepam:* May increase impairment of cognition and motor skills

▲ *MAOIs:* Possible serotonin syndrome (hyperthermia, autonomic instability, seizures, death)

SPECIAL CONSIDERATIONS

- Chemical structure unrelated to TCAs, SSRIs, MAOIs
- Shown to be an effective antidepressant in several trials but place in therapy not yet determined
- Manufacturer recommends stopping MAOI 14 days before initiating therapy secondary to interactions between MAOIs and other antidepressants

PATIENT/FAMILY EDUCATION

- Take mirtazapine as a single bedtime dose
- Avoid alcohol and other sedating medications during therapy
- Avoid tasks that require mental alertness or motor skills until response to the drug has been established

MONITORING PARAMETERS

- Assess appearance, behavior, level of interest, mood, and sleep pattern to determine the drug's therapeutic effect
- Closely supervise suicidal patients during early therapy; as depression lessens, the patient's energy level improves, increasing the suicide potential
- Monitor for signs and symptoms of hypotension and arrhythmias

misoprostol

(mye-soe-prost'-ol)

Rx: Cytotec

Combinations

Rx: with diclofenac (Arthrotec)

Chemical Class: Prostaglandin E_1 analog

Therapeutic Class: Abortifacient; gastrointestinal protectant

CLINICAL PHARMACOLOGY

Mechanism of Action: A prostaglandin that inhibits basal, nocturnal gastric acid secretion via direct action on parietal cells. ***Therapeutic Effect:*** Increases production of protective gastric mucus.

Pharmacokinetics

Rapidly absorbed from gastrointestinal (GI) tract. Rapidly converted to active metabolite. Primarily excreted in urine. ***Half-life:*** 20-40 min.

INDICATIONS AND DOSAGES

Prevention of NSAID-induced gastric ulcer

PO

Adults: 200 mcg 4 times/day with food (last dose at bedtime). Continue for duration of NSAID therapy. May reduce dosage to 100 mcg if 200 mcg dose is not tolerable.

Elderly: 100-200 mcg 4 times/day with food.

AVAILABLE FORMS

- *Tablets:* 100 mcg, 200 mcg (Cytotec).

UNLABELED USES: Treatment of duodenal ulcer

CONTRAINDICATIONS: Pregnancy (produces uterine contractions), hypersensitivity to misoprostol or any component of the formulation

PREGNANCY AND LACTATION: Pregnancy category X; do not use in breast-feeding (possible diarrhea in infant)

SIDE EFFECTS

Frequent

Abdominal pain, diarrhea

Occasional

Nausea, flatulence, dyspepsia, headache

Rare

Vomiting, constipation

SERIOUS REACTIONS

- Overdosage may produce sedation, tremor, convulsions, dyspnea, palpitations, hypotension, and bradycardia.

INTERACTIONS

Drugs

3 *Antacids:* May decrease misoprostol effectiveness

3 *Phenylbutazone:* Increase in adverse effects (headache, flushes, dizziness, nausea)

SPECIAL CONSIDERATIONS

- Reserve use for those patients at high risk for NSAID-induced ulcer (e.g., elderly, history of previous ulcer)
- Does not prevent NSAID-associated GI pain or discomfort

PATIENT/FAMILY EDUCATION

- Avoid magnesium-containing antacids
- Warn women of childbearing potential that they must not be pregnant before or during medication therapy (may result in hospitalization, surgery, infertility, fetal death)

MONITORING PARAMETERS

- Female patients for pregnancy
- Therapeutic response to therapy

modafinil

(moe-daf'-ih-nil)

Rx: Provigil

Chemical Class: Benzhydrylsulfinylacetamide compound

Therapeutic Class: Central nervous system stimulant

CLINICAL PHARMACOLOGY

Mechanism of Action: An $alpha_1$-agonist that may bind to dopamine reuptake carrier sites, increasing alpha activity and decreasing delta, theta, and beta brain wave activity. ***Therapeutic Effect:*** Reduces the number of sleep episodes and total daytime sleep.

Pharmacokinetics

Well absorbed. Protein binding: 60%. Widely distributed. Metabolized in the liver. Excreted by the kidneys. Unknown if removed by hemodialysis. ***Half-life:*** 8-10 hr.

INDICATIONS AND DOSAGES

Narcolepsy, other sleep disorders

PO

Adults, Elderly. 200 mg/day.

AVAILABLE FORMS

• *Tablets:* 100 mg, 200 mg.

UNLABELED USES: Treatment of attention deficit hyperactivity disorder, brain injury–related underarousal, depression, endozepine stupor, multiple sclerosis–related fatigue, parkinson-related fatigue, seasonal affective disorder

CONTRAINDICATIONS: None known.

PREGNANCY AND LACTATION: Pregnancy category C; no mutagenic or clastogenic potential in several *in vitro* assays; *in vivo* mouse bone marrow micronucleus assays were also negative for mutagenicity; not fully evaluated; breast milk excretion unknown

SIDE EFFECTS

Frequent

Anxiety, insomnia, nausea

Occasional

Anorexia, diarrhea, dizziness, dry mouth or skin, muscle stiffness, polydipsia, rhinitis, paraesthesia, tremor, headache, vomiting

SERIOUS REACTIONS

• Agitation, excitation, hypertension, and insomnia may occur.

INTERACTIONS

3 *Cyclosporine, oral contraceptives, theophylline:* Reduces plasma concentrations of these drugs

3 *Phenytoin, propranolol, tricyclic antidepressants, warfarin:* May increase plasma concentrations of these drugs

3 *Other CNS stimulants:* May increase CNS stimulation

3 *Triazolam:* Reduces triazolam plasma concentrations; reduces hypnotic effect

SPECIAL CONSIDERATIONS

• Comparisons of modafinil with agents that have proven effective in narcolepsy, including methylphenidate, pemoline, and dextroamphetamine, are needed to clarify its relative safety and efficacy, and place in therapy

PATIENT/FAMILY EDUCATION

• Do not increase the drug dose without physician approval

• Avoid tasks that require mental alertness or motor skills until response to the drug has been established

• Use a nonhormonal contraceptive method during modafinil therapy and for 1 mo afterward; modafinil decreases the effectiveness of hormonal contraceptives

• Take sips of tepid water and chew sugarless gum to relieve dry mouth

MONITORING PARAMETERS

• *Efficacy:* Daytime sleepiness, daytime sleep episodes, and overall daily performance

• *Toxicity:* Blood pressure

moexipril hydrochloride

(moe-ex'-i-pril hye-droe-klor'-ide)

Rx: Univasc

Combinations

Rx: with hydrochlorothiazide (Uniretic)

Chemical Class: Angiotensin-converting enzyme (ACE) inhibitor, nonsulfhydryl

Therapeutic Class: Antihypertensive

CLINICAL PHARMACOLOGY

Mechanism of Action: An angiotensin-converting enzyme (ACE) inhibitor that suppresses the renin-angiotensin-aldosterone system and prevents conversion of angiotensin I to angiotensin II, a potent vasoconstrictor; may also inhibit angiotensin II at local vascular and renal sites. ***Therapeutic Effect:*** Reduces peripheral arterial resistance and lowers BP.

Pharmacokinetics

Route	Onset	Peak	Duration
PO	1 hr	3-6 hrs	24 hrs

Incompletely absorbed from the GI tract. Food decreases drug absorption. Rapidly converted to active metabolite. Protein binding: 50%. Primarily recovered in feces, partially excreted in urine. Unknown if removed by dialysis. ***Half-life:*** 1 hr, metabolite 2-9 hrs.

INDICATIONS AND DOSAGES

Hypertension

PO

Adults, Elderly. For patients not receiving diuretics, initial dose is 7.5 mg once a day 1 hr before meals. Adjust according to BP effect. Maintenance: 7.5-30 mg a day in 1-2 divided doses 1 hr before meals.

Hypertension in patients with impaired renal function

PO

Adults, Elderly. 3.75 mg once a day in patients with creatinine clearance of 40 ml/min. Maximum: May titrate up to 15 mg/day.

AVAILABLE FORMS

• *Tablets:* 7.5 mg, 15 mg.

CONTRAINDICATIONS: History of angioedema from previous treatment with ACE inhibitors

PREGNANCY AND LACTATION: Pregnancy category C (D if used in second or third trimesters); ACE inhibitors can cause fetal and neonatal morbidity and death when administered to pregnant women; when pregnancy is detected, discontinue ACE inhibitors as soon as possible

SIDE EFFECTS

Occasional

Cough, headache (6%); dizziness (4%); fatigue (3%)

Rare

Flushing, rash, myalgia, nausea, vomiting

SERIOUS REACTIONS

• Excessive hypotension ("first-dose syncope") may occur in patients with CHF and in those who are severely salt or volume depleted.

• Angioedema (swelling of face and lips) and hyperkalemia occur rarely.

• Agranulocytosis and neutropenia may be noted in those with collagen vascular disease, including scleroderma and systemic lupus erythematosus, and impaired renal function.

• Nephrotic syndrome may be noted in those with history of renal disease.

INTERACTIONS

Drugs

3 *Alcohol:* May increase the effects of moexipril

2 *Allopurinol:* Combination may predispose to hypersensitivity reactions

3 *α-adrenergic blockers:* Exaggerated first-dose hypotensive reactions when added to moexipril

3 *Aspirin:* May reduce hemodynamic effects of moexipril; less likely at doses under 236 mg; less likely with nonacetylated salicylates

3 *Azathioprine:* Increased myelosuppression

3 *Cyclosporine:* Combination may cause renal insufficiency

3 *Insulin:* Moexipril may enhance insulin sensitivity

3 *Iron:* Moexipril may increase chance of systemic reaction to IV iron

3 *Lithium:* Reduced lithium clearance

3 *Loop diuretics:* Initiation of moexipril may cause hypotension and renal insufficiency in patients taking loop diuretics

3 *NSAIDs:* May reduce hemodynamic effects of moexipril

3 *Potassium-sparing diuretics:* Increased risk of hyperkalemia

3 *Trimethoprim:* Additive risk of hyperkalemia, especially in patient predisposed to renal insufficiency

Labs

- ACE inhibition can account for approximately 0.5 mEq/L rise in serum potassium

SPECIAL CONSIDERATIONS

PATIENT/FAMILY EDUCATION

- Caution with salt substitutes containing potassium chloride
- Rise slowly to sitting/standing position to minimize orthostatic hypotension
- Dizziness, fainting, lightheadedness may occur during first few days of therapy
- May cause altered taste perception or cough; persistent dry cough usually does not subside unless medication is stopped; notify clinician if these symptoms persist
- Do not abruptly discontinue the drug
- Notify the physician if chest pain, cough, difficulty breathing, fever, sore throat, or swelling of the eyes, face, feet, hands, lips, or tongue occurs

MONITORING PARAMETERS

- BUN, creatinine, potassium within 2 wk after initiation of therapy (increased levels may indicate acute renal failure)
- Blood pressure, WBC count

molindone hydrochloride

(moe-lin′-done hye-droe-klor′-ide)

Rx: Moban

Chemical Class: Dihydroindolone derivative

Therapeutic Class: Antipsychotic

CLINICAL PHARMACOLOGY

Mechanism of Action: An indole derivative of dihydroindole compounds that reduces spontaneous locomotion and aggressiveness. ***Therapeutic Effect:*** Suppresses behavioral response in psychosis.

Pharmacokinetics

Rapidly absorbed from the gastrointestinal (GI) tract. Metabolized in liver. Excreted in feces, and a small amount excreted via lungs as carbon dioxide. Not removed by dialysis. ***Half-life:*** Unknown.

INDICATIONS AND DOSAGES

Schizophrenia

PO

Adults, Children 12 yrs and older. Initially, 50-75 mg/day, increased to 100 mg/day in 3-4 days. Maintenance: 5-15 mg 3-4 times/day (mild psychosis). Maintenance: 10-25 mg 3-4 times/day (moderate psychosis). Maintenance: 225 mg/day maximum in divided doses (severe psychosis).

Elderly. Start at a lower dose.

AVAILABLE FORMS

- *Oral Solutions:* 20 mg/ml (Moban).
- *Tablets:* 5 mg, 10 mg, 25 mg, 50 mg, 100 mg (Moban).

CONTRAINDICATIONS: Severe central nervous system (CNS) depression, hypersensitivity to molindone or any component of the formulation

PREGNANCY AND LACTATION: Pregnancy category C

SIDE EFFECTS

Frequent

Blurred vision, constipation, drowsiness, headache, extrapyramidal symptoms

Occasional

Mental depression

Rare

Skin rash, hot and dry skin, inability to sweat, muscle weakness, confusion, jaundice, convulsions

SERIOUS REACTIONS

- Neuroleptic malignant syndrome or tardive dyskinesia has been reported.

INTERACTIONS

Drugs

3 *Alcohol, CNS depressants:* Increased CNS depression

3 *Barbiturates:* Reduce serum levels of molindone

3 *Benztropine:* May inhibit therapeutic response to molindone

3 *Bromocriptine:* May inhibit therapeutic response to molindone; molindone may inhibit therapeutic effect of bromocriptine on hyperprolactinemia

3 *Carbamazepine:* Reduces serum levels of molindone

3 *Fluoxetine:* Increases serum levels of molindone

3 *Guanethidine:* Reduced antihypertensive effect of guanethidine

3 *Indomethacin:* May increase risk of CNS side effects of molindone

2 *Levodopa:* Molindone reduces antiparkinsonian effects of levodopa

3 *Lithium:* May reduce serum levels of lithium

3 *Orphenadrine:* Reduces serum levels of molindone

3 *Paroxetine:* Increases serum levels of molindone

3 *Quinidine:* Increases serum levels of molindone

3 *Trihexyphenidyl:* May inhibit therapeutic response to molindone

SPECIAL CONSIDERATIONS

- Neuroleptic structurally different from the phenothiazines, thioxanthenes, and butyrophenones
- High potency with high incidence of EPS, but a low incidence of sedation, anticholinergic effects, and cardiovascular effects

PATIENT/FAMILY EDUCATION

- Do not abruptly discontinue molindone after long-term therapy
- Notify the physician if high fever, muscle stiffness, fast or irregular heartbeat, unexplained weakness or tiredness, muscle spasms, twitching, or uncontrolled tongue occurs
- Drowsiness usually subsides with continued therapy
- Avoid alcohol and CNS depressants

MONITORING PARAMETERS

- CBC
- Liver and renal function tests

mometasone furoate monohydrate

(mo-met'-a-zone fyoo-roe'-ate)

Rx: Elocon, Nasonex

Chemical Class: Corticosteroid, synthetic

Therapeutic Class: Corticosteroid, topical

CLINICAL PHARMACOLOGY

Mechanism of Action: An adrenocorticosteroid that inhibits the release of inflammatory cells into nasal tissue, preventing early activation of the allergic reaction. ***Therapeutic Effect:*** Decreases response to seasonal and perennial rhinitis.

Pharmacokinetics

Undetectable in plasma. Protein binding: 98%-99%. The swallowed portion undergoes extensive metabolism. Excreted primarily through bile and, to a lesser extent, urine. ***Half-life:*** 5.8 hr (nasal).

INDICATIONS AND DOSAGES

Allergic rhinitis

Nasal Spray

Adults, Elderly, Children 12 yrs and older. 2 sprays in each nostril once a day.

Children 2-11 yrs. 1 spray in each nostril once a day.

Asthma

Inhalation

Adults, Elderly, Children 12 yrs and older. Initially, inhale 220 mcg (1 puff) once a day. Maximum: 880 mcg once a day.

Skin disease

Topical

Adults, Elderly, Children 12 yrs and older. Apply cream, lotion, or ointment to affected area once a day.

Nasal polyp

Nasal spray

Adults, Elderly. 2 sprays in each nostril twice a day.

AVAILABLE FORMS

- *Nasal Spray (Nasonex):* 50 mcg/spray.
- *Cream (Elocon):* 0.1%.
- *Lotion (Elocon):* 0.1%.
- *Ointment (Elocon):* 0.1%.
- *Oral Inhaler (Asmanex Twisthaler):* 220 mcg.

CONTRAINDICATIONS: Hypersensitivity to any corticosteroid, persistently positive sputum cultures for *Candida albicans,* status asthmaticus (inhalation), systemic fungal infections, untreated localized infection involving nasal mucosa.

PREGNANCY AND LACTATION: Pregnancy category C; systemic corticosteroids are excreted into breast milk in quantities not likely to have deleterious effects in breastfeeding infants; no information on topical steroids

SIDE EFFECTS

Occasional

Inhalation: Headache, allergic rhinitis, upper respiratory infection, muscle pain, fatigue

Nasal: Nasal irritation, stinging

Topical: Burning

Rare

Inhalation: Abdominal pain, dyspepsia, nausea

Nasal: Nasal or pharyngeal candidiasis

Topical: Pruritus

SERIOUS REACTIONS

- An acute hypersensitivity reaction, including urticaria, angioedema, and severe bronchospasm, occurs rarely.
- Transfer from systemic to local steroid therapy may unmask previously suppressed bronchial asthma condition.

INTERACTIONS

Labs

- *Interference:* With adrenal function as assessed by corticotropin stimulation, 24-hr urine-free cortisol measurements; plasma cortisol

SPECIAL CONSIDERATIONS

PATIENT/FAMILY EDUCATION

- Symptoms should start to improve within 2 days of the first dose but the drug's maximum benefit may take up to 2 wks to appear
- Notify the physician of nasal irritation or if symptoms, such as sneezing, fail to improve

MONITORING PARAMETERS

- Pulse rate and quality, ABG levels, and respiratory rate, depth, rhythm and type

monobenzone

(mon-oh-benz'-one)

Rx: Benoquin

Chemical Class: Hydroquinone derivative

Therapeutic Class: Depigmenting agent

CLINICAL PHARMACOLOGY

Mechanism of Action: The mechanism of action is not fully understood. Monobenzone may be converted to hydroquinone, which inhibits the enzymatic oxidation of tyrosine to DOPA; it may have a direct action on tyrosinase; or, it may act as an antioxidant to prevent SH-group oxidation so that more SH groups are available to inhibit tyrosinase. ***Therapeutic Effect:*** Depigmentation in extensive vitiligo.

Pharmacokinetics

Not fully understood. Initial response occurs in 1-4 mos.

INDICATIONS AND DOSAGES

Vitiligo

Topical

Adults, Elderly. Apply 2-3 times/day to affected area.

AVAILABLE FORMS

• *Cream:* 20% (Benoquin).

CONTRAINDICATIONS: History of hypersensitivity to monobenzone or any of its components.

PREGNANCY AND LACTATION: Pregnancy category C; excretion into breast milk unknown

SIDE EFFECTS

Occasional

Irritation, burning sensation, dermatitis

SERIOUS REACTIONS

• None known.

SPECIAL CONSIDERATIONS

PATIENT/FAMILY EDUCATION

• Drug is not a mild cosmetic bleach; treated areas should not be exposed to sunlight (protect with a topical sunscreen)

• Notify the physician of irritation or burning

• Monobenzone is for external use only

MONITORING PARAMETERS

• Skin for irritation

montelukast sodium

(mon-te'-loo-kast soe'-dee-um)

Rx: Singulair

Chemical Class: Cyclopropaneacetic acid derivative

Therapeutic Class: Antiasthmatic; leukotriene receptor antagonist

CLINICAL PHARMACOLOGY

Mechanism of Action: An antiasthmatic that binds to cysteinyl leukotriene receptors, inhibiting the effects of leukotrienes on bronchial smooth muscle. ***Therapeutic Effect:*** Decreases bronchoconstriction, vascular permeability, mucosal edema, and mucus production.

Pharmacokinetics

Route	*Onset*	*Peak*	*Duration*
PO	N/A	N/A	24 hrs
PO (chewable)	N/A	N/A	24 hrs

Rapidly absorbed from the GI tract. Protein binding: 99%. Extensively metabolized in the liver. Excreted almost exclusively in feces. ***Half-life:*** 2.7-5.5 hrs (slightly longer in the elderly).

INDICATIONS AND DOSAGES

Bronchial asthma, perennial allergic rhinitis, seasonal allergic rhinitis

PO

Adults, Elderly, Adolescents older than 14 yr. One 10-mg tablet a day, taken in the evening.

Children 6-14 yrs. One 5-mg chewable tablet a day, taken in the evening.
Children 1-5 yrs. One 4-mg chewable tablet a day, taken in the evening.

AVAILABLE FORMS
- *Oral Granules:* 4 mg.
- *Tablets:* 10 mg.
- *Tablets (Chewable):* 4 mg, 5 mg.

CONTRAINDICATIONS: None known.

PREGNANCY AND LACTATION: Pregnancy category B; excretion into breast milk unknown; use caution in nursing mothers

SIDE EFFECTS
Adults, Adolescents 15 yrs and older
Frequent (18%)
Headache
Occasional (4%)
Influenza
Rare (3%-2%)
Abdominal pain, cough, dyspepsia, dizziness, fatigue, dental pain
Children 6-14 years
Rare (less than 2%)
Diarrhea, laryngitis, pharyngitis, nausea, otitis media, sinusitis, viral infection

SERIOUS REACTIONS
- None known.

INTERACTIONS
3 *Phenobarbital, rifampin:* May decrease montelukast's duration of action
3 *Prednisone:* May decrease the bioavailability of montelukast

SPECIAL CONSIDERATIONS

PATIENT/FAMILY EDUCATION
- Take regularly, even during symptom-free periods
- Do not alter the dosage or abruptly discontinue other asthma medications
- Montelukast is not intended to treat acute asthma attacks
- Drink plenty of fluids to decrease the thickness of lung secretions
- Patients with aspirin sensitivity should avoid aspirin and NSAIDs while taking montelukast

MONITORING PARAMETERS
- Pulmonary function tests
- Pulse rate and quality as well as respiratory depth, rate, rhythm, and type
- Auscultate the patient's breath sounds for crackles, rhonchi, and wheezing
- Observe the patient's fingernails and lips for a blue or dusky color in light-skinned patients and a gray color in dark-skinned patients, which may be signs of hypoxemia

moricizine hydrochloride

(mor-i'-siz-een hye-droe-klor'-ide)

Rx: Ethmozine

Chemical Class: Phenothiazine derivative

Therapeutic Class: Antiarrhythmic, class IA

CLINICAL PHARMACOLOGY
Mechanism of Action: An antiarrhythmic that prevents sodium current across myocardial cell membranes. Has potent local anesthetic activity and membrane stabilizing effects. Slows AV and His-Purkinje conduction and decreases action potential duration and effective refractory period. ***Therapeutic Effect:*** Suppresses ventricular arrhythmias.
Pharmacokinetics
Almost completely absorbed from the GI tract. Protein binding: 92%-95%. Extensively metabolized in liver. Excreted in urine. ***Half-life:*** 2 hr.

INDICATIONS AND DOSAGES
Arrhythmias
PO
Adults, Elderly. 200-300 mg q8h. May increase by 150 mg/day at no less than 3-day intervals.

AVAILABLE FORMS
• *Tablets:* 200 mg, 250 mg, 300 mg.

UNLABELED USES: Atrial arrhythmias, complete and non-sustained ventricular arrhythmias, premature ventricular contractions (PVCs)

CONTRAINDICATIONS: Cardiogenic shock, preexisting second- or third-degree AV block or right bundle-branch block without pacemaker

PREGNANCY AND LACTATION: Pregnancy category B; secreted into breast milk (1 patient); potential for serious adverse effects exists

SIDE EFFECTS
Frequent (15%-6%)
Dizziness, nausea, headache, fatigue, dyspnea
Occasional (5%-2%)
Nervousness, paraesthesia, sleep disturbances, dyspepsia, vomiting, diarrhea

SERIOUS REACTIONS
• Moricizine may worsen existing arrhythmias or produce new ones.
• Jaundice with hepatitis occurs rarely.
• Overdosage produces vomiting, lethargy, syncope, hypotension, conduction disturbances, exacerbation of CHF, MI, and sinus arrest.

INTERACTIONS
Drugs
3 *Cimetidine:* Increases serum moricizine concentrations
3 *Theophylline:* Reduces serum theophylline levels by increasing clearance

SPECIAL CONSIDERATIONS
• Antidysrhythmic therapy has not been proven to be beneficial in terms of improving survival among patients with asymptomatic or mildly symptomatic ventricular dysrhythmias
• Studied in the CAST (Cardiac Arrhythmia Suppression Trial, I and II) with findings of excessive cardiac mortality and no benefit on long-term survival compared to placebo
• Initiate therapy in facilities capable of providing continuous ECG monitoring and managing life-threatening dysrhythmias

PATIENT/FAMILY EDUCATION
• Do not abruptly discontinue the drug
• Notify the physician if chest pain or irregular heartbeats occurs

MONITORING PARAMETERS
• EKG for cardiac changes, especially increase in PR and QRS intervals
• Pulse rate for quality and irregularity
• Electrolytes, intake and output
• Liver and renal function

morphine sulfate
(mor'-feen sul'-fate)
Rx: Astramorph PF, Avinza, DepoDur, Duramorph PF, Infumorph, Kadian, M-Eslon, MS Contin, MSIR, MS/S, Oramorph SR, Rapi-Ject, RMS, Roxanol, Roxanol-T
Chemical Class: Natural opium alkaloid; phenanthrene derivative
Therapeutic Class: Narcotic analgesic
DEA Class: Schedule II

CLINICAL PHARMACOLOGY
Mechanism of Action: An opioid agonist that binds with opioid receptors in the CNS. ***Therapeutic Effect:***

M

Alters the perception of and emotional response to pain; produces generalized CNS depression.

Pharmacokinetics

Route	Onset	Peak	Duration
Oral Solution	N/A	1 hr	3-5 hrs
Tablets	N/A	1 hr	3-5 hrs
Tablets (ER)	N/A	3-4 hrs	8-12 hrs
IV	Rapid	0.3 hrs	3-5 hrs
IM	5-30 mins	0.5-1 hr	3-5 hrs
Epidural	N/A	1 hr	12-20 hrs
Subcutaneous	N/A	1.1-5 hrs	3-5 hrs
Rectal	N/A	0.5-1 hr	3-7 hrs

Variably absorbed from the GI tract. Readily absorbed after IM or subcutaneous administration. Protein binding: 20%-35%. Widely distributed. Metabolized in the liver. Primarily excreted in urine. Removed by hemodialysis. ***Half-life:*** 2-3 hrs (increased in patients with hepatic disease).

INDICATIONS AND DOSAGES:

Alert: Dosage should be titrated to desired effect.

Analgesia

PO (Prompt-Release)

Adults, Elderly. 10-30 mg q3-4h as needed.

Children. 0.2-0.5 mg/kg q3-4h as needed.

Alert: For the Avinza dosage below, be aware that this drug is to be administered once a day only.

Alert: For the Kadian dosage information below, be aware that this drug is to be administered q12h or once a day only.

Alert: Be aware that pediatric dosages of extended-release preparations Kadian and Avinza have not been established.

Alert: For the MSContin and Oramorph SR dosage information below, be aware that the daily dosage is divided and given q8h or q12h.

PO (Extended-Release [Avinza])

Adults, Elderly. Dosage requirement should be established using prompt-release formulations and is based on total daily dose. Avinza is given once a day only.

PO (Extended-Release [Kadian])

Adults, Elderly. Dosage requirement should be established using prompt-release formulations and is based on total daily dose. Dose is given once a day or divided and given q12h.

PO (Extended-Release [MSContin, Oramorph SR])

Adults, Elderly. Dosage requirement should be established using prompt-release formulations and is based on total daily dose. Daily dose is divided and given q8h or q12h.

Children. 0.3-0.6 mg/kg/dose q12h.

IV

Adults, Elderly. 2.5-5 mg q3-4h as needed. Note: Repeated doses (e.g., 1-2 mg) may be given more frequently (e.g., every hour) if needed.

Children. 0.05-0.1 mg/kg q3-4h as needed.

IV (Continuous Infusion)

Adults, Elderly. 0.8-10 mg/h. Range: Up to 80 mg/h.

Children. 10-30 mcg/kg/hr.

IM

Adults, Elderly. 5-10 mg q3-4h as needed.

Children. 0.1 mg/kg q3-4h as needed.

Epidural

Adults, Elderly. Initially, 1-6 mg bolus, infusion rate: 0.1-1 mg/h. Maximum: 10 mg/24 h.

Intrathecal

Adults, Elderly. One-tenth of the epidural dose: 0.2-1 mg/dose.

PCA

IV

Adults, Elderly. Loading dose: 5-10 mg. Intermittent bolus: 0.5-3 mg. Lockout interval: 5-12 min. Continuous infusion: 1-10 mg/hr. 4-hr limit: 20-30 mg.

AVAILABLE FORMS

- *Capsules (Extended-Release):* 20 mg (Kadian), 30 mg (Avinza, Kadian), 50 mg (Kadian), 60 mg (Avinza, Kadian), 90 mg (Avinza), 100 mg (Kadian), 120 mg (Avinza).
- *Capsules (MSIR):* 15 mg, 30 mg.
- *Solution for Injection:* 0.5 mg/ml, 1 mg/ml, 2 mg/ml, 4 mg/ml, 5 mg/ml, 8 mg/ml, 10 mg/ml, 15 mg/ml, 25 mg/ml, 50 mg/ml.
- *Solution for Injection:* 5% dextrose-20 mg morphine/100 ml, 5% dextrose-100 mg morphine/100 ml.
- *Solution for Injection (Preservative-Free):* 0.5 mg/ml (Astramorph PF, Duramorph PF), 1 mg/ml (Astramorph PF, Duramorph PF), 10 mg/ml (Infumorph), 15 mg/ml, 25 mg/ml (Infumorph), 50 mg/ml.
- *Epidural and Intrathecal via Infusion Device (Infumorph):* 10 mg/ml, 25 mg/ml.
- *Oral Solution:* 10 mg/ml (MSIR), 20 mg/ml (MSIR, Roxanol), 100 mg/ml (Roxanol).
- *Suppositories (RMS):* 5 mg, 10 mg, 20 mg, 30 mg.
- *Tablets (MSIR):* 15 mg, 30 mg.
- *Tablets (Extended-Release):* 15 mg (MS Contin, Oramorph SR), 30 mg (MS Contin, Oramorph SR), 60 mg (MS Contin, Oramorph SR), 100 mg (MS Contin, Oramorph SR), 200 mg (MS Contin).
- *Liposomal Injection (DepoDur):* 10 mg/ml, 15 mg/1.5 ml, 20 mg/2 ml.

CONTRAINDICATIONS: Acute or severe asthma, GI obstruction, paralytic ileus, severe hepatic or renal impairment, severe respiratory depression

PREGNANCY AND LACTATION: Pregnancy category C (D if used for prolonged periods or at high dosages at term); trace amounts enter breast milk; compatible with breast-feeding

Controlled Substance: Schedule II

SIDE EFFECTS

Frequent

Sedation, decreased BP (including orthostatic hypotension), diaphoresis, facial flushing, constipation, dizziness, somnolence, nausea, vomiting

Occasional

Allergic reaction (rash, pruritus), dyspnea, confusion, palpitations, tremors, urine retention, abdominal cramps, vision changes, dry mouth, headache, decreased appetite, pain or burning at injection site

Rare

Paralytic ileus

SERIOUS REACTIONS

- Overdose results in respiratory depression, skeletal muscle flaccidity, cold or clammy skin, cyanosis, and extreme somnolence progressing to seizures, stupor, and coma.
- The patient who uses morphine repeatedly may develop a tolerance to the drug's analgesic effect and physical dependence.
- The drug may have a prolonged duration of action and cumulative effect in those with hepatic and renal impairment.

INTERACTIONS

Drugs

3 *Amitryptyline:* Additive respiratory and CNS depressant effects

3 *Antihistamines, chloral hydrate, glutethimide, methocarbamol:* Enhanced depressant effects

3 *Barbiturates:* Additive respiratory and CNS depressant effects

3 *Cimetidine:* Increased respiratory and CNS depression
3 *Cloimpramine:* Additive respiratory and CNS depressant effects
3 *Ethanol, other CNS depressants:* Additive CNS effects
3 *MAOIs:* Markedly potentiate the actions of morphine
3 *Nortriptyline:* Additive respiratory and CNS depressant effects
3 *Rifampin:* Reduces the concentration of morphine
3 *Somatostatin:* Inhibits the analgesic effect of morphine
3 *Trovafloxacin:* Intravenous morphine reduces the serum concentration of orally administered trovafloxacin; reduced antibiotic efficacy may result

Labs
- *Increase:* Urine glucose, urine 17-ketosteroids
- False elevations of amylase and lipase

SPECIAL CONSIDERATIONS
- *Treatment of overdose:* Naloxone (Narcan) 0.2-0.8 mg IV
- Remains the strong analgesic of choice for acute, severe pain, acute MI pain, and the agent of choice for chronic cancer pain
- 200-mg Sus Action tablet for use only in opioid-tolerant patients
- Do not administer agonist/antagonist analgesics (i.e., pentazocine, nalbuphine, butorphanol, dezocine, buprenorphine) to patient who has received a prolonged course of morphine (a pure agonist). In opioid-dependent patients, mixed agonist/anagonist analgesics may precipitate withdrawal symptoms

PATIENT/FAMILY EDUCATION
- Change position slowly to avoid orthostasis
- Avoid alcohol and other CNS depressants
- Physical dependency may result
- Do not chew or crush Sus Action preparations
- Injection of morphine may cause discomfort
- Avoid tasks that require mental alertness or motor skills until response to the drug has been established

MONITORING PARAMETERS
- Vital signs for 5-10 mins after IV administration and 15-30 mins after IM or subcutaneous injection
- Pattern of daily bowel activity and stool consistency
- Clinical improvement, and record the onset of pain relief

moxifloxacin hydrochloride

(mox-ee-flox'-a-sin hye-droe-klor'-ide)

Rx: Avelox, Avelox IV, Vigamox

Chemical Class: Fluoroquinolone derivative

Therapeutic Class: Antibiotic

CLINICAL PHARMACOLOGY

Mechanism of Action: A fluoroquinolone that inhibits two enzymes, topoisomerase II and IV, in susceptible microorganisms. ***Therapeutic Effect:*** Interferes with bacterial DNA replication. Prevents or delays emergence of resistant organisms. Bactericidal.

Pharmacokinetics

Well absorbed from the GI tract after PO administration. Protein binding: 50%. Widely distributed throughout body with tissue concentration often exceeding plasma concentration. Metabolized in liver. Primarily excreted in urine with a lesser amount in feces. ***Half-life:*** 10.7-13.3 hr.

INDICATIONS AND DOSAGES

Acute bacterial sinusitis

PO, IV

Adults, Elderly. 400 mg q24h for 10 days.

Acute bacterial exacerbation of chronic bronchitis

PO, IV

Adults, Elderly. 400 mg q24h for 5 days.

Community-acquired pneumonia

IV, PO

Adults, Elderly. 400 mg q24h for 7-14 days.

Skin and skin-structure infection

PO, IV

Adults, Elderly. 400 mg once a day for 7 days.

Topical treatment of bacterial conjunctivitis due to susceptible strains of bacteria

Ophthalmic

Adults, Elderly, Children older than 1 yr. 1 drop 3 times a day for 7 days.

AVAILABLE FORMS

- *Tablets (Avelox):* 400 mg.
- *Injection (Avelox IV):* 400 mg.
- *Ophthalmic Solution (Vigamox):* 0.5%.

CONTRAINDICATIONS: Hypersensitivity to quinolones

PREGNANCY AND LACTATION: Pregnancy category C; excreted into breast milk, safety not established; allow 48 hr to elapse after last dose before resuming breast-feeding

SIDE EFFECTS

Frequent (8%-6%)

Nausea, diarrhea

Occasional (3%-2%)

Dizziness, headache, abdominal pain, vomiting

Ophthalmic (6%-1%): conjunctival irritation, reduced visual acuity, dry eye, keratitis, eye pain, ocular itching, swelling of tissue around cornea, eye discharge, fever, cough, pharyngitis, rash, rhinitis

Rare (1%)

Change in sense of taste, dyspepsia (heartburn, indigestion), photosensitivity

SERIOUS REACTIONS

- Pseudomembranous colitis as evidenced by fever, severe abdominal cramps or pain, and severe watery diarrhea may occur.
- Superinfection manifested as anal or genital pruritus, moderate to severe diarrhea, and stomatitis may occur.

INTERACTIONS

Drugs

3 *Aluminum:* Reduced absorption of moxifloxacin; do not take within 4 hr of dose

3 *Antacids:* Reduced absorption of moxifloxacin; do not take within 4 hr of dose

3 *Antipyrine:* Inhibits metabolism of antipyrine; increased plasma antipyrine level

3 *Calcium:* Reduced absorption of moxifloxacin; do not take within 4 hr of dose

3 *Diazepam:* Inhibits metabolism of diazepam; increased plasma diazepam level

3 *Didanosine:* Markedly reduced absorption of moxifloxacin; take moxifloxacin 2 hr before didanosine

3 *Foscarnet:* Coadministration increases seizure risk

3 *Iron:* Reduced absorption of moxifloxacin; do not take within 4 hr of dose

3 *Magnesium:* Reduced absorption of moxifloxacin; do not take within 4 hr of dose

3 *Metoprolol:* Inhibits metabolism of metoprolol; increased plasma metoprolol level

3 *Morphine:* Reduced absorption of moxifloxacin; do not take within 2 hr of dose

3 *Pentoxifylline:* Inhibits metabolism of pentoxifylline; increased plasma pentoxifylline level

3 *Phenytoin:* Inhibits metabolism of phenytoin; increased plasma phenytoin level

3 *Propranolol:* Inhibits metabolism of propranolol; increased plasma propranolol level

3 *Ropinirole:* Inhibits metabolism of ropinirole; increased plasma ropinirole level

3 *Sodium bicarbonate:* Reduced absorption of moxifloxacin; do not take within 4 hr of dose

3 *Sucralfate:* Reduced absorption of moxifloxacin; do not take within 4 hr of dose

3 *Warfarin:* Inhibits metabolism of warfarin; increases hypoprothrombinemic response to warfarin

3 *Zinc:* Reduced absorption of moxifloxacin; do not take within 4 hr of dose

2 *Ziprasidone:* Prolongs the QTc interval; theoretically, could increase the risk of ventricular arrhythmias

SPECIAL CONSIDERATIONS

PATIENT/FAMILY EDUCATION

- May be taken with or without meals
- Should be taken at least 4 hr before or 8 hr after multivitamins (containing iron or zinc), antacids (containing magnesium, calcium, or aluminum), sucralfate, or didanosine chewable/buffered tablets
- Discontinue treatment, rest and refrain from exercise, and inform prescriber if pain, inflammation, or rupture of a tendon occur
- Test reaction to this drug before operating an automobile or machinery or engaging in activities requiring mental alertness or coordination
- Drink plenty of fluids
- Avoid exposure to direct sunlight as this may cause a photosensitivity reaction
- Take for the full course of therapy

MONITORING PARAMETERS

- WBC count
- Signs of infection
- Pattern of daily bowel activity and stool consistency
- Evaluate for abdominal pain, altered sense of taste, dyspepsia (heartburn, indigestion), headache, and vomiting

---

mupirocin

(myoo-pye'-roe-sin)

Rx: Bactroban

Chemical Class: Pseudomonic acid derivative

Therapeutic Class: Antibiotic, topical

CLINICAL PHARMACOLOGY

Mechanism of Action: An antibacterial agent that inhibits bacterial protein, RNA synthesis. Less effective on DNA synthesis. Nasal: Eradicates nasal colonization of MRSA. ***Therapeutic Effect:*** Prevents bacterial growth and replication. Bacteriostatic.

Pharmacokinetics

Metabolized in skin to inactive metabolite. Transported to skin surface; removed by normal skin desquamation.

INDICATIONS AND DOSAGES

Impetigo, infected traumatic skin lesions

Topical

Adults, Elderly, Children. Apply 3 times/day (may cover w/gauze).

Nasal colonization of resistant Staphylococcus aureus

Intranasal

Adults, Elderly, Children 12 yrs and older. Apply 2 times/day for 5 days.

AVAILABLE FORMS

- *Ointment:* 2% (Bactroban).
- *Nasal ointment:* 2% (Bactroban).

UNLABELED USES: Treatment of infected eczema, folliculitis, minor bacterial skin infections.

CONTRAINDICATIONS: Hypersensitivity to mupirocin or any component of the formulation

PREGNANCY AND LACTATION: Pregnancy category B; excretion into breast milk unknown

SIDE EFFECTS

Frequent

Nasal: Headache, rhinitis, upper respiratory congestion, pharyngitis, altered taste

Occasional

Nasal: Burning, stinging, cough

Topical: Pain, burning, stinging, itching

Rare

Nasal: Pruritis, diarrhea, dry mouth, epistaxis, nausea, rash

Topical: Rash, nausea, dry skin, contact dermatitis

SERIOUS REACTIONS

- Superinfection may result in bacterial or fungal infections, especially with prolonged or repeated therapy.

SPECIAL CONSIDERATIONS

- Comparable efficacy to systemic semisynthetic penicillins and erythromycin in impetigo and infected wounds

PATIENT/FAMILY EDUCATION

- For external use only
- Notify the physician if skin reaction or irritation occurs
- If there is no improvement in 3-5 days, see the physician to be reevaluated

MONITORING PARAMETERS

- Skin for irritation

mycophenolate mofetil

(mye-koe-fen′-oh-late)

Rx: CellCept, Myfortic

Chemical Class: Mycophenolic acid derivative

Therapeutic Class: Immunosuppressant

CLINICAL PHARMACOLOGY

Mechanism of Action: An immunologic agent that suppresses the immunologically mediated inflammatory response by inhibiting inosine monophosphate dehydrogenase, an enzyme that deprives lymphocytes of nucleotides necessary for DNA and RNA synthesis, thus inhibiting the proliferation of T and B lymphocytes. ***Therapeutic Effect:*** Prevents transplant rejection.

Pharmacokinetics

Rapidly and extensively absorbed after PO administration (food decreases drug plasma concentration but does not affect absorption). Protein binding: 97%. Completely hydrolyzed to active metabolite mycophenolic acid. Primarily excreted in urine. Not removed by hemodialysis. ***Half-life:*** 17.9 hr.

INDICATIONS AND DOSAGES

Prevention of renal transplant rejection

PO, IV (Cellcept)

Adults, Elderly. 1 g twice a day.

PO (Myfortic)

Adults, Elderly. 720 mg twice a day.

Children 5-16 yr. 400 mg/m^2 twice a day. Maximum: 720 mg twice a day.

Prevention of heart transplant rejection

PO, IV (Cellcept)

Adults, Elderly. 1.5 g twice a day.

Prevention of liver transplant rejection
PO (Cellcept)
Adults, Elderly. 1.5 g twice a day.
IV (Cellcept)
Adults, Elderly. 1 g twice a day.
Usual pediatric dosage
PO (Cellcept)
Children. 600 mg/m^2/dose twice a day. Maximum: 2 g/day.

AVAILABLE FORMS
- *Capsules (Cellcept):* 250 mg.
- *Oral Suspension (Cellcept):* 200 mg/ml.
- *Tablets (Cellcept):* 500 mg.
- *Tablets (Delayed-Release [Myfortic]):* 180 mg, 360 mg.
- *Injection (Cellcept):* 500 mg.

UNLABELED USES: Treatment of liver transplantation rejection, mild heart transplant rejection, moderate to severe psoriasis

CONTRAINDICATIONS: Hypersensitivity to mycophenolic acid or polysorbate 80 (IV formulation)

PREGNANCY AND LACTATION: Pregnancy category C; mycophenolic acid excreted in milk; not recommended during breast-feeding

SIDE EFFECTS
Frequent (37%-20%)
UTI, hypertension, peripheral edema, diarrhea, constipation, fever, headache, nausea
Occasional (18%-10%)
Dyspepsia; dyspnea; cough; hematuria; asthenia; vomiting; edema; tremors; abdominal, chest, or back pain; oral candidiasis; acne
Rare (9%-6%)
Insomnia, respiratory tract infection, rash, dizziness

SERIOUS REACTIONS
- Significant anemia, leukopenia, thrombocytopenia, neutropenia, and leukocytosis may occur, particularly in those undergoing renal transplant rejection.
- Sepsis and infection occur occasionally.
- GI tract hemorrhage occurs rarely.
- Patients receiving mycophenolate have an increased risk of developing neoplasms.
- Immunosuppression may result in an increased susceptibility to infection and the development of lymphoma.

INTERACTIONS
Drugs
3 *Acyclovir:* Increased serum acyclovir and mycophenolate concentrations possible
3 *Antacids with magnesium and aluminum hydroxides:* Decreased mycophenolate bioavailability; separate administration times
3 *Azathioprine:* Due to potential bone marrow suppression, concomitant administration not recommended
3 *Cholestyramine:* Decreased mycophenolate bioavailability due to interruption of enterohepatic recirculation
2 *Echinacea:* May decrease the effects of mycophenolate
3 *Food:* May decrease mycophenolate plasma concentration
3 *Ganciclovir:* Increased serum ganciclovir and mycophenolate concentrations possible
3 *Live vaccines:* Use of live attenuated vaccines should be avoided; vaccines may be less effective
3 *Probenecid:* Increased serum mycophenolate concentrations

SPECIAL CONSIDERATIONS
- Drug can be given concurrently with cyclosporine, which may enable reduced cyclosporine doses and lower toxicity, or potential cyclosporine substitute in patients developing cyclosporine toxicity
- Drug is less likely than azathioprine to induce severe bone marrow depression, and may replace aza-

thioprine in conventional maintenance immunosuppression regimens
• IV can be administered for up to 14 days; switch to PO as soon as possible

PATIENT/FAMILY EDUCATION
• Women of childbearing potential should use effective contraception before and during therapy and 6 wks after therapy has stopped
• Notify the physician if abdominal pain, fever, sore throat, or unusual bleeding or bruising occurs
• Regular laboratory tests during mycophenolate therapy is essential
• Malignancies may occur; be prepared to answer questions and provide additional information

MONITORING PARAMETERS
• CBC qwk × 1 mo, then q2wk × 2 mo, then monthly
• Reduce the dosage or discontinue the drug if the patient experiences a rapid fall in WBC count

nabumetone

(na-byoo′-me-tone)
Rx: Relafen
Chemical Class: Acetic acid derivative
Therapeutic Class: NSAID; antipyretic; nonnarcotic analgesic

CLINICAL PHARMACOLOGY
Mechanism of Action: An NSAID that produces analgesic and antiinflammatory effects by inhibiting prostaglandin synthesis. ***Therapeutic Effect:*** Reduces the inflammatory response and intensity of pain.
Pharmacokinetics
Readily absorbed from the GI tract. Protein binding: 99%. Widely distributed. Metabolized in the liver to active metabolite. Primarily excreted in urine. Not removed by hemodialysis. ***Half-life:*** 22-30 hr.

INDICATIONS AND DOSAGES
Acute or chronic rheumatoid arthritis and osteoarthritis
PO
Adults, Elderly. Initially, 1000 mg as a single dose or in 2 divided doses. May increase up to 2000 mg/day as a single or in 2 divided doses.

AVAILABLE FORMS
• *Tablets (Relafen):* 500 mg, 750 mg.

CONTRAINDICATIONS: Active peptic ulcer disease, chronic inflammation of GI tract, GI bleeding or ulceration, history of hypersensitivity to aspirin or NSAIDs, history of significant renal impairment

PREGNANCY AND LACTATION: Pregnancy category C (D if used in third trimester or near delivery); excretion into breast milk unknown; not recommended for use in nursing mothers

SIDE EFFECTS
Frequent (14%-12%)
Diarrhea, abdominal cramps or pain, dyspepsia
Occasional (9%-4%)
Nausea, constipation, flatulence, dizziness, headache
Rare (3%-1%)
Vomiting, stomatitis, confusion

SERIOUS REACTIONS
• Overdose may result in acute hypotension and tachycardia.
• Rare reactions with long-term use include peptic ulcer disease, GI bleeding, gastritis, nephrotoxicity (dysuria, cystitis, hematuria, proteinuria, nephrotic syndrome), severe hepatic reactions (cholestasis, jaundice), and severe hypersensitivity reactions (bronchospasm, angioedema).

INTERACTIONS

Drugs

3 *Aminoglycosides:* Reduced clearance with elevated aminoglycoside levels and potential for toxicity (especially indomethacin in premature infants; other NSAIDs probably)

3 *Antihypertensives:* (α-blockers, angiotensin-converting enzyme inhibitors, angiotensin II receptor blockers, β-blockers, diuretics) inhibition of antihypertensive and other favorable hemodynamic effects

3 *Aspirin, other salicylates:* May increase the risk of GI side effects such as bleeding

3 *Bone marrow depressants:* May increase the risk of hematologic reactions

3 *Corticosteroids:* Increased risk of GI ulceration

3 *Cyclosporine:* Increased nephrotoxicity risk

3 *Feverfew:* May decrease the effects of feverfew

3 *Ginkgo biloba:* May increase the risk of bleeding

3 *Lithium:* Decreased clearance of lithium (mediated via prostaglandins) resulting in elevated serum lithium levels and risk of toxicity

3 *Methotrexate:* Decreased renal secretion of methotrexate resulting in elevated methotrexate levels and risk of toxicity

3 *Phenylpropanolamine:* Possible acute hypertensive reaction

3 *Potassium-sparing diuretics:* Additive hyperkalemia potential

3 *Triamterene:* Acute renal failure reported with addition of indomethacin; caution with other NSAIDs

2 *Warfarin:* Transient increase in prothrombin time due to displaced protein binding; increased risk of GI bleeding although likely less risky than other NSAIDs due to preferential action on COX-2

SPECIAL CONSIDERATIONS

- No significant advantage over other NSAIDs; cost should govern use

PATIENT/FAMILY EDUCATION

- Take nabumetone with food if GI upset occurs
- Nabumetone may cause serious GI bleeding with or without pain; avoid aspirin during nabumetone therapy because it increases the risk of GI bleeding
- Nabumetone may cause confusion or dizziness; avoid performing tasks that require mental alertness or motor skills until response to the drug has been established
- The female patient should inform the physician if she is or plans to become pregnant

MONITORING PARAMETERS

- Initial hemogram and fecal occult blood test within 3 mos of starting regular chronic therapy; repeat every 6-12 mos (more frequently in high risk patients (>65 yrs, peptic ulcer disease, concurrent steroids or anticoagulants); electrolytes, creatinine, and BUN within 3 mos of starting regular chronic therapy; repeat every 6-12 mos
- Pattern of daily bowel activity
- Therapeutic response, such as improved grip strength, increased joint mobility, and decreased pain, tenderness, stiffness, and swelling

nadolol

(nay-doe'-lole)

Rx: Corgard

Combinations

Rx: With Bendroflumenthiazide (Corzide)

Chemical Class: β-adrenergic blocker, nonselective

Therapeutic Class: Antianginal; antiglaucoma agent; antihypertensive

CLINICAL PHARMACOLOGY

Mechanism of Action: A nonselective beta-blocker that blocks $beta_1$- and $beta_2$-adrenergenic receptors. Large doses increase airway resistance. ***Therapeutic Effect:*** Slows sinus heart rate, decreases cardiac output and BP. Decreases myocardial ischemia severity by decreasing oxygen requirements.

Pharmacokinetics

Variable absorption after PO administration. Protein binding: 28%-30%. Not metabolized. Excreted unchanged in feces. ***Half-life:*** 20-24 hr.

INDICATIONS AND DOSAGES

Mild to moderate hypertension, angina

PO

Adults. Initially, 40 mg/day. May increase by 40-80 mg at 3-7 day intervals. Maximum: 240-360 mg/day.

Elderly. Initially, 20 mg/day. May increase gradually. Range: 20-240 mg/day.

Dosage in renal impairment

Dosage is modified based on creatinine clearance.

Creatinine Clearance	*% Usual Dosage*
10-50 ml/mins	50
less than 10 ml/mins	25

AVAILABLE FORMS

• *Tablets:* 20 mg, 40 mg, 80 mg, 120 mg, 160 mg.

UNLABELED USES: Treatment of arrhythmias, hypertrophic cardiomyopathy, MI, mitral valve prolapse syndrome, neuroleptic-induced akathisia, pheochromocytoma, tremors, thyrotoxicosis, vascular headaches

CONTRAINDICATIONS: Bronchial asthma, cardiogenic shock, CHF secondary to tachyarrhythmias, chronic obstructive pulmonary disease (COPD), patients receiving MAOI therapy, second- or third-degree heart block, sinus bradycardia, uncontrolled cardiac failure

PREGNANCY AND LACTATION: Pregnancy category C (D if used in second or third trimester); similar drug, atenolol, frequently used in the third trimester for treatment of hypertension (many studies of efficacy and safety of atenolol in pregnancy-induced hypertension); long-term use has been associated with intrauterine growth retardation; mean milk: plasma ratio, 0.80 in one study; quantity of drug ingested by breast-feeding infant unlikely to be therapeutically significant

SIDE EFFECTS

Nadolol is generally well tolerated, with transient and mild side effects.

Frequent

Diminished sexual ability, drowsiness, unusual fatigue or weakness

Occasional

Bradycardia, difficulty breathing, depression, cold hands or feet, diarrhea, constipation, anxiety, nasal congestion, nausea, vomiting

Rare

Altered taste, dry eyes, itching

SERIOUS REACTIONS

• Overdose may produce profound bradycardia and hypotension.

• Abrupt withdrawal of nadolol may result in diaphoresis, palpitations, headache, tremors, exacerbation of angina, MI, and ventricular arrhythmias.
• Nadolol administration may precipitate CHF and MI in patients with cardiac disease; thyroid storm in those with thyrotoxicosis; and peripheral ischemia in those with existing peripheral vascular disease.
• Hypoglycemia may occur in patients with previously controlled diabetes.

INTERACTIONS

Drugs

3 *Adenosine:* Bradycardia aggravated
3 *α_1-adrenergic blockers:* Potential enhanced first-dose response (marked initial drop in blood pressure, particularly on standing (especially prazocin).
3 *Amiodarone:* Symptomatic bradycardia and sinus arrest; caution in patients with bradycardia, sick sinus syndrome, or partial AV block when either amiodarone or β-blocking drug is used
3 *Ampicillin:* Reduced nadolol bioavailability
3 *Antacids:* Reduced nadolol absorption
3 *Calcium channel blockers:* See dihydropyridine and verapamil
3 *Cimetidine:* May increase blood concentration
3 *Clonidine:* Exacerbation of rebound hypertension upon discontinuation of clonidine
3 *Digoxin:* Additive prolongation of atrioventricular (AV) conduction time
3 *Dihydropyridine calcium channel blockers:* Severe hypotension or impaired cardiac performance; most prevalent with impaired left ventricular function, cardiac arrhythmias, or aortic stenosis
3 *Diuretics, other antihypertensives:* May increase hypotensive effect
3 *Diltiazem:* Potentiates β-adrenergic effects; hypotension, left ventricular failure, and AV conduction disturbances problematic in elderly, patients with left ventricular dysfunction, aortic stenosis, or with large doses of either drug
3 *Dipyridamole:* Bradycardia aggravated
3 *Hypoglycemic agents:* Masked hypoglycemia, hyperglycemia
3 *Lidocaine:* Increased serum lidocaine concentrations possible
3 *Neostigmine:* Bradycardia aggravated
3 *NSAIDs:* Reduced antihypertensive effect of nadolol
3 *Physostigmine:* Bradycardia aggravated
3 *Prazosin:* First-dose response to prazosin may be enhanced by β-blockade
3 *Sympathomimetics, xanthines:* May mutually inhibit effects
3 *Tacrine:* Bradycardia aggravated
2 *Theophylline:* Antagonistic pharmacodynamic effects
3 *Verapamil:* Potentiates β-adrenergic effects; hypotension, left ventricular failure, and AV conduction disturbances problematic in elderly, patients with left ventricular dysfunction, aortic stenosis, or with large doses of either drug

SPECIAL CONSIDERATIONS

• No unique advantage over less expensive β-blockers

PATIENT/FAMILY EDUCATION

• Do **not** discontinue abruptly; may require taper; rapid withdrawal may produce rebound hypertension or angina
• Notify the physician if confusion, depression, difficulty breathing, dizziness, fever, night cough, rash,

slow pulse, sore throat, swelling of arms and legs, or unusual bleeding or bruising occurs
• Avoid tasks that require mental alertness or motor skills until response to the drug has been established

MONITORING PARAMETERS
• *Angina:* Reduction in nitroglycerin usage; frequency, severity, onset, and duration of angina pain; heart rate
• *Arrhythmias:* Heart rate
• *Congestive heart failure:* Functional status, cough, dyspnea on exertion, paroxysmal nocturnal dyspnea, exercise tolerance, and ventricular function
• *Hypertension:* Blood pressure
• *Migraine headache:* Reduction in the frequency, severity, and duration of attacks
• *Post myocardial infarction:* Left ventricular function, lower resting heart rate
• *Toxicity:* Blood glucose, bronchospasm, hypotension, bradycardia, depression, confusion, hallucination, sexual dysfunction

nafarelin acetate
(naf'-a-rel-in ass'-e-tate)
Rx: Synarel
Chemical Class: Gonadotropin-releasing hormone analog
Therapeutic Class: Antiendometriosis agent

CLINICAL PHARMACOLOGY
Mechanism of Action: A gonadotropin inhibitor that initially stimulates the release of the pituitary gonadotropins, luteinizing hormone and follicle-stimulating hormone, then decreases secretion of gonadal steroids. ***Therapeutic Effect:*** Temporarily increases ovarian steroidogenesis, abolishes the stimulatory effect on the pituitary gland, decreases secretion of gonadal steroids.
Pharmacokinetics
Rapidly absorbed after nasal administration. Protein binding: 78%-84%, binds primarily to albumin. Metabolism: unknown. Excreted in urine. ***Half-life:*** 3 hrs.

INDICATIONS AND DOSAGES
Endometriosis
Intranasal
Adults. 400 mcg/day: 200 mcg (1 spray) into 1 nostril in morning, 1 spray into other nostril in evening. For patients with persistent regular menstruation after months of treatment, increase dose to 800 mcg/day (1 spray into each nostril in morning and evening).
Central precocious puberty
Intranasal
Children. 1600 mcg/day: 400 mcg (2 sprays into each nostril in morning and evening; total 8 sprays).

AVAILABLE FORMS
• *Nasal Spray:* 2 mg/ml (Synarel).

CONTRAINDICATIONS: Pregnancy, other agonist analogs, undiagnosed abnormal vaginal bleeding, hypersensitivity to nafarelin or any component of the formulation

PREGNANCY AND LACTATION: Pregnancy category X; not recommended in nursing mothers

SIDE EFFECTS
Frequent
Hot flashes. muscle pain, decreased breast size, myalgia
Occasional
Nasal irritation, decreased libido, vaginal dryness, headache, emotional lability, acne
Rare
Insomnia, edema, weight gain, seborrhea, depression

SERIOUS REACTIONS
• None reported.

INTERACTIONS

Drugs

3 *Decongestants, nasal/topical:* Potential interference with absorption; allow 30 min after use of nafarelin before applying a topical decongestant

Labs

• *Interference:* Gonadal and gonadotropic function tests conducted during treatment and for 4-8 wk after treatment may be misleading

SPECIAL CONSIDERATIONS

• Alternative to danazol and oophorectomy in the treatment of endometriosis; more tolerable adverse effect profile compared to danazol for some patients
• Agent of choice in patients concerned about future fertility
• Benefits are temporary

PATIENT/FAMILY EDUCATION

• Use nonhormonal contraceptives during therapy
• Do not take this drug if pregnancy is suspected
• Take for the full length of therapy

MONITORING PARAMETERS

• Inquire about menstrual cessation

nafcillin sodium

(naf-sill'-in soe'-dee-um)

Rx: Nafcil, Nallpen, Unipen

Chemical Class: Penicillin derivative, penicillinase-resistant

Therapeutic Class: Antibiotic

CLINICAL PHARMACOLOGY

Mechanism of Action: A penicillin that acts as a bactericidal in susceptible microorganisms. ***Therapeutic Effect:*** Inhibits bacterial cell wall synthesis. Bactericidal.

Pharmacokinetics

Poorly absorbed from gastrointestinal (GI) tract. Protein binding: 87%-90%. Metabolized in liver. Primarily excreted in urine. Not removed by hemodialysis. ***Half-life:*** 10.5-1 hr (half-life increased with impaired renal function, neonates).

INDICATIONS AND DOSAGES

Staphylococcal infections

IV

Adults, Elderly. 3-6 g/24 hr in divided doses.

Children. 25 mg/kg 2 times/day.

Neonates 7 days and older. 75 mg/kg/day in 4 divided doses.

Neonates less than 7 days old. 50 mg/kg/day in 2-3 divided doses.

Neonates less than 7 days old. 50 mg/kg/day in 2-3 divided doses.

IM

Adults, Elderly. 500 mg q4-6h.

Children. 25 mg/kg 2 times/day.

Neonates 7 days and older. 75 mg/kg/day in 4 divided doses.

Neonates 7 days and older. 75 mg/kg/day in 4 divided doses.

PO

Adults, Elderly. 250 mg-1 g q4-6h.

Children. 25-50 mg/kg/day in 4 divided doses.

AVAILABLE FORMS

• *Tablets:* 500 mg (Unipen).
• *Capsules:* 250 mg (Unipen).
• *Powder for Injection:* 1 g, 2 g, 10 g (Nafcil, Nallpen, Unipen).

UNLABELED USES: Surgical prophylaxis

CONTRAINDICATIONS: Hypersensitivity to any penicillin

PREGNANCY AND LACTATION: Pregnancy category B; excreted into breast milk

SIDE EFFECTS

Frequent

Mild hypersensitivity reaction (fever, rash, pruritus), GI effects (nausea, vomiting, diarrhea) more frequent w/oral administration

Occasional

Hypokalemia with high IV doses, phlebitis, thrombophlebitis (more common in elderly)

Rare
Extravasation with IV administration

SERIOUS REACTIONS

• Superinfections, potentially fatal antibiotic-associated colitis may result from altered bacterial balance.
• Hematologic effects (especially involving platelets, WBCs), severe hypersensitivity reactions, and anaphylaxis occur rarely.

INTERACTIONS

Drugs

3 *Chloramphenicol:* Inhibited antibacterial activity of nafcillin; administer nafcillin 3 hr before chloramphenicol
3 *Cyclosporine:* Reduced serum cyclosporine concentrations
3 *Macrolide antibiotics:* Inhibited antibacterial activity of nafcillin; administer nafcillin 3 hr before macrolides
3 *Methotrexate:* Increased serum methotrexate concentrations
2 *Nifedipine:* Results in a large reduction in the plasma concentration of nifedipine; loss of efficacy is likely to result
3 *Oral contraceptives:* Occasional impairment of oral contraceptive efficacy; consider use of supplemental contraception during cycles in which nafcillin is used
3 *Tacrolimus:* Reduced serum tacrolimus concentrations
3 *Tetracyclines:* Inhibited antibacterial activity of nafcillin; administer nafcillin 3 hr before tetracyclines
3 *Warfarin:* May inhibit hypoprothrombinemic response to warfarin

Labs

• *Increase:* Serum protein

SPECIAL CONSIDERATIONS

PATIENT/FAMILY EDUCATION

• Take for the full length of treatment
• Notify the physician if diarrhea, rash, or other new symptoms occur

MONITORING PARAMETERS

• Oral nafcillin absorption is erratic (consider alternate oral penicillinase-resistant penicillins)
• CBC, creatinine and UA for eosinophils during therapy to monitor for adverse effects
• Be alert for superinfection such as increased fever, onset sore throat, vomiting, diarrhea, ulceration/changes of oral mucosa, and anal/genital pruritus

---

naftifine hydrochloride

(naf'-ti-feen hye-droe-klor'-ide)
Rx: Naftin
Chemical Class: Allylamine derivative
Therapeutic Class: Antifungal

N

CLINICAL PHARMACOLOGY

Mechanism of Action: An antifungal that selectively inhibits the enzyme squalene epoxidase in a dose-dependent manner, which results in the primary sterol, ergosterol, within the fungal membrane not being synthesized. ***Therapeutic Effect:*** Results in fungal cell death. Fungistatic and fungicidal.

Pharmacokinetics

Minimal systemic absorption. Metabolized in the liver. Excreted in the urine as well as the feces and bile. ***Half-life:*** 48-72 hrs.

INDICATIONS AND DOSAGES

Tinea pedis, t. cruris, t. corporis

Topical
Adults, Elderly, Children 12 yrs and older. Apply cream 1 time a day for 4 wks or until signs and symptoms significantly improve. Apply gel 2

times a day for 4 wks or until signs and symptoms significantly improve.

AVAILABLE FORMS

- *Gel:* 1% (Naftin).
- *Cream:* 1% (Naftin).

UNLABELED USES: Trichomycosis

CONTRAINDICATIONS: Hypersensitivity to naftifine or any of its components

PREGNANCY AND LACTATION: Pregnancy category B; excretion into breast milk unknown

SIDE EFFECTS

Frequent

Burning, stinging

Occasional

Erythema, itching, dryness, irritation

SERIOUS REACTIONS

- Excessive irritation may indicate hypersensitivity reaction.

SPECIAL CONSIDERATIONS

- First of a new class of antifungals (allylamine derivatives) unrelated to imidazoles
- Because of fungicidal activity at low concentrations may provide quicker onset of healing, enhance patient compliance with qd therapy

PATIENT/FAMILY EDUCATION

- Wash hands after application
- Do not use occlusive dressings unless directed to do so

MONITORING PARAMETERS

- Skin for signs of therapeutic response

nalbuphine hydrochloride

(nal'-byoo-feen)

Rx: Nubain

Chemical Class: Opiate derivative; phenanthrene derivative

Therapeutic Class: Narcotic agonist-antagonist analgesic

CLINICAL PHARMACOLOGY

Mechanism of Action: A narcotic agonist-antagonist that binds with opioid receptors in the CNS. May displace opioid agonists and competitively inhibit their action; may precipitate withdrawal symptoms. ***Therapeutic Effect:*** Alters the perception of and emotional response to pain.

Pharmacokinetics

Route	*Onset*	*Peak*	*Duration*
IV	2-3 mins	30 mins	3-6 hrs
IM	less than 15 mins	60 mins	3-6 hrs
Subcutaneous	less than 15 mins	N/A	3-6 hrs

Well absorbed after IM or subcutaneous administration. Protein binding: 50%. Metabolized in the liver. Primarily eliminated in feces by biliary secretion. ***Half-life:*** 3.5-5 hrs.

INDICATIONS AND DOSAGES

Analgesia

IV, IM, Subcutaneous

Adults, Elderly. 10 mg q3-6h as needed. Do not exceed maximum single dose of 20 mg or daily dose of 160 mg. For patients receiving long-term narcotic analgesics of similar duration of action, give 25% of usual dose.

Children. 0.1-0.15 mg/kg q3-6h as needed.

Supplement to anesthesia

IV

Adults, Elderly. Induction: 0.3-3 mg/kg over 10-15 min. Maintenance: 0.25-0.5 mg/kg as needed.

AVAILABLE FORMS

• *Injection:* 10 mg/ml, 20 mg/ml.

CONTRAINDICATIONS: Respiratory rate less than 12 breaths/minute

PREGNANCY AND LACTATION: Pregnancy category B (D if used for prolonged periods or at high dosages at term)

SIDE EFFECTS

Frequent (35%)

Sedation

Occasional (9%-3%)

Diaphoresis, cold and clammy skin, nausea, vomiting, dizziness, vertigo, dry mouth, headache

Rare (less than 1%)

Restlessness, emotional lability, paresthesia, flushing, paradoxical reaction

SERIOUS REACTIONS

• Abrupt withdrawal after prolonged use may produce symptoms of narcotic withdrawal, such as abdominal cramping, rhinorrhea, lacrimation, anxiety, fever, and piloerection (goose bumps).

• Overdose results in severe respiratory depression, skeletal muscle flaccidity, cyanosis, and extreme somnolence progressing to seizures, stupor, and coma.

• Repeated use may result in drug tolerance and physical dependence.

INTERACTIONS

Drugs

3 *Alcohol, other CNS depressants:* May increase CNS or respiratory depression and hypotension

3 *Barbiturates:* Additive respiratory and CNS depression

3 *Buprenorphine:* May decrease the effects of nalbuphine

3 *Cimetidine:* Inhibition of narcotic hepatic metabolism; additive CNS effects

3 *MAOIs:* May produce a severe, possibly fatal reaction; plan to administer 25% of the usual nalbuphine dose

3 *Rifampin:* May reduce narcotic concentrations and precipitate withdrawal

Labs

• *Increase:* Amylase

SPECIAL CONSIDERATIONS

• Proposed, but not significant, advantages include low abuse potential, low respiratory depressant effects, low incidence of psychomimetic toxicity, and a lower incidence of hemodynamic toxicity

PATIENT/FAMILY EDUCATION

• The patient should alert the physician as soon as pain occurs and should not wait until the pain is unbearable because nalbuphine is more effective when given at the onset of pain

• Nalbuphine may be habit-forming

• Avoid alcohol and CNS depressants

• Avoid tasks that require mental alertness or motor skills until response to the drug has been established

• Nalbuphine may cause dry mouth

MONITORING PARAMETERS

• Blood pressure, pulse rate, respiratory rate

• Pattern of daily bowel activity and stool consistency

• Clinical improvement, record the onset of relief of pain

nalmefene hydrochloride

(nal'-me-feen hye-droe-klor'-ide)

Rx: Revex

Chemical Class: Thebaine derivative

Therapeutic Class: Antidote, opiate

CLINICAL PHARMACOLOGY

Mechanism of Action: A narcotic antagonist that binds to opioid receptors. ***Therapeutic Effect:*** Prevents and reverses effects of opioids (respiratory depression, sedation, hypotension).

Pharmacokinetics

Well absorbed. Protein binding: 45%. Metabolized primarily via glucuronidation. Excreted in urine and feces. ***Half-life:*** 8.5-10.8 hrs.

INDICATIONS AND DOSAGES

Solution for Injection: 100 mcg/ml ([blue label] Revex), 1000 mcg/ml ([green label] Revex)

IV/IM/Subcutaneous

Adults. Initially, 0.25 mcg/kg followed by additional 0.25-mcg doses at 2-5-min intervals until desired response. Cumulative doses >1 mcg/kg do not provide additional therapeutic effect.

Known or suspected opioid overdose

IV/IM/Subcutaneous

Adults. Initially, 0.5 mg/70 kg. May give 1 mg/70 kg in 2-5 min. If physical opioid dependence suspected, initial dose is 0.1 mg/70 kg.

AVAILABLE FORMS

- *Solution for Injection:* 100 mcg/ml ([blue label] Revex), 1000 mcg/ml ([green label] Revex)

CONTRAINDICATIONS: Hypersensitivity to nalmefene

PREGNANCY AND LACTATION: Pregnancy category B; excretion into breast milk unknown; use caution in nursing mothers

SIDE EFFECTS

Frequent

Nausea, headache, hypertension

Occasional

Postop pain, fever, dizziness, headache, chills, hypotension, vasodilation

SERIOUS REACTIONS

- Signs and symptoms of opioid withdrawal include stuffy or runny nose, tearing, yawning, sweating, tremor, vomiting, piloerection, feeling of temperature change, joint, bone or muscle pain, abdominal cramps, and feeling of skin crawling.

SPECIAL CONSIDERATIONS

- Longer duration of action than naloxone at fully reversing doses; agent of choice in instances where prolonged opioid effects are predicted, including overdose with longer-acting opioids (e.g., methadone, propoxyphene), patients given large doses of opioids, and those with liver disease or renal failure (eliminating the need for continuous infusions of naloxone and prolonged observation periods after outpatient procedures)

PATIENT/FAMILY EDUCATION

- Notify the physician of abdominal pain, dark-colored urine, white bowel movements, or yellow of the whites of the eyes

MONITORING PARAMETERS

- Observe patient until there is no reasonable risk of recurrent respiratory depression

naloxone hydrochloride

(nal-oks'-one hye-droe-klor'-ide)

Rx: Narcan

Combinations

Rx: with pentazocine (Talwin NX); with buprenorphine (Suboxone)

Chemical Class: Thebaine derivative

Therapeutic Class: Antidote, opiate

CLINICAL PHARMACOLOGY

Mechanism of Action: A narcotic antagonist that displaces opioids at opioid-occupied receptor sites in the CNS. ***Therapeutic Effect:*** Reverses opioid-induced sleep or sedation, increases respiratory rate, raises BP to normal range.

Pharmacokinetics

Route	Onset	Peak	Duration
IV	1-2 mins	N/A	20-60 mins
IM	2-5 mins	N/A	20-60 mins
Subcutaneous	2-5 mins	N/A	20-60 mins

Well absorbed after IM or subcutaneous administration. Metabolized in the liver. Primarily excreted in urine. ***Half-life:*** 60-100 mins.

INDICATIONS AND DOSAGES

Opioid toxicity

IV, IM, Subcutaneous

Adults, Elderly. 0.4-2 mg q2-3min as needed. May repeat q20-60min.

Children 5 yrs and older and weighing 20 kg and more. 2 mg/dose; if no response, may repeat q2-3min. May need to repeat dose q20-60min.

Children younger than 5 yrs and weighing less than 20 kg. 0.1 mg/kg; if no response, repeat q2-3min. May need to repeat dose q20-60min.

Postanesthesia narcotic reversal

IV

Children. 0.01 mg/kg; may repeat q2-3min.

Neonatal opioid-induced depression

IV

Neonates. May repeat q2-3min as needed. May need to repeat dose q1-2h.

AVAILABLE FORMS

- *Injection:* 0.02 mg/ml, 0.4 mg/ml, 1 mg/ml.

UNLABELED USES: Treatment of ethanol ingestion, *Pneumocystitis carinii* pneumonia (PCP)

CONTRAINDICATIONS: Respiratory depression due to nonopioid drugs

PREGNANCY AND LACTATION: Pregnancy category B; excretion into breast milk unknown, use caution in nursing mothers

SIDE EFFECTS

None known; little or no pharmacologic effect in absence of narcotics.

SERIOUS REACTIONS

- Too-rapid reversal of narcotic-induced respiratory depression may result in nausea, vomiting, tremors, increased BP, and tachycardia.
- Excessive dosage in postoperative patients may produce significant excitement, tremors, and reversal of analgesia.
- Patients with cardiovascular disease may experience hypotension or hypertension, ventricular tachycardia and fibrillation, and pulmonary edema.

INTERACTIONS

Drugs

3 *Butorphanol, nalbuphine, opioid agonist analgesics, pentazocine:* Reverses the analgesic and adverse effects of these drugs and may precipitate withdrawal symptoms

SPECIAL CONSIDERATIONS
• Duration of action of some narcotics may exceed that of naloxone; repeat doses prn

PATIENT/FAMILY EDUCATION
• Notify the physician if pain or increased sedation occurs

MONITORING PARAMETERS
• ECG, blood pressure, respiratory rate, mental status, pupil dilation
• Continue to monitor the patient even after a satisfactory response has been achieved. If the duration of action of the opioid exceeds that of naloxone, respiratory depression may recur

naltrexone hydrochloride

(nal-trex'-one)

Rx: ReVia

Chemical Class: Thebaine derivative

Therapeutic Class: Alcohol deterrent; antidote, opiate

CLINICAL PHARMACOLOGY

Mechanism of Action: A narcotic antagonist that displaces opioids at opioid-occupied receptor sites in the CNS. ***Therapeutic Effect:*** Blocks physical effects of opioid analgesics; decreases craving for alcohol and relapse rate in alcoholism.

Pharmacokinetics

Well absorbed following oral administration. Metabolized in liver; undergoes first pass metabolism. Excreted primarily in urine; partial elimination in feces. ***Half-life:*** 4 hr.

INDICATIONS AND DOSAGES

Naloxone challenge test to determine if patient is opioid dependent

IV

Alert: Expect to perform the naloxone challenge test if there is any question that the patient is opioid dependent. Do not administer naltrexone until the naloxone challenge test is negative.

Adults, Elderly. Draw 2 ml (0.8 mg) of naloxone into syringe. Inject 0.5 ml (0.2 mg); while needle is still in vein, observe patient for 30 sec for withdrawal signs or symptoms. If no evidence of withdrawal, inject remaining 1.5 ml (0.6 mg); observe patient for additional 20 min for withdrawal signs or symptoms.

Subcutaneous

Adults, Elderly. Inject 2 ml (0.8 mg) of naloxone; observe patient for 45 min for withdrawal signs or symptoms.

Treatment of opioid dependence in patients who have been opioid free for at least 7-10 days

PO

Adults, Elderly. Initially, 25 mg. Observe patient for 1 hr. If no withdrawal signs or symptoms appear, give another 25 mg. May be given as 100 mg every other day or 150 mg every 3 days.

Adjunctive treatment of alcohol dependence

PO

Adults, Elderly. 50 mg once a day.

AVAILABLE FORMS
• *Tablets:* 50 mg.

UNLABELED USES: Treatment of eating disorders, post-concussional syndrome unresponsive to other treatments

CONTRAINDICATIONS: Acute hepatitis, acute opioid withdrawal, failed naloxone challenge test, hepatic failure, history of hypersensitivity to naltrexone, opioid dependence, positive urine screen for opioids

PREGNANCY AND LACTATION: Pregnancy category C

SIDE EFFECTS

Frequent

Alcoholism (10%-7%): Nausea, headache, depression

Narcotic addiction (10%-5%): Insomnia, anxiety, nervousness, headache, low energy, abdominal cramps, nausea, vomiting, arthralgia, myalgia

Occasional

Alcoholism (4%-2%): Dizziness, nervousness, fatigue, insomnia, vomiting, anxiety, suicidal ideation

Narcotic addiction (5%-2%): Irritability, increased energy, dizziness, anorexia, diarrhea or constipation, rash, chills, increased thirst

SERIOUS REACTIONS

- Signs and symptoms of opioid withdrawal include stuffy or runny nose, tearing, yawning, diaphoresis, tremor, vomiting, piloerection, feeling of temperature change, bone pain, arthralgia, myalgia, abdominal cramps, and feeling of skin crawling.
- Accidental naltrexone overdose produces withdrawal symptoms within 5 mins of ingestion that may last for up to 48 hrs. Symptoms include confusion, visual hallucinations, somnolence, and significant vomiting and diarrhea.
- Hepatocellular injury may occur with large doses.

INTERACTIONS

Drugs

3 *Opioid-containing products (including analgesics, antidiarrheals, and antitussives):* Blocks the therapeutic effects of these drugs

3 *Thioridazine:* May produce lethargy and somnolence

SPECIAL CONSIDERATIONS

PATIENT/FAMILY EDUCATION

- Wear ID tag indicating naltrexone use
- Do not try to overcome reversal of opiate effects by self-administration of large doses of narcotic
- Do not exceed recommended dose
- Take naltrexone tablets with antacids, after meals, or with food to avoid GI upset
- Notify the physician if abdominal pain that lasts longer than 3 days, dark urine, white stools, or yellowing of the whites of the eyes occurs

MONITORING PARAMETERS

- Liver function tests
- Creatinine clearance

nandrolone decanoate

(nan'-droe-lone)

Rx: Deca-Durabolin, Durabolin

Chemical Class: Anabolic steroid; testosterone derivative

Therapeutic Class: Androgen; antineoplastic

DEA Class: Schedule III

CLINICAL PHARMACOLOGY

Mechanism of Action: An anabolic steroid that promotes tissue-building processes, increases production of erythropoietin, causes protein anabolism, and increases hemoglobin and red blood cell volume. ***Therapeutic Effect:*** Controls metastatic breast cancer and helps manage anemia of renal insufficiency.

Pharmacokinetics

Well absorbed after IM administration (about 77%). Metabolized in liver. Primarily excreted in urine. ***Half-life:*** 6-8 days.

INDICATIONS AND DOSAGES

Breast cancer

IM

Adults, Elderly. 50-100 mg/week.

Anemia of renal insufficiency
IM
Adults, Elderly (male). 100-200 mg/week.
Adults, Elderly (female). 50-100 mg/week.
Children, 2-13 yr. 25-50 mg every 3-4 wks.

AVAILABLE FORMS
- *Injection, as decanoate (in sesame oil):* 100 mg/ml, 200 mg/ml (Deca-Durabolin).

UNLABELED USES: Hyperlipidemia, lung cancer, male contraception, malnutrition, postmenopausal osteoporosis, rheumatoid arthritis, Sjogren's syndrome, trauma/surgery

CONTRAINDICATIONS: Nephrosis, pregnancy, carcinoma of breast or prostate, not for use in infants, hypersensitivity to nandrolone or any component of the formulation such as sesame oil

PREGNANCY AND LACTATION: Pregnancy category X; use extreme caution in nursing mothers
Controlled Substance: Schedule III

SIDE EFFECTS
Frequent
Male, postpubertal: Gynecomastia, acne, bladder irritability, priapism
Male, prepubertal: Acne, virilism
Females: Virilism
Occasional
Male, postpubertal/prepubertal: Insomnia, chills, decreased libido, hepatic dysfunction, nausea, diarrhea, prostatic hyperplasia (elderly), iron-deficiency anemia, suppression of clotting factors
Male, prepubertal: Chills, insomnia, hyperpigmentation, diarrhea, nausea, iron deficiency anemia, suppression of clotting factors
Female: Chills, insomnia, hypercalcemia, nausea, diarrhea, iron deficiency anemia, suppression of clotting factors, hepatic dysfunction
Rare
Hepatic necrosis, heptocellular carcinoma

SERIOUS REACTIONS
- Peliosis hepatitis of liver, spleen replaced with blood-filled cysts, hepatic neoplasms and hepatocellular carcinoma have been associated with prolonged high-dosage, anaphylactic reactions.

INTERACTIONS
Drugs
3 *Antidiabetic agents:* Enhanced hypoglycemic effects
❷ *Cyclosporine:* Increased cyclosporine concentrations, potential for toxicity
3 *HMG CoA reductase inhibitors (lovastatin, pravastatin):* Myositis risk increased
❷ *Oral anticoagulants:* Enhanced hypoprothrombinemic response
3 *Tacrolimus:* Increased tacrolimus concentrations, potential for toxicity

SPECIAL CONSIDERATIONS
- Anabolic steroids have potential for abuse, especially in the athlete

PATIENT/FAMILY EDUCATION
- Do not take any other medications, including OTC drugs, without first consulting the physician
- Weigh oneself each day
- Notify the physician if acne, nausea, pedal edema, or vomiting occurs
- Female patients should report deepening of voice, hoarseness, and menstrual irregularities
- Male patients should report difficulty urinating, frequent erections, and gynecomastia

MONITORING PARAMETERS
- Women should be observed for signs of virilization
- Liver function tests, lipids, Hct
- Growth rate in children (X-rays for bone age q6mo)
- Blood pressure

- Intake and output
- Sleep patterns

naproxen/naproxen sodium

(na-prox'-en)

Rx: (naproxen) EC-Naprosyn, Naprelan, Naprelan 375, Naprelan 500

Rx: (naproxen sodium) Aflaxen, Aleve, Anaprox, Anaprox DS, Pamprin

Combinations

Rx: with lansoprazole (NapraPAC)

Chemical Class: Propionic acid derivative

Therapeutic Class: NSAID; antipyretic; nonnarcotic analgesic

CLINICAL PHARMACOLOGY

Mechanism of Action: An NSAID that produces analgesic and antiinflammatory effects by inhibiting prostaglandin synthesis. ***Therapeutic Effect:*** Reduces the inflammatory response and intensity of pain.

Pharmacokinetics

Route	Onset	Peak	Duration
PO (analgesic)	less than 1 hr	N/A	7 hrs or less
PO (antirheumatic)	less than 14 days	2-4 wks	N/A

Completely absorbed from the GI tract. Protein binding: 99%. Metabolized in the liver. Primarily excreted in urine. Not removed by hemodialysis. ***Half-life:*** 13 hr.

INDICATIONS AND DOSAGES

Rheumatoid arthritis, osteoarthritis, ankylosing spondylitis

PO

Adults, Elderly. 250-500 mg naproxen (275-550 mg naproxen sodium) twice a day or 250 mg naproxen (275 mg naproxen sodium) in morning and 500 mg naproxen (550 mg naproxen sodium) in evening. Naprelan: 750-1000 mg once a day.

Acute gouty arthritis

PO

Adults, Elderly. Initially, 750 mg naproxen (825 mg naproxen sodium), then 250 mg naproxen (275 mg naproxen sodium) q8h until attack subsides. Naprelan: Initially, 1000-1500 mg, then 1000 mg once a day until attack subsides.

Mild to moderate pain, dysmenorrhea, bursitis, tendinitis

PO

Adults, Elderly. Initially, 500 mg naproxen (550 mg naproxen sodium), then 250 mg naparoxen (275 mg naproxen sodium) q6-8h as needed. Maximum: 1.25 g/day naproxen (1.375 g/day naproxen sodium). Naprelan: 1000 mg once a day.

Juvenile rheumatoid arthritis

PO (naproxen only)

Children. 10-15 mg/kg/day in 2 divided doses. Maximum: 1000 mg/day.

OTC uses

PO

Adults 65 yrs and younger, Children 12 yrs and older. 220 mg (200 mg naproxen sodium) q8-12h. May take 440 mg (200 mg naproxen sodium) as initial dose.

Adults older than 65 yrs. 220 mg (200 mg naproxen sodium) q12h.

AVAILABLE FORMS

- *Gelcaps (Aleve):* 220 mg naproxen sodium (equivalent to 200 mg naproxen).
- *Oral Suspension (Naprosyn):* 125 mg/5 ml naproxen.
- *Tablets:* 220 mg naproxen (Aleve), 250 mg (Naprosyn), 275 mg naproxen sodium (equivalent to 250 mg naproxen) (Anaprox), 550 mg

naproxen sodium (equivalent to 500 mg naproxen) (Aflaxen, Anaprox DS).

• *Tablets (Controlled-Release):* 375 mg naproxen (EC-Naprosyn), 421 mg naproxen (Naprelan), 500 mg naproxen (EC-Naprosyn), 550 mg naproxen sodium (equivalent to 500 mg naproxen) (Naprelan).

UNLABELED USES: Treatment of vascular headaches

CONTRAINDICATIONS: Hypersensitivity to aspirin, naproxen, or other NSAIDs

PREGNANCY AND LACTATION: Pregnancy category B (category D if used in third trimester or near delivery); could cause constriction of the ductus arteriosus *in utero,* persistent pulmonary hypertension of the newborn, or prolonged labor; passes into breast milk in small quantities; compatible with breast-feeding

SIDE EFFECTS

Frequent (9%-4%)

Nausea, constipation, abdominal cramps or pain, heartburn, dizziness, headache, somnolence

Occasional (3%-1%)

Stomatitis, diarrhea, indigestion

Rare (less than 1%)

Vomiting, confusion

SERIOUS REACTIONS

• Rare reactions with long-term use include peptic ulcer disease, GI bleeding, gastritis, severe hepatic reactions (cholestasis, jaundice), nephrotoxicity (dysuria, hematuria, proteinuria, nephrotic syndrome), and a severe hypersensitivity reaction (fever, chills, bronchospasm).

INTERACTIONS

Drugs

3 *Aminoglycosides:* Reduced clearance with elevated aminoglycoside levels and potential for toxicity (especially indomethacin in premature infants; other NSAIDs probably)

3 *Anticoagulants:* Excessive hypoprothrombinemia, decreased platelet aggregation with increased risk of GI bleeding

3 *Antihypertensives (α-blockers, angiotensin-converting enzyme inhibitors, angiotensin II receptor blockers, β-blockers, diuretics):* Inhibition of antihypertensive and other favorable hemodynamic effects

3 *Aspirin, other salicylates:* May increase the risk of GI side effects such as bleeding

3 *Bone marrow depressants:* May increase the risk of GI side effects such as bleeding

3 *Corticosteroids:* Increased risk of GI ulceration

3 *Cyclosporine:* Increased nephrotoxicity risk

3 *Feverfew:* May decrease the effects of feverfew

3 *Ginkgo biloba:* May increase the risk of bleeding

3 *Lithium:* Decreased clearance of lithium (mediated via prostaglandins) resulting in elevated serum lithium levels and risk of toxicity

3 *Methotrexate:* Decreased renal secretion of methotrexate resulting in elevated methotrexate levels and risk of toxicity

3 *Phenylpropanolamine:* Possible acute hypertensive reaction

3 *Potassium-sparing diuretics:* Additive hyperkalemia potential

3 *Probenecid:* May increase naproxen blood concentration

3 *Triamterene:* Acute renal failure reported with addition of indomethacin; caution with other NSAIDs

Labs

• *False increase:* Serum bicarbonate, urine 5-HIAA

SPECIAL CONSIDERATIONS

• No significant advantage over other NSAIDs; cost should govern use

PATIENT/FAMILY EDUCATION

- Avoid concurrent use of aspirin and alcoholic beverages
- Take with food, milk, or antacids to decrease GI upset
- Notify clinician if edema, black stools, or persistent headache occur
- Avoid tasks that require mental alertness or motor skills until response to the drug has been established
- The female patient should inform the physician if she is or plans to become pregnant

MONITORING PARAMETERS

- Initial hemogram and fecal occult blood test within 3 mo of starting regular chronic therapy; repeat every 6-12 mo (more frequently in high-risk patients (>65 years, peptic ulcer disease, concurrent steroids or anticoagulants); electrolytes, creatinine, and BUN within 3 mo of starting regular chronic therapy; repeat every 6-12 mo
- CBC (particularly Hgb, Hct, and platelet count)
- Serum alkaline phosphatase, bilirubin, AST (SGOT), and ALT (SGPT) levels to assess hepatic and renal function
- Pattern of daily bowel activity and stool consistency
- Therapeutic response, such as improved grip strength, increased joint mobility, and decreased pain, tenderness, stiffness, and swelling

naratriptan hydrochloride

(nar-a-trip′-tan hye-droe-klor′-ide)

Rx: Amerge

Chemical Class: Serotonin derivative

Therapeutic Class: Antimigraine agent

CLINICAL PHARMACOLOGY

Mechanism of Action: A serotonin receptor agonist that binds selectively to vascular receptors producing a vasoconstrictive effect on cranial blood vessels. ***Therapeutic Effect:*** Relieves migraine headache.

Pharmacokinetics

Well absorbed after PO administration. Protein binding: 28%-31%. Metabolized by the liver to inactive metabolite. Eliminated primarily in urine and, to a lesser extent, in feces. ***Half-life:*** 6 hr (increased in hepatic or renal impairment).

INDICATIONS AND DOSAGES

Acute migraine attack

PO

Adults. 1 mg or 2.5 mg. If headache improves but then returns, dose may be repeated after 4 hr. Maximum: 5 mg/24 hr.

Dosage in mild to moderate hepatic or renal impairment

A lower starting dose is recommended. Do not exceed 2.5 mg/24 hr.

AVAILABLE FORMS

- *Tablets:* 1 mg, 2.5 mg.

CONTRAINDICATIONS: Basilar or hemiplegic migraine, cerebrovascular or peripheral vascular disease, coronary artery disease, ischemic heart disease (including angina pectoris, history of MI, silent ischemia, and Prinzmetal's angina), severe hepatic impairment (Child-Pugh grade C), severe renal impairment (serum creatinine less than 15 ml/min), uncontrolled hypertension, use within 24 hrs of ergotamine-containing preparations or another serotonin receptor agonist, use within 14 days of MAOIs

PREGNANCY AND LACTATION: Pregnancy category C; use caution in nursing mothers

SIDE EFFECTS

Occasional (5%)

Nausea

Rare (2%)

Paresthesia; dizziness; fatigue; somnolence; jaw, neck, or throat pressure

SERIOUS REACTIONS

- Corneal opacities and other ocular defects may occur.
- Cardiac reactions (including ischemia, coronary artery vasospasm, and MI) and noncardiac vasospasm-related reactions (such as hemorrhage and cerebrovascular accident [CVA]), occur rarely, particularly in patients with hypertension, diabetes, or a strong family history of coronary artery disease; obese patients; smokers; males older than 40 yrs; and postmenopausal women.

INTERACTIONS

Drugs

▲ *Ergotamine-containing drugs:* Increased vasoconstriction

3 *Fluoxetine, fluvoxamine, paroxetine, sertraline:* May produce hyperreflexia, incoordination, and weakness

▲ *MAO inhibitors:* Potential for decreased metabolism of naratriptan

❷ *Sibutramine:* Increased risk of serotonin syndrome

SPECIAL CONSIDERATIONS

- Longer acting than sumatriptan and zolmitriptan so recurrent headaches requiring a second dose less likely; slower onset than sumatriptan and zolmitriptan; should probably be reserved for patients who get recurrent headaches
- Safety of treating, on average, more than 4 headaches in a 30-day period has not been established

PATIENT/FAMILY EDUCATION

- Use only to treat migraine headache, not for prevention
- Swallow tablets whole with water; do not to crush or chew them
- Take another dose of naratriptan, if needed, 4 hrs after the first dose for a maximum of 5 mg/24 hrs
- May cause dizziness, drowsiness, and fatigue
- Avoid tasks that require mental alertness or motor skills until response to the drug has been established
- Notify the physician if anxiety, chest pain, palpitations, or tightness in the throat
- The female patient of childbearing age should use contraceptives during therapy and should notify the physician immediately if she suspects she is pregnant
- Lie down in dark, quiet room for additional benefit after taking naratriptan

MONITORING PARAMETERS

- Assess for relief of migraines and associated symptoms, including nausea and vomiting, photophobia, and phonophobia (sound sensitivity)

natamycin

(na-ta-mye'-sin)

Rx: Natacyn

Chemical Class: Tetraene polyene derivative

Therapeutic Class: Ophthalmic antifungal

CLINICAL PHARMACOLOGY

Mechanism of Action: A polyene antifungal agent that increases cell membrane permeability in susceptible fungi. ***Therapeutic Effect:*** Fungicidal.

Pharmacokinetics

Minimal systemic absorption. Adheres to cornea and retained in conjunctival fornices.

INDICATIONS AND DOSAGES

Fungal keratitis, ophthalmic fungal infections

Ophthalmic

Adults, Elderly. Instill 1 drop in conjunctival sac every 1-2 hrs. After 3-4 days, reduce to 1 drop 6-8 times daily. Usual course of therapy is 2-3 wks.

AVAILABLE FORMS

• *Ophthalmic Suspension:* 5% (Natacyn).

UNLABELED USES: Oral and vaginal candidiasis, onychomycosis, pulmonary aspergillosis

CONTRAINDICATIONS: Hypersensitivity to natamycin or any component of the formulation

PREGNANCY AND LACTATION: Pregnancy category C

SIDE EFFECTS

Occasional (10%-3%)

Blurred vision, eye irritation, eye pain, photophobia

SERIOUS REACTIONS

• Vomiting and diarrhea have occurred with large doses in the treatment of systemic mycoses.

SPECIAL CONSIDERATIONS

PATIENT/FAMILY EDUCATION

• Shake well before using
• Do not touch dropper to eye
• Notify the physician if the condition worsens or does not improve after 3-4 days

MONITORING PARAMETERS

• Failure of keratitis to improve following 7-10 days of administration suggests infection not susceptible to natamycin

nateglinide

(na-teg'-lin-ide)

Rx: Starlix

Chemical Class: Amino acid derivative; meglitinide

Therapeutic Class: Antidiabetic; hypoglycemic

CLINICAL PHARMACOLOGY

Mechanism of Action: An antihyperglycemic that stimulates release of insulin from beta cells of the pancreas by depolarizing beta cells, leading to an opening of calcium channels. Resulting calcium influx induces insulin secretion. ***Therapeutic Effect:*** Lowers blood glucose concentration.

Pharmacokinetics

Absolute bioavailability is approximately 73%. Protein binding: 98%. Extensive metabolism in liver. Primarily excreted in urine; minimal elimination in feces. ***Half-life:*** 1.5 hr.

INDICATIONS AND DOSAGES

Diabetes mellitus

PO

Adult, Elderly. 120 mg 3 times a day before meals. Initially, 60 mg may be given.

AVAILABLE FORMS

• *Tablets:* 60 mg, 120 mg.

CONTRAINDICATIONS: Diabetic ketoacidosis, type 1 diabetes mellitus

PREGNANCY AND LACTATION: Pregnancy category C (no adequate and well-controlled studies in pregnant women); excretion into human breast milk unknown

SIDE EFFECTS

Frequent (10%)

Upper respiratory tract infection

Occasional (4%-3%)

Back pain, flu symptoms, dizziness, arthropathy, diarrhea

Rare (3% or less)

Bronchitis, cough

SERIOUS REACTIONS

• Hypoglycemia occurs in less than 2% of patients.

INTERACTIONS

Drugs

3 *β-blockers:* Antagonistic glycemic effects, prolong hypoglycemia, mask hypoglycemia symptoms

3 *Corticosteroids, thiazide diuretics, thyroid medication, sympathomimetics:* May decrease hypoglycemic effect of nateglinide

3 *Diazoxide:* Antagonistic effects (diazoxide causes hyperglycemia)

3 *Epinephrine:* Antagonistic effects; combination may decrease hypoglycemic efficacy

3 *MAOIs:* MAOIs stimulate insulin secretion; additive effects; increased risk of hypoglycemia

3 *Hypoglycemics (bioguanides, insulin):* Combination increases risk of hypoglycemia

3 *Isoniazid:* Antagonistic effects; combination may decrease hypoglycemic efficacy

3 *Liquid meal:* Peak plasma levels may be significantly reduced if administered 10 mins before a liquid meal

3 *Niacin:* Antagonistic effects; combination may decrease hypoglycemic efficacy

3 *NSAIDs:* May increase hypoglycemic effect of nateglinide

Labs

• *Uric acid:* Increased

SPECIAL CONSIDERATIONS

• *Pharmacodynamics* (60-120 mg tid ac for 24 wks): HbA1c change −0.5%; fasting plasma glucose change −15 mg/dL; weight change −0.3-0.9 kg

PATIENT/FAMILY EDUCATION

• Review signs and symptoms and management of hypoglycemia

• Drug administration timing (i.e., before meals)

• The prescribed diet is a principal part of treatment

• Carry candy, sugar packets, or other sugar supplements for immediate response to hypoglycemia and wear medical alert identification stating that he or she has diabetes

• Consult the physician when glucose demands are altered, such as with fever, heavy physical activity, infection, stress, or trauma

MONITORING PARAMETERS

• Home/self blood glucose monitoring, HbA1c, signs and symptoms of hyper/hypoglycemia, complete blood count, routine blood chemistry

nedocromil sodium

(ne doe kroe' mil)

Rx: *Oral:* Tilade

Rx: *Ophth:* Alocril

Chemical Class: Mast cell stabilizer; pyranoquinoline dicarboxylic acid derivative

Therapeutic Class: Antiasthmatic; inhaled antiinflammatory

CLINICAL PHARMACOLOGY

Mechanism of Action: A mast cell stabilizer that prevents the activation and release of inflammatory mediators, such as histamine, leukotrienes, mast cells, eosinophils, and monocytes. ***Therapeutic Effect:*** Prevents both early and late asthmatic responses.

Pharmacokinetics

The extent of absorption is 7%-9% of a single inhaled dose of 3.5-4 mg and 17% of multiple inhaled doses, with absorption largely from the respiratory tract. Although most of the inhaled dose is subsequently swallowed, only 2%-3% is absorbed from the GI tract. Less than 4% of the total dose is systemically absorbed following multiple doses of ophthalmic solution. Protein binding: 89%. Not metabolized. Excreted in urine. ***Half-life:*** 1.5-3.3 hr.

INDICATIONS AND DOSAGES

Mild to moderate asthma

Oral Inhalation

Adults, Elderly, Children 6 yr and older. 2 inhalations 4 times a day. May decrease to 3 times a day, then twice a day as asthma becomes controlled.

Allergic conjunctivitis

Ophthalmic

Adults, Elderly, Children 3 yr and older. 1-2 drops in each eye twice a day.

AVAILABLE FORMS

- *Aerosol for Inhalation (Tilade):* 1.75 mg/activation.
- *Ophthalmic Solution (Alocril):* 2%.

UNLABELED USES: Prevention of bronchospasm in patients with reversible obstructive airway disease

CONTRAINDICATIONS: None known.

PREGNANCY AND LACTATION: Pregnancy category B; excretion into breast milk unknown

SIDE EFFECTS

Frequent (10%-6%)

Inhalation: Cough, pharyngitis, bronchospasm, headache, altered taste

Ophthalmic: Burning sensation in eye

Occasional (5%-1%)

Inhalation: Rhinitis, upper respiratory tract infection, abdominal pain, fatigue

Rare (less than 1%)

Inhalation: Diarrhea, dizziness

Ophthalmic: Conjunctivitis, light intolerance

SERIOUS REACTIONS

- None known.

SPECIAL CONSIDERATIONS

PATIENT/FAMILY EDUCATION

- Must be used regularly to achieve benefit, even during symptom-free periods
- Therapeutic effect may take up to 4 wk
- Not to be used to treat acute asthmatic symptoms
- Administer nedocromil at regular intervals, even when symptom-free, to achieve optimal results
- Rinse mouth with water immediately after inhalation to help relieve unpleasant taste
- Drink plenty of fluids to decrease the thickness of lung secretions

MONITORING PARAMETERS

- Therapeutic response, such as less frequent or severe asthmatic attacks or reduced dependence on antihistamines

nefazodone hydrochloride

(neh-faz'-oh-doan hye-droe-klor'-ide)

Rx: Serzone

Chemical Class: Phenylpiperazine derivative

Therapeutic Class: Antidepressant

CLINICAL PHARMACOLOGY

Mechanism of Action: Exact mechanism is unknown. Appears to inhibit neuronal uptake of serotonin and norepinephrine and to antagonize $alpha_1$-adrenergic receptors. ***Therapeutic Effect:*** Relieves depression.

Pharmacokinetics

Rapidly and completely absorbed from the GI tract; food delays absorption. Protein binding: 99%. Widely distributed in body tissues, including CNS. Extensively metabolized to active metabolites. Excreted in urine and eliminated in feces. Unknown if removed by hemodialysis. ***Half-life:*** 2-4 hr.

INDICATIONS AND DOSAGES

Depression, prevention of relapse of acute depressive episode

PO

Adults. Initially, 200 mg/day in 2 divided doses. Gradually increase by 100-200 mg/day at intervals of at least 1 wk. Range: 300-600 mg/day.

Elderly. Initially, 100 mg/day in 2 divided doses. Subsequent dosage titration based on clinical response. Range: 200-400 mg/day.

Children. 300-400 mg/day.

AVAILABLE FORMS

- *Tablets:* 50 mg, 100 mg, 150 mg, 200 mg, 250 mg.

CONTRAINDICATIONS: Coadministration of terfenadine, astemizole, cisapride, pimozide, or carbamazepine; hypersensitivity to other phenylpiperazine antidepressants; those who were withdrawn from nefazodone due to evidence of hepatic injury; use within 14 days of MAOIs

PREGNANCY AND LACTATION: Pregnancy category C; excretion into breast milk unknown; use caution in nursing mothers

SIDE EFFECTS

Frequent

Headache (36%); dry mouth, somnolence (25%); nausea (22%); dizziness (17%); constipation (14%); insomnia, asthenia, lightheadedness (10%).

Occasional

Dyspepsia, blurred vision (9%); diarrhea, infection (8%); confusion, abnormal vision (7%); pharyngitis (6%); increased appetite (5%); orthostatic hypotension, flushing, feeling of warmth (4%); peripheral edema, cough, flu-like symptoms (3%).

SERIOUS REACTIONS

Alert: Cases of life-threatening hepatic failures have been reported.

- Serious reactions, such as hyperthermia, rigidity, myoclonus, extreme agitation, delirium, and coma, will occur if the patient takes an MAOI concurrently or fails to let enough time elapse when switching from an MAOI to nefazodone or vice versa.

INTERACTIONS

Drugs

❷ *Alprazolam:* Significant increase in serum alprazolam concentrations; if coadministered reduce alprazolam dose by 50%

3 *Atorvastatin, lovastatin, simvastatin:* Potential for development of myositis with rhabdomyolysis
3 *Buspirone:* Significant increase in serum buspirone concentrations
❷ *Carbamazepine:* 95% decrease in serum nefazodone concentrations; concomitant use contraindicated
⚠ *Cisapride, pimozide:* Theoretical potential for QT prolongation and dysrhythmia; concomitant use contraindicated
3 *Cyclosporine, tacrolimus:* Toxic blood levels of immunosuppressives have been reported; monitor levels and adjust immunosuppressive dosage as needed
3 *Digoxin:* Increased serum digoxin concentrations
❷ *Triazolam:* Significant increase in serum triazolam concentrations; if coadministered reduce triazolam dose by 75%
❷ *MAOIs:* Serious adverse reactions possible including hyperthermia, rigidity, myoclonus, autonomic instability, mental status changes, seizures; observe a 14-day washout period between discontinuing one drug and starting the other
3 *Paroxetine:* Increased risk of developing serotonin syndrome
3 *St. John's Wort:* May increase the risk of adverse effects

SPECIAL CONSIDERATIONS

- Priapism has been reported; educate and monitor appropriately

PATIENT/FAMILY EDUCATION

- Therapeutic effect may not be apparent for several weeks
- Drug may cause drowsiness, use caution driving or performing other tasks where alertness is required
- Notify the physician if headache, nausea, or visual disturbances occurs
- Avoid tasks that require mental alertness or motor skills until response to the drug has been established
- Avoid alcohol while taking nefazodone
- Take sips of tepid water or chew sugarless gum to help relieve dry mouth

MONITORING PARAMETERS

- Blood pressure and pulse rate
- Pattern of daily bowel activity and stool consistency
- Assess appearance, behavior, level of interest, mood, and sleep pattern before and during therapy

nelfinavir mesylate

(nel-fin'-a-veer mes'-sil-ate)

Rx: Viracept
Chemical Class: Protease inhibitor, HIV
Therapeutic Class: Antiretroviral

CLINICAL PHARMACOLOGY

Mechanism of Action: Inhibits the activity of HIV-1 protease, the enzyme necessary for the formation of infectious HIV. ***Therapeutic Effect:*** Formation of immature noninfectious viral particles rather than HIV replication.

Pharmacokinetics

Well absorbed after PO administration (absorption increased with food). Protein binding: 98%. Metabolized in the liver. Highly bound to plasma proteins. Eliminated primarily in feces. Unknown if removed by hemodialysis. ***Half-life:*** 3.5-5 hr.

INDICATIONS AND DOSAGES

HIV infection

PO

Adults. 750 mg (three 250-mg tablets) 3 times a day or 1250 mg twice

a day in combination with nucleoside analogs (enhances antiviral activity).
Children 2-13 yr. 45-55 mg/kg twice a day or 25-30 mg/kg 3 times a day. Maximum: 2500 mg/day.

AVAILABLE FORMS

- *Powder for Oral Suspension:* 50 mg/g.
- *Tablets:* 250 mg, 625 mg.

UNLABELED USES: HIV, postexposure prophylaxis

CONTRAINDICATIONS: Concurrent administration with midazolam, rifampin, or triazolam

PREGNANCY AND LACTATION: Pregnancy category B; excreted in breast milk; breast-feeding not recommended for HIV-infected women

SIDE EFFECTS

Frequent (20%)
Diarrhea
Occasional (7%-3%)
Nausea, rash
Rare (2%-1%)
Flatulence, asthenia

SERIOUS REACTIONS

- Diabetes mellitus and hyperglycemia occur rarely.

INTERACTIONS

Drugs

3 *Barbiturates:* Increased clearance of nelfinavir; reduced clearance of barbiturates
2 *Carbamazepine:* Increased clearance of nelfinavir; reduced clearance of carbamazepine
⚠ *Cisapride:* Increased plasma levels of cisapride
⚠ *Ergot alkaloids:* Increased plasma levels of ergot alkaloids
3 *Erythromycin:* Reduced clearance of nelfinavir; nelfinavir reduces clearance of erythromycin
⚠ *Lovastatin:* Nelfinavir reduces clearance of lovastatin
3 *Methadone:* Reduces methadone concentrations
⚠ *Midazolam:* Increased plasma levels of midazolam and prolonged effect
3 *Nevirapine:* Reduces plasma nelfinavir levels; increase nelfinavir dose to 1000 mg tid
3 *Oral contraceptives:* Nelfinavir may reduce efficacy
3 *Phenytoin:* Increased clearance of nelfinavir; reduced clearance of phenytoin
2 *Rifabutin:* Increased clearance of nelfinavir; reduced clearance of rifabutin—reduce rifabutin dose to 150 mg qd and increase nelfinavir dose to 1000 mg tid
⚠ *Rifampin:* Increased clearance of nelfinavir
3 *Ritonavir:* Decreased clearance of nelfinavir; decrease nelfinavir dose to 750 mg bid
3 *Saquinavir:* Decreased clearance of saquinavir; reduce dose of Fortovase (saquinavir soft gel capsule) to 800 mg tid
3 *Sildenafil:* Increases sildenafil plasma concentrations
⚠ *Simvastatin:* Nelfinavir reduces clearance of simvastatin
⚠ *Triazolam:* Increased plasma levels of triazolam and prolonged effect

SPECIAL CONSIDERATIONS

- Positive results of treatment are based on surrogate markers only
- Take with meal or snack

PATIENT/FAMILY EDUCATION

- Contains phenylalanine, take with food
- Space drug doses evenly around the clock and take the drug every day as prescribed
- Do not alter the dose or discontinue the drug without first notifying the physician
- Nelfinavir is not a cure for HIV infection, nor does it reduce the risk of transmitting HIV to others; the pa-

tient may continue to experience illnesses associated with advanced HIV infection, including opportunistic infections

MONITORING PARAMETERS

- CBC, electrolytes, renal function, liver enzymes, CPK
- Pattern of daily bowel activity and stool consistency
- Signs and symptoms of opportunistic infections, such as chills, cough, fever, and myalgia

neomycin sulfate

(nee-oh-mye'-sin)

Rx: Myciguent, Neo-Fradin, Neo-Rx, Neo-Tab

Combinations

Rx: with polymyxin B (Neosporin G.U. irrigant)

OTC: with polymyxin B, bacitracin (Neosporin, Mycitracin)

Chemical Class: Aminoglycoside

Therapeutic Class: Antibiotic

CLINICAL PHARMACOLOGY

Mechanism of Action: An aminoglycoside antibiotic that binds to bacterial microorganisms. ***Therapeutic Effect:*** Interferes with bacterial protein synthesis.

Pharmacokinetics

Poorly absorbed from the GI tract following PO administration. Protein binding: low. Primarily eliminated unchanged in the feces; minimal excretion in urine. Removed by hemodialysis. ***Half-life:*** 3 hr.

INDICATIONS AND DOSAGES

Preoperative bowel antisepsis

PO

Adults, Elderly. 1 g/hr for 4 doses; then 1 g q4h for 5 doses or 1 g at 1 p.m., 2 p.m., and 10 p.m. (with erythromycin) on day before surgery.

Children. 90 mg/kg/day in divided doses q4h for 2 days or 25 mg/kg at 1 p.m., 2 p.m., and 10 p.m. on day before surgery.

Hepatic encephalopathy

PO

Adults, Elderly. 4-12 g/day in divided doses q4-6h.

Children. 2.5-7 g/m^2/day in divided doses q4-6h.

Diarrhea caused by *Escherichia coli*

PO

Adults, Elderly. 3 g/day in divided doses q6h.

Children. 50 mg/kg/day in divided doses q6h.

Minor skin infections

Topical

Adults, Elderly, Children. Usual dosage, apply to affected area 1-3 times a day.

AVAILABLE FORMS

- *Tablets (Neo-Tab):* 500 mg.
- *Ointment (Myciguent):* 0.5%.
- *Cream (Myciguent):* 0.5%.
- *Oral Solution (Neo-Fradin):* 125 mg/5 ml.
- *Powder for Compounding (Neo-Rx):* 100%.

CONTRAINDICATIONS: Hypersensitivity to neomycin, other aminoglycosides (cross-sensitivity), or their components

PREGNANCY AND LACTATION: Pregnancy category D; ototoxicity has not been reported as an effect of *in utero* exposure; eighth cranial nerve toxicity in the fetus is well known following exposure to other aminoglycosides and could potentially occur with neomycin

SIDE EFFECTS

Frequent

Systemic: Nausea, vomiting, diarrhea, irritation of mouth or rectal area

Topical: Itching, redness, swelling, rash

Rare

Systemic: Malabsorption syndrome, neuromuscular blockade (difficulty breathing, drowsiness, weakness)

SERIOUS REACTIONS

- Nephrotoxicity (as evidenced by increased BUN and serum creatinine levels and decreased creatinine clearance) may be reversible if the drug is stopped at the first sign of nephrotoxic symptoms.
- Irreversible ototoxicity (manifested as tinnitus, dizziness, and impaired hearing) and neurotoxicity (as evidenced by headache, dizziness, lethargy, tremor, and visual disturbances) occur occasionally.
- Severe respiratory depression and anaphylaxis occur rarely.
- Superinfections, particularly fungal infections, may occur.

INTERACTIONS

Drugs

3 *Digitalis glycosides:* Reduced serum digoxin concentration

❷ *Ethacrynic acid:* Increased risk of ototoxicity, especially in patients with renal impairment

3 *Oral anticoagulants:* Enhanced hypoprothrombinemic response; more common with large doses of neomycin, dietary vitamin K deficiency, impaired hepatic function

▲ *Methotrexate:* Oral absorption of methotrexate reduced 30%-50%

3 *Penicillin V:* Reduced concentrations of penicillin V, possible reduced efficacy

3 *Warfarin:* Enhanced hypoprothrombinemic response

SPECIAL CONSIDERATIONS

- Inform patient and family about possible toxic effects on the eighth cranial nerve; monitor for loss of hearing, ringing or roaring in ears, or a feeling of fullness in head

PATIENT/FAMILY EDUCATION

- Drink plenty of fluids
- Continue taking neomycin for the full course of treatment and space doses evenly around the clock
- Notify the physician if dizziness, impaired hearing, or ringing in the ears occurs
- The patient using topical neomycin should clean the affected area gently before applying the drug and should notify the physician if itching or redness occurs

MONITORING PARAMETERS

- Renal function, audiometric testing during extended therapy or with application to extensive burns or large surface area
- Evaluate the patient for signs and symptoms of a hypersensitivity reaction. With topical application, symptoms may include a rash, redness, or itching
- Watch the patient for signs and symptoms of superinfection, particularly diarrhea, genital or anal pruritus, and stomatitis

---

neostigmine bromide

(nee-oh-stig′-meen)

Rx: Prostigmin, Prostigmin Bromide

Chemical Class: Cholinesterase inhibitor; quaternary ammonium derivative

Therapeutic Class: Cholinergic

CLINICAL PHARMACOLOGY

Mechanism of Action: A cholinergic that prevents destruction of acetylcholine by inhibiting the enzyme acetylcholinesterase, thus enhancing impulse transmission across the myoneural junction. ***Therapeutic Effect:*** Improves intestinal and skeletal muscle tone; stimulates salivary and sweat gland secretions.

Pharmacokinetics

Poorly absorbed from the GI tract following oral administration. Partially eliminated in urine. ***Half-life:*** 52 min.

INDICATIONS AND DOSAGES

Myasthenia gravis

PO

Adults, Elderly. Initially, 15-30 mg 3-4 times a day. Increase as necessary. Maintenance: 150 mg/day (range of 15-375 mg).

Children. 2 mg/kg/day or 60 mg/m^2/day divided q3-4h.

IV, IM, Subcutaneous

Adults. 0.5-2.5 mg as needed.

Children. 0.01-0.04 mg/kg q2-4h.

Diagnosis of myasthenia gravis

IM

Adults, Elderly. 0.022 mg/kg. If cholinergic reaction occurs, discontinue tests and administer 0.4-0.6 mg or more atropine sulfate IV.

Children. 0.025-0.04 mg/kg preceded by atropine sulfate 0.011 mg/kg subcutaneously.

Prevention of postoperative urinary retention

IM, Subcutaneous

Adults, Elderly. 0.25 mg q4-6h for 2-3 days.

Postoperative abdomonial distention and urine retention

IM, Subcutaneous

Adults, Elderly. 0.5-1 mg. Catheterize patient if voiding does not occur within 1 hr. After voiding, administer 0.5 mg q3h for 5 injections.

Reversal of neuromuscular blockade

IV

Adults, Elderly. 0.5-2.5 mg given slowly.

Children. 0.025-0.08 mg/kg/dose.

Infants. 0.025-0.1 mg/kg/dose.

AVAILABLE FORMS

- *Tablets (Prostigmin Bromide):* 15 mg.
- *Injection (Prostigmin):* 0.25 mg/ml, 0.5 mg/ml, 1 mg/ml.

CONTRAINDICATIONS: GI or GU obstruction, history of hypersensitivity reaction to bromides, peritonitis

PREGNANCY AND LACTATION: Pregnancy category C; transient muscle weakness occurred in 20% of infants born to mothers using neostigmine and similar drugs; ionized at physiologic pH, would not be expected to be excreted in breast milk

SIDE EFFECTS

Frequent

Muscarinic effects (diarrhea, diaphoresis, increased salivation, nausea, vomiting, abdominal cramps or pain)

Occasional

Muscarinic effects (urinary urgency or frequency, increased bronchial secretions, miosis, lacrimation)

SERIOUS REACTIONS

- Overdose produces a cholinergic crisis manifested as abdominal discomfort or cramps, nausea, vomiting, diarrhea, flushing, facial warmth, excessive salivation, diaphoresis, lacrimation, pallor, bradycardia or tachycardia, hypotension, bronchospasm, urinary urgency, blurred vision, miosis, and fasciculation (involuntary muscular contractions visible under the skin).

INTERACTIONS

Drugs

3 *Anticholinergics:* Reverse or prevent the effects of neostigmine

3 *Cholinesterase inhibitors:* May increase the risk of toxicity

3 *Neuromuscular blockers:* Antagonizes the effects of these drugs

3 *Procainamide, quinidine:* May antagonize the action of neostigmine

3 *Propranolol:* May slow heart rate

3 *Tacrine:* Increased cholinergic effects

SPECIAL CONSIDERATIONS

PATIENT/FAMILY EDUCATION

- Notify the physician if diarrhea, difficulty breathing, increased salivation, irregular heartbeat, muscle weakness, nausea and vomiting, severe abdominal pain, or increased sweating occurs
- Log energy level and muscle strength as a guide for drug dosing

MONITORING PARAMETERS

- Vital signs
- Intake and output

Myasthenia gravis

- *Therapeutic response:* Increased muscle strength, improved gait, absence of labored breathing
- *Toxicity:* Narrow margin between first appearance of side effects and serious toxicity

nesiritide

(ni-sir'-i-tide)

Rx: Natrecor

Chemical Class: Recombinant human peptide

Therapeutic Class: Vasodilator

CLINICAL PHARMACOLOGY

Mechanism of Action: A brain natriuretic peptide that facilitates cardiovascular homeostasis and fluid status through counterregulation of the renin-angiotensin-aldosterone system, stimulating cyclic guanosine monophosphate, thereby leading to smooth-muscle cell relaxation. ***Therapeutic Effect:*** Promotes vasodilation, natriuresis, and diuresis, correcting CHF.

Pharmacokinetics

Route	*Onset*	*Peak*	*Duration*
IV	15-30 mins	1-2 hrs	4 hrs

Excreted primarily in the heart by the left ventricle. Metabolized by the natriuretic neutral endopeptidase enzymes on the vascular luminal surface. ***Half-life:*** 18-23 mins.

INDICATIONS AND DOSAGES

Treatment of acutely decompensated CHF in patients with dyspnea at rest or with minimal activity

IV bolus

Adults, Elderly. 2 mcg/kg followed by a continuous IV infusion of 0.01 mcg/kg/min. At intervals of 3 hrs or longer, may be increased by 0.005 mcg/kg/min (preceded by a bolus of 1 mcg/kg), up to a maximum of 0.03 mcg/kg/min.

AVAILABLE FORMS

- *Injection Powder for Reconstitution:* 1.5 mg/5-ml vial.

CONTRAINDICATIONS: Cardiogenic shock, systolic BP less than 90 mm Hg

PREGNANCY AND LACTATION: Pregnancy category C (neither animal or human studies have been done); breast milk data unavailable

SIDE EFFECTS

Frequent (11%)

Hypotension

Occasional (8%-2%)

Headache, nausea, bradycardia

Rare (1% or less)

Confusion, paresthesia, somnolence, tremor

SERIOUS REACTIONS

- Ventricular arrhythmias, including ventricular tachycardia, atrial fibrillation, AV node conduction abnormalities, and angina pectoris occur rarely.

INTERACTIONS

Drugs

3 *Angiotensin-converting enzyme inhibitors:* Added hypotensive effects

3 *Arsenic trioxide:* May increase the risk of QT prolongation

❷ *Bumetanide:* Physically and/or chemically incompatible; should not be coadministered as infusions

❷ *Enalaprilat:* Physically and/or chemically incompatible; should not be coadministered as infusions

❷ *Ethacrynic acid:* Physically and/or chemically incompatible; should not be coadministered as infusions

❷ *Furosemide:* Physically and/or chemically incompatible; should not be coadministered as infusions

❷ *Heparin:* Physically and/or chemically incompatible; should not be coadministered as infusions

❷ *Hydralazine:* Physically and/or chemically incompatible; should not be coadministered as infusions

❷ *Insulin:* Physically and/or chemically incompatible; should not be coadministered as infusions

❷ *Sodium metabisulfite (preservative):* Incompatible; flush line between administration

SPECIAL CONSIDERATIONS

- Limited experience in administration for longer than 48 hr
- If hypotension occurs, discontinue and subsequently restart at dose reduced dose by 30% (no bolus) once patient has stabilized

PATIENT/FAMILY EDUCATION

- Nesiritide is not a cure for CHF but it will help relieve symptoms
- Immediately report chest pain or palpitations

MONITORING PARAMETERS

- Plasma brain natriuretic peptide concentrations, plasma aldosterone, heart failure hemodynamic measurements, clinical symptoms of heart failure, routine blood chemistries, blood pressure for hypotension and pulse rate for abnormalities (hypotension is dose-limiting/dose-dependent)

---

nevirapine

(ne-vye'-ra-peen)

Rx: Viramune

Chemical Class: Dipyridodiazepinone derivative; non-nucleoside reverse transcriptase inhibitor

Therapeutic Class: Antiretroviral

CLINICAL PHARMACOLOGY

Mechanism of Action: A non-nucleoside reverse transcriptase inhibitor that binds directly to HIV-1 reverse transcriptase, thus changing the shape of this enzyme and blocking RNA- and DNA-dependent polymerase activity. ***Therapeutic Effect:*** Interferes with HIV replication, slowing the progression of HIV infection.

Pharmacokinetics

Readily absorbed after PO administration. Protein binding: 60%. Widely distributed. Extensively metabolized in the liver. Excreted primarily in urine. ***Half-life:*** 45 hr (single dose), 25-30 hr (multiple doses).

INDICATIONS AND DOSAGES

HIV infection

PO

Adults. 200 mg once a day for 14 days (to reduce the risk of rash). Maintenance: 200 mg twice a day in combination with nucleoside analogs.

Children older than 8 yr. 4 mg/kg once a day for 14 days; then 4 mg/kg twice a day. Maximum: 400 mg/day.

N

Children 2 mos-8 yrs. 4 mg/kg once a day for 14 days; then 7 mg/kg twice a day.

AVAILABLE FORMS

- *Tablets:* 200 mg.
- *Oral Suspension:* 50 mg/5 ml.

UNLABELED USES: To reduce the risk of transmitting HIV from infected mother to newborn

CONTRAINDICATIONS: None known.

PREGNANCY AND LACTATION: Pregnancy category C; excreted in breast milk, breast-feeding not recommended

SIDE EFFECTS

Frequent (8%-3%)

Rash, fever, headache, nausea, granulocytopenia (more common in children)

Occasional (3%-1%)

Stomatitis (burning, erythema, or ulceration of the oral mucosa; dysphagia)

Rare (less than 1%)

Paresthesia, myalgia, abdominal pain

SERIOUS REACTIONS

- Hepatitis and rash may become severe and life-threatening.

INTERACTIONS

Drugs

3 *Clarithromycin:* 26% increase in plasma nevirapine level by clarithromycin; 30% decrease in plasma clarithromycin level by nevirapine; dose adjustment not recommended

3 *Erythromycin:* Mild increase in plasma nevirapine level by erythromycin; dose adjustment not recommended

3 *Indinavir:* 28% decrease in indinavir AUC by nevirapine; dose adjustment not recommended

❷ *Ketoconazole:* 63% reduction in plasma ketoconazole level by nevirapine; 15%-30% increase in plasma nevirapine level by ketoconazole; coadministration not recommended

3 *Methadone:* Marked decrease in methadone level by nevirapine; dose adjustment recommended

3 *Nelfinavir:* 10% increase in nelfinavir AUC by nevirapine; dose adjustment not recommended

3 *Oral contraceptives:* May decrease the plasma concentrations of oral contraceptives

3 *Rifabutin:* 16% reduction in plasma nevirapine level by rifabutin

❷ *Rifampin:* 37% reduction in plasma nevirapine level by rifampin; coadministration not recommended

3 *Ritonavir:* 11% decrease in ritonavir AUC by nevirapine; dose adjustment not recommended

3 *Saquinavir:* 25% decrease in saquinavir AUC by nevirapine; dose adjustment not recommended

3 *St. John's wort:* May decrease blood concentration and effects of nevirapine

3 *Troleandomycin:* Mild increase in plasma nevirapine level by troleandomycin; dose adjustment not recommended

SPECIAL CONSIDERATIONS

- 2-wk lead in period with qd dosing decreases the potential for development of rash; stop therapy in any patient developing a severe rash or rash with constitutional symptoms

PATIENT/FAMILY EDUCATION

- Space drug doses evenly around the clock and continue nevirapine therapy for the full course of treatment
- If the patient fails to take nevirapine for longer than 7 days, instruct him or her to restart therapy by taking one 200-mg tablet each day for the first 14 days, and then one 200-mg tablet twice a day

• Stop therapy and notify the physician if a rash occurs
• Nevirapine is not a cure for HIV infection, nor does it reduce the risk of transmitting HIV to others

MONITORING PARAMETERS

• CBC, ALT, AST, renal function
• Closely monitor for evidence of rash, which usually appears on the extremities, face, or trunk within the first 6 wks of drug therapy
• Evaluate for a rash accompanied by blistering, conjunctivitis, fever, general malaise, muscle or joint aches, oral lesions, and edema, which may indicate a severe, life-threatening skin or hypersensitivity reaction

niacin, nicotinic acid

(nye'-a-sin)

Rx: Cardene, Niacor, Niaspan ER

Combinations

Rx: with lovastatin (Advicor)

Chemical Class: Vitamin B complex

Therapeutic Class: Antilipemic; vitamin

CLINICAL PHARMACOLOGY

Mechanism of Action: An antihyperlipidemic, water-soluble vitamin that is a component of two coenzymes needed for tissue respiration, lipid metabolism, and glycogenolysis. Inhibits synthesis of VLDLs. ***Therapeutic Effect:*** Reduces total, LDL, and VLDL cholesterol levels and triglyceride levels; increases HDL cholesterol concentration.

Pharmacokinetics

Readily absorbed from the GI tract. Widely distributed. Metabolized in the liver. Primarily excreted in urine. ***Half-life:*** 45 min.

INDICATIONS AND DOSAGES

Hyperlipidemia

PO (Immediate-Release)

Adults, Elderly. Initially, 50-100 mg twice a day for 7 days. Increase gradually by doubling dose qwk up to 1-1.5 g/day in 2-3 doses. Maximum: 3 g/day.

Children. Initially, 100-250 mg/day (maximum: 10 mg/kg/day) in 3 divided doses. May increase by 100 mg/wk or 250 mg q2-3wk. Maximum: 2250 mg/day.

PO (Timed-Release)

Adults, Elderly. Initially, 500 mg/day in 2 divided doses for 1 week; then increase to 500 mg twice a day. Maintenance: 2 g/day.

Nutritional supplement

PO

Adults, Elderly. 10-20 mg/day. Maximum: 100 mg/day.

Pellegra

PO

Adults, Elderly. 50-100 mg 3-4 times a day. Maximum: 500 mg/day.

Children. 50-100 mg 3 times a day.

AVAILABLE FORMS

- *Capsules (Timed-Release):* 125 mg, 250 mg, 400 mg, 500 mg.
- *Tablets (Niacor):* 50 mg, 100 mg, 250 mg, 500 mg.
- *Tablets (Timed-Release [Slo-Niacin]):* 250 mg, 500 mg, 750 mg.
- *Tablets (Timed-Release [Niaspan]):* 500 mg, 750 mg, 1000 mg.
- *Elixir (Nicotinex):* 50 mg/5 ml.

CONTRAINDICATIONS: Active peptic ulcer disease, arterial hemorrhaging, hepatic dysfunction, hypersensitivity to niacin or tartrazine (frequently seen in patients sensitive to aspirin), severe hypotension

PREGNANCY AND LACTATION: Pregnancy category A (category C if used in doses greater than recommended daily allowance); actively excreted in human breast milk; recommended daily allowance during lactation is 18-20 mg

SIDE EFFECTS

Frequent

Flushing (especially of the face and neck) occurring within 20 mins of drug administration and lasting for 30-60 mins, GI upset, pruritus

Occasional

Dizziness, hypotension, headache, blurred vision, burning or tingling of skin, flatulence, nausea, vomiting, diarrhea

Rare

Hyperglycemia, glycosuria, rash, hyperpigmentation, dry skin

SERIOUS REACTIONS

- Arrhythmias occur rarely.

INTERACTIONS

Drugs

3 *Lovastatin, pravastatin, simvastatin:* Isolated cases of myopathy and rhabdomyolysis have occurred, causality not established

Labs

- *Interference:* Plasma and urine catecholamines, urine glucose with Benedict's reagent

SPECIAL CONSIDERATIONS

- In 1-g doses: 10%-20% reduction of total plus LDL-cholesterol, 30%-70% reduction in triglycerides, and a 20%-35% increase in HDL-cholesterol
- Increased risk of hepatotoxicity with sustained-release products

PATIENT/FAMILY EDUCATION

- Gradual dosage titration lessens flushing, adverse effects
- Avoid alcohol and hot beverages (increases flushing)
- Administer with meals and 2 glasses of water
- 125-350 mg of aspirin 20-30 min prior to dose may lessen flushing
- Do not miss any doses (flushing may return)
- If dizziness occurs, avoid sudden posture changes and activities that require steady and alert responses
- Flushing may decrease with continued therapy

MONITORING PARAMETERS

- Liver function tests, blood glucose, uric acid regularly
- Fasting lipid profile q3-6mo
- Pattern of bowel activity
- Skin for rash or dryness

nicardipine hydrochloride

(nye-kar'-de-peen)

Rx: Cardene, Cardene IV, Cardene SR

Chemical Class: Dihydropyridine

Therapeutic Class: Antianginal; antihypertensive; calcium channel blocker

CLINICAL PHARMACOLOGY

Mechanism of Action: An antianginal and antihypertensive agent that inhibits calcium ion movement across cell membranes, depressing contraction of cardiac and vascular smooth muscle. ***Therapeutic Effect:*** Increases heart rate and cardiac output. Decreases systemic vascular resistance and BP.

Pharmacokinetics

Route	*Onset*	*Peak*	*Duration*
PO	N/A	1-2 hr	8 hr

Rapidly, completely absorbed from the GI tract. Protein binding: 95%. Undergoes first-pass metabolism in the liver. Primarily excreted in urine. Not removed by hemodialysis. ***Half-life:*** 2-4 hr.

INDICATIONS AND DOSAGES

Chronic stable (effort-associated) angina

PO

Adults, Elderly. Initially, 20 mg 3 times a day. Range: 20-40 mg 3 times a day.

Essential hypertension

PO

Adults, Elderly. Initially, 20 mg 3 times a day. Range: 20-40 mg 3 times a day.

PO (Sustained-Release)

Adults, Elderly. Initially, 30 mg twice a day. Range: 30-60 mg twice a day.

Short-term treatment of hypertension when oral therapy is not feasible or desirable (substitute for oral nicardipine)

IV

Adults, Elderly. 0.5 mg/hr (for patient receiving 20 mg PO q8h); 1.2 mg/hr (for patient receiving 30 mg PO q8h); 2.2 mg/hr (for patient receiving 40 mg PO q8h).

Patients not already receiving nicardipine

IV

Adults, Elderly (gradual BP decrease). Initially, 5 mg/hr. May increase by 2.5 mg/hr q15min. After BP goal is achieved, decrease rate to 3 mg/hr.

Adults, Elderly (rapid BP decrease). Initially, 5 mg/hr. May increase by 2.5 mg/hr q5min. Maximum: 15 mg/hr until desired BP attained. After BP goal achieved, decrease rate to 3 mg/hr.

Changing from IV to oral antihypertensive therapy

Adults, Elderly. Begin antihypertensives other than nicardipine when IV has been discontinued; for nicardipine, give first dose 1 hr before discontinuing IV.

Dosage in hepatic impairment

For adults and elderly patients, initially give 20 mg twice a day; then titrate.

Dosage in renal impairment

For adults and elderly patients, initially give 20 mg q8h (30 mg twice a day [sustained-release capsules]); then titrate.

AVAILABLE FORMS

- *Capsules (Cardene):* 20 mg, 30 mg.
- *Capsules (Sustained-Release [Cardene SR]):* 30 mg, 45 mg, 60 mg.
- *Injection (Cardene IV):* 2.5 mg/ml.

UNLABELED USES: Treatment of associated neurologic deficits, Raynaud's phenomenon, subarachnoid hemorrhage, vasospastic angina

CONTRAINDICATIONS: Atrial fibrillation or flutter associated with accessory conduction pathways, cardiogenic shock, CHF, second- or third-degree heart block, severe hypotension, sinus bradycardia, ventricular tachycardia, within several hours of IV beta-blocker therapy

PREGNANCY AND LACTATION: Pregnancy category C; significant excretion into rat maternal milk

SIDE EFFECTS

Frequent (10%-7%)

Headache, facial flushing, peripheral edema, light-headedness, dizziness

Occasional (6%-3%)

Asthenia (loss of strength, energy), palpitations, angina, tachycardia

Rare (less than 2%)

Nausea, abdominal cramps, dyspepsia, dry mouth, rash

SERIOUS REACTIONS

• Overdose produces confusion, slurred speech, somnolence, marked hypotension, and bradycardia.

INTERACTIONS

Drugs

3 *Cyclosporine, tacrolimus:* Increased blood concentrations of these drugs, increased risk of toxicity

3 *Digoxin:* May increase nicardipine blood concentration

3 *Histamine H_2-antagonists:* Increased blood levels of nicardipine with cimetidine and ranitidine

3 *Hypokalemia-producing agents (such as furosemide and certain other diuretics):* May increase the risk of arrhythmias

3 *Fentanyl:* Severe hypotension or increased fluid volume requirements

3 *Neuromuscular blocking agents:* Prolongation of neuromuscular blockade

3 *Procainamide, quinidine:* May increase the risk of QT-interval prolongation

3 *Propranolol:* Increases propranolol concentrations; an increase in B-blocker effect may occur

SPECIAL CONSIDERATIONS

PATIENT/FAMILY EDUCATION

• Take nicardipine's sustained-release form with food and do not crush or open the capsules

• Avoid alcohol and limit caffeine

• Notify the physician if anginal pain is not relieved by the medication or if constipation, dizziness, irregular heartbeat, nausea, shortness of breath, swelling, or symptoms of hypotension such as light-headedness occurs

MONITORING PARAMETERS

• Blood pressure

• Liver function test

• EKG and pulse for tachycardia

• Skin for dermatitis, facial flushing, or rash

---

nicotine

(nik'-oh-teen)

Rx: NicoDerm CQ, NicoDerm CQ Clear, Nicorette, Nicotrol, Nictrol Inhaler, Nicotrol NS

Chemical Class: Pyridine alkaloid

Therapeutic Class: Smoking deterrent

CLINICAL PHARMACOLOGY

Mechanism of Action: A cholinergic-receptor agonist that binds to acetylcholine receptors, producing both stimulating and depressant effects on the peripheral and central nervous systems. ***Therapeutic Effect:*** Provides a source of nicotine during nicotine withdrawal and reduces withdrawal symptoms.

Pharmacokinetics

Absorbed slowly after transdermal administration. Protein binding: 5%. Metabolized in the liver. Excreted primarily in urine. ***Half-life:*** 4 hr.

INDICATIONS AND DOSAGES

Smoking cessation aid to relieve nicotine withdrawal symptoms

PO (Chewing gum)

Adults, Elderly. Usually, 10-12 pieces/day. Maximum: 30 pieces/day.

PO (Lozenge)

Alert: For those who smoke the first cigarette within 30 min of waking, administer the 4 mg-lozenge; otherwise administer the 2-mg lozenge.

Adults, Elderly. One 4-mg or 2-mg lozenge q1-2h for the first 6 wks; one lozenge q2-4h for wk 7-9; and one lozenge q4-8h for wk 10-12. Maximum: one lozenge at a time, 5 lozenges/6 hr, 20 lozenges/day.

Transdermal

Adults, Elderly who smoke 10 cigarettes or more per day. Follow the guidelines below.

Step 1: 21 mg/day for 4-6 wks.

Step 2: 14 mg/day for 2 wks.

Step 3: 7 mg/day for 2 wks.

Adults, Elderly who smoke less than 10 cigarettes per day. Follow the guidelines below.

Step 1: 14 mg/day for 6 wks.

Step 2: 7 mg/day for 2 wks.

Patients weighing less than 100 lb, patients with a history of cardiovascular disease. Initially, 14 mg/day for 4-6 wks, then 7 mg/day for 2-4wks.

Transdermal (Nicotrol)

Adults, Elderly. One patch a day for 6 wks.

Nasal

Adults, Elderly. 1-2 doses/hr (1 dose = 2 sprays [1 in each nostril] = 1 mg). Maximum: 5 doses (5 mg)/hr; 40 doses (40 mg)/day.

Inhaler (Nicotrol)

Adults, Elderly. Puff on nicotine cartridge mouthpiece for about 20 min as needed.

AVAILABLE FORMS

- *Chewing Gum (Nicorette):* 2 mg, 4 mg.
- *Lozenge (Commit):* 2 mg, 4 mg.
- *Transdermal Patch (NicoDerm CQ, Nicotrol):* 5 mg/16 hr, 7 mg/24 hr, 10 mg/16 hr, 14 mg/24 hr, 21 mg/24 hr mg.
- *Nasal Spray (Nicotrol NS):* 0.5 mg/spray.
- *Inhalation (Nicotrol Inhaler):* 10-mg cartridge.

CONTRAINDICATIONS: Immediate post MI period, life-threatening arrhythmias, severe or worsening angina

PREGNANCY AND LACTATION: Pregnancy category D; use of nicotine gum during last trimester has been associated with decreased fetal breathing movements; passes freely into breast milk; however, lower concentrations in milk can be expected with transdermal systems than cigarette smoking when used as directed

SIDE EFFECTS

Frequent

All forms: Hiccups, nausea

Gum: Mouth or throat soreness, nausea, hiccups

Transdermal: Erythema, pruritus, or burning at application site

Occasional

All forms: Eructation, GI upset, dry mouth, insomnia, diaphoresis, irritability

Gum: Hiccups, hoarseness
Inhaler: Mouth or throat irritation, cough
Rare
All forms: Dizziness, myalgia, arthralgia
SERIOUS REACTIONS
• Overdose produces palpitations, tachyarrhythmias, seizures, depression, confusion, diaphoresis, hypotension, rapid or weak pulse, and dyspnea. Lethal dose for adults is 40-60 mg. Death results from respiratory paralysis.
INTERACTIONS
Drugs
3 *Adenosine:* Increased hemodynamic and AV blocking effects of adenosine
3 *β-blockers, bronchodilators (such as theophylline), insulin, propoxyphene:* May increase the effects of these drugs
3 *Cimetidine:* Increased blood nicotine concentration, may reduce the amount of gum or patches needed
3 *Coffee, cola:* Reduced absorption of nicotine from chewing gum
SPECIAL CONSIDERATIONS
• Drugs that may require dosage reduction with smoking cessation: acetaminophen, caffeine, imipramine, oxazepam, pentazocine, propranolol, theophylline, insulin, prazocin, labetalol
• Drugs that may require an increase in dose with smoking cessation: isoproterenol, phenylephrine
PATIENT/FAMILY EDUCATION
• Chew gum slowly until burning or tingling sensation is felt, then park gum between cheek and gum until tingling sensation goes away
• Chew <30 min/piece
• Avoid coffee and cola drinks while chewing gum or using inhaler
• Do not smoke while utilizing nicotine replacement therapy
• Apply new transdermal system daily
• Rotate sites; apply to non-hairy area on upper torso
• Notify the physician if itching or a persistent rash occurs during treatment with the transdermal patch
MONITORING PARAMETERS
• Blood pressure, pulse rate
• If the transdermal system is used, monitor the application site for burning, erythema, and pruritus

nifedipine

(nye-fed′-i-peen)
Rx: Adalat CC, Procardia, Procardia XL
Chemical Class: Dihydropyridine
Therapeutic Class: Antianginal; antihypertensive; calcium channel blocker

CLINICAL PHARMACOLOGY
Mechanism of Action: An antianginal and antihypertensive agent that inhibits calcium ion movement across cell membranes, depressing contraction of cardiac and vascular smooth muscle. ***Therapeutic Effect:*** Increases heart rate and cardiac output. Decreases systemic vascular resistance and BP.
Pharmacokinetics

Route	*Onset*	*Peak*	*Duration*
Sublingual	1-5 mins	N/A	N/A
PO	20-30 mins	N/A	4-8 hrs
PO (extended release)	2 hrs	N/A	24 hrs

Rapidly, completely absorbed from the GI tract. Protein binding: 92%-98%. Undergoes first-pass metabolism in the liver. Primarily excreted in urine. Not removed by hemodialysis. ***Half-life:*** 2-5 hrs.

INDICATIONS AND DOSAGES

Prinzmetal's variant angina, chronic stable (effort-associated) angina

PO

Adults, Elderly. Initially, 10 mg 3 times a day. Increase at 7- to 14-day intervals. Maintenance: 10 mg 3 times a day up to 30 mg 4 times a day.

PO (Extended-Release)

Adults, Elderly. Initially, 30-60 mg/day. Maintenance: Up to 120 mg/day.

Essential hypertension

PO (Extended-Release)

Adults, Elderly. Initially, 30-60 mg/day. Maintenance: Up to 120 mg/day.

AVAILABLE FORMS

- *Capsules (Procardia):* 10 mg.
- *Tablets (Extended-Release):* 30 mg (Adalat CC, Nifedical XL, Procardia XL), 60 mg (Adalat CC, Nifedical XL, Procardia XL), 90 mg (Adalat CC, Procardia XL).

UNLABELED USES: Treatment of Raynaud's phenomenon

CONTRAINDICATIONS: Advanced aortic stenosis, severe hypotension

SIDE EFFECTS

Frequent (30%-11%)

Peripheral edema, headache, flushed skin, dizziness

Occasional (12%-6%)

Nausea, shakiness, muscle cramps and pain, somnolence, palpitations, nasal congestion, cough, dyspnea, wheezing

Rare (5%-3%)

Hypotension, rash, pruritus, urticaria, constipation, abdominal discomfort, flatulence, sexual difficulties

SERIOUS REACTIONS

- Nifedipine may precipitate CHF and MI in patients with cardiac disease and peripheral ischemia.
- Overdose produces nausea, somnolence, confusion, and slurred speech.

INTERACTIONS

Drugs

3 *Barbiturates, rifampin, rifabutin:* Reduced plasma concentrations of nifedipine

3 *β-blockers:* Enhanced effects of β-blockers, hypotension; increased metoprolol and propanolol concentrations; additive negative effects on myocardial contractility

3 *Cimetidine, ranitidine, famotidine:* Increased nifedipine concentrations possible

3 *Digitalis glycosides:* Increased digitalis levels; increased risk of toxicity

3 *Diltiazem:* Increased serum concentrations of nifedipine

3 *Doxazosin:* Enhanced hypotensive effects

3 *Fentanyl:* Severe hypotension or increased fluid volume requirements

3 *Food:* Increased absorption of Adalat CC

3 *Grapefruit juice:* Increased serum nifedipine concentrations

3 *Histamine H_2-antagonists:* Increased blood levels of nifedipine with cimetidine

3 *Lansoprazole:* Increased nifedipine absorption

3 *Magnesium:* Potential for transient hypotensive effect

3 *Phenytoin:* Increased phenytoin concentration

3 *Quinidine:* Reduced blood concentrations of quinidine

3 *Quinupristin/Dalfopristin:* Increased plasma concentration of nifedipine; reduced doses of nifedipine may be necessary

3 *St. John's Wort:* Reduces the plasma concentration of nifedipine

3 *Tacrolimus:* Reduced the dosage requirements of tacrolimus; dosage supplements may be required

3 *Vincristine:* Marked increase in vincristine half-life, clinical significance unknown

SPECIAL CONSIDERATIONS

- Given the seriousness of the reported adverse events and the lack of any clinical documentation attesting to a benefit, the use of nifedipine capsules for hypertensive urgencies or emergencies should be abandoned (*JAMA* 1996; 276:1328-1331)

PATIENT/FAMILY EDUCATION

- Administer Adalat CC on an empty stomach
- Do not crush or chew sustained release dosage forms
- Empty Procardia XL tablets may appear in stool; this is no cause for concern
- Rise slowly from a lying to a sitting position and permit legs to dangle from bed momentarily before standing to reduce nifedipine's hypotensive effect
- Notify the physician if irregular heartbeat, prolonged dizziness, nausea, or shortness of breath occurs
- Avoid alcohol, grapefruit, and grapefruit juice

MONITORING PARAMETERS

- Skin for flushing
- Liver function tests

nimodipine

(nye-moe'-di-peen)

Rx: Nimotop

Chemical Class: Dihydropyridine

Therapeutic Class: Calcium channel blocker; cerebral vasodilator

CLINICAL PHARMACOLOGY

Mechanism of Action: A cerebral vasospasm agent that inhibits movement of calcium ions across vascular smooth-muscle cell membranes. ***Therapeutic Effect:*** Produces favorable effect on severity of neurologic deficits due to cerebral vasospasm. Exerts greatest effect on cerebral arteries; may prevent cerebral spasm.

Pharmacokinetics

Rapidly absorbed from the GI tract. Protein binding: 95%. Metabolized in the liver. Excreted in urine; eliminated in feces. Not removed by hemodialysis. ***Half-life:*** terminal, 3 hr.

INDICATIONS AND DOSAGES

Improvement of neurologic deficits after subarachnoid hemorrhage from ruptured congenital aneurysms

PO

Adults, Elderly. 60 mg q4h for 21 days. Begin within 96 hr of subarachnoid hemorrhage.

AVAILABLE FORMS

- *Capsules:* 30 mg.

UNLABELED USES: Treatment of chronic and classic migraine, chronic cluster headaches

CONTRAINDICATIONS: Atrial fibrillation or flutter, cardiogenic shock, CHF, heart block, sinus bradycardia, ventricular tachycardia, within several hours of IV beta-blocker therapy

PREGNANCY AND LACTATION: Pregnancy category C

SIDE EFFECTS

Occasional (6%-2%)

Hypotension, peripheral edema, diarrhea, headache

Rare (less than 2%)

Allergic reaction (rash, hives), tachycardia, flushing of skin

SERIOUS REACTIONS

• Overdose produces nausea, weakness, dizziness, somnolence, confusion, and slurred speech.

INTERACTIONS

Drugs

3 *β-blockers:* May prolong SA and AV conduction, which may lead to severe hypotension, bradycardia, and cardiac failure

3 *Cimetidine:* Increased serum nimodipine concentrations

3 *Erythromycin, itraconazole, ketoconazole, protease inhibitors:* May inhibit the metabolism of nimodipine

3 *Omeprazole:* Increased serum nimodipine concentrations

3 *Rifabutin, rifampin:* May increase the metabolism of nimodipine

3 *Valproic acid:* Increased oral bioavailability of nimodipine

SPECIAL CONSIDERATIONS

PATIENT/FAMILY EDUCATION

• Do not crush or chew capsules

• Notify the physician if constipation, dizziness, irregular heartbeat, nausea, shortness of breath, or swelling occurs

MONITORING PARAMETERS

• Blood pressure

• CNS response

• Heart rate for signs and symptoms of CHF and hypotension

nisoldipine

(nye-sole'-di-peen)

Rx: Sular

Chemical Class: Dihydropyridine

Therapeutic Class: Antihypertensive; calcium channel blocker

CLINICAL PHARMACOLOGY

Mechanism of Action: A calcium channel blocker that inhibits calcium ion movement across cell membrane, depressing contraction of cardiac and vascular smooth muscle. ***Therapeutic Effect:*** Increases heart rate and cardiac output. Decreases systemic vascular resistance and blood pressure (BP).

Pharmacokinetics

Poor absorption from the gastrointestinal (GI) tract. Food increases bioavailability. Protein binding: more than 99%. Metabolism occurs in the gut wall. Primarily excreted in urine. Not removed by hemodialysis. ***Half-life:*** 7-12 hrs.

INDICATIONS AND DOSAGES

Hypertension

PO

Adults. Initially, 20 mg once daily, then increase by 10 mg per week, or longer intervals until therapeutic BP response is attained.

Elderly. Initially, 10 mg once daily. Increase by 10 mg per week to therapeutic response. Maintenance: 20-40 mg once daily. Maximum: 60 mg once daily.

AVAILABLE FORMS

• *Tablets (Extended-Release):* 10 mg, 20 mg, 30 mg, 40 mg (Sular).

UNLABELED USES: Stable angina pectoris, CHF

CONTRAINDICATIONS: Sick-sinus syndrome/second- or third-degree AV block (except in presence of pacemaker), hypersensitivity to nisoldipine or any component of the formulation

PREGNANCY AND LACTATION: Pregnancy category C

SIDE EFFECTS

Frequent

Giddiness, dizziness, lightheadedness, peripheral edema, headache, flushing, weakness, nausea

Occasional

Transient hypotension, heartburn, muscle cramps, nasal congestion, cough, wheezing, sore throat, palpitations, nervousness, mood changes

Rare

Increase in frequency, intensity, duration of anginal attack during initial therapy

SERIOUS REACTIONS

- May precipitate congestive heart failure (CHF) and myocardial infarction (MI) in patients with cardiac disease and peripheral ischemia.
- Overdose produces nausea, drowsiness, confusion, and slurred speech.

INTERACTIONS

Drugs

3 *β-adrenergic blockers:* Increased propranolol concentration

3 *Cimetidine, famotidine, nizatidine, omeprazole, ranitidine:* Increased nisoldipine concentrations possible

3 *Fentanyl:* Severe hypotension or increased fluid volume requirements

3 *Food:* Increased absorption with high-fat meal or grapefruit juice

SPECIAL CONSIDERATIONS

- No significant advantages over other dihydropyridine calcium channel blockers

PATIENT/FAMILY EDUCATION

- Do not take with high-fat meal or grapefruit juice
- Rise slowly from lying to sitting position and permit legs to dangle from bed momentarily before standing to reduce the drug's hypotensive effect

MONITORING PARAMETERS

- Blood pressure

nitazoxanide

(nye-ta-zox'-ah-nide)

Rx: Alinia

Chemical Class: Benzamide derivative

Therapeutic Class: Antiprotozoal

CLINICAL PHARMACOLOGY

Mechanism of Action: An antiparasitic that interferes with the body's reaction to pyruvate ferredoxin oxidoreductase, an enzyme essential for anaerobic energy metabolism. ***Therapeutic Effect:*** Produces antiprotozoal activity, reducing or terminating diarrheal episodes.

Pharmacokinetics

Rapidly hydrolyzed to an active metabolite. Protein binding: 99%. Excreted in the urine, bile, and feces. ***Half-life:*** 2-4 hrs.

INDICATIONS AND DOSAGES

Diarrhea caused by C. parvum

PO

Children 4-11 yrs. 200 mg q12h for 3 days.

Children 12-47 mos. 100 mg q12h for 3 days.

Diarrhea caused by G. lambia

PO

Adults, Elderly, Children 12 yrs and older. 500 mg q12h for 3 days.

Children 4-11 yrs. 200 mg q12h for 3 days.

Children 12-47 mos. 100 mg q12h for 3 days.

AVAILABLE FORMS

- *Powder for Oral Suspension:* 100 mg/5 ml.
- *Tablets:* 500 mg.

CONTRAINDICATIONS: History of sensitivity to aspirin and salicylates

PREGNANCY AND LACTATION: Pregnancy category B; excretion into breast milk unknown; use caution in nursing mothers

SIDE EFFECTS

Occasional (8%)

Abdominal pain

Rare (2%-1%)

Diarrhea, vomiting, headache

SERIOUS REACTIONS

- None known.

SPECIAL CONSIDERATIONS

- Efficacy in adults or immunocompromised patients not known
- Efficacy for *Cryptosporidium parvum* 88% (38% for placebo in controlled trial)
- Efficacy for *Giardia lamblia* 90% (equal to metronidazole)

PATIENT/FAMILY EDUCATION

- Take with food
- Tell parents of children with diabetes mellitus that the oral suspension of nitazoxanide contains 1.48 g of sucrose per 5 ml
- Nitazoxanide therapy should significantly improve diarrhea

MONITORING PARAMETERS

- Blood glucose level in the patient with diabetes
- Electrolyte levels for abnormalities that may have been caused by diarrhea
- Weigh each day and encourage patient to maintain adequate fluid intake
- Bowel sounds for peristalsis; pattern of daily bowel activity and stool consistency

nitrofurantoin sodium

(nye-troe-fyoor-an′-toyn)

Rx: Furadantin, Macrobid, Macrodantin, Nitro Macro

Combinations

Rx: Nitrofurantoin macrocrystals with nitrofurantoin monohydrate (Macrobid)

Chemical Class: Nitrofuran derivative

Therapeutic Class: Antibiotic

CLINICAL PHARMACOLOGY

Mechanism of Action: An antibacterial UTI agent that inhibits the synthesis of bacterial DNA, RNA, proteins, and cell walls by altering or inactivating ribosomal proteins. ***Therapeutic Effect:*** Bacteriostatic (bactericidal at high concentrations).

Pharmacokinetics

Microcrystalline form rapidly and completely absorbed; macrocrystalline form more slowly absorbed. Food increases absorption. Protein binding: 40%. Primarily concentrated in urine and kidneys. Metabolized in most body tissues. Primarily excreted in urine. Removed by hemodialysis. ***Half-life:*** 20-60 min.

INDICATIONS AND DOSAGES

UTIs

PO (Furadantin, Macrodantin)

Adults, Elderly. 50-100 mg q6h. Maximum: 400 mg/day.

Children. 5-7 mg/kg/day in divided doses q6h. Maximum: 400 mg/day.

PO (Macrobid)

Adults, Elderly. 100 mg twice a day. Maximum: 400 mg/day.

Long-term prevention of UTIs

PO

Adults, Elderly. 50-100 mg at bedtime.

Children. 1-2 mg/kg/day as a single dose. Maximum: 100 mg/day.

AVAILABLE FORMS

• *Capsules (Macrocrystalline, Monohydrate [Macrobid]):* 100 mg.

• *Capsules (Macrocrystalline [Macrodantin, Nitro Macro]):* 25 mg, 50 mg, 100 mg

• *Oral Suspension (Microcrystalline [Furadantin]):* 25 mg/5 ml.

UNLABELED USES: Prevention of bacterial UTIs

CONTRAINDICATIONS: Anuria, oliguria, substantial renal impairment (creatinine clearance less than 40 ml/min); infants younger than 1 mo old because of the risk of hemolytic anemia

PREGNANCY AND LACTATION: Pregnancy category B; compatible with breast-feeding in infants >1 mo

SIDE EFFECTS

Frequent

Anorexia, nausea, vomiting, dark urine

Occasional

Abdominal pain, diarrhea, rash, pruritus, urticaria, hypertension, headache, dizziness, drowsiness

Rare

Photosensitivity, transient alopecia, asthmatic exacerbation in those with history of asthma

SERIOUS REACTIONS

• Superinfection, hepatotoxicity, peripheral neuropathy (may be irreversible), Stevens-Johnson syndrome, permanent pulmonary function impairment, and anaphylaxis occur rarely.

INTERACTIONS

Drugs

3 *Hemolytics:* May increase the risk of nitrofurantoin toxicity

3 *Neurotoxic medications:* May increase the risk of neurotoxicity

3 *Probenecid:* May increase blood concentration and toxicity of nitrofurantoin

Labs

• *Interference:* Urine alkaline phosphatase, urine lactate dehydrogenase

• *False positive:* Urine glucose (not with glucose enzymatic tests)

• *False increase:* Serum bilirubin, serum creatinine

• *False decrease:* Serum unconjugated bilirubin

SPECIAL CONSIDERATIONS

PATIENT/FAMILY EDUCATION

• Food or milk may decrease GI upset

• May cause brown discoloration of urine

• Continue taking nitrofurantoin for the full course of therapy

• Avoid exposure to the sun and ultraviolet light and use sunscreen and wear protective clothing when outdoors

• Notify the physician if chest pain, cough, difficult breathing, fever, or numbness and tingling of fingers or toes occurs

• Hair loss may occur but is only temporary

MONITORING PARAMETERS

• Periodic liver function tests during prolonged therapy

• CBC with differential and platelets during prolonged therapy

• Pulmonary review of systems

• Intake and output and renal function test results

• Pattern of daily bowel activity and stool consistency

• Be alert for signs and symptoms of peripheral neuropathy, such as numbness or tingling, especially in the lower extremities

nitrofurazone

(nye-troe-fyoor'-a-zone)

Rx: Furacin

Chemical Class: Nitrofuran derivative

Therapeutic Class: Antibiotic, topical

CLINICAL PHARMACOLOGY

Mechanism of Action: A synthetic nitrofuran that inhibits bacterial enzymes involved in carbohydrate metabolism. ***Therapeutic Effect:*** Inhibits a variety of enzymes. Bactericidal.

Pharmacokinetics

Not known.

INDICATIONS AND DOSAGES

Burns, catheter-related urinary tract infection, skin grafts

Topical

Adults. Apply directly on lesion with spatula or place on a piece of gauze first. Use of a bandage is optional. Preparation should remain on lesion for at least 24 hrs. Dressing may be changed several times daily or left on the lesion for a longer period.

AVAILABLE FORMS

- *Cream:* 0.2% (Furacin).
- *Ointment:* 0.2% (Furacin).
- *Solution:* 0.2% (Furacin).

UNLABELED USES: Fire and ant bites, scabies, urethritis, vaginal malodor, vasectomy, wounds

CONTRAINDICATIONS: Hypersensitivity to nitrofurazone or any of its components

PREGNANCY AND LACTATION: Pregnancy category C; excretion into breast milk unknown

SIDE EFFECTS

Occasional

Itching, rash, swelling

SERIOUS REACTIONS

- Use of nitrofurazone may result in bacterial or fungal overgrowth of nonsusceptible pathogens, which may lead to secondary infection.

INTERACTIONS

Labs

- *False increase:* Urine creatinine, urine glucose via Benedict's reagent

SPECIAL CONSIDERATIONS

PATIENT/FAMILY EDUCATION

- Avoid contact with eye
- Notify the physician if irritation, inflammation, or rash occurs

MONITORING PARAMETERS

- Skin for irritation

nitroglycerin

(nye-troe-gli'-ser-in)

Rx: Minitran, Nitrek, Nitro-Bid, Nitro-Bid IV, Nitrocot, Nitro-Dur, Nitrogard, Nitroglyn E-R, Nitrol Appli-Kit, Nitrolingual, Nitrong, NitroQuick, Nitrostat, Nitro-Tab, Nitro TD Patch-A, Nitro-Time, Tridil

Chemical Class: Nitrate, organic

Therapeutic Class: Antianginal; vasodilator

CLINICAL PHARMACOLOGY

Mechanism of Action: A nitrate that decreases myocardial oxygen demand. Reduces left ventricular preload and afterload. ***Therapeutic Effect:*** Dilates coronary arteries and improves collateral blood flow to ischemic areas within myocardium. IV form produces peripheral vasodilation.

Pharmacokinetics

Route	Onset	Peak	Duration
Sublingual	1-3 mins	4-8 mins	30-60 mins
Translingual Spray	2 mins	4-10 mins	30-60 mins
Buccal Tablet	2-5 mins	4-10 mins	2 hrs
PO (Extended-Release)	20-45 mins	45-120 mins	4-8 hrs
Topical	15-60 mins	30-120 mins	2-12 hrs
Transdermal Patch	40-60 mins	60-180 mins	18-24 hrs
IV	1-2 mins	Immediate	3-5 mins

Well absorbed after PO, sublingual, and topical administration. Undergoes extensive first-pass metabolism. Metabolized in the liver and by enzymes in the bloodstream. Primarily excreted in urine. Not removed by hemodialysis. ***Half-life:*** 1-4 mins.

INDICATIONS AND DOSAGES

Acute relief of angina pectoris, acute prophylaxis

Lingual Spray

Adults, Elderly. 1 spray onto or under tongue q3-5min until relief is noted (no more than 3 sprays in 15-min period).

Sublingual

Adults, Elderly. 0.4 mg q5min until relief is noted (no more than 3 doses in 15-min period). Use prophylactically 5-10 min before activities that may cause an acute attack.

Long-term prophylaxis of angina

PO (Extended-Release)

Adults, Elderly. 2.5-9 mg 2-4 times a day. Maximum: 26 mg 4 times a day.

Topical

Adults, Elderly. Initially, ½ inch q8h. Increase by ½ inch with each application. Range: 1-2 inches q8h up to 4-5 inches q4h.

Transdermal Patch

Adults, Elderly. Initially, 0.2-0.4 mg/hr. Maintenance: 0.4-0.8 mg/hr. Consider patch on for 12-14 hr, patch off for 10-12 hr (prevents tolerance).

CHF associated with acute MI

IV

Adults, Elderly. Initially, 5 mcg/min via infusion pump. Increase in 5-mcg/min increments at 3- to 5-min intervals until BP response is noted or until dosage reaches 20 mcg/min; then increase as needed by 10 mcg/min. Dosage may be further titrated according to clinical, therapeutic response up to 200 mcg/min.

Children. Initially, 0.25-0.5 mcg/kg/min; titrate by 0.5-1 mcg/kg/min up to 20 mcg/kg/min.

AVAILABLE FORMS

- *Capsules (Extended-Release [NitroBid, Nitrocot, Nitroglyn E-R, Nitro-Time]):* 2.5 mg, 6.5 mg, 9 mg.
- *Tablets (Extended-Release, Oral Transmucosal):* 1 mg (Nitrogard), 2.6 mg (Nitrong), 3 mg (Nitrogard), 6.5 mg (Nitrong).
- *Tablets (Sublingual [Nitroquick, Nitrostat, Nitro-Tab]):* 0.3 mg, 0.4 mg, 0.6 mg.
- *Spray (Translingual [Nitrolingual]):* 0.4 mg/spray.
- *Infusion Solution:* 0.1 mg/ml, 0.2 mg/ml, 0.4 mg/ml.
- *Intravenous Solution (Nitro-Bid IV, Tridil):* 5 mg/ml.
- *Intravenous Solution:* 5% dextrose-10 mg nitroglycerin/100 ml, 5% dextrose-20 mg nitroglycerin/100 ml, 5% dextrose-40 mg nitroglycerin/100 ml.
- *Topical Ointment (Nitro-Bid, Nitrol, Nitrol Appl-Kit):* 2%.
- *Transdermal Patch (Minitran):* 0.1 mg/h (Minitran, Nitro-Dur), 0.2 mg/h (Minitran, Nitrek, Nitro-Dur), 0.3 mg/h (Minitran, Nitro-Dur), 0.4

mg/h (Minitran, Nitrek, Nitro-Dur), 0.6 mg/h (Nitrek, Nitro-Dur), 0.8 mg/h (Nitro-Dur).

CONTRAINDICATIONS: Allergy to adhesives (transdermal), closed-angle glaucoma, constrictive pericarditis (IV), early MI (sublingual), GI hypermotility or malabsorption (extended-release), head trauma, hypotension (IV), inadequate cerebral circulation (IV), increased intracranial pressure (ICP), nitrates, orthostatic hypotension, pericardial tamponade (IV), severe anemia, uncorrected hypovolemia (IV)

PREGNANCY AND LACTATION: Pregnancy category C; use of SL for angina during pregnancy without fetal harm has been reported

SIDE EFFECTS

Frequent

Headache (possibly severe; occurs mostly in early therapy, diminishes rapidly in intensity, and usually disappears during continued treatment), transient flushing of face and neck, dizziness (especially if patient is standing immobile or is in a warm environment), weakness, orthostatic hypotension

Sublingual: Burning, tingling sensation at oral point of dissolution

Ointment: Erythema, pruritus

Occasional

GI upset

Transdermal: Contact dermatitis

SERIOUS REACTIONS

- Nitroglycerin should be discontinued if blurred vision or dry mouth occurs.
- Severe orthostatic hypotension may occur, manifested by fainting, pulselessness, cold or clammy skin, and diaphoresis.
- Tolerance may occur with repeated, prolonged therapy; minor tolerance may occur with intermittent use of sublingual tablets.
- High doses of nitroglycerin tend to produce severe headache.

INTERACTIONS

Drugs

❷ *Ergot alkaloids:* Opposition to coronary vasodilatory effects of nitrates

3 *Ethanol:* Additive vasodilation could cause hypotension

3 *Metronidazole:* Ethanol, other antihypertensives, vasodilators contained in IV nitroglycerine preparations could cause disulfiram-like reaction in some patients

3 *Sildenafil, tadalafil, vardenafil:* Excessive hypotensive effects

Labs

- *False increase:* Serum triglycerides

SPECIAL CONSIDERATIONS

- 10-12-hrs drug-free intervals prevent development of tolerance
- Remove the transdermal patch before cardioversion or defibrillation because the electrical current may cause arcing, which can burn the patient and damage the paddles

PATIENT/FAMILY EDUCATION

- Avoid alcohol
- Notify clinician if persistent headache occurs
- Take oral nitrates on empty stomach with full glass of water
- Keep tablets and capsules in original container, keep container closed tightly
- Dissolve SL tablets under tongue, lack of burning does not indicate loss of potency, use when seated, take at first sign of anginal attack, activate emergency response system if no relief after 3 tablets spaced 5 min apart
- Spray translingual spray onto or under tongue, do not inhale spray
- Place buccal tablets under upper lip or between cheek and gum, permit to dissolve slowly over 3-5 min, do not chew or swallow

• Spread thin layer of ointment on skin using applicator or dose-measuring papers, do not use fingers, do not rub or massage
• Apply transdermal systems to non-hairy area on upper torso, remove for 10-12 hr/day (usually hs)

MONITORING PARAMETERS
• Blood pressure, heart rate at peak effect times
• EKG during IV administration
• Examine the patient for facial or neck flushing

nitroprusside sodium

(nye-troe-pruss'-ide)
Rx: Nitropress
Chemical Class: Cyanonitrosylferrate derivative
Therapeutic Class: Antihypertensive

CLINICAL PHARMACOLOGY
Mechanism of Action: A potent vasodilator used to treat emergent hypertensive conditions; acts directly on arterial and venous smooth muscle. Decreases peripheral vascular resistance, preload and afterload; improves cardiac output. ***Therapeutic Effect:*** Dilates coronary arteries, decreases oxygen consumption, and relieves persistent chest pain.
Pharmacokinetics

Route	Onset	Peak	Duration
IV	1-10 mins	Dependent on infusion rate	Dissipates rapidly after stopping IV

Reacts with Hgb in erythrocytes, producing cyanmethemoglobin, and cyanide ions. Primarily excreted in urine. ***Half-life:*** less than 10 mins.

INDICATIONS AND DOSAGES
Immediate reduction of BP in hypertensive crisis; to produce controlled hypotension in surgical procedures to reduce bleeding; treatment of acute CHF
IV Infusion
Adults, Elderly. Initially, 0.3-0.5 mcg/kg/min. May increase by 0.5 mcg/kg/min to desired hemodynamic effect or appearance of headache or nausea. Usual dose: 3 mcg/kg/min. Maximum: 10 mcg/kg/min.

AVAILABLE FORMS
• *Injection:* 25 mg/ml.
• *Powder for Injection:* 50 mg.

UNLABELED USES: Control of paroxysmal hypertension before and during surgery for pheochromocytoma, peripheral vasospasm caused by ergot alkaloid overdose, treatment adjunct for MI, valvular regurgitation

CONTRAINDICATIONS: Compensatory hypertension (atrioventricular [AV] shunt or coarctation of aorta), congenital (Leber's) optic atrophy, inadequate cerebral circulation, moribund patients, tobacco amblyopia

PREGNANCY AND LACTATION: Pregnancy category C; excretion into breast milk is unknown; use caution in nursing mothers

SIDE EFFECTS
Occasional
Flushing of skin, increased intracranial pressure, rash, pain or redness at injection site

SERIOUS REACTIONS
• A too-rapid IV infusion rate reduces BP too quickly.
• Nausea, vomiting, diaphoresis, apprehension, headache, restlessness, muscle twitching, dizziness, palpitations, retrosternal pain, and abdominal pain may occur. Symp-

toms disappear rapidly if rate of administration is slowed or drug is temporarily discontinued.

- Overdose produces metabolic acidosis and tolerance to therapeutic effect.

INTERACTIONS

Drugs

3 *Clonidine:* Severe hypotensive reactions have been reported

3 *Diltiazem:* Reduction in the dose of nitroprusside required to produce hypotension

3 *Dobutamine:* May increase cardiac output and decrease pulmonary wedge pressure

3 *Guanabenz, guanfacine:* Potential for severe hypotensive reactions

SPECIAL CONSIDERATIONS

PATIENT/FAMILY EDUCATION

- Immediately report dizziness, headache, nausea, palpitations, or other unusual signs or symptoms

MONITORING PARAMETERS

- Blood pressure, arterial blood gases, oxygen saturation, cyanide and thiocyanate concentrations, anion gap, lactate levels
- Intake and output
- Monitor the rate of infusion frequently
- Therapeutic response—expect to discontinue nitroprusside if the therapeutic response is not achieved within 10 mins after IV infusion at 10 mcg/kg/mins is initiated

nizatidine

(nye-za'-ti-deen)

Rx: Axid

OTC: Axid AR

Chemical Class: Ethenediamine derivative

Therapeutic Class: Antiulcer agent

CLINICAL PHARMACOLOGY

Mechanism of Action: An antiulcer agent and gastric acid secretion inhibitor that inhibits histamine action at $histamine_2$ receptors of parietal cells. ***Therapeutic Effect:*** Inhibits basal and nocturnal gastric acid secretion.

Pharmacokinetics

Rapidly, well absorbed from the GI tract. Protein binding: 35%. Metabolized in the liver. Primarily excreted in urine. Not removed by hemodialysis. ***Half-life:*** 1-2 hr (increased with impaired renal function).

INDICATIONS AND DOSAGES

Active duodenal ulcer

PO

Adults, Elderly. 300 mg at bedtime or 150 mg twice a day.

Prevention of duodenal ulcer recurrence

PO

Adults, Elderly. 150 mg at bedtime.

Gastroesophageal reflux disease

PO

Adults, Elderly. 150 mg twice a day.

Active benign gastric ulcer

PO

Adults, Elderly. 150 mg twice a day or 300 mg at bedtime.

PO, oral solution

Children 12 yr and older. 2 tsp twice a day.

Dyspepsia
PO
Adults, Elderly. 75 mg 30-60 min before meals; no more than 2 tablets a day.
Dosage in renal impairment
Dosage adjustment is based on creatinine clearance.

Creatinine Clearance	*Active Ulcer*	*Maintenance Therapy*
20-50 ml/min	150 mg at bedtime	150 mg every other day
less than 20 ml/min	150 mg every other day	150 mg q3 days

AVAILABLE FORMS
• *Capsules:* 75 mg (Axid AR), 150 mg (Axid), 300 mg (Axid).
• *Oral Solution (Axid):* 15 mg/ml.
UNLABELED USES: Gastric hypersecretory conditions, multiple endocrine adenoma, Zollinger-Ellison syndrome, weight gain reduction in patients taking Zyprexa
CONTRAINDICATIONS: Hypersensitivity to other H_2-antagonists
PREGNANCY AND LACTATION: Pregnancy category B; excreted in breast milk (0.1% of dose)
SIDE EFFECTS
Occasional (2%)
Somnolence, fatigue
Rare (1%)
Diaphoresis, rash
SERIOUS REACTIONS
• Asymptomatic ventricular tachycardia, hyperuricemia not associated with gout, and nephrolithiasis occur rarely.
INTERACTIONS
Drugs
3 *Antacids:* May decrease the absorption of nazatidine
3 *Cefpodoxime, cefuroxime; enoxacin; ketoconazole:* Reduction in gastric acidity reduces absorption, decreases plasma levels, potential for therapeutic failure
3 *Glipizide, glyburide tolbutamide:* Increased absorption of these drugs, potential for hypoglycemia
3 *Nifedipine, nitrendipine, nisoldipine:* Increased concentrations of these drugs
SPECIAL CONSIDERATIONS
• No advantage over other agents of this class, base selection on cost
PATIENT/FAMILY EDUCATION
• Stagger doses of nizatidine and antacids
• Avoid tasks that require mental alertness or motor skills until response to the drug has been established
• Avoid alcohol, aspirin, and smoking during nizatidine therapy
• Notify the physician if acid indigestion, gastric distress, or heartburn occurs after 2 wks of continuous nizatidine therapy
MONITORING PARAMETERS
• Serum alkaline phosphatase, bilirubin, AST (SGOT), and ALT (SGPT) levels
• Assess the patient for abdominal pain and GI bleeding. Observe for overt blood in emesis or stool and for tarry stools

norepinephrine bitartrate
(nor-ep-i-nef′-rin bi-tar′-trate)
Rx: Levophed
Chemical Class: Catecholamine, synthetic
Therapeutic Class: Vasopressor; α- and β-adrenergic sympathomimetic

CLINICAL PHARMACOLOGY
Mechanism of Action: A sympathomimetic that stimulates $beta_1$-adrenergic receptors and alpha-adrenergic receptors, increasing peripheral resistance. Enhances contractile

myocardial force, increases cardiac output. Constricts resistance and capacitance vessels. ***Therapeutic Effect:*** Increases systemic BP and coronary blood flow.

Pharmacokinetics

Route	*Onset*	*Peak*	*Duration*
IV	Rapid	1-2 min	N/A

Localized in sympathetic tissue. Metabolized in the liver. Primarily excreted in urine.

INDICATIONS AND DOSAGES

Acute hypotension unresponsive to fluid volume replacement

IV

Adults, Elderly. Initially, administer at 0.5-1 mcg/min. Adjust rate of flow to establish and maintain desired BP (40 mm Hg below preexisting systolic pressure). Average maintenance dose: 8-30 mcg/min.

Children. Initially, 0.05-0.1 mcg/kg/min; titrate to desired effect. Maximum: 1-2 mcg/kg/min. Range: 0.5-3 mcg/min.

AVAILABLE FORMS

- *Injection:* 1-mg/ml ampules.

CONTRAINDICATIONS: Hypovolemic states (unless as an emergency measure), mesenteric or peripheral vascular thrombosis, profound hypoxia

PREGNANCY AND LACTATION: Pregnancy category C

SIDE EFFECTS

Norepinephrine produces less pronounced and less frequent side effects than epinephrine.

Occasional (5%-3%)

Anxiety, bradycardia, palpitations

Rare (2%-1%)

Nausea, anginal pain, shortness of breath, fever

SERIOUS REACTIONS

- Extravasation may produce tissue necrosis and sloughing.
- Overdose is manifested as severe hypertension with violent headache (which may be the first clinical sign of overdose), arrhythmias, photophobia, retrosternal or pharyngeal pain, pallor, excessive sweating, and vomiting.
- Prolonged therapy may result in plasma volume depletion. Hypotension may recur if plasma volume is not restored.

INTERACTIONS

Drugs

❷ *Amitriptyline, desipramine, imipramine, protriptyline:* Marked enhancement of pressor response to norepinephrine

❸ *β-blockers:* May have mutually inhibitory effects

❸ *Digoxin:* May increase the risk of arrhythmias

❸ *Guanadrel, guanethidine:* Exaggerated pressor response to norepinephrine

❸ *MAOIs:* Slight increase in the pressor response to norepinephrine

❸ *Methyldopa:* Prolongation in the pressor response to norepinephrine

❸ *Tricyclic antidepressants:* May increase cardiovascular effects

SPECIAL CONSIDERATIONS

- Antidote for extravasation ischemia: infiltrate with 10-15 ml of saline containing 5-10 mg of phentolamine

PATIENT/FAMILY EDUCATION

- Immediately report burning, pain, or coolness at the IV site

MONITORING PARAMETERS

- Blood pressure, heart rate, ECG, urine output, peripheral perfusion
- Assess the patient for extravasation. If extravasation occurs, expect to infiltrate the affected area with 10-15 ml sterile saline containing 5-10 mg phentolamine. Know that phentolamine does not alter the pressor effects of norepinephrine

N

norethindrone

(nor-eth-in'-drone)

Rx: Aygestin, Camila, Errin, Jolivette, Micronor, Nora-BE, Nor-QD

Combinations

Rx: with ethinyl estradiol (see oral contraceptives)

Chemical Class: 19-nortestosterone derivative; progestin derivative

Therapeutic Class: Contraceptive; progestin

CLINICAL PHARMACOLOGY

Mechanism of Action: A synthetic progestin that is used as a single agent or in combination with estrogens for the treatment of gynecologic disorders. It inhibits secretion of pituitary gonadotropin (LH), which prevents follicular maturation and ovulation. ***Therapeutic Effect:*** Transforms endometrium from proliferative to secretory in an estrogen-primed endometrium, promotes mammary gland development, relaxes uterine smooth muscle.

Pharmacokinetics

Rapidly absorbed from the gastrointestinal (GI) tract. Widely distributed. Protein binding: 61%. Metabolized in liver. Excreted in urine and feces. ***Half-life:*** 4-13 hrs.

INDICATIONS AND DOSAGES

Contraception

PO

Adults. 1 tablet/day.

Amenorrhea and abnormal uterine bleeding

PO

Adults. 5-20 mg/day cyclically (21 days on; 7 days off or continuously) or for acetate salt formulation, 2.5-10 mg cyclically.

Endometriosis

PO

Adults. 10 mg/day for 2 wks, increase at increments of 5 mg/day every 2 wks until 30 mg/day; continue for 6-9 mos or until breakthrough bleeding demands temporary termination. For acetate salt formulation, 5 mg/day for 14 days, increase at increments of 2.5 mg/day every 2 wks up to 15 mg/day; continue for 6-9 mos or until breakthrough bleeding demands temporary termination.

AVAILABLE FORMS

- *Tablets:* 0.35 mg (Camila, Errin, Jolivette, Micronor, Nora-BE, Nor-QD).
- *Tablets, as norethindrone acetate:* 5 mg (Aygestin).

UNLABELED USES: Treatment of corpus luteum dysfunction

CONTRAINDICATIONS: Acute liver disease, benign or malignant liver tumors, hypersensitivity to norethindrone and any component of the formulation, known or suspected carcinoma of the breast, known or suspected pregnancy, undiagnosed abnormal genital bleeding

PREGNANCY AND LACTATION: Pregnancy category X; compatible with breast-feeding

SIDE EFFECTS

Occasional

Breast tenderness, dizziness, headache, breakthrough bleeding, amenorrhea, menstrual irregularity, nausea, weakness

Rare

Mental depression, fever, insomnia, rash, acne, increased breast tenderness, weight gain/loss, changes in cervical erosion and secretions, cholestatic jaundice

SERIOUS REACTIONS

• Thrombophlebitis, cerebrovascular disorders, retinal thrombosis, cholestatic jaundice, and pulmonary embolism occur rarely.

INTERACTIONS

Drugs

3 *Hepatic enzyme-inducing drugs (e.g., phenytoin, carbamazepine, barbiturates, rifampin):* May decrease the effectiveness of norethindrone

SPECIAL CONSIDERATIONS

PATIENT/FAMILY EDUCATION

• Missed dose: one tablet—take as soon as remembered, or take 2 tablets at next regular time

• Missed 2 consecutive tablets—take 2 tablets at next 2 regular times

• Three missed tablets—discontinue, restart after menses appear or pregnancy is ruled out

NOTE: Use an additional method of contraception if 2 or more tablets are missed until menses appear or pregnancy ruled out

• Progestin-only pills have slightly higher failure rate than combination oral contraceptives

• When used as contraceptive, menstrual cycle may be disrupted and irregular and unpredictable bleeding or spotting may result

• Notify the physician of abnormal vaginal bleeding or other symptoms

• Stop smoking tobacco

MONITORING PARAMETERS

• Weight

• Blood pressure

norfloxacin

(nor-flox'-a-sin)

Rx: Noroxin

Chemical Class: Fluoroquinolone derivative

Therapeutic Class: Antibiotic

CLINICAL PHARMACOLOGY

Mechanism of Action: A quinolone that inhibits DNA gyrase in susceptible microorganisms, interfering with bacterial cell replication and repair. ***Therapeutic Effect:*** Bactericidal.

Pharmacokinetics

Well absorbed following oral administration. Protein binding: 10%-15%. Eliminated through metabolism, biliary excretion, and renal excretion. ***Half-life:*** 3-4 hr.

INDICATIONS AND DOSAGES

UTIs

PO

Adults, Elderly. 400 mg twice a day for 3-21 days.

Prostatitis

PO

Adults. 400 mg twice a day for 28 days.

Uncomplicated gonococcal infections

PO

Adults. 800 mg as a single dose.

Dosage in renal impairment

Dosage and frequency are modified based on creatinine clearance.

Creatinine Clearance	*Dosage*
30 ml/min or higher	400 mg twice a day
less than 30 ml/min	400 mg once a day

AVAILABLE FORMS

• *Tablets:* 400 mg.

CONTRAINDICATIONS: Children younger than 18 yrs because of risk of arthropathy; hypersensitivity to other quinolones or their components

N

PREGNANCY AND LACTATION: Pregnancy category C; excretion into breast milk unknown; due to the potential for arthropathy and osteochondrosis use extreme caution in nursing mothers

SIDE EFFECTS

Frequent

Nausea, headache, dizziness

Rare

Vomiting, diarrhea, dry mouth, bitter taste, nervousness, drowsiness, insomnia, photosensitivity, tinnitus, crystalluria, rash, fever, seizures

SERIOUS REACTIONS

• Superinfection, anaphylaxis, Stevens-Johnson syndrome, and arthropathy occur rarely.

• Hypersensitivity reactions, including photosensitivity (as evidenced by rash, pruritus, blisters, edema, and burning skin), have occurred in patients receiving fluoroquinolones.

INTERACTIONS

Drugs

3 *Aluminum:* Reduced absorption of norfloxacin; do not take within 4 hr of dose

3 *Antithyroid agents:* May increase the risk of agranulocytosis

3 *Antacids:* Reduced absorption of norfloxacin; do not take within 4 hr of dose

3 *Antipyrine:* Inhibits metabolism of antipyrine; increased plasma antipyrine level

3 *Caffeine:* Inhibits metabolism of caffeine; increased plasma caffeine level

3 *Calcium:* Reduced absorption of norfloxacin; do not take within 4 hr of dose

3 *Diazepam:* Inhibits metabolism of diazepam; increased plasma diazepam level

3 *Didanosine:* Markedly reduced absorption of norfloxacin; take norfloxacin 2 hr before didanosine

3 *Foscarnet:* Coadministration increase seizure risk

3 *Iron:* Reduced absorption of norfloxacin; do not take within 4 hr of dose

3 *Magnesium:* Reduced absorption of norfloxacin; do not take within 4 hr of dose

3 *Metoprolol:* Inhibits metabolism of metoprolol; increased plasma metoprolol level

3 *Pentoxifylline:* Inhibits metabolism of pentoxifylline; increased plasma pentoxifylline level

3 *Phenytoin:* Inhibits metabolism of phenytoin; increased plasma phenytoin level

3 *Propranolol:* Inhibits metabolism of propranolol; increased plasma propranolol level

3 *Ropinirole:* Inhibits metabolism of ropinirole; increased plasma ropinirole level

3 *Sodium bicarbonate:* Reduced absorption of norfloxacin; do not take within 4 hr of dose

3 *Sucralfate:* Reduced absorption of norfloxacin; do not take within 4 hr of dose

3 *Theobromine:* Inhibits metabolism of theobromine; increased plasma theobromine level

3 *Theophylline:* Inhibits metabolism of theophylline; cut maintenance theophylline dose in half during therapy with norfloxacin

3 *Warfarin:* Inhibits metabolism of warfarin; increases hypoprothrombinemic response to warfarin

3 *Zinc:* Reduced absorption of norfloxacin; do not take within 4 hr of dose

Labs

• *False increase:* Uroporphyrin

SPECIAL CONSIDERATIONS

PATIENT/FAMILY EDUCATION

• Administer on an empty stomach (1 hr before or 2 hr after meals)

• Drink fluids liberally

• Do not take antacids containing magnesium or aluminum or products containing iron or zinc within 4 hr before or 2 hr after dosing
• Avoid excessive exposure to sunlight
• Take for the full course of therapy
• May cause dizziness or drowsiness
• Take sips of tepid water or chew sugarless gum to relieve dry mouth

MONITORING PARAMETERS

• Assess the patient for chest pain, dizziness, headache, joint pain, and nausea
• Evaluate the patient's food tolerance

norgestrel

(nor-jes´-trel)

Rx: Ovrette

Combinations

Rx: with ethinyl estradiol (see oral contraceptives)

Chemical Class: 19-nortestosterone derivative; progestin derivative

Therapeutic Class: Contraceptive; progestin

CLINICAL PHARMACOLOGY

Mechanism of Action: A progestin that inhibits secretion of pituitary gonadotropin (LH), which prevents follicular maturation and ovulation. ***Therapeutic Effect:*** Transforms endometrium from proliferative to secretory in an estrogen-primed endometrium, promotes mammary gland development, relaxes uterine smooth muscle.

Pharmacokinetics

Well absorbed from the gastrointestinal (GI) tract. Widely distributed. Protein binding: 97%. Metabolized in liver via reduction and conjugation. Primarily excreted in urine. ***Half-life:*** 20 hrs.

INDICATIONS AND DOSAGES

Contraception, female

PO

Adults. 0.075 mg/day.

AVAILABLE FORMS

• *Tablets:* 0.075 mg (Ovrette).

UNLABELED USES: Endometrial protection, endometriosis, menorrhagia

CONTRAINDICATIONS: Hypersensitivity to norgestrel or any component of the formulation, hypersensitivity to tartrazine, thromboembolic disorders, severe hepatic disease, breast cancer, undiagnosed vaginal bleeding, pregnancy

PREGNANCY AND LACTATION: Pregnancy category X; compatible with breast-feeding

SIDE EFFECTS

Frequent

Breakthrough bleeding or spotting at beginning of therapy, amenorrhea, change in menstrual flow, breast tenderness

Occasional

Edema, weight gain or loss, rash, pruritus, photosensitivity, skin pigmentation

Rare

Pain or swelling at injection site, acne, mental depression, alopecia, hirsutism

SERIOUS REACTIONS

• Thrombophlebitis, cerebrovascular disorders, retinal thrombosis, and pulmonary embolism occur rarely.

SPECIAL CONSIDERATIONS

PATIENT/FAMILY EDUCATION

• Missed dose: one tablet—take as soon as remembered, take next tablet at regular time; two consecutive tablets—take 1 of the missed tablets, discard the other
• Three missed tablets—discontinue

• Use an additional method of contraception if 2 or more tablets are missed until menses appear or pregnancy ruled out.
• Progestin-only pills have slightly higher failure rate than combination oral contraceptives
• Take with food if GI upset occurs
• Menstrual cycle may be disrupted and irregular and unpredictable bleeding or spotting can result
• Based on WHO study, norgestrel (levonorgestrel)-only pills preferred emergency contraception; equal efficacy and 50% less nausea, vomiting compared to combined regimen
• Notify the physician of abnormal vaginal bleeding or other symptoms

MONITORING PARAMETERS

• Blood pressure
• Weight

nortriptyline hydrochloride

(noor-trip'-ti-leen hye-droe-klor'-ide)

Rx: Aventyl, Pamelor

Chemical Class: Dibenzocycloheptene derivative; secondary amine

Therapeutic Class: Antidepressant, tricyclic

CLINICAL PHARMACOLOGY

Mechanism of Action: A tricyclic antidepressant that blocks reuptake of the neurotransmitters norepinephrine and serotonin at neuronal presynaptic membranes, increasing their availability at postsynaptic receptor sites. ***Therapeutic Effect:*** Relieves depression.

Pharmacokinetics

Well absorbed from the GI tract. Protein binding: 86%-95%. Metabolized in the liver. Primarily excreted in urine. ***Half-life:*** 17.6 hr.

INDICATIONS AND DOSAGES

Depression

PO

Adults. 75-100 mg/day in 1-4 divided doses until therapeutic response is achieved. Reduce dosage gradually to effective maintenance level.

Elderly. Initially, 10-25 mg at bedtime. May increase by 25 mg every 3-7 days. Maximum: 150 mg/day.

Children 12 yrs and older. 30-50 mg/day in 3-4 divided doses. Maximum: 150 mg/day.

Children 6-11 yrs. 10-20 mg/day in 3-4 divided doses.

Enuresis

PO

Children 12 yrs and older. 25-35 mg/day.

Children 8-11 yrs. 10-20 mg/day.

Children 6-7 yrs. 10 mg/day.

AVAILABLE FORMS

• *Capsules (Aventyl):* 10 mg, 25 mg.
• *Capsules (Pamelor):* 10 mg, 25 mg, 50 mg, 75 mg.
• *Oral Solution (Aventyl, Pamelor):* 10 mg/5 ml.

UNLABELED USES: Treatment of neurogenic pain, panic disorder; prevention of migraine headache

CONTRAINDICATIONS: Acute recovery period after MI, use within 14 days of MAOIs

PREGNANCY AND LACTATION: Pregnancy category D; effect on nursing infant unknown but may be of concern, especially after prolonged exposure

SIDE EFFECTS

Frequent

Somnolence, fatigue, dry mouth, blurred vision, constipation, delayed micturition, orthostatic hypotension, diaphoresis, impaired concentration, increased appetite, urine retention

Occasional
GI disturbances (nausea, GI distress, metallic taste), photosensitivity
Rare
Paradoxical reactions (agitation, restlessness, nightmares, insomnia), extrapyramidal symptoms (particularly fine hand tremor)

SERIOUS REACTIONS

• Overdose may produce seizures; cardiovascular effects, such as severe orthostatic hypotension, dizziness, tachycardia, palpitations, and arrhythmias; and altered temperature regulation, such as hyperpyrexia or hypothermia.

• Abrupt discontinuation after prolonged therapy may produce headache, malaise, nausea, vomiting, and vivid dreams.

INTERACTIONS

Drugs

3 *Anticholinergics:* Excessive anticholinergic effects
3 *Antithyroid agents:* May increase the risk of agranulocytosis
3 *Barbiturates:* Reduced serum concentrations of cyclic antidepressants
3 *Carbamazepine, rifampin:* Reduced cyclic antidepressant serum concentrations
3 *Chlorpropamide:* Enhanced by hypoglycemic effects of chlorpropamide
3 *Cimetidine:* Increased serum nortriptyline concentrations
3 *Clonidine:* Reduced antihypertensive response to clonidine; enhanced hypertensive response with abrupt clonidine withdrawal
2 *Epinephrine:* Markedly enhanced pressor response to IV epinephrine
3 *Ethanol:* Additive impairment of motor skills; abstinent alcoholics may eliminate cyclic antidepressants more rapidly than non-alcoholics
3 *Fluoxetine:* Marked increases in cyclic antidepressant plasma concentrations
2 *Guanethidine:* Inhibited antihypertensive response to guanethidine
2 *Moclobemide:* Potential association with fatal or non-fatal serotonin syndrome
▲ *MAOIs:* Excessive sympathetic response, mania or hyperpyrexia possible
3 *Neuroleptics:* Increased therapeutic and toxic effects of both drugs
2 *Norepinephrine:* Markedly enhanced pressor response to norepinephrine
3 *Phenylephrine:* Enhanced pressor response to IV phenylephrine
3 *Propoxyphene:* Enhanced effect of cyclic antidepressants
3 *Quinidine:* Increased cyclic antidepressant serum concentrations

Labs

• *False increase:* Serum carbamazepine

SPECIAL CONSIDERATIONS

PATIENT/FAMILY EDUCATION

• Therapeutic effects may take 2-3 wk
• Avoid rising quickly from sitting to standing, especially in elderly
• Avoid alcohol and other CNS depressants
• Do not discontinue abruptly after long-term use
• Wear sunscreen or large hat to prevent sunburn
• Avoid tasks that require mental alertness or motor skills until response to the drug has been established
• Notify the physician of visual disturbances

N

• Take sips of tepid water or chew sugarless gum to relieve dry mouth

MONITORING PARAMETERS

• CBC, weight, ECG, mental status (mood, sensorium, affect, suicidal tendencies)

• Determination of nortriptyline plasma concentrations is not routinely recommended but may be useful in identifying toxicity, drug interactions, or noncompliance (adjustments in dosage should be made according to clinical response not plasma concentrations), therapeutic range 50-150 ng/ml

• Blood pressure, pulse rate

• Pattern of daily bowel activity and stool consistency

nystatin

(nye-stat'-in)

Rx: Bio-Statin, Mycostatin, Mycostatin Pastilles, Mycostatin Topical, Nyaderm, Nystat-Rx, Nystex, Nystop, Pedi-Dri

Combinations

Rx: *Topical:* with triamcinolone (Mycolog-II, Mycomer, Mycasone, Myco Biotic II, Tri-Statin II, Mytrex, Myco-Triacet II, Mycogen II)

Chemical Class: Amphoteric polyene macrolide

Therapeutic Class: Antifungal

CLINICAL PHARMACOLOGY

Mechanism of Action: A fungistatic antifungal that binds to sterols in the fungal cell membrane. ***Therapeutic Effect:*** Increases fungal cell-membrane permeability, allowing loss of potassium and other cellular components.

Pharmacokinetics

PO: Poorly absorbed from the GI tract. Eliminated unchanged in feces. Topical: Not absorbed systemically from intact skin.

INDICATIONS AND DOSAGES

Intestinal infections

PO

Adults, Elderly. 500,000-1,000,000 units q8h.

Oral candidiasis

PO

Adults, Elderly, Children. 400,000-600,000 units 4 times/day.

Infants. 200,000 units 4 times/day.

Vaginal infections

Vaginal

Adults, Elderly, Adolescents. 1 tablet/day at bedtime for 14 days.

Cutaneous candidal infections

Topical

Adults, Elderly, Children. Apply 2-4 times/day.

AVAILABLE FORMS

• *Oral Suspension (Mycostatin):* 100,000 units/ml.

• *Tablets (Mycostatin):* 500,000 units.

• *Capsules (Bio-Statin):* 500,000 units, 1,000,000 units.

• *Oral Lozenge (Mycostatin Pastilles):* 200,000 units.

• *Vaginal Tablets:* 100,000 units.

• *Cream (Mycostatin Topical):* 100,000 units/g.

• *Ointment:* 100,000 units/g.

• *Topical Powder (Mycostatin Topical, Nystop, Pedi-Dri):* 100,000 units/g.

• *Powder (Compounding):* 50,000,000 units (Nystat-Rx), 150,000,000 units (Bio-Statin, Nystat-Rx), 500,000,000 units (Nystat-Rx), 1,000,000,000 units, 2,000,000,000 units (Bio-Statin, Nystat-Rx).

UNLABELED USES: Prophylaxis and treatment of oropharyngeal candidiasis, tinea barbae, tinea capitis

CONTRAINDICATIONS: None known.

PREGNANCY AND LACTATION: Pregnancy category C; due to poor bioavailability, serum and breast milk levels do not occur

SIDE EFFECTS

Occasional

PO: None known

Topical: Skin irritation

Vaginal: Vaginal irritation

SERIOUS REACTIONS

- High dosages of oral form may produce nausea, vomiting, diarrhea, and GI distress.

SPECIAL CONSIDERATIONS

PATIENT/FAMILY EDUCATION

- Do not use troches in child <5 yrs
- Do not miss a dose and complete the full course of treatment
- Swish the oral suspension in the mouth for as long as possible before swallowing
- Insert the vaginal form high into the vagina and continue using the drug during menstruation
- Do not let the topical form come in contact with the eyes
- Rub the topical form well into affected areas, keep affected areas clean and dry, and wear light clothing for ventilation

MONITORING PARAMETERS

- Assess the patient for increased irritation with topical application or increased vaginal discharge with vaginal application

octreotide acetate

(ok-tree'-oh-tide)

Rx: Sandostatin, Sandostatin Lar Depot

Chemical Class: Somatostatin analog

Therapeutic Class: Acromegaly agent; antidiarrheal

CLINICAL PHARMACOLOGY

Mechanism of Action: An antidiarrheal and growth hormone suppressant that suppresses the secretion of serotonin and gastroenteropancreatic peptides and enhances fluid and electrolyte absorption from the GI tract. ***Therapeutic Effect:*** Prolongs intestinal transit time.

Pharmacokinetics

Route	*Onset*	*Peak*	*Duration*
Subcutaneous	N/A	N/A	Up to 12 hr

Rapidly and completely absorbed from injection site. Excreted in urine. Removed by hemodialysis. ***Half-life:*** 1.5 hr.

INDICATIONS AND DOSAGES

Diarrhea

IV (Sandostatin)

Adults, Elderly. Initially, 50-100 mcg q8h. May increase by 100 mcg/dose q48h. Maximum: 500 mcg q8h.

Subcutaneous (Sandostatin)

Adults, Elderly. 50 mcg 1-2 times a day.

IV, Subcutaneous (Sandostatin)

Children. 1-10 mcg/kg q12h.

Carcinoid tumors

IV, Subcutaneous (Sandostatin)

Adults, Elderly. 100-600 mcg/day in 2-4 divided doses.

IM (Sandostatin LAR)

Adults, Elderly. 20 mg q4wk.

Vipomas
IV, Subcutaneous (Sandostatin)
Adults, Elderly. 200-300 mcg/day in 2-4 divided doses.
IM (Sandostatin LAR)
Adults, Elderly. 20 mg q4wk.
Esophageal varices
IV (Sandostatin)
Adults, Elderly. Bolus of 25-50 mcg followed by IV infusion of 25-50 mcg/hr for 48 hr.
Acromegaly
IV, Subcutaneous (Sandostatin)
Adults, Elderly. 50 mcg 3 times a day. Increase as needed. Maximum: 500 mcg 3 times a day.
IM (Sandostatin LAR Depot)
Adults, Elderly. 20 mg q4wk for 3 mo. Maximum: 40 mg q4wk.

AVAILABLE FORMS
- *Injection (Sandostatin):* 0.05 mg/ml, 0.1 mg/ml, 0.2 mg/ml, 0.5 mg/ml, 1 mg/ml.
- *Suspension for Injection (Sandostatin LAR Depot):* 10-mg, 20-mg, 30-mg vials.

UNLABELED USES: Control of bleeding esophageal varices, treatment of AIDS-associated secretory diarrhea, chemotherapy-induced diarrhea, insulinomas, small-bowel fistulas, control of bleeding esophageal varices

CONTRAINDICATIONS: None known.

PREGNANCY AND LACTATION: Pregnancy category B; breast milk excretion unknown

SIDE EFFECTS
Frequent (10%-6%, 58%-30% in acromegaly patients)
Diarrhea, nausea, abdominal discomfort, headache, injection site pain
Occasional (5%-1%)
Vomiting, flatulence, constipation, alopecia, facial flushing, pruritus, dizziness, fatigue, arrhythmias, ecchymosis, blurred vision
Rare (less than 1%)
Depression, diminished libido, vertigo, palpitations, dyspnea

SERIOUS REACTIONS
- Patients using octreotide may develop cholelithiasis or, with prolonged high dosages, hypothyroidism.
- GI bleeding, hepatitis, and seizures occur rarely.

INTERACTIONS
Drugs
❷ *Cyclosporine:* Decreased serum cyclosporine concentrations
❸ *Oral hypoglycemic agents, insulin:* Octreotide can alter glycemic control, dose adjustment of antidiabetic agents may be necessary

SPECIAL CONSIDERATIONS
- Octreotide is incompatible in TPN solutions
- Patient tolerance to ocreotide should be determined with 2 wks SC/IV therapy before switching to depot therapy
- Only give depot intragluteally, avoid deltoid injections due to pain at injection site
- Withdraw octreotide yearly for 4 wk in acromegaly patients who have received irradiation to assess disease activity
- Notify the physician about any unusual signs or symptoms, such as palpitations or unusual bleeding
- Weigh patient daily; and report a weight gain of more than 5 lb per week

MONITORING PARAMETERS
- Thyroid function, serum glucose (especially in drug-treated diabetics), vitamin B_{12} levels
- Heart rate (especially in persons taking β-blockers and calcium channel blockers)
- Periodic zinc levels in patients receiving TPN
- Blood pressure
- Weight

ofloxacin

(oh-floks'-a-sin)

Rx: Floxin, Floxin Otic, Ocuflox

Chemical Class: Fluoroquinolone derivative

Therapeutic Class: Antibiotic

CLINICAL PHARMACOLOGY

Mechanism of Action: A fluoroquinolone antibiotic that inhibits DNA gyrase in susceptible microorganisms, interfering with bacterial cell replication and repair. ***Therapeutic Effect:*** Bactericidal.

Pharmacokinetics

Rapidly and well absorbed from the GI tract. Protein binding: 20%-25%. Widely distributed (including to cerebrospinal fluid [CSF]). Metabolized in the liver. Primarily excreted in urine. Removed by hemodialysis. ***Half-life:*** 4.7-7 hr (increased in impaired renal function, cirrhosis, and the elderly).

INDICATIONS AND DOSAGES

UTIs

PO

Adults. 200 mg q12h.

Pelvic inflammatory disease (PID)

PO

Adults. 400 mg q12h for 10-14 days.

Lower respiratory tract, skin and skin-structure infections

PO

Adults. 400 mg q12h for 10 days.

Prostatitis, sexually transmitted diseases (cervicitis, urethritis)

PO

Adults. 300 mg q12h.

Acute, uncomplicated gonorrhea

PO

Adults. 400 mg 1 time.

Usual elderly dosage

PO

Elderly. 200-400 mg q12-24h for 7 days up to 6 wk.

Bacterial conjunctivitis

Ophthalmic

Adults, Elderly. 1-2 drops q2-4h for 2 days, then 4 times a day for 5 days.

Corneal ulcers

Ophthalmic

Adults. 1-2 drops q30min while awake for 2 days, then q60min while awake for 5-7 days, then 4 times a day.

Acute otitis media

Otic

Children 1-12 yr. 5 drops into the affected ear 2 times/day for 10 days.

Otitis externa

Otic

Adults, Elderly, Children 12 yr and older. 10 drops into the affected ear once a day for 7 days.

Children 6 mo-11 yr. 5 drops into the affected ear once a day for 7 days.

Dosage in renal impairment

After a normal initial dose, dosage and frequency are based on creatinine clearance.

Creatinine Clearance	*Adjusted Dose*	*Dosage Interval*
greater than 50 ml/min	None	q12h
10-50 ml/min	None	q24h
less than 10 ml/min	½	q24h

AVAILABLE FORMS

- *Tablets (Floxin):* 200 mg, 300 mg, 400 mg.
- *Ophthalmic Solution (Ocuflox):* 0.3%.
- *Otic Solution (Floxin):* 0.3%.

CONTRAINDICATIONS: Children 18 yrs and younger, hypersensitivity to any quinolones

PREGNANCY AND LACTATION: Pregnancy category C; excreted into breast milk in quantities approximating maternal plasma concentrations; due to the potential for arthropathy and osteochondrosis, use extreme caution in nursing mothers

SIDE EFFECTS

Frequent (10%-7%)

Nausea, headache, insomnia

Occasional (5%-3%)

Abdominal pain, diarrhea, vomiting, dry mouth, flatulence, dizziness, fatigue, drowsiness, rash, pruritus, fever

Rare (less than 1%)

Constipation, paraesthesia

SERIOUS REACTIONS

- Antibiotic-associated colitis and other superinfections may occur from altered bacterial balance.
- Hypersensitivity reactions, including photosensitivity (as evidenced by rash, pruritus, blisters, edema, and burning skin), have occurred in patients receiving fluoroquinolones.
- Arthropathy (swelling, pain, and clubbing of fingers and toes, degeneration of stress-bearing portion of a joint) may occur if the drug is given to children.
- There is a risk of peripheral neuropathy, tendon rupture, and torsades de pointes.

INTERACTIONS

Drugs

3 *Aluminum:* Reduced absorption of ofloxacin; do not take within 4 hr of dose

3 *Antacids:* Reduced absorption of ofloxacin; do not take within 4 hr of dose

3 *Caffeine:* May increase the effects of caffeine

3 *Calcium:* Reduced absorption of ofloxacin; do not take within 4 hr of dose

3 *Iron:* Reduced absorption of ofloxacin; do not take within 4 hr of dose

3 *Magnesium:* Reduced absorption of ofloxacin; do not take within 4 hr of dose

3 *Procainamide:* Ofloxacin competitively inhibits renal tubular excretion of procainamide

3 *Sodium bicarbonate:* Reduced absorption of ofloxacin; do not take within 4 hr of dose

3 *Sucralfate:* Reduced absorption of ofloxacin; do not take within 4 hr of dose

3 *Theophylline:* May increase theophylline blood concentration and risk of toxicity

3 *Warfarin:* Inhibits metabolism of warfarin; increases hypoprothrombinemic response to warfarin

3 *Zinc:* Reduced absorption of ofloxacin; do not take within 4 hr of dose

Labs

- *False increase:* Uroporphyrin

SPECIAL CONSIDERATIONS

PATIENT/FAMILY EDUCATION

- Administer on an empty stomach (1 hr before or 2 hr after meals)
- Drink fluids liberally
- Do not take antacids containing magnesium or aluminum or products containing iron or zinc within 4 hr before or 2 hr after dosing
- Avoid excessive exposure to sunlight
- Ofloxacin may cause dizziness, drowsiness, headache, and insomnia
- Avoid tasks requiring mental alertness or motor skills until response to ofloxacin is established

MONITORING PARAMETERS

- Signs and symptoms of infection
- Mental status and WBC count
- Skin for rash; withhold the drug and promptly notify the physician at the first sign of a rash or another allergic reaction
- Pattern of daily bowel activity and stool consistency

• Evaluate the patient for dizziness, headache, tremors, and visual difficulties
• Be alert for signs of superinfection, such as anal or genital pruritus, fever, stomatitis, and vaginitis

olanzapine

(oh-lan'-zah-peen)

Rx: Zyprexa, Zyprexa Intramuscular, Zyprexa Zydis

Combinations

Rx: with fluoxetine (Symbyax)

Chemical Class: Thienbenzodiazepine derivative

Therapeutic Class: Antipsychotic

CLINICAL PHARMACOLOGY

Mechanism of Action: A thienobenzodiazepine derivative that antagonizes alpha$_1$-adrenergic, dopamine, histamine, muscarinic, and serotonin receptors. Produces anticholinergic, histaminic, and CNS depressant effects. ***Therapeutic Effect:*** Diminishes manifestations of psychotic symptoms.

Pharmacokinetics

Well absorbed after PO administration. Protein binding: 93%. Extensively distributed throughout the body. Undergoes extensive first-pass metabolism in the liver. Excreted primarily in urine and, to a lesser extent, in feces. Not removed by dialysis. ***Half-life:*** 21-54 hr.

INDICATIONS AND DOSAGES

Schizophrenia

PO

Adults. Initially, 5-10 mg once daily. May increase by 10 mg/day at 5-7-day intervals. If further adjustments are indicated, may increase by 5-10 mg/day at 7-day intervals. Range: 10-30 mg/day.

Elderly. Initially, 2.5 mg/day. May increase as indicated. Range: 2.5-10 mg/day.

Children. Initially, 2.5 mg/day. Titrate as necessary up to 20 mg/day.

Bipolar mania

PO

Adults. Initially, 10-15 mg/day. May increase by 5 mg/day at intervals of at least 24 hr. Maximum: 20 mg/day.

Children. Initially, 2.5 mg/day. Titrate as necessary up to 20 mg/day.

Dosage for elderly or debilitated patients and those predisposed to hypotensive reactions

The initial dosage for these patients is 5 mg/day.

Control agitation in schizophrenic or bipolar patients

IM

Adults, Elderly. 2.5-10 mg. May repeat 2h after first dose and 4h after second dose. Maximum: 30 mg/day.

AVAILABLE FORMS

• *Tablets (Zyprexa):* 2.5 mg, 5 mg, 7.5 mg, 10 mg, 15 mg, 20 mg.
• *Tablets (Orally Disintegrating [Zyprexa Zydis]):* 5 mg, 10 mg, 15 mg, 20 mg.
• *Injection (Zyprexa Intramuscular):* 10 mg.

UNLABELED USES: Treatment of anorexia, apathy, borderline personality disorder, Huntington's disease; maintenance of long-term treatment response in schizophrenic patients; nausea; vomiting

CONTRAINDICATIONS: None known.

PREGNANCY AND LACTATION: Pregnancy category C; excretion into human breast milk unknown; excreted in the milk of treated rats

SIDE EFFECTS

Frequent

Somnolence (26%), agitation (23%), insomnia (20%), headache (17%), nervousness (16%), hostility (15%), dizziness (11%), rhinitis (10%)

Occasional

Anxiety, constipation (9%); nonaggressive atypical behavior (8%); dry mouth (7%); weight gain (6%); orthostatic hypotension, fever, arthralgia, restlessness, cough, pharyngitis, visual changes (dim vision) (5%)

Rare

Tachycardia; back, chest, abdominal, or extremity pain; tremor

SERIOUS REACTIONS

- Rare reactions include seizures and neuroleptic malignant syndrome, a potentially fatal syndrome characterized by hyperpyrexia, muscle rigidity, irregular pulse or BP, tachycardia, diaphoresis, and cardiac arrhythmias.
- Extrapyramidal symptoms and dysphagia may also occur.
- Overdose (300 mg) produces drowsiness and slurred speech.

INTERACTIONS

Drugs

3 *Alcohol, other CNS depressants:* May increase CNS depressant effects

3 *Antihypertensives:* May increase the hypotensive effects of these drugs

3 *Carbamazepine:* Decreased olanzapine concentrations

3 *Cigarette smoking:* Reduces olanzapine plasma concentrations; smoking cessation may increase the risk of olanzapine toxicity

3 *Ciprofloxacin, fluvoxamine:* May increase the olanzapine blood concentration

3 *Imipramine, theophylline:* May inhibit the metabolism of these drugs

3 *Levodopa:* Antagonism of the effects of levodopa due to dopamine receptor blockade

3 *Ritonavir:* Reduces olanzapine serum concentrations

SPECIAL CONSIDERATIONS

PATIENT/FAMILY EDUCATION

- Avoid exposure to extreme heat
- Take olanzapine as ordered; do not abruptly discontinue the drug or increase the dosage
- Drowsiness generally subsides with continued therapy
- Avoid tasks requiring mental alertness or motor skills until response to the drug has been established
- The female patient should notify the physician if she becomes pregnant or intends to become pregnant during olanzapine therapy
- Take sips of tepid water and chew sugarless gum to help relieve dry mouth
- Maintain a healthy diet and exercise program to prevent weight gain

MONITORING PARAMETERS

- Periodic assessment of liver transaminases in patients with significant hepatic disease
- Blood pressure
- Closely supervise suicidal patients during early therapy; as depression lessens, the patient's energy level improves, which increases the suicide potential
- Assess for evidence of a therapeutic response, such as improvement in self-care, increased interest in surroundings and ability to concentrate, and relaxed facial expression
- Assess the patient's sleep pattern

• Monitor the patient for extrapyramidal symptoms, and notify the physician if they occur

olsalazine sodium

(ole-sal'-a-zeen soe'-dee-um)

Rx: Dipentum

Chemical Class: Salicylate derivative

Therapeutic Class: Gastrointestinal antiinflammatory

CLINICAL PHARMACOLOGY

Mechanism of Action: A salicylic acid derivative that is converted to mesalamine in the colon by bacterial action. Blocks prostaglandin production in bowel mucosa. ***Therapeutic Effect:*** Reduces colonic inflammation in inflammatory bowel disease.

Pharmacokinetics

Small amount absorbed. Protein binding: 99%. Metabolized by bacteria in the colon. Minimal elimination in urine and feces. ***Half-life:*** 0.9 hr.

INDICATIONS AND DOSAGES

Maintenance of controlled ulcerative colitis

PO

Adults, Elderly. 1 g/day in 2 divided doses, preferably q12h.

AVAILABLE FORMS

• *Capsules:* 250 mg.

UNLABELED USES: Treatment of inflammatory bowel disease

CONTRAINDICATIONS: History of hypersensitivity to salicylates

PREGNANCY AND LACTATION: Pregnancy category C; mesalamine has produced adverse effects in a nursing infant and should be used with caution during breast-feeding, observe nursing infant closely for changes in stool consistency

SIDE EFFECTS

Frequent (10%-5%)

Headache, diarrhea, abdominal pain or cramps, nausea

Occasional (5%-1%)

Depression, fatigue, dyspepsia, upper respiratory tract infection, decreased appetite, rash, itching, arthralgia

Rare (1%)

Dizziness, vomiting, stomatitis

SERIOUS REACTIONS

• Sulfite sensitivity may occur in susceptible patients, manifested by cramping, headache, diarrhea, fever, rash, hives, itching, and wheezing. Discontinue drug immediately.

• Excessive diarrhea associated with extreme fatigue is noted rarely.

SPECIAL CONSIDERATIONS

PATIENT/FAMILY EDUCATION

• Take with food. Notify clinician if diarrhea occurs

• Notify physician if persistent or increasing cramping, diarrhea, fever, pruritus, and rash occur

• Maintain adequate fluid intake

MONITORING PARAMETERS

• BUN, urinalysis, serum creatinine in patients with preexisting renal disease

• Pattern of daily bowel activity and stool consistency; record time of evacuation

• Skin for hives and rash

omalizumab

(oh-mah-lye-zoo'-mab)

Rx: Xolair

Chemical Class: Monoclonal antibody

Therapeutic Class: Antiasthmatic

CLINICAL PHARMACOLOGY

Mechanism of Action: A monoclonal antibody that selectively

O

binds to human immunoglobulin E (IgE), preventing it from binding to the surface of mast cells and basophiles. ***Therapeutic Effect:*** Prevents or reduces the number of asthmatic attacks.

Pharmacokinetics

Absorbed slowly after subcutaneous administration, with peak concentration in 7-8 days. Excreted in the liver, reticuloendothelial system, and endothelial cells. ***Half-life:*** 26 days.

INDICATIONS AND DOSAGES

Moderate to severe persistent asthma in patients who are reactive to a perennial allergen and whose asthma symptoms have been inadequately controlled with inhaled corticosteroids

Subcutaneous

Adults, Elderly, Children 12 yr and older. 150-375 mg every 2 or 4 wk; dose and dosing frequency are individualized based on weight and pretreatment immunoglobulin E (IgE) level (as shown below).

4-week dosing table

Pre-treatment serum IgE levels (units/ml)	*Weight 30-60 kg*	*Weight 61-70 kg*	*Weight 71-90 kg*	*Weight 91-150 kg*
30-100	150 mg	150 mg	150 mg	300 mg
101-200	300 mg	300 mg	300 mg	See next table
201-300	300 mg	See next table	See next table	See next table

2-week dosing table

Pre-treatment serum IgE levels (units/ml)	*Weight 30-60 kg*	*Weight 61-70 kg*	*Weight 71-90 kg*	*Weight 91-150 kg*
101-200	see preceding table	see preceding table	see preceding table	225 mg
201-300	See previous table	225 mg	225 mg	300 mg
301-400	225 mg	225 mg	300 mg	Do not dose
401-500	300 mg	300 mg	375 mg	Do not dose
501-600	300 mg	375 mg	Do not dose	Do not dose
601-700	375 mg	Do not dose	Do not dose	Do not dose

AVAILABLE FORMS

• *Powder for Injection:* 202.5 mg/1.2 ml or 150 mg/1.2 ml after reconstitution.

UNLABELED USES: Treatment of seasonal allergic rhinitis

CONTRAINDICATIONS: None known.

PREGNANCY AND LACTATION: Pregnancy category B; while omalizumab presence in human milk has not been studied, IgG is excreted in human milk and therefore it is expected that omalizumab will be present in human milk; the potential harm to the infant is unknown; caution should be exercised when administering to nursing mothers

SIDE EFFECTS

Frequent (45%-11%)

Injection site ecchymosis, redness, warmth, stinging, and urticaria; viral infections; sinusitis; headache; pharyngitis

Occasional (8%-3%)

Arthralgia, leg pain, fatigue, dizziness

Rare (2%)
Arm pain, earache, dermatitis, pruritus

SERIOUS REACTIONS

• Anaphylaxis occurs within 2 hrs of the first dose or subsequent doses in 0.1% of patients.

• Malignant neoplasms occur in 0.5% of patients.

INTERACTIONS

Labs

• Serum total IgE levels increase following administration due to formation of omalizumab:IgE complexes; elevated serum total IgE levels may persist for up to 1 yr following discontinuation

SPECIAL CONSIDERATIONS

• In clinical studies, a reduction of asthma exacerbations was not observed in omalizumab-treated patients who had FEV_1 >80% at the time of randomization; reductions in exacerbations were not seen in patients who required oral steroids as maintenance therapy

PATIENT/FAMILY EDUCATION

• Systemic or inhaled corticosteroids should not be abruptly discontinued upon initiation of omalizumab therapy

• Do not decrease the dose of, or stop taking any other asthma medications unless otherwise instructed by clinician

• Immediate improvement in asthma symptoms may not be apparent after beginning omalizumab therapy

• Because the solution is slightly viscous, the injection may take 5-10 sec to administer

• Should be stored under refrigerated conditions 2-8°C (36-46°F)

• Drink plenty of fluids to decrease the thickness of lung secretions

MONITORING PARAMETERS

• Patients should be observed after injection of omalizumab, and medications for the treatment of severe hypersensitivity reactions, including anaphylaxis, should be available

• Total IgE levels are elevated during treatment and remain elevated for up to 1 yr after the discontinuation of treatment; retesting of IgE levels during omalizumab treatment cannot be used as a guide for dose determination; dose determination after treatment interruptions lasting <1 yr should be based on serum IgE levels obtained at the initial dose determination

• Doses should be adjusted for significant changes in body weight

• Pulse rate and quality as well as respiratory rate, depth, rhythm, and type

• Observe fingernails and lips for cyanosis characterized by a blue or dusky color in light-skinned patients or a gray color in dark-skinned patients

omeprazole

(oh-me'-pray-zol)

Rx: Prilosec, Zegerid

OTC: Prilosec OTC

Chemical Class: Benzimidazole derivative

Therapeutic Class: Antiulcer agent; gastrointestinal antisecretory agent

CLINICAL PHARMACOLOGY

Mechanism of Action: A benzimidazole that is converted to active metabolites that irreversibly bind to and inhibit hydrogen-potassium adenosine triphosphatase, an enzyme on the surface of gastric parietal cells. Inhibits hydrogen ion transport into gastric lumen. ***Therapeutic Effect:*** Increases gastric pH, reduces gastric acid production.

Pharmacokinetics

Route	Onset	Peak	Duration
PO	1 hr	2 hr	72 hr

Rapidly absorbed from the GI tract. Protein binding: 99%. Primarily distributed into gastric parietal cells. Metabolized extensively in the liver. Primarily excreted in urine. Unknown if removed by hemodialysis. ***Half-life:*** 0.5-1 hr (increased in patients with hepatic impairment).

INDICATIONS AND DOSAGES

Erosive esophagitis, poorly responsive gastroesophageal reflux disease, active duodenal ulcer, prevention and treatment of NSAID-induced ulcers

PO

Adults, Elderly. 20 mg/day.

To maintain healing of erosive esophagitis

PO

Adults, Elderly. 20 mg/day.

Pathologic hypersecretory conditions

PO

Adults, Elderly. Initially, 60 mg/day up to 120 mg 3 times a day.

H. pylori duodenal ulcer

PO

Adults, Elderly. 20 mg once daily or 40 mg/day as a single or in 2 divided doses in combination therapy with antibiotics. Dose varies with regimen used.

Active benign gastric ulcer

PO

Adults, Elderly. 40 mg/day for 4-8 wk.

OTC use (frequent heartburn)

PO

Adults, Elderly. 20 mg/day for 14 days. May repeat after 4 mo if needed.

Usual pediatric dosage

Children older than 2 yr, weighing 20 kg and more. 20 mg/day.

Children older than 2 yr, weighing less than 20 kg. 10 mg/day.

AVAILABLE FORMS

- *Capsules (Delayed-Release [Prilosec]):* 10 mg, 20 mg, 40 mg.
- *Oral Suspension (Zegerid):* 20 mg, 40 mg.

UNLABELED USES: *H. pylori*–associated duodenal ulcer (with amoxicillin and clarithromycin), prevention and treatment of NSAID-induced ulcers, treatment of active benign gastric ulcers

CONTRAINDICATIONS: None known.

PREGNANCY AND LACTATION: Pregnancy category C; excretion into breast milk unknown, suppression of gastric acid secretion is potential effect in nursing infant, clinical significance unknown, use with caution in nursing mothers

SIDE EFFECTS

Frequent (7%)

Headache

Occasional (3%-2%)

Diarrhea, abdominal pain, nausea

Rare (2%)

Dizziness, asthenia or loss of strength, vomiting, constipation, upper respiratory tract infection, back pain, rash, cough

SERIOUS REACTIONS

- Pancreatitis, hepatotoxicity, and interstitial nephritis have been reported.

INTERACTIONS

Drugs

3 *Benzodiazepines, carbamazepine, cyclosporine, digoxin, nifedipine, nimodipine, nisoldipine:* Increased concentrations of these drugs

3 *Ampicillin esters, cefpodoxime, cefuroxime, cyanocobalamin, enoxacin, iron salts, itraconazole, ketoconazole:* Decreased concentrations of these drugs

3 *Glipizide, glyburide, tolbutamide:* Increased absorption of these drugs, potential of hypoglycemia

3 *Methotrexate:* Case report of elevated methotrexate concentration

3 *Phenytoin:* Increased phenytoin concentration

3 *Voriconazole:* Increases omeprazole plasma concentrations

SPECIAL CONSIDERATIONS

• Some patients on maintenance therapy may respond to 10 mg qd or 20 mg qod

PATIENT/FAMILY EDUCATION

• Take before eating

• Swallow capsule whole; do not open, chew, or crush

• Notify the physician if headache occurs during omeprazole therapy

MONITORING PARAMETERS

• Therapeutic response (relief of GI symptoms)

ondansetron hydrochloride

(on-dan-seh′-tron hye-droe-klor′-ide)

Rx: Zofran, Zofran ODT

Chemical Class: Carbazole derivative

Therapeutic Class: Antiemetic

CLINICAL PHARMACOLOGY

Mechanism of Action: An antiemetic that blocks serotonin, both peripherally on vagal nerve terminals and centrally in the chemoreceptor trigger zone. ***Therapeutic Effect:*** Prevents nausea and vomiting.

Pharmacokinetics

Readily absorbed from the GI tract. Protein binding: 70%-76%. Metabolized in the liver. Primarily excreted in urine. Unknown if removed by hemodialysis. ***Half-life:*** 4 hr.

INDICATIONS AND DOSAGES

Chemotherapy-induced emesis

IV

Adults, Elderly. 0.15 mg/kg 3 times a day beginning 30 mins before chemotherapy or 0.45 mg/kg once daily or 8-10 mg 1-2 times/day or 24-32 mg once daily.

Children 4-18 yr. 0.15 mg/kg 3 times a day beginning 30 mins before chemotherapy and again 4 and 8 hrs after first dose or 0.45 mg/kg as a single dose.

PO

Adults, Elderly. (highly emetogenic) 24 mg 30 mins before start of chemotherapy, (moderately emetogenic) 8 mg q12h beginning 30 mins before chemotherapy and continuing for 1-2 days after completion of chemotherapy.

Prevention of postoperative nausea and vomiting

IV, IM

Adults, Elderly. 4 mg as a single dose

Children 2-12 yr, weighing more than 40 kg. 4 mg.

Children 2-12 yr, weighing 40 kg and less. 0.1 mg/kg.

PO

Adults, Elderly. 16 mg 1 hr before induction of anesthesia.

Prevention of radiation-induced nausea and vomiting

PO

Adults, Elderly. (total body irradiation) 8 mg 1-2 hrs daily before each fraction of radiotherapy, (single high-dose radiotherapy to abdomen) 8 mg 1-2 hrs before irradiation, then 8 mg q8h after first dose for 1-2 days after completion of radiotherapy, (daily fractionated radiotherapy to abdomen) 8 mg 1-2 hrs before irradiation, then 8 mg 8 hrs after first dose for each day of radiotherapy.

AVAILABLE FORMS

- *Oral Solution (Zofran):* 4 mg/5 ml.
- *Tablets (Zofran):* 4 mg, 8 mg, 24 mg.
- *Tablets (Orally Disintegrating [Zofran ODT]):* 4 mg, 8 mg.
- *Injection (Zofran):* 2 mg/ml.
- *Injection (Premix):* 32 mg/50 ml.

UNLABELED USES: Treatment of postoperative nausea and vomiting

CONTRAINDICATIONS: None known.

PREGNANCY AND LACTATION: Pregnancy category B; has been used in the treatment of hyperemesis gravidarum

SIDE EFFECTS

Frequent (13%-5%)

Anxiety, dizziness, somnolence, headache, fatigue, constipation, diarrhea, hypoxia, urine retention

Occasional (4%-2%)

Abdominal pain, xerostomia, fever, feeling of cold, redness and pain at injection site, paresthesia, asthenia

Rare (1%)

Hypersensitivity reaction (including rash and pruritus), blurred vision

SERIOUS REACTIONS

- Overdose may produce a combination of CNS stimulant and depressant effects.

INTERACTIONS

Drugs

3 *Rifampin:* Increases the metabolism of ondansetron; a loss of antiemetic activity may result

SPECIAL CONSIDERATIONS

PATIENT/FAMILY EDUCATION

- Nausea and vomiting should be relieved shortly after drug administration; notify the physician if vomiting persists
- Ondansetron may cause dizziness or drowsiness
- Avoid alcohol and barbiturates while taking ondansetron
- Use other methods of reducing nausea and vomiting, including lying quietly and avoiding strong odors
- Avoid performing tasks that require mental alertness or motor skills until response to ondansetron has been established

MONITORING PARAMETERS

- Pattern of daily bowel activity and stool consistency

opium tincture

(oh′-pee-um)

Rx: Opium Tincture

Combinations

Rx: with belladonna alkaloids (B&O Suppositories)

Chemical Class: Natural alkaloid

Therapeutic Class: Antidiarrheal; narcotic analgesic

DEA Class: Schedule II

CLINICAL PHARMACOLOGY

Mechanism of Action: An opioid agonist that contains many narcotic alkaloids including morphine. It inhibits gastric motility due to its morphine content. ***Therapeutic Effect:*** Decreases digestive secretions, increases in gastrointestinal (GI) muscle tone, and reduces GI propulsion.

Pharmacokinetics

Duration of action is 4-5 hrs. Variably absorbed from the GI tract. Protein binding: unknown. Metabolized in liver. Primarily excreted in urine. Unknown if removed by hemodialysis. ***Half-life:*** Unknown.

INDICATIONS AND DOSAGES

Analgesia

PO

Adults, Elderly. 0.6-1.5 ml q3-4h. Maximum: 6 ml/day.

Children. 0.01-0.02 ml/kg/dose q3-4h. Maximum: 6 doses/day.

Antidiarrheal

PO

Adults, Elderly. 0.3-1 ml q2-6h. Maximum: 6 ml/day.

Children. 0.005-0.01 ml/kg/dose q3-4h. Maximum: 6 doses/day.

AVAILABLE FORMS

• *Liquid:* 10%.

UNLABELED USES: Narcotic withdrawal symptoms in neonates

CONTRAINDICATIONS: Hypersensitivity to morphine sulfate or any component of the formulation, increased intracranial pressure, severe respiratory depression, severe hepatic or renal insufficiency, pregnancy (prolonged use or high dosages near term)

PREGNANCY AND LACTATION: Pregnancy category B (category D if used for prolonged periods or in high doses at term); compatible with breast-feeding

Controlled Substance: Schedule II

SIDE EFFECTS

Frequent

Constipation, drowsiness, nausea, vomiting

Occasional

Paradoxical excitement, confusion, pounding heartbeat, facial flushing, decreased urination, blurred vision, dizziness, dry mouth, headache, hypotension, decreased appetite, redness, burning, pain at injection site

Rare

Hallucinations, depression, stomach pain, insomnia

SERIOUS REACTIONS

• Overdosage results in cold or clammy skin, confusion, convulsions, decreased blood pressure (BP), restlessness, pinpoint pupils, bradycardia, respiratory depression, decreased level of consciousness (LOC), and severe weakness.

• Tolerance to analgesic effect and physical dependence may occur with repeated use.

INTERACTIONS

Drugs

3 *Barbiturates:* Additive CNS depression

3 *Cimetidine:* Increased effect of narcotic analgesics

3 *Ethanol:* Additive CNS effects

3 *Neuroleptics:* Hypotension and excessive CNS depression

Labs

• *False increase:* Amylase and lipase

SPECIAL CONSIDERATIONS

• Opium has been replaced by safer, more effective analgesics and sedative/hypnotics for diagnostic or operative medication; useful as an antidiarrheal

• Do not administer agonist/antagonist analgesics (i.e., pentazocine, nalbuphine, butorphanol, dezocine, buprenorphine) to patient who has received a prolonged course of opium (a pure agonist). In opioid-dependent patients, mixed agonist/antagonist analgesics may precipitate withdrawal symptoms

PATIENT/FAMILY EDUCATION

• Drug may be addictive if used for prolonged periods

• Do not exceed the prescribed dose

• Change positions slowly

• Avoid tasks that require mental alertness or motor skills until response to the drug is established

• Avoid alcohol

MONITORING PARAMETERS

• Daily pattern of bowel activity and stool consistency

• Clinical improvement

orlistat

(or'-li-stat)

Rx: Xenical

Chemical Class: Lipase inhibitor

Therapeutic Class: Weight loss

CLINICAL PHARMACOLOGY

Mechanism of Action: A gastric and pancreatic lipase inhibitor that inhibits absorption of dietary fats by inactivating gastric and pancreatic enzymes. ***Therapeutic Effect:*** Resulting caloric deficit may positively affect weight control.

Pharmacokinetics

Minimal absorption after administration. Protein binding: 99%. Primarily eliminated unchanged in feces. Unknown if removed by hemodialysis. ***Half-life:*** 1-2 hr.

INDICATIONS AND DOSAGES

Weight reduction

PO

Adults, Elderly, Children 12-16 yr. 120 mg 3 times a day with each main meal containing fat (omit if meal is occasionally missed or contains no fat).

AVAILABLE FORMS

• *Capsules:* 120 mg.

UNLABELED USES: Type 2 diabetes

CONTRAINDICATIONS: Cholestasis, chronic malabsorption syndrome

PREGNANCY AND LACTATION: Pregnancy category B

SIDE EFFECTS

Frequent (30%-20%)

Headache, abdominal discomfort, flatulence, fecal urgency, fatty or oily stool

Occasional (14%-5%)

Back pain, menstrual irregularity, nausea, fatigue, diarrhea, dizziness

Rare (less than 4%)

Anxiety, rash, myalgia, dry skin, vomiting

SERIOUS REACTIONS

• Hypersensitivity reaction occurs rarely.

INTERACTIONS

Drugs

❷ *Cyclosporine:* Reduces cyclosporine blood concentrations; avoid concurrent therapy

❷ *Fat-soluble vitamins:* pharmacokinetic interaction resulting in 30%-60% reduction in beta-carotene, vitamin E

❸ *Pravastatin:* May increase the blood concentration of pravastatin and risk of rhabdomyolysis

❷ *Warfarin:* Because fat-soluble vitamins may be depleted, an exaggerated hypoprothrombinemic effect is possible

SPECIAL CONSIDERATIONS

• Standard weight loss maintained over 2 yrs is approximately 10% of initial weight

PATIENT/FAMILY EDUCATION

• If a meal contains no fat, the dose of orlistat can be omitted

• Supplement with fat-soluble vitamin, vitamin D, and beta-carotene

• Psyllium laxative may decrease GI adverse effects

• Unpleasant side effects, such as flatulence and urgency, should diminish with time

MONITORING PARAMETERS

• Lipids, weight, plasma levels of vitamins A, D, E

• Blood glucose

orphenadrine citrate

(or-fen′-a-dreen sih′-trayt)

Rx: Antiflex, Banflex, Mio-rel, Myotrol, Norflex, Orfro, Orphenate

Combinations

Rx: with aspirin, caffeine (Norgesic, Norgesic Forte, Orphengesic, Orphengesic Forte)

Chemical Class: Tertiary amine

Therapeutic Class: Skeletal muscle relaxant

CLINICAL PHARMACOLOGY

Mechanism of Action: A skeletal muscle relaxant that is structurally related to diphenhydramine and may thought to indirectly affect skeletal muscle by central atropine-like effects. ***Therapeutic Effect:*** Relieves musculoskeletal pain.

Pharmacokinetics

Well absorbed after PO and IM absorption. Protein binding: low. Metabolized in liver. Primarily excreted in urine and feces. ***Half-life:*** 14 hrs.

INDICATIONS AND DOSAGES

Musculoskeletal pain

IM/IV

Adults, Elderly. 60 mg 2 times/day. Switch to oral form for maintenance.

PO

Adults, Elderly. 100 mg 2 times/day.

AVAILABLE FORMS

• *Injection:* 30 mg/ml (Norflex).

• *Tablets, Extended-Release:* 100 mg (Norflex).

UNLABELED USES: Drug-induced extrapyramidal reactions

CONTRAINDICATIONS: Angle-closure glaucoma, myasthenia gravis, pyloric or duodenal obstruction, stenosing peptic ulcer, prostatic hypertrophy, obstruction of the bladder neck, achalasia, cardiospasm (megaesophagus), hypersensitivity to orphenadrine or any component of the formulation

PREGNANCY AND LACTATION: Pregnancy category C; excretion into breast milk unknown, use caution in nursing mothers

SIDE EFFECTS

Frequent

Drowsiness, dizziness, muscular weakness, hypotension, dry mouth, nose, throat, and lips, urinary retention, thickening of bronchial secretions

Elderly

Frequent

Sedation, dizziness, hypotension

Occasional

Flushing, visual or hearing disturbances, paresthesia, diaphoresis, chill

SERIOUS REACTIONS

• Hypersensitivity reaction, such as eczema, pruritus, rash, cardiac disturbances, and photosensitivity, may occur.

• Overdosage may vary from CNS depression, including sedation, apnea, hypotension, cardiovascular collapse, or death to severe paradoxical reaction, such as hallucinations, tremor, and seizures.

INTERACTIONS

Drugs

3 *Neuroleptics:* Lower serum neuroleptic concentrations, excessive anticholinergic effects

SPECIAL CONSIDERATIONS

PATIENT/FAMILY EDUCATION

• Drowsiness usually diminishes with continued therapy

• Avoid tasks that require mental alertness or motor skills until response to the drug is established

- Avoid alcohol
- Notify the physician if bloody or tarry stools, continued weakness, diarrhea, fatigue, itching, nausea, or skin rash occurs

MONITORING PARAMETERS

- Therapeutic response

oseltamivir phosphate

(os-el-tam'-i-vir foss'-fate)

Rx: Tamiflu

Chemical Class: Carboxylic acid ethyl ester

Therapeutic Class: Antiviral

CLINICAL PHARMACOLOGY

Mechanism of Action: A selective inhibitor of influenza virus neuraminidase, an enzyme essential for viral replication. Acts against both influenza A and B viruses. ***Therapeutic Effect:*** Suppresses the spread of infection within the respiratory system and reduces the duration of clinical symptoms.

Pharmacokinetics

Readily absorbed. Protein binding: 3%. Extensively converted to active drug in the liver. Primarily excreted in urine. ***Half-life:*** 6-10 hr.

INDICATIONS AND DOSAGES

Influenza

PO

Adults, Elderly. 75 mg 2 times a day for 5 days.

Children weighing more than 40 kg. 75 mg twice a day.

Children weighing 24-40 kg. 60 mg twice a day.

Children weighing 15-23 kg. 45 mg twice a day.

Children weighing less than 15 kg. 30 mg twice a day.

Prevention of influenza

PO

Adults, Elderly, Children 13 yr and older. 75 mg once daily for at least 7 days.

Dosage in renal impairment

PO

For adult and elderly patients, dosage is decreased to 75 mg once a day for at least 7 days and possibly up to 6 wk.

AVAILABLE FORMS

- *Capsules:* 75 mg.
- *Oral Suspension:* 12 mg/ml.

CONTRAINDICATIONS: None known.

PREGNANCY AND LACTATION: Pregnancy category C; excreted in breast milk of animals

SIDE EFFECTS

Frequent (10%-7%)

Nausea, vomiting, diarrhea

Rare (2%-1%)

Abdominal pain, bronchitis, dizziness, headache, cough, insomnia, fatigue, vertigo

SERIOUS REACTIONS

- Colitis, pneumonia, tympanic membrane disorder, and pyrexia occur rarely.

SPECIAL CONSIDERATIONS

PATIENT/FAMILY EDUCATION

- May administer without regard for food
- When started within 40 hr of onset of symptoms, there was a 1.3 day reduction in the median time to improvement in influenza-infected subjects receiving osteltamivir compared to subjects receiving placebo

MONITORING PARAMETERS

- Renal function
- Blood glucose levels of diabetic patients

oxacillin

(ox-a-sill'-in soe'-dee-um)

Rx: Bactocill

Chemical Class: Penicillin derivative, penicillinase-resistant

Therapeutic Class: Antibiotic

CLINICAL PHARMACOLOGY

Mechanism of Action: A penicillin that binds to bacterial membranes. ***Therapeutic Effect:*** Bactericidal.

Pharmacokinetics

Rapid and incomplete absorption following PO administration. Protein binding: 94%. Rapidly excreted as unchanged drug in urine. ***Half-life:*** 30 min.

INDICATIONS AND DOSAGES

Upper respiratory tract, skin, and skin-structure infections

IV, IM

Adults, Elderly, Children weighing 40 kg or more. 250-500 mg q4-6h.

Children weighing less than 40 kg. 50 mg/kg/day in divided doses q6h. Maximum: 12 g/day.

Lower respiratory tract and other serious infections

IV, IM

Adults, Elderly, Children weighing 40 kg or more. 1 g q4-6h. Maximum: 12 g/day.

Children weighing less than 40 kg. 100 mg/kg/day in divided doses q4-6h.

Mild to moderate infections

PO

Adults, Elderly, Children weighing 40 kg and more. 500 mg q4-6h.

Children weighing less than 40 kg. 50 mg/kg/day in divided doses q6h.

Severe infections

PO

Adults, Elderly, Children weighing 40 kg and more. 1 g q4-6h.

Children weighing less than 40 kg. 100 mg/kg/day in divided doses q4-6h.

AVAILABLE FORMS

- *Capsules:* 250 mg, 500 mg.
- *Powder for Reconstitution (Oral):* 250 mg/5 ml.
- *Powder for Injection:* 500-mg vials, 1-g vials, 2-g vials, 4-g vials, 10-g vials.
- *Intravenous Solution:* 1 g/50 ml.

CONTRAINDICATIONS: Hypersensitivity to any penicillin

PREGNANCY AND LACTATION: Pregnancy category B; potential exists for modification of bowel flora in nursing infant, allergy or sensitization, and interference with interpretation of culture results if fever workup required

SIDE EFFECTS

Frequent

Mild hypersensitivity reaction (fever, rash, pruritus), GI effects (nausea, vomiting, diarrhea)

Occasional

Phlebitis, thrombophlebitis (more common in elderly), hepatotoxicity (with high IV dosage)

SERIOUS REACTIONS

- Antibiotic-associated colitis and other superinfections may result from altered bacterial balance.
- A mild to severe hypersensitivity reaction may occur in those allergic to penicillins.

INTERACTIONS

Drugs

3 *Chloramphenicol:* Inhibited antibacterial activity of oxacillin, ensure adequate amounts of both agents are given and administer oxacillin a few hours before chloramphenicol

3 *Methotrexate:* Increased serum methotrexate concentrations

3 *Probenecid:* May increase oxacillin blood concentration and risk of toxicity

3 *Tetracyclines:* Inhibited antibacterial activity of oxacillin, ensure adequate amounts of both agents are given and administer oxacillin a few hours before tetracycline

SPECIAL CONSIDERATIONS

- Sodium content of 1 g = 2.8-3.1 mEq

PATIENT/FAMILY EDUCATION

- Administer on an empty stomach (1 hr before or 2 hr after meals)
- Report burning or pain at IV site
- Immediately report signs of an allergic reaction, such as shortness of breath, chest tightness, or hives
- Practice good oral hygiene

MONITORING PARAMETERS

- Urinalysis, BUN, serum creatinine, CBC with differential, periodic liver function tests
- Withhold oxacillin as prescribed, and promptly notify the physician if the patient experiences a rash or diarrhea with abdominal pain, blood or mucus in stools, fever
- Assess the patient for signs and symptoms of superinfection, such as anal or genital pruritus, black hairy tongue, oral ulceration or pain, diarrhea, increased fever, sore throat, and vomiting

oxaliplatin

(ox-al'-i-pla-tin)

Rx: Eloxatin

Chemical Class: Organoplatinum complex

Therapeutic Class: Antineoplastic

CLINICAL PHARMACOLOGY

Mechanism of Action: A platinum-containing complex that cross-links with DNA strands, preventing cell division. Cell cycle–phase nonspecific. ***Therapeutic Effect:*** Inhibits DNA replication.

Pharmacokinetics

Rapidly distributed. Protein binding: 90%. Undergoes rapid, extensive nonenzymatic biotransformation. Excreted in urine. ***Half-life:*** 70 hr.

INDICATIONS AND DOSAGES

Metastatic colon or rectal cancer in patients whose disease has recurred or progressed during or within 6 mos of completing first-line therapy with bolus 5-fluorouracil (5-FU), leucovorin, and irinotecan.

IV

Adults. Day 1: Oxaliplatin 85 mg/m^2 in 250-500 ml D_5W and leucovorin 200 mg/m^2, both given simultaneously over more than 2 hr in separate bags using a Y-line, followed by 5-FU 400 mg/m^2 IV bolus given over 2-4 min, followed by 5-FU 600 mg/m^2 in 500 ml D_5W as a 22-hr continuous IV infusion. Day 2: Leucovorin 200 mg/m^2 IV infusion given over more than 2 hr, followed by 5-FU 400 mg/m^2 IV bolus given over 2-4 min, followed by 5-FU 600 mg/m^2 in 500 ml D_5W as a 22-hr continuous IV infusion.

Ovarian cancer

IV

Adults. Cisplatin 100 mg/m^2 and oxaliplatin 130 mg/m^{2}q3wk.

AVAILABLE FORMS

- *Injection Solution:* 50-mg, 100-mg vials 5 mg/ml.

UNLABELED USES: Treatment of germ cell cancer, ovarian cancer, pancreatic cancer, renal cell cancer, solid tumors

CONTRAINDICATIONS: History of allergy to other platinum compounds

PREGNANCY AND LACTATION: Pregnancy category D; excretion into breast milk unknown; breast-feeding not recommended

SIDE EFFECTS

Frequent (76%-20%)

Peripheral or sensory neuropathy (usually occurs in hands, feet, perioral area, and throat but may present as jaw spasm, abnormal tongue sensation, eye pain, chest pressure, or difficulty walking, swallowing, or writing), nausea (64%), fatigue, diarrhea, vomiting, constipation, abdominal pain, fever, anorexia

Occasional (14%-10%)

Stomatitis, earache, insomnia, cough, difficulty breathing, backache, edema

Rare (7%-3%)

Dyspepsia, dizziness, rhinitis, flushing, alopecia

SERIOUS REACTIONS

- Peripheral or sensory neuropathy can occur, sometimes precipitated or exacerbated by drinking or holding a glass of cold liquid during the IV infusion.
- Pulmonary fibrosis, characterized by a nonproductive cough, dyspnea, crackles, and radiologic pulmonary infiltrates, may require drug discontinuation.
- Hypersensitivity reaction (rash, urticaria, pruritus) occurs rarely.

INTERACTIONS

Drugs

3 *Live-virus vaccines:* May potentiate virus replication, increase vaccine side effects, and decrease the patient's antibody response to the vaccine

3 *Nephrotic medications:* May decrease the clearance of oxaliplatin

SPECIAL CONSIDERATIONS

- Extravasation may lead to tissue necrosis

PATIENT/FAMILY EDUCATION

- Neurotoxicity may be acute and aggravated by exposure to cold
- Promptly report easy bruising, fever, signs of local infection, sore throat, or unusual bleeding from any site
- Do not receive vaccinations during therapy and avoid contact with anyone who has recently received an oral polio vaccine

MONITORING PARAMETERS

- CBC with platelets, hepatic and renal function
- Intake and output
- Evaluate for diarrhea and signs of GI bleeding, such as bright red or tarry stools
- Signs and symptoms of stomatitis, including erythema of the oral mucosa, sore throat, and ulceration of the lips or mouth

oxandrolone

(ox-an'-droe-lone)

Rx: Oxandrin

Chemical Class: Anabolic steroid; testosterone derivative

Therapeutic Class: Androgen

DEA Class: Schedule III

CLINICAL PHARMACOLOGY

Mechanism of Action: A synthetic testosterone derivative that promotes growth and development of male sex organs, maintains secondary sex characteristics in androgen-deficient males. ***Therapeutic Effect:*** Androgenic and anabolic actions.

Pharmacokinetics

Well absorbed from the gastrointestinal (GI) tract. Protein binding: 94%-97%. Metabolized in liver. Primarily excreted in urine. Unknown if removed by hemodialysis. ***Half-life:*** 5-13 hrs.

INDICATIONS AND DOSAGES

Weight gain

Adults, Elderly. 2.5-20 mg in divided doses 2-4 times/day usually for 2-4 wks. Course of therapy is based on individual response. Repeat intermittently as needed.

Children. Total daily dose is 0.1 mg/kg. Repeat intermittently as needed.

AVAILABLE FORMS

• *Tablets:* 2.5 mg, 10 mg (Oxandrin).

UNLABELED USES: AIDS wasting syndrome, alcoholic hepatitis, athletic performance enhancement, burns, growth hormone deficiency, hyperlipidemia, Turner syndrome

CONTRAINDICATIONS: Nephrosis, carcinoma of breast or prostate hypercalcemia, pregnancy, hypersensitivity to oxandrolone or any component of the formulation

PREGNANCY AND LACTATION: Pregnancy category X; use extreme caution in nursing mothers

Controlled Substance: Schedule III

SIDE EFFECTS

Frequent

Gynecomastia, acne, amenorrhea, other menstrual irregularities

Females: Hirsutism, deepening of voice, clitoral enlargement that may not be reversible when drug is discontinued

Occasional

Edema, nausea, insomnia, oligospermia, priapism, male pattern of baldness, bladder irritability, hypercalcemia in immobilized patients or those with breast cancer, hypercholesterolemia

Rare

Polycythemia with high dosage

SERIOUS REACTIONS

• Peliosis hepatitis of the liver, spleen replaced with blood-filled cysts, hepatic neoplasms and hepatocellular carcinoma have been associated with prolonged high-dosage, anaphylactic reactions.

INTERACTIONS

Drugs

3 *Adrenal steroids, ACTH:* May increase the risk of edema

3 *Antidiabetic agents:* Enhanced hypoglycemic effects

❷ *Cyclosporine:* Increased cyclosporine concentrations, toxicity

3 *HMG CoA reductase inhibitors (lovastatin, pravastatin):* Myositis risk increased

3 *Tacrolimus:* Increased tacrolimus concentrations, toxicity

❷ *Oral anticoagulants:* Enhanced hypoprothrombinemic response

SPECIAL CONSIDERATIONS

• Anabolic steroids have potential for abuse, especially in the athlete

PATIENT/FAMILY EDUCATION

• Adequate dietary intake of calories and protein essential for successful treatment

• Reduce salt intake

• Notify the physician if acne, nausea, pedal edema, or vomiting occurs

• The female patient should promptly report deepening of voice, hoarseness, and menstrual irregularities

• The male patient should report difficulty urinating, frequent erections, and gynecomastia

MONITORING PARAMETERS

• LFTs, lipids

• Growth rate in children (X-rays for bone age q6mo)

• Serum calcium in breast cancer patients

• Weight

• Intake and output

• Sleep patterns

• Blood pressure

oxaprozin

(ox-a-proe'-zin)

Rx: Daypro

Chemical Class: Propionic acid derivative

Therapeutic Class: NSAID; antipyretic; nonnarcotic analgesic

CLINICAL PHARMACOLOGY

Mechanism of Action: An NSAID that produces analgesic and antiinflammatory effects by inhibiting prostaglandin synthesis. ***Therapeutic Effect:*** Reduces the inflammatory response and intensity of pain.

Pharmacokinetics

Well absorbed from the GI tract. Protein binding: 99%. Widely distributed. Metabolized in the liver. Primarily excreted in urine; partially eliminated in feces. Not removed by hemodialysis. ***Half-life:*** 42-50 hr.

INDICATIONS AND DOSAGES

Osteoarthritis

PO

Adults, Elderly. 1200 mg once a day (600 mg in patients with low body weight or mild disease). Maximum: 1800 mg/day.

Rheumatoid arthritis

PO

Adults, Elderly. 1200 mg once a day. Range: 600-1800 mg/day.

Juvenile rheumatoid arthritis

Children weighing more than 54 kg. 1200 mg/day.

Children weighing 32-54 kg. 900 mg/day.

Children weighing 22-31 kg. 600 mg/day.

Dosage in renal impairment

For adults and elderly patients with renal impairment, the recommended initial dose is 600 mg/day; may be increased up to 1200 mg/day.

AVAILABLE FORMS

- *Tablets:* 600 mg.

CONTRAINDICATIONS: Active peptic ulcer disease, chronic inflammation of GI tract, GI bleeding or ulceration, history of hypersensitivity to aspirin or NSAIDs

PREGNANCY AND LACTATION: Pregnancy category C (category D if used in third trimester); could cause constriction of the ductus arteriosus in utero, persistent pulmonary hypertension of the newborn, or prolonged labor

SIDE EFFECTS

Occasional (9%-3%)

Nausea, diarrhea, constipation, dyspepsia, edema

Rare (less than 3%)

Vomiting, abdominal cramps or pain, flatulence, anorexia, confusion, tinnitus, insomnia, somnolence

SERIOUS REACTIONS

- Hypertension, acute renal failure, respiratory depression, GI bleeding, and coma occur rarely.

INTERACTIONS

Drugs

3 *Aminoglycosides:* Reduced clearance with elevated aminoglycoside levels and potential for toxicity (especially indomethacin in premature infants; other NSAIDs probably)

3 *Anticoagulants:* Excessive hypoprothrombinemia, decreased platelet aggregation with increased risk of GI bleeding

3 *Antihypertensives (α-blockers, angiotensin-converting enzyme inhibitors, angiotensin II receptor blockers, β-blockers, diuretics):* Inhibition of antihypertensive and other favorable hemodynamic effects

3 *Aspirin, other salicylates:* May increase the risk of GI side effects such as bleeding

3 *Bone marrow depressants:* May increase the risk of hematologic reactions

3 *Corticosteroids:* Increased risk of GI ulceration

3 *Cyclosporine:* Increased nephrotoxicity risk

3 *Feverfew:* May increase the risk of bleeding

3 *Ginkgo biloba:* May increase the risk of bleeding

3 *Lithium:* Decreased clearance of lithium (mediated via prostaglandins) resulting in elevated serum lithium levels and risk of toxicity

3 *Methotrexate:* Decreased renal secretion of methotrexate resulting in elevated methotrexate levels and risk of toxicity

3 *Phenylpropanolamine:* Possible acute hypertensive reaction

3 *Potassium-sparing diuretics:* Additive hyperkalemia potential

3 *Probenecid:* May increase the oxaprozin blood concentration

3 *Triamterene:* Acute renal failure reported with addition of indomethacin; caution with other NSAIDs

SPECIAL CONSIDERATIONS

- No significant advantage over other NSAIDs; cost should govern use

PATIENT/FAMILY EDUCATION

- Avoid aspirin and alcoholic beverages
- Take with food, milk, or antacids to decrease GI upset
- Avoid performing tasks that require mental alertness or motor skills until response to the drug has been established
- Notify the physician if persistent GI effects, especially black, tarry stools occur
- The female patient should inform the physician if she is or plans to become pregnant

MONITORING PARAMETERS

- Initial hemogram and fecal occult blood test within 3 mo of starting regular chronic therapy; repeat every 6-12 mo (more frequently in high-risk patients [>65 years, peptic ulcer disease, concurrent steroids or anticoagulants]); electrolytes, creatinine, and BUN within 3 mo of starting regular chronic therapy; repeat every 6-12 mo
- Therapeutic response, such as improved grip strength, increased joint mobility, and decreased pain, tenderness, stiffness, and swelling

oxazepam

(ox-a'-ze-pam)

Rx: Serax

Chemical Class: Benzodiazepine

Therapeutic Class: Anxiolytic

DEA Class: Schedule IV

CLINICAL PHARMACOLOGY

Mechanism of Action: A benzodiazepine that potentiates the effects of gamma-aminobutyric acid and other inhibitory neurotransmitters by binding to specific receptors in the CNS. ***Therapeutic Effect:*** Produces anxiolytic effect and skeletal muscle relaxation.

Pharmacokinetics

Well absorbed from the GI tract. Protein binding: 97%. Metabolized in the liver. Primarily excreted in urine. Not removed by hemodialysis. ***Half-life:*** 5-20 hr.

INDICATIONS AND DOSAGES

Anxiety

PO

Adults. 10-30 mg 3-4 times a day.

Elderly. 10 mg 2-3 times a day.

Children. 1 mg/kg/day.

Alcohol withdrawal

PO

Adults, Elderly. 15-30 mg 3-4 times a day.

AVAILABLE FORMS

- *Capsules:* 10 mg, 15 mg, 30 mg.
- *Tablets:* 15 mg.

CONTRAINDICATIONS: Angle-closure glaucoma; preexisting CNS depression; severe, uncontrolled pain

PREGNANCY AND LACTATION: Pregnancy category D; may cause fetal damage when administered during pregnancy; excreted into breast milk; may accumulate in breast-fed infants and is therefore not recommended

Controlled Substance: Schedule IV

SIDE EFFECTS

Frequent

Mild, transient somnolence at beginning of therapy

Occasional

Dizziness, headache

Rare

Paradoxical CNS reactions, such as hyperactivity or nervousness in children and excitement or restlessness in the elderly or debilitated (generally noted during the first 2 wks of therapy)

SERIOUS REACTIONS

- Abrupt or too-rapid withdrawal may result in pronounced restlessness, irritability, insomnia, hand tremor, abdominal or muscle cramps, diaphoresis, vomiting, and seizures.
- Overdose results in somnolence, confusion, diminished reflexes, and coma.

INTERACTIONS

Drugs

3 *Ethanol:* Enhanced adverse psychomotor effects of benzodiazepines

3 *Kava kava, valerian:* May increase CNS depression

Labs

- *False increase:* Serum glucose

SPECIAL CONSIDERATIONS

- Niche compared to other benzodiazepines: treatment of anxiety in patients with hepatic disease; consider for alcohol withdrawal
- Tablet form contains tartrazine; risk of allergic-type reactions, especially in patients with aspirin hypersensitivity

PATIENT/FAMILY EDUCATION

- Avoid alcohol and other CNS depressants
- Do not discontinue abruptly after prolonged therapy
- Inform clinician if planning to become pregnant, pregnant, or become pregnant while taking this medicine
- Oxazepam may cause drowsiness. Avoid tasks requiring mental alertness or motor skills until response to the drug has been established
- May be habit forming

MONITORING PARAMETERS

- Periodic CBC, UA, blood chemistry analyses during prolonged therapy
- Hepatic and renal function periodically
- Therapeutic response, such as a calm facial expression and decreased restlessness and diminished insomnia
- The therapeutic serum level for oxazepam is 0.2-1.4 mcg/ml; the toxic serum level is not established

oxcarbazepine

(ox-car-baz'-e-peen)

Rx: Trileptal

Chemical Class: Dibenzazepine derivative

Therapeutic Class: Anticonvulsant

CLINICAL PHARMACOLOGY

Mechanism of Action: An anticonvulsant that blocks sodium channels, resulting in stabilization of hyperexcited neural membranes, inhibition of repetitive neuronal firing, and diminishing synaptic impulses. ***Therapeutic Effect:*** Prevents seizures.

Pharmacokinetics

Completely absorbed from GI tract and extensively metabolized in the liver to active metabolite. Protein binding: 40%. Primarily excreted in urine. ***Half-life:*** 2 hr; metabolite, 6-10 hr.

INDICATIONS AND DOSAGES

Adjunctive treatment of seizures

PO

Adults, Elderly. Initially, 600 mg/day in 2 divided doses. May increase by up to 600 mg/day at weekly intervals. Maximum: 2400 mg/day.

Children 4-16 yr. 8-10 mg/kg. Maximum: 600 mg/day. Maintenance (based on weight): 1800 mg/day for children weighing more than 39 kg; 1200 mg/day for children weighing 29.1-39 kg; and 900 mg/day for children weighing 20-29 kg.

Conversion to monotherapy

PO

Adults, Elderly. 600 mg/day in 2 divided doses (while decreasing concomitant anticonvulsant over 3-6 wk). May increase by 600 mg/day at weekly intervals up to 2400 mg/day.

Children. Initially, 8-10 mg/kg/day in 2 divided doses with simultaneous initial reduction of dose of concomitant antiepileptic.

Initiation of monotherapy

PO

Adults, Elderly. 600 mg/day in 2 divided doses. May increase by 300 mg/day every 3 days up to 1200 mg/day.

Children. Initially, 8-10 mg/kg/day in 2 divided doses. Increase at 3-day intervals by 5 mg/kg/day to achieve maintenance dose by weight; (70 kg): 1500-2100 mg/day; (60-69 kg): 1200-2100 mg/day; (50-59 kg): 1200-1800 mg/day; (41-49 kg): 1200-1500 mg/day; (35-40 kg): 900-1500 mg/day; (25-34 kg): 900-1200 mg/day; (20-24 kg): 600-900 mg/day.

Dosage in renal impairment

For patients with creatinine clearance less than 30 ml/min, give 50% of normal starting dose, then titrate slowly to desired dose.

AVAILABLE FORMS

- *Oral Suspension:* 300 mg/5 ml.
- *Tablets:* 150 mg, 300 mg, 600 mg.

UNLABELED USES: Atypical panic disorder, bipolar disorders, neuralgia/neuropathy

CONTRAINDICATIONS: None known.

PREGNANCY AND LACTATION: Pregnancy category C; increased incidence of fetal structural abnormalities and other manifestation of developmental toxicity have been observed in the offspring of animals; no adequate and well-controlled data in humans; oxcarbazepine and MHD both excreted in human breast milk; milk:plasma ratio: 0.5 (both)

SIDE EFFECTS

Frequent (22%-13%)

Dizziness, nausea, headache

Occasional (7%-5%)
Vomiting, diarrhea, ataxia, nervousness, heartburn, indigestion, epigastric pain, constipation
Rare (4%)
Tremor, rash, back pain, epistaxis, sinusitis, diplopia

SERIOUS REACTIONS

• Clinically significant hyponatremia may occur.

INTERACTIONS

Drugs

• *Note:* Oxcarbazepine is an inhibitor of CYP2C19 and an inducer of CYP3A4 and CYP3A5

3 *Alcohol:* Additive CND depression and psychomotor impairment

3 *Barbiturates:* Decreases oxcarbazepine levels

3 *Benzodiazepines:* Additive CNS effects

3 *Calcium channel blockers (dihydropyridines):* Induction of antihypertensive metabolism; decreased antihypertensive efficacy

3 *Estradiol, oral contraceptives:* Induction of hepatic metabolism; decreased hormonal efficacy

3 *Medroxyprogesterone:* Induction of hepatic metabolism; decreased hormonal efficacy

3 *Lamotrigine:* Induction of hepatic metabolism; decreased lamotrigine levels by 30%

3 *Phenytoin:* Alterations in hepatic metabolism resulting in increases in phenytoin levels/risk of toxicity and decreases in oxcarbazepine

3 *Verapamil:* Decreased plasma oxcarbazepine concentrations

Labs

• *Thyroid levels:* Decreased

• *Serum sodium:* Decreased; increased risk of hyponatremia

SPECIAL CONSIDERATIONS

• Considered an alternative to carbamazepine in intolerant patients

PATIENT/FAMILY EDUCATION

• Review and reinforce prevalence of CNS adverse effects early in treatment (reason for gradual titration regimens) with tolerance developing with continued adherence

• Risk of recurrent seizures with missed doses

• Periodic blood tests are necessary

MONITORING PARAMETERS

• Seizure frequency and electroencephalogram changes in patients with seizure disorder; a reduction or elimination of pain in patients with trigeminal neuralgia; therapeutic serum levels not adequately established—estimates of therapeutic serum concentrations of the active metabolite (MHD) in the 50-110 μmol range; serum electrolytes (especially sodium), LFTs, blood counts, serum lipids

oxiconazole nitrate

(ox-i-kon′-a-zole nye′-trate)
Rx: Oxistat
Chemical Class: Imidazole derivative
Therapeutic Class: Antifungal

CLINICAL PHARMACOLOGY

Mechanism of Action: An antifungal agent that inhibits ergosterol synthesis. ***Therapeutic Effect:*** Destroys cytoplasmic membrane integrity of fungi. Fungicidal.

Pharmacokinetics

Low systemic absorption. Absorbed and distributed in each layer of the dermis. Excreted in the urine.

INDICATIONS AND DOSAGES

Tinea pedis

Topical

Adults, Elderly, Children 12 yrs and older. Apply 1-2 times daily for 1 mo or until signs and symptoms significantly improve.

Tinea cruris, tinea corporis
Topical
Adults, Elderly, Children 12 yrs and older. Apply 1-2 times daily for 2 wks or until signs and symptoms significantly improve.

AVAILABLE FORMS
- *Cream:* 1% (Oxistat).
- *Lotion:* 1% (Oxistat).

CONTRAINDICATIONS: Not for ophthalmic use, hypersensitivity to oxiconazole or any other azole fungals

PREGNANCY AND LACTATION: Pregnancy category B; excreted in breast milk

SIDE EFFECTS
Occasional
Itching, local irritation, stinging, dryness

SERIOUS REACTIONS
- Hypersensitivity reactions characterized by rash, swelling, pruritus, maceration, and a sensation of warmth may occur.

SPECIAL CONSIDERATIONS
- *Niche:* once daily imadazole; base choice on cost and convenience

PATIENT/FAMILY EDUCATION
- For external use only, avoid contact with eyes or vagina
- Separate personal items that come in contact with affected areas
- Rub topical form well into the affected and surrounding area
- Notify the physician if skin irritation occurs

MONITORING PARAMETERS
- Therapeutic response
- Skin for irritation

oxtriphylline
(ox-trye'-fi-lin)
Rx: Choledyl SA
Chemical Class: Xanthine derivative (64% theophylline)
Therapeutic Class: COPD agent; antiasthmatic; bronchodilator

CLINICAL PHARMACOLOGY
Mechanism of Action: A choline salt of theophylline acts as a bronchodilator by directly relaxing smooth muscle of the bronchial airway and pulmonary blood vessels. ***Therapeutic Effect:*** Relieves bronchospasm, increases vital capacity. Produces cardiac skeletal muscle stimulation.

Pharmacokinetics
Absorbed slowly due to extended release formulation. Protein binding: 40%. Distributed rapidly into peripheral non-adipose tissues and body water, including cerebrospinal fluid (CSF). Metabolized in liver. Eliminated in urine. ***Half-life:*** Adults, 6-12 hrs; Children, 1.2-7 hrs.

INDICATIONS AND DOSAGES
Asthma
PO
Adults, Elderly, Children. 400-600 mg q12h.
Children (younger than 5 yrs). 24-36 mg/kg/day given in divided doses.
Children (5-9 yrs). 200-400 mg/day given in divided doses.
Children (10-14 yrs). 400-800 mg/day given in divided doses.

AVAILABLE FORMS
- *Tablet (Extended Release):* 400 mg, 600 mg (Choledyl SA).

CONTRAINDICATIONS: Active peptic ulcer disease, seizure disorder (unless receiving appropriate anticonvulsant medication), history of hypersensitivity to xanthines

PREGNANCY AND LACTATION: Pregnancy category C; pharmacokinetics of theophylline may be altered during pregnancy, monitor serum concentrations carefully; excreted into breast milk, may cause irritability in the nursing infant; otherwise compatible with breastfeeding

SIDE EFFECTS

Frequent

Headache, shakiness, restlessness, tachycardia, trembling

Occasional

Nausea, vomiting, epigastric pain, diarrhea, headache, mild diuresis, insomnia

Rare

Alopecia, hyperglycemia, SIADH, rash

SERIOUS REACTIONS

• Nausea, vomiting, seizures and coma can result from overdosage.

INTERACTIONS

Drugs

3 *Adenosine:* Inhibited hemodynamic effects of adenosine

3 *Allopurinol, amiodarone, cimetadine, ciprofloxacin, disulfiram, erythromycin, interferon alfa, isoniazid, methimazole, metoprolol, norfloxacin, oral contraceptives, pefloxacin, pentoxifylline, propafenone, propylthiouracil, radioactive iodine, tacrine, thiabendazole, ticlopidine, verapamil:* Increased theophylline concentrations

3 *Aminoglutethimide, barbiturates, carbamazepine, moricizine, phenytoin, rifampin, ritonavir, thyroid hormone:* Reduced theophylline concentrations; decreased serum phenytoin concentrations

2 *Enoxacin, fluvoxamine, mexiletine, propanolol, troleandomycin:* Increased theophylline concentrations

3 *Imipenem:* Some patients on oxtriphylline have developed seizures following the addition of imipenem

3 *Lithium:* Reduced lithium concentrations

3 *Smoking:* Increased oxtriphylline dosing requirements

Labs

• *False increase:* Serum barbiturate concentrations, urinary uric acid

• *False decrease:* Serum bilirubin

• *Interference:* Plasma somatostatin

SPECIAL CONSIDERATIONS

• Touted to produce less GI side effects; if dosed equipotently based on theophylline equivalents (oxtriphylline = 64% theophylline) no difference; compare costs as well as other characteristics

PATIENT/FAMILY EDUCATION

• Avoid large amounts of caffeine-containing products (tea, coffee, chocolate, colas)

• Increase fluid intake

• Smoking and charcoal-broiled food may decrease drug level

MONITORING PARAMETERS

• Serum theophylline concentrations (therapeutic level is 8-20 mcg/ml); toxicity may occur with small increase above 20 mcg/ml, especially in the elderly

• Rate, depth, rhythm, and type of breathing

• ABGs

oxybutynin

(ox-i-byoo′-ti-nin)

Rx: Ditropan, Ditropan XL, Oxytro, Urotrol

Chemical Class: Tertiary amine

Therapeutic Class: Antispasmodic; gastrointestinal; genitourinary muscle relaxant

CLINICAL PHARMACOLOGY

Mechanism of Action: An anticholinergic that exerts antispasmodic (papaverine-like) and antimuscarinic (atropine-like) action on the detrusor smooth muscle of the bladder. ***Therapeutic Effect:*** Increases bladder capacity and delays desire to void.

Pharmacokinetics

Route	*Onset*	*Peak*	*Duration*
PO	0.5-1 hr	3-6 hrs	6-10 hrs

Rapidly absorbed from the GI tract. Metabolized in the liver. Primarily excreted in urine. Unknown if removed by hemodialysis. ***Half-life:*** 1-2.3 hrs.

INDICATIONS AND DOSAGES

Neurogenic bladder

PO

Adults. 5 mg 2-3 times a day up to 5 mg 4 times a day.

Elderly. 2.5-5 mg twice a day. May increase by 2.5 mg/day every 1-2 days.

Children 5 yrs and older. 5 mg twice a day up to 5 mg 4 times a day.

Children 1-4 yrs. 0.2 mg/kg/dose 2-4 times a day.

PO (Extended-Release)

Adults, Elderly. 5-10 mg/day up to 30 mg/day.

Children 6 yrs and older. Initially, 5-10 mg once daily. May increase in 5-10 mg increments. Maximum: 30 mg/day.

Transdermal

Adults. 3.9 mg applied twice a week. Apply every 3-4 days.

AVAILABLE FORMS

- *Syrup (Ditropan):* 5 mg/5 ml.
- *Tablets (Ditropan, Urotrol):* 5 mg.
- *Tablets (Extended-Release [Ditropan XL]):* 5 mg, 10 mg, 15 mg.
- *Transdermal (Oxytrol):* 3.9 mg.

CONTRAINDICATIONS: GI or GU obstruction, glaucoma, myasthenia gravis, toxic megacolon, ulcerative colitis

PREGNANCY AND LACTATION: Pregnancy category B; may suppress lactation

SIDE EFFECTS

Frequent

Constipation, dry mouth, somnolence, decreased perspiration

Occasional

Decreased lacrimation or salivation, impotence, urinary hesitancy and retention, suppressed lactation, blurred vision, mydriasis, nausea or vomiting, insomnia

SERIOUS REACTIONS

- Overdose produces CNS excitation (including nervousness, restlessness, hallucinations, and irritability), hypotension or hypertension, confusion, tachycardia, facial flushing, and respiratory depression.

INTERACTIONS

Drugs

3 *Anticholinergic agents (such as antihistamines):* May increase the anticholinergic effects of oxybutynin

SPECIAL CONSIDERATIONS

- Reported anticholinergic side effects not clinically or significantly different from other agents (i.e., propantheline); compare costs

PATIENT/FAMILY EDUCATION

- Avoid prolonged exposure to hot environments, heat prostration may result

• Use caution in driving or other activities requiring alertness
• Swallow extended release tablets whole; do not chew or crush
• Extended release tablet shell not absorbable
• Apply patch to dry, intact skin on abdomen, hip, or buttock; select new side with each new patch to avoid reapplication to the same site within 7 days
• May cause drowsiness and dry mouth
• Avoid alcohol

MONITORING PARAMETERS

• Intake and output
• Pattern of daily bowel activity and stool consistency
• Symptomatic relief

oxycodone hydrochloride

(ox-i-koe'-done hye-droe-klor'-ide)

Rx: M-Oxy, OxyContin, Oxydose, OxyFast, OxyIR, Percolone, Roxicodone, Roxicodone Intensol

Combinations

Rx: with aspirin (Percodan, Endodan, Roxiprin); with acetaminophen (Percocet, Endocet, Tylox, Roxicet, Roxilox)

Chemical Class: Opiate derivative; phenanthrene derivative
Therapeutic Class: Narcotic analgesic
DEA Class: Schedule II

CLINICAL PHARMACOLOGY

Mechanism of Action: An opioid analgesic that binds with opioid receptors in the CNS. ***Therapeutic Effect:*** Alters the perception of and emotional response to pain.

Pharmacokinetics

Route	*Onset*	*Peak*	*Duration*
PO, Immediate-Release	N/A	N/A	4-5 hrs
PO, Controlled-Release	N/A	N/A	12 hrs

Moderately absorbed from the GI tract. Protein binding: 38%-45%. Widely distributed. Metabolized in the liver. Excreted in urine. Unknown if removed by hemodialysis. ***Half-life:*** 2-3 hr (3.2 hr controlled-release).

INDICATIONS AND DOSAGES

Analgesia

PO (Controlled-Release)

Adults, Elderly. Initially, 10 mg q12h. May increase every 1-2 days by 25%-50%. Usual: 40 mg/day (100 mg/day for cancer pain).

PO (Immediate-Release)

Adults, Elderly. Initially, 5 mg q6h as needed. May increase up to 30 mg q4h. Usual: 10-30 mg q4h as needed.

Children. 0.05-0.15 mg/kg/dose q4-6h.

AVAILABLE FORMS

• *Capsules (Immediate-Release [OxyIR]):* 5 mg.
• *Oral Concentrate (Oxydose, OxyFast, Roxicodone Intensol):* 20 mg/ml.
• *Oral Solution (Roxicodone):* 5 mg/5ml.
• *Tablets (M-Oxy, Percolone, Roxicodone):* 5 mg, 15 mg, 30 mg.
• *Tablets (Extended-Release [OxyContin]):* 10 mg, 20 mg, 40 mg, 80 mg, 160 mg.

CONTRAINDICATIONS: Acute bronchial asthma or hypercarbia, paralytic ileus, respiratory depression

PREGNANCY AND LACTATION: Pregnancy category B (category D if used for prolonged periods or in high doses at term); excreted into breast milk

Controlled Substance: Schedule II

SIDE EFFECTS

Frequent

Somnolence, dizziness, hypotension (including orthostatic hypotension), anorexia

Occasional

Confusion, diaphoresis, facial flushing, urine retention, constipation, dry mouth, nausea, vomiting, headache

Rare

Allergic reaction, depression, paradoxical CNS hyperactivity or nervousness in children, paradoxical excitement and restlessness in elderly or debilitated patients

SERIOUS REACTIONS

- Overdose results in respiratory depression, skeletal muscle flaccidity, cold or clammy skin, cyanosis, and extreme somnolence progressing to seizures, stupor, and coma.
- Hepatotoxicity may occur with overdose of the acetaminophen component of fixed-combination products.
- The patient who uses oxycodone repeatedly may develop a tolerance to the drug's analgesic effect and physical dependence.

INTERACTIONS

Drugs

3 *Amitriptyline:* Additive respiratory and CNS depressant effects

3 *Antihistamines, chloral hydrate, glutethimide, methocarbamol:* Enhanced depressant effects

3 *Barbiturates:* Additive respiratory and CNS depressant effects

3 *Cimetidine:* Increased respiratory and CNS depression

3 *Clomipramine:* Additive respiratory and CNS depressant effects

3 *Ethanol, other CNS depressants:* Additive CNS effects

3 *MAOIs:* Markedly potentiate the actions of morphine

3 *Nortriptyline:* Additive respiratory and CNS depressant effects

3 *Protease inhibitors:* Increased CNS and respiratory depression

Labs

- *False increase:* Amylase and lipase

SPECIAL CONSIDERATIONS

PATIENT/FAMILY EDUCATION

- Physical dependency may result when used for extended periods
- Change position slowly, orthostatic hypotension may occur
- Do not administer agonist/antagonist analgesics (i.e., pentazocine, nalbuphine, butorphanol, dezocine, buprenorphine) to patient who has received a prolonged course of oxycodone (a pure agonist). In opioid-dependent patients, mixed agonist/antagonist analgesics may precipitate withdrawal symptoms
- Do not break, chew, or crush controlled-release tablets (OxyContin)
- Take oxycodone before the pain returns
- Avoid performing tasks that require mental alertness or motor skills until response to the drug has been established
- Avoid alcohol

MONITORING PARAMETERS

- Blood pressure, respiratory rate
- Mental status
- Pattern of daily bowel activity and stool consistency
- Clinical improvement and onset of pain relief

oxymetazoline

(ox-i-met-az'-oh-leen)

OTC: Afrin, Afrin 12-Hour, Afrin Children's Strength Nose Drops, Ocuclear, Sinex 12 Hour Long-Acting

Chemical Class: Imidazoline derivative

Therapeutic Class: Decongestant

CLINICAL PHARMACOLOGY

Mechanism of Action: A direct-acting sympathomimetic amine that acts on alpha-adrenergic receptors in arterioles of the nasal mucosa to produce constriction. ***Therapeutic Effect:*** Causes vasoconstriction resulting in decreased blood flow and decreased nasal congestion.

Pharmacokinetics

Onset of action is about 10 mins, and a duration of action is 7 hrs or more. Absorption occurs from the nasal mucosa and can produce systemic effects, primarily following overdose or excessive use. Excreted mostly in the urine as well as the feces. ***Half-life:*** 5-8 hrs.

INDICATIONS AND DOSAGES

Rhinitis

Intranasal

Adults, Elderly, Children older than 6 yrs. 2-3 drops/sprays (0.05% nasal solution) in each nostril q12h.

Children (2-5 yrs). 2-4 drops/sprays (0.025% nasal solution) in each nostril q12h for up to 3 days.

Conjunctivitis

Ophthalmic

Adults, Elderly, Children older than 6 yrs. 1-2 drops (0.025% ophthalmic solution) q6h for 3-4 days.

AVAILABLE FORMS

- *Eye Drops:* 0.025% (Ocuclear).
- *Nasal Drops:* 0.025% (Afrin Children's Strength Nose Drops), 0.05% (Afrin).
- *Nasal Spray:* 0.05% (Afrin, Afrin 12-Hour, Sinex 12 Hour Long-Acting).

UNLABELED USES: Otitis media surgical procedures

CONTRAINDICATIONS: Narrow-angle glaucoma or hypersensitivity to oxymetazoline or other adrenergic agents

PREGNANCY AND LACTATION: Pregnancy category C

SIDE EFFECTS

Occasional

Burning, stinging, drying nasal mucosa, sneezing, rebound congestion, insomnia, nervousness

SERIOUS REACTIONS

- Large doses may produce tachycardia, hypertension, arrhythmias, palpitations, lightheadedness, nausea, and vomiting.

SPECIAL CONSIDERATIONS

- Manage rebound congestion by stopping oxymetazoline: one nostril at a time, substitute systemic decongestant, substitute inhaled steroid

PATIENT/FAMILY EDUCATION

- Do not use for > 3-5 days or rebound congestion may occur
- Do not discontinue if slow, irregular heartbeat, trouble breathing, or seizures occurs

MONITORING PARAMETERS

- Monitor for rebound nasal congestion

oxymetholone

(ox-i-meth'-oh-lone)

Rx: Anadrol-50

Chemical Class: Anabolic steroid; testosterone derivative

Therapeutic Class: Androgen; hematopoietic agent

DEA Class: Schedule III

CLINICAL PHARMACOLOGY

Mechanism of Action: An androgenic-anabolic steroid that is a synthetic derivative of testosterone synthesized to accentuate anabolic as opposed to androgenic effects. ***Therapeutic Effect:*** Improves nitrogen balance in conditions of unfavorable protein metabolism with adequate caloric and protein intake, stimulates erythropoiesis, suppresses gonadotropic functions of pituitary and may exert a direct effect upon the testes.

Pharmacokinetics

The pharmacokinetics of oxymetholone has been studied. Metabolized in the liver via reduction and oxidation. Unchanged oxymetholone and its metabolites are excreted in urine. ***Half-life:*** Unknown.

INDICATIONS AND DOSAGES

Anemia, chronic renal failure, acqured aplastic anemia, chemotherapy-induced myelosuppresion, Fanconi's anemia, red cell aplasia

PO

Adults, Elderly, Children. 1-5 mg/kg/day. Response is not immediate and a minimum of 3-6 mos should be given.

AVAILABLE FORMS

• *Tablets:* 50 mg (Anadrol).

UNLABELED USES: Amegakaryocytic thrombocytopenia, familial antithrombin III deficiency, hereditary angioedema, HIV wasting, metastatic breast cancer in women, relief of bone pain associated with osteoporosis, neutropenia, Turner's syndrome, xeroderma pigmentosum

CONTRAINDICATIONS: Cardiac impairment, hypercalcemia, pregnancy/lactation, prostatic or breast cancer in males, metastatic breast cancer in women with active hypercalcemia, nephrosis or nephritic phase nephritis, severe liver disease, hypersensitivity to oxymetholone or any of its components

PREGNANCY AND LACTATION: Pregnancy category X; use extreme caution in nursing mothers

Controlled Substance: Schedule III

SIDE EFFECTS

Frequent

Gynecomastia, acne, amenorrhea, menstrual irregularities

Females: Hirsutism, deepening of voice, clitoral enlargement that may not be reversible when drug is discontinued

Occasional

Edema, nausea, insomnia, oligospermia, priapism, male pattern of baldness, bladder irritability, hypercalcemia in immobilized patients or those with breast cancer, hypercholesterolemia, inflammation and pain at IM injection site

Transdermal: Itching, erythema, skin irritation

Rare

Liver damage, hypersensitivity

SERIOUS REACTIONS

• Cholestatic jaundice, hepatic necrosis and death occur rarely but have been reported in association with long-term androgenic-anabolic steroid use.

INTERACTIONS

Drugs

3 *Antidiabetic agents:* Enhanced hypoglycemic effects

❷ *Cyclosporine:* Increased cyclosporine concentrations, toxicity

❸ *HMG CoA reductase inhibitors (lovastatin, prevastatin):* Myositis risk increased

❸ *Tacrolimus:* Increased tacrolimus concentrations, potential for toxicity

❷ *Oral anticoagulants:* Enhanced hypoprothrombinemic response

SPECIAL CONSIDERATIONS

- Anabolic steroids have potential for abuse, especially in the athlete
- Comparative advantages include less potential for virilization in women, convenience of oral administration; disadvantage includes increased risk of hepatotoxicity

PATIENT/FAMILY EDUCATION

- Hematologic response is often not immediate, needs minimum trial of 3-6 mo
- Notify the physician if acne, nausea, pedal edema, or vomiting occurs. Female patients should promptly report deepening of voice, hoarseness, and menstrual irregularities. Male patients should report difficulty urinating, frequent erections, and gynecomastia
- Avoid alcohol

MONITORING PARAMETERS

- LFTs, lipids, Hct
- Serum calcium in breast cancer patients
- Growth rate in children (X-rays for bone age q6mo)
- Weight
- Blood pressure
- Signs of virilization

oxymorphone hydrochloride

(ox-ee-mor′-fone)

Rx: Numorphan

Chemical Class: Opiate derivative; phenanthrene derivative

Therapeutic Class: Narcotic analgesic

DEA Class: Schedule II

CLINICAL PHARMACOLOGY

Mechanism of Action: An opioid agonist, similar to morphine, that binds at opiate receptor sites in the central nervous system (CNS). ***Therapeutic Effect:*** Reduces intensity of pain stimuli incoming from sensory nerve endings, altering pain perception and emotional response to pain; suppresses cough reflex.

Pharmacokinetics

Route	*Onset*	*Peak*	*Duration*
Subcutaneous	5-10 mins	30-90 mins	4-6 hrs
IM	5-10 mins	30-60 mins	3-6 hrs
IV	5-10 mins	15-30 mins	3-6 hrs
Rectal	15-30 mins	N/A	3-6 hrs

Well absorbed from the gastrointestinal (GI) tract, after IM administration. Widely distributed. Metabolized in liver via glucuronidation. Excreted in urine. ***Half-life:*** 1-2 hrs.

INDICATIONS AND DOSAGES

Analgesic, anxiety, preanesthesia

IV

Adults, Elderly, Children 12 yrs and older. Initially 0.5 mg.

SC/IM

Adults, Elderly, Children 12 yrs and older. 1-1.5 mg IM or SC q4-6h as needed.

Rectal

Adults, Elderly, Children 12 yrs and older. 0.5-1 mg q4-6h.

O

Obstetric analgesic
IM
Adults, Elderly, Children 12 yrs and older. 0.5-1 mg IM during labor.

AVAILABLE FORMS

- *Injection:* 1 mg/ml, 1.5 mg/ml (Numorphan).
- *Suppository:* 5 mg (Numorphan).

UNLABELED USES: Cancer pain, intractable pain in narcotic-tolerant patients

CONTRAINDICATIONS: Paralytic ileus, acute asthma attack, pulmonary edema secondary to chemical respiratory irritant, severe respiratory depression, upper airway obstruction

PREGNANCY AND LACTATION: Pregnancy category B (category D if used for prolonged periods or in high doses at term); use during labor produces neonatal respiratory depression
Controlled Substance: Schedule II

SIDE EFFECTS

Frequent
Drowsiness, dizziness, hypotension, decreased appetite, tolerance or dependence

Occasional
Confusion, diaphoresis, facial flushing, urinary retention, constipation, dry mouth, nausea, vomiting, headache, pain at injection site, abdominal cramps

Rare
Allergic reaction, depression

SERIOUS REACTIONS

- Hypotension, paralytic ileus, respiratory depression, and toxic megacolon rarely occur.
- Overdosage results in respiratory depression, skeletal muscle flaccidity, cold or clammy skin, cyanosis, extreme somnolence progressing to seizures, stupor, and coma.
- Tolerance to analgesic effect and physical dependence may occur with repeated use.
- Prolonged duration of action and cumulative effect may occur in patients with impaired liver or renal function.

INTERACTIONS

Drugs

3 *Barbiturates:* Additive CNS depression

3 *Cimetidine:* Increased effect of narcotic analgesics

❷ *Ethanol, other CNS depressants:* Additive CNS effects

3 *Neuroleptics:* Hypotension and excessive CNS depression

Labs

- *False increase:* Amylase and lipase

SPECIAL CONSIDERATIONS

- Do not administer agonist/antagonist analgesics (i.e., pentazocine, nalbuphine, butorphanol, dezocine, buprenorphine) to patient who has received a prolonged course of oxymorphone (a pure agonist). In opioid-dependent patients, mixed agonist/antagonist analgesics may precipitate withdrawal symptoms.

PATIENT/FAMILY EDUCATION

- Physical dependency may result when used for extended periods
- Change position slowly, orthostatic hypotension may occur
- Avoid alcohol
- Avoid tasks that require mental alertness and motor skills until response to the drug is established

MONITORING PARAMETERS

- Vital signs
- Pattern of daily bowel activity and stool consistency
- Clinical improvement, onset of relief of cough or pain

oxytetracycline hydrochloride

(ox'-ee-tet-tra-sye'-kleen hye-droe-klor'-ide)

Rx: Terramycin IM

Combinations

Rx: with polymyxin (Terek); with phenazopyridine, sulfamethizole (Urobiotic-250, Tija)

Chemical Class: Tetracycline derivative

Therapeutic Class: Antibiotic

CLINICAL PHARMACOLOGY

Mechanism of Action: A tetracycline antibiotic that inhibits bacterial protein synthesis by binding to ribosomes. Cell wall synthesis is not affected. ***Therapeutic Effect:*** Prevents bacterial cell growth. Bacteriostatic.

Pharmacokinetics

Poorly absorbed after IM administration. Protein binding: 27%-35%. Metabolized in liver. Excreted in urine. Eliminated in feces via biliary system. Not removed by hemodialysis. ***Half-life:*** 8.5-9.6 hrs (half-life is increased with impaired renal function).

INDICATIONS AND DOSAGES

Treatment of inflammatory acne, anthrax, gonorrhea, skin infections, urinary tract infection (UTI)

IM

Adults, Elderly. 250 mg/day or 300 mg/day divided q8-12h.

Children 8 yrs and older. 15-25 mg/kg/day in divided doses q8-12h. Maximum: 250 mg/dose.

Dosage in renal impairment

Creatinine Clearance	*Dosage Interval*
less than 10 ml/min	q24h

AVAILABLE FORMS

- *Injection, solution:* 5% (Terramycin IM).

UNLABELED USES: Chlamydia, non-specific urethritis, peptic ulcer

CONTRAINDICATIONS: Hypersensitivity to tetracyclines or any component of the formulation, children 8 yrs and younger

PREGNANCY AND LACTATION: Pregnancy category D; excreted into breast milk; milk:plasma ratio: 0.6-0.8; theoretically, may cause dental staining, but usually undetectable in infant serum (<0.05 mcg/ml)

SIDE EFFECTS

Frequent

Dizziness, lightheadedness, diarrhea, nausea, vomiting, stomach cramps, increased sensitivity of skin to sunlight

Occasional

Pigmentation of skin, mucous membranes, itching in rectal or genital area, sore mouth or tongue, increased BUN, irritation at injection site

SERIOUS REACTIONS

- Superinfection (especially fungal), anaphylaxis, and increased intracranial pressure may occur.
- Bulging fontanelles occur rarely in infants.

INTERACTIONS

Drugs

❷ *Antacids:* Reduced absorption of oxytetracycline

③ *Bismuth salts:* Reduced absorption of oxytetracycline

③ *Calcium:* See antacids

③ *Food:* Reduced absorption of oxytetracycline

③ *Iron:* Reduced absorption of oxytetracycline

③ *Magnesium:* See antacids

❷ *Methoxyflurane:* Increased risk of nephrotoxicity

3 *Oral contraceptives:* Interruption of enterohepatic circulation of estrogens, reduced oral contraceptive effectiveness

3 *Zinc:* Reduced absorption of oxytetracycline

Labs

- *False negative:* Urine glucose with Clinistix or TesTape
- *Interference:* Uroporphyrin
- *False increase:* Urinary and plasma catecholamines, serum bilirubin, CFS protein, urine glucose, serum uric acid, urine vanillylmandelic acid

SPECIAL CONSIDERATIONS

- Offers no significant advantage over tetracycline; shares similar spectrum of activity (may be slightly less active than tetracycline and has longer dosage interval)

PATIENT/FAMILY EDUCATION

- Avoid milk products, take with a full glass of water
- Take for the full length of treatment and space doses around the clock
- Notify the physician if diarrhea, rash, or any other new symptoms occur
- Protect skin from sun exposure and avoid overexposure to sun or ultraviolet light to prevent photosensitivity reactions

MONITORING PARAMETERS

- Blood pressure
- Pattern of daily bowel activity and stool consistency
- Skin for rash

oxytocin

(ox-i-toe′-sin)

Rx: Pitocin

Chemical Class: Polypeptide hormone

Therapeutic Class: Galactokinetic; oxytocic

CLINICAL PHARMACOLOGY

Mechanism of Action: An oxytocic that affect uterine myofibril activity and stimulates mammary smooth muscle. ***Therapeutic Effect:*** Contracts uterine smooth muscle. Enhances lactation.

Pharmacokinetics

Route	*Onset*	*Peak*	*Duration*
IV	Immediate	N/A	1 hr
IM	3-5 mins	N/A	2-3 hrs

Rapidly absorbed through nasal mucous membranes. Protein binding: 30%. Distributed in extracellular fluid. Metabolized in the liver and kidney. Primarily excreted in urine. ***Half-life:*** 1-6 mins.

INDICATIONS AND DOSAGES

Induction or stimulation of labor

IV

Adults. 0.5-1 milliunit/min. May gradually increase in increments of 1-2 milliunit/min. Rates of 9-10 milliunit/min are rarely required.

Abortion

IV

Adults. 10-20 milliunit/min. Maximum: 30 unit/12h dose.

Control of postpartum bleeding

IV Infusion

Adults. 10-40 units in 1000 ml IV fluid at a rate sufficient to control uterine atony.

IM

Adults. 10 units (total dose) after delivery.

AVAILABLE FORMS

- *Injection:* 10 units/ml.
- *Nasal Spray*: 40 units/ml.

CONTRAINDICATIONS: Adequate uterine activity that fails to progress, cephalopelvic disproportion, fetal distress without imminent delivery, grand multiparity, hyperactive or hypertonic uterus, obstetric emergencies that favor surgical intervention, prematurity, unengaged fetal head, unfavorable fetal position or presentation, when vaginal delivery is contraindicated, such as active genital herpes infection, placenta previa, or cord presentation

PREGNANCY AND LACTATION: Pregnancy category X; nasal oxytocin contraindicated during pregnancy; only minimal amounts pass into breast milk

SIDE EFFECTS

Occasional

Tachycardia, premature ventricular contractions, hypotension, nausea, vomiting

Rare

Nasal: Lacrimation or tearing, nasal irritation, rhinorrhea, unexpected uterine bleeding or contractions

SERIOUS REACTIONS

- Hypertonicity may occur with tearing of the uterus, increased bleeding, abruptio placentae, and cervical and vaginal lacerations.
- In the fetus, bradycardia, CNS or brain damage, trauma due to rapid propulsion, low Apgar score at 5 mins, and retinal hemorrhage occur rarely.
- Prolonged IV infusion of oxytocin with excessive fluid volume has caused severe water intoxication with seizures, coma, and death.

INTERACTIONS

Drugs

3 *Caudal block anesthetics, vasopressors:* May increase pressor effects

3 *Other oxytocics:* May cause cervical lacerations, uterine hypertonus, or uterine rupture

SPECIAL CONSIDERATIONS

- Routinely used for the induction of labor at term and postpartum for the control of uterine bleeding; not the drug of choice for induction of labor for abortion

PATIENT/FAMILY EDUCATION

- The drug will be present in breast milk, breast-feeding is not recommended
- Inform the patient and family about the progress of labor
- Oxytocin can be used during the first postpartal week to promote milk ejection but its use beyond the first postpartal week is not recommended

MONITORING PARAMETERS

- Continuous monitoring necessary for IV use (length, intensity, duration of contractions); fetal heart rate—acceleration, deceleration, fetal distress
- Notify the physician of uterine contractions that last longer than 1 min, occur more frequently than every 2 mins, or stop
- Blood pressure, respiration rates
- Intake and output
- Monitor for unexpected or increased blood loss

palonosetron hydrochloride

(pal-oh-noe'-se-tron hye-droe-klor'-ide)

Rx: Aloxi

Chemical Class: Isoquinoline derivative

Therapeutic Class: Antiemetic

CLINICAL PHARMACOLOGY

Mechanism of Action: A 5-HT_3 receptor antagonist that acts centrally in the chemoreceptor trigger zone and peripherally at the vagal nerve terminals. ***Therapeutic Effect:*** Prevents nausea and vomiting associated with chemotherapy.

Pharmacokinetics

Protein binding: 52%. Metabolized in liver. Eliminated in urine. ***Half-life:*** 40 hr.

INDICATIONS AND DOSAGES

Chemotherapy-induced nausea and vomiting

IV

Adults, Elderly. 0.25 mg as a single dose 30 min before starting chemotherapy.

AVAILABLE FORMS

- *Injection:* 0.25 mg/5 ml.

UNLABELED USES: Prevention of postoperative bleeding

CONTRAINDICATIONS: None known.

PREGNANCY AND LACTATION: Pregnancy category B; excretion into breast milk unknown, use caution in nursing mothers

SIDE EFFECTS

Occasional (9%-5%)

Headache, constipation

Rare (less than 1%)

Diarrhea, dizziness, fatigue, abdominal pain, insomnia

SERIOUS REACTIONS

- Overdose may produce a combination of CNS stimulant and depressant effects.
- Cardiac dysrhythmia has been reported.

INTERACTIONS

Drugs

3 *Antiarrhythmics, diuretics, cumulative high-dose anthracycline therapy, drugs that prolong QTc interval:* Increased potential for arrhythmia

SPECIAL CONSIDERATIONS

- Clinical superiority over other 5-HT_3 receptor antagonists (e.g., ondansetron, dolasetron) has not been adequately demonstrated

PATIENT/FAMILY EDUCATION

- Nausea and vomiting should be relieved shortly after drug administration; notify the physician if vomiting persists
- Avoid alcohol and barbiturates during palonosetron therapy
- Other methods of reducing nausea and vomiting include lying quietly and avoiding strong odors

MONITORING PARAMETERS

- Pattern of daily bowel activity and stool consistency and record time of evacuation

pamidronate disodium

(pa-mi-droe'-nate)

Rx: Aredia, Pamidronate Disodium Novaplus

Chemical Class: Pyrophosphate analog

Therapeutic Class: Bisphosphonate; bone resorption inhibitor

CLINICAL PHARMACOLOGY

Mechanism of Action: A bisphosphate that binds to bone and inhibits osteoclast-mediated calcium resorption. ***Therapeutic Effect:*** Lowers serum calcium concentrations.

Pharmacokinetics

Route	Onset	Peak	Duration
IV	24-48 hrs	5-7 days	N/A

After IV administration, rapidly absorbed by bone. Slowly excreted unchanged in urine. Unknown if removed by hemodialysis. ***Half-life:*** bone, 300 days; unmetabolized, 2.5 hrs.

INDICATIONS AND DOSAGES

Hypercalcemia

IV Infusion

Adults, Elderly. Moderate hypercalcemia (corrected serum calcium level 12-13.5 mg/dl): 60-90 mg. Severe hypercalcemia (corrected serum calcium level greater than 13.5 mg/dl): 90 mg.

Paget's disease

IV Infusion

Adults, Elderly. 30 mg/day for 3 days.

Osteolytic bone lesion

IV Infusion

Adults, Elderly. 90 mg over 2-4 hrs once a month.

AVAILABLE FORMS

• *Powder for Injection (Aredia, Pamidronate Disodium Novaplus):* 30 mg, 90 mg.

• *Injection Solution:* 3 mg/ml, 6 mg/ml, 9 mg/ml.

CONTRAINDICATIONS: Hypersensitivity to other bisphosphonates, such as etidronate, tiludronate, risedronate, and alendronate

PREGNANCY AND LACTATION: Pregnancy category D; caution with administration to a nursing mother

SIDE EFFECTS

Frequent (greater than 10%)

Temperature elevation (at least 1°C) 24-48 hr after administration (27%); redness, swelling, induration, pain at catheter site with in patients receiving 90 mg (18%); anorexia, nausea, fatigue

Occasional (10%-1%)

Constipation, rhinitis

SERIOUS REACTIONS

• Hypophosphatemia, hypokalemia, hypomagnesemia, and hypocalcemia occur more frequently with higher dosages.

• Anemia, hypertension, tachycardia, atrial fibrillation, and somnolence occur more frequently with 90-mg doses.

• GI hemorrhage occurs rarely.

INTERACTIONS

Drugs

3 *Calcium-containing medications, vitamin D:* May antagonize the effects of pamidronate in treatment of hypercalcemia

SPECIAL CONSIDERATIONS

• "Second-generation" bisphosphonate that offers potential advantages over etidronate (as does alendronate) in that it inhibits bone resorption at doses that do not impair bone mineralization, and is less likely than etidronate to produce osteomalacia

• Allow at least 7 days between initial treatment for patients requiring retreatment for hypercalcemia

PATIENT/FAMILY EDUCATION

• Avoid drugs containing calcium and vitamin D, such as antacids, because they might antagonize the effects of pamidronate

MONITORING PARAMETERS

• Hct, Hgb, and serum magnesium and creatinine levels
• Fluid intake and output carefully
• Examine lungs for crackles and dependent body parts for edema
• Blood pressure, pulse, temperature

pancreatin/ pancrelipase

(pan-kree-ah'-tin/pan-kre-li'-pase)

Rx: (pancreatin) Ku-Zyme, Pancreatin

Rx: (pancrelipase) Cotazym-S, Creon 5, Creon 10, Creon 20, Ilozyme, Kutrase, Ku-Zyme, Ku-Zyme HP, Lipram, Lipram-CR, Lipram-CR 5, Lipram-CR 20, Lipram-PN, Lipram-UL 12, Lipram-UL 18, Lipram-UL 20, Panase, Pancrease, Pancrease MT 4, Pancrease MT 20, Pancreatic EC, Pancreatil-UL 12, Pancrecarb MS-4, Pancrecarb MS-8, Pangestyme CN 10, Pangestyme CN 20, Pangestyme EC, Pangestyme MT 16, Pangestyme NL 18, Panokase, Plaretase, Protilase, Ultrase, Ultrase MT 12, Ultrase MT 18, Ultrase MT 20, Viokase, Viokase 8, Viokase 16, Zymase

Chemical Class: Pancreatic enzymes

Therapeutic Class: Digestant

CLINICAL PHARMACOLOGY

Mechanism of Action: Digestive enzymes that replace endogenous pancreatic enzymes. ***Therapeutic Effect:*** Assist in digestion of protein, starch, and fats.

Pharmacokinetics

Not absorbed systemically. Released at the duodenojejunal junction.

INDICATIONS AND DOSAGES

Pancreatic enzyme replacement or supplement when enzymes are absent or deficient, such as with chronic pancreatitis, cystic fibro-

sis, or ductal obstruction from cancer of the pancreas or common bile duct; to reduce malabsorption; treatment of steatorrhea associated with bowel resection or postgastrectomy syndrome

PO

Adults, Elderly. 1-3 capsules or tablets before or with meals or snacks. May increase to 8 tablets/dose.

Children. 1-2 tablets with meals or snacks.

AVAILABLE FORMS

• *Capsules:* 15,000 units-12,000 units-15,000 units (Ku-Zyme), 30,000 units-24,000 units-30,000 units (Kutrase), 30,000 units-8000 units-30,000 units (Panokase, Cotazym, Ku-Zyme HP).

• *Capsules (Extended-Release):* 33,200 units-10,000 units-37,500 units (Creon 10, Lipram-CR), 30,000 units-10,000 units-30,000 units (Pangestyme CN 10, Lipram, Pancrease MT 10), 39,000 units-12,000 units-39,000 units (Lipram-UL 12, Pancreatil-UL 12, Ultrase MT 12), 12,000 units-4000 units-12,000 units (Pancrease MT 4), 48,000 units-16,000 units-48,000 units (Lipram-PN, Pancrease MT 16, Pangestyme MT 16), 16,600 units-5000 units-18,750 units (Creon 5, Lipram-CR5), 59,000 units-18,000 units-59,000 units (Pangestyme NL 18, Lipram-UL 18, Ultrase MT 18), 20,000 units-5000 units-20,000 units (Cotazym-S), 66,400 units-20,000 units-75,000 units (Creon 20, Lipram-CR 20), 20,000 units-4500 units-25,000 units (Lipram, Pancrease, Pangestyme EC, Ultrase), 56,000 units-20,000 units-44,000 units (Lipram-PN, Pancrease MT 20), 65,000 units-20,000 units-65,000 units (Lipram-UL 20, Pangestyme NL 18, Pangestyme CN 20, Ultrase MT 20), 20,000 units-4000 units-25,000 units (Panase, Pancreatic EC, Protilase), 25,000 units-4000 units-25,000 units (Pancrecarb MS-4), 40,000 units-8000 units-45,000 units (Pancrecarb MS-8).

• *Powder for Reconstitution, oral (Viokase):* 70,000 units-16,800 units-70,000 units/0.7 gm.

• *Tablets:* 30,000 units-11,000 units-30,000 units (Ilozyme), 60,000 units-16,000 units-60,000 units (Viokase 16), 30,000 units-8000 units-30,000 units (Panokase, Plaretase, Viokase 8).

UNLABELED USES: Treatment of occluded feeding tubes

CONTRAINDICATIONS: Acute pancreatitis, exacerbation of chronic pancreatitis, hypersensitivity to pork protein

PREGNANCY AND LACTATION: Pregnancy category C

SIDE EFFECTS

Rare

Allergic reaction, mouth irritation, shortness of breath, wheezing

SERIOUS REACTIONS

• Excessive dosage may produce nausea, cramping, and diarrhea.

• Hyperuricosuria and hyperuricemia have occurred with extremely high dosages.

INTERACTIONS

Drugs

3 *Antacids:* May decrease the effects of pancreatin and pancrelipase

3 *Iron supplements:* May decrease the absorption of iron supplements

SPECIAL CONSIDERATIONS

• Substitution at dispensing should be avoided

• Enteric-coated pancreatic enzymes are more effective than regular formulations; individual variations may require trials with several enzymatic preparations

P

• For patients who do not respond appropriately, adding antacid or H_2-antagonist may provide better results
• Preparations high in lipase concentration seem to be more effective for reducing steatorrhea

PATIENT/FAMILY EDUCATION
• Advise patient to take before or with meals
• Protect enteric coating; advise patient not to crush or chew microspheres in caps or tabs
• Do not spill Viokase powder on the hands because it may irritate the skin
• Avoid inhaling powder because it may irritate mucous membranes and produce bronchospasm
• Do not change brands of the drug without first consulting the physician

MONITORING PARAMETERS
• Growth curves in children
• Therapeutic response

pantoprazole sodium

(pan-toe-pra'-zole soe'-dee-um)

Rx: Protonix, Protonix IV

Chemical Class: Benzimidazole derivative

Therapeutic Class: Antiulcer agent

CLINICAL PHARMACOLOGY

Mechanism of Action: A benzimidazole that is converted to active metabolites that irreversibly bind to and inhibit hydrogen-potassium adenosine triphosphate, an enzyme on the surface of gastric parietal cells. Inhibits hydrogen ion transport into gastric lumen. ***Therapeutic Effect:*** Increases gastric pH and reduces gastric acid production.

Pharmacokinetics

Route	*Onset*	*Peak*	*Duration*
PO	N/A	N/A	24 hrs

Rapidly absorbed from the GI tract. Protein binding: 98%. Primarily distributed into gastric parietal cells. Metabolized extensively in the liver. Primarily excreted in urine. Not removed by hemodialysis. ***Half-life:*** 1 hr.

INDICATIONS AND DOSAGES

Erosive esophagitis

PO

Adults, Elderly. 40 mg/day for up to 8 wk. If not healed after 8 wk, may continue an additional 8 wk.

IV

Adults, Elderly. 40 mg/day for 7-10 days.

Hypersecretory conditions

PO

Adults, Elderly. Initially, 40 mg twice a day. May increase to 240 mg/day.

IV

Adults, Elderly. 80 mg twice a day. May increase to 80 mg q8h.

AVAILABLE FORMS
• *Tablets (Delayed-Release [Protonix]):* 20 mg, 40 mg.
• *Powder for Injection (Protonix IV):* 40 mg.

UNLABELED USES: Peptic ulcer disease, active ulcer bleeding (injection), adjunct in treatment of *H. pylori*

CONTRAINDICATIONS: None known.

PREGNANCY AND LACTATION: Pregnancy category B; excretion into breast milk unknown; use caution in nursing mothers

SIDE EFFECTS

Rare (less than 2%)

Diarrhea, headache, dizziness, pruritus, rash

SERIOUS REACTIONS
• Hyperglycemia occurs rarely.

INTERACTIONS

Drugs

3 *Ketoconazole:* Decreased bioavailability of ketoconazole

SPECIAL CONSIDERATIONS

PATIENT/FAMILY EDUCATION

- Caution patients not to split, crush or chew delayed-release tablets; swallow whole
- Notify the physician if headache occurs during pantoprazole therapy
- Take tablets before eating

MONITORING PARAMETERS

- Symptom relief, mucosal healing

---

paregoric

(par-e-gor′-ik)

Rx: Paregoric

Chemical Class: Opiate (most preparations also contain camphor and ethanol)

Therapeutic Class: Antidiarrheal

DEA Class: Schedule III

CLINICAL PHARMACOLOGY

Mechanism of Action: An opioid agonist that contains many narcotic alkaloids including morphine. It inhibits gastric motility due to its morphine content. ***Therapeutic Effect:*** Decreases digestive secretions, increases in gastrointestinal (GI) muscle tone, and reduces GI propulsion.

Pharmacokinetics

Variably absorbed from the GI tract. Protein binding: low. Metabolized in liver. Primarily excreted in urine primarily as morphine glucuronide conjugates and unchanged drug—morphine, codeine, papaverine, etc. Unknown if removed by hemodialysis. ***Half-life:*** 2-3 hrs.

INDICATIONS AND DOSAGES

Antidiarrheal

PO

Adults, Elderly. 5-10 ml 1-4 times/day.

Children. 0.25-0.5 ml/kg/dose 1-4 times/day.

AVAILABLE FORMS

- *Tincture:* 2 mg/5 ml (Paregoric).

UNLABELED USES: Narcotic withdrawal symptoms in neonates

CONTRAINDICATIONS: Diarrhea caused by poisoning until the toxic material is removed, hypersensitivity to morphine sulfate or any component of the formulation, pregnancy (prolonged use or high dosages near term)

PREGNANCY AND LACTATION: Pregnancy category B, D; excreted in breast milk

Controlled Substance: Schedule III

SIDE EFFECTS

Frequent

Constipation, drowsiness, nausea, vomiting

Occasional

Paradoxical excitement, confusion, pounding heartbeat, facial flushing, decreased urination, blurred vision, dizziness, dry mouth, headache, hypotension, decreased appetite, redness, burning, pain at injection site

Rare

Hallucinations, depression, stomach pain, insomnia

SERIOUS REACTIONS

- Overdosage results in cold or clammy skin, confusion, convulsions, decreased blood pressure (BP), restlessness, pinpoint pupils, bradycardia, respiratory depression, decreased level of consciousness (LOC), and severe weakness.
- Tolerance to analgesic effect and physical dependence may occur with repeated use.

INTERACTIONS

Drugs

3 *Alcohol, other CNS depressants:* Additive depressant effects

3 *Barbiturates, rifampin:* Increased metabolism of paregoric

3 *Cimetidine:* Decreased metabolism of paregoric

SPECIAL CONSIDERATIONS

• Contains ethanol

PATIENT/FAMILY EDUCATION

• Avoid performing tasks that require mental alertness or motor skills until response to the drug has been established

• Avoid alcohol

• Drug dependence or tolerance may occur with prolonged use of high dosages

MONITORING PARAMETERS

• Pattern of bowel activity and stool consistency

---

paricalcitol

(par-i-kal'-si-trole)

Rx: Zemplar

Chemical Class: Vitamin D analog

Therapeutic Class: Vitamin

CLINICAL PHARMACOLOGY

Mechanism of Action: A fat-soluble vitamin that is essential for absorption, utilization of calcium phosphate, and normal calcification of bone. ***Therapeutic Effect:*** Stimulates calcium and phosphate absorption from small intestine, promotes secretion of calcium from bone to blood, promotes renal tubule phosphate resorption, acts on bone cells to stimulate skeletal growth and on parathyroid gland to suppress hormone synthesis and secretion.

Pharmacokinetics

Protein binding: more than 99%. Metabolized in liver. Primarily eliminated in feces; minimal excretion in urine. Not removed by hemodialysis. ***Half-life:*** 14-15 hrs.

INDICATIONS AND DOSAGES

Hypoparathyroidism

IV

Adults, Elderly, Children. 0.04-0.1 mcg/kg (2.8-7 mcg) given as a bolus dose no more frequently than every other day at any time during dialysis; dose as high as 0.24 mcg/kg (16.8 mcg) have been administered safely. Usually start with 0.04 mcg/kg 3 times/wk as a bolus, increased by 0.04 mcg/kg every 2 wks. Dose adjust based on serum PTH levels:

Same or increasing serum PTH level: Increase dose

Serum PTH level decreased by <30%: Increase dose

Serum PTH level decreased by >30% and <60%: Maintain dose

Serum PTH level decrease by >60%: Decrease dose

Serum PTH level 1.5-3 times upper limit of normal: Maintain dose

AVAILABLE FORMS

• *Injection:* 5 mcg/ml (Zemplar).

CONTRAINDICATIONS: Hypercalcemia, malabsorption syndrome, vitamin D toxicity, hypersensitivity to other vitamin D products or analogs

PREGNANCY AND LACTATION: Pregnancy category C; use caution in nursing mothers

SIDE EFFECTS

Occasional

Edema, nausea, vomiting, headache, dizziness

Rare

Palpitations

SERIOUS REACTIONS

- Early signs of overdosage are manifested as weakness, headache, somnolence, nausea, vomiting, dry mouth, constipation, muscle and bone pain, and metallic taste sensation.
- Later signs of overdosage are evidenced by polyuria, polydipsia, anorexia, weight loss, nocturia, photophobia, rhinorrhea, pruritus, disorientation, hallucinations, hyperthermia, hypertension, and cardiac arrhythmias.
- Hypercalcemia occurs rarely.

INTERACTIONS

Drugs

3 *Digoxin:* Hypercalcemia produced by paricalcitol may potentiate digoxin toxicity

SPECIAL CONSIDERATIONS

- Phosphate-binding compounds may be needed to control serum phosphorus levels

PATIENT/FAMILY EDUCATION

- Adhere to a dietary regimen of calcium supplementation and phosphorus restriction; avoid excessive use of aluminum-containing compounds
- Consume foods rich in vitamin D, including eggs, leafy vegetables, margarine, meats, milk, vegetable oils, and vegetable shortening
- Drink plenty of fluids

MONITORING PARAMETERS

- Serum calcium and phosphorus twice weekly during initial phase of therapy, then at least monthly once dosage has been established; if an elevated calcium level or a Ca × P product > 75 is noted, immediately reduce or interrupt dosage until parameters are normalized, then reinitiate at lower dose; intact PTH assay every 3 mo (target range in CRF patients ≤ 1.5-3 × the nonuremic upper limit of normal)
- Serum alkaline phosphatase, BUN, serum creatinine

paromomycin sulfate

(par-oh-moe-mye'-sin)

Rx: Humatin

Chemical Class: Aminoglycoside

Therapeutic Class: Amebicide; antibiotic

CLINICAL PHARMACOLOGY

Mechanism of Action: An antibacterial agent that acts directly on amoebas and against normal and pathogenic organisms in the GI tract. Interferes with bacterial protein synthesis by binding to 30S ribosomal subunits. ***Therapeutic Effect:*** Produces amoebicidal effects.

Pharmacokinetics

Poorly absorbed from the gastrointestinal (GI) tract and most of the dose is eliminated unchanged in feces.

INDICATIONS AND DOSAGES

Intestinal amebiasis

PO

Adults, Elderly, Children. 25-35 mg/kg/day q8h for 5-10 days.

Hepatic coma

PO

Adults, Elderly. 4 g/day q6-12h for 5-6 days.

AVAILABLE FORMS

- *Capsules:* 250 mg (Humantin).

UNLABELED USES: Cryptosporidiosis, giardiasis, leishmaniasis, microsporidiosis, mycobacterial infections, tapeworm infestation, trichomoniasis, typhoid carriers

CONTRAINDICATIONS: Intestinal obstruction, renal failure, hypersensitivity to paromomycin or any of its components

PREGNANCY AND LACTATION: Pregnancy category C; poor oral bioavailability and lipid solubility limit passage into breast milk

SIDE EFFECTS

Occasional

Diarrhea, abdominal cramps, nausea, vomiting, heartburn

Rare

Rash, pruritus, vertigo

SERIOUS REACTIONS

- Overdosage may result in nausea, vomiting, and diarrhea.

SPECIAL CONSIDERATIONS

PATIENT/FAMILY EDUCATION

- Report any audio disturbances
- Do not skip doses

MONITORING PARAMETERS

- Skin for rash
- Renal function

paroxetine hydrochloride

(par-ox'-e-teen hye-droe-klor'-ide)

Rx: Paxeva, Paxil, Paxil CR

Chemical Class: Phenylpiperidine derivative

Therapeutic Class: Antidepressant, selective serotonin reuptake inhibitor (SSRI)

CLINICAL PHARMACOLOGY

Mechanism of Action: An antidepressant, anxiolytic, and antiobsessional agent that selectively blocks uptake of the neurotransmitter serotonin at neuronal presynaptic membranes, thereby increasing its availability at postsynaptic receptor sites. ***Therapeutic Effect:*** Relieves depression, reduces obsessive-compulsive behavior, decreases anxiety.

Pharmacokinetics

Well absorbed from the GI tract. Protein binding: 95%. Widely distributed. Metabolized in the liver. Excreted in urine. Not removed by hemodialysis. ***Half-life:*** 24 hr.

INDICATIONS AND DOSAGES

Depression

PO

Adults. Initially, 20 mg/day. May increase by 10 mg/day at intervals of more than 1 wk. Maximum: 50 mg/day.

PO (Controlled-Release)

Adults. Initially, 25 mg/day. May increase by 12.5 mg/day at intervals of more than 1 wk. Maximum: 62.5 mg/day.

Generalized anxiety disorder

PO

Adults. Initially, 20 mg/day. May increase by 10 mg/day at intervals of more than 1 wk. Range: 20-50 mg/day.

Obsessive-compulsive disorder

PO

Adults. Initially, 20 mg/day. May increase by 10 mg/day at intervals of more than 1 wk. Range: 20-60 mg/day.

Panic disorder

PO

Adults. Initially, 10-20 mg/day. May increase by 10 mg/day at intervals of more than 1 wk. Range: 10-60 mg/day.

Social anxiety disorder

PO

Adults. Initially, 20 mg/day. Range: 20-60 mg/day.

Posttraumatic stress disorder

PO

Adults. Initially, 20 mg/day. May increase by 10 mg/day at intervals of more than 1 wk. Range: 20-50 mg/day.

Premenstrual dysphoric disorder

PO (Paxil CR)

Adults. Initially, 12.5 mg/day. May increase by 12.5 mg at weekly intervals to a maximum of 25 mg/day.

Usual elderly dosage

PO: Initially, 10 mg/day. May increase by 10 mg/day at intervals of more than 1 wk. Maximum: 40 mg/day.

PO (Controlled-Release): Initially, 12.5 mg/day. May increase by 12.5 mg/day at intervals of more than 1 wk. Maximum: 50 mg/day.

AVAILABLE FORMS

- *Oral Suspension (Paxil):* 10 mg/5 ml.
- *Tablets (Paxil, Pexeva):* 10 mg, 20 mg, 30 mg, 40 mg.
- *Tablets (Controlled-Release [Paxil CR]):* 12.5 mg, 25 mg, 37.5 mg.

UNLABELED USES: Eating disorders, impulse disorders, menopause symptoms, premenstrual disorders, treatment of depression and OCD in children

CONTRAINDICATIONS: Use within 14 days of MAOIs

PREGNANCY AND LACTATION: Pregnancy category C; limited information; milk concentrations similar to plasma following a single oral dose; thus <1% of the daily dose would be transferred to a breast-feeding infant

SIDE EFFECTS

Frequent

Nausea (26%); somnolence (23%); headache, dry mouth (18%); asthenia (15%); constipation (15%); dizziness, insomnia (13%); diarrhea (12%); diaphoresis (11%); tremor (8%)

Occasional

Decreased appetite, respiratory disturbance (such as increased cough) (6%); anxiety, nervousness (5%); flatulence, paresthesia, yawning (4%); decreased libido, sexual dysfunction, abdominal discomfort (3%)

Rare

Palpitations, vomiting, blurred vision, altered taste, confusion

SERIOUS REACTIONS

- Abnormal bleeding, hyponatremia, seizures, hypomania, and suicidal thoughts have been reported.

INTERACTIONS

Drugs

3 *β-blockers (metroprolol, propranolol, sotalol):* Inhibition of metabolism (CYP2D6) leads to increased plasma concentrations of selective β-blockers and potential cardiac toxicity; atenolol may be safer choice

3 *Cimetidine:* Increased plasma paroxetine concentrations

3 *Cyproheptadine:* Serotonin antagonist may partially reverse antidepressant and other effects

2 *Dexfenfluramine:* Duplicate effects on inhibition of serotonin reuptake; inhibition of dexfenfluramine metabolism (CYP2D6) exaggerates effect; both mechanisms increase risk of serotonin syndrome

3 *Dextromethorphan:* Inhibition of dextromethorphan's metabolism (CYP2D6) by paroxetine and additive serotonergic effects

3 *Diuretics, loop (bumetanide, furosemide, torsemide):* Possible additive hyponatremia; two fatal case reports with furosemide and paroxetine

2 *Fenfluramine:* Duplicate effects on inhibition of serotonin reuptake; inhibition of dexfenfluramine metabolism (CYP2D6) exaggerates effect; both mechanisms increase risk of serotonin syndrome

▲ *Furazolidone:* Increased risk of serotonin syndrome

3 *Haloperidol:* Inhibition of haloperidol's metabolism (CYP2D6) may increase risks of extrapyramidal symptoms

3 *Lithium:* Neurotoxicity (tremor, confusion, ataxia, dizziness, dysarthria, and absence seizures) reported in patients receiving this combination; mechanism unknown

⚠ *MAOI's (isocarboxazid, phenelzine, tranylcypromine):* Increased CNS serotonergic effects have been associated with severe or fatal reactions with this combination

3 *Phenobarbital:* Decreased plasma paroxetine concentrations

3 *Phenytoin:* Decreased plasma paroxetine concentrations

3 *Risperidone:* May increase risperidone blood concentration and cause extrapyramidal symptoms

⚠ *Selegiline:* Sporadic cases of mania and hypertension

3 *St. John's Wort:* May increase paroxetine's pharmacologic effects and risk of toxicity

3 *Sumatriptan (and other "triptans"):* Increased incidence of adverse effects, including serotonin syndrome

3 *Theophylline:* Elevated theophylline levels have been reported

⚠ *Thioridazine:* Increased plasma thioridazine concentrations; increased risk of ventricular arrhythmias

3 *Tramadol:* Increased risk of serotonin syndrome

3 *Tricyclic antidepressants (clomipramine, desipramine, doxepin, imipramine, nortriptyline, trazodone):* Marked increases in tricyclic antidepressant levels due to inhibition of metabolism (CYP2D6)

2 *Tryptophan:* Additive serotonergic effects

3 *Warfarin:* Increased risk of bleeding

SPECIAL CONSIDERATIONS

• Somewhat sedating compared to fluoxetine and sertraline

PATIENT/FAMILY EDUCATION

• Avoid alcohol
• May take 1-4 wks to see improvement of symptoms
• Do not abruptly discontinue paroxetine
• Avoid tasks that require mental alertness or motor skills until response to the drug has been established
• The female patient should notify the physician if she is or intends to become pregnant
• Take sips of tepid water or chew sugarless gum to help relieve dry mouth

MONITORING PARAMETERS

• CBC and hepatic and renal function tests periodically, as ordered, for patients on long-term therapy
• Closely supervise suicidal patients during early therapy; as depression lessens, energy level improves, increasing the suicide potential
• Assess appearance, behavior, level of interest, mood, and sleep pattern to determine the drug's therapeutic effect

---

pegfilgrastim

(peg-fil-gra'-stim)

Rx: Neulasta

Chemical Class: Amino acid glycoprotein

Therapeutic Class: Hematopoietic agent

CLINICAL PHARMACOLOGY

Mechanism of Action: A colony-stimulating factor that regulates production of neutrophils within bone marrow. Also a glycoprotein that primarily affects neutrophil progenitor proliferation, differentiation, and selected end-cell functional activation. ***Therapeutic Effect:*** Increases phagocytic ability and antibody-dependent destruction; decreases incidence of infection.

Pharmacokinetics

Readily absorbed after subcutaneous administration. ***Half-life:*** 15-80 hrs.

INDICATIONS AND DOSAGES

Myelosuppression

Subcutaneous

Adults, Elderly. Give as a single 6-mg injection once per chemotherapy cycle.

AVAILABLE FORMS

• *Solution for Injection:* 6 mg/0.6 ml syringe.

CONTRAINDICATIONS: Hypersensitivity to *Escherichia coli*–derived proteins, do not administer within 14 days before and 24 hrs after cytotoxic chemotherapy

PREGNANCY AND LACTATION: Pregnancy category C; breast milk excretion unknown; use caution in nursing mothers

SIDE EFFECTS

Frequent (72%-15%)

Bone pain, nausea, fatigue, alopecia, diarrhea, vomiting, constipation, anorexia, abdominal pain, arthralgia, generalized weakness, peripheral edema, dizziness, stomatitis, mucositis, neutropenic fever

SERIOUS REACTIONS

• Allergic reactions, such as anaphylaxis, rash, and urticaria, occur rarely.

• Cytopenia resulting from an antibody response to growth factors occurs rarely.

• Splenomegaly occurs rarely; assess for left upper abdominal or shoulder pain.

• Adult respiratory distress syndrome (ARDS) may occur in patients with sepsis.

• Severe sickle cell crisis has been reported.

INTERACTIONS

Drugs

3 *Lithium:* Enhanced leukocytosis

SPECIAL CONSIDERATIONS

• Do not administer in the period between 14 days before and 24 hr after administration of cytotoxic chemotherapy

• Reduces duration of severe neutropenia from 6 days to 2 days, and incidence of febrile neutropenia from 30%-40% to 10%-20%

PATIENT/FAMILY EDUCATION

• Compliance is important, including regular monitoring of blood counts

• Be aware of signs and symptoms of allergic reactions that may occur with pegfilgrastim

MONITORING PARAMETERS

• CBC with platelets

• Monitor for allergic reactions

• Examine for peripheral edema, particularly behind the medial malleolus, which is usually the first area to show peripheral edema

• Assess mucous membranes for evidence of mucositis (such as red mucous membranes, white patches, and extreme mouth soreness), and stomatitis

• Evaluate muscle strength

• Pattern of daily bowel activity and stool consistency

• Evaluate patients with sepsis for signs and symptoms of ARDS, such as dyspnea

peginterferon alfa-2a

(peg-in-ter-feer'-on alfa-2a)

Rx: Pegasys

Chemical Class: Recombinant interferon

Therapeutic Class: Antiviral

CLINICAL PHARMACOLOGY

Mechanism of Action: An immunomodulator that binds to specific membrane receptors on the cell surface, inhibiting viral replication in virus-infected cells, suppressing cell proliferation, and producing reversible decreases in leukocyte and platelet counts. ***Therapeutic Effect:*** Inhibits hepatitis C virus.

Pharmacokinetics

Readily absorbed after subcutaneous administration. Excreted by the kidneys. ***Half-life:*** 80 hr.

INDICATIONS AND DOSAGES

Hepatitis C

Subcutaneous

Adults 18 yr and older, Elderly. 180 mcg (1 ml) injected in abdomen or thigh once weekly for 48 wk.

Dosage in renal impairment

For patients who require hemodialysis, dosage is 135 mg injected in abdomen or thigh once weekly for 48 wk.

Dosage in hepatic impairment

For patients with progressive ALT increases above baseline values, dosage is 90 mcg injected in abdomen or thigh once weekly for 48 wk.

AVAILABLE FORMS

- *Injection Solution:* 180 mcg/ml.
- *Injection, Prefilled Syringe:* 180 mcg/0.5 ml.

CONTRAINDICATIONS: Autoimmune hepatitis, decompensated hepatic disease, infants, neonates

PREGNANCY AND LACTATION: Pregnancy category C (category X when used with ribavirin); breast milk excretion unknown

SIDE EFFECTS

Frequent (54%)

Headache

Occasional (23%-13%)

Alopecia, nausea, insomnia, anorexia, dizziness, diarrhea, abdominal pain, flu-like symptoms, psychiatric reactions (depression, irritability, anxiety), injection site reaction

Rare (8%-5%)

Impaired concentration, diaphoresis, dry mouth, nausea, vomiting

SERIOUS REACTIONS

- Serious, acute hypersensitivity reactions, such as urticaria, angioedema, bronchoconstriction, and anaphylaxis, may occur. Other rare reactions include pancreatitis, colitis, endocrine disorders (e.g., diabetes mellitus), hyperthyroidism or hypothyroidism, ophthalmologic neuropsychiatric, autoimmune, ischemic, infectious, and pulmonary disorders.

INTERACTIONS

Drugs

- *Note that additional interactions occur when peginterferon is combined with ribavirin; see ribavirin monograph*

3 *Theophylline:* Peginterferon increases plasma theophylline level by up to 25%

3 *Bone marrow depressants:* May increase myelosuppression

SPECIAL CONSIDERATIONS

- Weekly administration of peginterferon alfa-2a equivalent to 3 times weekly administration of interferon alfa-2a for hepatitis C
- Sustained viral response rates substantially better when combined with ribavirin (genotype 1:

40%-50%; genotype 2 or 3: 70%-80% for combination therapy; overall response rate 40% for monotherapy)

PATIENT/FAMILY EDUCATION

• Effective contraception required; when used with ribavirin, effective contraception also required in female partners of male patients undergoing treatment

• The drug's therapeutic effect should appear in 1-3 mos

• Flu-like symptoms tend to diminish with continued therapy

• Immediately notify the physician if depression or suicidal thoughts occur

• Avoid performing tasks requiring mental alertness or motor skills until response to the drug has been established

MONITORING PARAMETERS

• Availability of expert consultation for management of toxicity is essential

• *Baseline tests:* CBC, hepatic function, pregnancy test, TSH, renal function, uric acid, HCV RNA level. Exclusions to treatment: platelet count <90,000 cells/mm^3 (as low as 75,000 cells/mm^3 in patients with cirrhosis); absolute neutrophil count <1500 cells/mm^3; serum creatinine concentration >1.5 × upper limit of normal; abnormal thyroid function

• CBC q2wks

• ALT, bilirubin q4wks; if ALT rises persistently above baseline values, reduce dose to 135 μg per week, if ALT increases are progressive despite dose reduction or accompanied by increased bilirubin or evidence of hepatic decompensation, therapy should be immediately discontinued

• TSH q12wks

• Depression, evaluated q2wks for weeks 1-8 of treatment; may require dose reduction

• All patients should receive an eye examination at baseline; patients with preexisting ophthalmologic disorders (e.g., diabetic or hypertensive retinopathy) should receive periodic ophthalmologic exams during interferon alpha treatment

• HCV RNA (early virologic response defined as HCV RNA undetectable or >2 $\log_{10}$ lower than baseline at 12 wks and 24 wks); for patients who lack an early viral response at 12 wks, chance of sustained viral response is 13%; for patients who lack an early viral response at 24 wks, chance of sustained viral response is near zero; in consultation with experts, consider stopping peginterferon therapy if virologic response absent at 12-24 wks

pemoline

(pem'-oh-leen)

Rx: Cylert, PemADD, PemADD CT

Chemical Class: Oxazolidinone derivative

Therapeutic Class: Anorexiant; central nervous system stimulant

DEA Class: Schedule IV

P

CLINICAL PHARMACOLOGY

Mechanism of Action: A CNS stimulant that blocks the reuptake mechanism present in dopaminergic neurons in the cerebral cortex and subcortical structures. ***Therapeutic Effect:*** Reduces motor restlessness and fatigue, increases alertness, elevates mood.

Pharmacokinetics

Rapidly absorbed from GI tract. Protein binding: 50%. Metabolized in liver. Primarily excreted in urine. ***Half-life:*** 12 hr.

INDICATIONS AND DOSAGES

ADHD

PO

Children 6 yrs and older. Initially, 37.5 mg/day as a single dose in morning. May increase by 18.75 mg at weekly intervals until therapeutic response is achieved. Range: 56.25-75 mg/day. Maximum: 112.5 mg/day.

AVAILABLE FORMS

- *Tablets (Cylert, PemADD):* 18.75 mg, 37.5 mg, 75 mg.
- *Tablets (Chewable [Cylert, PemADD CT]):* 37.5 mg.

CONTRAINDICATIONS: Family history of Tourette's syndrome, hepatic impairment, motor tics

PREGNANCY AND LACTATION: Pregnancy category B

Controlled Substance: Schedule IV

SIDE EFFECTS

Frequent

Anorexia, insomnia

Occasional

Nausea, abdominal discomfort, diarrhea, headache, dizziness, somnolence

SERIOUS REACTIONS

- Visual disturbances, rash, and dyskinetic movements of the tongue, lips, face, and extremities have occurred.
- Large doses of pemoline may produce extreme nervousness and tachycardia.
- Hepatic effects, such as hepatitis and jaundice, appear to be reversible when the drug is discontinued.
- Prolonged administration to children with ADHD may temporarily delay growth.

INTERACTIONS

Drugs

3 *Other CNS stimulants:* May increase CNS stimulation

SPECIAL CONSIDERATIONS

PATIENT/FAMILY EDUCATION

- Avoid tasks that require mental alertness or motor skills until response to the drug has been established
- May be habit forming
- Do not abruptly discontinue the drug
- Notify the physician if dark urine, GI complaints, loss of appetite, or yellow skin occurs
- Avoid alcohol and caffeine during pemoline therapy

MONITORING PARAMETERS

- LFTs periodically
- Height and weight

penbutolol sulfate

(pen-byoo'-toe-lole sul'-fate)

Rx: Levatol

Chemical Class: β-adrenergic blocker, nonselective

Therapeutic Class: Antianginal; antihypertensive

CLINICAL PHARMACOLOGY

Mechanism of Action: An antihypertensive that possesses nonselective beta-blocking. Has moderate intrinsic sympathomimetic activity.

Therapeutic Effect: Reduces cardiac output, decreases blood pressure (BP), increases airway resistance, and decreases myocardial ischemia severity.

Pharmacokinetics

Rapidly and extensively absorbed from the gastrointestinal (GI) tract. Protein binding: 80%-90%. Metabolized in liver. Excreted primarily via urine. ***Half-life:*** 17-26 hrs.

INDICATIONS AND DOSAGES
Hypertension
PO
Adults. Initially, 20 mg/day as a single dose. May increase to 40-80 mg/day.
Elderly. Initially, 10 mg/day.
AVAILABLE FORMS
• *Tablets:* 20 mg (Levatol).
CONTRAINDICATIONS: Bronchial asthma or related bronchospastic conditions, cardiogenic shock, pulmonary edema, second- or third-degree atrioventricular (AV) block, severe bradycardia, overt cardiac failure, hypersensitivity to penbutolol or any component of the formulation
PREGNANCY AND LACTATION: Pregnancy category C
SIDE EFFECTS
Frequent
Decreased sexual ability, drowsiness, trouble sleeping, unusual tiredness/weakness
Occasional
Diarrhea, bradycardia, depression, cold hands/feet, constipation, anxiety, nasal congestion, nausea, vomiting
Rare
Altered taste, dry eyes, itching, numbness of fingers, toes, scalp
SERIOUS REACTIONS
• Abrupt withdrawal may result in sweating, palpitations, headache, and tremulousness.
• Hypoglycemia may occur in patients with previously controlled diabetes.
INTERACTIONS
Drugs
3 *Adenosine:* Bradycardia aggravated
3 *Amiodarone:* Bradycardia, cardiac arrest, ventricular arrhythmia risk after initiation of penbutolol
3 *Antacids:* Reduced penbutolol absorption
3 *Calcium channel blockers:* See dihydropyridine calcium channel blockers and verapamil
3 *Clonidine, guanabenz, guanfacine:* Exacerbation of rebound hypertension upon discontinuation of clonidine
3 *Cocaine:* Cocaine-induced vasoconstriction potentiated; reduced coronary blood flow
3 *Contrast media:* Increased risk of anaphylaxis
3 *Digitalis:* Enhances bradycardia
3 *Dihydropyridine, calcium channel blockers:* Additive pharmacodynamic effects
3 *Dipyridamole:* Bradycardia aggravated
2 *Epinephrine, isoproterenol, phenylephrine:* Potentiates pressor response; resultant hypertension and bradycardia
3 *Flecainide:* Additive negative inotropic effects
3 *Fluoxetine:* Increased β-blockade activity
3 *Fluoroquinolones:* Reduced clearance of penbutolol
2 *Glimepiride, glipizide, glyburide:* Prolong hypoglycemia reactions
2 *Insulin:* Altered response to hypoglycemia; increased blood glucose concentrations; impaired peripheral circulation
3 *Lidocaine:* Increased serum lidocaine concentrations possible
3 *Neostigmine:* Bradycardia aggravated
3 *Neuroleptics:* Both drugs inhibit each other's metabolism; additive hypotension
3 *NSAIDs:* Reduced antihypertensive effect of penbutolol
3 *Physostigmine:* Bradycardia aggravated
3 *Prazosin:* First-dose response to prazosin may be enhanced by β-blockade

3 *Tacrine:* Bradycardia aggravated

2 *Terbutaline:* Antagonized bronchodilating effects of terbutaline

2 *Theophylline:* Antagonistic pharmacodynamic effects

3 *Verapamil:* Enhanced effects of both drugs; particularly AV nodal conduction slowing; reduced penbutolol clearance

SPECIAL CONSIDERATIONS

- Exacerbation of ischemic heart disease following abrupt withdrawal due to rebound sensitivity to catecholamines possible
- Comparative trials indicate that penbutolol is as effective as propranolol and atenolol in the treatment of hypertension; may have fewer adverse CNS effects than propranolol

PATIENT/FAMILY EDUCATION

- The full antihypertensive effect of penbutolol will be noted in 1-2 wks
- Do not abruptly discontinue penbutolol; compliance with the therapy regimen is essential to control hypertension
- Avoid tasks that require mental alertness or motor skills until response to the drug is established
- Notify the physician if excessive fatigue or prolonged dizziness occurs
- Do not take nasal decongestants and OTC cold preparations, especially those containing stimulants, without physician approval
- Limit alcohol and salt intake

MONITORING PARAMETERS

- Blood pressure, pulse
- EKG for arrhythmias
- Daily bowel activity and stool consistency
- Skin for rash

penciclovir

(pen-sye'-kloe-veer)

Rx: Denavir

Chemical Class: Acyclic purine nucleoside analog

Therapeutic Class: Antiviral

CLINICAL PHARMACOLOGY

Mechanism of Action: Penciclovir triphosphate inhibits HSV polymerase competitively with deoxyguanosine triphosphate. Consequently, herpes viral DNA synthesis and, therefore, replication are selectively inhibited. ***Therapeutic Effect:*** An antiviral compound that has inhibitory activity against herpes simplex virus types 1 (HSV-1) and 2 (HSV-2).

Pharmacokinetics

Measurable penciclovir concentrations were not detected in plasma or urine. The systemic absorption of penciclovir following topical administration has not been evaluated.

INDICATIONS AND DOSAGES

Herpes labialis (cold sores)

Topical

Adolescents, Adults. Penciclovir should be applied every 2 hrs during waking hours for a period of 4 days. Treatment should be started as early as possible (i.e., during the prodrome or when lesions appear).

AVAILABLE FORMS

- *Cream:* 10 mg/g.

UNLABELED USES: Varicella-zoster virus

CONTRAINDICATIONS: Hypersensitivity to penciclovir or any of its components.

PREGNANCY AND LACTATION: Pregnancy category B; no data in nursing mothers, but milk concentrations should be low due to apparent lack of systemic absorption

SIDE EFFECTS

Frequent

Headache

Occasional

Change in sense of taste; decreased sensitivity of skin, particularly to touch; redness of the skin; skin rash (maculopapular, erythematous) local edema, skin discoloration; pruritis; hypoesthesia; parathesias; parosmia; urticaria; oral/pharyngeal edema

Rare

Mild pain, burning, or stinging

SPECIAL CONSIDERATIONS

• In clinical trials, shortened the duration of lesions by approximately ½ day compared to placebo (4½ vs. 5 days); duration of pain was also shortened by approximately ½ day

PATIENT/FAMILY EDUCATION

• Avoid exposure of cold sores to direct sunlight

MONITORING PARAMETERS

• Therapeutic response

---

penicillamine

(pen-i-sill'-a-meen)

Rx: Cuprimine, Depen

Chemical Class: Thiol derivative

Therapeutic Class: Antidote, heavy metal; disease-modifying antirheumatic drug (DMARD)

CLINICAL PHARMACOLOGY

Mechanism of Action: A heavy metal antagonist that chelates copper, iron, mercury, and lead to form complexes, promoting excretion of copper. Combines with cystine-forming complex, thus reducing concentration of cystine to below levels for formation of cystine stones. Exact mechanism for rheumatoid arthritis is unknown. May decrease cell-mediated immune response. May inhibit collagen formation. ***Therapeutic Effect:*** Promotes excretion of copper, prevents renal calculi, dissolves existing stones, acts as anti-inflammatory drug.

Pharmacokinetics

Moderately absorbed from the gastrointestinal (GI) tract. Protein binding: 80% to albumin. Metabolized in small amounts in liver. Excreted unchanged in urine. ***Half-life:*** 1.7-3.2 hrs.

INDICATIONS AND DOSAGES

Wilson's disease

PO

Adults, Elderly, Children. Initially, 250 mg 4 times/day (some pts may begin at 250 mg/day; gradually increase). Dosages of 750-1500 mg/day that produce initial 24-hr cupruresis >2 mg should be continued for 3 mos. Maintenance: Based on serum-free copper concentration (<10 mcg/dL indicative of adequate maintenance). Maximum: 2 g/day.

Cystinuria

PO

Adults, Elderly. Initially, 250 mg/day. Gradually increase dose. Maintenance: 2 g/day. Range: 1-4 g/day.

Children. 30 mg/kg/day.

Rheumatoid arthritis

PO

Adults, Elderly. Initially, 125-250 mg/day. May increase by 125-250 mg/day at 1-3-mo intervals. Maintenance: 500-750 mg/day. After 2-3 mos with no improvement or toxicity, may increase by 250 mg/day at 2-3-mo intervals until remission or toxicity. Maximum: 1 g up to 1.5 g/day.

AVAILABLE FORMS

• *Capsules:* 125 mg, 250 mg (Cuprimine).

• *Tablets:* 250 mg (Depen).

UNLABELED USES: Treatment of rheumatoid vasculitis, heavy metal toxicity.

CONTRAINDICATIONS: History of penicillamine-related aplastic anemia or agranulocytosis, rheumatoid arthritis patients with history or evidence of renal insufficiency, pregnancy, breast-feeding

PREGNANCY AND LACTATION: Pregnancy category D (continued therapy in Wilson's disease and cystinuria probably OK, not rheumatoid arthritis)

SIDE EFFECTS

Frequent

Rash (pruritic, erythematous, maculopapular, morbilliform), reduced/altered sense of taste (hypogeusia), GI disturbances (anorexia, epigastric pain, nausea, vomiting, diarrhea), oral ulcers, glossitis

Occasional

Proteinuria, hematuria, hot flashes, drug fever

Rare

Alopecia, tinnitus, pemphigoid rash (water blisters)

SERIOUS REACTIONS

- Aplastic anemia, agranulocytosis, thrombocytopenia, leukopenia, myasthenia gravis, bronchiolitis, erythematous-like syndrome, evening hypoglycemia, skin friability at sites of pressure/trauma producing extravasation or white papules at venipuncture, surgical sites reported.
- Iron deficiency (particularly children, menstruating women) may develop.

INTERACTIONS

Drugs

3 *Antacids:* Magnesium-aluminum hydroxides reduce bioavailability

3 *Digoxin:* Reduced digoxin concentrations

3 *Iron:* Oral iron substantially reduces plasma penicillamine concentration, with reduced therapeutic response

Labs

- *Cholesterol:* Decreased serum levels
- *Fructoseamine:* Decreased serum levels
- *Iron:* Decreased serum levels
- *Ketones:* Increased false-positive reactions with legal reaction

SPECIAL CONSIDERATIONS

- Because penicillamine can cause severe adverse reactions, restrict its use in rheumatoid arthritis to patients who have severe, active disease and who have failed to respond to an adequate trial of conventional therapy

PATIENT/FAMILY EDUCATION

- Should be administered on empty stomach, ½-1 hr before meals or at least 2 hr after meals
- Urine may become discolored (red)
- Patients with cystinuria should drink large amounts of water
- Therapeutic effect may take 1-3 mo
- Promptly report any missed menstrual periods

MONITORING PARAMETERS

- Hepatic, renal studies: CBC, urinalysis, skin for rash
- Urinary copper excretion
- WBC

penicillin

(pen-i-sill'-in)

Rx: *Penicillin G (Aqueous Pen G:)* Pfizerpen

Rx: *Penicillin G:* Pentids

Rx: *Penicillin V:* (Phenoxy-methyl Penicillin), Beepen VK, Pen-V, Pen-Vee K, Truxcillin VK, Veetids

Rx: *Penicillin G Benzathine:* Bicillin L-A, Permapen

Rx: *Penicillin G Procaine:* Crysticillin, Wycillin

Rx: *Penicillin G Benzathine and Procaine combined:* Bicillin C-R

Combinations

Rx: amoxicillin, ampicillin, bacampicillin, carbenicillin, cloxacillin, dicloxacillin, flucloxacillin, methicillin, mezlocillin, nafcillin, oxacillin, penicillin G benzathine, penicillin G potassium, penicillin V potassium, piperacillin, pivampicillin, pivmecillinam, ticarcillin; penicillin and beta-lactamase inhibitors; amoxicillin/clavulanate potassium, ampicillin/sulbactam sodium, piperacillin sodium/tazobactam sodium, ticarcillin disodium/clavulanate potassium

Chemical Class: Penicillin, natural

Therapeutic Class: Antibiotic

CLINICAL PHARMACOLOGY

Mechanism of Action: Penicillins bind to bacterial cell wall, inhibiting bacterial cell wall synthesis. ***Therapeutic Effect:*** Inhibits bacterial cell wall synthesis.

Beta-lactamase inhibitors: inhibit the action of bacterial beta-lactamase. ***Therapeutic Effect:*** Protects the penicillin from enzymatic degradation.

Pharmacokinetics

Penicillins are generally well absorbed from the gastrointestinal (GI) tract after oral administration. Widely distributed to most tissues and body fluids. Protein binding: 20%. Partially metabolized in liver. Primarily excreted in urine. ***Half-life:*** Varies (half-life increased in reduced renal function).

INDICATIONS AND DOSAGES: Penicillins may be used to treat a large number of infections, including pneumonia and other respiratory diseases, urinary tract infections, septicemia, meningitis, intraabdominal infections, gonorrhea, syphilis, and bone and joint infections.

Doses vary depending on the drug used. In general, penicillins should be taken on an empty stomach. Patients with impaired renal function may required dose adjustment.

AVAILABLE FORMS

- Penicillins are available in tablets, chewable tablets, capsules, powder for oral suspension, powder for injection, prefilled syringes for injection, premixed dextrose solutions for injection, and solutions for infusion.

UNLABELED USES: Some penicillins, such as amoxicillin, have been use in the treatment of Lyme disease and typhoid fever.

CONTRAINDICATIONS: Hypersensitivity to any penicillin, infectious mononucleosis

PREGNANCY AND LACTATION: Pregnancy category B; may cause diarrhea, candidiasis, or allergic response in nursing infant

SIDE EFFECTS

Frequent

Gastrointestinal (GI) disturbances (mild diarrhea, nausea, or vomiting), headache, oral or vaginal candidiasis

Occasional

Generalized rash, urticaria

SERIOUS REACTIONS

- Altered bacterial balance may result in potentially fatal superinfections and antibiotic-associated colitis as evidenced by abdominal cramps, watery or severe diarrhea, and fever.
- Severe hypersensitivity reactions, including anaphylaxis and acute interstitial nephritis, occur rarely.

INTERACTIONS

Drugs

3 *Chloramphenicol:* Inhibited antibacterial activity of penicillin; administer penicillin 3 hr before chloramphenicol

3 *Macrolide antibiotics:* Inhibited antibacterial activity of penicillin; administer penicillin 3 hr before macrolides

3 *Methotrexate:* Penicillin in large doses may increase serum methotrexate concentrations

3 *Oral contraceptives:* Occasional impairment of oral contraceptive efficacy; consider use of supplemental contraception during cycles in which penicillin is used

3 *Probenecid:* May increase penicillin blood concentration and risk of toxicity

3 *Tetracyclines:* Inhibited antibacterial activity of penicillin; administer penicillin 3 hr before tetracyclines

Labs

- *Albumin:* Decreased serum levels at very high penicillin levels
- *Aminoglycosides:* Decreased serum levels if specimen stored for a prolonged period of time
- *Folate:* Decreased serum levels
- *17-ketogenic steroids:* Increased urine concentrations
- *17-ketosteroids:* Increased urine concentrations
- *Protein:* Increased CSF concentrations
- *Protein electrophoresis:* False positives; causes bisalbuminemia
- *Sugar:* False positive with copper reduction procedures
- *Piperacillin:* False positive in the presence of penicillin V
- *Amdinocillin:* False positive in the presence of penicillin G
- *Methicillin:* False positive in the presence of penicillin G

SPECIAL CONSIDERATIONS

- Cross-reactivity with cephalosporins is approx 10%

PATIENT/FAMILY EDUCATION

- Space doses evenly around the clock and continue taking the drug for the full course of treatment
- Immediately notify the physician if bleeding, bruising, diarrhea, a rash, or any other new symptoms occur

MONITORING PARAMETERS

- Intake and output, renal function, urinalysis for signs of nephrotoxicity
- Blood Hgb levels
- Severe diarrhea with abdominal pain, fever, and mucus or blood in stools may indicate antibiotic-associated colitis
- Be alert for signs and symptoms of superinfection, including anal or genital pruritus, vaginal discharge, diarrhea, increased fever, nausea and vomiting, sore throat, and stomatitis
- Check for signs of bleeding, including ecchymosis, overt bleeding, and swelling of tissue

pentamidine isethionate

(pen-tam'-i-deen)

Rx: NebuPent, Pentam 300

Chemical Class: Aromatic diamidine derivative

Therapeutic Class: Antiprotozoal

CLINICAL PHARMACOLOGY

Mechanism of Action: An antiinfective that interferes with nuclear metabolism and incorporation of nucleotides, inhibiting DNA, RNA, phospholipid, and protein synthesis. ***Therapeutic Effect:*** Produces antibacterial and antiprotozoal effects.

Pharmacokinetics

Well absorbed after IM administration; minimally absorbed after inhalation. Widely distributed. Primarily excreted in urine. Minimally removed by hemodialysis. ***Half-life:*** 6.5 hr (increased in impaired renal function).

INDICATIONS AND DOSAGES

Pneumocystis carinii pneumonia (PCP)

IV, IM

Adults, Elderly. 4 mg/kg/day once a day for 14-21 days.

Children. 4 mg/kg/day once a day for 10-14 days.

Prevention of PCP

Inhalation

Adults, Elderly. 300 mg once q4wk.

Children 5 yrs and older. 300 mg q3-4wk.

Children younger than 5 yrs. 8 mg/kg/dose once q3-4wk.

AVAILABLE FORMS

- *Injection (Pentam-300):* 300 mg.
- *Powder for Nebulization (Nebupent):* 300 mg.

UNLABELED USES: Treatment of African trypanosomiasis, cutaneous or visceral leishmaniasis

CONTRAINDICATIONS: Concurrent use with didanosine

PREGNANCY AND LACTATION: Pregnancy category C; since aerosolized pentamidine results in very low systemic concentrations, fetal exposure to the drug is probably negligible; breast milk levels following aerosolized administration are likely nil

SIDE EFFECTS

Frequent

Injection (greater than 10%): Abscess, pain at injection site

Inhalation (greater than 5%): Fatigue, metallic taste, shortness of breath, decreased appetite, dizziness, rash, cough, nausea, vomiting, chills

Occasional

Injection (10%-1%): Nausea, decreased appetite, hypotension, fever, rash, altered taste, confusion

Inhalation (5%-1%): Diarrhea, headache, anemia, muscle pain

Rare

Injection (less than 1%): Neuralgia, thrombocytopenia, phlebitis, dizziness

SERIOUS REACTIONS

- Rare reactions include life-threatening or fatal hypotension, arrhythmias, hypoglycemia, leukopenia, nephrotoxicity or renal failure, anaphylactic shock, Stevens-Johnson syndrome, and toxic epidural necrolysis.
- Hyperglycemia and insulin-dependent diabetes mellitus (often permanent) may occur even months after therapy has stopped.

INTERACTIONS

Drugs

3 *Blood dyscrasia-producing medications, bone marrow depressants:* May increase the abnormal hematologic effects of pentamidine

3 *Didanosine:* May increase the risk of pancreatitis

P

3 *Foscarnet:* May increase the risk of hypocalcemia, hypomagnesemia, and nephrotoxicity of pentamidine

3 *Nephrotoxic medications:* May increase the risk of nephrotoxicity

SPECIAL CONSIDERATIONS

• Considered second line for *P. carinii* pneumonia, following cotrimoxazole (unresponsive to or intolerant of cotrimoxazole)

PATIENT/FAMILY EDUCATION

• Remain flat in bed during pentamidine administration and get up slowly and with assistance only when blood pressure becomes stable
• Notify the nurse immediately if light-headedness, palpitations, shakiness, or sweating occurs
• Drowsiness, decreased appetite, and increased thirst and urination may develop in the months following therapy
• Drink plenty of water to maintain adequate hydration
• Avoid consuming alcohol during therapy

MONITORING PARAMETERS

• BUN, serum creatinine, blood glucose daily
• CBC and platelets; liver function tests, including bilirubin, alkaline phosphatase, AST, and ALT; and serum calcium before, during, and after therapy
• ECG at regular intervals
• Skin for rash

pentazocine lactate

(pen-taz'-oh-seen)

Rx: Talwin

Combinations

Rx: with ASA (Talwin Compound) with APAP (Talacen)

Chemical Class: Benzomorphan; opiate derivative

Therapeutic Class: Narcotic agonist-antagonist analgesic

DEA Class: Schedule IV

CLINICAL PHARMACOLOGY

Mechanism of Action: An opioid antagonist that binds with opioid receptors within CNS. ***Therapeutic Effect:*** Alters processes affecting pain perception, emotional response to pain.

Pharmacokinetics

Well absorbed after administration. Widely distributed including CSF. Metabolized in liver via oxidative and glucuronide conjugation pathways, extensive first-pass effect. Excreted in small amounts as unchanged drug. ***Half-life:*** 2-3 hrs, prolonged with hepatic impairment.

INDICATIONS AND DOSAGES

Analgesia

PO

Adults. 50 mg q3-4h. May increase to 100 mg q3-4h, if needed. Maximum: 600 mg/day.

Elderly. 50 mg q4h.

Subcutaneous/IM/IV

Adults. 30 mg q3-4h. Do not exceed 30 mg IV or 60 mg subcutaneous/IM per dose. Maximum: 360 mg/day.

IM

Elderly. 25 mg q4h.

Obstetric labor

IM

Adults. 30 mg as a single dose.

IV

Adults. 20 mg when contractions are regular. May repeat 2-3 times q2-3h.

AVAILABLE FORMS

• *Tablets:* 12.5 mg and 325 mg aspirin (Talwin Compound), 25 mg and 650 mg acetaminophen (Talacen), 50 mg pentazocine and 0.5 mg naloxone (Talwin NX), 50 mg (Talwin).

• *Injection:* 30 mg (Talwin).

CONTRAINDICATIONS: Hypersensitivity to pentazocine or any component of the formulation

PREGNANCY AND LACTATION: Pregnancy category B (category D if used for prolonged periods or in high doses at term); use during labor may produce neonatal respiratory depression

SIDE EFFECTS

Frequent

Drowsiness, euphoria, nausea, vomiting

Occasional

Allergic reaction, histamine reaction (decreased BP, increased sweating, flushing, wheezing), decreased urination, altered vision, constipation, dizziness, dry mouth, headache, hypotension, pain/burning at injection site

SERIOUS REACTIONS

• Overdosage results in severe respiratory depression, skeletal muscle flaccidity, cyanosis, extreme somnolence progressing to convulsions, stupor, and coma.

• Abrupt withdrawal after prolonged use may produce symptoms of narcotic withdrawal (abdominal cramps, rhinorrhea, lacrimation, nausea, vomiting, restlessness, anxiety, increased temperature, piloerection).

INTERACTIONS

Drugs

3 *Aspirin:* Increased risk of papillary necrosis

3 *Barbiturates:* Additive CNS depression

3 *Phenothiazines:* Additive CNS depression

Labs

• *Increase:* Amylase

SPECIAL CONSIDERATIONS

• Naloxone 0.5 mg added to oral tablets to discourage misuse via parenteral inj

• Less effective compared to morphine, but less respiratory depression and opposite cardiovascular pharmacodynamics; increases pulmonary, arterial, and central venous pressure

PATIENT/FAMILY EDUCATION

• Report any symptoms of CNS changes, allergic reactions

• Physical dependency may result when used for extended periods

• Change position slowly, orthostatic hypotension may occur

• Avoid hazardous activities if drowsiness or dizziness occurs

• Avoid alcohol, other CNS depressants unless directed by clinician

MONITORING PARAMETERS

• Degree of pain relief

P

pentobarbital sodium

(pen-toe-bar'-bi-tal soe'-dee-um)

Rx: Nembutal

Chemical Class: Barbituric acid derivative

Therapeutic Class: Anticonvulsant; sedative/hypnotic

DEA Class: Schedule II; Schedule III

CLINICAL PHARMACOLOGY

Mechanism of Action: A barbiturate that binds at the GABA receptor complex, enhancing GABA activity. ***Therapeutic Effect:*** Depresses central nervous system (CNS) activity and reticular activating system.

Pharmacokinetics
Well absorbed after PO, parenteral administration. Protein binding: 35%-55%. Rapidly, widely distributed. Metabolized in liver. Primarily excreted in urine. Removed by hemodialysis. ***Half-life:*** 15-48 hrs.

INDICATIONS AND DOSAGES
Preanesthetic
PO
Adults, Elderly. 100 mg.
Children. 2-6 mg/kg. Maximum: 100 mg/dose.
IM
Adults, Elderly. 150-200 mg.
Children. 2-6 mg/kg. Maximum: 100 mg/dose.
Rectal
Children 12-14 yrs. 60 or 120 mg.
Children 5-12 yrs. 60 mg.
Children 1-4 yrs. 30-60 mg.
Children 1 yr-2 mos. 30 mg.
Hypnotic
PO
Adults, Elderly. 100 mg at bedtime.
IM
Adults, Elderly. 150-200 mg at bedtime.
Children. 2-6 mg/kg. Maximum: 100 mg/dose at bedtime.
IV
Adults, Elderly. 100 mg initially then, after 1 min, may give additional small doses at 1-min intervals, up to 500 mg total.
Children. 50 mg initially then, after 1 min, may give additional small doses at 1-min intervals, up to desired effect.
Rectal
Adults, Elderly. 120-200 mg at bedtime.
Children 12-14 yrs. 60 or 120 mg at bedtime.
Children 5-12 yrs. 60 mg at bedtime.
Children 1-4 yrs. 30-60 mg at bedtime.
Children 2 mos-1 yr. 30 mg at bedtime.
Anticonvulsant
IV
Adults, Elderly. 2-15 mg/kg loading dose given slowly over 1-2 hrs. Maintenance infusion: 0.5-5 mg/kg/hr.
Children. 5-15 mg/kg loading dose given slowly over 1-2 hrs. Maintenance infusion: 0.5-3 mg/kg/hr.

AVAILABLE FORMS
- *Capsules:* 50 mg, 100 mg.
- *Injection:* 50 mg/ml.
- *Suppositories:* 30 mg, 120 mg, 200 mg.

UNLABELED USES: Intracranial hypertension, psychiatric interviews, sedative withdrawal, drug abuse withdrawal

CONTRAINDICATIONS: Porphyria, hypersensitivity to barbiturates

PREGNANCY AND LACTATION: Pregnancy category D; excreted in breast milk; effect on nursing infant unknown

Controlled Substance: Schedule II (capsules, injection), Schedule III (suppositories)

SIDE EFFECTS
Occasional
Agitation, confusion, dizziness, somnolence
Rare
Confusion, paradoxical CNS hyperactivity or nervousness in children, excitement or restlessness in elderly

SERIOUS REACTIONS
- Agranulocytosis, megaloblastic anemia, apnea, hypoventilation, bradycardia, hypotension, syncope, hepatic damage, and Stevens-Johnson syndrome occur rarely.
- Abrupt withdrawal after prolonged therapy may produce effects ranging from markedly increased dreaming, nightmares or insomnia, tremor, sweating and vomiting, to hallucinations, delirium, seizures, and status epilepticus.

- Skin eruptions appear as hypersensitivity reactions.
- Overdosage produces cold or clammy skin, hypothermia, severe CNS depression, cyanosis, and rapid pulse.

INTERACTIONS

Drugs

3 *Acetaminophen:* Enhanced hepatotoxic potential of acetaminophen overdoses

3 *Antidepressants, cyclic:* Reduced serum concentrations of cyclic antidepressants

3 *β-adrenergic blockers:* Reduced serum concentrations of β-blockers, which are extensively metabolized

3 *Calcium channel blockers:* Reduced serum concentrations of verapamil and dihydropyridines

3 *Chloramphenicol:* Increased barbiturate concentrations; reduced serum chloramphenicol concentrations

3 *Corticosteroids:* Reduced serum concentrations of corticosteroids; may impair therapeutic effect

3 *Cyclosporine:* Reduced serum concentration of cyclosporine

3 *Digitoxin:* Reduced serum concentration of digitoxin

3 *Disopyramide:* Reduced serum concentration of disopyramide

3 *Doxycycline:* Reduced serum doxycycline concentrations

3 *Estrogen:* Reduced serum concentration of estrogen

3 *Ethanol:* Excessive CNS depression

3 *Griseofulvin:* Reduced griseofulvin absorption

3 *Methoxyflurane:* Enhanced nephrotoxic effect

3 *MAOIs:* Prolonged effect of barbiturates

3 *Narcotic analgesics:* Increased toxicity of meperidine; reduced effect of methadone; additive CNS depression

3 *Neuroleptics:* Reduced effect of either drug

2 *Oral anticoagulants:* Decreased hypoprothrombinemic response to oral anticoagulants

3 *Oral contraceptives:* Reduced efficacy of oral contraceptives

3 *Phenytoin:* Unpredictable effect on serum phenytoin levels

3 *Propafenone:* Reduced serum concentration of propafenone

3 *Quinidine:* Reduced quinidine plasma concentration

3 *Tacrolimus:* Reduced serum concentration of tacrolimus

3 *Theophylline:* Reduced serum theophylline concentrations

3 *Valproic acid:* Increased serum concentrations of amobarbital

3 *Warfarin:* See oral anticoagulants

SPECIAL CONSIDERATIONS

PATIENT/FAMILY EDUCATION

- Avoid driving or other activities requiring alertness
- Avoid alcohol ingestion or CNS depressants
- Do not discontinue medication abruptly after long-term use
- Limit caffeine intake
- May be habit forming
- Avoid tasks that require mental alertness or motor skills until response to the drug is established
- Notify the physician of feelings of depression or thoughts of suicide

MONITORING PARAMETERS

- Excessive usage; hypnotic hangover
- Blood pressure, heart rate, respiratory rate
- Liver and renal function
- CNS status

pentosan polysulfate sodium

(pen-toe-san)

Rx: Elmiron

Chemical Class: Glycosaminoglycan, sulfated; heparin derivative

Therapeutic Class: Anticoagulant; fibrinolytic

CLINICAL PHARMACOLOGY

Mechanism of Action: A negatively charged synthetic sulfated polysaccharide with heparin-like properties that appears to adhere to bladder wall mucosal membrane, may act as a buffering agent to control cell permeability preventing irritating solutes in the urine. Has anticoagulant/fibrinolytic effects. ***Therapeutic Effect:*** Relieves bladder pain.

Pharmacokinetics

Poorly and erratically absorbed from the gastrointestinal tract. Distributed in uroepithelium of GU tract with lesser amount found in the liver, spleen, lung, skin, periosteum, and bone marrow. Metabolized in liver and kidney (secondary). Eliminated in the urine. ***Half-life:*** 4.8 hrs.

INDICATIONS AND DOSAGES

Interstitial cystitis

PO

Adults, Elderly. 100 mg 3 times/day.

AVAILABLE FORMS

• *Capsules:* 100 mg (Elmiron).

UNLABELED USES: Urolithiasis

CONTRAINDICATIONS: Hypersensitivity to pentosan polysulfate sodium or structurally related compounds

PREGNANCY AND LACTATION: Pregnancy category B; no data in nursing mothers

SIDE EFFECTS

Frequent

Alopecia areata (a single area on the scalp), diarrhea, nausea, headache, rash, abdominal pain, dyspepsia.

Occasional

Dizziness, depression, increased liver function tests.

SERIOUS REACTIONS

• Ecchymosis, epistaxis, gum hemorrhage have been reported (drug produces weak anticoagulant effect).

• Overdose may produce liver function abnormalities.

INTERACTIONS

Drugs

3 *Anticoagulants:* May increase the risk of bleeding

SPECIAL CONSIDERATIONS

PATIENT/FAMILY EDUCATION

• Take with water

• Notify the physician if any unusual bleeding occurs

MONITORING PARAMETERS

• CBC, aPTT, PT, liver and renal function

pentoxifylline

(pen-tox-i′-fi-leen)

Rx: Pentopak, Pentoxil, Trental

Chemical Class: Dimethylxanthine derivative

Therapeutic Class: Hemorrheologic agent

CLINICAL PHARMACOLOGY

Mechanism of Action: A blood viscosity-reducing agent that alters the flexibility of RBCs; inhibits production of tumor necrosis factor, neutrophil activation, and platelet aggregation. ***Therapeutic Effect:*** Reduces blood viscosity and improves blood flow.

Pharmacokinetics
Well absorbed after oral administration. Undergoes first-pass metabolism in the liver. Primarily excreted in urine. Unknown if removed by hemodialysis. ***Half-life:*** 24-48 min; metabolite, 60-90 min.

INDICATIONS AND DOSAGES
Intermittent claudication
PO
Adults, Elderly. 400 mg 3 times a day. Decrease to 400 mg twice a day if GI or CNS adverse effects occur. Continue for at least 8 wk.

AVAILABLE FORMS
• *Tablets (Controlled-Release [Pentopak, Pentoxil, Trental]):* 400 mg.

UNLABELED USES: Diabetic neuropathy, gangrene, hemodialysis shunt thrombosis, septic shock, sickle cell syndrome, vascular impotence

CONTRAINDICATIONS: History of intolerance to xanthine derivatives, such as caffeine, theophylline, or theobromine; recent cerebral or retinal hemorrhage

PREGNANCY AND LACTATION: Pregnancy category C; excreted in breast milk

SIDE EFFECTS
Occasional (5%-2%)
Dizziness, nausea, altered taste, dyspepsia, marked by heartburn, epigastric pain, and indigestion
Rare (less than 2%)
Rash, pruritus, anorexia, constipation, dry mouth, blurred vision, edema, nasal congestion, anxiety

SERIOUS REACTIONS
• Angina and chest pain occur rarely and may be accompanied by palpitations, tachycardia, and arrhythmias.
• Signs and symptoms of overdose, such as flushing, hypotension, nervousness, agitation, hand tremor, fever, and somnolence, appear 4-5 hrs after ingestion and last for 12 hrs.

INTERACTIONS
Drugs
3 *Antihypertensives:* May increase the effects of antihypertensives
3 *Fluoroquinolones (ciprofloxin, enoxacin, norfloxacin, pefloxacin, pipemidic acid):* Increased pentoxyphylline concentrations with subsequent side effects
3 *Theophylline:* Increased plasma theophylline concentrations

SPECIAL CONSIDERATIONS
• Statistically, but not always, clinically significant effects in intermittent claudication; however, other drugs less impressive; will not replace surgical options

PATIENT/FAMILY EDUCATION
• Therapeutic effect may require 2-4 wk
• Stop smoking
• Avoid tasks requiring mental alertness or motor skills until response to the drug has been established
• Limit caffeine intake

MONITORING PARAMETERS
• Assess for hand tremor
• Monitor the patient for relief of signs and symptoms of intermittent claudication. Symptoms generally occur while walking or exercising or with weight bearing in the absence of walking or exercising

pergolide mesylate
(per'-go-lide mes'-sil-ate)
Rx: Permax
Chemical Class: Ergoline derivative
Therapeutic Class: Anti-Parkinson's agent; dopaminergic

CLINICAL PHARMACOLOGY
Mechanism of Action: A centrally active dopamine agonist that directly stimulates dopamine recep-

tors. ***Therapeutic Effect:*** Decreases signs and symptoms of Parkinson's disease.

Pharmacokinetics

Well absorbed from the GI tract. Protein binding: 90%. Undergoes extensive first-pass metabolism in the liver. Primarily excreted in urine. Unknown if removed by hemodialysis.

INDICATIONS AND DOSAGES

Parkinsonism

PO

Adults, Elderly. Initially, 0.05 mg/day for 2 days. May increase by 0.1-0.15 mg/day every 3 days over the next 12 days; afterward may increase by 0.25 mg/day every 3 days. Range: 2-3 mg/day in 3 divided doses. Maximum: 5 mg/day.

AVAILABLE FORMS

- *Tablets:* 0.05 mg, 0.25 mg, 1 mg.

UNLABELED USES: Chronic motor or vocal tic disorder, Tourette syndrome

CONTRAINDICATIONS: Hypersensitivity to other ergot derivatives

PREGNANCY AND LACTATION: Pregnancy category B; may interfere with lactation

SIDE EFFECTS

Frequent (24%-10%)

Nausea, dizziness, hallucinations, constipation, rhinitis, dystonia, confusion, somnolence

Occasional (9%-3%)

Orthostatic hypotension, insomnia, dry mouth, peripheral edema, anxiety, diarrhea, dyspepsia, abdominal pain, headache, abnormal vision, anorexia, tremor, depression, rash

Rare (less than 2%)

Urinary frequency, vivid dreams, neck pain, hypotension, vomiting

SERIOUS REACTIONS

- Symptoms of overdose may vary from CNS depression, characterized by sedation, apnea, cardiovascular collapse, and death, to severe paradoxical reactions, such as hallucinations, tremor, and seizures.

INTERACTIONS

Drugs

3 *Hypotension-producing medications:* May increase the hypotensive effect

3 *Lisinopril:* Additive hypotension

3 *Neuroleptics:* Potentially antagonistic pharmacodynamic effects

SPECIAL CONSIDERATIONS

- Adjunct to levodopa/carbidopa in Parkinson's disease; longer acting than bromocriptine

PATIENT/FAMILY EDUCATION

- Hypotensive cautions
- Avoid tasks that require mental alertness or motor skills until response to the drug has been established
- Avoid alcohol

MONITORING PARAMETERS

- Blood pressure, EKG
- Assess the patient for relief of parkinsonian symptoms, such as improvement of masklike facial expression, muscular rigidity, shuffling gait, and resting tremors of the hands and head
- Overdose may require supportive measures to maintain BP. Plan to monitor cardiac function, obtain vital signs, and check ABG and serum electrolyte levels
- Activated charcoal may be more effective than emesis or lavage for overdose

perindopril erbumine

(per-in'-doe-pril-er-byoo'-meen)

Rx: Aceon

Chemical Class: Angiotensin-converting enzyme (ACE) inhibitor, nonsulfhydryl

Therapeutic Class: Antihypertensive

CLINICAL PHARMACOLOGY

Mechanism of Action: An angiotensin-converting enzyme (ACE) inhibitor that suppresses the renin-angiotensin-aldosterone system and prevents conversion of angiotensin I to angiotensin II, a potent vasoconstrictor; may also inhibit angiotensin II at local vascular and renal sites. ***Therapeutic Effect:*** Reduces peripheral arterial resistance and BP.

Pharmacokinetics

Rapidly absorbed from the GI tract. Protein binding: 60%. Extensively metabolized in liver. Excreted in urine. ***Half-life:*** 0.8-1 hr.

INDICATIONS AND DOSAGES

Hypertension

PO

Adults, Elderly. 2-8 mg/day as single dose or in 2 divided doses. Maximum: 16 mg/day.

AVAILABLE FORMS

- *Tablets:* 2 mg, 4 mg, 8 mg.

UNLABELED USES: Management of heart failure, hypertension, and/or renal crisis in scleroderma

CONTRAINDICATIONS: History of angioedema from previous treatment with ACE inhibitors

PREGNANCY AND LACTATION: Pregnancy category C (first trimester); category D (second and third trimesters); associated with fetal and neonatal injury including hypotension, neonatal skull hypoplasia, anuria, reversible or irreversible renal effects and death; oligohydramnios; possibly hypoplastic lung development, IUGR, PDA

SIDE EFFECTS

Occasional (5%-1%)

Cough, back pain, sinusitis, upper extremity pain, dyspepsia, fever, palpitations, hypotension, dizziness, fatigue, syncope

SERIOUS REACTIONS

- Excessive hypotension ("first-dose syncope") may occur in patients with CHF and in those who are severely salt or volume depleted.
- Angioedema (swelling of face and lips) and hyperkalemia occur rarely.
- Agranulocytosis and neutropenia may be noted in those with collagen vascular disease, including scleroderma and systemic lupus erythematosus, and impaired renal function.
- Nephrotic syndrome may be noted in those with history of renal disease.

INTERACTIONS

Drugs

3 *Alcohol:* Increases the effects of perindopril

3 *Azathioprine:* Increased myelosuppression

3 *Cyclosporine, tacrolimus:* Additive effects; increased risk of hyperkalemia, nephrotoxicity

3 *Diuretics:* Excessive hypotension, hypoperfusion

3 *Heparin:* Hyperkalemia

3 *Insulin, sulfonylureas:* Additive hypoglycemia

3 *Lithium:* Increase lithium levels

3 *Nonsteroidal antiinflammatory drugs:* Decreased antihypertensive efficacy, increased risk of nephrotoxicity

2 *Potassium supplements, potassium-sparing diuretics, potassium salt substitutes:* Hyperkalemia

3 *Trimethoprim:* Additive risk of hyperkalemia, especially in patient predisposed to renal insufficiency
3 *Interferon alfa 2a:* Increased myelosupression

Labs

• ACE inhibition can account for an approximately 0.5 mEq/L rise in serum potassium

SPECIAL CONSIDERATIONS

PATIENT/FAMILY EDUCATION

• Caution with salt substitutes containing potassium chloride
• Rise slowly to sitting/standing position to minimize orthostatic hypotension
• Dizziness, fainting, lightheadedness may occur during first few days of therapy
• May cause altered taste perception or cough; persistent dry cough usually does not subside unless medication is stopped; notify clinician if these symptoms persist
• Warnings regarding angioedema (swelling of face, extremities, eyes, lips, tongue, hoarseness, or difficulty swallowing or breathing), especially following first dose
• Skipping doses or voluntarily discontinuing the drug may produce severe, rebound hypertension

MONITORING PARAMETERS

• Baseline electrolytes, renal function tests, and urinalysis baseline and at least BUN, creatinine, potassium within 2 wks after initiation of therapy (increased levels may indicate acute renal failure)
• Serial orthostatic blood pressures and pulse rates
• Pattern of daily bowel activity and stool consistency

permethrin

(per-meth'-rin)

Rx: Acticin, Elimite

Chemical Class: Pyrethroid derivative

Therapeutic Class: Pediculicide; scabicide

CLINICAL PHARMACOLOGY

Mechanism of Action: An antiparasitic agent that inhibits sodium influx through nerve cell membrane channels. ***Therapeutic Effect:*** Results in delayed repolarization, paralysis, and death of parasites.

Pharmacokinetics

Less than 2% absorption after topical application. Detected in residual amounts on hair for at least 10 days following treatment. Metabolized by liver to inactive metabolites. Excreted in urine.

INDICATIONS AND DOSAGES

Head lice

Shampoo

Adults, Elderly, Children 2 mos and older. Shampoo hair, towel dry, apply to scalp, leave on for 10 mins and rinse. Remove nits with nit comb. Repeat application if live lice present 7 days after initial treatment.

Scabies

Topical

Adults, Elderly, Children 2 mos and older. Apply from head to feet, leave on for 8-14 hrs. Wash with soap and water. Repeat application if living mites present 14 days after initial treatment.

AVAILABLE FORMS

• *Cream:* 5% (Acticin).
• *Liquid, topical:* 1% (Nix).
• *Shampoo:* 0.33% (A200 Lice).
• *Solution:* 0.25% (Nix), 0.5% (A200 Lice, RID).

UNLABELED USES: Demodicidosis, insect bite prophylaxis, leishmaniasis prophylaxis, malaria prophylaxis

CONTRAINDICATIONS: Infants less than 2 mos of age, hypersensitivity to pyrethyroid, pyrethrin, chrysanthemums, or any component of the formulation

PREGNANCY AND LACTATION: Pregnancy category B; excretion into breast milk unknown

SIDE EFFECTS

Occasional

Burning, pruritus, stinging, erythema, rash, swelling

SERIOUS REACTIONS

- Shortness of breath and difficulty breathing have been reported.

SPECIAL CONSIDERATIONS

PATIENT/FAMILY EDUCATION

- For external use only; shake well
- Avoid contact with eyes, mucous membranes
- Itching may be temporarily aggravated following application
- Do not repeat administration sooner than 1 wk
- Itching from allergic reaction caused by mite may persist for several weeks even though infestation is cured
- Disinfect clothing, bedding, combs, and brushes

MONITORING PARAMETERS

- After treatment with permethrin, patients should be observed for the presence of live lice. If live lice are detected 14 days after the initial application of permethrin, retreatment is indicated
- Check skin for local burning, itching, and irritation

perphenazine

(per-fen'-a-zeen)

Rx: Trilafon

Chemical Class: Piperidine phenothiazine derivative

Therapeutic Class: Antiemetic; antipsychotic

CLINICAL PHARMACOLOGY

Mechanism of Action: An antipsychotic agent and antiemetic that blocks postsynaptic dopamine receptor sites in the brain. ***Therapeutic Effect:*** Suppresses behavioral response in psychosis, and relieves nausea and vomiting.

Pharmacokinetics

Well absorbed following oral administration. Protein binding: greater than 90%. Metabolized in liver. Excreted in urine. ***Half-life:*** 9-12 hr.

INDICATIONS AND DOSAGES

Severe schizophrenia

PO

Adults. 4-16 mg 2-4 times a day. Maximum: 64 mg/day.

Elderly. Initially, 2-4 mg/day. May increase at 4-7-day intervals by 2-4 mg/day up to 32 mg/day.

Severe nausea and vomiting

PO

Adults. 8-16 mg/day in divided doses up to 24 mg/day.

AVAILABLE FORMS

- *Oral Concentrate:* 16 mg/5 ml.
- *Tablets:* 2 mg, 4 mg, 8 mg, 16 mg.

CONTRAINDICATIONS: Coma, myelosuppression, hypersensitivity to other piperazine phenothiazines, severe cardiovascular disease, severe CNS depression, subcortical brain damage

PREGNANCY AND LACTATION: Pregnancy category C; has been used as an antiemetic during normal labor without producing any observable effect on newborn; excreted

P

into human breast milk; effects on nursing infant unknown, but may be of concern

SIDE EFFECTS

Occasional

Marked photosensitivity, somnolence, dry mouth, blurred vision, lethargy, constipation or diarrhea, nasal congestion, peripheral edema, urine retention

Rare

Ocular changes, altered skin pigmentation, hypotension, dizziness, syncope

SERIOUS REACTIONS

• Extrapyramidal symptoms appear to be dose-related and are divided into 3 categories: akathisia (characterized by inability to sit still, tapping of feet), parkinsonian symptoms (including masklike face, tremors, shuffling gait, hypersalivation), and acute dystonias (such as torticollis, opisthotonos, and oculogyric crisis).

• Tardive dyskinesia occurs rarely.

• Abrupt withdrawal after long-term therapy may precipitate nausea, vomiting, gastritis, dizziness, and tremors.

INTERACTIONS

Drugs

3 *Amodiaquine, chloroquine, sulfadoxine-pyrimethamine:* Increased neuroleptic concentrations

3 *Anticholinergics:* May inhibit neuroleptic response; excess anticholinergic effects

3 *Antidepressants:* Potential for increased therapeutic and toxic effects from increased levels of both drugs

3 *Antithyroid agents:* May increase the risk of agranulocytosis

3 *Apple juice, caffeine- or tannic-containing beverages (such as tea):* Do not mix oral concentrate with these beverages

3 *Barbiturates:* Decreased neuroleptic levels

3 *Clonidine, guanadrel, granethidine:* Severe hypotensive episodes possible

3 *Epinephrine:* Blunted pressor response to epinephrine

3 *Ethanol, other CNS depressants:* Additive CNS depression

3 *Extrapyramidal symptom–producing medications:* May increase the severity and frequency of extrapyramidal symptoms

2 *Levodopa:* Inhibited antiparkinsonian effect of levodopa

3 *Lithium:* Lowered levels of both drugs, rarely neurotoxicity in acute mania

3 *Narcotic analgesics:* Hypotension and increased CNS depression

3 *Orphenadrine:* Lowered neuroleptic concentrations, excessive anticholinergic effects

3 *Propranolol:* Increased plasma

Labs

• *Creatinine:* Decreased serum levels

SPECIAL CONSIDERATIONS

PATIENT/FAMILY EDUCATION

• Arise slowly from reclining position

• Do not discontinue abruptly

• Use a sunscreen during sun exposure to prevent burns, take special precautions to stay cool in hot weather

• Concentrate may be diluted just prior to administration with distilled water, acidified tap water, orange or grape juice

• Drowsiness generally subsides during continued therapy

MONITORING PARAMETERS

• Observe closely for signs of tardive dyskinesia (abnormal involuntary movement scale)

• Periodic CBC with platelets, hepatic and renal function during prolonged therapy

- Blood pressure for hypotension
- Therapeutic response, such as increased ability to concentrate and interest in surroundings, improvement in self-care, and a relaxed facial expression

phenazopyridine hydrochloride

(fen-az'-o-peer'-i-deen hye-droe-klor'-ide)

Rx: Azo-Gesic, Azo-Standard, Eridium, Prodium, Pyridiate, Pyridium, Uristat, Urodol, Urogesic

Combinations

Rx: with sulfamethoxazole (Azo-Gantanol); with sulfisoxazole (Azo-Gantrisin)

Chemical Class: Azo dye

Therapeutic Class: Urinary tract analgesic

CLINICAL PHARMACOLOGY

Mechanism of Action: An interstitial cystitis agent that exerts topical analgesic effect on urinary tract mucosa. ***Therapeutic Effect:*** Relieves urinary pain, burning, urgency, and frequency.

Pharmacokinetics

Well absorbed from the GI tract. Partially metabolized in the liver. Primarily excreted in urine. ***Half-life:*** Unknown.

INDICATIONS AND DOSAGES

Urinary analgesic

PO

Adults. 100-200 mg 3-4 times a day.

Children 6 yrs and older. 12 mg/kg/day in 3 divided doses for 2 days.

Dosage in renal impairment

Dosage interval is modified based on creatinine clearance.

Creatinine Clearance	*Interval*
50-80 ml/min	Usual dose q8-16h
less than 50 ml/min	Avoid use

AVAILABLE FORMS

- *Tablets:* 95 mg (Pyridium), 100 mg (Azo-Gesic, Azo-Standard, Prodium, Uristat), 200 mg (Azo-Gesic, Azo-Standard, Prodium, Uristat).

CONTRAINDICATIONS: Hepatic or renal insufficiency

PREGNANCY AND LACTATION: Pregnancy category B

SIDE EFFECTS

Occasional

Headache, GI disturbance, rash, pruritus

SERIOUS REACTIONS

- Overdose may lead to hemolytic anemia, nephrotoxicity, or hepatotoxicity. Patients with renal impairment or severe hypersensitivity to the drug may also develop these reactions.
- A massive and acute overdose may result in methemoglobinemia.

INTERACTIONS

Labs

- *Albumin:* Increased serum concentrations
- *Bacteria:* False negatives on Microstix
- *Bile:* False positive with Ictotest, BiliLabstix
- *Bilirubin, conjugated:* False elevations in serum
- *Bilirubin, unconjugated:* False serum concentration elevations
- *BSP retention:* False negatives
- *Cholinesterase:* Adds 34% negative bias to Ectachem method
- *Urine:* Yellow-orange color
- *Feces:* Orange-red color
- *Glucose:* Decreased serum levels
- *17-ketogenic steroids:* False positives in urine

• *Ketones:* Nitroprusside reactions masked by color; false negatives
• *17-ketosteroids:* Increase in urine
• *Porphyrins:* False positive
• *Pregnanediol:* Increased urine levels
• *Protein:* Increased serum levels
• *PSP excretion:* False positive in alkaline pH
• *Urobilinogen:* False positive urine test
• *Vanillylmandelic acid:* Increased urine concentrations
• *Xylose excretion:* Increased urine concentrations

SPECIAL CONSIDERATIONS

PATIENT/FAMILY EDUCATION

• May cause GI upset
• Take after meals
• May cause reddish-orange discoloration of urine; may stain fabric; may also stain contact lenses

MONITORING PARAMETERS

• Assess the patient for a therapeutic response: relief of urinary frequency, pain, and burning

phendimetrazine tartrate

(fen-dye-me'-tra-zeen tar'-trate)

Rx: Adipost, Bontril PDM, Bontril Slow-Release, Melfiat, Obezine, Phendiet, Phendiet-105, Plegine, Prelu-2

Chemical Class: Morpholine
Therapeutic Class: Anorexiant
DEA Class: Schedule III; Schedule IV

CLINICAL PHARMACOLOGY

Mechanism of Action: A phenylalkylamine sympathomimetic with activity similar to amphetamines that stimulates the central nervous system (CNS) and elevates blood pressure (BP) most likely mediated via norepinephrine and dopamine metabolism. Causes stimulation of the hypothalamus. ***Therapeutic Effect:*** Decreases appetite.

Pharmacokinetics

The pharmacokinetics of phendimetrazine tartrate has not been well established. Metabolized to active metabolite, phendimetrazine. Excreted in urine. ***Half-life:*** 2-4 hrs.

INDICATIONS AND DOSAGES

Obesity

PO

Adults, Elderly. 105 mg/day in the morning or before the morning meal (sustained-release); 35 mg 2-3 times/day (immediate-release). Maximum: 70 mg 3 times/day.

AVAILABLE FORMS

• *Tablets:* 35 mg (Bontril PDM, Obezine, Phendiet, Plegine).
• *Capsules (Extended-Release):* 105 mg (Adipost, Bontril Slow-Release, Melfiat, Phendiet-105, Prelu-2).

CONTRAINDICATIONS: Advanced arteriosclerosis, agitated states, glaucoma, history of drug abuse, history of hypersensitivity to sympathomimetic amines, hyperthyroidism, moderate to severe hypertension, symptomatic cardiovascular disease, use within 14 days of discontinuation of MAOI, hypersensitivity to phendimetrazine or sympathomimetics

PREGNANCY AND LACTATION: Pregnancy category C

SIDE EFFECTS

Occasional

Constipation, nausea, diarrhea, dry mouth, dysuria, libido changes, flushing, hypertension, insomnia, nervousness, headache, dizziness, irritability, agitation, restlessness, palpitations, increased heart rate, sweating, tremor, urticaria

SERIOUS REACTIONS

- Multivalvular heart disease, primary pulmonary hypertension, and arrhythmias occur rarely.
- Overdose may produce flushing, arrhythmias, and psychosis.
- Abrupt withdrawal following prolonged administration of high doses may produce extreme fatigue and depression.

SPECIAL CONSIDERATIONS

PATIENT/FAMILY EDUCATION

- May cause insomnia; avoid taking late in the day
- Weight reduction requires strict adherence to caloric restriction
- Do not discontinue abruptly
- Swallow capsules whole
- Take 1 hr before meal, usually the first meal of the day
- Avoid performing tasks that require mental alertness or motor skills until response to the drug is established
- Notify the physician if palpitations, dizziness, dry mouth, or pronounced nervousness occurs

MONITORING PARAMETERS

- Blood pressure, heart rate
- Weight
- CNS overstimulation

phenelzine sulfate

(fen'-el-zeen sul'-fate)

Rx: Nardil

Chemical Class: Hydrazine derivative

Therapeutic Class: Antidepressant, monoamine oxidase inhibitor (MAOI)

CLINICAL PHARMACOLOGY

Mechanism of Action: An MAOI that inhibits the activity of the enzyme monoamine oxidase at CNS storage sites, leading to increased levels of the neurotransmitters epinephrine, norepinephrine, serotonin, and dopamine at neuronal receptor sites. ***Therapeutic Effect:*** Relieves depression.

Pharmacokinetics

Well absorbed from GI tract. Metabolized in the liver. Primarily excreted in urine. ***Half-life:*** 1.2 hr.

INDICATIONS AND DOSAGES

Depression refractory to other antidepressants or electroconvulsive therapy

PO

Adults. 15 mg 3 times a day. May increase to 60-90 mg/day.

Elderly. Initially, 7.5 mg/day. May increase by 7.5-15 mg/day q3-4wk up to 60 mg/day in divided doses.

AVAILABLE FORMS

- *Tablets:* 15 mg.

UNLABELED USES: Treatment of panic disorder, selective mutism, vascular or tension headaches

CONTRAINDICATIONS: Cardiovascular or cerebrovascular disease, hepatic or renal impairment, pheochromocytoma

PREGNANCY AND LACTATION: Pregnancy category C

SIDE EFFECTS

Frequent

Orthostatic hypotension, restlessness, GI upset, insomnia, dizziness, headache, lethargy, asthenia, dry mouth, peripheral edema

Occasional

Flushing, diaphoresis, rash, urinary frequency, increased appetite, transient impotence

Rare

Visual disturbances

SERIOUS REACTIONS

- Hypertensive crisis occurs rarely and is marked by severe hypertension, occipital headache radiating frontally, neck stiffness or soreness, nausea, vomiting, diaphoresis, fever or chilliness, clammy skin, dilated pupils, palpitations, tachycardia or bradycardia, and constricting chest pain.

• Intracranial bleeding has been reported in association with severe hypertension.

INTERACTIONS

Drugs

▲ *Amphetamines, alcoholic beverages containing tyramine, metaraminol, phenylephrine, phenylpropanolamine, pseudoephedrine, tyramine, caffeine, chocolate:* Severe hypertensive reaction

❷ *Antidepressants, cyclic:* Excessive sympathetic response, mania, hyperpyrexia

③ *Antidiabetic agents:* May increase the effects of these drugs

③ *Barbiturates:* Prolonged effect of some barbiturates

▲ *Buspirone:* May increase blood pressure

▲ *Clomipramine:* Death

▲ *Dexfenfluramine, dextromethorphan, fenfluramine, meperidine:* Agitation, blood pressure changes, hyperpyrexia, convulsions

▲ *Dopamine, tryptophan:* May increase sudden, severe hypertension

▲ *Fluoxetine, sertraline:* Hypomania, confusion, hypertension, tremor

▲ *Food:* Foods containing large amounts of tyramine can result in hypertensive reactions

③ *Guanadrel, guanethidine:* May inhibit antihypertensive effects

③ *Levodopa:* Severe hypertensive reaction

❷ *Lithium:* Malignant hyperpyrexia

▲ *Methylphenidate:* May increase the CNS stimulant effects of methylphenidate

③ *Neuromuscular blocking agents:* Prolonged muscle relaxation caused by succinylcholine

③ *Reserpine:* Hypertensive reaction

▲ *Sibutramine, venlafaxine:* Increased risk of serotonin syndrome

③ *Sumatriptan:* Increased sumatriptan plasma concentrations

Labs

• *Aspartate aminotransferase:* Increased serum levels

• *Bilirubin:* False-positive increases in serum

• *Uric acid:* False-positive increases in serum

SPECIAL CONSIDERATIONS

PATIENT/FAMILY EDUCATION

• Avoid tyramine-containing foods, beverages, and OTC products containing decongestants or dextromethorphan and products such as diet aids

• Avoid foods that require bacteria or molds for their preparation or preservation (such as yogurt and aged cheese)

• May cause drowsiness, dizziness, blurred vision

• Use caution driving or performing other tasks requiring alertness

• Arise slowly from reclining position

• Therapeutic effect may require 4-8 wk

• Notify the physician if headache or neck soreness or stiffness occurs

MONITORING PARAMETERS

• Blood pressure, heart rate

• Weight

• Diet

• Behavior, level of interest, mood, and sleep pattern

• Monitor the patient for occipital headache radiating frontally and neck stiffness or soreness, which may be the first symptoms of an impending hypertensive crisis. If hypertensive crisis occurs, administer phentolamine 5-10 mg IV, as prescribed

phenobarbital

(fee-noe-bar'-bi-tal)

Rx: Luminal

Combinations

Rx: with atropine, hyoscyamine, scopolamine (Donnatal); with belladonna, ergotamine (Bellergal Spacetabs)

Chemical Class: Barbituric acid derivative

Therapeutic Class: Anticonvulsant; sedative/hypnotic

DEA Class: Schedule IV

CLINICAL PHARMACOLOGY

Mechanism of Action: A barbiturate that enhances the activity of gamma-aminobutyric acid (GABA) by binding to the GABA receptor complex. ***Therapeutic Effect:*** Depresses CNS activity.

Pharmacokinetics

Route	*Onset*	*Peak*	*Duration*
PO	20-60 min	N/A	6-10 hr
IV	5 min	30 min	4-10 hr

Well absorbed after PO or parenteral administration. Protein binding: 35%-50%. Rapidly and widely distributed. Metabolized in the liver. Primarily excreted in urine. Removed by hemodialysis. ***Half-life:*** 53-118 hr.

INDICATIONS AND DOSAGES

Status epilepticus

IV

Adults, Elderly. Initially, 300-800 mg, then 120-240 mg/dose at 20-min intervals until seizures are controlled or total dose of 1-2 g administered.

Children, Infants. 10-20 mg/kg. May administer additional 5 mg/kg/dose q15-30min until seizures controlled or total dose of 40 mg/kg administered.

Seizure control

PO, IV

Adults, Elderly, Children older than 12 yrs. 1-3 mg/kg/day. Or 50-100 mg 2-3 times a day.

Children 6-12 yrs. 4-6 mg/kg/day.

Children 1-5 yrs. 6-8 mg/kg/day.

Children younger than 1 yr. 5-6 mg/kg/day.

Neonates. 3-4 mg/kg/day.

Sedation

PO, IM

Adults, Elderly. 30-120 mg/day in 2-3 divided doses.

Children. 2 mg/kg 3 times a day.

Hypnotic

PO, IV, IM, Subcutaneous

Adults, Elderly. 100-320 mg at bedtime.

Children. 3-5 mg/kg at bedtime.

AVAILABLE FORMS

- *Elixir:* 15 mg/5 ml, 20 mg/5 ml.
- *Tablets:* 15 mg, 30 mg, 32.4 mg, 60 mg, 64.8 mg, 97.2 mg, 100 mg.
- *Injection:* 30 mg/ml, 60 mg/ml, 65 mg/ml, 130 mg/ml.

UNLABELED USES: Prevention and treatment of febrile seizures in children and hyperbilirubinemia, management of sedative or hypnotic withdrawal

CONTRAINDICATIONS: Hypersensitivity to other barbiturates, porphyria, preexisting CNS depression, severe pain, severe respiratory disease

PREGNANCY AND LACTATION: Pregnancy category D; risks to fetus include minor congenital defects, hemorrhage at birth, addiction; risk to mother may be greater if seizure control is lost due to stopping drug; use at lowest possible level to control seizures; excreted into breast milk; has caused major adverse effects in some nursing infants; use caution in nursing women

Controlled Substance: Schedule IV

SIDE EFFECTS

Occasional (3%-1%)

Somnolence

Rare (less than 1%)

Confusion; paradoxical CNS reactions, such as hyperactivity or nervousness in children and excitement or restlessness in the elderly (generally noted during first 2 wks of therapy, particularly in presence of uncontrolled pain)

SERIOUS REACTIONS

- Abrupt withdrawal after prolonged therapy may produce increased dreaming, nightmares, insomnia, tremor, diaphoresis, and vomiting, hallucinations, delirium, seizures, and status epilepticus.
- Skin eruptions may be a sign of a hypersensitivity reaction.
- Blood dyscrasias, hepatic disease, and hypocalcemia occur rarely.
- Overdose produces cold or clammy skin, hypothermia, severe CNS depression, cyanosis, tachycardia, and Cheyne-Stokes respirations.
- Toxicity may result in severe renal impairment.

INTERACTIONS

Drugs

3 *Acetaminophen:* Enhanced hepatotoxic potential of acetaminophen overdoses

3 *Antidepressants:* Reduced serum concentrations of cyclic antidepressants

3 *β-blockers:* Reduced serum concentrations of β-blockers, which are extensively metabolized (metoprolol, propranolol, sotalol)

3 *Calcium channel blockers:* Reduced concentrations of verapamil and nifedipine

3 *Chloramphenicol:* Increased barbiturate concentrations; reduced serum chloramphenicol concentrations

3 *Corticosteroids:* Reduced serum concentrations of corticosteroids, may impair therapeutic effect

3 *Cyclosporine:* Reduced serum concentration of cyclosporine

3 *Digitoxin:* Reduced serum concentration of digitoxin

3 *Disopyramide:* Reduced serum concentration of disopyramide

3 *Doxycycline:* Reduced serum doxycycline concentrations

3 *Estrogen:* Reduced serum concentration of estrogen

3 *Ethanol:* Excessive CNS depression

3 *Felbamate:* Increased phenobarbital concentrations; increased risk of toxicity

3 *Furosemide:* Decreased diuretic effect

3 *Griseofulvin:* Reduced griseofulvin absorption

3 *Lamotrigine:* Lower lamotrigine plasma levels and decreased elimination $t_{1/2}$

3 *Methoxyflurane:* Enhanced nephrotoxic effect

3 *Narcotic analgesics:* Increased toxicity of meperidine; reduced effect of methadone; additive CNS depression

3 *Neuroleptics:* Reduced effect of either drug

2 *Oral anticoagulants:* Decreased hypoprothrombinemic response to oral anticoagulants

3 *Oral contraceptives:* Reduced efficacy of oral contraceptives

3 *Phenytoin:* Unpredictable effect on serum phenytoin levels

3 *Primidone:* Excessive phenobarbital concentrations

3 *Propafenone:* Reduced serum concentration of propafenone

3 *Quinidine:* Reduced quinidine plasma concentration

3 *Tacrolimus:* Reduced serum concentration of tacrolimus

3 *Theophylline:* Reduced serum theophylline concentrations
3 *Valproic acid:* Increased serum phenobarbital concentrations

Labs

- *Amino acids:* Increase in urine collection measurements
- *Calcium:* False increases with Technicon SRA-2000
- *Glucose:* False negatives with Clinistix, Diastix
- *5-Hydroxyindoleacetic acid:* False high colorimetric values
- *Lactate dehydrogenase:* Increased serum levels
- *Protein:* False elevations at high concentrations

SPECIAL CONSIDERATIONS

PATIENT/FAMILY EDUCATION

- Avoid driving or other activities requiring alertness
- Avoid alcohol ingestion or CNS depressants
- Do not discontinue medication abruptly after long-term use
- May be habit-forming

MONITORING PARAMETERS

- Periodic CBC, liver and renal function tests, serum folate, vitamin D during prolonged therapy
- Serum phenobarbital concentration (therapeutic range for seizure disorders 20-40 mcg/ml)
- Blood pressure, heart rate, respiratory rate
- CNS status
- Seizure activity

phenoxybenzamine hydrochloride

(fen-ox-ee-ben'-za-meen hye-droe-klor'-ide)

Rx: Dibenzyline

Chemical Class: Haloalkylamine derivative

Therapeutic Class: Pheochromocytoma agent; sympatholytic

CLINICAL PHARMACOLOGY

Mechanism of Action: An antihypertensive that produces long-lasting noncompetitive alpha-adrenergic blockade of postganglionic synapses in exocrine glands and smooth muscles. Relaxes urethra and increases opening of the bladder. ***Therapeutic Effect:*** Controls hypertension.

Pharmacokinetics

Well absorbed from the gastrointestinal (GI) tract. Distributed into fatty tissue. Metabolized in liver. Eliminated in urine and feces. Not removed by hemodialysis. ***Half-life:*** 24 hrs.

INDICATIONS AND DOSAGES

Pheochromocytoma

PO

Adults. Initially, 10 mg twice daily. May increase dose every other day to 20-40 mg 2-3 times/day.

Children. 1-2 mg/kg/day in divided doses.

AVAILABLE FORMS

- *Tablets:* 10 mg (Dibenzyline).

UNLABELED USES: Bladder instability, complex regional pain syndrome (CRPS), contraception, prostatic obstruction, Raynaud's disease

CONTRAINDICATIONS: Any condition compromised by hypotension, hypersensitivity to phenoxybenzamine or any component of the formulation

PREGNANCY AND LACTATION: Pregnancy category C; indicated in hypertension secondary to pheochromocytoma during pregnancy, especially after 24 wk gestation when surgical intervention is associated with high rates of maternal and fetal mortality; no adverse fetal effects due to this treatment have been observed

SIDE EFFECTS

Frequent

Headache, lethargy, confusion, fatigue

Occasional

Nausea, postural hypotension, syncope, dry mouth

Rare

Palpitations, diarrhea, constipation, inhibition of ejaculation, weakness, altered vision, dizziness

SERIOUS REACTIONS

• Overdosage produces severe hypotension, irritability, lethargy, tachycardia, dizziness, and shock.

INTERACTIONS

Drugs

3 *Compounds that stimulate both alpha- and beta-adrenergic receptors (e.g., epinephrine):* May produce an exaggerated hypotensive response and tachycardia

SPECIAL CONSIDERATIONS

PATIENT/FAMILY EDUCATION

• Avoid alcohol; avoid sudden changes in posture, dizziness may result

• Avoid cough, cold, or allergy medications containing sympathomimetics

• Avoid driving or other activities requiring alertness

MONITORING PARAMETERS

• Blood pressure

phentermine hydrochloride

Rx: Adipex-P, Fastin, Ionamin, Oby-Cap, Phentercot, Pro-Fast HS, Pro-Fast SA, Pro-Fast SR, T-Diet, Teramine, Zantryl

Chemical Class: Phenethylamine analog (amphetamine-like)

Therapeutic Class: Anorexiant

DEA Class: Schedule IV

CLINICAL PHARMACOLOGY

Mechanism of Action: A sympathomimetic amine structurally similar to dextroamphetamine and is most likely mediated via norephinephrine and dopamine metabolism. Causes stimulation of the hypothalamus. ***Therapeutic Effect:*** Decreased appetite.

Pharmacokinetics

Well absorbed from the gastrointestinal (GI) tract; resin absorbed slower. Excreted unchanged in urine. ***Half-life:*** 20 hrs.

INDICATIONS AND DOSAGES

Obesity

PO

Adults, Children older than 16 yrs.

Adipex-P: 37.5 mg as a single daily dose or in divided doses.

Ionamin: 15-37.5 mg/day before breakfast or 1-2 hrs. after breakfast.

Fastin: 30 mg/day taken in the morning.

AVAILABLE FORMS

• *Capsules (as hydrochloride):* 15 mg, 18.75 mg, 30 mg (Fastin), 37.5 mg (Adipex-P).

• *Capsules (as resin complex):* 15 mg (Ionamin), 30 mg (Ionamin).

• *Tablets (as hydrochloride):* 8 mg, 37.5 mg (Adipex-P).

CONTRAINDICATIONS: Advanced arteriosclerosis, agitated states, cardiovascular disease, concurrent use or within 14 days of discontinuation of MAOI therapy, glaucoma, history of drug abuse, hypertension (moderate-to-severe), hyperthyroidism, hypersensitivity to phentermine or sympathomimetic amines

PREGNANCY AND LACTATION: Pregnancy category B

Controlled Substance: Schedule IV

SIDE EFFECTS

Occasional

Restlessness, insomnia, tremor, palpitations, tachycardia, elevation in blood pressure, headache, dizziness, dry mouth, unpleasant taste, diarrhea or constipation, changes in libido

SERIOUS REACTIONS

- Primary pulmonary hypertension (PPH), psychotic episodes, and valvular heart disease rarely occur.
- Anorectic agents have been associated with regurgitant multivalvular heart disease involving mitral, aortic, and/or tricuspid valves.
- Prolonged use may cause physical or psychologic dependence.

INTERACTIONS

Drugs

3 *Furazolidone:* Increased pressor response

3 *Guanethidine:* Decreased hypotensive effect

▲ *MAOIs:* Increased pressor response

3 *Tricyclic antidepressants:* Decreased anorexiant effect

Labs

- *Drugs of abuse:* Urine screen; false positive for amphetamines
- *Phenmetrazine:* False positive urine
- *Quinine:* False positive urine

SPECIAL CONSIDERATIONS

PATIENT/FAMILY EDUCATION

- May cause insomnia, avoid taking late in the day
- Weight reduction is facilitated by adherence to caloric restriction and exercise
- Avoid tasks that require mental alertness or motor skills until response to the drug is established
- May be habit-forming
- Notify the physician if fast, pounding, or irregular heartbeat occurs

MONITORING PARAMETERS

- Blood pressure
- Weight

phentolamine mesylate

(fen-tole'-a-meen)

Rx: Regitine

Chemical Class: Imidazoline derivative

Therapeutic Class: Pheochromocytoma agent; sympatholytic

CLINICAL PHARMACOLOGY

Mechanism of Action: An alpha-adrenergic blocking agent that produces peripheral vasodilation and cardiac stimulation. ***Therapeutic Effect:*** Decreases blood pressure (BP).

Pharmacokinetics

Poorly absorbed from the gastrointestinal (GI) tract. Protein binding: 72%. Metabolized in liver. Eliminated in urine and feces. Not removed by hemodialysis. ***Half-life:*** 19 min.

INDICATIONS AND DOSAGES

Extravasation—norepinephrine

SC

Adults, Elderly. Infiltrate area with a small amount (1 ml) of solution (made by diluting 5-10 mg in 10 ml

of NS) within 12 hrs of extravasation. Do not exceed 0.1-0.2 mg/kg or 5 mg total. If dose is effective, normal skin color should return to the blanched area within 1 hr.
Children. Infiltrate area with a small amount (1 ml) of solution (made by diluting 5-10 mg in 10 ml of NS) within 12 hrs of extravasation. Do not exceed 0.1-0.2 mg/kg or 5 mg total.

Diagnosis of pheochromocytoma
IM/IV
Adults, Elderly. 5 mg as a single dose.
Children. 0.05-0.1 mg/kg/dose. Maximum single dose: 5 mg.

Surgery for pheochromocytoma: Hypertension
IM/IV
Adults, Elderly. 5 mg given 1-2 hrs before procedure and repeated as needed every 2-4 hrs.
Children. 0.05-0.1 mg/kg/dose given 1-2 hrs before procedure. Repeat as needed every 2-4 hrs until hypertension is controlled. Maximum single dose: 5 mg.

Hypertensive crisis
IV
Adults, Elderly. 5-20 mg as a single dose.

AVAILABLE FORMS
• *Injection:* 5 mg/ml (Regitine).

UNLABELED USES: Treatment of pralidoxime-induced hypertension, arrhythmias, asthma, bladder instability, cardiac diseases, diabetes mellitus, erectile dysfunction, extravasation (dopamine and epinephrine), hyperhidrosis, myocardial infarction, Raynaud's phenomenon, surgery, sympathetic pain

CONTRAINDICATIONS: Renal impairment; coronary or cerebral arteriosclerosis; concurrent use with phosphodiesterase-5 (PDE-5) inhibitors including sildenafil (>25 mg), tadalafil, or vardenafil; hypersensitivity to phentolamine or related compounds.

PREGNANCY AND LACTATION: Pregnancy category C

SIDE EFFECTS
Occasional
Hypotension, tachycardia, arrhythmia, flushing, orthostatic hypotension, weakness, dizziness, nausea, vomiting, diarrhea, nasal congestion, pulmonary hypertension

SERIOUS REACTIONS
• Symptoms of overdosage include tachycardia, shock, vomiting, and dizziness.
• Mixed agents, such as epinephrine, may cause more hypotension.

INTERACTIONS
Drugs
3 *Epinepherine, ephedrine:* Vasoconstricting and hypertensive effects of these drugs are antagonized
Labs
• *5-hydroxyindoleacetic acid:* Urine, falsely high colorimetric values

SPECIAL CONSIDERATIONS
• Urinary catecholamines preferred over phentolamine for screening for pheochromocytoma

PATIENT/FAMILY EDUCATION
• Notify the physician if dizziness or palpitations occurs
• Avoid tasks that require mental alertness or motor skills until response to drug is established

MONITORING PARAMETERS
• Blood pressure

phenylephrine (systemic)

(fen-ill-ef'-rin)

Rx: Neofrin; Neo-Synephrine Ophthalmic; Ocu-Phrin; Phenoptic; Rectasol

Combinations

Rx: with chlorpheniramine (Ed A-Hist, Prehist, Histatab); with brompheniramine (Dimetane); with chlorpheniramine, phenylpropanolamine (Hista-Vadrin); with chlorpheniramine, phenyltoloxamine (Comhist); with brompheniramine, phenylpropanolamine (Bromophen T.D., Tamine S.R.); with chlorpheniramine, phenyltoloxamine, phenylpropanolamine (Decongestabs, Naldecon, Nalgest, Tri-phen, Uni-decon); with chlorpheniramine, pyrilamine, phenylpropanolamine (Vanex, Histalet); with chlorpheniramine, pyrilamine (R-tannate, Rhinatate, R-tannamine, Rynatan, Tanoral, Triotann, Tritan, Tri-tannate)

Chemical Class: Substituted phenylethylamine

Therapeutic Class: Vasopressor

CLINICAL PHARMACOLOGY

Mechanism of Action: Phenylephrine is a powerful postsynaptic alpha-receptor stimulant with little effect on the beta receptors of the heart, lacking chronotropic and inotropic actions on the heart. ***Therapeutic Effect:*** Vasoconstriction, decreases heart rate, increases stroke output, increases blood pressure.

Pharmacokinetics

Phenylephrine is irregularly absorbed from and readily metabolized in the GI tract. After IV administration, a pressor effect occurs almost immediately and persists for 15-20 mins. After IM administration, a pressor effect occurs within 10-15 mins and persists for 50 mins-1 hr. After oral inhalation of phenylephrine in combination with isoproterenol, pulmonary effects occur within a few minutes and persist for about 3 hrs. The pharmacologic effects of phenylephrine are terminated at least partially by the uptake of the drug into the tissues. Phenylephrine is metabolized in the liver and intestine by the enzyme monoamine oxidase (MAO). The metabolites and their route and rate of excretion have not been identified.

INDICATIONS AND DOSAGES

Paroxysmal supraventricular tachycardia (PSVT)

Adults. The initial dose, given by rapid IV injection, should not exceed 0.5 mg. Subsequent doses may be increased in increments of 0.1-0.2 mg. Maximum single dose is 1 mg IV.

Children. 5-10 mcg/kg IV over 20-30 sec.

Mild to moderate hypotension

SC/IM

Adults. 2-5 mg IM or SC (range 1-10 mg), repeated no more than every 10-15 mins. Maximum initial IM or SC dose is 5 mg.

Children. 0.1 mg/kg IM or SC every 1-2 hrs as needed. Maximum dose is 5 mg.

IV

Adults. 0.2 mg IV (range 0.1-0.5 mg), given no more frequently than every 10-15 mins. Maximum initial IV dose is 0.5 mg.

Severe hypotension or shock

IV

Adults. Initially, 100-180 mcg/min IV infusion, with dose titration to the desired MAP and SVR. A maintenance infusion rate of 40-60 mcg/min IV is usually adequate after blood pressure stabilizes. If necessary to produce the desired pressor response, additional phenylephrine in increments of 10 mg or more may be added to the infusion solution and the rate of flow adjusted according to the response of the patient.

Children. 5-20 mcg/kg IV bolus, followed by an initial IV infusion of 0.1-0.5 mcg/kg/min, titrated to desired effect. Doses up to 3-5 mcg/kg/min IV may be required.

Hypotensive emergencies during spinal anesthesia

IV

Adults. Initially, 0.2 mg IV. Subsequent doses should not exceed the previous dose by more than 0.1-0.2 mg. Maximum of 0.5 mg per dose.

Hypotension during spinal anesthesia in children

IM/SC

Children. A dose of 0.044-0.088 mg/kg IM or SC is recommended by the manufacturer.

Hypotension prophylaxis during spinal anesthesia

IM/SC

Adults. 2-3 mg SC or IM, 3 or 4 mins before anesthesia. A dose of 2 mg SC or IM is usually adequate with low spinal anesthesia; 3 mg IM or SC may be necessary with high spinal anesthesia.

Vasoconstriction in regional anesthesia

IV

Adults. The manufacturer states that the optimum concentration of phenylephrine HCl is 0.05 mg/ml (1:20,000). Solutions may be prepared for regional anesthesia by adding 1 mg of phenylephrine HCl to each 20 ml of local anesthesia solution. Some pressor response can be expected when at least 2 mg is injected.

Prolongation of spinal anesthesia.

IV

Adults. The addition of 2-5 mg added to the anesthetic solution increases the duration of motor block by as much as 50% without an increase in the incidence of complications such as nausea, vomiting, or blood pressure disturbances.

Hypotension during special anesthesia in children.

IM/SC

Children. A dose of 0.5-1 mg per 25 lbs body weight, administered subcutaneously or IM, is recommended.

AVAILABLE FORMS

- *Solution (Ophthalmic):* 2.5%, 10%.
- *Solution (Nasal):* 0.125%, 0.16%, 0.25%, 0.5%.
- *Solution (Injection):* 10 mg/ml.
- *Solution (Oral):* 5 mg/ml.
- *Suppository (Rectal):* 0.25%.

CONTRAINDICATIONS: Phenylephrine HCl injection should not be used with patients with severe hypertension, ventricular tachycardia or fibrillation, acute myocardial infarction (MI), atrial flutter or fibrillation, cardiac arrhythmias, cardiac disease, cardiomyopathy, closed-angle glaucoma, coronary artery disease, women who are in labor, during obstetric delivery, or in patients who have a known hypersensitivity to phenylephrine, sulfites, or to any one of its components.

PREGNANCY AND LACTATION: Pregnancy category C; unknown if excreted in breast milk

SIDE EFFECTS

Occasional

Headache, reflex bradycardia, excitability, restlessness, and rarely arrhythmias.

SERIOUS REACTIONS

• Overdose may induce ventricular extrasystoles and short paroxysms of ventricular tachycardia, a sensation of fullness in the head, and tingling of the extremities. Should an excessive elevation of blood pressure occur, it may be immediately relieved by an α-adrenergic blocking agent (e.g., phentolamine). The oral LD_{50} in the rat is 350 mg/kg, in the mouse 120 mg/kg.

INTERACTIONS

Drugs

3 *β-blockers (non-selective):* Predisposed to hypertensive episodes

3 *Digoxin:* Increased risk of arrhythmias

3 *Ergonovine, oxytocin:* May increase vasoconstriction

3 *Guanethidine:* Enhanced pupillary response to phenylephrine

3 *Imipramine:* Enhanced pressor response

1 *MAOIs:* Hypertensive episodes

3 *Methyldopa:* May decrease the effects of methyldopa

Labs

• *Amino acids:* Increased in urine

• *Metanephrines, total:* Increased in urine

SPECIAL CONSIDERATIONS

• *Antidote to extravasation:* 5-10 ml phentolamine in 10-15 ml saline infiltrated throughout ischemic area

• Not indicated for hypotension secondary to hypovolemia

• As not bioavailable orally (see pharmacokinetics), combination products essentially lack decongestant. Only available by prescription, as lack effectiveness data required by FDA OTC panels

PATIENT/FAMILY EDUCATION

• Immediately contact the physician and discontinue the drug if dizziness, feeling of irregular heartbeat, insomnia, tremor, or weakness occurs

MONITORING PARAMETERS

• Blood pressure, heart rate

---

phenylephrine (topical)

(fen-ill-ef'-rin)

Rx: AK-Dilate; Mydfrin; Neofrin; Neo-Synephrine Ophthalmic; Ocu-Phrin; Phenoptic; Rectasol

Combinations

Rx: (Nasal): with zinc (Zincfrin); with pheniramine (Dristan Nasal);

Rx: (Ophthalmic); with tropicamide (Diophenyl-t); with pyrilamine (Prefrin-A)

Chemical Class: Substituted phenylethylamine

Therapeutic Class: Decongestant; mydriatic

CLINICAL PHARMACOLOGY

Mechanism of Action: Phenylephrine HCl is an alpha-receptor sympathetic agonist used in local ocular disorders because of its vasoconstrictor and mydriatic action. It exhibits rapid and moderately prolonged action, and it produces little rebound vasodilatation. Systemic side effects are uncommon. ***Therapeutic Effect:*** Vasoconstriction and pupil dilation.

Pharmacokinetics

Some absorption systemically. The duration of action of intranasal administration ranges from 30 mins to 4 hrs. The duration of the mydriatic effect is roughly 3 hrs after administration of the 2.5% solution but may be as long as 7 hrs after the 10% solution.

INDICATIONS AND DOSAGES

Mydriasis induction (ophthalmic)

Topical

Adults, Adolescents, Elderly. Instill 1 or 2 drops of a 2.5% or 10% solution in eye before procedure. May be repeated in 10-60 mins if needed. In general, the 2.5% solution is preferred in the elderly to avoid cardiac reactions.

Children. Instill 1 or 2 drops of a 2.5% solution in the eye before procedure. May be repeated in 10-60 mins if needed.

Infants < 1 yr. 1 drop of 2.5% solution 15-30 mins before procedure.

Uveitis (posterior synechia)

Topical

Adults, Elderly. Instill 1 drop of 10% solution in eye 3 or more times daily with atropine sulfate. In general, the 2.5% solution is preferred in elderly to avoid adverse cardiac reactions.

Adults and children over age 12 (intranasal): Apply 2-3 drops or 1-2 sprays of a 0.25%-0.5% solution instilled in each nostril or a small quantity of 0.5% nasal jelly applied into each nostril. Apply every 4 hrs as needed. The 1% solution may be used in adults with severe congestion.

Children 6-12 yrs (intranasal): 2-3 drops of the 0.25% solution in each nostril every 4 hrs as needed.

Children < 6 yrs (intranasal): Apply 2-3 drops or sprays of a 0.125% or 0.16% solution in each nostril every 4 hrs as needed.

Infants > 6 mos (intranasal): 1-2 drops of the 0.16% solution in each nostril every 3 hrs.

Conjunctival congestion

Topical

Adults, Elderly: 1-2 drops of a 0.12% to 0.25% solution applied to the conjunctiva every 3-4 hrs as needed. In general, the 2.5% solution is preferred in elderly to avoid cardiac reactions.

Postoperative malignant glaucoma

Topical

Adults, Elderly. Instill 1 drop of a 10% solution with 1 drop of a 1%-4% solution 3 or more times per day. In general, the 2.5% solution is preferred in elderly to avoid cardiac reactions.

Vasoconstriction and pupil dilatation

Topical

Adults. A drop of a suitable topical anesthetic may be applied, followed in a few minutes by 1 drop of the on the upper limbus.

Surgery

Topical

Adults. When a short-acting mydriatic is needed for wide dilatation of the pupil before intraocular surgery, phenylephrine HCl 2.5% (or the 10%) may be applied topically from 30-60 mins before the operation.

Cycloplegia

Topical

Adults. One drop of the preferred cycloplegic is placed in each eye, followed in 5 mins by 1 drop of phenylephrine HCl 2.5%.

Children. For a "one application method," phenylephrine HCl 2.5% may be combined with one of the preferred rapid-acting cycloplegics to produce adequate cycloplegia.

Ophthalmoscopic examination
Topical
Adults. One drop of phenylephrine HCl 2.5% is placed in each eye.
Blanching test
Topical
Adults. One or two drops of phenylephrine HCl 2.5% should be applied to the injected eye.
Glaucoma
Topical
Adults. In certain patients with glaucoma, temporary reduction of intraocular tension may be attained by producing vasoconstriction of the intraocular vessels; this may be accompanied by placing 1 drop of the 10% solution on the upper surface of the cornea. This treatment may be repeated as often as necessary.
Nasal congestion
Intranasal
Adults, Children 12 and older. Use 2 or 3 drops or sprays of a 0.25%-0.5% solution in the nose every 4 hrs as needed
Children 6-12 yrs. Use 2 or 3 drops or sprays of a 0.25% solution in the nose every 4 hrs as needed.
Children 2-6 yrs. Use 2 or 3 drops of a 0.125%-0.16% solution in the nose every 4 hrs as needed.

AVAILABLE FORMS

- *Solution (ophthalmic):* 2.5%, 10%.
- *Solution (nasal):* 0.125%, 0.16%, 0.25%, 0.5%.
- *Solution (injection):* 10 mg/ml.
- *Solution (oral):* 5 mg/ml.
- *Suppository (rectal):* 0.25%.

CONTRAINDICATIONS: Ophthalmic solutions, (both strengths), of phenylephrine HCl are contraindicated in patients with anatomically narrow angles or narrow angle glaucoma, some low birth weight infants, and some elderly adults with severe arteriosclerotic cardiovascular or cerebrovascular disease, use during intraocular operative procedures when the corneal epithelial barrier has been disturbed, and in persons with a known sensitivity to phenylephrine, sulfites, or any of its components, including preservatives. The 10% solution is contraindicated in infants and in patients with aneurysms.

PREGNANCY AND LACTATION: Pregnancy category C; no breast-feeding data; use caution

SIDE EFFECTS

Frequent

Burning or stinging or eyes, headache or browache, sensitivity to light, watering of the eyes, increase in runny or stuffy nose, burning, stinging, dryness of inside the nose

Rare

Irritation, dizziness, fast and/or irregular and/or pounding heartbeat, increased sweating, increase in blood pressure, paleness, trembling, headache, nervousness, trouble sleeping

SERIOUS REACTIONS

- There have been reports associating the use of phenylephrine HCl 10% ophthalmic solutions with the development of serious cardiovascular reactions, including ventricular arrhythmias and myocardial infarctions. These episodes, some ending fatally, have usually occurred in elderly patients with preexisting cardiovascular diseases.

INTERACTIONS

- See interactions under systemic phenylephrine; interactions less likely than with systemic administration if given in proper dosage

SPECIAL CONSIDERATIONS

- Do not administer for more than 3-5 days (nasal product) or 2-3 days (ocular product used as decongestant) due to rebound congestion

PATIENT/FAMILY EDUCATION
• Burning or stinging of the eyes, headache, browache, sensitivity of eyes to light, and watering of eyes may occur

MONITORING PARAMETERS
• Blood pressure, heart rate

phenytoin/ fosphenytoin

(fen'-i-toy-in/fos-fen'-i-toy-in)

Rx: Dilantin, Epamin
Rx: Dilantin
Rx: Cerebyx

Chemical Class: Hydantoin derivative

Therapeutic Class: Anticonvulsant

CLINICAL PHARMACOLOGY

Mechanism of Action: An anticonvulsant and antiarrhythmic agent that stabilizes neuronal membranes in motor cortex, and decreases abnormal ventricular automaticity. ***Therapeutic Effect:*** Limits spread of seizure activity. Stabilizes threshold against hyperexcitability. Decreases posttetanic potentiation and repetitive discharge. Shortens refractory period, QT interval, and action potential duration.

Pharmacokinetics

Phenytoin: Slowly, variably absorbed after PO administration; slow but completely absorbed after IM administration. Protein binding: 90%-95%. Widely distributed. Metabolized in liver. Primarily excreted in urine. Not removed by hemodialysis. ***Half-life:*** 22 hrs.

Fosphenytoin: Completely absorbed after IM administration. Protein binding: 95%-99%. After IM or IV administration, rapidly and completely hydrolyzed to phenytoin. Time of complete conversion to phenytoin: IM: 4 hrs after injection; IV: 2 hrs after the end of infusion. ***Half-life*** for conversion to phenytoin: 8-15 min.

INDICATIONS AND DOSAGES

Status epilepticus (Phenytoin)

IV

Adults, Elderly, Children. Loading dose: 15-18 mg/kg. Maintenance dose: 300 mg/day in 2-3 divided doses.

Children 10-16 yrs. Loading dose: 15-18 mg/kg. Maintenance dose: 6-7 mg/kg/day.

Children 7-9 yrs. Loading dose: 15-18 mg/kg. Maintenance dose: 7-8 mg/kg/day.

Children 4-6 yrs. Loading dose: 15-18 mg/kg. Maintenance dose: 7.5-9 mg/kg/day.

Children 6 mos-3 yrs. Loading dose 15-18 mg/kg. Maintenance dose: 8-10 mg/kg/day.

Neonates. Loading dose: 15-20 mg/kg. Maintenance dose: 5-8 mg/kg/day.

Status epilepticus (Fosphenytoin)

IV

Adults. Loading dose: 15-20 mg PE/kg infused at rate of 100-150 mg PE/min.

Nonemergent seizures

IV

Adults. Loading dose: 10-20 mg PE/kg. Maintenance: 4-6 mg PE/kg/day.

Anticonvulsant

PO

Adults, Elderly, Children. Loading dose: 15-20 mg/kg in 3 divided doses 2-4 hrs apart. Maintenance dose: Same as above.

Arrhythmias

IV

Adults, Elderly, Children. Loading dose: 1.25 mg/kg q5min. May repeat up to total dose of 15 mg/kg.

PO
Adults, Elderly. Maintenance Dose: 250 mg 4 times/day for 1 day, then 250 mg 2 times/day for 2 days, then 300-400 mg/day in divided doses 1-4 times/day.
PO/IV
Children. Maintenance dose: 5-10 mg/kg/day in 2-3 divided doses.

AVAILABLE FORMS

Phenytoin

- *Capsules:* 30 mg, 100 mg (Dilantin).
- *Tablets (chewable):* 50 mg (Dilantin).
- *Oral Suspension:* 125 mg/5 ml (Dilantin).
- *Injection, as sodium:* 50 mg/ml (Dilantin).

Fosphenytoin

- *Injection:* 75 mg/ml, equivalent to 50 mg/ml phenytoin, or 50 mg phenytoin equivalent/ml (Cerebyx).

UNLABELED USES

Phenytoin: Adjunct in treatment of tricyclic antidepressant toxicity, muscle relaxant in treatment of muscle hyperirritability, treatment of digoxin-induced arrhythmias and trigeminal neuralgia

CONTRAINDICATIONS: Hydantoin hypersensitivity, seizures due to hypoglycemia, Adam-Stokes syndrome, second- and third-degree heart block, sinoatrial block, sinus bradycardia

PREGNANCY AND LACTATION: Pregnancy category D (risk of congenital defects increased 2-3 times; fetal hydantoin syndrome includes craniofacial abnormalities, hypoplasia, ossification of distal phalanges; may also be transplacental carcinogen); compatible with breast-feeding

SIDE EFFECTS

Frequent
Drowsiness; lethargy; confusion; slurred speech; irritability; gingival hyperplasia; hypersensitivity reaction; including fever, rash, and lymphadenopathy; constipation; dizziness; nausea
Occasional
Headache, hair growth, insomnia, muscle twitching

SERIOUS REACTIONS

- Abrupt withdrawal may precipitate status epilepticus.
- Blood dyscrasias, lymphadenopathy, and osteomalacia, caused by interference of vitamin D metabolism, may occur.
- Toxic phenytoin blood concentration of 25 mcg/ml may produce ataxia, characterized by muscular incoordination, nystagmus or rhythmic oscillation of eyes, and double vision. As level increases, extreme lethargy to comatose states occur.

INTERACTIONS

Drugs

3 *Acetaminophen:* Enhances the hepatotoxic potential of acetaminophen overdoses; may reduce the therapeutic response to acetaminophen

3 *Acetazolamide:* Osteomalacia

3 *Alcohol, other CNS depressants:* Increases CNS depression

3 *Amiodarone:* Increased phenytoin levels; decreased amiodarone levels

3 *Antacids:* May decrease phenytoin absorption

3 *Azole-antifungals (fluconazole):* Phenytoin induces metabolism (CYP3A4), reducing antifungal effects

3 *Benzodiazepines (alprazolam, diazepam, midazolam, triazolam):* Enhanced metabolism (CYP3A4) phenytoin reduces benzodiazepine effects

3 *Carbamazepine:* Combined use usually decreases levels of both drugs

P

3 *Chloramphenicol, disulfiram, fluoxetine, isoniazid, omeprazole, sulfonamides:* Increased phenytoin levels
3 *Cimetidine, cisplatin, diazoxide, folate, rifampin:* Decreased phenytoin levels
3 *Clozapine:* Reduced levels via phenytoin induced enhanced metabolism
3 *Corticosteroids:* Decreased therapeutic effect of steroids
3 *Cyclic antidepressants:* Increased antidepressant levels
3 *Cyclosporine:* Reduced cyclosporine levels
3 *Dicumarol:* Increased anticoagulant effect, increased phenytoin levels
3 *Digitalis glycosides:* Lower digitalis levels
3 *Disopyramide:* Reduced efficacy, increased toxicity of disopyramide
3 *Dopamine:* More susceptible to hypotension after IV phenytoin
3 *Doxycycline:* Reduced doxycycline concentrations
3 *Felbamate:* Felbamate consistently increases phenytoin levels
3 *Furosemide:* Decreased diuretic effect
2 *Itraconazole:* Phenytoin induces metabolism (CYP3A4), reducing antifungal effects
3 *Lamotrigine:* Phenytoin stimulates metabolism-lower plasma levels; decreased $t_{1/2}$
3 *Levodopa:* Decreased antiparkinsonian effect
3 *Lidocaine, propranolol:* May increase cardiac depressant effects
3 *Lithium:* Increased risk of lithium intoxication; causal explanation not known
2 *Mebendazole in high doses:* Decreased mebendazole levels
2 *Methadone:* Withdrawal
3 *Metyrapone:* Invalidates test
3 *Mexiletine:* Decreased mexiletine levels
3 *Oral contraceptives:* Decreased contraceptive effect
3 *Primidone:* Enhanced conversion to phenobarbital
3 *Pyridoxine:* Large doses may decrease phenytoin levels
3 *Quinidine:* Decreased quinidine levels
3 *Quinolone antibiotics (ciprofloxacin, enoxacin, norfloxacin):* Elevates phenytoin concentrations
3 *Sucralfate:* Phenytoin reduces GI absorption
3 *Tacrolimus:* Reduced tacrolimus levels
3 *Theophylline:* Reduced theophylline levels
3 *Thyroid hormone:* Increased thyroid replacement dose requirements
3 *Tolbutamide:* Phenytoin inhibits insulin release, may result in hyperglycemia; tolbutamide displaces phenytoin from protein-binding sites; monitor for alterations in glucose control
3 *Trimethoprim:* Increased phenytoin concentrations
3 *Valproic acid:* Variable effects on phenytoin levels; decreased valproic acid levels
3 *Warfarin:* Transient increased hypoprothrombinemic response followed by inhibition of hypoprothrombinemic response
3 *Xanthine:* May increase the metabolism of these drugs

Labs

- *False positive:* Barbiturates, urine
- *Increased:* Cholesterol, serum; thyroxine, serum

SPECIAL CONSIDERATIONS

- Pro-drug, fosphenytoin rapidly converted to phenytoin *in vivo:* minimal activity before conversion; water soluble, thus more suitable for parenteral applications: does not require cardiac monitoring; can be administered at faster rate; no IV filter required; compatible with both saline and dextrose mixtures; requires refrigeration

PATIENT/FAMILY EDUCATION

• Do not abruptly discontinue phenytoin after long-term use because doing so may precipitate seizures; strict maintenance of drug therapy is essential for control of seizures and arrhythmias
• IV injection may cause pain
• Maintain good oral hygiene, including gum massage and regular dental visits, to prevent gingival hyperplasia, marked by bleeding, swelling, and tenderness of gums
• Undergo a CBC every month for 1 yr after the maintenance dose is established and every 3 mos thereafter
• Avoid tasks that require mental alertness or motor skills until response to the drug is established; drowsiness usually diminishes with continued therapy
• Notify the physician if fever, swollen glands, sore throat, a skin reaction, or signs of hematologic toxicity (such as a bleeding tendency, bruising, fatigue, or fever) occurs
• Avoid alcohol while taking phenytoin

MONITORING PARAMETERS

• Therapeutic range 10-20 mcg/ml; nystagmus appears at 20 mcg/ml, ataxia at 30 mcg/ml, dysarthria and lethargy at levels above 40 mcg/ml; lethal dose 2-5 g
• Blood pressure (with IV use), CBC, and renal and hepatic function
• Be alert for signs of IV phenytoin toxicity, such as cardiovascular collapse and CNS depression
• Signs of clinical improvement, such as a decrease in the frequency or intensity of seizures

phosphorated carbohydrate solution

Rx: Emetrol
Chemical Class: Hyperosmolar carbohydrate with phosphoric acid
Therapeutic Class: Antiemetic

CLINICAL PHARMACOLOGY

Mechanism of Action: An antiemetic whose mechanism of action has not been determined. Phosphorated carbohydrate solution consists of fructose, dextrose, and phosphoric acid, and may directly act on the wall of the gastrointestinal (GI) tract and reduce smooth muscle contraction and delays gastric emptying time through high osmotic pressure exerted by the solution of simple sugars. ***Therapeutic Effect:*** Relieves nausea and vomiting.

Pharmacokinetics

Fructose Fructose is slowly absorbed from the GI tract. Metabolized in liver by phosphorylation and partly converted to liver glycogen and glucose. Excreted in urine.
Dextrose: Dextrose is rapidly absorbed from GI tract. Distributed and stored throughout tissues. Metabolized in liver to carbon dioxide and water.

INDICATIONS AND DOSAGES

Antiemetic

PO

Adults, Elderly. 15-30 ml initially. May repeat dose every 15 mins until distress subsides. Maximum: 5 doses in a 1-hr period
Children 3 yrs and older. 5-15 ml initially. May repeat dose every 15 mins until distress subsides. Maximum: 5 doses in a 1-hr period

P

AVAILABLE FORMS

• *Solution:* 1.87 g fructose/1.87 g dextrose/21.5 mg phosphoric acid/5 ml (Emetrol).

CONTRAINDICATIONS: Symptoms of appendicitis or inflamed bowel, hereditary fructose intolerance, hypersensitivity to any component of the formulation

PREGNANCY AND LACTATION: Pregnancy category NR

SIDE EFFECTS

Frequent

Diarrhea, abdominal pain

SERIOUS REACTIONS

• Fructose intolerance includes symptoms of fainting; swelling of face, arms, and legs; unusual bleeding; vomiting; weight loss; and yellow eyes and skin.

SPECIAL CONSIDERATIONS

PATIENT/FAMILY EDUCATION

• Seek medical attention if symptoms are not relieved or recur frequently

• Notify the physician if headache or persistent vomiting occurs

MONITORING PARAMETERS

• Bowel sounds for peristalsis; pattern of daily bowel activity and stool consistency

---

physostigmine

(fi-zoe-stig'-meen)

Rx: Antilirium

Chemical Class: Alkaloid; cholinesterase inhibitor; tertiary ammonium compound

Therapeutic Class: Antiglaucoma agent; cholinergic; miotic; ophthalmic cholinergic

---

CLINICAL PHARMACOLOGY

Mechanism of Action: A cholinergic that inhibits destruction of acetylcholine by enzyme acetylcholinesterase, thus enhancing impulse transmission across the myoneural junction. ***Therapeutic Effect:*** Improves skeletal muscle tone, stimulates salivary and sweat gland secretions.

Pharmacokinetics

Penetrates blood-brain barrier. Rapidly hydrolyzed by cholinesterases. Small amount eliminated in urine; largely destroyed in body by hydrolysis. ***Half-life:*** Unknown.

INDICATIONS AND DOSAGES

To reverse CNS effects of anticholinergic drugs and tricyclic antidepressants

IV, IM

Adults, Elderly. Initially, 0.5-2 mg. If no response, repeat q20min until response or adverse cholinergic effects occur. If initial response occurs, may give additional doses of 1-4 mg q30-60min as life-threatening signs, such as arrhythmias, seizures, and deep coma, recur.

Children. 0.01-0.03 mg/kg. May give additional doses q5-10min until response or adverse cholinergic effects occur or total dose of 2 mg given.

AVAILABLE FORMS

• *Injection:* 1 mg/ml.

UNLABELED USES: Treatment of hereditary ataxia

CONTRAINDICATIONS: Active uveal inflammation, angle-closure glaucoma before iridectomy, asthma, cardiovascular disease, concurrent use of ganglionic-blocking agents, diabetes, gangrene, glaucoma associated with iridocyclitis, hypersensitivity to cholinesterase inhibitors or their components, mechanical obstruction of intestinal or urogenital tract, vagotonic state

PREGNANCY AND LACTATION: Pregnancy category C; no data on breast-feeding available

SIDE EFFECTS

Expected

Miosis, increased GI and skeletal muscle tone, bradycardia

Occasional

Marked drop in BP (hypertensive patients)

Rare

Allergic reaction

SERIOUS REACTIONS

• Parenteral overdose produces a cholinergic crisis manifested as abdominal discomfort or cramps, nausea, vomiting, diarrhea, flushing, facial warmth, excessive salivation, diaphoresis, urinary urgency, and blurred vision. If overdose occurs, stop all anticholinergic drugs and immediately and administer 0.6-1.2 mg atropine sulfate IM or IV for adults, or 0.01 mg/kg for infants and children younger than 12 yrs.

INTERACTIONS

Drugs

3 *β-blockers:* Additive bradycardia

3 *Cholinesterase agents, including bethanechol and carbachol:* May increase the effects of these drugs

3 *Succinylcholine:* May prolong the action of succinylcholine

SPECIAL CONSIDERATIONS

• Atropine is antidote

PATIENT/FAMILY EDUCATION

• The drug's adverse effects usually subside after the first few days of therapy

• Avoid driving at night and activities requiring visual acuity in dim light during physostigmine therapy

MONITORING PARAMETERS

• Vital signs immediately before and every 15-30 mins after physostigmine administration

• Monitor the patient for cholinergic reactions, such as abdominal pain, dyspnea, hypotension, arrhythmias, muscle weakness, and diaphoresis, after drug administration

phytonadione (vitamin K_1)

(fye-toe-na-dye'one)

Rx: AquaMEPHYTON, Mephyton, Vitamin K_1

Chemical Class: Naphthoquinone derivative

Therapeutic Class: Antihemorrhagic; vitamin

CLINICAL PHARMACOLOGY

Mechanism of Action: A fat-soluble vitamin that promotes hepatic formation of coagulation factors II, VII, IX, and X. ***Therapeutic Effect:*** Essential for normal clotting of blood.

Pharmacokinetics

Readily absorbed from the GI tract (duodenum) after IM or subcutaneous administration. Metabolized in the liver. Excreted in urine; eliminated by biliary system. ***Onset of action:*** with PO form, 6-10 hr; with parenteral form, hemorrhage controlled in 3-6 hr and PT returns to normal in 12-14 hr.

INDICATIONS AND DOSAGES

Oral anticoagulant overdose

PO, IV, Subcutaneous

Adults, Elderly. 2.5-10 mg/dose. May repeat in 12-48 hr if given orally and in 6-8 hr if given by IV or subcutaneous route.

Children. 0.5-5 mg depending on need for further anticoagulation and severity of bleeding.

Vitamin K deficiency

PO

Adults, Elderly. 2.5-25 mg/24 hr.

Children. 2.5-5 mg/24 hr.

IV, IM, Subcutaneous
Adults, Elderly. 10 mg/dose.
Children. 1-2 mg/dose.
Hemorrhagic disease of newborn
IM, Subcutaneous
Neonate. Treatment: 1-2 mg/dose/day. Prophylaxis: 0.5-1 mg within 1 hr of birth; may repeat in 6-8 hr if necessary.

AVAILABLE FORMS
- *Tablets (Mephyton):* 5 mg.
- *Injection (AquaMEPHYTON, Vitamin K_1):* 1 mg/0.5 ml, 10 mg/ml.

CONTRAINDICATIONS: None known.

PREGNANCY AND LACTATION: Pregnancy category C; oral supplementation of women on anticonvulsants during last 2 wks of pregnancy has been done to prevent HDN, but effectiveness unproven; compatible with breast-feeding

SIDE EFFECTS
Occasional
Pain, soreness, and swelling at IM injection site; pruritic erythema (with repeated injections); facial flushing; unusual taste

SERIOUS REACTIONS
- Newborns (especially premature infants) may develop hyperbilirubinemia.
- A severe reaction (cramp-like pain, chest pain, dyspnea, facial flushing, dizziness, rapid or weak pulse, rash, diaphoresis, hypotension progressing to shock, cardiac arrest) occurs rarely just after IV administration.

INTERACTIONS
Drugs
3 *Oral anticoagulants:* Decreased anticoagulant effect

SPECIAL CONSIDERATIONS
- IV doses should be diluted and infused slowly over 20-30 min

PATIENT/FAMILY EDUCATION
- Avoid taking any other medications, including OTC preparations, without the physician's approval because they may interfere with platelet aggregation
- Use an electric razor and soft toothbrush to prevent bleeding
- Consuming foods high in vitamin K, including milk, egg yolks, leafy green vegetables, meat, tomatoes, and vegetable oil, is encouraged
- Notify the physician of abdominal or back pain, severe headache, black or red stool, coffee-ground vomitus, red or dark urine, or red-speckled mucus from a cough

MONITORING PARAMETERS
- PT and international normalized ration, Hct, platelet count
- Stool and urine specimens for occult blood

pilocarpine hydrochloride

(pye-loe-kar′-peen hye-droe-klor′-ide)

Rx: Adsorbocarpine, Akarpine, Isopto Carpine, Ocu-Carpine, Ocusert, Pilagan with C Cap, Pilocar, Pilopine-HS, Piloptic-HS, Piloptic-1, Piloptic-1/2, Piloptic-2, Piloptic-3, Piloptic-4, Piloptic-6, Pilostat

Combinations

Rx: with epinephrine (E-Pilo-6)

Chemical Class: Choline ester

Therapeutic Class: Antiglaucoma agent; miotic; ophthalmic cholinergic; salivation stimulant

CLINICAL PHARMACOLOGY

Mechanism of Action: A cholinergic parasympathomimetic that increases exocrine gland secretions by stimulating cholinergic receptors. Acts through direct stimulation of muscarinic neuroreceptors and smooth muscles such as the iris and secretory glands. Contracts the iris sphincter, causing increased tension on the scleral spur and opening of the trabecular mesh work spaces to facilitate outflow of aqueous humor. ***Therapeutic Effect:*** Improves symptoms of dry mouth in patients with salivary gland hypofunction. Produces miosis. Lowers intraocular pressure (IOP).

Pharmacokinetics

Route	*Onset*	*Peak*	*Duration*
PO	20 mins	1 hr	3-5 hrs
Ophthalmic	10-30 mins	75 mins-2 hrs	4-14 hrs

Absorption decreased if taken with a high-fat meal. Inactivation of pilocarpine thought to occur at neuronal synapses and probably in plasma. Excreted in urine. ***Half-life:*** 4-12 hr.

INDICATIONS AND DOSAGES

Dry mouth associated with radiation treatment for head and neck cancer

PO

Adults, Elderly. 5 mg three times a day. Range: 15-30 mg/day. Maximum: 2 tablets/dose.

Dry mouth associated with Sjögren's syndrome

PO

Adults, Elderly. 5 mg four times a day. Range: 20-40 mg/day.

Glaucoma

Ophthalmic

Adults, Elderly. 1-2 drops to affected eye(s) up to 4 times a day.

Miosis induction

Ophthalmic

Adults, Elderly. 1-2 drops to affected eye(s) up to 4 times a day.

Dosage in hepatic impairment

Dosage decreased to 5 mg twice a day for adults and elderly with hepatic impairment.

AVAILABLE FORMS

- *Tablets (Salagen):* 5 mg.
- *Ophthalmic Gel (Pilopine-HS):* 4%.
- *Ophthalmic Solution:* 0.25% (Isopto Carpine), 0.5% (Ocu-Carpine, Pilostat, Piloptic-1/2, Pilocar), 1% (Ocu-Carpine, Pilocar, Piloptic-1, Pilostat), 2% (Akarpine, Ocu-Carpine, Pilocar, Piloptic-2), 3% (Ocu-Carpine, Pilocar, Piloptic-3, Pilostat), 4% (Akarpine, Isopto-Carpine, Ocu-Carpine, Pilocar, Piloptic-4, Pilostat), 5% (Isopto Carpine, Ocu-Carpine), 6% (Isopto Carpine, Ocu-Carpine, Pilocar, Piloptic-6, Pilostat), 8% (Isopto Carpine).

• *Ophthalmic Solution, Nitrate (Pilagan with C Cap):* 1%, 4%.

CONTRAINDICATIONS: Conditions in which miosis is undesirable, such as acute iritis and angle-closure glaucoma; uncontrolled asthma

PREGNANCY AND LACTATION: Pregnancy category C

SIDE EFFECTS

Frequent

Oral: Diaphoresis

Ophthalmic: Stinging, burning

Occasional

Oral: Headache, dizziness, urinary frequency, flushing, dyspepsia, nausea, asthenia, lacrimation, visual disturbances

Ophthalmic: Blurred vision, itching of eye

Rare

Oral: Diarrhea, abdominal pain, peripheral edema, chills

Ophthalmic: Lens opacity

SERIOUS REACTIONS

• Patients with diaphoresis who do not drink enough fluids may develop dehydration.

• Retinal detachment has been reported.

INTERACTIONS

Drugs

3 *Anticholinergics:* May antagonize the effects of anticholinergics

3 *β-blockers:* May produce conduction disturbances

SPECIAL CONSIDERATIONS

• Antidote is atropine

PATIENT/FAMILY EDUCATION

• Miotics cause poor dark adaptation; use caution with night driving

• Drink plenty of fluids

• Avoid tasks that require mental alertness or motor skills until response to the drug has been established

MONITORING PARAMETERS

• Pattern of daily bowel activity and stool consistency

• Urinary frequency

• Monitor for signs of dehydration, such as decreased skin turgor, and dizziness

pimecrolimus

(pim-e-kroe'-li-mus)

Rx: Elidel

Chemical Class: Ascomycin derivative

Therapeutic Class: Immunosuppressant

CLINICAL PHARMACOLOGY

Mechanism of Action: An immunomodulator that inhibits release of cytokine, an enzyme that produces an inflammatory reaction. ***Therapeutic Effect:*** Produces antiinflammatory activity.

Pharmacokinetics

Minimal systemic absorption with topical application. Metabolized in liver. Excreted in feces.

INDICATIONS AND DOSAGES

Atopic dermatitis (eczema)

Topical

Adults, Elderly, Children 2-17 yrs. Apply to affected area twice daily for up to 3 wks (up to 6 wks in adolescents, children 2-17 yrs). Rub in gently and completely.

AVAILABLE FORMS

• *Cream:* 1% (Elidel).

UNLABELED USES: Allergic contact dermatitis, irritant contact dermatitis, psoriasis

CONTRAINDICATIONS: Hypersensitivity to pimecrolimus or any component of the formulation, Netherton's syndrome (potential for increased systemic absorption), application to active cutaneous viral infections.

PREGNANCY AND LACTATION: Pregnancy category C; excretion into breast milk unknown; use caution in nursing mothers

SIDE EFFECTS

Rare

Transient application-site sensation of burning or feeling of heat

SERIOUS REACTIONS

• Lymphadenopathy and phototoxicity occur rarely.

INTERACTIONS

Drugs

3 *Erythromycin, itraconazole, ketoconazole, fluconazole, calcium channel blockers, cimetidine:* Theoretic increase in pimecrolimus concentrations

SPECIAL CONSIDERATIONS

• May be associated with increased risk of varicella-zoster virus infection, herpes simplex virus infection, or eczema herpeticum

PATIENT/FAMILY EDUCATION

• Do not use with occlusive dressings

• Wash hands after application

• Minimize exposure to artificial sunlight or tanning beds

MONITORING PARAMETERS

• Therapeutic response

---

pimozide

(pi'-moe-zide)

Rx: Orap

Chemical Class: Diphenylbutylpiperidine derivative

Therapeutic Class: Antipsychotic

CLINICAL PHARMACOLOGY

Mechanism of Action: A diphenylbutylpiperidine that blocks dopamine at postsynaptic receptor sites in the brain. ***Therapeutic Effect:*** Suppresses behavioral response in psychosis.

INDICATIONS AND DOSAGES

Tourette syndrome

PO

Adults, Elderly. 1-2 mg/day in divided doses 3 times/day. Maximum: 10 mg/day.

Children older than 12 yrs. Initially, 0.5 mg/kg/day. Maximum: 10 mg/day.

AVAILABLE FORMS

• *Tablets:* 1 mg, 2 mg (Orap).

CONTRAINDICATIONS: Aggressive schizophrenics when sedation is required; concurrent administration of pemoline, methylphenidate or amphetamines; concurrent administration with dofetilide, sotalol, quinidine, other Class IA and III antiarrhythmics, mesoridazine, thioridazine, chlorpromazine, droperidol, sparfloxacin, gatifloxacin, moxifloxacin, halofantrine, mefloquine, pentamidine, arsenic trioxide, levomethadyl acetate, dolasetron mesylate, probucol, tacrolimus, ziprasidone, sertraline, macrolide antibiotics, drugs that cause QT prolongation, and less potent inhibitors of CYP3A; congenital or drug-induced long QT syndrome; doses greater than 10 mg daily/day; history of cardiac arrhythmias; Parkinson's disease; patients with known hypokalemia or hypomagnesemia; severe central nervous system depression; simple tics or tics not associated with Tourette's syndrome; hypersensitivity to pimozide or any of its components

PREGNANCY AND LACTATION: Pregnancy category C

SIDE EFFECTS

Occasional

Akathisia, dystonic extrapyramidal effects, parkinsonian extrapyramidal effects, tardive dyskinesia, blurred vision, ocular changes, constipation, decreased sweating, dry mouth, nasal congestion, dizziness, drowsiness, orthostatic hypotension, urinary retention, somnolence

Rare

Rash, cholestatic jaundice, priapism

SERIOUS REACTIONS

• Serious reactions such as blood dyscrasias, agranulocytosis, leukocytopenia, thrombocytopenia, cholestatic jaundice, neuroleptic malignant syndrome (NMS), constipation or paralytic ileus, priapism, QT prolongation and torsades de pointes, seizure, systemic lupus erythematosus-like syndrome, and temperature regulation dysfunction (heatstroke or hypothermia) occur rarely.

• Abrupt withdrawal following long-term therapy may precipitate nausea, vomiting, gastritis, dizziness, and tremors.

INTERACTIONS

Drugs

3 *Anticholinergics (benztropine, trihexyphenidyl):* Antagonistic pharmacodynamic effects; excessive anticholinergic effects

2 *Azole antifungals (itraconazole, ketoconazole):* QT prolongation

3 *Bromocriptine:* Antagonistic pharmacodynamic effects

3 *Carbamazepine:* Decreased antipsychotic drug concentrations; decreased therapeutic response

3 *Clonidine:* Exaggerated hypotension

3 *Fluoxetine:* Increased risk of extrapyramidal symptoms

3 *Indomethacin:* Exaggerated side effects: drowsiness, tiredness, confusion

2 *Levodopa:* Antagonistic effects on the antiparkinsonian effects

3 *Lithium:* Reduced serum concentrations of both drugs; neurotoxic reactions reported in manic patients (delirium, seizures, encephalopathy, extrapyramidal symptoms)

3 *Macrolide antibiotics (clarithromycin, erythrmycin, azithromycin, dirithromycin):* QT prolongation

3 *Meperidine:* Excessive hypotension and CNS depression

3 *Paroxetine:* Increased risk of extrapyramidal symptoms

3 *Phenobarbital:* Reduced pimozide concentrations; increased risk of hyperthermia associated with phenobarbital withdrawal

3 *Protease inhibitors (ritonavir, saquinavir, indinivir, nelfinavir):* QT prolongation

3 *Quinidine:* Increased pimozide concentrations and risk or subsequent toxicity

▲ *Sertraline:* Increases pimozide plasma concentrations; elevated pimozide concentrations can be life-threatening

▲ *Thioridazine:* Produces additive prolongation of the QT interval; may increase the risk of ventricular arrhythmias

3 *Trazodone:* Additive hypotension

2 *Verapamil:* Elevated pimozide concentrations and cardiac arrhythmias may occur

2 *Ziprasidone:* Prolong the QT interval; may increase the risk of ventricular arrhythmias

SPECIAL CONSIDERATIONS

PATIENT/FAMILY EDUCATION

• Notify the physician if fast or irregular heartbeat, fast breathing, fever, sever muscle stiffness, muscle spasms, twitching, or uncontrolled tongue or jaw movement occurs

• Do not abruptly discontinue the drug after long-term therapy

• Drowsiness usually subsides during continued therapy

• Avoid alcohol

MONITORING PARAMETERS

• EKG

• Blood pressure

pindolol

(pin′-doe-loll)

Rx: Visken

Chemical Class: β-adrenergic blocker, nonselective

Therapeutic Class: Antianginal; antihypertensive

CLINICAL PHARMACOLOGY

Mechanism of Action: A nonselective beta blocker that blocks $beta_1$- and $beta_2$-adrenergic receptors. ***Therapeutic Effect:*** Slows heart rate, decreases cardiac output, decreases blood pressure (BP), and exhibits antiarrhythmic activity. Decreases myocardial ischemia severity by decreasing oxygen requirements.

Pharmacokinetics

Completely absorbed from GI tract. Metabolized in liver. Primarily excreted in urine. ***Half-life:*** 3-4 hrs (half-life increased with impaired renal function, elderly).

INDICATIONS AND DOSAGES

Mild to moderate hypertension

PO

Adults. Initially, 5 mg 2 times/day. Gradually increase dose by 10 mg/day at 2-4-wk intervals. Maintenance: 10-30 mg/day in 2-3 divided doses. Maximum: 60 mg/day.

Usual elderly dosage:

PO

Initially, 5 mg/day. May increase by 5 mg q3-4wks.

AVAILABLE FORMS

• *Capsules:* 5 mg, 10 mg (Visken).

UNLABELED USES: Treatment of chronic angina pectoris, hypertrophic cardiomyopathy, tremors, and mitral valve prolapse syndrome. Increases antidepressant effect with fluoxetine and other SSRIs.

CONTRAINDICATIONS: Bronchial asthma, COPD, uncontrolled cardiac failure, sinus bradycardia, heart block greater than first degree, cardiogenic shock, CHF, unless secondary to tachyarrhythmias

PREGNANCY AND LACTATION: Pregnancy category B; similar drug, atenolol, frequently used in the third trimester for treatment of hypertension (many studies of efficacy and safety of atenolol in pregnancy-induced hypertension); long-term use has been associated with intrauterine growth retardation; enters breast milk in measurable amounts; observe for signs of β-blockade

SIDE EFFECTS

Frequent

Decreased sexual ability, drowsiness, trouble sleeping, unusual tiredness/weakness

Occasional

Bradycardia, depression, cold hands/feet, diarrhea, constipation, anxiety, nasal congestion, nausea, vomiting

Rare

Altered taste, dry eyes, itching, numbness of fingers, toes, and scalp

SERIOUS REACTIONS

• Overdosage may produce profound bradycardia and hypotension.

• Abrupt withdrawal may result in sweating, palpitations, headache, and tremulousness.

• May precipitate congestive heart failure (CHF) or myocardial infarction (MI) in patients with heart disease; thyroid storm in those with thyrotoxicosis; or peripheral ischemia in those with existing peripheral vascular disease.

• Hypoglycemia may occur in previously controlled diabetics.

• Signs of thrombocytopenia, such as unusual bleeding or bruising, occur rarely.

INTERACTIONS

Drugs

3 *Adenosine:* Bradycardia aggravated

3 *Amiodarone:* Additive prolongation of atrioventricular (AV) conduction time; symptomatic bradycardia and sinus arrest

3 *Antacids:* Reduced pindolol absorption

3 *Calcium channel blockers:* See dihydropyridine calcium channel blockers and verapamil

3 *Cimetidine:* Renal clearance reduced; AUC increased with cimetidine coadministration

3 *Clonidine, guanabenz, guanfacine:* Exacerbation of rebound hypertension upon discontinuation of clonidine

3 *Cocaine:* Cocaine-induced vasoconstriction potentiated; reduced coronary blood flow

3 *Contrast media:* Increased risk of anaphylaxis

3 *Digitalis:* Enhances bradycardia:

3 *Digoxin:* Additive prolongation of atrioventricular (AV) conduction time

3 *Dihydropyridine calcium channel blockers:* Additive pharmacodynamic effects:

3 *Disopyramide:* Additive decreases in cardiac output

3 *Dipyridamole:* Bradycardia aggravated

3 *Diltiazem:* Potentiates pharmacologic effects of β-adrenergic blocker; hypotension, left ventricular failure, and AV conduction disturbances reported; more likely in the elderly and in patients with left ventricular dysfunction, aortic stenosis, or large doses

3 *Epinephrine, isoproterenol, phenylephrine:* Potentiates pressor response; resultant hypertension and bradycardia

3 *Flecainide:* Additive negative inotropic effects

3 *Fluoxetine:* Increased β-blockade activity

3 *Fluoroquinolones:* Reduced clearance of pindolol

3 *Insulin:* Altered response to hypoglycemia; increased blood glucose concentrations; impair peripheral circulation

3 *Lidocaine:* Increased serum lidocaine concentrations possible

3 *Neostigmine:* Bradycardia aggravated

3 *Neuroleptics:* Both drugs inhibit each other's metabolism; additive hypotension

3 *NSAIDs:* Reduced antihypertensive effect of pindolol

3 *Physostigmine:* Bradycardia aggravated

3 *Prazosin:* First-dose response to prazosin may be enhanced by β-blockade

3 *Prazosin, terazosin, doxazosin:* Potential enhanced first-dose response (marked initial drop in blood pressure), particularly on standing (especially prazosin)

3 *Tacrine:* Bradycardia aggravated

❷ *Terbutaline:* Antagonized bronchodilating effects of terbutaline

❷ *Theophylline:* Antagonistic pharmacodynamic effects

3 *Verapamil:* Enhanced effects of both drugs, particularly AV nodal conduction slowing; reduced pindolol clearance

Labs

- *Alkaline phosphatase:* Increased serum levels
- *Aspartate aminotransferase:* Decreased serum levels
- *Bilirubin:* Decreased serum level
- *Creatine kinase:* Decreased serum level

SPECIAL CONSIDERATIONS

- Abrupt discontinuation may precipitate angina; taper over 1-2 wk
- Effective antihypertensive and probably antianginal agent (though not approved for this indication), especially for patients who develop symptomatic bradycardia with β-blockade

PATIENT/FAMILY EDUCATION

- Do not abruptly discontinue the drug
- Report excessive fatigue, headache, prolonged dizziness, shortness of breath, or weight gain
- Avoid nasal decongestants or OTC cold preparations (stimulants) without physician approval
- Avoid salt and alcohol intake

MONITORING PARAMETERS

- *Angina:* Reduction in nitroglycerin usage; frequency, severity, onset, and duration of angina pain; heart rate
- *Hypertension:* Blood pressure
- *Toxicity:* Blood glucose, bronchospasm, hypotension, bradycardia, depression, confusion, hallucination, sexual dysfunction

pioglitazone hydrochloride

(pye-oh-gli'-ta-zone hye-droe-klor'-ide)

Rx: Actos

Chemical Class: Thiazolidinedione

Therapeutic Class: Antidiabetic; hypoglycemic; insulin resistance reducer

CLINICAL PHARMACOLOGY

Mechanism of Action: An antidiabetic that improves target-cell response to insulin without increasing pancreatic insulin secretion. Decreases hepatic glucose output and increases insulin-dependent glucose utilization in skeletal muscle. ***Therapeutic Effect:*** Lowers blood glucose concentration.

Pharmacokinetics

Rapidly absorbed. Highly protein bound (99%), primarily to albumin. Metabolized in the liver. Excreted in urine. Unknown if removed by hemodialysis. ***Half-life:*** 16-24 hr.

INDICATIONS AND DOSAGES

Diabetes mellitus, combination therapy

PO

Adults, Elderly. With insulin: Initially, 15-30 mg once a day. Initially, continue current insulin dosage; then decrease insulin dosage by 10%-25% if hypoglycemia occurs or plasma glucose level decreases to less than 100 mg/dl. Maximum: 45 mg/day. With sulfonylureas: Initially, 15-30 mg/day. Decrease sulfonylurea dosage if hypoglycemia occurs. With metformin: Initially, 15-30 mg/day. As monotherapy: Monotherapy is not to be used if patient is well controlled with diet and exercise alone. Initially, 15-30 mg/day. May increase dosage in increments until 45 mg/day is reached.

AVAILABLE FORMS

- *Tablets:* 15 mg, 30 mg, 45 mg.

CONTRAINDICATIONS: Active hepatic disease; diabetic ketoacidosis; increased serum transaminase levels, including ALT greater than 2.5 times normal serum level; type 1 diabetes mellitus

PREGNANCY AND LACTATION: Pregnancy category C; abnormally high glucose levels during pregnancy associated with higher incidence of congenital anomalies, morbidity, and mortality; insulin monotherapy or sulfonylurea preferred agents; breast milk excretion unknown

SIDE EFFECTS

Frequent (13%-9%)

Headache, upper respiratory tract infection

Occasional (6%-5%)

Sinusitis, myalgia, pharyngitis, aggravated diabetes mellitus

SERIOUS REACTIONS

• Hepatotoxicity occurs rarely.

INTERACTIONS

Drugs

3 *Combination oral contraceptives:* May reduce estrogen and progestin levels (another thiazolidinedione reduced both hormones 30%)

3 *Fenugreek, ginseng, glucomannan, guar gum:* Pharmacodynamic interaction as both pioglitazone and listed natural products both possess hypoglycemic effects

3 *Gemfibrozil:* May increase the effects and toxicity of pioglitazone

3 *Ketoconazole:* May significantly inhibit metabolism of pioglitazone

Labs

• Possible elevations of AST, ALT, bilirubin, LDH; increases in LDL cholesterol (15%) and HDL cholesterol (15%); decreased in hematocrit, hemoglobin; decreased alkaline phosphatase

SPECIAL CONSIDERATIONS

• Expected hypoglycemic effects: Decreases in serum glucose: 50-75 mg/dL; decreases in hemoglobin A1c: 1.2%-1.5%

PATIENT/FAMILY EDUCATION

• Caloric restriction, weight loss, and exercise are essential adjuvant therapy

• Blood draws for LFT monitoring along with routine diabetes mellitus labs. Review symptoms of hepatitis (unexplained nausea, vomiting, abdominal pain, fatigue, anorexia, or dark urine)

• Notify clinician for rapid increases in weight or edema or symptoms of heart failure (shortness of breath, nocturia)

• Review hypoglycemia risks and symptoms when added to other hypoglycemic agents

• Avoid alcohol

• The prescribed diet is a principal part of treatment

MONITORING PARAMETERS

• Diabetes mellitus symptoms, periodic serum glucose and HbA1c measurements; LFT (AST, ALT) prior to initiation of therapy and periodically thereafter; hemoglobin/hematocrit, signs and symptoms of heart failure

---

piperacillin sodium/tazobactam sodium

(pi-per'-a-sill-in; pi-per'-a-sill-in/ta-zoe-bak'-tam)

Rx: *Piperacillin:* Pipracil

Rx: *Piperacillin/tazobactam:* Zosyn

Chemical Class: Penicillin derivative, extended-spectrum; β-lactamase inhibitor (tazobactam)

Therapeutic Class: Antibiotic

CLINICAL PHARMACOLOGY

Mechanism of Action: Piperacillin inhibits cell wall synthesis by binding to bacterial cell membranes. Tazobactam inactivates bacterial beta-lactamase. ***Therapeutic Effect:*** Piperacillin is bactericidal in susceptible organisms. Tazobactam protects piperacillin from enzymatic degradation, extends its spectrum of activity, and prevents bacterial overgrowth.

Pharmacokinetics

Protein binding: 16%-30%. Widely distributed. Primarily excreted unchanged in urine. Removed by hemodialysis. ***Half-life:*** 0.7-1.2 hr (increased in hepatic cirrhosis and impaired renal function).

INDICATIONS AND DOSAGES

Severe infections

IV

Adults, Elderly, Children 12 yr and older. 4 g/0.5 g q8h or 3 g/0.375 g q6h. Maximum: 18 g/2.25 g daily.

Moderate infections

IV

Adults, Elderly, Children 12 yr and older. 2 g/0.225 g q6-8h.

Dosage in renal impairment

Dosage and frequency are modified based on creatinine clearance.

Creatinine Clearance	*Dosage*
20-40 ml/min	8 g/1 g/day (2.25 g q6h)
less than 20 ml/min	6 g/0.75 g/day (2.25 g q8h)

Dosage in hemodialysis patients

IV

Adults, Elderly. 2.25 g q8h with additional dose of 0.75 g after each dialysis session.

AVAILABLE FORMS

• **Alert:** Piperacillin/tazobactam is a combination product in an 8:1 ratio of piperacillin to tazobactam.

• *Powder for Injection:* 2.25 g, 3.375 g, 4.5 g.

• *Premix Ready to Use:* 2.25 g, 3.375 g, 4.5 g.

CONTRAINDICATIONS: Hypersensitivity to any penicillin, cephalosporins, or beta-lactamase inhibitors

PREGNANCY AND LACTATION: Pregnancy category B; excreted in breast milk in small concentrations

SIDE EFFECTS

Frequent

Diarrhea, headache, constipation, nausea, insomnia, rash

Occasional

Vomiting, dyspepsia, pruritus, fever, agitation, candidiasis, dizziness, abdominal pain, edema, anxiety, dyspnea, rhinitis

SERIOUS REACTIONS

• Antibiotic-associated colitis and other superinfections may result from altered bacterial balance.

• Seizures and other neurologic reactions are more likely to occur in patients with renal impairment and those who have received an overdose.

• Severe hypersensitivity reactions, including anaphylaxis, occur rarely.

INTERACTIONS

Drugs

3 *Aminoglycosides:* Carbenicillin and other piperacillins can inactivate aminoglycosides in vitro and in certain patients with renal dysfunction

3 *Chloramphenicol:* Inhibited antibacterial activity of piperacillin; administer piperacillin 3 hr before chloramphenicol

3 *Macrolide antibiotics:* Inhibited antibacterial activity of piperacillin; administer piperacillin 3 hr before macrolides

3 *Methotrexate:* Piperacillin in large doses may increase serum methotrexate concentrations

3 *Oral contraceptives:* Occasional impairment of oral contraceptive efficacy; consider use of supplemental contraception during cycles in which piperacillin is used

3 *Probenecid:* May increase piperacillin blood concentration and risk of toxicity

3 *Tetracyclines:* Inhibited antibacterial activity of piperacillin; administer piperacillin 3 hr before tetracyclines

Labs

- *Cephalothin:* False positive serum
- *Penicillin G:* False positive serum
- *Protein:* False positive urine

SPECIAL CONSIDERATIONS

- Preferred over mezlocillin, more effective against *Pseudomonas,* reserve for carbenicillin- or ticarcillin-resistant *P. aeruginosa* infections in combination with an aminoglycoside

PATIENT/FAMILY EDUCATION

- Notify the physician if severe diarrhea occurs and avoid taking antidiarrheals until directed to do so
- Notify the physician if pain, redness, or swelling occurs at the infusion site
- Reduce salt intake because piperacillin contains sodium

MONITORING PARAMETERS

- Electrolyte levels (especially potassium), intake and output, renal function test results, and urinalysis results
- Pattern of daily bowel activity and stool consistency; mild GI effects may be tolerable, but severe symptoms may indicate the onset of antibiotic-associated colitis
- Be alert for signs and symptoms of superinfection, including abdominal pain, moderate to severe diarrhea, severe anal or genital pruritus, and stomatitis

pirbuterol acetate

(peer-byoo'-ter-ole ass'-eh-tayte)

Rx: Maxair, Maxair Autohaler

Chemical Class: Sympathomimetic amine; β_2-adrenergic agonist

Therapeutic Class: Antiasthmatic; bronchodilator

CLINICAL PHARMACOLOGY

Mechanism of Action: A sympathomimetic, adrenergic agonist that stimulates beta$_2$-adrenergic receptors in the lungs, resulting in relaxation of bronchial smooth muscle. ***Therapeutic Effect:*** Relieves bronchospasm, reduces airway resistance.

Pharmacokinetics

Absorbed from bronchi following inhalation. Metabolized in liver. Primarily excreted in urine. Unknown if removed by hemodialysis. ***Half-life:*** 2-3 hrs.

INDICATIONS AND DOSAGES

Prevention of bronchospasm

Inhalation

Adults, Elderly, Children 12 yrs and older. 2 inhalations q4-6h. Maximum: 12 inhalations daily.

Treatment of bronchospasm

Inhalation

Adults, Elderly, Children 12 yrs and older. 2 inhalations separated by at least 1-3 mins, followed by a third inhalation. Maximum: 12 inhalations daily.

AVAILABLE FORMS

- *Oral Inhalation:* 0.2 mg/actuation (Autohaler).

CONTRAINDICATIONS: History of hypersensitivity to pirbuterol, albuterol, or any of its components

PREGNANCY AND LACTATION: Pregnancy category C

SIDE EFFECTS

Occasional (7%-1%)

Nervousness, tremor, headache, palpitations, nausea, dizziness, tachycardia, cough

SERIOUS REACTIONS

• Excessive sympathomimetic stimulation may produce palpitations, extrasystoles, tachycardia, chest pain, slight increases in BP followed by a substantial decrease, chills, sweating, and blanching of skin.

• Too-frequent or excessive use may lead to loss of bronchodilating effectiveness and severe, paradoxical bronchoconstriction.

INTERACTIONS

Drugs

❷ *β-blockers:* Decreased action of pirbuterol, cardioselective agents preferable if concurrent use necessary

❸ *Furosemide:* Potential for additive hypokalemia

❸ *MAOIs, tricyclic antidepressants:* May potentiate cardiovascular effects

SPECIAL CONSIDERATIONS

• No significant advantage over other selective β_2-agonists

PATIENT/FAMILY EDUCATION

• Initial and periodic reviews of metered dose inhaler technique

• Increase fluid intake to decrease the viscosity of pulmonary secretions

• Rinse mouth immediately after inhalation to prevent mouth and throat dryness

• Avoid excessive use of caffeine derivatives, such as chocolate, cocoa, coffee, cola, and tea

MONITORING PARAMETERS

• Depth, rate, rhythm, and type of respirations

• Quality and rate of pulse

piroxicam

(peer-ox′-i-kam)

Rx: Feldene

Chemical Class: Oxicam derivative

Therapeutic Class: NSAID; antipyretic; nonnarcotic analgesic

CLINICAL PHARMACOLOGY

Mechanism of Action: An NSAID that produces analgesic and antiinflammatory effects by inhibiting prostaglandin synthesis. ***Therapeutic Effect:*** Reduces inflammatory response and intensity of pain.

Pharmacokinetics

Well absorbed following oral administration. Protein binding: 99%. Extensively metabolized in liver. Primarily excreted in urine; small amount eliminated in feces. ***Half-life:*** 50 hr.

INDICATIONS AND DOSAGES

Acute or chronic rheumatoid arthritis and osteoarthritis

PO

Adults, Elderly. Initially, 10-20 mg/day as a single dose or in divided doses. Some patients may require up to 30-40 mg/day.

Children. 0.2-0.3 mg/kg/day. Maximum: 15 mg/day.

AVAILABLE FORMS

• *Capsules:* 10 mg, 20 mg.

UNLABELED USES: Treatment of acute gouty arthritis, ankylosing spondylitis, dysmenorrhea

CONTRAINDICATIONS: Active peptic ulcer disease, chronic inflammation of the GI tract, GI bleeding or ulceration, history of hypersensitivity to aspirin or NSAIDs

PREGNANCY AND LACTATION: Pregnancy category C (D if used in third trimester or near delivery); excreted into breast milk; approximately 1% of mother's serum levels; should not present a risk to nursing infant

SIDE EFFECTS

Frequent (9%-4%)

Dyspepsia, nausea, dizziness

Occasional (3%-1%)

Diarrhea, constipation, abdominal cramps or pain, flatulence, stomatitis

Rare (less than 1%)

Hypertension, urticaria, dysuria, ecchymosis, blurred vision, insomnia, phototoxicity

SERIOUS REACTIONS

• Rare reactions with long-term use include peptic ulcer disease, GI bleeding, gastritis, severe hepatic reaction (cholestasis, jaundice), nephrotoxicity (dysuria, hematuria, proteinuria, nephrotic syndrome), hematologic sensitivity (anemia, leukopenia, eosinophilia, thrombocytopenia), and a severe hypersensitivity reaction (fever, chills, bronchospasm).

INTERACTIONS

Drugs

3 *Aminoglycosides:* Reduced clearance with elevated aminoglycoside levels and potential for toxicity (especially indomethacin in premature infants; other NSAIDs probably)

3 *Anticoagulants:* Excessive hypoprothrombinemia, decreased platelet aggregation with increased risk of GI bleeding

3 *Antihypertensives (α-blockers, angiotensin-converting enzyme inhibitors, angiotensin II receptor blockers, β-blockers, diuretics):* Inhibition of antihypertensive and other favorable hemodynamic effects

3 *Aspirin, other salicylates:* May increase the risk of GI side effects

3 *Bone marrow depressants:* May increase the risk of hematologic reactions

3 *Corticosteroids:* Increased risk of GI ulceration

3 *Cyclosporine:* Increased nephrotoxicity risk

3 *Lithium:* Decreased clearance of lithium (mediated via prostaglandins) resulting in elevated serum lithium levels and risk of toxicity

3 *Methotrexate:* Decreased renal secretion of methotrexate resulting in elevated methotrexate levels and risk of toxicity

3 *Phenylpropanolamine:* Possible acute hypertensive reaction

3 *Potassium-sparing diuretics:* Additive hyperkalemia potential

3 *Probenecid:* May increase the piroxicam blood concentration

3 *Triamterene:* Acute renal failure reported with addition of indomethacin; caution with other NSAIDs

SPECIAL CONSIDERATIONS

• Similar in efficacy to the other NSAIDs but has the advantage and disadvantage of an extended $t_{1/2}$; high GI toxicity potential

PATIENT/FAMILY EDUCATION

• Take piroxicam with food, milk, or antacids if GI upset occurs

• Avoid tasks that require mental alertness or motor skills until response to the drug has been established

• Avoid alcohol and aspirin during piroxicam therapy because these substances increase the risk of GI bleeding

• The female patient should inform the physician if she is or plans to become pregnant

MONITORING PARAMETERS

• Initial hemogram and fecal occult blood test within 3 mo of starting regular chronic therapy; repeat every 6-12 mo (more frequently in high-risk patients [>65 years, pep-

tic ulcer disease, concurrent steroids or anticoagulants]); electrolytes, creatinine, and BUN within 3 mo of starting regular chronic therapy; repeat every 6-12 mo
• Therapeutic response, such as improved grip strength, increased joint mobility, and decreased pain, tenderness, stiffness, and swelling
• Pattern of daily bowel activity and stool consistency

plicamycin

(plye-ka-mye'-sin)
Rx: Mithracin
Chemical Class: Crystalline aglycone
Therapeutic Class: Antihypercalcemic; antineoplastic

CLINICAL PHARMACOLOGY
Mechanism of Action: An antibiotic that forms complexes with DNA, inhibiting DNA-directed RNA synthesis. May inhibit parathyroid hormone effect on osteoclasts and inhibit bone resorption. ***Therapeutic Effect:*** Lowers serum calcium and phosphate levels. Blocks hypercalcemic action of vitamin D and action of parathyroid hormone. Decreases serum calcium.
Pharmacokinetics

Route	Onset	Peak	Duration
IV	1-2 days	2-3 days	3-15 days

Protein binding: none. Greatest concentrations in liver, kidney, and formed bone surfaces. Crosses the blood-brain barrier and enters CSF. Primarily excreted in urine.

INDICATIONS AND DOSAGES
Testicular tumors
IV
Adults, Elderly. 25-30 mcg/kg/day for 8-10 days. Repeat at monthly intervals.
Hypercalcemia, hyperuricemia
IV
Adults, Elderly. 25 mcg/kg as a single dose; may repeat in 48 hr if no response occurs. Or give 25 mcg/kg/day for 3-4 days or 25-50 mcg/kg/dose every other day for 3-8 doses.
Paget's disease
IV
Adults, Elderly. 15 mcg/kg/day for 10 days.

AVAILABLE FORMS
• *Powder for Injection:* 2500 mcg.

UNLABELED USES: Treatment of Paget's disease refractory to other therapy

CONTRAINDICATIONS: Preexisting coagulation disorders, thrombocytopathy, thrombocytopenia, impaired bone marrow function, or tendency to hemorrhage

PREGNANCY AND LACTATION: Pregnancy category X

SIDE EFFECTS
Frequent
Nausea, vomiting, anorexia, diarrhea, stomatitis
Occasional
Fever, drowsiness, weakness, lethargy, malaise, headache, depression, nervousness, dizziness, rash, acne

SERIOUS REACTIONS
• The risk of hematologic toxicity (characterized by marked facial flushing, persistent nosebleeds, hemoptysis, purpura, ecchymosis, leukopenia, and thrombocytopenia) increases with administration of high dosages or more than 10 doses.
• Electrolyte imbalances may occur.

INTERACTIONS
Drugs
3 *Bisphosphonates, calcitonin, foscarnet, glucagon:* Additive hypocalcemic effect

3 *Bone marrow depressants, hepatotoxic, nephrotoxic medications:* May increase toxicity

3 *Live-virus vaccines:* May potentiate virus replication, increase vaccine side effects, and decrease patient's antibody response to the vaccine

3 *NSAIDs, aspirin, dipyridamole, sulfinpyrazone, valproic acid:* May increase the risk of hemorrhage

3 *Oral anticoagulants, heparin, thrombolytics:* May increase the effects of these drugs

SPECIAL CONSIDERATIONS

- Effective but also toxic; use is therefore limited; additive with other calcium-lowering therapies

PATIENT/FAMILY EDUCATION

- Maintain fastidious oral hygiene
- Do not have immunizations without physician's approval (drug lowers body's resistance)
- Avoid crowds, those with infection
- Promptly report fever, sore throat, signs of local infection, easy bruising, and unusual bleeding from any site
- Contact physician if nausea/vomiting continues at home
- Use nonhormonal contraception

MONITORING PARAMETERS

- CBC, differential, platelet count qwk; withhold drug if WBC is $<4000/mm^3$ or platelet count is $<50,000/mm^3$
- Renal function studies: BUN, serum uric acid, urine CrCl, electrolytes, input and output ratio
- Liver function tests: bilirubin, AST, ALT, alk phosphatase before and during therapy
- Monitor for stomatitis (burning/erythema of oral mucosa at inner margin of lips, sore throat, difficulty swallowing, oral ulceration)
- Monitor for thrombocytopenia (bleeding from gums, tarry stool, petechiae, small subcutaneous hemorrhages)

podofilox

(po-doe-fil'-ox)

Rx: Condylox

Chemical Class: Podophyllum derivative

Therapeutic Class: Keratolytic

CLINICAL PHARMACOLOGY

Mechanism of Action: An active component of podophyllin resin that binds to tubulin to prevent formation of microtubules, resulting in mitotic arrest. Exercises many biologic effects, such as damages endothelium of small blood vessels, attenuates nucleoside transport, suppresses immune responses, inhibits macrophage metabolism, induces interleukin-1 and interleukin-2, decreases lymphocytes response to mitogens, and enhances macrophage growth. ***Therapeutic Effect:*** Removes genital warts.

Pharmacokinetics

Time to peak occurs in 1-2 hrs. Some degree of absorption. ***Half-life:*** 1-4.5 hrs.

INDICATIONS AND DOSAGES

Anogenital warts

Topical

Adults. Apply 0.5% gel for 3 days, then withhold for 4 days. Repeat cycle up to 4 times.

Genital warts (condylomata acuminate)

Topical

Adults. Apply 0.5% solution or gel q12h in the morning and evening for 3 days, then withhold for 4 days. Repeat cycle up to 4 times.

AVAILABLE FORMS
• *Gel:* 0.5% (Condylox).
• *Solution:* 0.5% (Condylox).
UNLABELED USES: Systemic: Treatment of fungal pneumonia, prostate cancer, septicemia
CONTRAINDICATIONS: Bleeding warts, moles, birthmarks or unusual warts with hair, diabetes, poor blood circulation, pregnancy, steroid use, hypersensitivity to podofilox or any component of its formulation
PREGNANCY AND LACTATION: Pregnancy category C
SIDE EFFECTS
Occasional
Erosion, inflammation, itching, pain, burning
Rare
Nausea, vomiting
SERIOUS REACTIONS
• Nausea and vomiting occur rarely and usually after cumulative doses.
SPECIAL CONSIDERATIONS
• Safety preferred over podophyllum resin
PATIENT/FAMILY EDUCATION
• Use a small amount of solution on the warts with a dry cotton-tipped swab
MONITORING PARAMETERS
• Skin for burning, itching, and irritation

podophyllum resin

(pode-oh-fill'-um rez'-in)
Rx: Podocon-25, Pododerm
Chemical Class: Podophyllum derivative
Therapeutic Class: Keratolytic

CLINICAL PHARMACOLOGY
Mechanism of Action: A cytotoxic agent that directly affects epithelial cell metabolism by arresting mitosis through binding to a protein subunit of spindle microtubules. ***Therapeutic Effect:*** Removes soft genital warts.
Pharmacokinetics
Topical podophyllum is systemically absorbed. Absorption may be increased if applied to bleeding, friable, or recently biopsied warts.
INDICATIONS AND DOSAGES
Genital warts (condylomata acuminate)
Topical
Adults, Elderly, Children. Apply 10%-25% solution in compound benzoin tincture to dry surface. Use 1 drop at a time allowing drying between drops until area is covered. Total volume should be limited to less than 0.5 ml per treatment session.
AVAILABLE FORMS
• *Liquid:* 25% (Podocon-25, Pododerm).
UNLABELED USES: Epitheliomatosis, laryngeal papilloma
CONTRAINDICATIONS: Diabetes mellitus, concomitant steroids therapy, circulation disorders, bleeding warts, moles, birthmarks or unusual warts with hair growing from them, pregnancy, hypersensitivity to podophyllum resin preparations
PREGNANCY AND LACTATION: Pregnancy category X; excretion into breast milk unknown; use caution in nursing mothers
SIDE EFFECTS
Occasional (10%-1%)
Pruritus, nausea, vomiting, abdominal pain, diarrhea
SERIOUS REACTIONS
• Paresthesia, polyneuritis, paralytic ileus, pyrexia, leukopenia, thrombocytopenia, coma, and death have been reported with podophyllum resin use.
SPECIAL CONSIDERATIONS
• Not to be dispensed to the patient, professional application only

• Because of the potential for toxicity, cryotherapy should be attempted first or podofilox substituted

PATIENT/FAMILY EDUCATION

• Avoid contact with eyes
• Notify the physician if painful urination, dizziness, lightheadedness, increased heart rate, constipation, or tingling in hands or feet occurs

MONITORING PARAMETERS

• Electrolytes, serum calcium
• Hgb concentrations

polymyxin B sulfate

(polly-mix-in B sul'-fate)

Rx: Aerosporin

Combinations

Rx: *Ophth:* with bacitracin (Polysporin); with dexamethasone, neomycin (Dexacidin, Maxitrol); with hydrocortisone, neomycin (Cortisporin); with neomycin, bacitracin (Neosporin, Ocutricin); with neomycin, gramicidin (Neosporin); with oxytetracycline (Terak); with prednisolone, neomycin (Poly-Pred); with trimethoprim (Polytrim)
Topical: with bacitracin, hydrocortisone, neomycin (Cortisporin); with dexamethasone, neomycin (Dioptrol, Maxitrol); with hydrocortisone, neomycin (Cortisporin)

OTC: *Topical:* with bacitracin (Bacimyxin, Polysporin); with bacitracin, neomycin (Neosporin, Triple Antibiotic); with bacitracin, neomycin, lidocaine (Lanabiotic, Spectrocin); with gramicidin (Polysporin); with gramicidin, lidocaine (Lidosporin, Polysporin Burn Formula); with gramicidin, neomycin (Neosporin)

Chemical Class: Polymyxin derivative
Therapeutic Class: Antibiotic; ophthalmic antibiotic

CLINICAL PHARMACOLOGY

Mechanism of Action: An antibiotic that alters cell membrane permeability in susceptible microorganisms. ***Therapeutic Effect:*** Bactericidal activity.

Pharmacokinetics
Negligible absorption. Protein binding: low. Excreted in urine. Poor removal in hemodialysis. ***Half-life:*** 6 hrs.

INDICATIONS AND DOSAGES

Mild to moderate infections

IV

Adults, Elderly, Children 2 yrs and older. 15,000-25,000 units/kg/day in divided doses q12h.

Infants. Up to 40,000 units/kg/day.

IM

Adults, Elderly, Children 2 yrs and older. 25,000-30,000 units/kg/day in divided doses q4-6h.

Infants. Up to 40,000 units/kg/day.

Usual irrigation dosage

Continuous bladder irrigation

Adults, Elderly. 1 ml urogenital concentrate (contains 200,000 units polymyxin B, 57 mg neomycin) added to 1000 ml 0.9% NaCl. Give each 1000 ml >24 hrs for up to 10 days (may increase to 2000 ml/day when urine output >2 L/day).

Usual ophthalmic dosage

Ophthalmic

Adults, Elderly, Children. 1 drop q3-4h.

AVAILABLE FORMS

- *Powder:* 500,000 (Aerosporin).

CONTRAINDICATIONS: Hypersensitivity to polymyxin B or any component of the formulation

PREGNANCY AND LACTATION: Pregnancy category B

SIDE EFFECTS

Frequent

Severe pain, irritation at IM injection sites, phlebitis, thrombophlebitis with IV administration

Occasional

Fever, urticaria

SERIOUS REACTIONS

- Nephrotoxicity, especially with concurrent/sequential use of other nephrotoxic drugs, renal impairment, concurrent/sequential use of muscle relaxants.
- Superinfection, especially with fungi, may occur.

INTERACTIONS

Drugs

❷ *Anesthetics, neuromuscular blockers (e.g., gallamine, pancuronium, succinylcholine, tubocurarine):* Increased skeletal muscle relaxation

SPECIAL CONSIDERATIONS

- Generally replaced by the aminoglycosides or extended-spectrum penicillins for serious infections; still used for bladder irrigation and gut decontamination; used in combination with other antibiotics and/or corticosteroids topically to treat infections of the eye and skin

PATIENT/FAMILY EDUCATION

- Continue for the full length of treatment
- Space doses evenly
- Discomfort may occur at IM injection site
- Report any increased irritation, inflammation, itching, or burning with ophthalmic therapy

MONITORING PARAMETERS

- Intake and output, BUN, creatinine, urinalysis

polythiazide

(poly-thi'-a-zide)

Rx: Renese

Combinations

Rx: with prazosin (Minizide); with reserpine (Renese-R)

Chemical Class: Sulfonamide derivative

Therapeutic Class: Antihypertensive; diuretic, thiazide

CLINICAL PHARMACOLOGY

Mechanism of Action: A sulfonamide derivative that acts as a thiaz-

P

ide diuretic and antihypertensive. As a diuretic blocks reabsorption of water, sodium and potassium at cortical diluting segment of distal tubule. As an antihypertensive it reduces plasma and extracellular fluid volume and decreases peripheral vascular resistance (PVR) by direct effect on blood vessels. ***Therapeutic Effect:*** Promotes diuresis, reduces blood pressure (BP).

Pharmacokinetics

Rapidly absorbed from the gastrointestinal (GI) tract. Primarily excreted unchanged in urine. Not removed by hemodialysis. ***Half-life:*** 25.7 hrs.

INDICATIONS AND DOSAGES

Edema

PO

Adults. 1-4 mg/day.

Hypertension

PO

Adults. 2-4 mg/day.

AVAILABLE FORMS

• *Tablets:* 1 mg, 2 mg, 4 mg (Renese).

UNLABELED USES: Prevention of calcium-containing renal stones

CONTRAINDICATIONS: Anuria, history of hypersensitivity to sulfonamides or thiazide diuretics, renal decompensation

PREGNANCY AND LACTATION: Pregnancy category D; therapy for preexisting hypertension can be continued throughout pregnancy with minimal risk; initiating for simple edema not recommended; few unequivocal indications for diuretic therapy in pregnancy except for pulmonary edema or congestive heart failure; excreted in breast milk in low concentrations; compatible with breast-feeding

SIDE EFFECTS

Expected

Increase in urine frequency and volume

Frequent

Potassium depletion

Occasional

Postural hypotension, headache, GI disturbances, photosensitivity reaction

SERIOUS REACTIONS

• Vigorous diuresis may lead to profound water loss and electrolyte depletion, resulting in hypokalemia, hyponatremia, and dehydration.

• Acute hypotensive episodes may occur.

• Hyperglycemia may be noted during prolonged therapy.

• GI upset, pancreatitis, dizziness, paresthesias, headache, blood dyscrasias, pulmonary edema, allergic pneumonitis, and dermatologic reactions occur rarely.

• Overdosage can lead to lethargy and coma without changes in electrolytes or hydration.

INTERACTIONS

Drugs

❷ *Angiotensin-converting enzyme inhibitors:* Risk of postural hypotension when added to ongoing diuretic therapy; more common with loop diuretics; first-dose hypotension possible in patients with sodium depletion or hypovolemia due to diuretics or sodium restriction; hypotensive response is usually transient; hold diuretic day of first dose

❸ *Calcium:* With large doses can result in milk-alkali syndrome

❸ *Carbenoxolone:* Additive potassium wasting; severe hypokalemia

❸ *Cholestyramine, colestipol:* Reduced absorption

❸ *Corticosteroids:* Concomitant therapy may result in excessive potassium loss

❸ *Diazoxide:* Hyperglycemia

❸ *Digitalis glycosides:* Diuretic-induced hypokalemia increases risk of digitalis toxicity

3 *Hypoglycemic agents:* Increased dosage requirements due to increased glucose levels
3 *Lithium:* Increased lithium levels, potential toxicity
3 *Methotrexate:* Additive bone marrow suppression
3 *Nonsteroidal antiinflammatory drugs:* Concurrent use may reduce diuretic and antihypertensive effects

Labs

• *False decrease:* Urine estriol

SPECIAL CONSIDERATIONS

• Doses above 1 mg provide no further blood pressure reduction, but are more likely to induce metabolic disturbance (i.e., hypokalemia, hyperuricemia)

• May protect against osteoporotic hip fractures

• Loop diuretics or metolazone more effective if CrCl <40-50 ml/min

PATIENT/FAMILY EDUCATION

• Will increase urination temporarily (approx. 3 wk); take early in the day to prevent sleep disturbance

• May cause sensitivity to sunlight; avoid prolonged exposure to the sun and other ultraviolet light

• May cause gout attacks; notify clinician if sudden joint pain occurs

• Rise slowly from lying to sitting position and permit legs to dangle momentarily before standing to reduce the drug's hypotensive effect

MONITORING PARAMETERS

• Weight, urine output, serum electrolytes, BUN, creatinine, CBC, uric acid, glucose, lipids

• Blood pressure

poractant alfa

(poor-ak'-tant)
Rx: Curosurf
Chemical Class: Phospholipid
Therapeutic Class: Lung surfactant, porcine

CLINICAL PHARMACOLOGY

Mechanism of Action: A pulmonary surfactant that reduces alveolar surface tension during ventilation and stabilizes the alveoli against collapse that may occur at resting transpulmonary pressures. ***Therapeutic Effect:*** Improves lung compliance and respiratory gas exchange.

Pharmacokinetics

The pharmacokinetics of poractant alfa are not fully understood.

INDICATIONS AND DOSAGES

Respiratory distress syndrome (RDS)

Intratracheal

Infants. Initially, 2.5 ml/kg of birth weight. May give up to 2 subsequent doses of 1.25 ml/kg of birth weight at 12-hr intervals. Maximum: 5 ml/kg (total dose).

AVAILABLE FORMS

• *Intratracheal Suspension:* 1.5 ml (120 mg), 3 ml (240 mg).

UNLABELED USES: Adult RDS due to viral pneumonia or near-drowning, *Pneumocystis carinii* pneumonia in HIV-infected patients, prevention of RDS

CONTRAINDICATIONS: None known.

PREGNANCY AND LACTATION: This drug is not indicated for use in pregnant women.

SIDE EFFECTS

Frequent

Transient bradycardia, oxygen (O_2) desaturation, increased carbon dioxide (CO_2) retention

Occasional
Endotracheal tube reflux
Rare
Hypotension or hypertension, pallor, vasoconstriction
SERIOUS REACTIONS
- Desaturation of blood, blocked endotracheal tube, apnea occur rarely.

SPECIAL CONSIDERATIONS
PATIENT/FAMILY EDUCATION
- Tell the parents the purpose of the treatment and the expected outcome

MONITORING PARAMETERS
- Continuous ECG and transcutaneous O_2 saturation; pCO_2; lung compliance; respiratory rate
- Heart rate
- Limit visitors during treatment, and monitor for hand washing and other infection control measures to minimize the risk of nosocomial infections

potassium salts

(poe-tass'-i-um)
Rx: (potassium bicarbonate-citrate) Effer K, Klor-Con EF, K-Lyte, K-Lyte DS
Rx: (potassium chloride) Cena K, Ed K+10, K+Care, K-8, K-10, Kaochlor, Kaon-Cl, Kaon-CL 10, Kaon-CL 20%, Kato, Kay Ciel, KCl-20, KCl-40, K-Dur, K-Dur 10, K-Dur 20, K-Lor, K-Lor-Con M 15, Klor-Con, Klor-Con 8, Klor-Con 10, Klor-Con/25, Klor-Con M10, Klor-Con M15, Klor-Con M20, Klotrix, K-Norm, K-Sol, K-Tab, Kaon-Cl, Micro-K, Micro-K 10, Rum-K
Rx: (potassium gluconate) Kaon
Chemical Class: Monovalent cation
Therapeutic Class: Electrolyte supplement

CLINICAL PHARMACOLOGY
Mechanism of Action: An electrolyte that is necessary for multiple cellular metabolic processes. Primary action is intracellular. ***Therapeutic Effect:*** Needed for nerve impulse conduction and contraction of cardiac, skeletal, and smooth muscle; maintains normal renal function and acid-base balance.
Pharmacokinetics
Well absorbed from the GI tract. Enters cells by active transport from extracellular fluid. Primarily excreted in urine.
INDICATIONS AND DOSAGES
Prevention of hypokalemia (in patients on diuretic therapy)
PO
Adults, Elderly. 20-40 mEq/day in 1-2 divided doses.

Children. 1-2 mEq/kg/day in 1-2 divided doses.

Treatment of hypokalemia

PO

Adults, Elderly. 40-80 mEq/day; further doses based on laboratory values.

Children. 2-5 mEq/day; further doses based on laboratory values.

IV

Adults, Elderly. 5-10 mEq/hr. Maximum: 400 mEq/day.

Children. 1 mEq/kg over 1-2 hr.

AVAILABLE FORMS

Potassium Acetate

• *Injection:* 2 mEq/ml.

Potassium Bicarbonate and Potassium Citrate

• *Tablets for Solution:* 25 mEq (Klor-Con EF, Effer-K, K-Lyte), 50 mEq (K-Lyte DS).

Potassium Chloride

• *Capsules (Controlled-Release [Micro-K]):* 8 mEq, 10 mEq.

• *Liquid:* 20 mEq/15 ml (Kaochlor), 40 mEq/15 ml (Kaon-Cl).

• *Powder for Oral Solution (K-Lor):* 20 mEq.

Powder for Reconstitution (K+Care): 20 mEq.

• *Injection:* 2 mEq/ml.

• *Tablets (Extended-Release):* 8 mEq (K-8, Klor-Con, Klor-Con 8, Klor-Con M10, Micro-K, Micro-K10), 10 mEq (K-8, Kaon-CL, Kaon-CL 10, K-Dur, Klor-Con, Klor-Con 8, Klor-Con M10,Klotrix, K-Tab, Micro-K, Micro-K 10), 20 mEq (K-Dur).

Potassium Gluconate

• *Elixir (Kaon):* 20 mEq/15 ml.

CONTRAINDICATIONS: Concurrent use of potassium-sparing diuretics, digitalis toxicity, heat cramps, hyperkalemia, postoperative oliguria, severe burns, severe renal impairment, shock with dehydration or hemolytic reaction, untreated Addison's disease

PREGNANCY AND LACTATION: Pregnancy category: C (A for potassium chloride)

SIDE EFFECTS

Occasional

Nausea, vomiting, diarrhea, flatulence, abdominal discomfort with distention, phlebitis with IV administration (particularly when potassium concentration of greater than 40 mEq/L is infused)

Rare

Rash

SERIOUS REACTIONS

• Hyperkalemia (more common in elderly patients and those with impaired renal function) may be manifested as paresthesia, feeling of heaviness in the lower extremities, cold skin, grayish pallor, hypotension, confusion, irritability, flaccid paralysis, and cardiac arrhythmias.

INTERACTIONS

Drugs

3 *ACE inhibitors:* Hyperkalemia

3 *Anticholinergics:* May increase the risk of GI lesions

3 *Disopyramide:* Increased potassium concentrations can enhance disopyramide effects

3 *Hypoglycemics:* Correction of hypokalemia may result in hypoglycemia

❷ *Potassium-sparing diuretics:* Hyperkalemia

❷ *Spironolactone:* Hyperkalemia

SPECIAL CONSIDERATIONS

• Avoid use of compressed tablets or enteric-coated tablets (i.e., non–sustained-release or effervescent tablets for sol) due to significant ulcerogenic tendency and propensity to cause significant local tissue destruction

• Sol, powder, and oral susp: dilute or dissove in 120 ml cold water or juice

P

• Extended release caps and tabs: do not crush; take with food; swallow with full glass of liquid
• Injectable potassium products must be diluted prior to administration; direct inj of potassium concentrate may be fatal
• Central line preferable for IV infusions concentrated >40 mEq/L

PATIENT/FAMILY EDUCATION

• List of foods rich in potassium, including apricots, avocados, bananas, beans, beef, broccoli, brussel sprouts, cantaloupe, chicken, dates, fish, ham, lentils, milk, molasses, potatoes, prunes, raisins, spinach, turkey, watermelon, veal, and yams
• Notify the physician if a feeling of heaviness in the lower extremities and paresthesia occurs

MONITORING PARAMETERS

• ECG monitoring advisable for IV infusion rate >10 mEq/hr
• Normal serum potassium level 3.5-5.0 mEq/L (higher, to 7.7 mEq/L in neonates)
• Intake and output diligently for diuresis; be alert for decreased urine output, which may be an indication of renal insufficiency
• Pattern of daily bowel activity and stool consistency
• Be alert for signs and symptoms of hyperkalemia, including cold skin, feeling of heaviness in lower extremities, paresthesia, and skin pallor

pralidoxime chloride

(pra-li-dox'-eem klor'-ide)

Rx: Protopam Chloride
Chemical Class: Quaternary ammonium derivative
Therapeutic Class: Antidote, anticholinesterase

CLINICAL PHARMACOLOGY

Mechanism of Action: Reactivates cholinesterase activity by 2-formyl-1-methylpyridinium ion. ***Therapeutic Effect:*** Restores cholinesterase activity following organophosphate anticholinesterase poisoning.

Pharmacokinetics

Onset of activity is 1 hr and duration of action is short, which may require readministration. Not protein bound. Excreted in urine. ***Half-life:*** 1.2-2.6 hrs.

INDICATIONS AND DOSAGES

Anticholinesterase overdosage

IV

Adults, Elderly. 1-2 g initially, followed by increments of 250 mg q5min until response is observed.

Organophosphate poisoning

IV

Adults, Elderly. 1-2 g initially in 100 ml 0.9 NaCl infused over 15-30 mins or 5% solution in sterile water for injection over not less than 5 mins. Repeat 1-2 g in 1 hr if muscle weakness persists.

Children. 25-50 mg/kg/dose. Repeat in 1-2 hrs if muscle weakness has not been relieved, then at 8-12-hrs intervals if cholinergic signs recur.

AVAILABLE FORMS

• *Injection, powder for reconstitution:* 1 g (Protopam Chloride).

CONTRAINDICATIONS: Use of aminophylline, morphine, therophylline and succinylcholine, hypersensitivity to pralidoxime or any of its components

PREGNANCY AND LACTATION: Pregnancy category C

SIDE EFFECTS

Occasional

Blurred vision, dizziness, headache, laryngospasm, hyperventilation, nausea, tachycardia, hypertension, pain at injection site

Rare

Rash, muscle rigidity, decreased renal function

SERIOUS REACTIONS

• Excessive doses may cause blurred vision, nausea, tachycardia and dizziness.

INTERACTIONS

Drugs

3 *Aminophylline, caffeine, theophylline, reserpine, phenothiazines:* May exacerbate the effects of organophosphate poisoning

3 *Atropine:* Atropinization (flushing, mydriasis, tachycardia, dryness of the mouth and nose) may occur

3 *Barbiturates:* May increase the effect of pralidoxime

3 *Succinylcholine:* May prolong respiratory paralysis

SPECIAL CONSIDERATIONS

PATIENT/FAMILY EDUCATIONs

• Avoid consuming an excessive amount of caffeine derivatives such as chocolate, cocoa, coffee, cola, or tea

• Immediately report any new symptoms such as weakness, dizziness, nausea, or tachycardia

MONITORING PARAMETERS

• CBC; plasma cholinesterase activity may help confirm diagnosis and follow course of illness

• Respiratory rate, heart rate

pramipexole dihydrochloride

(pra-mi-pex'-ole dye-hye-droe-klor'-ide)

Rx: Mirapex

Chemical Class: Benzothiazolamine derivative

Therapeutic Class: Anti-Parkinson's agent; dopaminergic

CLINICAL PHARMACOLOGY

Mechanism of Action: An antiparkinson agent that stimulates dopamine receptors in the striatum. ***Therapeutic Effect:*** Relieves signs and symptoms of Parkinson's disease.

Pharmacokinetics

Rapidly and extensively absorbed after PO administration. Protein binding: 15%. Widely distributed. Steady-state concentrations achieved within 2 days. Primarily eliminated in urine. Not removed by hemodialysis. ***Half-life:*** 8 hr (12 hr in patients older than 65 yr).

INDICATIONS AND DOSAGES

Parkinson's disease

PO

Adults, Elderly. Initially, 0.375 mg/day in 3 divided doses. Do not increase dosage more frequently than every 5-7 days. Maintenance: 1.5-4.5 mg/day in 3 equally divided doses.

Dosage in renal impairment

Dosage and frequency are modified based on creatinine clearance.

Creatinine Clearance	*Initial Dose*	*Maximum Dose*
Greater than 60 ml/min	0.125 mg 3 times a day	1.5 mg 3 times a day
35-59 ml/min	0.125 mg twice a day	1.5 mg twice a day
15-34 ml/min	0.125 mg once a day	1.5 mg once a day

AVAILABLE FORMS

• *Tablets:* 0.125 mg, 0.25 mg, 0.5 mg, 1 mg, 1.5 mg.

P

UNLABELED USES: Depression (due to bipolar disorder), fibromyalgia, restless legs syndrome

CONTRAINDICATIONS: History of hypersensitivity to pramipexole

PREGNANCY AND LACTATION: Pregnancy category C; inhibits prolactin secretion; excretion into breast milk unknown

SIDE EFFECTS

Frequent

Early Parkinson's disease (28%-10%): Nausea, asthenia, dizziness, somnolence, insomnia, constipation

Advanced Parkinson's disease (53%-17%): Orthostatic hypotension, extrapyramidal reactions, insomnia, dizziness, hallucinations

Occasional

Early Parkinson's disease (5%-2%): Edema, malaise, confusion, amnesia, akathisia, anorexia, dysphagia, peripheral edema, vision changes, impotence

Advanced Parkinson's disease (10%-7%): Asthenia, somnolence, confusion, constipation, abnormal gait, dry mouth

Rare

Advanced Parkinson's disease (6%-2%): General edema, malaise, chest pain, amnesia, tremor, urinary frequency or incontinence, dyspnea, rhinitis, vision changes

SERIOUS REACTIONS

• Vascular disease, MI, angina pectoris, atrial fibrillation, heart failure, arrhythmia, atrial arrhythmia, and pulmonary embolism have been reported.

INTERACTIONS

Drugs

3 *Cimetidine:* 50% increase in pramipexole AUC and 40% increase in $t_{1/2}$

3 *Diltiazem, quinidine, quinine, ranitidine, triamterene, verapamil:* May decrease pramipexole clearance

3 *Dopamine antagonists (phenothiazines, butyrophenones, thioxanthenes, metoclopropamide):* May diminish effectiveness of pramipexole

3 *Levodopa:* 40% increase in levodopa concentrations

SPECIAL CONSIDERATIONS

• At least as effective as bromocriptine in the treatment of advanced parkinsonian patients with levodopa-related motor fluctuations; adverse effects similar in incidence and severity; appears to lack some of the toxicity seen with bromocriptine, pergolide, and cabergoline (e.g., pleuropulmonary disease); may be a useful alternative in patients with intolerable adverse effects due to ergot derivatives

PATIENT/FAMILY EDUCATION

• Take pramipexole with food if nausea is a problem

• Do not abruptly discontinue pramipexole

• The drug may cause hallucinations

• Orthostatic hypotension occurs more commonly during initial therapy

• Avoid tasks that require mental alertness or motor skills until response to the drug has been established

MONITORING PARAMETERS

• United Parkinson's Disease Rating Scale (UPDRS) useful for monitoring efficacy endpoints

• Relief of symptoms, such as improvement of masklike facial expression, muscular rigidity, shuffling gait, and resting tremors of the hands and head

• Assess for constipation

pramoxine hydrochloride

(pra-mox'-een hye-droe-klor'-ide)

Rx: Analpram-HC, Anusol, Enzone, Epifoam, Pramosome, Prax, Procotcream, Rectocort, Tronolane, Zone-A

Chemical Class: Morpholine derivative

Therapeutic Class: Anesthetic, topical

CLINICAL PHARMACOLOGY

Mechanism of Action: A surface or local anesthetic that is not chemically related to the "caine" types of local anesthetics. Decreases the neuronal membranes permeability to sodium ions, blocking both initiation and conduction of nerve impulses, therefore inhibiting depolarization of the neuron. ***Therapeutic Effect:*** Temporarily relieves pain and itching associated with anogenital pruritus or irritation.

Pharmacokinetics

Onset of action occurs within a few mins of application. Peak effect is reached in 3-5 mins. Duration is several days.

INDICATIONS AND DOSAGES

Anogenital pruritus or irritation, dermatosis, minor burns, hemorrhoids

Topical

Adults, Elderly: Apply to affected area 3 or 4 times daily.

AVAILABLE FORMS

- *Foam:* 1% (Proctofoam NS).
- *Cream:* 1% (Tranolane).
- *Gel:* 1% (Itch-X).
- *Lotion:* 1% (Prax).
- *Ointment:* 1% (Anusol).
- *Solution:* 1% (Itch-X).
- *Suppository:* 1% (Tronolane).

CONTRAINDICATIONS: Hypersensitivity to any component of the product.

PREGNANCY AND LACTATION: Pregnancy category C; excretion into breast milk unknown

SIDE EFFECTS

Occassional

Angioedema, contact dermatitis, burning, itching, irritation, stinging

Rare

Dryness, folliculitis, hypopigmentation, perioral dermatitis, maceration of the skin, secondary infection, skin atrophy, striae, miliaria

SERIOUS REACTIONS

- None known.

SPECIAL CONSIDERATIONS

- Cross-sensitization with other local anesthetics unlikely

PATIENT/FAMILY EDUCATION

- Do not use near eyes or nose
- Contact clinician if condition fails to improve after 3-4 days or worsens
- Do not apply to large areas
- Do not apply to unaffected areas
- Notify the physician if bleeding at affected area, hoarseness, hives, rash, severe itching, difficulty breathing or swallowing, or swelling of the face, throat, lips, eyes, hands, feet, or ankles occurs
- Wash hands before and after administration

MONITORING PARAMETERS

- Therapeutic response
- Skin for irritation

pravastatin

(pra'-va-stat-in soe'-dee-um)

Rx: Pravachol

Chemical Class: Substituted hexahydronaphthalene

Therapeutic Class: HMG-CoA reductase inhibitor; antilipemic

CLINICAL PHARMACOLOGY

Mechanism of Action: An HMG-CoA reductase inhibitor that interferes with cholesterol biosynthesis by preventing the conversion of HMG-CoA reductase to mevalonate, a precursor to cholesterol. ***Therapeutic Effect:*** Lowers serum LDL and VLDL cholesterol and plasma triglyceride levels; increases serum HDL concentration.

Pharmacokinetics

Poorly absorbed from the GI tract. Protein binding: 50%. Metabolized in the liver (minimal active metabolites). Primarily excreted in feces via the biliary system. Not removed by hemodialysis. ***Half-life:*** 2.7 hr.

INDICATIONS AND DOSAGES

Hyperlipidemia, primary and secondary prevention of cardiovascular events in patient with elevated cholesterol levels

PO

Adults, Elderly. Initially, 40 mg/day. Titrate to desired response. Range: 10-80 mg/day.

Children 14-18 yr. 40 mg/day.

Children 8-13 yr. 20 mg/day.

Dosage in hepatic and renal impairment

For adults, give 10 mg/day initially. Titrate to desired response.

AVAILABLE FORMS

• *Tablets:* 10 mg, 20 mg, 40 mg, 80 mg.

CONTRAINDICATIONS: Active hepatic disease or unexplained, persistent elevations of liver function test results

PREGNANCY AND LACTATION: Pregnancy category X; small amounts excreted in breast milk; should probably not be used by women who are nursing

SIDE EFFECTS

Pravastatin is generally well tolerated. Side effects are usually mild and transient.

Occasional (7%-4%)

Nausea, vomiting, diarrhea, constipation, abdominal pain, headache, rhinitis, rash, pruritus

Rare (3%-2%)

Heartburn, myalgia, dizziness, cough, fatigue, flu-like symptoms

SERIOUS REACTIONS

• Malignancy and cataracts may occur.

• Hypersensitivity occurs rarely.

• Myopathy and rhabdomyolysis have been reported.

INTERACTIONS

Drugs

❷ *Azole antifungals (fluconazole, itraconazole, ketoconazole, miconazole):* Increased plasma pravastatin levels via inhibition of metabolism with increased risk of rhabdomyolysis

❸ *Cholestyramine, colestipol:* Reduced bioavailability of pravastatin; give pravastatin 1 hr before or 4 hr following a bile acid sequestrant

❸ *Clarithromycin:* Increased plasma pravastain levels via inhibition of metabolism with increased risk of rhabdomyolysis

❷ *Clofibrate:* Small increased risk of myopathy with combination

❸ *Cyclosporine:* Concomitant administration increases risk of severe myopathy or rhabdomyolysis; if used together, initiate pravastatin at 10 mg qhs and titrate cautiously, usual max is 20 mg/day

3 *Danazol:* Increased plasma pravastatin levels via inhibition of metabolism with increased risk of rhabdomyolysis

3 *Erythromycin:* Increased pravastatin levels via inhibition of metabolism with increased risk of rhabdomyolysis

3 *Fluoxetine:* Increased pravastatin levels via inhibition of metabolism with increased risk of rhabdomyolysis

❷ *Gemfibrozil:* Small increased risk of myopathy with combination, especially at high doses of statin

3 *Isradipine:* May decrease pravastatin plasma concentrations

3 *Niacin:* Concomitant administration increases risk of severe myopathy or rhabdomyolysis

3 *Nefazodone:* May inhibit hepatic metabolism of pravastatin with risk of rhabdomyolysis

3 *Troleandomycin:* Increased pravastatin levels via inhibition of metabolism with increased risk of rhabdomyolysis

SPECIAL CONSIDERATIONS

- Statin selection based on lipid-lowering prowess, cost, and availability

PATIENT/FAMILY EDUCATION

- Avoid prolonged exposure to sunlight and other UV light
- Promptly report any unexplained muscle pain, tenderness, or weakness, especially if accompanied by fever or malaise
- Strictly adhere to low cholesterol diet
- Take daily doses in the evening for increased effect
- Periodic laboratory tests are an essential part of therapy
- Avoid tasks that require mental alertness or motor skills until response to the drug is established
- Women of childbearing years should use nonhormonal contraceptives while taking pravastatin; pravastatin is pregnancy risk category X

MONITORING PARAMETERS

- ALT and AST at baseline, and at 12 wks of therapy. If no change at 12 wks, no further monitoring necessary (discontinue if elevations persist at >3 times upper limit of normal)
- CPK in any patient complaining of diffuse myalgia, muscle tenderness, or weakness
- Fasting lipid profile
- Pattern of daily bowel activity and stool consistency
- Skin for rash
- Assess the patient for malaise and muscle cramping or weakness. If these conditions occur and are accompanied by fever, expect that pravastatin may be discontinued

praziquantel

(pray-zih-kwon′-tel)

Rx: Biltricide

Chemical Class: Pyrazinoisoquinoline derivative

Therapeutic Class: Antihelmintic

CLINICAL PHARMACOLOGY

Mechanism of Action: An antihelmintic that increases cell permeability in susceptible helminths, resulting in loss of intracellular calcium, massive contractions and paralysis of their musculature, followed by attachment of phagocytes to the parasites. ***Therapeutic Effect:*** Vermicidal. Dislodges the dead and dying worms.

Pharmacokinetics
Well absorbed from gastrointestinal (GI) tract. Protein binding: 80%. Widely distributed, including CSF. Metabolized in liver. Primarily excreted in urine. Not removed by hemodialysis. ***Half-life:*** 4-5 hrs.

INDICATIONS AND DOSAGES
Schistosomiasis
PO
Adults, Elderly. 3 doses of 20 mg/kg as 1-day treatment. Do not give doses less than 4 hrs or more than 6 hrs apart.
Clonorchiasis/opisthorchiasis
PO
Adults, Elderly. 3 doses of 25 mg/kg as 1-day treatment.

AVAILABLE FORMS
• *Tablets:* 600 mg (Biltricide).

CONTRAINDICATIONS: Ocular cysticercosis, hypersensitivity to praziquantel or any component of the formulation

PREGNANCY AND LACTATION: Pregnancy category B; do not nurse on day of treatment and during the subsequent 72 hr

SIDE EFFECTS
Frequent
Headache, dizziness, malaise, abdominal pain
Occasional
Anorexia, vomiting, diarrhea, severe cramping abdominal pain may occur within 1 hr of administration w/fever, sweating, bloody stools
Rare
Giddiness, urticaria

SERIOUS REACTIONS
• Overdose should be treated with fast-acting laxative.

INTERACTIONS
Drugs
3 *Chloroquine and hydroxychloroquine:* Reduces plasma level of praziquantel
3 *Cimetidine:* Increases plasma level of praziquantel
❷ *Rifampin:* Reduces praziquantel plasma concentrations; loss of therapeutic effect may occur

SPECIAL CONSIDERATIONS

PATIENT/FAMILY EDUCATION
• Swallow tablets unchewed with some liquid during meals
• May cause drowsiness
• Use caution driving or performing other tasks requiring alertness
• Take for the full course of therapy
• Notify the physician if symptoms do not improve in a few days

MONITORING PARAMETERS
• Collect stool and urine specimens to monitor effectiveness
• Check hematology results for anemia

---

prazosin hydrochloride
(pra'-zoe-sin hye-droe-klor'-ide)
Rx: Minipress
Combinations
Rx: with polythiazide (Minizide)
Chemical Class: Quinazoline derivative
Therapeutic Class: Antihypertensive; α_1-adrenergic blocker

CLINICAL PHARMACOLOGY
Mechanism of Action: An antidote, antihypertensive, and vasodilator that selectively blocks alpha$_1$-adrenergic receptors, decreasing peripheral vascular resistance. ***Therapeutic Effect:*** Produces vasodilation of veins and arterioles, decreases total peripheral resistance, and relaxes smooth muscle in bladder, neck, and prostate.

Pharmacokinetics
Well absorbed following oral administration. Protein binding: 92%-97%. Metabolized in liver. Primarily excreted in feces. ***Half-life:*** 2-4 hr.

INDICATIONS AND DOSAGES
Mild to moderate hypertension
PO
Adults, Elderly. Initially, 1 mg 2-3 times a day. Maintenance: 3-15 mg/day in divided doses. Maximum: 20 mg/day.
Children. 5 mcg/kg/dose q6h. Gradually increase up to 25 mcg/kg/dose.

AVAILABLE FORMS
- *Capsules:* 1 mg, 2 mg, 5 mg.

UNLABELED USES: Treatment of benign prostate hyperplasia, CHF, ergot alkaloid toxicity, pheochromocytoma, Raynaud's phenomenon

CONTRAINDICATIONS: Hypersensitivity to quinazolines

PREGNANCY AND LACTATION: Pregnancy category C

SIDE EFFECTS
Frequent (10%-7%)
Dizziness, somnolence, headache, asthenia (loss of strength, energy)
Occasional (5%-4%)
Palpitations, nausea, dry mouth, nervousness
Rare (less than 1%)
Angina, urinary urgency

SERIOUS REACTIONS
- First-dose syncope (hypotension with sudden loss of consciousness) may occur 30-90 minutes following initial dose of more than 2 mg, a too-rapid increase in dosage, or addition of another antihypertensive agent to therapy. First-dose syncope may be preceded by tachycardia (pulse rate of 120-160 beats/minute).

INTERACTIONS
Drugs
3 *ACE inhibitors:* Exaggerated first-dose response to prazosin
3 *β-adrenergic blockers:* Exaggerated first-dose response to prazosin
3 *Estrogen, other sympathomimetics:* May decrease the effects of prazosin
3 *Hypotension-producing medications, such as antihypertensives and diuretics:* May increase the effects of prazosin
3 *Licorice:* Causes sodium and water retention and potassium loss
3 *NSAIDs:* Inhibits antihypertensive response to prazosin
3 *Verapamil:* Reduces first-pass metabolism of prazosin
Labs
- False positive urinary metabolites of norepinephrine and VMA
- No effect on prostate specific antigen (PSA)

SPECIAL CONSIDERATIONS
- The doxazosin arm of the ALLHAT study was stopped early; the doxazosin group had a 25% greater risk of combined cardiovascular disease events, which was primarily accounted for by a doubled risk of CHF vs the chlorthalidone group; doxazosin was also found to be less effective at controlling systolic BP an average of 3 mm Hg; may want to consider primary antihypertensives in addition to α-blockers for BPH symptoms
- Use as single antihypertensive agent limited by tendency to cause sodium and water retention and increased plasma volume

PATIENT/FAMILY EDUCATION
- Alert patients to the possibility of syncopal and orthostatic symptoms, especially with the first dose ("first-dose syncope")

• Initial dose should be administered at bedtime in the smallest possible dose
• Avoid tasks that require mental alertness or motor skills until response to the drug is established
• Notify the physician if dizziness or palpitations become bothersome

MONITORING PARAMETERS

• Blood pressure, pulse
• Pattern of daily bowel activity and stool consistency

prednisolone

(pred-niss'-oh-lone)

Rx: AK-Pred, Cotolone, Depo-Predate, Hydeltrasol, Inflamase Forte, Inflamase Mild, Key-Pred, Key-Pred SP, Orapred, Pediapred, Predacort 50, Predaject-50, Predate-50, Pred Forte, Pred-Ject-50, Pred Mild, Prednisolone Acetate, Prelone

Chemical Class: Glucocorticoid, synthetic

Therapeutic Class: Corticosteroid, ophthalmic; corticosteroid, systemic

CLINICAL PHARMACOLOGY

Mechanism of Action: An adrenocortical steroid that inhibits accumulation of inflammatory cells at inflammation sites, phagocytosis, lysosomal enzyme release and synthesis, and release of mediators of inflammation. ***Therapeutic Effect:*** Prevents or suppresses cell-mediated immune reactions. Decreases or prevents tissue response to inflammatory process.

Pharmacokinetics

Well absorbed from the GI tract. Protein binding: 90%-95%. Widely distributed. Metabolized in the liver. Primarily excreted in urine. Not removed by hemodialysis. ***Half-life:*** 2.6-3 hr.

INDICATIONS AND DOSAGES

Substitution therapy for deficiency states: acute or chronic adrenal insufficiency, congenital adrenal hyperplasia, and adrenal insufficiency secondary to pituitary insufficiency; nonendocrine disorders: arthritis; rheumatic carditis; allergic, collagen, intestinal tract, liver, ocular, renal, skin diseases; bronchial asthma; cerebral edema; malignancies

PO

Adults, Elderly. 5-60 mg/day in divided doses.

Children. 0.1-2 mg/kg/day in 1-4 divided doses.

Intraarticular, intralesional (acetate)

Adults, Elderly. 4-100 mg, repeated as needed.

Intraarticular, intralesional (sodium phosphate)

Adults, Elderly. 2-30 mg, repeated at 3-day to 3-wk intervals, as needed.

IM (acetate, sodium phosphate)

Adults, Elderly. 4-60 mg a day.

Treatment of conjuctivitis and corneal injury

Ophthalmic

Adults, Elderly. 1-2 drops every hr during day and q2h during night. After response, decrease dosage to 1 drop q4h, then 1 drop 3-4 times a day.

AVAILABLE FORMS

• *Tablets:* 5 mg.
• *Syrup:* 5 mg/5 ml (Prelone), 15 mg/5 ml (Prednisolone Acetate, Prelone).
• *Oral Liquid, Sodium Phosphate:* 5 mg/5 ml (Orapred, Pediapred), 15 mg/5 ml (Orapred).

• *Injectable Solution, Sodium Phosphate (Hydeltrasol, Key-Pred SP):* 20 mg/ml.

• *Injectable Suspension, Acetate:* 25 mg/ml (Cotolone, Key-Pred), 40 mg/ml (Depo-Predate), 50 mg/ml (Cotolone, Predacort 50, Predaject-50, Predate-50, Pred-Ject-50), 80 mg/ml (Depo-Predate).

• *Ophthalmic Solution, Sodium Phosphate:* 0.125% (Inflamase Mild), 1% (AK-Pred, Inflamase Forte).

• *Ophthalmic Suspension, Acetate:* 0.12% (Pred Mild), 1% (Pred Forte).

CONTRAINDICATIONS: Acute superficial herpes simplex keratitis, systemic fungal infections, varicella

PREGNANCY AND LACTATION: Pregnancy category C (D if used in first trimester); compatible with breast-feeding

SIDE EFFECTS

Frequent

Insomnia, heartburn, nervousness, abdominal distention, increased sweating, acne, mood swings, increased appetite, facial flushing, delayed wound healing, increased susceptibility to infection, diarrhea or constipation

Occasional

Headache, edema, change in skin color, frequent urination

Rare

Tachycardia, allergic reaction (such as rash and hives), psychologic changes, hallucinations, depression

Ophthalmic: stinging or burning, posterior subcapsular cataracts

SERIOUS REACTIONS

• Long-term therapy may cause hypocalcemia, hypokalemia, muscle wasting (especially in the arms and legs), osteoporosis, spontaneous fractures, amenorrhea, cataracts, glaucoma, peptic ulcer disease, and CHF.

• Abruptly withdrawing the drug after long-term therapy may cause anorexia, nausea, fever, headache, severe or sudden joint pain, rebound inflammation, fatigue, weakness, lethargy, dizziness, and orthostatic hypotension.

• Suddenly discontinuing prednisolone may be fatal.

INTERACTIONS

Drugs

3 *Aminoglutethamide:* Increased clearance of prednisolone; doubling of dose may be required

3 *Amphotericin:* May increase hypokalemia

3 *Antidiabetics:* Increased blood glucose

3 *Barbiturates:* Increased clearance of prednisolone

3 *Cholestyramine, colestipol:* Reduced absorption of prednisolone

3 *Clarithromycin, erythromycin, troleandomycin, ketoconazole:* Possible enhanced steroid effect

3 *Digoxin:* May increase the risk of digoxin toxicity caused by hypokalemia

3 *Diuretics, potassium supplements:* May decrease the effects of these drugs

3 *Estrogens, oral contraceptives:* Enhanced effects of corticosteroids

3 *Hepatic enzyme inducers:* May decrease the effects of prednisolone

3 *Intrauterine devices:* Decreased contraceptive effect (possibly secondary inhibition of inflammatory reaction)

3 *Isoniazid:* Reduced plasma concentrations of isoniazid; (rapid isoniazid acetylators at increased risk)

3 *Live-virus vaccines:* May decrease the patient's antibody response to vaccine, increase vaccine side effects, and potentiate virus replication

3 *NSAIDs:* Increased risk GI ulceration

3 *Rifampin:* May reduce hepatic clearance of prednisolone

3 *Salicylates:* Increased salicylate clearance

Labs

- *False increase:* Cortisol, digoxin, theophylline
- *False decrease:* Urine glucose (Clinistix, Diastix only, Testape no effect)
- *False negative:* Skin allergy tests

SPECIAL CONSIDERATIONS

PATIENT/FAMILY EDUCATION

- May cause GI upset
- Take single daily doses in a.m.
- Increased dose of rapidly acting corticosteroids may be necessary in patients subjected to unusual stress
- Signs of adrenal insufficiency include fatigue, anorexia, nausea, vomiting, diarrhea, weight loss, weakness, dizziness, and low blood sugar
- Avoid abrupt withdrawal of therapy following high-dose or long-term therapy. Relative insufficiency may exist for up to 1 yr after discontinuation
- Patients on chronic steroid therapy should wear medical alert bracelet
- Do not give live-virus vaccines to patients on prolonged therapy
- Avoid exposure to chickenpox or measles
- Avoid alcohol and limit caffeine intake

MONITORING PARAMETERS

- Potassium and blood sugar during long-term therapy
- Edema, blood pressure, cardiac symptoms, mental status, weight
- Observe growth and development of infants and children on prolonged therapy
- Check intraocular pressure and lens frequently during prolonged use of ophthalmic preparations
- Be alert to signs and symptoms of infection, such as fever, sore throat, and vague symptoms
- Check mouth for signs and symptoms of candidal infection, such as white patches and painful mucous membranes and tongue

prednisone

(pred′-ni-sone)

Rx: Deltasone, Liquid Pred, Meticorten, Prednicen-M, Prednicot, Prednisone Intensol, Sterapred, Sterapred DS

Chemical Class: Glucocorticoid, synthetic

Therapeutic Class: Corticosteroid, systemic

CLINICAL PHARMACOLOGY

Mechanism of Action: An adrenocortical steroid that inhibits accumulation of inflammatory cells at inflammation sites, phagocytosis, lysosomal enzyme release and synthesis, and release of mediators of inflammation. ***Therapeutic Effect:*** Prevents or suppresses cell-mediated immune reactions. Decreases or prevents tissue response to inflammatory process.

Pharmacokinetics

Well absorbed from the GI tract. Protein binding: 70%-90%. Widely distributed. Metabolized in the liver and converted to prednisolone. Primarily excreted in urine. Not removed by hemodialysis. ***Half-life:*** 3.4-3.8 hrs.

INDICATIONS AND DOSAGES

Substitution therapy in deficiency states: acute or chronic adrenal insufficiency, congenital adrenal hyperplasia, and adrenal insufficiency secondary to pituitary insufficiency; nonendocrine disorders:

arthritis; rheumatic carditis; allergic, collagen, intestinal tract, liver, ocular, renal, skin diseases; bronchial asthma; cerebral edema; malignancies

PO

Adults, Elderly. 5-60 mg/day in divided doses.

Children. 0.05-2 mg/kg/day in 1-4 divided doses.

AVAILABLE FORMS

• *Oral Concentrate (Prednisone Intensol):* 5 mg/ml.

• *Oral Solution (Liquid Pred):* 5 mg/5 ml.

• *Tablets:* 1 mg (Sterapred), 2.5 mg (Deltasone), 5 mg (Deltasone, Prednicen-M, Sterapred), 10 mg (Deltasone, Sterapred), 20 mg (Deltasone), 50 mg (Deltasone).

CONTRAINDICATIONS: Acute superficial herpes simplex keratitis, systemic fungal infections, varicella

PREGNANCY AND LACTATION: Pregnancy category C (D if used in first trimester)

SIDE EFFECTS

Frequent

Insomnia, heartburn, nervousness, abdominal distention, increased sweating, acne, mood swings, increased appetite, facial flushing, delayed wound healing, increased susceptibility to infection, diarrhea or constipation

Occasional

Headache, edema, change in skin color, frequent urination

Rare

Tachycardia, allergic reaction (including rash and hives), psychologic changes, hallucinations, depression

SERIOUS REACTIONS

• Long-term therapy may cause muscle wasting in the arms and legs, osteoporosis, spontaneous fractures, amenorrhea, cataracts, glaucoma, peptic ulcer disease, and CHF.

• Abruptly withdrawing the drug following long-term therapy may cause anorexia, nausea, fever, headache, sudden or severe joint pain, rebound inflammation, fatigue, weakness, lethargy, dizziness, and orthostatic hypotension.

• Suddenly discontinuing prednisone may be fatal.

INTERACTIONS

Drugs

3 *Aminoglutethamide:* Increased clearance of prednisone; doubling of dose may be necessary

3 *Amphotericin:* May increase hypokalemia

3 *Antidiabetics:* Increased blood glucose

3 *Barbiturates, carbamazepine:* Increased clearance of prednisone

3 *Cholestyramine, colestipol:* Possible reduced absorption of corticosteroids

3 *Cyclosporine:* Possible increased concentration of both drugs, seizures

3 *Digoxin:* May increase the risk of digoxin toxicity caused by hypokalemia

3 *Diuretics, potassium supplements:* May decrease the effects of these drugs

3 *Erythromycin, troleandomycin, clarithromycin, ketoconazole:* Possible enhanced steroid effect

3 *Estrogens, oral contraceptives:* Enhanced effects of corticosteroids

3 *Hepatic enzyme inducers:* May decrease the effects of prednisone

3 *IUDs:* Inhibition of inflammation may decrease contraceptive effect

3 *Isoniazid:* Reduced plasma concentrations of isoniazid

3 *Live-virus vaccines:* May decrease the patient's antibody response to vaccine, increase vaccine side effects, and potentiate virus replication
3 *NSAIDs:* Increased risk GI ulceration
3 *Rifampin:* May reduce hepatic clearance of prednisone
3 *Salicylates:* Increased salicylate clearance

Labs

- *False increase:* Cortisol, digoxin, theophylline
- *False decrease:* Urine glucose (Clinistix, Diastix only, Testape no effect)
- *False negative:* Skin allergy tests

SPECIAL CONSIDERATIONS

PATIENT/FAMILY EDUCATION

- May cause GI upset, teach patient to take with meals or snacks
- May mask infections
- Take single daily doses in a.m.
- Increased dose of rapidly acting corticosteroids may be necessary in patients subjected to unusual stress
- Signs of adrenal insufficiency include fatigue, anorexia, nausea, vomiting, diarrhea, weight loss, weakness, dizziness, and low blood sugar
- Avoid abrupt withdrawal of therapy following high-dose or long-term therapy; relative insufficiency may exist for up to 1 yr after discontinuation
- Patients on chronic steroid therapy should wear medical alert bracelet
- Do not give live-virus vaccines to patients on prolonged therapy
- Avoid exposure to chickenpox or measles
- Avoid alcohol and limit caffeine intake

MONITORING PARAMETERS

- Serum K and glucose
- Edema, blood pressure, CHF symptoms, mental status, weight
- Growth in children on prolonged therapy
- Be alert to signs and symptoms of infection, such as fever, sore throat, and vague symptoms
- Check mouth for signs and symptoms of candidal infection, such as white patches and painful mucous membranes and tongue

primaquine phosphate

(prim-a-kween)

Rx: Primaquine

Chemical Class: 8-aminoquinoline derivative

Therapeutic Class: Antimalarial

CLINICAL PHARMACOLOGY

Mechanism of Action: An antimalarial and antirheumatic that eliminates tissue exoerythrocytic forms of *Plasmodium falciparum*. Disrupts mitochondria and binds to DNA. ***Therapeutic Effect:*** Inhibits parasite growth.

Pharmacokinetics

Well absorbed. Metabolized in the liver to the active metabolite, carboxyprimaquine. Excreted in the urine in small amounts as unchanged drug. ***Half-life:*** 4-6 hrs.

INDICATIONS AND DOSAGES

Treatment of malaria

PO

Adults, Elderly. 15 mg base daily for 14 days.

Children. 0.3 mg base/kg/wk once daily for 14 days.

Malaria prophylaxis

Adults, Elderly. 30 mg base daily. Begin 1 day before departure and continue for 7 days after leaving malarious area.

AVAILABLE FORMS

• *Tablets:* 26.3 mg (Primaquine phosphate).

CONTRAINDICATIONS: Concomitant medications that cause bone marrow suppression, rheumatoid arthritis, lupus erythematosus, glucose-6-phosphate dehydrogenase (G-6-PD) deficiency, pregnancy, hypersensitivity to primaquine or any of its components

PREGNANCY AND LACTATION: Pregnancy category C; if possible, withhold until after delivery; however, if prophylaxis or treatment is required, primaquine should not be withheld

SIDE EFFECTS

Frequent

Abdominal pain, nausea, vomiting

Rare

Leukopenia, hemolytic anemia, methemoglobinemia

SERIOUS REACTIONS

• Leukopenia, hemolytic anemia, methemoglobinemia occur rarely.

• Overdosage includes symptoms of abdominal cramps, vomiting, burning epigastric distress, central nervous system and cardiovascular disturbances, cyanosis, methemoglobinemia, moderate leukocytosis or leukopenia, and anemia.

• Acute hemolysis occurs, but patients recover completely if the dosage is discontinued.

SPECIAL CONSIDERATIONS

PATIENT/FAMILY EDUCATION

• Take with food if GI upset occurs, notify clinician if GI distress continues

• Urine may turn brown

• Take for the full length of treatment

• Notify the physician if unexplained fever, sore throat, or weakness occurs

MONITORING PARAMETERS

• CBC periodically during therapy, discontinue if marked darkening of urine or sudden decrease in hemoglobin concentrations or leukocyte count occurs

primidone

(pri'-mi-done)

Rx: Mysoline

Chemical Class: Pyrimidinedione

Therapeutic Class: Anticonvulsant

DEA Class: Schedule IV

CLINICAL PHARMACOLOGY

Mechanism of Action: A barbiturate that decreases motor activity from electrical and chemical stimulation and stabilizes the seizure threshold against hyperexcitability. ***Therapeutic Effect:*** Reduces seizure activity.

Pharmacokinetics

Rapidly and usually completely absorbed following oral administration. Protein binding: 20%-30%. Extensively metabolized in liver to phenobarbital and phenylethylmalonamide (PEMA). Minimal excretion in urine. ***Half-life:*** 3.3-7 hr.

INDICATIONS AND DOSAGES

Seizure control

PO

Adults, Elderly, Children 8 yrs and older. 125-150 mg/day at bedtime. May increase by 125-250 mg/day every 3-7 days. Maximum: 2 g/day.

Children younger than 8 yrs. Initially, 50-125 mg/day at bedtime. May increase by 50-125 mg/day every 3-7 days. Usual dose: 10-25 mg/kg/day in divided doses.

Neonates. 12-20 mg/kg/day in divided doses.

P

AVAILABLE FORMS

- *Tablets:* 50 mg, 250 mg.
- *Oral Suspension:* 250 mg/5 ml.

UNLABELED USES: Treatment of essential tremor

CONTRAINDICATIONS: History of bronchopneumonia, hypersensitivity to phenobarbital, porphyria

PREGNANCY AND LACTATION: Pregnancy category D; reported association between use of other anticonvulsants (phenobarbital and phenytoin) and increased incidence of birth defects; should not be discontinued abruptly in patients who become pregnant when the drug is being used to prevent major seizures because of possibility of precipitating status epilepticus with attendant hypoxia and threat to life; the majority of mothers on anticonvulsant medication deliver normal infants; neonatal hemorrhage, with a coagulation defect resembling vitamin K deficiency, has been described in newborns whose mothers were taking primidone; pregnant women on primidone should receive prophylactic vitamin K_1 therapy for 1 mo before, and during, delivery; excreted in breast milk in percentages of maternal serum concentration as high as 106.9% for primidone and 56.9% for phenobarbital

SIDE EFFECTS

Frequent

Ataxia, dizziness

Occasional

Anorexia, drowsiness, mental changes, nausea, vomiting, paradoxical excitement

Rare

Rash

SERIOUS REACTIONS

- Abrupt withdrawal after prolonged therapy may produce effects ranging from increased dreaming, nightmares, insomnia, tremor, diaphoresis, and vomiting to hallucinations, delirium, seizures, and status epilepticus.
- Skin eruptions may be a sign of a hypersensitivity reaction.
- Blood dyscrasias, hepatic disease, and hypocalcemia occur rarely.
- Overdose produces cold or clammy skin, hypothermia, and severe CNS depression, followed by high fever and coma.

INTERACTIONS

Drugs

3 *Acetazolamide:* Decreased absorption, hence decreased anticonvulsant efficacy

2 *Anticoagulants (anisindione, dicumarol, warfarin):* Decreased anticoagulant effectiveness

2 *Barbiturates:* Additive CNS and respiratory depressant effects

2 *Benzodiazepines:* Additive CNS and respiratory depressant effects

3 *Betamethasone:* Decreased betamethasone effectiveness

3 *Cannabis:* Increased CNS depression

3 *Carbamazepine:* Decreased carbamazepine effectiveness with loss of seizure control

3 *Centrally acting muscle relaxants:* Additive respiratory depression

2 *Chloral hydrate:* Additive respiratory depression

3 *Cortisone:* Decreased cortisone effectiveness

3 *Dexamethasone:* Decreased dexamethasone effectiveness

2 *Dexmethylphenidate:* Inhibits metabolism; increased primidone plasma concentrations

3 *Digoxin:* May decrease the effects of these drugs

3 *Estradiol:* Estrogen effects decreased; increased doses of estrogen may be needed

3 *Ethanol:* Excessive CNS depression

3 *Ethchlorvynol:* Additive CNS and respiratory effects
2 *Ethinyl estradiol:* Decreased contraceptive effectiveness
3 *Fosphenytoin:* Increased phenobarbital levels
3 *Ginkgo:* Decreased effectiveness of primidone due to presence of seizure-provoking contaminant in some ginkgo preparations
3 *Hydrocortisone:* Decreased hydrocortisone effectiveness
3 *Isoniazid:* Isoniazid inhibits primidone metabolism with elevations of primidone plasma concentrations as well as prolonging $t_{1/2}$
3 *Lamotrigine:* Decreased lamotrigine efficacy (40% decreases in lamotrigine concentrations)
3 *Leucovorin:* Antiepileptic effect counteracted; decreased primidone efficacy
2 *Levonorgestrel:* Decreased contraceptive effectiveness
3 *Mesoridazine:* Decreased levels of antipsychotic via induced metabolism (25%-40%)
2 *Mestranol:* Decreased contraceptive effectiveness
3 *Methylprednisolone:* Decreased methylprednisolone effectiveness
3 *Methsuximide:* Competitive inhibition of hydroxylation; increased phenobarbital and primidone plasma concentrations
3 *Norethindrone:* Decreased contraceptive effectiveness
3 *Norgestrel:* Decreased contraceptive effectiveness
3 *Opioid analgesics:* Additive CNS and respiratory effects
3 *Phenytoin:* Increased phenobarbital levels
3 *Prednisolone, prednisone:* Decreased corticosteroid effectiveness
3 *Rifabutin:* Reduced primidone effectiveness
3 *Sodium oxybate:* Additive CNS and respiratory depression
2 *Theophylline:* Decreased serum levels and concentration of theophylline via hepatic microsomal enzyme induction
3 *Triamcinolone:* Decreased triamcinolone effectiveness
3 *Tricyclic antidepressants:* Decreased tricyclic antidepressant serum concentrations
2 *Valproic acid:* Additive respiratory and CNS depression
2 *Warfarin:* Decreased anticoagulant effectiveness

SPECIAL CONSIDERATIONS

- Second-line anticonvulsant for treatment of generalized tonic-clonic seizures (or alternative to phenobarbital, which probably accounts for most of the anticonvulsant activity)
- Most effective anti-essential tremor medication, but sedative side effects troublesome; usually used second line to β-adrenergic blocking agents (non-selective)

PATIENT/FAMILY EDUCATION

- Importance of effective contraception, and considerations surrounding pregnancy
- Importance of adherence to regimen and risk associated with abrupt discontinuance of anticonvulsant
- Sedative liabilities regarding driving and operating heavy machinery
- Avoid alcohol

MONITORING PARAMETERS

- Therapeutic drug concentration for seizure control: 5-12 mcg/ml; serum concentrations should also include phenobarbital determinations (therapeutic: 20-40 mcg/ml)
- Periodic CBC, liver and renal function tests, serum folate, vitamin D during prolonged therapy

probenecid

(proe-ben'-e-sid)

Rx: Probalan

Combinations

Rx: with colchicine (Colbenemid Proben-C); with ampicillin (Polycillin-PRB, Probampacin)

Chemical Class: Sulfonamide derivative

Therapeutic Class: Antigout agent; uricosuric

CLINICAL PHARMACOLOGY

Mechanism of Action: A uricosuric that competitively inhibits reabsorption of uric acid at the proximal convoluted tubule. Also, inhibits renal tubular secretion of weak organic acids, such as penicillins. ***Therapeutic Effect:*** Promotes uric acid excretion, reduces serum uric acid level, and increases plasma levels of penicillins and cephalosporins.

Pharmacokinetics

Rapidly and completely absorbed following oral administration. Protein binding: high. Extensively metabolized in liver. Excreted in urine. Excretion is dependent upon urinary pH and is increased in alkaline urine. ***Half-life:*** 3-8 hr (dose-dependent).

INDICATIONS AND DOSAGES

Gout

PO

Adults, Elderly. Initially, 250 mg twice a day for 1 wk; then 500 mg twice a day. May increase by 500 mg q4wk. Maximum: 2-3 g/day. Maintenance: Dosage that maintains normal uric acid level.

As adjunct to penicillin or cephalosporin therapy to prolong antibiotic plasma levels

PO

Adults, Elderly. 2 g/day in divided doses.

Children weighing more than 50 kg. Receive adult dosage.

Children 2-14 yrs. Initially, 25 mg/kg. Maintenance: 40 mg/kg/day in 4 divided doses.

Gonorrhea

PO

Adults, Elderly. 1 g 30 min before penicillin, ampicillin, or amoxicillin.

Children weighing less than 45 kg. 25 mg/kg 30 min before penicillin, ampicillin, amoxicillin. Maximum: 1 g.

AVAILABLE FORMS

- *Tablets:* 500 mg.

CONTRAINDICATIONS: Blood dyscrasias, children younger than 2 yrs, concurrent high-dose aspirin therapy, severe renal impairment, uric acid calculi

PREGNANCY AND LACTATION: Pregnancy category C; has been used during pregnancy without causing adverse effects in fetus or infant

SIDE EFFECTS

Frequent (10%-6%)

Headache, anorexia, nausea, vomiting

Occasional (5%-1%)

Lower back or side pain, rash, hives, itching, dizziness, flushed face, frequent urge to urinate, gingivitis

SERIOUS REACTIONS

- Severe hypersensitivity reactions, including anaphylaxis, occur rarely and usually within a few hours after administration following previous use. If severe hypersensitivity reactions develop, discontinue the drug immediately and contact the physician.
- Pruritic maculopapular rash, possibly accompanied by malaise, fever, chills, arthralgia, nausea, vomit-

ing, leukopenia, and aplastic anemias should be considered a toxic reaction.

INTERACTIONS

Drugs

3 *Alcohol:* May increase serum urate level

3 *Antineoplastics:* May increase the risk of uric acid nephropathy

3 *Cephalosporins, nitrofurantoin, NSAIDs, penicillins:* May increase blood concentrations of these drugs

3 *Dapsone:* Increased serum dapsone concentrations

3 *Dyphylline:* Increased serum dyphylline concentrations

3 *Heparin:* May increase and prolong the effects of heparin

2 *Methotrexate:* Marked increases in serum methotrexate concentrations

3 *Salicylates:* Inhibition of uricosuric effect if used regularly

3 *Thiopental:* Prolonged anesthesia

3 *Zidovudine:* Increased plasma zidovudine concentrations

Labs

- *False positive:* Urine glucose (Ames Clinitest tablet, no effect on Ames Keto-Diastix, Diastix, Multistix, Clinistix)
- *False increase:* Free T_4 (Boehringer-Mannheim Enzymum procedure)

SPECIAL CONSIDERATIONS

PATIENT/FAMILY EDUCATION

- Avoid aspirin or other salicylates
- Take with food or antacids
- Drink 48-64 oz water daily to prevent development of kidney stones
- Avoid alcohol
- Avoid eating high-purine foods, such as anchovies, kidneys, liver, meat extracts, sardines, and sweetbreads
- Full therapeutic response may take more than 1 wk
- Discontinue if rash or other evidence of an allergic reaction occurs

MONITORING PARAMETERS

- Serum uric acid concentrations: continue the probenecid dose that maintains normal concentrations
- Renal function tests
- CBC
- Encourage the patient to maintain a high fluid intake (3000 ml/day). Monitor the patient's intake and urine output. Output should be at least 2000 ml/day
- Therapeutic response, including improved joint range of motion and reduced joint tenderness, redness, and swelling

procainamide hydrochloride

(proe-kane'-a-mide hye-droe-klor'-ide)

Rx: Procanbid, Procan-SR, Procan SR, Pronestyl, Pronestyl-SR

Chemical Class: Para-aminobenzoic acid derivative

Therapeutic Class: Antiarrhythmic, class IA

CLINICAL PHARMACOLOGY

Mechanism of Action: An antiarrhythmic that increases the electrical stimulation threshold of the ventricles and His-Purkinje system. Decreases myocardial excitability and conduction velocity and depresses myocardial contractility. Exerts direct cardiac effects. ***Therapeutic Effect:*** Suppresses arrhythmias.

Pharmacokinetics

Rapidly, completely absorbed from the GI tract. Protein binding: 15%-20%. Widely distributed. Metabolized in the liver to active metabolite. Primarily excreted in urine. Removed by hemodialysis. ***Half-life:*** 2.5-4.5 hr; metabolite, 6 hr.

INDICATIONS AND DOSAGES

Maintenance of normal sinus rhythm after conversion of atrial fibrillation or flutter; treatment of premature ventricular contractions, paroxysmal atrial tachycardia, atrial fibrillation, and ventricular tachycardia

PO

Adults, Elderly. 250-500 mg of immediate-release tablets q3-6h. 0.5-1 g of extended-release tablets q6h. 1-2 g of Procanbid q12h.

Children. 15-50 mg/kg/day of immediate-release tablets in divided doses q3-6h. Maximum: 4 g/day.

IV

Adults, Elderly. Loading dose: 50-100 mg. May repeat q5-10min or 15-18 mg/kg (maximum: 1-1.5 g). Then maintenance infusion of 3-4 mg/min. Range: 1-6 mg/min.

Children. Loading dose: 3-6 mg/kg over 5 min (maximum: 100 mg). May repeat q5-10min to maximum total dose of 15 mg/kg. Then maintenance dose of 20-80 mcg/kg/min. Maximum: 2 g/day.

Dosage in renal impairment

Dosag interval is modified based on creatinine clearance.

Creatinine Clearance	*Dosage Interval*
10-50 ml/min	q6-12h
less than 10 ml/min	q8-24h

AVAILABLE FORMS

• *Capsules (Pronestyl):* 250 mg, 500 mg.

• *Tablets (Pronestyl):* 250 mg, 375 mg, 500 mg.

• *Tablets (Extended-Release [Pronestyl-SR]):* 500 mg.

• *Tablest (Extended-Release [Procanbid]):* 500 mg, 750 mg, 1000 mg.

• *Injection (Pronestyl):* 100 mg/ml, 500 mg/ml.

UNLABELED USES: Conversion and management of atrial fibrillation

CONTRAINDICATIONS: Complete heart block, myasthenia gravis, preexisting QT prolongation, second-degree heart block, systemic lupus erythematosus, torsades de pointes

PREGNANCY AND LACTATION: Pregnancy category C; compatible with breast-feeding; long-term effects in nursing infant unknown

SIDE EFFECTS

Frequent

PO: Abdominal pain or cramping, nausea, diarrhea, vomiting

Occasional

Dizziness, giddiness, weakness, hypersensitivity reaction (rash, urticaria, pruritus, flushing)

IV: Transient, but at times, marked hypotension

Rare

Confusion, mental depression, psychosis

SERIOUS REACTIONS

• Paradoxical, extremely rapid ventricular rate may occur during treatment of atrial fibrillation or flutter.

• Systemic lupus erythematosus-like syndrome (fever, myalgia, pleuritic chest pain) may occur with prolonged therapy.

• Cardiotoxic effects occur most commonly with IV administration and appear as conduction changes (50% widening of QRS complex, frequent ventricular premature contractions, ventricular tachycardia, and complete AV block).

• Prolonged PR and QT intervals and flattened T waves occur less frequently.

INTERACTIONS

Drugs

3 *Amiodarone, cimetidine, trimethoprim:* Increased procainamide concentrations

3 *Antihypertensives (IV procainamide), neuromuscular blockers:* May increase the effects of these drugs; may decrease antimyasthenic effect on skeletal muscle

3 *Cholinergic drugs:* Antagonism of cholinergic actions on skeletal muscle

3 *Other antiarrhythmics, pimozide:* May increase cardiac effects

3 *Procaine:* Interferes with procainamide concentration assay

3 *Quinidine:* Increases procainamide serum concentrations

2 *Thioridazine:* May produce additive prolongation of the QT interval

Labs

- *False decrease:* Cholinesterase
- *False increase:* Potassium

SPECIAL CONSIDERATIONS

PATIENT/FAMILY EDUCATION

- Strict compliance to dosage schedule imperative
- Empty wax core from sustained-release tablets may appear in stool; this is harmless
- Initiate therapy in facilities capable of providing continuous ECG monitoring and managing life-threatening dysrhythmias
- Do not abruptly discontinue the drug
- Do not take nasal decongestants or OTC cold preparations, especially those containing stimulants, without physician approval
- Avoid performing tasks that require mental alertness or motor skills until response to the drug is established

MONITORING PARAMETERS

- CBC with differential and platelets qwk for first 3 mo, periodically thereafter
- ECG: R/O overdosage if QRS widens >25% or QT prolongation occurs; reduce dosage if QRS widens >50%
- ANA titer increases may precede clinical symptoms of lupoid syndrome
- Serum creatinine, urea nitrogen
- Plasma procainamide concentration (therapeutic range 3-10 mcg/ml; 10-30 mcg/ml NAPA)
- Check blood pressure every 5-10 mins during IV infusion. If a fall in blood presure exceeds 15 mm Hg, discontinue infusion and contact the physician
- Pulse rate for quality and irregularity
- Intake and output
- Serum electrolyte levels, including chloride, potassium, and sodium
- Pattern of daily bowel activity and stool consistency
- Skin for hypersensitivity reaction, especially in patients receiving high-dose therapy

procaine hydrochloride

(proe'-kane hye-droe-klor'-ide)

Rx: Novocain, Mericaine

Chemical Class: Benzoic acid derivative

Therapeutic Class: Anesthetic, local

CLINICAL PHARMACOLOGY

Mechanism of Action: Procaine causes a reversible blockade of nerve conduction by decreasing nerve membrance permeability to sodium. ***Therapeutic Effect:*** Local anesthesia.

Pharmacokinetics

Highly plasma protein-bound and distributed to all body tissues. Excreted in the urine (80%). ***Half-life:*** 40 ± 9 secs in adults, 84 ± 30 secs in neonates.

INDICATIONS AND DOSAGES

Spinal anesthesia

Intrathecal

Adults. 0.5-1 ml of a 10% solution (50-100 mg) mixed with an equal volume of diluent injected into the third or fourth lumber interspace (perineum and lower extremeties). 2 ml of a 10% solution (200 mg) mixed with 1 ml of diluent injected into the second, third, or fourth interspace.

Infiltration anesthesia, dental anesthesia, control of severe pain (post-herpatic neuralgia, cancer pain, or burns)

Topical

Adults. A single dose of 350-600 mg using a 0.25% or 0.5% solution. Use 0.9% sodium chloride for dilution.

Children. 15 mg/kg of a 0.5% solution is the maximum recommended dose.

Peripheral or sympathetic nerve block (regional anesthesia)

Topical

Adults. Up to 200 ml of a 0.5% solution (1 g), 100 ml of a 1% solution (1 g), or 50 ml of a 2% solution (1 g). The 2% solution should only be used when a small volume of anesthetic is required.

AVAILABLE FORMS

• *Solution:* 0.25%, 0.5%, 10% (Novocaine).

UNLABELED USES: Severe pain

CONTRAINDICATIONS: Hypersensitivity to ester local anesthetics, sulfites, PABA, patients on anticoagulant therapy, and in patients with coagulopathy, infection, thrombocytopenia. Should not be given intraarterial, intrathecal, or intravenous.

PREGNANCY AND LACTATION: Pregnancy category C; use caution in nursing mothers

SIDE EFFECTS

Frequent

Numbness or tingling of the face or mouth, pain at the injection site, dizziness, drowsiness, lightheadedness, nausea, vomiting, back pain, headache

Rare

Anxiety, restlessness, difficulty breathing, shortness of breath, seizures (convulsions), skin rash, itching (hives), slow irregular heartbeat (palpitations), swelling of the face or mouth, tremors, QT prolongation, PR prolongation, atrial fibrillation, sinus bradycardia, hypotension, angina, cardiovascular collapse, fecal or urinary incontinence, loss of perineal sensation and sexual function, persistent motor, sensory, and/or autonomic (sphincter control) deficit

SERIOUS REACTIONS

• Procaine-induced CNS toxicity usually presents with symptoms of stimulation such as anxiety, apprehension, restlessness, nervousness, disorientation, confusion, dizziness, blurred vision, tremor, nausea/vomiting, shivering, or seizures. Subsequently, depressive symptoms can occur including drowsiness, unconsciousness, and respiratory arrest.

• If higher concentrations are introduced into the blood stream, depression of cardiac excitability and contractility may cause AV block, ventricular arrhythmias, or cardiac arrest. CNS toxicity, including dizziness, tongue numbness, visual impairment and disturbances, and muscular twitching appear to occur before cardiotoxic effects.

Alert: Procaine should be used with caution in patients that have asthma since there is the increased risk of anaphylactoid reactions, including bronchospasm and status asthmaticus.

Alert: Local anesthetics can cause varying degrees of maternal, fetal, and neonatal toxicities during labor and obstetric delivery. Fetal heart rate should be monitored, as well as the presence of symptoms indicating fetal bradycardia, fetal acidosis, and maternal hypotension. Epidural procaine may cause decreased uterine contractility or maternal expulsion efforts and alter the forces of parturition.

Alert: Unintentional fetal intracranial injection of procaine occurring during pudenal or paracervical block has been shown to lead to neonatal depression at birth and can lead to seizures within 6 hours as a result of high serum concentrations.

INTERACTIONS

Drugs

3 *β-blockers:* Acute discontinuation of β-blockers before local anesthesia increases the risk of hypertensive reactions

3 *Ergot-type oxytocic drugs:* May cause severe, persistent hypertension or cerebrovascular accidents

3 *MAOIs, tricyclic antidepressants:* May produce severe, prolonged hypertension

Labs

- *False increase:* CSF protein, urine porphobilinogen, urobilinogen

SPECIAL CONSIDERATIONS

- Esther-type local anesthetic

PATIENT/FAMILY EDUCATION

- A burning sensation may occur at the site of injection

MONITORING PARAMETERS

- Blood pressure, pulse, respiration during treatment, ECG
- Fetal heart tones if used during labor

prochlorperazine

(proe-klor-per′-a-zeen)

Rx: Compazine, Compazine Spansule, Compro, Procot

Chemical Class: Piperazine phenothiazine derivative

Therapeutic Class: Antiemetic; antipsychotic

CLINICAL PHARMACOLOGY

Mechanism of Action: A phenothiazine that acts centrally to inhibit or block dopamine receptors in the chemoreceptor trigger zone and peripherally to block the vagus nerve in the GI tract. ***Therapeutic Effect:*** Relieves nausea and vomiting and improves psychotic conditions.

Pharmacokinetics

Route	*Onset**	*Peak*	*Duration*
Tablets, Oral Solution	30-40 mins	N/A	3-4 hrs
Capsules (Extended-Release)	30-40 mins	N/A	10-12 hrs
Rectal	60 mins	N/A	3-4 hrs

* As an antiemetic

Variably absorbed after PO administration. Widely distributed. Metabolized in the liver and GI mucosa. Primarily excreted in urine. Unknown if removed by hemodialysis. ***Half-life:*** 23 hrs.

INDICATIONS AND DOSAGES

Nausea and vomiting

PO

Adults, Elderly. 5-10 mg 3-4 times a day.

Children. 0.4 mg/kg/day in 3-4 divided doses.

PO (Extended-Release)

Adults, Elderly. 10 mg twice a day or 15 mg once a day.

IV
Adults, Elderly. 2.5-10 mg. May repeat q3-4h.
IM
Adults, Elderly. 5-10 mg q3-4h.
Children. 0.1-0.15 mg/kg/dose q8-12h. Maximum: 40 mg/day.
Rectal
Adults, Elderly. 25 mg twice a day.
Children. 0.4 mg/kg/day in 3-4 divided doses.

Psychosis
PO
Adults, Elderly. 5-10 mg 3-4 times a day. Maximum: 150 mg/day.
Children. 2.5 mg 2-3 times a day. Maximum: 25 mg for children 6-12 yr; 20 mg for children 2-5 yr.
IM
Adults, Elderly. 10-20 mg q4h.
Children. 0.13 mg/kg/dose.

AVAILABLE FORMS
- *Capsules (Extended-Release [Compazine Spansule]):* 10 mg, 15 mg.
- *Oral Solution (Compazine):* 5 mg/5 ml.
- *Tablets (Compazine):* 5 mg, 10 mg.
- *Suppositories (Compazine):* 2.5 mg, 5 mg, 25 mg.
- *Injection (Compazine, Procot):* 5 mg/ml.

UNLABELED USES: Behavior syndromes in dementia

CONTRAINDICATIONS: Angle-closure glaucoma, CNS depression, coma, myelosuppression, severe cardiac or hepatic impairment, severe hypotension or hypertension

PREGNANCY AND LACTATION: Pregnancy category C; majority of evidence indicates safety for both mother and fetus if used occasionally in low doses; excretion into breast milk should be expected; sedation is a possible effect in nursing infant

SIDE EFFECTS
Frequent
Somnolence, hypotension, dizziness, fainting (commonly occurring after first dose, occasionally after subsequent doses, and rarely with oral form)
Occasional
Dry mouth, blurred vision, lethargy, constipation, diarrhea, myalgia, nasal congestion, peripheral edema, urine retention

SERIOUS REACTIONS
- Extrapyramidal symptoms appear to be dose related and are divided into three categories: akathisia (marked by inability to sit still, tapping of feet), parkinsonian symptoms (including mask-like face, tremors, shuffling gait, hypersalivation), and acute dystonias (such as torticollis, opisthotonos, and oculogyric crisis. A dystonic reaction may also produce diaphoresis or pallor.
- Tardive dyskinesia, manifested as tongue protrusion, puffing of the cheeks, and puckering of the mouth, is a rare reaction that may be irreversible.
- Abrupt withdrawal after long-term therapy may precipitate nausea, vomiting, gastritis, dizziness, and tremors.
- Blood dyscrasias, particularly agranulocytosis and mild leukopenia, may occur.
- Prochlorperazine use may lower the seizure threshold.

INTERACTIONS
Drugs
3 *Anticholinergics:* Inhibited therapeutic response to antipsychotic; enhanced anticholinergic side effects
3 *Antidepressants:* Increased serum concentrations of some cyclic antidepressants
3 *Antihypertensives:* May increase hypotension

3 *Antithyroid agents:* May increase the risk of agranulocytosis
3 *Attapulgite:* Inhibition of phenothiazine absorption
3 *Barbiturates:* Reduced effect of antipsychotic
3 *Bromocriptine, lithium:* Reduced effects of both drugs
3 *β-blockers:* Enhanced effects of both drugs (interaction less likely with atenolol, nadolol)
3 *Chloroquine, amodiaquine, pyrimethamine:* Possible increased phenothiazine concentrations
3 *Cigarettes:* Possible enhanced metabolism of neuroleptic
3 *Clonidine:* Possible enhanced hypotensive effect
3 *Epinephrine:* Reversed pressor response to epinephrine
3 *Ethanol:* Enhanced ethanol effects
3 *Extrapyramidal symptom–producing medications:* May increase extrapyramidal symptoms
3 *Guanethidine:* Inhibited antihypertensive response to guanethidine
3 *Indomethacin:* Possible increased CNS effects, other NSAIDs less likely to have effect
3 *Narcotic analgesics:* Excessive CNS depression, hypotension, respiratory depression
2 *Levodopa:* Inhibited effect of levodopa on Parkinson's disease
3 *Orphenadrine:* Reduced serum neuroleptic concentrations, excessive anticholinergic effects
3 *Procarbazine:* Increased sedation, EPS effects
3 *SSRIs:* Increased risk EPS effects
3 *Trazadone:* Possible increased risk of hypotension

Labs

• *False positive:* Phenylketones

SPECIAL CONSIDERATIONS

PATIENT/FAMILY EDUCATION

• Arise slowly from reclining position
• Do not discontinue abruptly
• Use a sunscreen during sun exposure to prevent burns; take special precautions to stay cool in hot weather
• May cause drowsiness
• Avoid alcohol and limit caffeine intake
• Avoid tasks that require mental alertness or motor skills until response to the drug has been established

MONITORING PARAMETERS

• Observe closely for signs of tardive dyskinesia
• Treat acute dystonic reactions with parenteral diphenhydramine (2 mg/kg to max 50 mg) or benztropine (2 mg)
• Periodic CBC with platelets during prolonged therapy
• Blood pressure for hypotension
• Therapeutic response, including improvement in self-care, increased ability to concentrate and interest in surroundings, and a relaxed facial expression

procyclidine hydrochloride

(proe-sye-kli-deen hye-droe-klor'-ide)

Rx: Kemadrin

Chemical Class: Tertiary amine
Therapeutic Class: Anti-Parkinson's agent; anticholinergic

CLINICAL PHARMACOLOGY

Mechanism of Action: An anticholinergic agent that exerts an atropine-like action and produces an antispasmodic effect on smooth muscle, is a potent mydriatic, and inhibits salivation. ***Therapeutic Effect:*** Relieves symptoms of Parkinson's disease and drug-induced extrapyramidal symptoms.

Pharmacokinetics
Well absorbed from the gastrointestinal (GI) tract. Protein binding: extensive. Metabolized in liver—undergoes extensive first-pass effect. Primarily excreted in urine. Unknown if removed by hemodialysis. ***Half-life:*** 7.7-16.1 hrs.

INDICATIONS AND DOSAGES
Drug-induced extrapyramidal reactions
PO
Adults, Elderly. Initially, 2.5 mg 3 times/day. May increase by 2.5 mg daily as needed. Maintenance: 10-20 mg/day in divided doses 3 times/day.
Parkinson's disease
PO
Adults, Elderly. Initially, 2.5 mg 3 times/day after meals. Maintenance: 2.5-5 mg mg/day in divided doses 3 times/day after meals.
Hepatic function impairment
PO
Adults, Elderly. 2.5-5 mg mg/day in divided doses twice a day after meals

AVAILABLE FORMS
- *Tablets:* 5 mg (Kemadrin).

CONTRAINDICATIONS: Angle-closure glaucoma

PREGNANCY AND LACTATION: Pregnancy category C; nursing infants may be particularly sensitive to anticholinergic effects

SIDE EFFECTS
Frequent
Blurred vision, mydriasis, disorientation, lightheadedness, nausea, vomiting, dry mouth, nose, throat, and lips

SERIOUS REACTIONS
- Overdosage may vary from severe anticholinergic effects, such as unsteadiness; severe drowsiness; severe dryness of mouth, nose, or throat; tachycardia; shortness of breath; and skin flushing.
- Also produces severe paradoxical reaction, marked by hallucinations, tremor, seizures, and toxic psychosis.

INTERACTIONS
Drugs
3 *Amantadine:* Potentiates CNS side effects of amantadine
3 *Anticholinergic:* Increased anticholinergic side effects
3 *Antipsychotic agents:* Possible worsening of psychosis, increased anticholinergic side effects
3 *Digoxin (slow dissolution tab):* Increased digoxin concentration
3 *Tacrine:* Reduced therapeutic effects of both drugs

SPECIAL CONSIDERATIONS

PATIENT/FAMILY EDUCATION
- Do not discontinue this drug abruptly
- Hard candy, frequent drinks, sugarless gum to relieve dry mouth
- Take with or after meals to prevent GI upset
- Use caution in hot weather, may increase susceptibility to heat stroke
- Avoid tasks that require mental alertness or motor skills until response to the drug is established
- Avoid alcohol

MONITORING PARAMETERS
- Blood pressure
- Clinical reversal of symptoms, such as improvement of mask-like facial expression, muscular rigidity, shuffling gait, and resting tremors of hands and head

progesterone

(proe-jes'-ter-one)

Rx: Crinone, First Progesterone MC10, First Progesterone MC5, Prochieve, Prometrium

Chemical Class: Progestin, natural

Therapeutic Class: Contraceptive; progestin

CLINICAL PHARMACOLOGY

Mechanism of Action: A natural steroid hormone that promotes mammary gland development and relaxes uterine smooth muscle. ***Therapeutic Effect:*** Decreases abnormal uterine bleeding; transforms endometrium from proliferative to secretory in an estrogen-primed endometrium.

Pharmacokinetics

Oral: Maximum serum concentrations attained within 3 hrs.

Protein binding: 96%-99%. Metabolized in liver. Excreted in bile and urine. ***Half-life:*** 18.3 hr.

IM: Rapidly absorbed. Undergoes rapid metabolism. ***Half-life:*** Few min.

Long-acting form: Approximately 10 wk.

Vaginal gel: Rate limited by absorption rather than by elimination.

Protein binding: 96%-99%. Undergoes both biliary and renal elimination. ***Half-life:*** 5-20 hr.

INDICATIONS AND DOSAGES

Amenorrhea

PO

Adults. 400 mg daily in evening for 10 days.

IM

Adults. 5-10 mg for 6-8 days. Withdrawal bleeding expected in 48-72 hrs if ovarian activity produced proliferative endometrium.

Vaginal

Adults. Apply 45 mg (4% gel) every other day for 6 or fewer doses.

Abnormal uterine bleeding

IM

Adults. 5-10 mg for 6 days. When estrogen given concomitantly, begin progesterone after 2 wk of estrogen therapy; discontinue when menstrual flow begins.

Prevention of endometrial hyperplasia

PO

Adults. 200 mg in evening for 12 days per 28-day cycle in combination with daily conjugated estrogen.

Infertility

Vaginal

Adults. 90 mg (8% gel) once a day (2 twice a day in women with partial or complete ovarian failure).

AVAILABLE FORMS

- *Capsules (Prometrium):* 100 mg, 200 mg.
- *Injection:* 50 mg/ml.
- *Vaginal Gel (Crinone, Prochieve):* 4% (45 mg), 8% (90 mg).
- *Topical Cream:* 5% (First Progesterone MC5), 10% (First Progesterone MC10).

UNLABELED USES: Treatment of corpus luteum dysfunction

CONTRAINDICATIONS: Allergy to peanut oil (oral), breast cancer, history of active cerebral apoplexy, thromboembolic disorders or thrombophlebitis, missed abortion, severe hepatic dysfunction, undiagnosed vaginal bleeding, use as a pregnancy test

PREGNANCY AND LACTATION: Pregnancy category D; possible increase in limb reduction defects, hypospadias in male fetuses and mild virilization of female fetuses

SIDE EFFECTS

Frequent

Breakthrough bleeding or spotting at beginning of therapy, amenorrhea, change in menstrual flow, breast tenderness

Gel: Drowsiness

Occasional

Edema, weight gain or loss, rash, pruritus, photosensitivity, skin pigmentation

Rare

Pain or swelling at injection site, acne, depression, alopecia, hirsutism

SERIOUS REACTIONS

• Thrombophlebitis, cerebrovascular disorders, retinal thrombosis, and pulmonary embolism occur rarely.

INTERACTIONS

Drugs

3 *Aminoglutethimide:* Possible decreased progestin effect

3 *Bromocriptine:* May interfere with the effects of bromocriptine

Labs

• *Increase:* Alk phosphatase, pregnanediol, liver function tests

• *Decrease:* Glucose tolerance test, HDL

SPECIAL CONSIDERATIONS

• Gel provides enhanced uterine delivery compared with IM administration

PATIENT/FAMILY EDUCATION

• Diabetic patients may note decreased glucose tolerance

• No evidence that use for habitual or threatened abortion is effective

• Notify clinician of abnormal or excessive bleeding, severe cramping, abnormal or odorous vaginal discharge, missed period (IUD)

• Cost and risk of infection (greatest in first months after insertion) less for nonhormonal IUDs (e.g., ParaGard)

• Use sunscreen and wear protective clothing until tolerance to sunlight and ultraviolet light has been determined

• Stop smoking tobacco

MONITORING PARAMETERS

• Weight

• Blood pressure

• Skin for rash

promethazine hydrochloride

(proe-meth'-a-zeen hye-droe-klor'-ide)

Rx: Adgan, Anergan 50, Antinaus 50, Pentazine, Phenadoz, Phenergan, Phenoject-50, Promacot, Promethegan

Combinations

Rx: with codeine (Phenergan with Codeine Syrup); with dextromethorphan (Phenergan with Dextromethorphan Syrup)

Chemical Class: Ethylamine phenothiazine derivative

Therapeutic Class: Antiemetic; antihistamine; antitussive; antivertigo agent; sedative

DEA Class: Schedule V

CLINICAL PHARMACOLOGY

Mechanism of Action: A phenothiazine that acts as an antihistamine, antiemetic, and sedative-hypnotic. As an antihistamine, inhibits histamine at histamine receptor sites. As an antiemetic, diminishes vestibular stimulation, depresses labyrinthine function, and acts on the chemoreceptor trigger zone. As a sedative-hypnotic, produces CNS depression by decreasing stimulation to the brainstem reticular formation. ***Therapeutic Effect:*** Prevents allergic responses mediated by histamine, such as rhinitis, urticaria, and pruritus. Prevents and relieves nausea and vomiting.

Pharmacokinetics

Route	Onset	Peak	Duration
PO	20 mins	N/A	2-8 hrs
IV	3-5 mins	N/A	2-8 hrs
IM	20 mins	N/A	2-8 hrs
Rectal	20 mins	N/A	2-8 hrs

Well absorbed from the GI tract after IM administration. Widely distributed. Metabolized in the liver. Primarily excreted in urine. Not removed by hemodialysis. ***Half-life:*** 16-19 hrs.

INDICATIONS AND DOSAGES:
Alert: Contraindicated in children 2 yr and younger.

Allergic symptoms

PO

Adults, Elderly. 6.25-12.5 mg 3 times a day plus 25 mg at bedtime.

Children. 0.1 mg/kg/dose (maximum: 12.5 mg) 3 times a day plus 0.5 mg/kg/dose (maximum: 25 mg) at bedtime.

IV, IM

Adults, Elderly. 25 mg. May repeat in 2 hr.

Motion sickness

PO

Adults, Elderly. 25 mg 30-60 min before departure; may repeat in 8-12 hrs, then every morning on rising and before evening meal.

Children. 0.5 mg/kg 30-60 min before departure; may repeat in 8-12 hrs, then every morning on rising and before evening meal.

Prevention of nausea and vomiting

PO, IV, IM, Rectal

Adults, Elderly. 12.5-25 mg q4-6h as needed.

Children. 0.25-1 mg/kg q4-6h as needed.

Preoperative and postoperative sedation; adjunct to analgesics

IV, IM

Adults, Elderly. 25-50 mg.

Children. 12.5-25 mg.

Sedative

PO, IV, IM, Rectal

Adults, Elderly. 25-50 mg/dose. May repeat q4-6h as needed.

Children. 0.5-1 mg/kg/dose q6h as needed. Maximum: 50 mg/dose.

AVAILABLE FORMS

- *Syrup (Pentazine, Phenergan):* 6.25 mg/ml.
- *Tablets (Phenergan, Promacot):* 12.5 mg, 25 mg, 50 mg.
- *Injection:* 25 mg/ml (Phenergan), 50 mg/ml (Adgan, Anergan 50, Antinaus 50, Phenergan, Phenoject-50, Promacot).
- *Suppositories:* 12.5 mg (Phenergan, Promethegan), 25 mg (Phenadoz, Phenergan, Promethegan), 50 mg (Phenergan, Promethegan).

CONTRAINDICATIONS: Angle-closure glaucoma, children 2 yr and younger, GI or GU obstruction, hypersensitivity to phenothiazines, severe CNS depression or coma

PREGNANCY AND LACTATION: Pregnancy category C; passage of drug into breast milk should be expected

SIDE EFFECTS

Expected

Somnolence, disorientation; in elderly, hypotension, confusion, syncope

Frequent

Dry mouth, nose, or throat; urine retention; thickening of bronchial secretions

Occasional

Epigastric distress, flushing, visual disturbances, hearing disturbances, wheezing, paresthesia, diaphoresis, chills

Rare
Dizziness, urticaria, photosensitivity, nightmares

SERIOUS REACTIONS

- Children may experience paradoxical reactions, such as excitation, nervousness, tremor, hyperactive reflexes, and seizures.
- Infants and young children have experienced CNS depression manifested as respiratory depression, sleep apnea, and sudden infant death syndrome.
- Long-term therapy may produce extrapyramidal symptoms, such as dystonia (abnormal movements), pronounced motor restlessness (most frequently in children), and parkinsonian (most frequently in elderly patients).
- Blood dyscrasias, particularly agranulocytosis, occur rarely.

INTERACTIONS

Drugs

3 *Alcohol, CNS depressants:* Additive sedative action

3 *Anticholinergics:* May increase anticholinergic effects

3 *MAOIs:* May intensify and prolong the anticholinergic and CNS depressant effects of promethazine

Labs

- *False increase:* Tricyclic antidepressant

SPECIAL CONSIDERATIONS

PATIENT/FAMILY EDUCATION

- Avoid prolonged exposure to sunlight
- Drowsiness and dry mouth are expected side effects of the drug. Drinking coffee or tea may help reduce drowsiness, and sipping tepid water and chewing sugarless gum may relieve dry mouth
- Avoid performing tasks that require mental alertness or motor skills until response to the drug has been established
- Notify the physician if visual disturbances occur
- Avoid alcohol

MONITORING PARAMETERS

- Blood pressure, pulse
- Electrolytes

propafenone hydrochloride

(proe-pa-feen'-one hye-droe-klor'-ide)

Rx: Rythmol, Rythmol SR
Chemical Class: 3-phenylpropiophenone derivative
Therapeutic Class: Antiarrhythmic, class IC

CLINICAL PHARMACOLOGY

Mechanism of Action: An antiarrhythmic that decreases the fast sodium current in Purkinje or myocardial cells. Decreases excitability and automaticity; prolongs conduction velocity and the refractory period. ***Therapeutic Effect:*** Suppresses arrhythmias.

Pharmacokinetics

Nearly completely absorbed following oral administration. Protein binding: 85%-97%. Metabolized in liver; undergoes first-pass metabolism. Primarily excreted in feces. ***Half-life:*** 2-10 hr.

INDICATIONS AND DOSAGES

Documented, life-threatening ventricular arrhythmias, such as sustained ventricular tachycardia

PO

Adults, Elderly. Initially, 150 mg q8h; may increase at 3-4-day intervals to 225 mg q8h, then to 300 mg q8h. Maximum: 900 mg/day.

PO (Extended-Release)

Adults, Elderly. Initially, 225 mg q12h. May increase at 5-day intervals. Maximum: 425 mg q12h.

AVAILABLE FORMS

• *Tablets (Rythmol):* 150 mg, 225 mg, 300 mg.

• *Capsules (Extended-Release [Rythmol SR]):* 225 mg, 325 mg, 425 mg.

UNLABELED USES: Treatment of supraventricular arrhythmias

CONTRAINDICATIONS: Bradycardia; bronchospastic disorders; cardiogenic shock; electrolyte imbalance; sinoatrial, AV, and intraventricular impulse generation or conduction disorders, such as sick sinus syndrome or AV block, without the presence of a pacemaker; uncontrolled CHF

PREGNANCY AND LACTATION: Pregnancy category C

SIDE EFFECTS

Frequent (13%-7%)

Dizziness, nausea, vomiting, altered taste, constipation

Occasional (6%-3%)

Headache, dyspnea, blurred vision, dyspepsia (heartburn, indigestion, epigastric pain)

Rare (less than 2%)

Rash, weakness, dry mouth, diarrhea, edema, hot flashes

SERIOUS REACTIONS

• Propafenone may produce or worsen existing arrhythmias.

• Overdose may produce hypotension, somnolence, bradycardia, and atrioventricular conduction disturbances.

INTERACTIONS

Drugs

3 *β-blockers:* Increased metoprolol or propranolol concentrations

3 *Cimetidine:* Increased propafenone concentrations

3 *Digitalis glycosides:* Increased serum digoxin concentrations

3 *Food:* Increased peak serum propafenone concentrations

3 *Oral anticoagulants:* Increased serum warfarin concentrations, prolonged protime

3 *Quinidine:* Increased propafenone concentrations but reduced concentrations of its active metabolite; net effect uncertain (toxicity vs reduced efficacy)

3 *Rifampin, phenobarbital, rifabutin:* Reduced serum propafenone concentrations

3 *Theophylline:* Increased plasma theophylline concentrations

2 *Thioridazine:* Increases thioridazine serum concentrations, and thus may increase the risk of ventricular arrhythmias

SPECIAL CONSIDERATIONS

PATIENT/FAMILY EDUCATION

• Signs of overdosage include hypotension, excessive drowsiness, decreased heart rate, or abnormal heartbeat

• Compliance is essential to control arrhythmias

• Altered taste sensation may occur

• Notify the physician if blurred vision or headache occurs

• Avoid tasks that require mental alertness or motor skills until response to the drug has been established

MONITORING PARAMETERS

• ECG, consider dose reduction in patients with significant widening of the QRS complex or second- or third-degree AV block

• ANA, carefully evaluate abnormal ANA test, consider discontinuation if persistent or worsening ANA titers are detected

• Electrolytes

• Pattern of daily bowel activity and stool consistency

• Hepatic enzymes

• Therapeutic serum level, which is 0.06-1 mcg/ml

propantheline bromide

(proe-pan-the-leen broe'-mide)

Rx: Pro-Banthine

Chemical Class: Quaternary ammonium derivative

Therapeutic Class: Antispasmodic; antiulcer agent (adjunct); gastrointestinal

CLINICAL PHARMACOLOGY

Mechanism of Action: A quaternary ammonium compound that has anticholinergic properties and inhibits action of acetylcholine at postganglionic parasympathetic sites. ***Therapeutic Effect:*** Reduces gastric secretions and urinary frequency, urgency and urge incontinence.

Pharmacokinetics

Onset occurs within 90 min but less than 50% is absorbed from gastrointestinal (GI) tract. Extensive hepatic metabolism. Excreted in the urine and feces. ***Half-life:*** 2.9 hrs.

INDICATIONS AND DOSAGES

Peptic ulcer

PO

Adults, Elderly. 15 mg 3 times/day 30 mins before meals and 30 mg at bedtime.

Children. 1-2 mg/kg/day, divided q4-6h and at bedtime.

AVAILABLE FORMS

• *Tablets:* 7.5 mg, 15 mg (Pro-Banthine).

CONTRAINDICATIONS: GI or genitourinary (GU) obstruction, myasthenia gravis, narrow-angle glaucoma, toxic megacolon, severe ulcerative colitis, unstable cardiovascular adjustment in acute hemorrhage, hypersensitivity to propantheline or other anticholinergics

PREGNANCY AND LACTATION: Pregnancy category C; excretion into breast milk unknown, although would be expected to be minimal due to quaternary structure

SIDE EFFECTS

Frequent

Dry mouth, decreased sweating, constipation

Occasional

Blurred vision, intolerance to light, urinary hesitancy, drowsiness, agitation, excitement

Rare

Confusion, increased intraocular pressure, orthostatic hypotension, tachycardia

SERIOUS REACTIONS

• Overdosage may produce temporary paralysis of ciliary muscle, pupillary dilation, tachycardia, palpitations, hot, dry, or flushed skin, absence of bowel sounds, hyperthermia, increased respiratory rate, EKG abnormalities, nausea, vomiting, rash over face or upper trunk, CNS stimulation, and psychosis, marked by agitation, restlessness, rambling speech, visual hallucinations, paranoid behavior, and delusions, followed by depression.

INTERACTIONS

Drugs

3 *Belladonna alkaloids, synthetic or semisynthetic anticholinergic agents, narcotic analgesics such as meperidine, Type 1 antiarrhythmic drugs (e.g., disopyramide, procainamide, or quinidine), antihistamines, phenothiazines, tricyclic antidepressants, or other psychoactive drugs:* Additive anticholinergic effects

3 *Digoxin:* May cause increased serum digoxin levels with slow-dissolving tablets of digoxin

Labs

• *False increase:* Bicarbonate, chloride

SPECIAL CONSIDERATIONS

PATIENT/FAMILY EDUCATION

- Avoid driving or other hazardous activities until stabilized on medication
- Avoid alcohol or other CNS depressants
- Avoid hot environments, heat stroke may occur
- Use sunglasses when outside to prevent photophobia, may cause blurred vision

MONITORING PARAMETERS

- Blood pressure, body temperature
- Bowel sounds for peristalsis

---

propoxyphene hydrochloride/ propoxyphene napsylate

(proe-pox'-i-feen hye-droe-klor'-ide)

Rx: (propoxyphene hydrochloride) Darvon

Rx: (propoxyphene napsylate) Darvon-N

Combinations

Rx: with acetaminophen (Darvocet, Propacet, Wygesic)

Chemical Class: Diphenylheptane derivative; opiate derivative

Therapeutic Class: Narcotic analgesic

DEA Class: Schedule IV

CLINICAL PHARMACOLOGY

Mechanism of Action: An opioid agonist that binds with opioid receptors in the CNS. ***Therapeutic Effect:*** Alters the perception of and emotional response to pain.

Pharmacokinetics

Route	Onset	Peak	Duration
PO	15-60 mins	N/A	4-6 hrs

Well absorbed from the GI tract. Protein binding: high. Widely distributed. Metabolized in the liver. Primarily excreted in urine. Not removed by hemodialysis. ***Half-life:*** 6-12 hr; metabolite: 30-36 hr.

INDICATIONS AND DOSAGES

Mild to moderate pain

PO (propoxyphene hydrochloride)

Adults, Elderly. 65 mg q4h as needed. Maximum: 390 mg/day.

PO (propoxyphene napsylate)

Adults, Elderly. 100 mg q4h as needed. Maximum: 600 mg/day.

AVAILABLE FORMS

- *Capsules (Hydrochloride):* 65 mg.
- *Tablets (Napsylate):* 100 mg.

CONTRAINDICATIONS: None known.

PREGNANCY AND LACTATION: Pregnancy category C (category D if used for prolonged periods or in high doses at term); withdrawal could theoretically occur in infants exposed *in utero* to prolonged maternal ingestion; compatible with breast-feeding

Controlled Substance: Schedule IV

SIDE EFFECTS

Frequent

Dizziness, somnolence, dry mouth, euphoria, hypotension (including orthostatic hypotension), nausea, vomiting, fatigue

Occasional

Allergic reaction (including decreased BP), diaphoresis, flushing, and wheezing), trembling, urine retention, vision changes, constipation, headache

Rare

Confusion, increased BP, depression, abdominal cramps, anorexia

SERIOUS REACTIONS

- Overdose results in respiratory depression, skeletal muscle flaccidity, cold or clammy skin, cyanosis, and extreme somnolence progressing to seizures, stupor, and coma.

• Hepatotoxicity may occur with overdose of the acetaminophen component of fixed-combination products.
• The patient who uses propoxyphene repeatedly may develop a tolerance to the drug's analgesic effect and physical dependence.

INTERACTIONS

Drugs

3 *Anticoagulants:* Potentiation of warfarin's anticoagulant effect
3 *Antidepressants:* Increased cyclic antidepressant serum concentrations
3 *Antihistamines, chloral hydrate, glutethimide, methocarbamol:* Enhanced depressant effects
3 *Barbiturates:* Additive respiratory and CNS depressant effects
3 *β-blockers:* Increased concentrations of highly metabolized β-blockers (metoprolol, propranolol)
3 *Buprenorphine:* May decrease the effects of propoxyphene
❷ *Carbamazepine:* Marked increases in plasma carbamazepine concentrations
3 *Ethanol, other CNS depressants:* Additive CNS effects
❷ *MAOIs:* May produce a severe, sometimes fatal reaction; plan to administer 25% of usual propoxyphene dose
3 *Protease inhibitors:* Increased respiratory and CNS depression

Labs

• *False increase:* Amylase and lipase

SPECIAL CONSIDERATIONS

PATIENT/FAMILY EDUCATION

• May cause drowsiness, dizziness, or blurred vision
• Use caution driving or engaging in other activities requiring alertness
• Avoid alcohol
• Take propoxyphene before the pain fully returns, within prescribed intervals
• Do not abruptly discontinue the drug
• May be habit-forming

MONITORING PARAMETERS

• Pattern of daily bowel activity and stool consistency
• Clinical improvement and onset of pain relief
• Therapeutic serum level of propoxyphene is 100-400 ng/ml, and the toxic serum level is over 500 ng/ml

propranolol hydrochloride

(proe-pran'-oh-lole hye-droe-klor'-ide)

Rx: Inderal, Inderal LA, InnoPran XL, Propranolol Intensol

Combinations

Rx: with HCTZ (Inderide)

Chemical Class: β-adrenergic blocker, nonselective

Therapeutic Class: Antianginal; antiarrhythmic, class II; antiglaucoma agent; antihypertensive; antimigraine agent

CLINICAL PHARMACOLOGY

Mechanism of Action: An antihypertensive, antianginal, antiarrhythmic, and antimigraine agent that blocks $beta_1$- and $beta_2$-adrenergic receptors. Decreases oxygen requirements. Slows AV conduction and increases refractory period in AV node. Large doses increase airway resistance. ***Therapeutic Effect:*** Slows sinus heart rate; decreases cardiac output, BP, and myocardial ischemia severity. Exhibits antiarrhythmic activity.

Pharmacokinetics

Route	*Onset*	*Peak*	*Duration*
PO	1-2 hrs	N/A	6 hrs

Well absorbed from the GI tract. Protein binding: 93%. Widely distributed. Metabolized in the liver. Primarily excreted in urine. Not removed by hemodialysis. ***Half-life:*** 3-5 hr.

INDICATIONS AND DOSAGES

Hypertension

PO

Adults, Elderly. Initially, 40 mg twice a day. May increase dose q3-7 days. Range: Up to 320 mg/day in divided doses. Maximum: 640 mg/day.

Children. Initially, 0.5-1 mg/kg/day in divided doses q6-12h. May increase at 3- to 5-day intervals. Usual dose: 1-5 mg/kg/day. Maximum: 16 mg/kg/day.

Angina

PO

Adults, Elderly. 80-320 mg/day in divided doses. (Long-acting): Initially, 80 mg/day. Maximum: 320 mg/day.

Arrhythmias

IV

Adults, Elderly. 1 mg/dose. May repeat q5min. Maximum: 5 mg total dose.

Children. 0.01-0.1 mg/kg. Maximum: infants, 1 mg; children, 3 mg.

PO

Adults, Elderly. Initially, 10-20 mg q6-8h. May gradually increase dose. Range: 40-320 mg/day.

Children. Initially, 0.5-1 mg/kg/day in divided doses q6-8h. May increase q3-5 days. Usual dosage: 2-4 mg/kg/day. Maximum: 16 mg/kg/day or 60 mg/day.

Life-threatening arrhythmias

IV

Adults, Elderly. 0.5-3 mg. Repeat once in 2 min. Give additional doses at intervals of at least 4 hr.

Children. 0.01-0.1 mg/kg.

Hypertrophic subaortic stenosis

PO

Adults, Elderly. 20-40 mg in 3-4 divided doses. Or 80-160 mg/day as extended-release capsule.

Adjunct to alpha-blocking agents to treat pheochromocytoma

PO

Adults, Elderly. 60 mg/day in divided doses with alpha-blocker for 3 days before surgery. Maintenance (inoperable tumor): 30 mg/day with alpha-blocker.

Migraine headache

PO

Adults, Elderly. 80 mg/day in divided doses. Or 80 mg once daily as extended-release capsule. Increase up to 160-240 mg/day in divided doses.

Children. 0.6-1.5 mg/kg/day in divided doses q8h. Maximum: 4 mg/kg/day.

Reduction of cardiovascular mortality and reinfarction in patients with previous MI

PO

Adults, Elderly. 180-240 mg/day in divided doses.

Essential tremor

PO

Adults, Elderly. Initially, 40 mg twice a day increased up to 120-320 mg/day in 3 divided doses.

AVAILABLE FORMS

- *Tablets (Inderal):* 10 mg, 20 mg, 40 mg, 60 mg, 80 mg.
- *Capsules (Extended-Release):* 60 mg (Inderal LA), 80 mg (Inderal LA, InnoPran XL), 120 mg (Inderal LA, InnoPran XL), 160 mg (Inderal LA).

• *Oral Solution (Inderal):* 20 mg/5 ml, 40 mg/5 ml.
• *Oral Concentrate (Propranolol Intensol):* 80 mg/ml.
• *Injection (Inderal):* 1 mg/ml.

UNLABELED USES: Treatment adjunct for anxiety, mitral valve prolapse syndrome, thyrotoxicosis

CONTRAINDICATIONS: Asthma, bradycardia, cardiogenic shock, chronic obstructive pulmonary disease (COPD), heart block, Raynaud's syndrome, uncompensated CHF

PREGNANCY AND LACTATION: Pregnancy category C (D if used in second or third trimester); similar drug, atenolol, frequently used in the third trimester for treatment of hypertension (many studies of efficacy and safety of atenolol in pregnancy-induced hypertension); long-term use has been associated with intrauterine growth retardation; milk levels approximately half of peak plasma levels; considered insignificant; compatible with breast-feeding

SIDE EFFECTS

Frequent

Diminished sexual ability, drowsiness, difficulty sleeping, unusual fatigue or weakness

Occasional

Bradycardia, depression, sensation of coldness in extremities, diarrhea, constipation, anxiety, nasal congestion, nausea, vomiting

Rare

Altered taste, dry eyes, pruritus, paresthesia

SERIOUS REACTIONS

• Overdose may produce profound bradycardia and hypotension.
• Abrupt withdrawal may result in sweating, palpitations, headache, and tremors.
• Propranolol administration may precipitate CHF and MI in patients with cardiac disease; thyroid storm in those with thyrotoxicosis; and peripheral ischemia in those with existing peripheral vascular disease.
• Hypoglycemia may occur in patients with previously controlled diabetes.

INTERACTIONS

Drugs

3 *α_1-adrenergic blockers:* Potential enhanced first-dose response (marked initial drop in blood pressure), particularly on standing (especially prazosin)

3 *Amiodarone:* Bradycardia, cardiac arrest, ventricular dysrhythmia shortly after initiation of β-blocker

3 *Antidiabetics:* Masked symptoms of hypoglycemia, prolonged recovery of normoglycemia

3 *Barbiturates, rifampin:* Reduced concentrations of propranolol

3 *Antipyrine:* Increased antipyrine concentrations

3 *β-agonists:* Antagonistic effects

3 *Calcium channel blockers:* Increased concentrations of propranolol; increased bioavailability of nifedipine

3 *Chlorpromazine:* Additive hypotensive effects and grand mal seizures; chlorpromazine decreases the clearance of oral propranolol by 25%-32%, resulting in increased propranolol bioavailability

3 *Cimetidine, etintidine, fluoxetine, propoxyphene, propafenone, quinidine, quinolones:* Increased propranolol concentrations

3 *Clonidine, guanabenz, guanfacine:* Exacerbation of hypertension upon withdrawal of clonidine

3 *Cocaine:* Potentiation of cocaine-induced coronary vasospasm

3 *Contrast media:* Increased risk of anaphylaxis

3 *Digitalis glycosides:* Increased digoxin concentrations

3 *Dihydroergotamine, ergotamine:* May result in excessive vasoconstriction

3 *Epinephrine:* Enhanced pressor response to epinephrine

3 *Fluvoxamine:* Increased propranolol serum concentrations; increased risk of bradycardia and hypotension

3 *Flecainide:* Increased propranolol and flecainide concentrations; additive negative inotropic effects

3 *Hydralazine:* Increases oral bioavailability of propranolol (high clearance and lipophilic β-blockers), increasing risk of adverse effects

3 *Hydrochlorothiazide:* Exaggerated hyperglycemic response

3 *Lidocaine:* Increased lidocaine concentrations

3 *Local anesthetics:* Enhanced sympathomimetic side effects of epinephrine-containing local anesthetics

3 *Neostigmine, physostigmine, tacrine:* Additive bradycardia

3 *Neuroleptics:* Increased plasma concentrations of both drugs

3 *NSAIDs:* Reduced hypotensive effect of propranolol

3 *Phenylephrine:* Predisposition to acute hypertensive episodes

2 *Theophylline:* Increased theophylline concentrations; antagonistic pharmacodynamic effects

Labs

- *False increase:* Bilirubin

SPECIAL CONSIDERATIONS

PATIENT/FAMILY EDUCATION

- Do not discontinue abruptly, may require taper; rapid withdrawal may produce rebound hypertension or angina
- If a dose is missed, take the next scheduled dose and do not double the dose
- Rise slowly from a lying to sitting position and wait momentarily before standing to avoid the drug's hypotensive effect
- Do not take nasal decongestants and OTC cold preparations, especially those containing stimulants, without physician approval
- Limit alcohol and salt intake

MONITORING PARAMETERS

- *Angina:* Reduction in nitroglycerin usage; frequency, severity, onset, and duration of angina pain; heart rate
- *Arrhythmias:* Heart rate
- *Congestive heart failure:* Functional status, cough, dyspnea on exertion, paroxysmal nocturnal dyspnea, exercise tolerance, and ventricular function
- *Hypertension:* Blood pressure
- *Migraine headache:* Reduction in the frequency, severity, and duration of attacks
- *Postmyocardial infarction:* Left ventricular function, lower resting heart rate
- *Toxicity:* Blood glucose, bronchospasm, hypotension, bradycardia, depression, confusion, hallucination, sexual dysfunction

P

propylthiouracil

(proe-pill-thye-oh-yoor′-a-sill)

Chemical Class: Thioamide derivative

Therapeutic Class: Antithyroid agent

CLINICAL PHARMACOLOGY

Mechanism of Action: A thiourea derivative that blocks oxidation of iodine in the thyroid gland and blocks synthesis of thyroxine and triiodothyronine. ***Therapeutic Effect:*** Inhibits synthesis of thyroid hormone.

Pharmacokinetics

Readily absorbed from GI tract. Protein binding: 80%. Metabolized in liver. Excreted in urine. ***Half-life:*** 1-4 hr.

INDICATIONS AND DOSAGES

Hyperthyroidism

PO

Adults, Elderly. Initially: 300-450 mg/day in divided doses q8h. Maintenance: 100-150 mg/day in divided doses q8-12h.

Children. Initially: 5-7 mg/kg/day in divided doses q8h. Maintenance: 33%-66% of initial dose in divided doses q8-12h.

Neonates. 5-10 mg/kg/day in divided doses q8h.

AVAILABLE FORMS

• *Tablets:* 50 mg.

CONTRAINDICATIONS: Breast-feeding mothers

PREGNANCY AND LACTATION: Pregnancy category D; considered drug of choice for medical treatment of hyperthyroidism during pregnancy; excreted into breast milk in low amounts; compatible with breast-feeding

SIDE EFFECTS

Frequent

Urticaria, rash, pruritus, nausea, skin pigmentation, hair loss, headache, paresthesia

Occasional

Somnolence, lymphadenopathy, vertigo

Rare

Drug fever, lupus-like syndrome

SERIOUS REACTIONS

• Agranulocytosis as long as 4 mos after therapy, pancytopenia, and fatal hepatitis have occurred.

INTERACTIONS

Drugs

3 *Amiodarone, iodinated glycerol, iodine, potassium iodide:* May decrease response of propylthiouracil

3 *Digoxin:* May increase digoxin blood concentration as patient becomes euthyroid

3 *I^{131}:* May decrease thyroid uptake of I^{131}

3 *Oral anticoagulants:* Reduced hypoprothrombinemic response to oral anticoagulants

3 *Theophylline:* Physiologic response to antithyroid drug will increase theophylline concentrations via decreased clearance

Labs

• *False increase:* Glucose

SPECIAL CONSIDERATIONS

PATIENT/FAMILY EDUCATION

• Notify clinician of fever, sore throat, unusual bleeding or bruising, rash, yellowing of skin, vomiting

• Space doses evenly around the clock

• Take resting pulse daily to monitor therapeutic results; report pulse rate of less than 60 beats per min

• Restrict consumption of iodine products and seafood

MONITORING PARAMETERS

• CBC periodically during therapy (especially during initial 3 mo), TSH

• Pulse

• Weight

• Be alert to signs and symptoms of hepatitis, including somnolence, jaundice, nausea, and vomiting

protamine sulfate

(proe′-ta-meen sul′-fate)
Chemical Class: Basic protein
Therapeutic Class: Antidote, heparin

CLINICAL PHARMACOLOGY
Mechanism of Action: A protein that complexes with heparin to form a stable salt. ***Therapeutic Effect:*** Reduces anticoagulant activity of heparin.
Pharmacokinetics
Metabolized by fibrinolysin. ***Half-life:*** 7.4 min.
INDICATIONS AND DOSAGES
Heparin overdose (antidote and treatment)
IV
Adults, Elderly. 1-1.5 mg protamine neutralizes 100 units heparin. Heparin disappears rapidly from circulation, reducing the dosage demand for protamine as time elapses.
AVAILABLE FORMS
• *Injection:* 10 mg/ml.
UNLABELED USES: Treatment of low-molecular-weight heparin toxicity
CONTRAINDICATIONS: None known.
PREGNANCY AND LACTATION: Pregnancy category C
SIDE EFFECTS
Frequent
Decreased BP, dyspnea
Occasional
Hypersensitivity reaction (urticaria, angioedema); nausea and vomiting, which generally occur in those sensitive to fish and seafood, vasectomized men, infertile men, those on isophane (NPH) insulin, or those previously on protamine therapy
Rare
Back pain
SERIOUS REACTIONS
• Too-rapid IV administration may produce acute hypotension, bradycardia, pulmonary hypertension, dyspnea, transient flushing, and feeling of warmth.
• Heparin rebound may occur several hours after heparin has been neutralized (usually 8-9 hrs after protamine administration). Heparin rebound occurs most often after arterial or cardiac surgery.
SPECIAL CONSIDERATIONS
• Will not reliably inactivate low-molecular-weight heparin
• Activated partial thromboplastin time (aPTT) or protamine activated clotting time (ACT) 15 min after dose, then in several hr
PATIENT/FAMILY EDUCATION
• Use an electric razor and soft toothbrush to prevent bleeding until coagulation studies normalize
• Report black or red stool, coffee-ground vomitus, dark or red urine, or red-speckled mucus from cough
MONITORING PARAMETERS
• Activated clotting time, aPTT, BP, cardiac function, and other coagulation tests

P

protriptyline hydrochloride

(proe-trip′-ti-leen hye-droe-klor′-ide)
Rx: *Vivactil*
Chemical Class: Dibenzocycloheptene derivative; secondary amine
Therapeutic Class: Antidepressant, tricyclic

CLINICAL PHARMACOLOGY
Mechanism of Action: A tricyclic antidepressant that increases synaptic concentration of norepinephrine and/or serotonin by inhibiting their

reuptake by presynaptic membranes. ***Therapeutic Effect:*** Produces antidepressant effect.

Pharmacokinetics

Well absorbed from the gastrointestinal (GI) tract. Protein binding: 92%. Widely distributed. Extensively metabolized in liver. Excreted in urine. Not removed by hemodialysis. ***Half-life:*** 54-92 hrs.

INDICATIONS AND DOSAGES

Depression

PO

Adults. 15-40 mg/day divided into 3-4 doses/day. Maximum: 600 mg/day.

Elderly. 5 mg 3 times/day. May increase gradually.

AVAILABLE FORMS

- *Tablets:* 5 mg, 10 mg (Vivactil).

UNLABELED USES: Narcolepsy, sleep apnea, sleep hypoxemia

CONTRAINDICATIONS: Acute recovery period after myocardial infarction, coadministration with cisapride, use of MAOIs within 14 days, hypersensitivity to protriptyline or any component of the formulation

PREGNANCY AND LACTATION: Pregnancy category C

SIDE EFFECTS

Frequent

Drowsiness, weight gain, fatigue, dry mouth, blurred vision, constipation, delayed micturition, postural hypotension, diaphoresis, disturbed concentration, increased appetite, urinary retention

Occasional

Gastrointestinal (GI) disturbances, such as nausea, diarrhea, GI distress, metallic taste sensation

Rare

Paradoxical reaction, marked by agitation, restlessness, nightmares, insomnia, extrapyramidal symptoms, particularly fine hand tremor

SERIOUS REACTIONS

- High dosage may produce confusion, seizures, severe drowsiness, arrhythmias, fever, hallucinations, agitation, shortness of breath, vomiting, and unusual tiredness or weakness.
- Abrupt withdrawal from prolonged therapy may produce severe headache, malaise, nausea, vomiting, and vivid dreams.

INTERACTIONS

Drugs

3 *Altretamine:* Orthostatic hypotension

3 *Amphetamines:* Theoretic increase in effect of amphetamines, clinical evidence lacking

3 *Antidiabetics:* Monitor for enhanced hypoglycemia

3 *Antithyroid agents:* May increase the risk of agranulocytosis

3 *Barbiturates, rifampin, carbamazepine:* Reduced cyclic antidepressant concentrations

3 *β-agonists (especially isoproterenol):* Cardiac arrhythmia risk increased

❷ *Bethanidine, clonidine, guanethidine, guanabenz, guanfacine, guanadrel, debrisoquen:* Reduced antihypertensive effect

❷ *Epinephrine, norepinephrine:* Markedly enhanced pressor response to IV administration

3 *Ethanol:* Additive impairment of motor skills; abstinent alcoholics may eliminate cyclic antidepressants more rapidly than non-alcoholics

3 *Fluoxetine, paroxetine:* Marked increases in cyclic antidepressant plasma concentrations

3 *H_2-blockers (especially cimetidine), calcium channel blockers:* Increased cyclic concentrations

3 *Lithium:* Increased risk of neurotoxicity (especially in elderly)

3 *MAOIs:* Excessive sympathetic response, mania, or hyperpyrexia possible

3 *Neuroleptics:* Increased therapeutic and toxic effects of both drugs

3 *Phenothiazines:* May increase the anticholinergic and sedative effects of protriptyline

3 *Phenylephrine:* Enhanced pressor response

3 *Phenytoin:* May decrease protriptyline blood concentration

3 *Propantheline:* Enhanced anticholinergic effects

3 *Propoxyphene:* Enhanced effect of cyclic antidepressants

3 *Quinidine:* Increased cyclic antidepressant serum concentrations

3 *Ritonavir, indinavir:* Possible increased cyclic concentrations, toxicity

3 *St. John's Wort:* May have additive effects

3 *Sympathomimetics:* May increase cardiac effects

Labs

- *Increase:* Serum bilirubin, blood glucose, alk phosphatase
- *Decrease:* VMA, 5-HIAA
- *False increase:* Urinary catecholamines

SPECIAL CONSIDERATIONS

PATIENT/FAMILY EDUCATION

- Therapeutic effects may take 2-3 wk
- Use caution in driving or other activities requiring alertness
- Avoid rising quickly from sitting to standing, especially in elderly
- Avoid alcohol and other CNS depressants
- Do not discontinue abruptly after long-term use
- Wear sunscreen or large hat to prevent photosensitivity
- Chew sugarless gum for dry mouth

MONITORING PARAMETERS

- CBC, weight, ECG, mental status (mood, sensorium, affect, suicidal tendencies)

pseudoephedrine hydrochloride

(soo-doe-e-fed′-rin hye-droe-klor′-ide)

OTC: Biofed, Cenafed, Decofed, Decofed, Dimetapp 12 Hour Non Drowsy Extentabs, Dimetapp Decongestant, Dimetapp Decongestant Infant Drops, Efidac Genaphed, PediaCare Infants' Decongestant, Seudotabs, Sudafed, Sudafed 12 Hour Caplets, Sudafed 24 Hour (Pseudoephedrine is available in many prescription and over-the-counter combinations; the following list is not all-inclusive)

Combinations

Rx: with azatadine (Trinalin Repetabs); brompheniramine (Bromfed); carbinoxamine (Rondec); chlorpheniramine (Deconamine SR, Novafed A); codeine (Nucofed); guaifenesin and codeine (Novagest Expectorant); loratadine (Claritin-D)

OTC: with acetaminophen (Dristan Cold); chlorpheniramine (Chlor-Trimeton 12 Hour Relief); dexbrompheniramine (Drixoral Cold and Allergy); dextromethorphan (Thera-Flu Non-Drowsy Formula); diphenhydramine (Actifed Allergy); ibuprofen (Advil Cold & Sinus, Dristan Sinus); triprolidine (Actifed)

Chemical Class: Sympathomimetic amine

Therapeutic Class: Decongestant

CLINICAL PHARMACOLOGY

Mechanism of Action: A sympathomimetic that directly stimulates alpha-adrenergic and beta-adrenergic receptors. ***Therapeutic Effect:*** Produces vasoconstriction of respiratory tract mucosa; shrinks nasal mucous membranes; reduces edema, and nasal congestion.

Pharmacokinetics

Route	*Onset*	*Peak*	*Duration*
PO (Tablets, Syrup)	15-30 mins	N/A	4-6 hrs
PO (Extended-Release)	N/A	N/A	8-12 hrs

Well absorbed from the GI tract. Partially metabolized in the liver. Primarily excreted in urine. Not removed by hemodialysis. ***Half-life:*** 9-16 hr (children, 3.1 hr).

INDICATIONS AND DOSAGES

Decongestant

PO

Adults, Children 12 yrs and older. 60 mg q4-6h. Maximum: 240 mg/day.

Children 6-11 yrs. 30 mg q6h. Maximum: 120 mg/day.

Children 2-5 yrs. 15 mg q6h. Maximum: 60 mg/day.

Children younger than 2 yrs. 4 mg/kg/day in divided doses q6h.

Elderly. 30-60 mg q6h as needed.

PO (Extended-Release)

Adults, Children 12 yrs and older. 120 mg q12h or 240 mg once daily.

AVAILABLE FORMS

- *Gelcaps (Dimetapp Decongestant):* 30 mg.
- *Liquid:* 15 mg/5 ml.
- *Oral Drops (Dimetapp Decongestant Infant Drops):* 7.5 mg/0.8 ml.
- *Syrup (Biofed, Decofed):* 30 mg/5 ml.

• *Tablets (Genaphed, Sudafed):* 30 mg.
• *Tablets (Chewable [Sudafed]):* 15 mg.
• *Tablets (Extended-Release):* 120 mg (Dimetapp 12 Hour Non Drowsy Extentabs, Sudafed 12 Hour), 240 mg (Sudafed 24 Hour).

CONTRAINDICATIONS: Breast-feeding women, coronary artery disease, severe hypertension, use within 14 days of MAOIs. Sustained release: children younger than 12 yrs.

PREGNANCY AND LACTATION: Pregnancy category C; not compatible with breast-feeding

SIDE EFFECTS

Occasional (10%-5%)
Nervousness, restlessness, insomnia, tremor, headache

Rare (4%-1%)
Diaphoresis, weakness

SERIOUS REACTIONS

• Large doses may produce tachycardia, palpitations (particularly in patients with cardiac disease), lightheadedness, nausea, and vomiting.
• Overdose in patients older than 60 yrs may result in hallucinations, CNS depression, and seizures.

INTERACTIONS

Drugs

3 *Antacids:* Sodium bicarbonate doses sufficient to alkalinize urine can inhibit elimination of pseudoephedrine

3 *Antihypertensives, β-blockers, diuretics:* May decrease the effects of these drugs

⚠ *MAOIs:* Hypertensive crisis

Labs

• *False increase:* Theophylline

SPECIAL CONSIDERATIONS

PATIENT/FAMILY EDUCATION

• May cause wakefulness or nervousness
• Take last dose 4-6 hr prior to hs, notify clinician of insomnia, dizziness, weakness, tremor, or irregular heartbeat
• Swallow extended-release tablets whole, do not chew or crush them
• Discontinue therapy and notify the physician if dizziness, insomnia, irregular or rapid heartbeat, tremors, or other side effects occurs

MONITORING PARAMETERS

• Therapeutic response

---

psyllium

(sil'-i-yum)

OTC: Fiberall, Hydrocil, Konsyl, Metamucil, Perdiem

Combinations

OTC: with senna (Perdiem)

Chemical Class: Psyllium colloid

Therapeutic Class: Laxative

CLINICAL PHARMACOLOGY

Mechanism of Action: A bulk-forming laxative that dissolves and swells in water, providing increased bulk and moisture content in stool. ***Therapeutic Effect:*** Promotes peristalsis and bowel motility.

Pharmacokinetics

Route	Onset	Peak	Duration
PO	12-24 hrs	2-3 days	N/A

Acts in small and large intestines.

INDICATIONS AND DOSAGES

Constipation, irritable bowel syndrome

PO

Alert: 3.4 g powder equals 1 rounded tsp, 1 packet, or 1 wafer.

Adults, Elderly. 2-5 capsules/dose 1-3 times a day. 1-2 tsp granules 1-2 times a day. 1 rounded tsp or 1 tbsp of powder 1-3 times a day. 2 wafers 1-3 times a day.

Children 6-11 yrs. One half-1 tsp powder in water 1-3 times a day.

AVAILABLE FORMS

- *Powder (Fiberall, Hydrocil, Konsyl, Metamucil).*
- *Wafer (Metamucil):* 3.4 g/dose.
- *Capsules (Metamucil):* 0.52 g.
- *Granules (Perdiem):* 4 g/5 ml.

CONTRAINDICATIONS: Fecal impaction, GI obstruction, undiagnosed abdominal pain

PREGNANCY AND LACTATION: Pregnancy category B; not systemically absorbed; exposure of fetus or nursing infant unlikely

SIDE EFFECTS

Rare

Some degree of abdominal discomfort, nausea, mild abdominal cramps, griping, faintness

SERIOUS REACTIONS

- Esophageal or bowel obstruction may occur if administered less than 250 ml of liquid.

INTERACTIONS

Drugs

3 *Digoxin, oral anticoagulants, salicylates:* May decrease the effects of digoxin, oral anticoagulants, and salicylates by decreasing absorption

3 *Potassium-sparing diuretics, potassium supplements:* May interfere with the effects of potassium-sparing diuretics and potassium supplements

SPECIAL CONSIDERATIONS

PATIENT/FAMILY EDUCATION

- Maintain adequate fluid consumption
- Do not use in presence of abdominal pain, nausea, or vomiting
- Avoid inhaling dust from powder preparations; can cause runny nose, watery eyes, wheezing
- Institute measures to promote defecation such as increasing fluid intake, exercising, and eating a high-fiber diet

MONITORING PARAMETERS

- Pattern of daily bowel activity and stool consistency; record time of evacuation
- Serum electrolyte levels

pyrantel pamoate

(pi-ran'-tel)

OTC: Antiminth, Pin-Rid, Pin-X, Reese's Pinworm

Chemical Class: Pyrimidine derivative

Therapeutic Class: Antihelmintic

CLINICAL PHARMACOLOGY

Mechanism of Action: A depolarizing neuromuscular blocking agent that causes the release of acetylcholine and inhibits cholinesterase. ***Therapeutic Effect:*** Results in a spastic paralysis of the worm and consequent expulsion from the host's intestinal tract.

Pharmacokinetics

Poorly absorbed through gastrointestinal (GI) tract. Time to peak occurs in 1-3 hrs. Partially metabolized in liver. Primarily excreted in feces; minimal elimination in urine.

INDICATIONS AND DOSAGES

Enterobiasis vermicularis (pinworm)

PO

Adults, Elderly, Children older than 2 yrs. 11 mg base/kg once. Repeat in 2 wks. Maximum: 1 g/day.

AVAILABLE FORMS

- *Caplets:* 180 mg (Reese's Pinworm Caplets).
- *Capsules:* 180 mg (Pin-Rid).
- *Liquid:* 50 mg/ml (Reese's Pinworm Medicine).
- *Suspension, oral:* 50 mg/ml (Antiminth, Pin-X).

CONTRAINDICATIONS: Hypersensitivity to pyrantel or any of its components

PREGNANCY AND LACTATION: Pregnancy category C

SIDE EFFECTS

Occasional

Nausea, vomiting, headache, dizziness, drowsiness, GI distress, weakness

SERIOUS REACTIONS

• Overdosage includes symptoms of anorexia, nausea, abdominal cramps, vomiting, diarrhea, and ataxia.

INTERACTIONS

Drugs

❷ *Piperazine:* Mutual antagonism

SPECIAL CONSIDERATIONS

PATIENT/FAMILY EDUCATION

• Take with food or milk
• Using a laxative to facilitate expulsion of worms is not necessary
• All family members in close contact with patient should be treated
• Strict hygiene is essential to prevent reinfection
• Shake suspension well before pouring
• Wash bedding and clothes to avoid being reinfected

MONITORING PARAMETERS

• Examine stool for presence of eggs or worms

---

pyrazinamide

(peer-a-zin'-a-mide)

Rx: Pyrazinamide

Chemical Class: Niacinamide derivative

Therapeutic Class: Antituberculosis agent

CLINICAL PHARMACOLOGY

Mechanism of Action: An antitubercular whose exact mechanism of action is unknown. ***Therapeutic Effect:*** Either bacteriostatic or bactericidal, depending on the drug's concentration at the infection site and the susceptibility of infecting bacteria.

Pharmacokinetics

Nearly completely absorbed from GI tract. Protein binding: 5%-10%. Excreted in urine. ***Half-life:*** 9-23 hr.

INDICATIONS AND DOSAGES

Tuberculosis (in combination with other antituberculars)

PO

Adults. 15-30 mg/kg/day in 1-4 doses. Maximum: 3 g/day.

Children. 20-40 mg/kg/day in 1 or 2 doses. Maximum: 2 g/day.

AVAILABLE FORMS

• *Tablets:* 500 mg.

CONTRAINDICATIONS: Severe hepatic dysfunction

PREGNANCY AND LACTATION: Pregnancy category C; excreted into human milk

SIDE EFFECTS

Frequent

Arthralgia, myalgia (usually mild and self-limiting)

Rare

Hypersensitivity reaction (rash, pruritus, urticaria), photosensitivity, gouty arthritis

SERIOUS REACTIONS

• Hepatotoxicity, gouty arthritis, thrombocytopenia, and anemia occur rarely.

INTERACTIONS

Drugs

❸ *Allopurinol, colchicine, probenecid, sulfinpyrazone:* May decrease the effects of these drugs

❸ *Cyclosporine:* Decreased concentrations of cyclosporine

❸ *Tacrolimus:* Decreased concentrations of tacrolimus

Labs

• *False positive:* Urine ketone tests

SPECIAL CONSIDERATIONS

PATIENT/FAMILY EDUCATION

- Compliance with full course is essential
- Notify clinician of fever, loss of appetite, malaise, nausea and vomiting, darkened urine, yellowish discoloration of skin and eyes, pain or swelling of joints
- Take with food to reduce GI upset
- Do not skip doses
- Follow-up physician office visits and laboratory tests are essential parts of treatment
- Avoid overexposure to the sun or ultraviolet light

MONITORING PARAMETERS

- Liver function tests, serum uric acid at baseline and periodically throughout therapy
- Blood glucose levels, especially in patients with diabetes mellitus, because pyrazinamide administration may make diabetes management difficult
- Skin for rash
- CBC for anemia and thrombocytopenia

pyridostigmine bromide

(peer-id-oh-stig′-meen broe′-mide)

Rx: Mestinon, Mestinon Timespan

Chemical Class: Cholinesterase inhibitor; quaternary ammonium derivative

Therapeutic Class: Cholinergic

CLINICAL PHARMACOLOGY

Mechanism of Action: A cholinergic that prevents destruction of acetylcholine by inhibiting the enzyme acetylcholinesterase, thus enhancing impulse transmission across the myoneural junction. ***Therapeutic Effect:*** Produces miosis; increases tone of intestinal, skeletal muscle tone; stimulates salivary and sweat gland secretions.

Pharmacokinetics

Not protein bound. Excreted unchanged in urine. ***Half-life:*** Unknown.

INDICATIONS AND DOSAGES

Myasthenia gravis

PO

Adults, Elderly. Initially, 60 mg 3 times a day. Dosage increased at 48-hr intervals. Maintenance: 60 mg-1.5 g a day.

PO (Extended-Release)

Adults, Elderly. 180-540 mg once or twice a day with at least a 6-hr interval between doses.

IV, IM

Adults, Elderly. 2 mg q2-3h.

Children, Neonates. 0.05-0.15 mg/kg/dose. Maximum single dose: 10 mg.

Reversal of nondepolarizing neuromuscular blockade

IV

Adults, Elderly. 10-20 mg with, or shortly after, 0.6-1.2 mg atropine sulfate or 0.3-0.6 mg glycopyrrolate.

Children. 0.1-0.25 mg/kg/dose preceded by atropine or glycopyrrolate.

AVAILABLE FORMS

- *Syrup (Mestinon):* 60 mg/5 ml.
- *Tablets (Mestinon):* 60 mg.
- *Tablets (Extended-Release [Mestinon Timespan]):* 180 mg.
- *Injection (Mestinon):* 5 mg/ml.

CONTRAINDICATIONS: Mechanical GI or urinary tract obstruction, hypersensitivity to anticholinesterase agents

PREGNANCY AND LACTATION: Pregnancy category C; would not be expected to cross the placenta because it is ionized at physiologic pH; although apparently safe for the fetus, may cause transient muscle weakness in the newborn; compatible with breast-feeding

SIDE EFFECTS

Frequent

Miosis, increased GI and skeletal muscle tone, bradycardia, constriction of bronchi and ureters, diaphoresis, increased salivation

Occasional

Headache, rash, temporary decrease in diastolic BP with mild reflex tachycardia, short periods of atrial fibrillation (in hyperthyroid patients), marked drop in BP (in hypertensive patients)

SERIOUS REACTIONS

• Overdose may produce a cholinergic crisis, manifested as increasingly severe muscle weakness that appears first in muscles involving chewing and swallowing and is followed by muscle weakness of the shoulder girdle and upper extremities, respiratory muscle paralysis, and pelvis girdle and leg muscle paralysis. If overdose occurs, stop all cholinergic drugs and immediately administer 1-4 mg atropine sulfate IV for adults or 0.01 mg/kg for infants and children younger than 12 yrs.

INTERACTIONS

Drugs

3 *Anticholinergics:* Prevent or reverse the effects of pyridostigmine

3 *β-blockers:* Additive bradycardia

3 *Cholinesterase inhibitors:* May increase the risk of toxicity

3 *Neuromuscular blockers:* Antagonizes the effects of these drugs

3 *Procainamide, quinidine:* May antagonize the action of pyridostigmine

3 *Tacrine:* Increased anticholinergic effects

Labs

• *False increase:* Serum bicarbonate, chloride

SPECIAL CONSIDERATIONS

PATIENT/FAMILY EDUCATION

• Do not crush or chew sustained-release preparations

• Notify the physician if diarrhea, difficulty breathing, profuse salivation or sweating, irregular heartbeat, muscle weakness, severe abdominal pain, or nausea and vomiting occurs

• Keep a log of energy level and muscle strength to help guide drug dosing

MONITORING PARAMETERS

• Therapeutic response: increased muscle strength, improved gait, absence of labored breathing (if severe)

• Appearance of side effects (narrow margin between first appearance of side effects and serious toxicity)

• Symptoms of increasing muscle weakness may be due to cholinergic crisis (overdosage) or myasthenic crisis (increased disease severity). If crisis is myasthenia, patient will improve after 1-2 mg edrophonium; if cholinergic, withdraw pyridostigmine and administer atropine

pyridoxine hydrochloride (vitamin B_6)

(peer-i-dox'-een hye-droe'-klor-ide)

Rx: Aminoxin, Beesix, Doxine, Nestrex, Pryi, Rodex, Vitabee 6, Vitamin B_6

Chemical Class: Vitamin B complex

Therapeutic Class: Antidote, hydralazine/isoniazid; vitamin

CLINICAL PHARMACOLOGY

Mechanism of Action: Acts as a coenzyme for various metabolic functions, including metabolism of proteins, carbohydrates, and fats. Aids in the breakdown of glycogen and in the synthesis of gamma-aminobutyric acid in the CNS. ***Therapeutic Effect:*** Prevents pyridoxine deficiency. Increases the excretion of certain drugs, such as isoniazid, that are pyridoxine antagonists.

Pharmacokinetics

Readily absorbed primarily in jejunum. Stored in the liver, muscle, and brain. Metabolized in the liver. Primarily excreted in urine. Removed by hemodialysis. ***Half-life:*** 15-20 days.

INDICATIONS AND DOSAGES

Pyridoxine deficiency

PO

Adults, Elderly. Initially, 2.5-10 mg/day; then 2.5 mg/day when clinical signs are corrected.

Children. Initially, 5-25 mg/day for 3 wk, then 1.5-2.5 mg/day.

Pyridoxine-dependent seizures

PO, IV, IM

Infants. Initially, 10-100 mg/day. Maintenance: PO: 50-100 mg/day.

Drug-induced neuritis

PO (treatment)

Adults, Elderly. 100-300 mg/day in divided doses

Children. 10-50 mg/day.

PO (prophylaxis)

Adults, Elderly. 25-100 mg/day.

Children. 1-2 mg/kg/day.

AVAILABLE FORMS

- *Capsules:* 250 mg.
- *Tablets:* 25 mg, 50 mg, 100 mg, 250 mg, 500 mg.
- *Tablets (Enteric-Coated [Aminoxin]):* 20 mg.
- *Injection (Vitamin B_6):* 100 mg/ml.

CONTRAINDICATIONS: None known.

PREGNANCY AND LACTATION: Pregnancy category A; deficiency during pregnancy is common in unsupplemented women; excreted in human breast milk; RDA for lactating women is 2.3-2.5 mg

SIDE EFFECTS

Occasional

Stinging at IM injection site

Rare

Headache, nausea, somnolence; sensory neuropathy (paresthesia, unstable gait, clumsiness of hands) with high doses

SERIOUS REACTIONS

- Long-term megadoses (2-6 g over more than 2 mo) may produce sensory neuropathy (reduced deep tendon reflexes, profound impairment of sense of position in distal limbs, gradual sensory ataxia). Toxic symptoms subside when drug is discontinued.
- Seizures have occurred after IV megadoses.

INTERACTIONS

Drugs

3 *Immunosuppressants, isoniazid, penicillamine:* May antagonize pyridoxine, causing anemia or peripheral neuritis

3 *Levodopa:* Inhibited antiparkinsonian effect of levodopa; concurrent use of carbidopa negates the interaction

3 *Phenytoin:* Reduced phenytoin concentrations

SPECIAL CONSIDERATIONS

PATIENT/FAMILY EDUCATION

- Avoid doses exceeding RDA unless directed by clinician
- IM injection may cause discomfort
- Eat foods rich in pyridoxine, including avocados, bananas, bran, carrots, eggs, organ meats, tuna, shrimp, hazelnuts, legumes, soybeans, sunflower seeds, and wheat germ

MONITORING PARAMETERS

- Respiratory rate, heart rate, blood pressure during large IV doses
- Observe the patient for improvement of deficiency symptoms, including CNS abnormalities (anxiety, depression, insomnia, motor difficulty, paresthesia and tremors) and skin lesions (glossitis, seborrhea-like lesions around eyes, mouth, nose)

---

pyrimethamine

(pye-ri-meth'-a-meen)

Rx: Daraprim

Combinations

Rx: with sulfadoxine (Fansidar)

Chemical Class: Aminopyrimidine derivative

Therapeutic Class: Antimalarial

CLINICAL PHARMACOLOGY

Mechanism of Action: An antiprotozoal with blood and some tissue schizonticidal activity against malaria parasites of humans. Highly selective activity against plasmodia and *Toxoplasma gondii*. ***Therapeutic Effect:*** Inhibition of tetrahydrofolic acid synthesis.

Pharmacokinetics

Well absorbed, peak levels occurring between 2-6 hrs following administration. Protein binding: 87%. Eliminated slowly. ***Half-life:*** approximately 96 hrs.

INDICATIONS AND DOSAGES

Toxoplasmosis

PO

Adults. Initially, 50-75 mg daily, with 1-4 g daily of a sulfonamide of the sulfapyrimidine type (e.g., sulfadoxine). Continue for 1-3 wks, depending on response of patient and tolerance to therapy then reduce dose to one-half that previously given for each drug and continue for additional 4-5 wks.

Children. 1 mg/kg/day divided into 2 equal daily doses; after 2-4 days reduce to one-half and continue for approximately 1 mo. The usual pediatric sulfonamide dosage is used in conjunction with pyrimethamine.

Acute malaria

PO

Adults (in combination with sulfonamide): 25 mg daily for 2 days with a sulfonamide.

Adults (without concomitant sulfonamide): 50 mg for 2 days.

Children 4-10 yrs: 25 mg daily for 2 days.

Chemoprophylaxis of malaria

PO

Adults and pediatric patients over 10 yrs: 25 mg once weekly.

Children 4-10 yrs: 12.5 mg once weekly.

Infants and children under 4 yrs: 6.25 mg once weekly.

AVAILABLE FORMS

- *Tablets:* 25 mg (Daraprim).

UNLABELED USES: Prophylaxis for first episode and recurrence of *Pneumocystis carinii* pneumonia and *Toxoplasma gondii* in HIV-infected patients.

CONTRAINDICATIONS: Hypersensitivity to pyrimethamine, megaloblastic anemia due to folate deficiency, monotherapy for treatment of acute malaria.

PREGNANCY AND LACTATION: Pregnancy category C; most studies have found pyrimethamine to be safe in pregnancy; folic acid supplementation should be given to prevent folate deficiency; compatible with breast-feeding

SIDE EFFECTS

Frequent

Anorexia, vomiting

Occasional

Hypersensitivity reactions, Stevens-Johnson syndrome, toxic epidermal necrolysis, erythema multiforme, anaphylaxis, hyperphenylalaninemia, megaloblastic anemia, leukopenia, thrombocytopenia, pancytopenia, atrophic glossitis, hematuria, and disorders of cardiac rhythm

Rare

Pulmonary eosinophilia

SERIOUS REACTIONS

• None known.

INTERACTIONS

Drugs

❷ *Folic acid:* Decreased efficacy of pyrimethamine

SPECIAL CONSIDERATIONS

• Discontinue if folate deficiency develops; administer leucovorin 5-15 mg IM qd for ≥3 days when recovery slow

PATIENT/FAMILY EDUCATION

• Take with food

• Discontinue at first sign of rash

• Take each dose with a full glass of water

MONITORING PARAMETERS

• CBC with platelets semi-weekly during therapy for toxoplasmosis, less frequently for malaria-related indications

quazepam

(kway'-ze-pam)

Rx: Doral

Chemical Class: Benzodiazepine

Therapeutic Class: Hypnotic

DEA Class: Schedule IV

CLINICAL PHARMACOLOGY

Mechanism of Action: A BZ-1 receptor selective benzodiazepine with sedative properties. ***Therapeutic Effect:*** Produces sedative effect from its central nervous system (CNS) depressant action.

Pharmacokinetics

Rapidly absorbed from gastrointestinal (GI) tract. Food increases absorption. Protein binding: 95%. Extensively metabolized in liver. Excreted in urine and feces. Unknown if removed by hemodialysis. ***Half-life:*** 25-41 hrs.

INDICATIONS AND DOSAGES

Insomnia

PO

Adults (older than 18 yrs). Initially, 15 mg at bedtime. Adjust dose up or down from 7.5 mg to 30 mg at bedtime depending on initial response.

Elderly, debilitated, liver disease. Initially, 7.5-15 mg at bedtime. Adjust dose depending on initial response.

AVAILABLE FORMS

• *Tablets:* 7.5 mg, 15 mg (Doral).

CONTRAINDICATIONS: Pregnancy, sleep apnea, hypersensitivity to quazepam or any component of the formulation

PREGNANCY AND LACTATION: Pregnancy category X; may cause fetal damage when administered during pregnancy; excreted into breast milk; may accumulate in breast-fed infants and is therefore not recommended
Controlled Substance: Schedule IV

SIDE EFFECTS

Frequent
Muscular incoordination (ataxia), lightheadedness, transient mild drowsiness, slurred speech (particularly in elderly or debilitated patients)

Occasional
Confusion, depression, blurred vision, constipation, diarrhea, dry mouth, headache, nausea

Rare
Behavioral problems such as anger, impaired memory, paradoxical reactions such as insomnia, nervousness, or irritability

SERIOUS REACTIONS

- Abrupt or too-rapid withdrawal may result in pronounced restlessness, irritability, insomnia, hand tremors, abdominal and muscle cramps, sweating, vomiting, and seizures.
- Overdosage results in somnolence, confusion, diminished reflexes, and coma.
- Blood dyscrasias have been reported rarely.

INTERACTIONS

Drugs

3 *Azole antifungals:* May inhibit liver metabolism and increase quazepam concentrations

3 *Cimetidine:* Increased plasma levels of quazepam

3 *Clozapine:* Isolated cases of cardiorespiratory collapse have been reported, causal relationship to benzodiazepines has not been established

3 *Disulfiram:* Increased serum quazepam concentrations

3 *Ethanol:* Enhanced adverse psychomotor side effects of benzodiazepines

3 *Levodopa:* Possible exacerbation of parkinsonism

3 *Neuroleptics:* Increased sedation, respiratory depression

3 *Omeprazole, macrolides, azole antifungals, isoniazid, digoxin, SSRIs, quinolones:* Possible increased benzodiazepine concentrations

3 *Rifampin:* Reduced serum quazepam concentrations

3 *Theophylline:* May decrease quazepam effectiveness

SPECIAL CONSIDERATIONS

PATIENT/FAMILY EDUCATION

- Avoid alcohol and other CNS depressants
- Do not discontinue abruptly after prolonged therapy
- May cause daytime sedation, use caution while driving or performing other tasks requiring alertness
- Inform clinician if planning to become pregnant, or are pregnant, or if you become pregnant while taking this medicine
- May be habit-forming
- Stop smoking

MONITORING PARAMETERS

- Hepatic and renal function
- Therapeutic response

quetiapine fumarate

(kwe-tye'-a-peen fyoo'-muh-rate)

Rx: Seroquel

Chemical Class: Dibenzothiazepine derivative

Therapeutic Class: Antipsychotic

CLINICAL PHARMACOLOGY

Mechanism of Action: A dibenzothiazepine derivative that antagonizes dopamine, serotonin, histamine, and alpha$_1$-adrenergic receptors. ***Therapeutic Effect:*** Diminishes manifestations of psychotic disorders. Produces moderate sedation, few extrapyramidal effects, and no anticholinergic effects.

Pharmacokinetics

Well absorbed after PO administration. Protein binding: 83%. Widely distributed in tissues; CNS concentration exceeds plasma concentration. Undergoes extensive first-pass metabolism in the liver. Primarily excreted in urine. ***Half-life:*** 6 hr.

INDICATIONS AND DOSAGES

To manage manifestations of psychotic disorders

PO

Adults, Elderly. Initially, 25 mg twice a day, then 25-50 mg 2-3 times a day on the second and third days, up to 300-400 mg/day in divided doses 2-3 times a day by the fourth day. Further adjustments of 25-50 mg twice a day may be made at intervals of 2 days or longer. Maintenance: 300-800 mg/day (adults); 50-200 mg/day (elderly).

Mania in bipolar disorder

PO

Adults, Elderly. Initially, 50 mg twice a day for 1 day. May increase in increments of 100 mg/day to 200 mg twice a day on day 4. May increase in increments of 200 mg/day to 800 mg/day on day 6. Range: 400-800 mg/day.

Dosage in hepatic impairment, elderly or debilitated patients, and those predisposed to hypotensive reactions

These patients should receive a lower initial dose and lower dosage increases.

AVAILABLE FORMS

- *Tablets:* 25 mg, 100 mg, 200 mg, 300 mg.

UNLABELED USES: Autism, psychosis (children)

CONTRAINDICATIONS: None known.

PREGNANCY AND LACTATION: Pregnancy category C; excretion into breast milk unknown; breast-feeding is not recommended

SIDE EFFECTS

Frequent (19%-10%)

Headache, somnolence, dizziness

Occasional (9%-3%)

Constipation, orthostatic hypotension, tachycardia, dry mouth, dyspepsia, rash, asthenia, abdominal pain, rhinitis

Rare (2%)

Back pain, fever, weight gain

SERIOUS REACTIONS

- Overdose may produce heart block hypotension, hypokalemia, and tachycardia.

INTERACTIONS

Drugs

3 *Antihypertensives:* Increased risk of hypotension

3 *CYP3A inhibitors (azole antifungals, macrolide antibiotics):* Increased plasma quetiapine concentrations

3 *Lorazepam:* Increased plasma lorazepam concentrations

3 *Phenytoin, carbamazepine, barbiturates, rifampin, glucocorticoids (enzyme inducers):* Decreased plasma quetiapine concentrations

3 *Thioridazine:* Decreased plasma quetiapine concentrations

SPECIAL CONSIDERATIONS

• Limited clinical experience, but similar to clozapine and risperidone; may be effective for negative symptoms of schizophrenia; so far no agranulocytosis reported with quetiapine

PATIENT/FAMILY EDUCATION

• Avoid alcohol

• Take quetiapine as ordered; do not abruptly discontinue the drug or increase the dosage

• Drowsiness generally subsides during continued therapy

• Avoid tasks that require mental alertness or motor skills until response to the drug has been established

• Change positions slowly to reduce the hypotensive effect of quetiapine

• Drink lots of fluids, especially during physical activity

MONITORING PARAMETERS

• Blood pressure for hypotension and pulse rate for tachycardia, especially if the drug dosage has been increased rapidly

• Pattern of daily bowel activity and stool consistency

• Assess for evidence of a therapeutic response, such as improvement in self-care, increased interest in surroundings and ability to concentrate, and relaxed facial expression

• Closely supervise suicidal patients during early therapy; as depression lessens, the patient's energy level improves, which increases the suicide potential

quinapril hydrochloride

(kwin'-a-pril hye-droe-klor'-ide)

Rx: Accupril

Chemical Class: Angiotensin-converting enzyme (ACE) inhibitor, nonsulfhydryl

Therapeutic Class: Antihypertensive

CLINICAL PHARMACOLOGY

Mechanism of Action: An angiotensin-converting enzyme (ACE) inhibitor that suppresses the renin-angiotensin-aldosterone system and prevents the conversion of angiotensin I to angiotensin II, a potent vasoconstrictor; may also inhibit angiotensin II at local vascular and renal sites. ***Therapeutic Effect:*** Reduces peripheral arterial resistance, BP, and pulmonary capillary wedge pressure; improves cardiac output.

Pharmacokinetics

Route	*Onset*	*Peak*	*Duration*
PO	1 hr	N/A	24 hrs

Readily absorbed from the GI tract. Protein binding: 97%. Metabolized in the liver, GI tract, and extravascular tissue to active metabolite. Primarily excreted in urine. Minimal removal by hemodialysis. ***Half-life:*** 1-2 hrs; metabolite, 3 hrs (increased in those with impaired renal function).

INDICATIONS AND DOSAGES

Hypertension (monotherapy)

PO

Adults. Initially, 10-20 mg/day. May adjust dosage at intervals of at least 2 wk or longer. Maintenance: 20-80 mg/day as single dose or 2 divided doses. Maximum: 80 mg/day.

Elderly. Initially, 2.5-5 mg/day. May increase by 2.5-5 mg q1-2wk.

Hypertension (combination therapy)
PO
Adults. Initially, 5 mg/day titrated to patient's needs.
Elderly. Initially, 2.5-5 mg/day. May increase by 2.5-5 mg q1-2wk.
Adjunct to manage heart failure
PO
Adults, Elderly. Initially, 5 mg twice a day. Range: 20-40 mg/day.
Dosage in renal impairment
Dosage is titrated to the patient's needs after the following initial doses:

Creatinine Clearance	*Initial Dose*
more than 60 ml/min	10 mg
30-60 ml/min	5 mg
10-29 ml/min	2.5 mg

AVAILABLE FORMS
• *Tablets:* 5 mg, 10 mg, 20 mg, 40 mg.
UNLABELED USES: Treatment of hypertension and renal crisis in scleroderma, treatment of left ventricular dysfunction following MI
CONTRAINDICATIONS: Bilateral renal artery stenosis, history of angioedema from previous treatment with ACE inhibitors
PREGNANCY AND LACTATION: Pregnancy category C (D if used in second or third trimester); ACE inhibitors can cause fetal and neonatal morbidity and death when administered to pregnant women; when pregnancy is detected, discontinue ACE inhibitors as soon as possible
SIDE EFFECTS
Frequent (7%-5%)
Headache, dizziness
Occasional (4%-2%)
Fatigue, vomiting, nausea, hypotension, chest pain, cough, syncope
Rare (less than 2%)
Diarrhea, cough, dyspnea, rash, palpitations, impotence, insomnia, drowsiness, malaise
SERIOUS REACTIONS
• Excessive hypotension ("first-dose syncope") may occur in patients with CHF and in those who are severely salt or volume depleted.
• Angioedema and hyperkalemia occur rarely.
• Agranulocytosis and neutropenia may be noted in those with collagen vascular disease, including scleroderma and systemic lupus erythematosus, and impaired renal function.
• Nephrotic syndrome may be noted in those with history of renal disease.
INTERACTIONS
Drugs
3 *Alcohol:* May increase the effects of quinapril
2 *Allopurinol:* Predisposition to hypersensitivity reactions
3 *α-adrenergic blockers:* Exaggerated first-dose hypotensive response
3 *Aspirin:* Reduced hemodynamic effects; less likely with nonacetylated salicylates
3 *Azathioprine:* Increased myelosuppression
3 *Cyclosporine:* Renal insufficiency
3 *Garlic:* May increase antihypertensive effect
3 *Ginseng, yohimbe:* May worsen hypertension
3 *Insulin:* Enhanced hypoglycemic response
3 *Iron (parenteral):* Increased risk systemic reaction
3 *Lithium:* Increased risk of serious lithium toxicity
3 *Loop diuretics:* Initiation of ACE inhibitor therapy may cause hypotension and renal insufficiency

3 *NSAIDs:* Inhibition of the antihypertensive response

3 *Potassium, potassium-sparing diuretics:* Increased risk for hyperkalemia

3 *Trimethoprim:* Additive risk of hyperkalemia, especially in patient predisposed to renal insufficiency

Labs

- ACE inhibition can account for approximately 0.5 mEq/L rise in serum potassium

SPECIAL CONSIDERATIONS

PATIENT/FAMILY EDUCATION

- Caution with salt substitutes containing potassium chloride
- Rise slowly to sitting/standing position to minimize orthostatic hypotension
- Dizziness, fainting, lightheadedness may occur during first few days of therapy
- May cause altered taste perception or cough; persistent dry cough usually does not subside unless medication is stopped; notify clinician if these symptoms persist
- Full therapeutic effect of quinapril may take 1-2 wks to appear
- Discontinuing the drug or skipping doses of quinapril may produce severe, rebound hypertension
- Avoid tasks that require mental alertness or motor skills until response to the drug has been established

MONITORING PARAMETERS

- BUN, creatinine, potassium within 2 wk after initiation of therapy (increased levels may indicate acute renal failure), WBC count

quinidine gluconate

(kwin'-i-deen glue'-kun-ate)

Rx: Apo-Quin-G, BioQuin Durules, Quinaglute Dura-Tabs, Quinidex Extentabs

Chemical Class: Quinine isomer, dextrorotatory

Therapeutic Class: Antiarrhythmic, class IA; antimalarial

CLINICAL PHARMACOLOGY

Mechanism of Action: An antiarrhythmic that decreases sodium influx during depolarization, potassium efflux during repolarization, and reduces calcium transport across the myocardial cell membrane. Decreases myocardial excitability, conduction velocity, and contractility. ***Therapeutic Effect:*** Suppresses arrhythmias.

Pharmacokinetics

Almost completely absorbed after PO administration. Protein binding: 80%-90%. Metabolized in liver. Excreted in urine. Removed by hemodialysis. ***Half-life:*** 6-8 hr.

INDICATIONS AND DOSAGES

Maintenance of normal sinus rhythm after conversion of atrial fibrillation or flutter; prevention of premature atrial, AV, and ventricular contractions; paroxysmal atrial tachycardia; paroxysmal AV junctional rhythm; atrial fibrillation; atrial flutter; paroxysmal ventricular tachycardia not associated with complete heart block

PO

Adults, Elderly: 100-600 mg q4-6h. (Long-acting): 324-972 mg q8-12h.

Children: 30 mg/kg/day in divided doses q4-6h.

IV

Adults, Elderly. 200-400 mg.

Children. 2-10 mg/kg.

AVAILABLE FORMS
- *Injection:* 80 mg/ml.
- *Tablets:* 200 mg, 300 mg.
- *Tablets (Extended-Release):* 300 mg (Quinidex Extentabs), 324 mg (Quinaglute Dura-Tabs).

UNLABELED USES: Treatment of malaria (IV only)

CONTRAINDICATIONS: Complete AV block, development of thrombocytopenic purpura during prior therapy with quinidine or quinine, intraventricular conduction defects (widening of QRS complex)

PREGNANCY AND LACTATION: Pregnancy category C; use during pregnancy has been classified in reviews of cardiovascular drugs as relatively safe for the fetus; high doses can produce oxytocic properties and potential for abortion; excreted in breast milk; compatible with breast-feeding

SIDE EFFECTS

Frequent

Abdominal pain and cramps, nausea, diarrhea, vomiting (can be immediate, intense)

Occasional

Mild cinchonism (ringing in ears, blurred vision, hearing loss) or severe cinchonism (headache, vertigo, diaphoresis, light-headedness, photophobia, confusion, delirium)

Rare

Hypotension (particularly with IV administration), hypersensitivity reaction (fever, anaphylaxis, photosensitivity reaction)

SERIOUS REACTIONS
- Cardiotoxic effects occur most commonly with IV administration, particularly at high concentrations, and are observed as conduction changes (50% widening of QRS complex, prolonged QT interval, flattened T waves, and disappearance of P wave), ventricular tachycardia or flutter, frequent premature ventricular contractions (PVCs), or complete AV block.
- Quinidine-induced syncope may occur with the usual dosage.
- Severe hypotension may result from high dosages.
- Patients with atrial flutter and fibrillation may experience a paradoxical, extremely rapid ventricular rate that may be prevented by prior digitalization.
- Hepatotoxicity with jaundice due to drug hypersensitivity may occur.

INTERACTIONS

Drugs

3 *Acetazolamide, antacids, sodium bicarbonate, thiazide diuretics:* Alkalinization of urine increases plasma quinidine concentrations

3 *Amiloride:* Increased risk of arrhythmias in patients with ventricular tachycardia

3 *Amiodarone, cimetidine, verapamil:* Increased plasma quinidine concentrations

3 *Azole antifungals:* Inhibition of quinidine metabolism (CYP3A4), increased concentrations

3 *Barbiturates, nifedipine, kaolin-pectin, phenytoin, rifampin, rifabutin:* Decreased plasma quinidine concentrations

3 *β-blockers:* Increased concentrations of metoprolol, propranolol, and timolol

3 *Cholinergic agents:* Reduced therapeutic effects of cholinergic drugs

2 *Codeine:* Inhibition of codeine to its active metabolite, diminished analgesia

3 *Cyclic antidepressants:* Increased imipramine, nortriptyline and desipramine concentrations

3 *Dextromethorphan:* Increased dextromethorphan concentrations, toxicity may result

3 *Digitalis glycosides:* Increased digoxin and digitoxin concentrations, toxicity may result
3 *Encainide:* Increased encainide serum concentrations in rapid encainide metabolizers
3 *Haloperidol:* Increased haloperidol concentrations, toxicity
3 *Macrolides:* Increased quinidine concentrations with erythromycin, troleandomycin, clarithromycin due to CYP34A inhibition
3 *Mexiletine:* Increased mexiletine concentrations
3 *Neuromuscular blocking agents:* Enhanced effects of neuromuscular blocking agents
3 *Nifedipine:* Increased serum nifedipine concentrations, decreased serum quinidine concentrations
3 *Procainamide:* Marked increased procainamide concentrations
3 *Propafenone:* Increased propafenone concentrations and decreased concentrations of its active metabolite; net effect unknown
⚠ *Thioridazine:* May increase thioridazine serum concentrations and produce additive prolongation of QT interval
3 *Warfarin:* Enhanced anticoagulant response
❷ *Ziprasidone:* May prolong QT interval

Labs

• *False increase:* Urine 17-ketosteroids

SPECIAL CONSIDERATIONS

• 267 mg gluconate=275 mg polygalacturonate=200 mg sulfate

PATIENT/FAMILY EDUCATION

• Take with food to decrease GI upset
• Do not crush or chew sustained-release tablets
• Notify the physician if fever, ringing in the ears, or visual disturbances occurs
• Avoid direct sunlight or artificial light

MONITORING PARAMETERS

• Plasma quinidine concentration (therapeutic range 2-6 mcg/ml)
• ECG
• Liver function tests during the first 4-8 wks
• CBC periodically during prolonged therapy
• Intake and output
• Renal function tests
• Serum potassium level

quinine sulfate

(kwye'-nine sul'-fate)

Rx: Quinine

Chemical Class: Cinchona alkaloid

Therapeutic Class: Antimalarial

CLINICAL PHARMACOLOGY

Mechanism of Action: A cinchona alkaloid that relaxes skeletal muscle by increasing the refractory period, decreasing excitability of motor end plates (curarelike), and affecting distribution of calcium with muscle fiber. Antimalaria: Depresses oxygen uptake, carbohydrate metabolism, elevates pH in intracellular organelles of parasites. ***Therapeutic Effect:*** Relaxes skeletal muscle; produces parasite death.

Pharmacokinetics

Rapidly absorbed mainly from upper small intestine. Protein binding: 70%-95%. Metabolized in liver. Excreted in feces, saliva, and urine. ***Half-life:*** 8-14 hrs (adults), 6-12 hrs (children).

Q

INDICATIONS AND DOSAGES

Nocturnal leg cramps

PO

Adults, Elderly. 260-300 mg at bedtime as needed.

Treatment of malaria

PO

Adults, Elderly. 260-650 mg 3 times a day for 6-12 days.

Children. 10 mg/kg q8h for 5-7 days.

Dosage in renal impairment

Creatinine Clearance	Dosage Interval
10-50 ml/min	75% of normal dose or q12h
Less than 10 ml/min	30%-50% of normal dose or q24h

AVAILABLE FORMS

- *Capsules:* 200 mg, 325 mg (Quinine).
- *Tablets:* 260 mg (Quinine).

CONTRAINDICATIONS: Hypersensitivity to quinine (possible cross-sensitivity to quinidine), G-6-PD deficiency, tinnitus, optic neuritis, history of thrombocytopenia during previous quinine therapy, blackwater fever

PREGNANCY AND LACTATION: Pregnancy category X; excreted into breast milk; compatible with breast-feeding; use caution in infants at risk for G-6-PD deficiency

SIDE EFFECTS

Frequent

Nausea, headache, tinnitus, slight visual disturbances (mild cinchonism)

Occasional

Extreme flushing of skin with intense generalized pruritus is most typical hypersensitivity reaction; also rash, wheezing, dyspnea, angioedema

Prolonged therapy: Cardiac conduction disturbances, decreased hearing

SERIOUS REACTIONS

- Overdosage (severe cinchonism) may result in cardiovascular effects, severe headache, intestinal cramps w/vomiting and diarrhea, apprehension, confusion, seizures, blindness, and respiratory depression.
- Hypoprothrombinemia, thrombocytopenic purpura, hemoglobinuria, asthma, agranulocytosis, hypoglycemia, deafness, and optic atrophy occur rarely.

INTERACTIONS

Drugs

3 *Digitalis glycosides:* Increased digoxin concentrations (especially at high quinine doses)

3 *Mefloquine:* May increase seizures and EKG abnormalities

3 *Smoking:* Reduced serum quinine concentrations

Labs

- *False increase:* 17-ketosteroids

SPECIAL CONSIDERATIONS

PATIENT/FAMILY EDUCATION

- Take with food
- May cause blurred vision, use caution driving
- Discontinue drug if flushing, itching, rash, fever, stomach pain, difficult breathing, ringing in ears, visual disturbances occur
- Use appropriate contraceptive measures (Pregnancy category X); use nonhormonal contraception
- Periodic lab tests are part of therapy

MONITORING PARAMETERS

- Check for hypersensitivity: flushing, rash/urticaria, itching, dyspnea, wheezing
- Assess level of hearing, visual acuity, presence of headache/tinnitus, nausea and report adverse effects promptly (possible cinchonism)
- CBC results for blood dyscrasias; be alert to infection (fever, sore throat) and bleeding/bruising or unusual tiredness/weakness

• Pulse, EKG for arrhythmias
• Fasting blood sugar levels and watch for hypoglycemia (cold sweating, tremors, tachycardia, hunger, anxiety)

quinupristin; dalfopristin

(kwin-yoo'-pris-tin; dal'-foh-pris-tin)

Rx: Synercid

Chemical Class: Streptogramin combination

Therapeutic Class: Antibiotic

CLINICAL PHARMACOLOGY

Mechanism of Action: Two chemically distinct compounds that, when given together, bind to different sites on bacterial ribosomes, inhibiting protein synthesis. ***Therapeutic Effect:*** Bactericidal.

Pharmacokinetics

After IV administration, both are extensively metabolized in the liver, with dalfopristin to active metabolite. Protein binding: quinupristin, 23%-32%; dalfopristin, 50%-56%. Primarily eliminated in feces. ***Half-life:*** quinupristin, 0.85 hr; dalfopristin, 0.7 hr.

INDICATIONS AND DOSAGES

Infections due to vancomycin-resistant Enterococcus faecium

IV

Adults, Elderly. 7.5 mg/kg/dose q8h.

Skin and skin-structure infections

IV

Adults, Elderly. 7.5 mg/kg/dose q12h.

AVAILABLE FORMS

• *Injection:* 500-mg vial (150 mg quinupristin/350 mg dalfopristin).

CONTRAINDICATIONS: Hypersensitivity to pristinamycin, virginiamycin

PREGNANCY AND LACTATION: Pregnancy category B; breast milk excretion unknown

SIDE EFFECTS

Frequent

Mild erythema, pruritus, pain, or burning at infusion site (with doses greater than 7 mg/kg)

Occasional

Headache, diarrhea

Rare

Vomiting, arthralgia, myalgia

SERIOUS REACTIONS

• Antibiotic-associated colitis and other superinfections may result from bacterial imbalance.
• Hepatic function abnormalities and severe venous pain and inflammation may occur.

INTERACTIONS

Drugs

❷ *Antihistamines (astemizole, terfenadine):* Reduced antihistamine metabolism by CYP3A4 inhibition, possible prolonged QT interval

③ *Antineoplastic agents (docetaxel, paclitaxel, vinca alkaloids):* Reduced antineoplastic metabolism by CYP3A4 inhibition

③ *Benzodiazepines (diazepam, midazolam):* Reduced benzodiazepine metabolism by CYP3A4 inhibition

③ *Calcium channel blockers (amlodipine, diltiazem, felodipine, isradipine, nicardipine, nifedipine, nimodipine, nisoldipine, verapamil):* Reduced calcium channel blocker metabolism by CYP3A4 inhibition

③ *Carbamazepine:* Reduced carbamazepine metabolism by CYP3A4 inhibition

❷ *Cisapride:* Reduced cisapride metabolism by CYP3A4 inhibition, possible prolonged QT interval

③ *Digoxin:* Decreased digoxin metabolism by GI bacteria may increase digoxin levels

❷ *Disopyramide:* Reduced disopyramide metabolism by CYP3A4 inhibition, possible prolonged QT interval

❸ *HMG-CoA reductase inhibitors (atorvastatin, fluvastatin, lovastatin, pravastatin, simvastatin):* Reduced statin metabolism by CYP3A4 inhibition

❷ *Immunosuppressives (cyclosporine, tacrolimus):* Reduced immunosuppressive metabolism by CYP3A4 inhibition

❸ *Non-nucleoside reverse transcriptase inhibitors (delavirdine, nevirapine):* Reduced NNRTI metabolism by CYP3A4 inhibition

❸ *Protease inhibitors (indinavir, ritonavir):* Reduced PI metabolism by CYP3A4 inhibition

❷ *Quinidine:* Reduced quinidine metabolism by CYP3A4 inhibition, possible prolonged QT interval

SPECIAL CONSIDERATIONS

- Most appropriate use is when vancomycin-resistant *Enterococcus faecium* infection is documented or strongly suspected, or for therapy of methicillin-resistant *Staphylococcus aureus* infection

PATIENT/FAMILY EDUCATION

- Due to high chance of drug interactions through inhibition of CYP3A4, use caution with any additional drugs
- Notify the physician if pain, redness, or swelling at the infusion site occurs
- Immediately notify the physician if severe diarrhea occurs and avoid taking antidiarrheals until instructed to do so

MONITORING PARAMETERS

- CBC, ALT, AST, bilirubin, renal function
- Withhold the drug and promptly inform the physician if diarrhea occurs; diarrhea with abdominal pain, fever, and mucus or blood in stools may indicate antibiotic-associated colitis
- Evaluate the IV site for redness, vein irritation, burning, pruritus, mild erythema, and pain
- Be alert for signs and symptoms of superinfection, such as anal or genital pruritus, diarrhea, increased fever, nausea and vomiting, sore throat, and stomatitis

rabeprazole sodium

(ra-be'-pray-zole soe'-dee-um)

Rx: Aciphex

Chemical Class: Benzimidazole derivative

Therapeutic Class: Antiulcer agent

CLINICAL PHARMACOLOGY

Mechanism of Action: A proton pump inhibitor that converts to active metabolites that irreversibly bind to and inhibit hydrogen-potassium adenosine triphosphate, an enzyme on the surface of gastric parietal cells. Actively secretes hydrogen ions for potassium ions, resulting in an accumulation of hydrogen ions in gastric lumen. ***Therapeutic Effect:*** Increases gastric pH, reducing gastric acid production.

Pharmacokinetics

Rapidly absorbed from the GI tract after passing through the stomach relatively intact. Protein binding: 96%. Metabolized extensively in the liver. Primarily excreted in urine. Unknown if removed by hemodialysis. ***Half-life:*** 1-2 hrs (increased with hepatic impairment).

INDICATIONS AND DOSAGES

Gastroesophageal reflux disease

PO

Adults, Elderly. 20 mg/day for 4-8 wks. Maintenance: 20 mg/day.

Duodenal ulcer
PO
Adults, Elderly. 20 mg/day after morning meal for 4 wk.
NSAID-induced ulcer
PO
Adults, Elderly. 20 mg/day.
Pathologic hypersecretory conditions
PO
Adults, Elderly. Initially, 60 mg once a day. May increase to 60 mg twice a day.
H. pylori infection
PO
Adults, Elderly. 20 mg twice a day for 7 days (given with amoxicillin 1000 mg and clarithromycin 500 mg)

AVAILABLE FORMS
• *Tablets (Delayed-Release):* 20 mg.

CONTRAINDICATIONS: None known.

PREGNANCY AND LACTATION: Pregnancy category B; excretion into breast milk unknown; use caution in nursing mothers

SIDE EFFECTS
Rare (less than 2%)
Headache, nausea, dizziness, rash, diarrhea, malaise

SERIOUS REACTIONS
• Hyperglycemia, hypokalemia, hyponatremia, and hyperlipemia occur rarely.

INTERACTIONS
Drugs
3 *Cyclosporine:* Potential for increased cyclosporine concentrations
3 *Digoxin:* Increased serum concentrations of digoxin possible
3 *Ketoconazole:* Decreased bioavailability of ketoconazole

SPECIAL CONSIDERATIONS
• Symptomatic response does not rule out gastric malignancy

PATIENT/FAMILY EDUCATION
• Sustained-action tablets should be swallowed whole; do not chew, crush, or split the tablets
• Notify the physician if headache occurs during rabeprazole therapy

MONITORING PARAMETERS
• Symptom relief, mucosal healing
• Assess the patient for diarrhea, GI discomfort, headache, nausea, and skin rash

raloxifene hydrochloride
(ral-ox'-i-feen hye-droe-klor'-ide)
Rx: Evista
Chemical Class: Benzothiophene derivative
Therapeutic Class: Antiosteoporotic; selective estrogen receptor modulator (SERM)

CLINICAL PHARMACOLOGY
Mechanism of Action: A selective estrogen receptor modulator that affects some receptors like estrogen. ***Therapeutic Effect:*** Like estrogen, prevents bone loss and improves lipid profiles.
Pharmacokinetics
Rapidly absorbed after PO administration. Highly bound to plasma proteins (greater than 95%) and albumin. Undergoes extensive first-pass metabolism in liver. Excreted mainly in feces and, to a lesser extent, in urine. Unknown if removed by hemodialysis. ***Half-life:*** 27.7 hr.

INDICATIONS AND DOSAGES
Prevention or treatment of osteoporosis
PO
Adults, Elderly. 60 mg a day.

AVAILABLE FORMS
• *Tablets:* 60 mg.

UNLABELED USES: Prevention of fractures, treatment of breast cancer in postmenopausal women

CONTRAINDICATIONS: Active or history of venous thromboembolic events, such as deep vein thrombosis (DVT), pulmonary embolism, and retinal vein thrombosis; women who are or may become pregnant

PREGNANCY AND LACTATION: Pregnancy category X; abortion and fetal anomalies noted in animal studies; unknown if excreted in milk.

SIDE EFFECTS

Frequent (25%-10%)

Hot flashes, flu-like symptoms, arthralgia, sinusitis

Occasional (9%-5%)

Weight gain, nausea, myalgia, pharyngitis, cough, dyspepsia, leg cramps, rash, depression

Rare (4%-3%)

Vaginitis, UTI, peripheral edema, flatulence, vomiting, fever, migraine, diaphoresis

SERIOUS REACTIONS

- Pneumonia, gastroenteritis, chest pain, vaginal bleeding, and breast pain occur rarely.

INTERACTIONS

Drugs

3 *Ampicillin:* Reduces raloxifene absorption

2 *Cholestyramine:* Decreased absorption and enterohepatic cycling of raloxifene

3 *Clofibrate, indomethacin, naproxen, ibuprofen, diazepam, diazoxide:* Possible displacement of these highly protein-bound drugs

3 *Hormone replacement therapy, systemic estrogen:* Do not use raloxifene concurrently with these drugs

3 *Warfarin:* Decreased PT

SPECIAL CONSIDERATIONS

- Shown to preserve bone mass, increase bone mineral density, and reduce fracture rate relative to calcium alone
- Ensure adequate dietary or supplemental calcium, vitamin D
- Not associated with endometrial proliferation; however, investigate uterine bleeding
- Risk of thromboembolic events greatest in first 4 mo, discontinue at least 72 hr prior to surgery involving immobilization. Resume when patient fully ambulatory

PATIENT/FAMILY EDUCATION

- May be taken without regard to meals
- Engage in weight-bearing exercises; do not smoke or use alcohol excessively
- Report leg pain or swelling, sudden chest pain, shortness of breath, vision changes
- Avoid restrictions of movement during travel. Discontinue if at bed rest.
- Take supplemental calcium and vitamin D if daily intake is inadequate

MONITORING PARAMETERS

- Bone density tests (e.g., DEXA scan)
- Platelet count, and serum levels of inorganic phosphate, calcium, total and LDL cholesterol, and protein

ramipril

(ra-mi′-pril)

Rx: Altace

Chemical Class: Angiotensin-converting enzyme (ACE) inhibitor, nonsulfhydryl

Therapeutic Class: Antihypertensive

CLINICAL PHARMACOLOGY

Mechanism of Action: An angiotensin-converting enzyme (ACE) inhibitor that suppresses the renin-angiotensin-aldosterone system. Decreases plasma angiotensin II, increases plasma renin activity, and decreases aldosterone secretion. ***Therapeutic Effect:*** Reduces peripheral arterial resistance and BP.

Pharmacokinetics

Route	Onset	Peak	Duration
PO	1-2 hrs	3-6 hrs	24 hrs

Well absorbed from the GI tract. Protein binding: 73%. Metabolized in the liver to active metabolite. Primarily excreted in urine. Not removed by hemodialysis. ***Half-life:*** 5.1 hr.

INDICATIONS AND DOSAGES

Hypertension (monotherapy)

PO

Adults, Elderly. Initially, 2.5 mg/day. Maintenance: 2.5-20 mg/day as single dose or in 2 divided doses.

Hypertension (in combination with other antihypertensives)

PO

Adults, Elderly. Initially, 1.25 mg/day titrated to patient's needs.

CHF

PO

Adults, Elderly. Initially, 1.25-2.5 mg twice a day. Maximum: 5 mg twice a day.

Risk reduction for MI stroke

PO

Adults, Elderly. Initially, 2.5 mg/day for 7 days, then 5 mg/day for 21 days, then 10 mg/day as a single dose or in divided doses.

Dosage in renal impairment

Creatinine clearance equal to or less than 40 ml/min. 25% of normal dose.

Hypertension. Initially, 1.25 mg/day titrated upward.

CHF. Initially, 1.25 mg/day, titrated up to 2.5 mg twice a day.

AVAILABLE FORMS

• *Capsules:* 1.25 mg, 2.5 mg, 5 mg, 10 mg.

UNLABELED USES: Treatment of hypertension and renal crisis in scleroderma

CONTRAINDICATIONS: Bilateral renal artery stenosis

PREGNANCY AND LACTATION: Pregnancy category D; ACE inhibitors can cause fetal and neonatal morbidity and death when administered to pregnant women; when pregnancy is detected, discontinue ACE inhibitors as soon as possible

SIDE EFFECTS

Frequent (12%-5%)

Cough, headache

Occasional (4%-2%)

Dizziness, fatigue, nausea, asthenia (loss of strength)

Rare (less than 2%)

Palpitations, insomnia, nervousness, malaise, abdominal pain, myalgia

SERIOUS REACTIONS

• Excessive hypotension ("first-dose syncope") may occur in patients with CHF and in those who are severely salt or volume depleted.

• Angioedema and hyperkalemia occur rarely.

• Agranulocytosis and neutropenia may be noted in those with collagen vascular disease, including scleroderma and systemic lupus erythematosus, and impaired renal function.

• Nephrotic syndrome may be noted in those with history of renal disease.

INTERACTIONS

Drugs

3 *Alcohol:* May increase the effects of ramipril

2 *Allopurinol:* Predisposition to hypersensitivity reactions

3 *α-adrenergic blockers:* Exaggerated first-dose hypotensive response

R

3 *Aspirin:* Reduced hemodynamic effects; less likely with nonacetylated salicylates
3 *Azathioprine:* Increased myelosuppression
3 *Cyclosporine:* Renal insufficiency
3 *Garlic:* May increase antihypertensive effect
3 *Ginseng, yohimbe:* May worsen hypertension
3 *Insulin:* Enhanced hypoglycemic response
3 *Iron (parenteral):* Increased risk of systemic reaction
3 *Lithium:* Increased risk of serious lithium toxicity
3 *Loop diuretics:* Initiation of ACE inhibitor therapy may cause hypotension and renal insufficiency
3 *NSAIDs:* Inhibition of the antihypertensive response to ACE inhibitors
3 *Potassium, potassium-sparing diuretics:* Increased risk for hyperkalemia
3 *Trimethoprim:* Additive risk of hyperkalemia, especially in patient predisposed to renal insufficiency

Labs

• ACE inhibition can account for approx 0.5 mEq/L rise in serum potassium

SPECIAL CONSIDERATIONS

PATIENT/FAMILY EDUCATION

• Caution with salt substitutes containing potassium chloride
• Rise slowly to sitting/standing position to minimize orthostatic hypotension
• Dizziness, fainting, lightheadedness may occur during first few days of therapy
• May cause altered taste perception or cough; persistent dry cough usually does not subside unless medication is stopped; notify clinician if these symptoms persist
• Do not discontinue the drug without physician approval
• Notify the physician if chest pain, cough, or palpitations occur
• Avoid tasks that require mental alertness or motor skills until response to the drug has been established

MONITORING PARAMETERS

• BUN, creatinine, potassium within 2 wk after initiation of therapy (increased levels may indicate acute renal failure)
• Potassium levels, although hyperkalemia rarely occurs
• WBC count
• Assess the patient for cough
• Assess the patient with CHF for crackles and wheezing
• Monitor urinalysis for proteinuria

ranitidine hydrochloride/ ranitidine bismuth citrate

(ra-ni'-ti-deen)

Rx: Zantac, Zantac-150, Zantac-300, Zantac EFFERdose, Zantac-25 EFFERdose, Zantac-150 EFFERdose

OTC: Zantac 75

Chemical Class: Aminoalkyl furan derivative

Therapeutic Class: Antiulcer agent

CLINICAL PHARMACOLOGY

Mechanism of Action: An antiulcer agent that inhibits histamine action at histamine$_2$ receptors of gastric parietal cells. ***Therapeutic Effect:*** Inhibits gastric acid secretion when fasting, at night, or when stimulated by food, caffeine, or insulin. Reduces volume and hydrogen ion concentration of gastric juice.

Pharmacokinetics

Rapidly absorbed from the GI tract. Protein binding: 15%. Widely distributed. Metabolized in the liver. Primarily excreted in urine. Not removed by hemodialysis. ***Half-life:*** PO, 2.5 hr; IV, 2-2.5 hr (increased with impaired renal function).

INDICATIONS AND DOSAGES

Duodenal ulcers, gastric ulcers, gastroesophageal reflux disease

PO

Adults, Elderly. 150 mg twice a day or 300 mg at bedtime. Maintenance: 150 mg at bedtime.

Children. 2-4 mg/kg/day in divided doses twice a day. Maximum: 300 mg/day.

Duodenal ulcers associated with H. pylori infection

PO

Adults, Elderly. 400 mg twice a day for 4 wks in combination with clarithromycin 500 mg 2-3 times a day for the first 2 wks.

Erosive esophagitis

PO

Adults, Elderly. 150 mg 4 times a day. Maintenance: 150 mg twice a day or 300 mg at bedtime.

Children. 4-10 mg/kg/day in 2 divided doses. Maximum: 600 mg/day.

Hypersecretory conditions

PO

Adults, Elderly. 150 mg twice a day. May increase up to 6 g/day.

OTC use

PO

Adults, Elderly. 75 mg 30-60 mins before eating food or drinking beverages that cause heartburn. Maximum: 150 mg per 24-hr period and/or longer than 14 days.

Usual parenteral dosage

IV, IM

Adults, Elderly. 50 mg/dose q6-8h. Maximum: 400 mg/day.

Children. 2-4 mg/kg/day in divided doses q6-8h. Maximum: 200 mg/day.

Usual neonatal dosage

PO

Neonates. 2 mg/kg/day in divided doses q12h.

IV

Neonates. Initially, 1.5 mg/kg/dose; then 1.5-2 mg/kg/day in divided doses q12h.

Dosage in renal impairment

For patients with creatinine clearance less than 50 ml/min, give 150 mg PO q24h or 50 mg IV or IM q18-24h.

AVAILABLE FORMS

- *Tablets (Effervescent):* 25 mg (Zantac-25 EFFERdose), 150 mg (Zantac-150 EFFERdose).
- *Capsules (Zantac):* 150 mg, 300 mg.
- *Granules (Zantac EFFERdose):* 150 mg.
- *Syrup (Zantac):* 15 mg/ml.
- *Tablets:* 75 mg (Zantac-75), 150 mg (Zantac-150, Zantac-150 Maximum Strength), 300 mg (Zantac-300).
- *Injection (Zantac):* 25 mg/ml.

UNLABELED USES: Prevention of aspiration pneumonia, treatment of recurrent postoperative ulcer, upper GI bleeding, prevention of acid aspiration pneumonitis during surgery, prevention of stress-induced ulcers.

CONTRAINDICATIONS: History of acute porphyria

PREGNANCY AND LACTATION: Pregnancy category B; compatible with breast-feeding

SIDE EFFECTS

Occasional (2%)

Diarrhea

Rare (1%)

Constipation, headache (may be severe)

SERIOUS REACTIONS

• Reversible hepatitis and blood dyscrasias occur rarely.

INTERACTIONS

Drugs

3 *Antacids:* May decrease the absorption of ranitidine

3 *Cefuroxine; cefpodoxime; enoxacin; ketoconazole:* Reduction in gastric acidity reduces absorption, decreased plasma levels, potential for therapeutic failure

3 *Glipizide; glyburide; tolbutamide:* Increased absorption of these drugs, potential for hypoglycemia

3 *Nifedipine, nitrendipine, nisoldipine:* Increased concentrations of these drugs

3 *Smoking:* Decreases the effectiveness of ranitidine

Labs

• *False positive:* Urine drugs of abuse screen

SPECIAL CONSIDERATIONS

• No advantage over other agents in this class, base selection on cost

PATIENT/FAMILY EDUCATION

• Stagger doses of ranitidine and antacids

• Dissolve effervescent tablets and granules in 6-8 oz water before drinking

• Smoking decreases the effectiveness of ranitidine

• Do not take ranitidine within 1 hr of magnesium- or aluminum-containing antacids

• Transient burning or itching may occur with IV administration

• Avoid alcohol and aspirin, both of which may cause GI distress, during ranitidine therapy

MONITORING PARAMETERS

• Intragastric pH when used for stress ulcer prophylaxis, titrate dose to maintain pH >4

• Serum alkaline phosphatase, bilirubin, AST and ALT levels

repaglinide

(re-pag'-lin-ide)

Rx: Prandin

Chemical Class: Meglitinide

Therapeutic Class: Antidiabetic; hypoglycemic

CLINICAL PHARMACOLOGY

Mechanism of Action: An antihyperglycemic that stimulates release of insulin from beta cells of the pancreas by depolarizing beta cells, leading to an opening of calcium channels. Resulting calcium influx induces insulin secretion. ***Therapeutic Effect:*** Lowers blood glucose concentration.

Pharmacokinetics

Rapidly, completely absorbed from the GI tract. Protein binding: 98%. Metabolized in the liver to inactive metabolites. Excreted primarily in feces with a lesser amount in urine. Unknown if removed by hemodialysis. ***Half-life:*** 1 hr.

INDICATIONS AND DOSAGES

Diabetes mellitus

PO

Adults, Elderly. 0.5-4 mg 2-4 times a day. Maximum: 16 mg/day.

AVAILABLE FORMS

• *Tablets:* 0.5 mg, 1 mg, 2 mg.

CONTRAINDICATIONS: Diabetic ketoacidosis, type 1 diabetes mellitus

PREGNANCY AND LACTATION: Pregnancy category C; excretion into breast milk unknown; due to the potential for hypoglycemia in the infant, use with caution in nursing mothers

SIDE EFFECTS

Frequent (10%-6%)

Upper respiratory tract infection, headache, rhinitis, bronchitis, back pain

Occasional (5%-3%)
Diarrhea, dyspepsia, sinusitis, nausea, arthralgia, UTI
Rare (2%)
Constipation, vomiting, paresthesia, allergy

SERIOUS REACTIONS

• Hypoglycemia occurs in 16% of patients.
• Chest pain occurs rarely.

INTERACTIONS

Drugs

3 *Aspirin, β-blockers, sulfa drugs, chloramphenicol, warfarin, MAO inhibitors:* Hypoglycemia

3 *Ketoconazole, miconazole, erythromycin, troglitazone, rifampicin, carbamazepine, phenobarbital, butalbital, secobarbital, or primidone:* Potential increased repaglinide metabolism secondary to cytochrome P450 enzyme induction

3 *Thiazide diuretics, calcium channel blockers, β-blockers, cough, cold, or hay fever medicines (sympathomimetics), estrogen, oral contraceptives, corticosteroids, thyroid medicine, phenytoin, isoniazid, or nicotinic acid:* Hyperglycemia

SPECIAL CONSIDERATIONS

PATIENT/FAMILY EDUCATION

• Skip the dose of this medication if you skip a meal; take an extra dose with extra meal
• Recognize and treat hypoglycemia; maintain ready supply of glucose (glucose tablets or gel)
• The prescribed diet is a principal part of treatment
• Be aware of the typical signs and symptoms of hypoglycemia and hyperglycemia
• Wear medical alert identification stating that he or she has diabetes
• Consult the physician when glucose demands are altered, such as with fever, heavy physical activity, infection, stress, or trauma
• Diabetes mellitus requires lifelong control
• Adhere to dietary instructions, a regular exercise program, and regular testing of urine or blood glucose
• If the patient is taking repaglinide with insulin or a sulfonylurea, always have a source of glucose available to treat symptoms of low blood sugar

MONITORING PARAMETERS

• Blood glucose—biggest effect noted on postprandial values (50-75 mg/dL reductions expected); minimal effect on fasting blood glucose
• Glycosylated hemoglobin (1%-2% reductions expected)
• Hyperglycemia/hypoglycemia signs and symptoms
• Be alert to conditions that alter blood glucose requirements, such as fever, increased activity, stress, or a surgical procedure

reserpine

(reh-zer'-peen)

Rx: Serpalan

Combinations

Rx: with thiazide diuretics: i.e., bendroflumethazide (flumethiazide), chlorothiazide, chlorthalidone (Regreton), hydrochlorothiazide (Hydropres, Hydroserpalan, Hydroserpine, Mallopress), hydroflumethiazide (Salutensin), polythiazide (Reneese), quinethazone (Hydromox R), trichloromethiazide (Metatensin, Naquival), hydrochlorothiazide and hydralazine (Hyserp, Lo-Ten, Marpres, Ser-A-Gen, Seralazide, Ser-Ap-Es, Unipres, Uni-Serp)

Chemical Class: Rauwolfia alkaloid

Therapeutic Class: Antihypertensive; antipsychotic; postganglionic adrenergic neuron inhibitor

CLINICAL PHARMACOLOGY

Mechanism of Action: An antihypertensive that depletes stores of catecholamines and 5-hydroxytryptamine in many organs, including the brain and adrenal medulla. Depression of sympathetic nerve function results in a decreased heart rate and a lowering of arterial blood pressure. Depletion of catecholamines and 5-hydroxytryptamine from the brain is thought to be the mechanism of the sedative and tranquilizing properties. ***Therapeutic Effects:*** Decreases blood pressure and heart rate; sedation.

Pharmacokinetics

Characterized by slow onset of action and sustained effects. Both cardiovascular and central nervous system effects may persist for a period of time following withdrawal of the drug. Mean maximum plasma levels were attained after a median of 3.5 hrs. Bioavailability was approximately 50% of that of a corresponding intravenous dose. Protein binding: 96%. ***Half life:*** 33 hrs.

INDICATIONS AND DOSAGES

Hypertension

PO

Adults: Usual initial dosage 0.5 mg daily for 1 or 2 wks. For maintenance, reduce to 0.1-0.25 mg daily.

Children: Reserpine is not recommended for use in children. If it is to be used in treating a child, the usual recommended starting dose is 20 μg/kg daily. The maximum recommended dose is 0.25 mg (total) daily.

Psychiatric disorders

PO

Adults: Initial dosage 0.5 mg daily, may range from 0.1-1.0 mg. Adjust dosage upward or downward according to response.

AVAILABLE FORMS

• *Tablets:* 0.25 mg, 0.1 mg (reserpine).

UNLABELED USES: Cerebral vasospasm, migraines, Raynaud's syndrome, reflex sympathetic dystrophy, refractory depression, tardive dyskinesia, thyrotoxic crisis

CONTRAINDICATIONS: Hypersensitivity, mental depression or history of mental depression (especially with suicidal tendencies), active peptic ulcer, ulcerative colitis, patients receiving electroconvulsive therapy

PREGNANCY AND LACTATION: Pregnancy category C; excreted into breast milk; no clinical reports of adverse effects in nursing infants have been located

SIDE EFFECTS

Occasional

Burning in the stomach, nausea, vomiting, diarrhea, dry mouth, nosebleed, stuffy nose, dizziness, headache, nervousness, nightmares, drowsiness, muscle aches, weight gain, redness of the eyes

Rare

Irregular heart beat, difficulty breathing, heart problems, feeling faint, swelling, gynecomastia, decreased libido

SERIOUS REACTIONS

• None known.

INTERACTIONS

Drugs

3 *Nonselective MAOIs:* Hypertensive reactions

Labs

• *False increase:* Serum bilirubin, urine creatinine

• *False positive:* Guiacols spot test

SPECIAL CONSIDERATIONS

• Only remaining rauwolfia derivative available

PATIENT/FAMILY EDUCATION

• May cause drowsiness or dizziness, use caution driving or participating in other activities requiring alertness

• Therapeutic effect may take 2-3 wk

• A low-salt diet should be followed

• Notify physician immediately if depression, nightmares, fainting, slow heartbeat, chest pain, or swollen ankles and feet occurs

MONITORING PARAMETERS

• Blood pressure, edema, drowsiness, despondency or self-depreciation, early morning insomnia, CNS depression, hypothermia, extrapyramidal tract effects

reteplase, recombinant

(re′-te-plays)

Rx: Retavase

Chemical Class: Tissue plasminogen activator (tPA)

Therapeutic Class: Thrombolytic

CLINICAL PHARMACOLOGY

Mechanism of Action: A tissue plasminogen activator that activates the fibrinolytic system by directly cleaving plasminogen to generate plasmin, an enzyme that degrades the fibrin of the thrombus. ***Therapeutic Effect:*** Exerts thrombolytic action.

Pharmacokinetics

Rapidly cleared from plasma. Eliminated primarily by the liver and kidney. ***Half-life:*** 13-16 mins.

INDICATIONS AND DOSAGES

Acute MI, CHF

IV Bolus

Adults, Elderly. 10 units over 2 min; repeat in 30 min.

AVAILABLE FORMS

• *Powder for Injection:* 10.4 units (18.1 mg).

UNLABELED USES: Occluded catheters

CONTRAINDICATIONS: Active internal bleeding, AV malformation or aneurysm, bleeding diathesis, history of cerebrovascular accident (CVA), intracranial neoplasm, recent intracranial or intraspinal surgery or trauma, severe uncontrolled hypertension

PREGNANCY AND LACTATION: Pregnancy category C

SIDE EFFECTS

Frequent

Bleeding at superficial sites, such as venous injection sites, catheter insertion sites, venous cutdowns, arte-

R

rial punctures, and sites of recent surgical procedures, gingival bleeding

SERIOUS REACTIONS

• Bleeding at internal sites may occur, including intracranial, retroperitoneal, GI, GU, and respiratory sites.

• Lysis or coronary thrombi may produce atrial or ventricular arrhythmias and stroke.

INTERACTIONS

Drugs

❷ *Heparin, oral anticoagulants, drugs that alter platelet function (i.e., aspirin, dipyridamole, abciximab, eptifibitide, tirofiban):* May increase the risk of bleeding

❸ *Ginkgo biloba:* May increase the risk of bleeding

SPECIAL CONSIDERATIONS

• No other IV medications should be administered in the same line

PATIENT/FAMILY EDUCATION

• Use an electric razor and soft toothbrush to prevent bleeding during drug therapy

• Report black or red stool, coffee-ground vomitus, dark or red urine, red-speckled mucus from cough, or other signs of bleeding

• Immediately report chest pain, headache, palpitations, or shortness of breath

MONITORING PARAMETERS

• Carefully monitor all needle puncture sites and catheter insertion sites for bleeding

• Continuous cardiac monitoring for arrhythmias, blood pressure, and pulse and respiration rates until patient is stable

• Evaluate breath sounds and peripheral pulses

• Monitor for relief of chest pain

ribavirin

(rye-ba-vye'-rin)

Rx: Copegus, Rebetol, Virazole

Combinations

Rx: with interferon alfa-2b (Rebetron)

Chemical Class: Nucleoside analog

Therapeutic Class: Antiviral

CLINICAL PHARMACOLOGY

Mechanism of Action: A synthetic nucleoside that inhibits influenza virus RNA polymerase activity and interferes with expression of messenger RNA. ***Therapeutic Effect:*** Inhibits viral protein synthesis and replication of viral RNA and DNA.

Pharmacokinetics

Rapidly absorbed from the GI tract following oral administration. A small amount is systemically absorbed following inhalation. Primarily excreted in urine. ***Half-life:*** 298 hr (oral); 9.5 hr (inhalation).

INDICATIONS AND DOSAGES

Chronic hepatitis C

PO (capsule or oral solution in combination with interferon alfa-2b)

Adults, Elderly. 1000-1200 mg/day in 2 divided doses.

Children weighing 60 kg or more. Use adult dosage. (51-60 kg): 400 mg 2 times/day. (37-50 kg): 200 mg in morning, 400 mg in evening. (24-36 kg): 200 mg 2 times/day.

PO (capsules in combination with peginterferon alfa-2b)

Adults, Elderly. 800 mg/day in 2 divided doses.

PO (tablets in combination with peginterferon alfa-2b)

Adults, Elderly. 800-1200 mg/day in 2 divided doses.

Severe lower respiratory tract infection caused by respiratory syncytial virus (RSV)
Inhalation
Children, Infants. Use with Viratek small-particle aerosol generator at a concentration of 20 mg/ml (6 g reconstituted with 300 ml sterile water) over 12-18 hr/day for 3-7 days.

AVAILABLE FORMS

- *Capsules (Rebetol, Rebetron Combination Therapy with alfa-2b injection):* 200 mg.
- *Tablets (Copegus):* 200 mg.
- *Powder for Reconstitution (Aerosol [Virazole]):* 6 g.
- *Oral Solution (Rebetol):* 40 mg/ml.

UNLABELED USES: Treatment of influenza A or B and west Nile virus

CONTRAINDICATIONS: Autoimmune hepatitis, creatinine clearance less than 50 ml/min, hemoglobinopathies, hepatic decompensation, hypersensitivity to ribavirin products, pregnancy, significant or unstable cardiac disease, women of childbearing age who do not use contraception reliably

PREGNANCY AND LACTATION: Pregnancy category X; teratogenic in animals; contraindicated in lactating women

SIDE EFFECTS

Frequent (greater than 10%)
Dizziness, headache, fatigue, fever, insomnia, irritability, depression, emotional lability, impaired concentration, alopecia, rash, pruritus, nausea, anorexia, dyspepsia, vomiting, decreased hemoglobin, hemolysis, arthralgia, musculoskeletal pain, dyspnea, sinusitis, flu-like symptoms

Occasional (1%-10%)
Nervousness, altered taste, weakness

SERIOUS REACTIONS

- Cardiac arrest, apnea and ventilator dependence, bacterial pneumonia, pneumonia, and pneumothorax occur rarely.
- Anemia may occur if ribavirin therapy exceeds 7 days.

INTERACTIONS

Drugs

3 *Didanosine:* May increase the risk of pancreatitis and peripheral neuropathy and decrease the effects of didanosine

3 *Nucleoside analogs (including adefovir, didanosine, lamivudine, stavudine, zalcitabine, zidovudine):* May increase the risk of lactic acidosis

3 *Warfarin:* Reduced anticoagulant effect

SPECIAL CONSIDERATIONS

PATIENT/FAMILY EDUCATION

- Female health care workers who are pregnant or may become pregnant should avoid exposure to ribavirin
- Immediately report difficulty breathing or itching, redness, or swelling of the eyes

MONITORING PARAMETERS

- Hematocrit
- Blood pressure, respirations
- Intake and output
- Be alert for impaired ventilation and gas exchange resulting from drug precipitate
- Periodically assess breath sounds and check the skin for a rash

rifabutin

(rif'-a-byoo-tin)

Rx: Mycobutin

Chemical Class: Rifamycin S derivative

Therapeutic Class: Antibiotic

CLINICAL PHARMACOLOGY

Mechanism of Action: An antitubercular that inhibits DNA-dependent RNA polymerase, an enzyme in susceptible strains of *Escherichia coli* and *Bacillus subtilis*. Rifabutin has a broad spectrum of antimicrobial activity, including against mycobacteria such as *Mycobacterium avium* complex (MAC). ***Therapeutic Effect:*** Prevents MAC disease.

Pharmacokinetics

Readily absorbed from the GI tract (high-fat meals delay absorption). Protein binding: 85%. Widely distributed. Crosses the blood-brain barrier. Extensive intracellular tissue uptake. Metabolized in the liver to active metabolite. Excreted in urine; eliminated in feces. Unknown if removed by hemodialysis. ***Half-life:*** 16-69 hr.

INDICATIONS AND DOSAGES

Prevention of MAC disease (first episode)

PO

Adults, Elderly. 300 mg as a single dose or in 2 divided doses if GI upset occurs.

Prevention of recurrent MAC disease

PO

Adults, Elderly. 300 mg/day (in combination)

Dosage in renal impairment

Dosage is modified based on creatinine clearance. If creatinine clearance is less than 30 ml/min, reduce dosage by 50%.

AVAILABLE FORMS

- *Capsules:* 150 mg.

UNLABELED USES: Part of multidrug regimen for treatment of MAC

CONTRAINDICATIONS: Active tuberculosis; hypersensitivity to other rifamycins, including rifampin

PREGNANCY AND LACTATION: Pregnancy category B

SIDE EFFECTS

Frequent (30%)

Red-orange or red-brown discoloration of urine, feces, saliva, skin, sputum, sweat, or tears

Occasional (11%-3%)

Rash, nausea, abdominal pain, diarrhea, dyspepsia, belching, headache, altered taste, uveitis, corneal deposits

Rare (less than 2%)

Anorexia, flatulence, fever, myalgia, vomiting, insomnia

SERIOUS REACTIONS

- Hepatitis and thrombocytopenia occur rarely. Anemia and neutropenia may also occur.

INTERACTIONS

Drugs

3 *Acetaminophen:* Enhanced hepatotoxicity (overdoses and possibly large therapeutic doses)

3 *Cyclosporine:* Reduced concentration of cyclosporine

3 *Delavirdine:* Reduced concentration of delavirdine

3 *Eprosartan:* Reduced concentration of eprosartan

3 *Nifedipine:* Reduced nifedipine concentrations

3 *Oral contraceptives:* Menstrual irregularities, contraceptive failure

3 *Oral hypoglycemics:* Reduced hypoglycemic activity

3 *Propafenone:* Lowered propafenone concentrations, loss of antiarrhythmic efficacy

❷ *Protease inhibitors:* Increased clearance (CYP3A4 induction) and decreased protease inhibitor efficacy

❸ *Quinidine:* Marked reduction quinidine levels

❸ *Tacrolimus:* Reduced concentration of tacrolimus

❸ *Zidovudine:* May decrease blood concentration of zidovudine

SPECIAL CONSIDERATIONS

- Has liver enzyme-inducing properties similar to rifampin although less potent
- Unlike rifampin, does not appear to alter the acetylation of isoniazid

PATIENT/FAMILY EDUCATION

- May discolor bodily secretions brown-orange, soft contact lenses may be permanently stained
- Avoid crowds
- Notify the physician promptly if dark urine, flu-like symptoms, nausea or vomiting, unusual bleeding or bruising, or any visual disturbances occurs

MONITORING PARAMETERS

- Periodic CBC with differential and platelets
- Liver function tests
- Hgb and Hct
- Body temperature

rifampin

(rif-am'-pin)

Rx: Rifadin, Rifadin IV, Rimactane

Chemical Class: Rifamycin B derivative

Therapeutic Class: Antituberculosis agent

CLINICAL PHARMACOLOGY

Mechanism of Action: An antitubercular that interferes with bacterial RNA synthesis by binding to DNA-dependent RNA polymerase, thus preventing its attachment to DNA and blocking RNA transcription. ***Therapeutic Effect:*** Bactericidal in susceptible microorganisms.

Pharmacokinetics

Well absorbed from the GI tract (food delays absorption). Protein binding: 80%. Widely distributed. Metabolized in the liver to active metabolite. Primarily eliminated by the biliary system. Not removed by hemodialysis. ***Half-life:*** 3-5 hr (increased in hepatic impairment).

INDICATIONS AND DOSAGES

Tuberculosis

PO, IV

Adults, Elderly. 10 mg/kg/day. Maximum: 600 mg/day.

Children. 10-20 mg/kg/day in divided doses q12-24h.

Prevention of meningococcal infections

PO, IV

Adults, Elderly. 600 mg q12h for 2 days.

Children 1 mo and older. 20 mg/kg/day in divided doses q12-24h. Maximum: 600 mg/dose.

Infants younger than 1 mo. 10 mg/kg/day in divided doses q12h for 2 days.

Staphylococcal infections

PO, IV

Adults, Elderly. 600 mg once a day.

Children. 15 mg/kg/day in divided doses q12h.

Staphylococcus aureus infections (in combination with other antiinfectives)

PO

Adults, Elderly. 300-600 mg twice a day.

Neonates. 5-20 mg/kg/day in divided doses q12h.

R

Prevention of Haemophilus influenzae infection
PO
Adults, Elderly. 600 mg/day for 4 days
Children 1 mo and older. 20 mg/kg/day in divided doses q12h for 5-10 days.
Children younger than 1 mo. 10 mg/kg/day in divided doses q12h for 2 days.

AVAILABLE FORMS
- *Capsules:* 150 mg (Rifadin), 300 mg (Rifadin, Rimactane).
- *Injection, Powder for Reconstitution (Rifadin IV):* 600 mg.

UNLABELED USES: Prophylaxis of *H. influenzae* type b infection; treatment of atypical mycobacterial infection and serious infections caused by *Staphylococcus* species

CONTRAINDICATIONS: Concomitant therapy with amprenavir, hypersensitivity to other rifamycins

PREGNANCY AND LACTATION: Pregnancy category C; compatible with breast-feeding

SIDE EFFECTS
Expected
Red-orange or red-brown discoloration of urine, feces, saliva, skin, sputum, sweat, or tears
Occasional (5%-2%)
Hypersensitivity reaction (such as flushing, pruritus, or rash)
Rare (2%-1%)
Diarrhea, dyspepsia, nausea, candida as evidenced by sore mouth or tongue

SERIOUS REACTIONS
- Rare reactions include hepatotoxicity (risk is increased when rifampin is taken with isoniazid), hepatitis, blood dyscrasias, Stevens-Johnson syndrome, and antibiotic-associated colitis.

INTERACTIONS
Drugs
3 *Acetaminophen:* Enhanced hepatotoxicity (overdoses and possibly large therapeutic doses)
3 *Aminosalicylic acid:* Reduced serum concentrations of rifampin
3 *Antidiabetics:* Diminished hypoglycemic activity of sulfonylureas
3 *Azole antifungals, barbiturates, benzodiazepines, β-blockers (except nadolol), calcium channel blockers, chloramphenicol, clofibrate, cyclic antidepressants, dapsone, digitalis glycosides, disopyramide, lorcainide, methadone, mexiletine, nortriptyline, phenytoin, pirmenol, propafenone, quinidine, tocainide, theophylline, zidovudine:* Reduced serum concentrations of these drugs
3 *Corticosteroids:* Reduced effect of corticosteroids
2 *Cyclosporine, tacrolimus:* Reduced concentrations of these drugs, possible therapeutic failure
3 *Isoniazid:* Increased hepatotoxic potential of isoniazid in slow acetylators or patients with preexisting liver disease
2 *Oral anticoagulants:* Reduced hypoprothrombinemic effect of oral anticoagulants
3 *Oral contraceptives:* Menstrual irregularities, contraceptive failure
2 *Protease inhibitors:* Increased clearance (CYP3A4 induction) and decreased protease inhibitor efficacy
3 *Ropivacaine:* Increased metabolism of ropivacaine; a reduction in anesthetic effect may occur
3 *Simvastatin:* Reduces simvastatin acid plasma concentrations; therapeutic failure is likely to occur
3 *Tamoxifen:* Reduces tamoxifen concentrations
3 *Thyroid:* Increased elimination, increased thyroid requirements

3 *Triazolam:* Reduces plasma concentrations of triazolam

3 *Zaleplon:* Reduces the concentration of zaleplon; loss of efficacy may result

3 *Zolpidem:* Reduces the plasma concentrations and effect of zolpidem

Labs

- *Increase:* Liver function tests, uric acid
- *Interference:* Folate, vitamin B_{12}, BSP, gallbladder studies
- *False decrease:* Serum bilirubin, ALT, AST (by some methods), cholesterol, triglycerides
- *False increase:* Serum bilirubin (some methods, may also be true physiologic increase), glucose, iron, LDH, uric acid, metronidazole, phosphate, tetracycline, trimethoprim
- *False positive:* Clindamycin, erythromycin, polymyxin

SPECIAL CONSIDERATIONS

PATIENT/FAMILY EDUCATION

- Take on empty stomach, at least 1 hr before or 2 hr after meals
- May cause reddish-orange discoloration of bodily secretions, may permanently discolor soft contact lenses
- Avoid consuming alcohol while taking this drug
- Do not take any other medications, including antacids, while taking rifampin without first consulting the physician; take rifampin at least 1 hr before taking an antacid
- Notify the physician immediately if fatigue, fever, flu-like symptoms, nausea, vomiting, unusual bleeding or bruising, weakness, yellow eyes and skin, or any other new symptoms occurs

MONITORING PARAMETERS

- Liver function tests at baseline and q2-4wk during therapy
- CBC with differential and platelets at baseline and periodically throughout treatment
- Pattern of daily bowel activity and stool consistency

rifapentine

(rif-a-pen'-teen)

Rx: Priftin

Chemical Class: Rifamycin B derivative

Therapeutic Class: Antituberculosis agent

CLINICAL PHARMACOLOGY

Mechanism of Action: An antitubercular that inhibits bacterial RNA synthesis by binding to DNA-dependent RNA polymerase in *Mycobacterium tuberculosis*. This action prevents the enzyme from attaching to DNA, thereby blocking RNA transcription. ***Therapeutic Effect:*** Bactericidal.

Pharmacokinetics

Rapidly and well absorbed from the GI tract. Protein binding: 97.7%. Metabolized in liver. Primarily eliminated in feces; partial excretion in urine. Not removed by hemodialysis. ***Half-life:*** 14-17 hr.

INDICATIONS AND DOSAGES

Tuberculosis

PO

Adults, Elderly. Intensive phase: 600 mg twice weekly for 2 mo (interval between doses no less than 3 days). Continuation phase: 600 mg weekly for 4 mo.

AVAILABLE FORMS

- *Tablets:* 150 mg.

CONTRAINDICATIONS: History of hypersensitivity to any rifamycins (e.g., rifampin and rifabutin)

PREGNANCY AND LACTATION: Pregnancy category C (teratogenic in rats); excreted in breast milk, but compatible with breast-feeding

SIDE EFFECTS

Rare (less than 4%)

Red-orange or red-brown discoloration of urine, feces, saliva, skin, sputum, sweat, or tears; arthralgia, pain, nausea, vomiting, headache, dyspepsia, hypertension, dizziness, diarrhea

SERIOUS REACTIONS

- Hyperuricemia, neutropenia, proteinuria, hematuria, and hepatitis occur rarely.

INTERACTIONS

Drugs

3 *Acetaminophen:* Enhanced hepatotoxicity

3 *Alcohol:* May increase the risk of hepatotoxicity

3 *Aminosalicylic acid:* Reduced plasma concentrations of rifapentine

3 *Azole antifungals, barbiturates, benzodiazepines, β-blockers, calcium channel blockers, chloramphenicol, clofibrate, cyclic antidepressants, dapsone, digitalis glycosides, disopyramide, lorcainide, methadone, mexiletine, phenytoin, pirmenol, propafenone, quinidine, tocainide, theophylline, zidovudine:* Reduced plasma concentrations of these drugs

3 *Corticosteroids:* Reduced effect of corticosteroids

❷ *Cyclosporine:* Reduced plasma concentration of cyclosporine

3 *Isoniazid:* Increased hepatotoxic potential of isoniazid in slow acetylators or patients with preexisting liver disease

3 *Oral contraceptives:* Reduced plasma levels of these drugs with menstrual irregularity and contraceptive failure

❷ *Protease inhibitors:* Increased clearance and decreased protease inhibitor efficacy

3 *Sulfonylureas:* Diminished hypoglycemic activity of sulfonylureas

❷ *Tacrolimus:* Reduced plasma concentration of tacrolimus

3 *Thyroid:* Increased clearance of thyroid hormone with increased dose requirement

❷ *Warfarin:* Reduced hypoprothrombinemic effect of warfarin

Labs

- *Interference:* Folate and vitamin B_{12} levels by microbiologic assay

SPECIAL CONSIDERATIONS

PATIENT/FAMILY EDUCATION

- Use an alternative method of contraception if taking oral contraceptives concurrently
- Avoid alcoholic beverages concurrently with this medication
- Rifapentine causes urine, stool, saliva, sputum, sweat, and tears to turn reddish-orange to reddish-brown and may also permanently discolor soft contact lenses; avoid wearing soft contact lenses
- Notify the physician if dark urine, decreased appetite, fever, nausea or vomiting, or pain or swelling of the joints occurs

MONITORING PARAMETERS

- ALT, AST, alkaline phosphate, bilirubin, and CBC prior to treatment and monthly during treatment
- Pattern of daily bowel activity and stool consistency

rifaximin

(rye-fax'-ih-min)

Rx: Xifaxan

Chemical Class: Semisynthetic rifamycin B derivative

Therapeutic Class: Antibiotic

CLINICAL PHARMACOLOGY

Mechanism of Action: An antiinfective that inhibits bacterial RNA synthesis by binding to a subunit of bacterial DNA-dependent RNA polymerase. ***Therapeutic Effect:*** Bactericidal.

Pharmacokinetics

Less than 0.4% absorbed after PO administration. Primarily eliminated in feces; minimal excretion in urine. ***Half-life:*** 5.85 hr.

INDICATIONS AND DOSAGES

Traveler's diarrhea

PO

Adults, Elderly, Children 12 yr and older. 200 mg 3 times a day for 3 days.

Hepatic encephalopathy

PO

Adults, Elderly. 1200 mg/day for 15-21 days.

AVAILABLE FORMS

• *Tablets:* 200 mg.

UNLABELED USES: Treatment of hepatic encephalopathy

CONTRAINDICATIONS: Hypersensitivity to other rifamycin antibiotics

PREGNANCY AND LACTATION: Pregnancy category C; breast milk excretion unknown, but probably compatible with breast-feeding as its absorption is less than 1%, and the parent compound, rifampin, is compatible with breast-feeding

SIDE EFFECTS

Occasional (11%-5%)

Flatulence, headache, abdominal discomfort, rectal tenesmus, defecation urgency, nausea

Rare (4%-2%)

Constipation, fever, vomiting

SERIOUS REACTIONS

• Hypersensitivity reactions, including dermatitis, angioneurotic edema, pruritus, rash, and urticaria may occur.

• Superinfection occurs rarely.

SPECIAL CONSIDERATIONS

• Has been used for diverticular disease and hepatic encephalopathy, but not FDA approved. Not effective for traveler's diarrhea due to bacteria other than enterotoxigenic *E. coli*

PATIENT/FAMILY EDUCATION

• Notify the physician if diarrhea worsens, a fever develops, or blood appears in the stool within 48 hrs

MONITORING PARAMETERS

• Bowel sounds for peristalsis; pattern of daily bowel activity and stool consistency

riluzole

(ril'-yoo-zole)

Rx: Rilutek

Chemical Class: Benzothiazolamine derivative

Therapeutic Class: Amyotrophic lateral sclerosis (ALS) agent

CLINICAL PHARMACOLOGY

Mechanism of Action: An amyotrophic lateral sclerosis (ALS) agent that inhibits presynaptic glutamate release in the CNS and intereferes postsynaptically with the effects of excitatory amino acids. ***Therapeutic Effect:*** Extends survival of ALS patients.

Pharmacokinetics

Well absorbed following PO administration. High-fat meals decrease absorption. Protein binding: 96%. Extensively metabolized in liver. Excreted in urine. ***Half-life:*** 12-14 hr.

INDICATIONS AND DOSAGES

ALS

PO

Adults, Elderly. 50 mg q12h.

AVAILABLE FORMS

- *Tablets:* 50 mg.

CONTRAINDICATIONS: None known.

PREGNANCY AND LACTATION: Pregnancy category C; excretion into breast milk unknown; use caution in nursing mothers

SIDE EFFECTS

Frequent (greater than 10%)

Nausea, asthenia, reduced respiratory function

Occasional (10%-1%)

Edema, tachycardia, headache, dizziness, somnolence, depression, vertigo, tremor, pruritus, alopecia, abdominal pain, diarrhea, anorexia, dyspepsia, vomiting, stomatitis, increased cough

SERIOUS REACTIONS

- Cardiac arrest, neutropenia, jaundice, and respiratory depression have been reported.

INTERACTIONS

Drugs

3 *Alcohol:* May increase CNS depression

3 *Caffeine, theophylline, amitriptyline, quinolones (CYP1A2 inhibitors):* Possible decreased riluzole elimination

3 *Cigarette smoking, rifampin, omeprazole (CYP1A2 inducers):* Possible increased riluzole elimination

3 *High-fat meals:* May decrease the absorption and effects of riluzole

SPECIAL CONSIDERATIONS

PATIENT/FAMILY EDUCATION

- Take riluzole at least 1 hr before or 2 hrs after a meal and at the same times each day
- Riluzole may cause drowsiness, dizziness, or vertigo
- Avoid tasks requiring mental alertness or motor skills until response to the drug has been established
- Avoid alcohol during therapy
- Notify the physician if fever develops

MONITORING PARAMETERS

- ALT, AST qmo for 3 mo, q3mo for 1 yr, then periodically thereafter; discontinue treatment if ALT or AST increases to >5 times upper limit of normal

rimantadine hydrochloride

(ri-man′-ti-deen hye-droe-klor′-ide)

Rx: Flumadine

Chemical Class: Tricyclic amine

Therapeutic Class: Antiviral

CLINICAL PHARMACOLOGY

Mechanism of Action: An antiviral that appears to exert an inhibitory effect early in the viral replication cycle. May inhibit uncoating of the virus. ***Therapeutic Effect:*** Prevents replication of influenza A virus.

Pharmacokinetics

Well absorbed following PO administration. Protein binding: 40%. Metabolized in liver. Excreted in urine. ***Half-life:*** 19-36 hr.

INDICATIONS AND DOSAGES

Influenza A virus

PO

Adults, Elderly. 100 mg twice a day for 7 days.

Elderly nursing home patients, patients with severe hepatic or renal impairment. 100 mg once a day for 7 days.

Prevention of influenza A virus

PO

Adults, Elderly, Children 10 yrs and older. 100 mg twice a day for at least 10 days after known exposure (usually for 6-8 wks).

Children younger than 10 yrs. 5 mg/kg once a day. Maximum: 150 mg.

Elderly nursing home patients, patients with severe hepatic or renal impairment. 100 mg once a day.

AVAILABLE FORMS

- *Syrup:* 50 mg/5 ml.
- *Tablets:* 100 mg.

CONTRAINDICATIONS: Hypersensitivity to amantadine

PREGNANCY AND LACTATION: Pregnancy category C; concentrated in breast milk

SIDE EFFECTS

Occasional (3%-2%)

Insomnia, nausea, nervousness, impaired concentration, dizziness

Rare (less than 2%)

Vomiting, anorexia, dry mouth, abdominal pain, asthenia, fatigue

SERIOUS REACTIONS

- None known.

INTERACTIONS

Drugs

3 *Acetaminophen, aspirin:* May decrease rimantadine blood concentration

3 *Anticholinergics, CNS stimulants:* May increase side effects of rimantadine

3 *Cimetidine:* May increase rimantadine blood concentration

3 *Triamterene:* Increased concentrations, toxicity of rimantadine

3 *Trihexyphenidyl:* Increased CNS effects

SPECIAL CONSIDERATIONS

• PRECAUTIONS

- Resistant strains may develop during treatment (10%-30%)
- Less CNS toxicity in at-risk populations

PATIENT/FAMILY EDUCATION

- Avoid contact with people who are at high risk for developing influenza A because a rimantadine-resistant virus may be shed during therapy
- Avoid performing tasks that require mental alertness or motor skills until response to the drug has been established
- Do not take acetaminophen, aspirin, or compounds containing these drugs
- Rimantadine may cause dry mouth

MONITORING PARAMETERS

- Assess for anxiety, nervousness, and insomnia

risedronate sodium

(rye-se-droe'-nate soe'-dee-um)

Rx: Actonel

Chemical Class: Pyrophosphate analog

Therapeutic Class: Antiosteoporotic; bisphosphonate; bone resorption inhibitor

CLINICAL PHARMACOLOGY

Mechanism of Action: A bisphosphonate that binds to bone hydroxyapatite and inhibits osteoclasts. ***Therapeutic Effect:*** Reduces bone turnover (the number of sites at which bone is remodeled) and bone resorption.

Pharmacokinetics

Rapidly absorbed following PO administration. Bioavailability is decreased when administered with food. Protein binding: 24%. Not metabolized. Excreted unchanged in urine and feces. Not removed by hemodialysis. ***Half-life:*** 1.5 hr (initial); 480 hr (terminal).

INDICATIONS AND DOSAGES

Paget's disease

PO

Adults, Elderly. 30 mg/day for 2 mo. Retreatment may occur after 2-mos post-treatment observation period.

Prevention and treatment of postmenopausal osteoporosis

PO

Adults, Elderly. 5 mg/day or 35 mg once weekly.

Glucocorticoid-induced osteoporosis

PO

Adults, Elderly. 5 mg/day.

AVAILABLE FORMS

• *Tablets:* 5 mg, 30 mg, 35 mg.

CONTRAINDICATIONS: Hypersensitivity to other bisphosphonates, including etidronate, tiludronate, risedronate, and alendronate; hypocalcemia; inability to stand or sit upright for at least 20 mins; renal impairment when serum creatinine clearance is greater than 5 mg/dL

PREGNANCY AND LACTATION: Pregnancy category C; breast milk excretion unknown

SIDE EFFECTS

Frequent (30%)

Arthralgia

Occasional (12%-8%)

Rash, flu-like symptoms, peripheral edema

Rare (5%-3%)

Bone pain, sinusitis, asthenia, dry eye, tinnitus

SERIOUS REACTIONS

• Overdose causes hypocalcemia, hypophosphatemia, and significant GI disturbances.

INTERACTIONS

Drugs

3 *Antacids, calcium:* Decreased absorption of risedronate

3 *Food:* Decreases bioavailability of risedronate by 50%

SPECIAL CONSIDERATIONS

PATIENT/FAMILY EDUCATION

• Administer 30 mins before the first food/beverage/medication of the day, with 6-8 oz plain water
• Taking risedronate with other beverages, including coffee, mineral water, and orange juice, significantly reduces the absorption of the drug
• Consider beginning weight-bearing exercises and modifying behavioral factors, such as avoiding alcohol consumption and cigarette smoking

MONITORING PARAMETERS

• Albumin-adjusted serum calcium; *N*-telopeptide, alkaline phosphatase, phosphorus, osteocalcin, DEXA scan, bone and joint pain, fractures on X-ray (osteoporosis, Paget's disease)
• Serum electrolytes, BUN, intake and output
• Serum creatinine in patients with renal impairment

risperidone

(ris-per'-i-done)

Rx: Risperdal, Risperdal Consta, Risperdol M-Tabs

Chemical Class: Benzisoxazole derivative

Therapeutic Class: Antipsychotic

CLINICAL PHARMACOLOGY

Mechanism of Action: A benzisoxazole derivative that may antagonize dopamine and serotonin receptors. ***Therapeutic Effect:*** Suppresses psychotic behavior.

Pharmacokinetics

Well absorbed from the GI tract; unaffected by food. Protein binding:

90%. Extensively metabolized in the liver to active metabolite. Primarily excreted in urine. ***Half-life:*** 3-20 hrs; metabolite: 21-30 hrs (increased in elderly).

INDICATIONS AND DOSAGES

Psychotic disorder

PO

Adults. 0.5-1 mg twice a day. May increase dosage slowly. Range: 2-6 mg/day.

Elderly. Initially, 0.25-2 mg/day in 2 divided doses. May increase dosage slowly. Range: 2-6 mg/day.

IM

Adults, Elderly. 25 mg q2wk. Maximum: 50 mg q2wk.

Mania

PO

Adults, Elderly. Initially, 2-3 mg as a single daily dose. May increase at 24-hr intervals of 1 mg/day. Range: 2-6 mg/day.

Dosage in renal impairment

Initial dosage for adults and elderly patients is 0.25-0.5 mg twice a day. Dosage is titrated slowly to desired effect.

AVAILABLE FORMS

- *Oral Solution (Risperdal):* 1 mg/ml.
- *Tablets (Risperdal):* 0.25 mg, 0.5 mg, 1 mg, 2 mg, 3 mg, 4 mg.
- *Tablets (Orally Disintegrating [Risperdal M-Tabs]):* 0.5 mg, 1 mg, 2 mg.
- *Injection (Risperdal Consta):* 25 mg, 37.5 mg, 50 mg.

UNLABELED USES: Autism in children, behavioral symptoms associated with dementia, Tourette's disorder

CONTRAINDICATIONS: None known.

PREGNANCY AND LACTATION: Pregnancy category C; excreted in breast milk

SIDE EFFECTS

Frequent (26%-13%)

Agitation, anxiety, insomnia, headache, constipation

Occasional (10%-4%)

Dyspepsia, rhinitis, somnolence, dizziness, nausea, vomiting, rash, abdominal pain, dry skin, tachycardia

Rare (3%-2%)

Visual disturbances, fever, back pain, pharyngitis, cough, arthralgia, angina, aggressive behavior, orthostatic hypotension, breast swelling

SERIOUS REACTIONS

- Rare reactions include tardive dyskinesia (characterized by tongue protrusion, puffing of the cheeks, and chewing or puckering of the mouth) and neuroleptic malignant syndrome (marked by hyperpyrexia, muscle rigidity, change in mental status, irregular pulse or BP, tachycardia, diaphoresis, cardiac arrhythmias, rhabdomyolysis, and acute renal failure).
- Hyperglycemia, in some cases extreme and associated with ketoacidosis or hyperosmolar coma or death, has been reported.

INTERACTIONS

Drugs

3 *Alcohol, other CNS depressants:* May increase CNS depression

3 *Carbamazepine:* May decrease the risperidone blood concentration

3 *Clozapine:* May increase the risperidone blood concentration

3 *Levodopa, dopamine agonists:* Risperidone may antagonize effect

3 *Paroxetine:* May increase the risperidone blood concentration and the risk of extrapyramidal symptoms

SPECIAL CONSIDERATIONS

PATIENT/FAMILY EDUCATION

- Risk of orthostatic hypotension, especially during the period of initial dose titration

• Do not operate machinery during dose titration period
• Notify the physician if altered gait, difficulty breathing, palpitations, pain or swelling in breasts, severe dizziness or fainting, trembling fingers, unusual movements, rash, or visual changes occur
• Avoid alcohol during risperidone therapy

MONITORING PARAMETERS

• Blood pressure, heart rate, liver function test results, EKG, and weight
• Observe the patient for fine tongue movement, which may be the first sign of irreversible tardive dyskinesia
• Closely supervise suicidal patients during early therapy; as depression lessens, energy level improves, which increases the suicide potential
• Therapeutic response, such as increased ability to concentrate and interest in surroundings, improvement in self-care, and relaxed facial expression
• Monitor for signs of neuroleptic malignant syndrome, such as altered mental status, fever, irregular blood pressure or pulse, and muscle rigidity

ritonavir

(ri-tone'-a-veer)

Rx: Norvir

Combinations

Rx: with lopinavir (Kaletra)

Chemical Class: Protease inhibitor, HIV

Therapeutic Class: Antiretroviral

CLINICAL PHARMACOLOGY

Mechanism of Action: Inhibits HIV-1 and HIV-2 proteases, rendering these enzymes incapable of processing the polypeptide precursors; this results in the production of noninfectious, immature HIV particles.
Therapeutic Effect: Impedes HIV replication, slowing the progression of HIV infection.

Pharmacokinetics

Well absorbed after PO administration (absorption increased with food). Protein binding: 98%-99%. Extensively metabolized in the liver to active metabolite. Primarily eliminated in feces. Unknown if removed by hemodialysis. ***Half-life:*** 2.7-5 hr.

INDICATIONS AND DOSAGES

HIV infection

PO

Adults, Children 12 yr and older. 600 mg twice a day. If nausea occurs at this dosage, give 300 mg twice a day for 1 day, 400 mg twice a day for 2 days, 500 mg twice a day for 1 day, then 600 mg twice a day thereafter.
Children younger than 12 yr. Initially, 250 mg/m^2/dose twice a day. Increase by 50 mg/m^2/dose up to 400 mg/m^2/dose. Maximum: 600 mg/dose twice a day.

Dosage adjustments in combination therapy

Amprenavir. Amprenavir 1200 mg and ritonavir 200 mg once a day or amprenavir 600 mg and ritonavir 100 mg twice a day.
Ampenavir and efavirenz. Amprenavir 1200 mg twice a day and ritonavir 200 mg twice a day with standard dose of efavirenz.
Indinavir. Indinavir 800 mg twice a day and ritonavir 100-200 mg twice a day or indinavir 400 mg twice a day and ritonavir 400 mg twice a day.
Nelfinavir or saquinavir. Ritonavir 400 mg twice a day.
Rifabutin. Decrease rifabutin dosage to 150 mg every other day.

AVAILABLE FORMS

- *Oral Solution:* 80 mg/ml.
- *Soft Gelatin Capsules:* 100 mg.

CONTRAINDICATIONS: Concurrent use of amiodarone, astemizole, bepridil, bupropion, cisapride, clozapine, encainide, flecainide, meperidine, piroxicam, propafenone, propoxyphene, quinidine, rifabutin, or terfenadine (increased risk of serious or life-threatening drug interactions, such as arrhythmias, hematologic abnormalities, and seizures); concurrent use of alprazolam, clorazepate, diazepam, estazolam, flurazepam, midazolam, triazolam, or zolpidem (may produce extreme sedation and respiratory depression)

PREGNANCY AND LACTATION: Pregnancy category B; breast milk excretion unknown; breast-feeding by HIV+ mothers not recommended

SIDE EFFECTS

Frequent

GI disturbances (abdominal pain, anorexia, diarrhea, nausea, vomiting), circumoral and peripheral paresthesias, altered taste, headache, dizziness, fatigue, asthenia

Occasional

Allergic reaction, flu-like symptoms, hypotension

Rare

Diabetes mellitus, hyperglycemia

SERIOUS REACTIONS

- Hepatitis and fatal cases of pancreatitis have been reported.

INTERACTIONS

Drugs

▲ *Amiodarone:* Increased plasma levels of amiodarone

❷ *Atorvastatin:* Increased risk of myopathy possible

▲ *Astemizole:* Increased plasma levels of astemizole

❸ *Barbiturates:* Increased clearance of ritonavir; reduced clearance of barbiturates

▲ *Bepredil:* Increased plasma levels of bepredil

▲ *Bupropion:* Increased plasma levels of bupropion

❷ *Carbamazepine:* Increased clearance of ritonavir; reduced clearance of carbamazepine

❷ *Cerivastatin:* Increased risk of myopathy possible

▲ *Cisapride:* Increased plasma levels of cisapride

❷ *Clarithromycin:* Reduced clearance of ritonavir; ritonavir reduces clearance of clarithromycin; reduce clarithromycin dose for renal insufficiency

▲ *Clorazepate:* Increased plasma levels of clorazepate

▲ *Clozapine:* Increased plasma levels of clozapine

❸ *Despiramine:* Ritonavir increases AUC of desipramine by 145%

▲ *Diazepam:* Increased plasma levels of diazepam

❸ *Didanosine:* Separate dosing by 2.5 hr to avoid formulation incompatibility

❷ *Disulfiram:* Ritonavir (gel capsules and solution) contain ethanol; disulfiram-like reaction possible

▲ *Encainide:* Increased plasma levels of encainide

▲ *Ergot alkaloids:* Increased plasma levels of ergot alkaloids

❸ *Erythromycin:* Reduced clearance of ritonavir; ritonavir reduces clearance of erythromycin

▲ *Estazolam:* Increases plasma levels of estazolam

▲ *Flecainide:* Increased plasma levels of flecainide

▲ *Flurazepam:* Increased plasma levels of flurazepam

❸ *Indinavir:* Increased plasma level of indinavir; reduce dose to 400 mg bid when ritonavir dose is 400 mg bid

3 *Ketoconazole:* Ritonavir reduces clearance of ketoconazole; reduce ketoconazole dose

▲ *Lovastatin:* Ritonavir reduces clearance of lovastatin

▲ *Meperidine:* Increased plasma levels of normeperidine, which has analgesic and CNS stimulant activity (seizures)

3 *Methadone:* Ritonavir reduces methadone plasma concentration by 37%

❷ *Metronidazole:* Ritonavir (gel capsules and solution) contain ethanol; disulfiram-like reaction possible

▲ *Midazolam:* Increased plasma levels of midazolam and prolonged effect

3 *Nelfinavir:* Increased plasma level of nelfinavir; reduce nelfinavir dose to 750 mg bid when ritonavir dose is 400 mg bid

3 *Oral contraceptives:* Ritonavir may reduce efficacy

3 *Phenytoin:* Increased clearance of ritonavir; reduced clearance of phenytoin

▲ *Pimozide:* Increased plasma levels of pimozide

▲ *Piroxicam:* Increased plasma levels of piroxicam

▲ *Propafenone:* Increased plasma levels of propafenone

▲ *Propoxyphene:* Increased plasma levels of propoxyphene

▲ *Quinidine:* Increased plasma levels of quinidine

❷ *Rifabutin:* Increased clearance of ritonavir; reduced clearance of rifabutin; reduce rifabutin dose to 150 mg qod

3 *Rifampin:* Increased clearance of ritonavir

▲ *St. John's Wort (hypericum perforatum):* Substantial decrease in plasma ritonavir concentrations with loss of virologic response

3 *Saquinavir:* Decreased clearance of saquinavir; reduce dose of saquinavir (Fortovase or Invirase) to 400 bid with ritonavir 400 mg bid

❷ *Sildenafil:* Substantial increases in serum sildenafil concentrations

▲ *Simvastatin:* Ritonavir reduces clearance of simvastatin

▲ *Terfenadine:* Increased plasma levels of terfenadine

3 *Theophylline:* Ritonavir reduces theophylline plasma concentration

▲ *Triazolam:* Increased plasma levels of triazolam and prolonged effect

3 *Troleandomycin:* Reduced clearance of ritonavir; ritonavir reduces clearance of troleandomycin

3 *Warfarin:* Decreased plasma warfarin concentrations

▲ *Zolpidem:* Increased plasma levels of zolpidem

SPECIAL CONSIDERATIONS

- As with other protease inhibitors, ritonavir will predominantly be used in combination regimens; the ability of ritonavir (alone or in combinations) to modify clinical endpoints (e.g., time to first AIDS-defining illness or death) will be important in determining the ultimate role of this agent in HIV; potential for drug interaction is troublesome; as with other protease inhibitors, resistance has been problematic after several mo of treatment

PATIENT/FAMILY EDUCATION

- Store capsules in the refrigerator until dispensed; refrigeration of capsules by patient not required if used within 30 days and stored below 77°F; store oral solution at room temperature, do not refrigerate, shake well; avoid exposure to excessive heat
- Take with food

• Space ritonavir doses evenly around the clock and continue taking the drug for the full course of treatment
• Notify the physician if abdominal pain, frequent urination, increased thirst, nausea, or vomiting occurs
• Ritonavir is not a cure for HIV infection, nor does it reduce the risk of transmitting HIV to others

MONITORING PARAMETERS
• *Therapeutic:* Serum HIV-1 RNA, and CD4+ cell counts (every 2-4 wk)
• *Toxicity:* Complete blood counts, routine blood chemistry, liver function tests, and serum lipid and lipoprotein profiles
• Closely monitor for signs and symptoms of GI or neurologic disturbances, particularly paresthesias

rivastigmine tartrate

(riv-a-stig'-meen tar'-trate)
Rx: Exelon
Chemical Class: Carbamate derivative; cholinesterase inhibitor
Therapeutic Class: Acetylcholinesterase inhibitor

CLINICAL PHARMACOLOGY
Mechanism of Action: A cholinesterase inhibitor that inhibits the enzyme acetylcholinesterase, thus increasing the concentration of acetylcholine at cholinergic synapses and enhancing cholinergic function in the CNS. ***Therapeutic Effect:*** Slows the progression of symptoms of Alzheimer's disease.
Pharmacokinetics
Rapidly and completely absorbed. Protein binding: 60%. Widely distributed throughout the body. Rapidly and extensively metabolized. Primarily excreted in urine. ***Half-life:*** 1.5 hr.

INDICATIONS AND DOSAGES
Alzheimer's disease
PO
Adults, Elderly. Initially, 1.5 mg twice a day. May increase at intervals of least 2 wk to 3 mg twice a day, then 4.5 mg twice a day, and finally 6 mg twice a day. Maximum: 6 mg twice a day.

AVAILABLE FORMS
• *Capsules:* 1.5 mg, 3 mg, 4.5 mg, 6 mg.
• *Oral Solution:* 2 mg/ml.

CONTRAINDICATIONS: Hypersensitivity to other carbamate derivatives

PREGNANCY AND LACTATION: Pregnancy category B; excretion into human breast milk unknown

SIDE EFFECTS
Frequent (47%-17%)
Nausea, vomiting, dizziness, diarrhea, headache, anorexia
Occasional (13%-6%)
Abdominal pain, insomnia, dyspepsia (heartburn, indigestion, epigastric pain), confusion, UTI, depression
Rare (5%-3%)
Anxiety, somnolence, constipation, malaise, hallucinations, tremor, flatulence, rhinitis, hypertension, flu-like symptoms, weight loss, syncope

SERIOUS REACTIONS
• Overdose may result in cholinergic crisis, characterized by severe nausea and vomiting, increased salivation, diaphoresis, bradycardia, hypotension, respiratory depression, and seizures.

INTERACTIONS
Drugs
3 *Anticholinergic drugs:* Interference with anticholinergic activity

3 *Cholinomimetics (cholinergics and other cholinesterase inhibitors i.e., bethanechol and succinylcholine):* Potential synergistic effects

3 *Clozapine:* Antagonistic effect on cholinesterase inhibitor activity

3 *Inhaled anesthetics:* Decreased neuromuscular blocking effects

3 *Local anesthetics:* Increased risk of local anesthetic toxicity (pseudocholinesterase competition)

3 *Neuromuscular blockers, nondepolarizing:* Antagonistic effects, reversal of neuromuscular blockade

SPECIAL CONSIDERATIONS

PATIENT/FAMILY EDUCATION

- Patient and caregiver should be advised of high incidence of gastrointestinal effects and directions for resource and resolution
- Take with morning and evening meals
- Swallow capsules whole; do not break, chew, or crush them
- If the patient is using the oral solution, explain that he or she should withdraw the prescribed amount of drug into the syringe and either sip it directly from the syringe or first mix it with a small glass of water, cold fruit juice, or soda and then stir and drink the mixture

MONITORING PARAMETERS

- Cognitive function (e.g., ADAS, Mini-Mental Status Exam [MMSE]), activities of daily living, global functioning, blood chemistry, complete blood counts, heart rate, blood pressure
- Monitor for a cholinergic reaction, including diaphoresis, dizziness, excessive salivation, facial warmth, abdominal cramps or discomfort, lacrimation, pallor, and urinary urgency

rizatriptan benzoate

(rye-za-trip′-tan)

Rx: Maxalt, Maxalt MLT

Chemical Class: Serotonin derivative

Therapeutic Class: Antimigraine agent

CLINICAL PHARMACOLOGY

Mechanism of Action: A serotonin receptor agonist that binds selectively to vascular receptors, producing a vasoconstrictive effect on cranial blood vessels. ***Therapeutic Effect:*** Relieves migraine headache.

Pharmacokinetics

Well absorbed after PO administration. Protein binding: 14%. Crosses the blood-brain barrier. Metabolized by the liver to inactive metabolite. Eliminated primarily in urine and, to a lesser extent, in feces. ***Half-life:*** 2-3 hr.

INDICATIONS AND DOSAGES

Acute migraine attack

PO

Adults older than 18 yr, Elderly. 5-10 mg. If headache improves, but then returns, dose may be repeated after 2 hr. Maximum: 30 mg/24 hr.

AVAILABLE FORMS

- *Tablets (Maxalt):* 5 mg, 10 mg.
- *Tablets (Orally Disintegrating [Maxalt-MLT]):* 5 mg, 10 mg.

CONTRAINDICATIONS: Basilar or hemiplegic migraine, coronary artery disease, ischemic heart disease (including angina pectoris, history of MI, silent ischemia, and Prinzmetal's angina), uncontrolled hypertension, use within 24 hrs of ergotamine-containing preparations or another serotonin receptor agonist, use within 14 days of MAOIs

PREGNANCY AND LACTATION: Pregnancy category C; use caution in nursing mothers

SIDE EFFECTS

Frequent (9%-7%)

Dizziness, somnolence, paresthesia, fatigue

Occasional (6%-3%)

Nausea, chest pressure, dry mouth

Rare (2%)

Headache; neck, throat, or jaw pressure; photosensitivity

SERIOUS REACTIONS

• Cardiac reactions (such as ischemia, coronary artery vasospasm, and MI) and noncardiac vasospasm-related reactions (including hemorrhage and cerebrovascular accident [CVA]), occur rarely, particularly in patients with hypertension, diabetes, or a strong family history of coronary artery disease; obese patients; smokers; males older than 40 yrs; and postmenopausal women.

INTERACTIONS

Drugs

⚠ *Ergotamine-containing drugs:* Increased vasoconstriction

3 *Fluoxetine, fluvoxamine, paroxetine, sertraline:* May produce hyperreflexia, incoordination, and weakness

⚠ *MAO inhibitors:* Potential for decreased metabolism of rizatriptan

3 *Propranolol:* Propranolol has been shown to increase the plasma concentrations of rizatriptan by 70%; patients receiving propranolol should use 5-mg tablets (max 15 mg/24 hr)

❷ *Sibutramine:* Increased risk of serotonin syndrome

SPECIAL CONSIDERATIONS

• Safety of treating, on average, more than 4 headaches in a 30-day period has not been established

• MLT does not provide faster absorption or onset of effect because almost the entire dose is swallowed with saliva and absorbed in the GI tract

PATIENT/FAMILY EDUCATION

• Use only to treat migraine headache, not for prevention

• MLT, administration with liquid is not necessary; orally disintegrating tablet is packaged in a blister within an outer aluminum pouch, do not remove the blister from the outer pouch until just prior to dosing; blister pack should then be peeled open with dry hands and the orally disintegrating tablet placed on the tongue, where it will dissolve and be swallowed with the saliva

• Avoid tasks that require mental alertness or motor skills until response to the drug has been established

• Notify the physician immediately if palpitations, pain or tightness in the chest or throat, or pain or weakness in the extremities occurs

• Protect against exposure to sunlight and ultraviolet rays by using sunscreen and wearing protective clothing

• Do not smoke during rizatriptan therapy

• Lie down in a dark, quiet room for additional benefit after taking the drug

MONITORING PARAMETERS

• Assess for relief of migraines and associated symptoms, including nausea and vomiting, photophobias, and phonophobia (sound sensitivity)

ropinirole hydrochloride

(ro-pin'-i-role hye-droe-klor'-ide)

Rx: ReQuip

Chemical Class: Dipropylaminoethyl indolone derivative

Therapeutic Class: Anti-Parkinson's agent; dopaminergic

CLINICAL PHARMACOLOGY

Mechanism of Action: An antiparkinson agent that stimulates dopamine receptors in the striatum. ***Therapeutic Effect:*** Relieves signs and symptoms of Parkinson's disease.

Pharmacokinetics

Rapidly absorbed after PO administration. Protein binding: 40%. Extensively distributed throughout the body. Extensively metabolized. Steady-state concentrations achieved within 2 days. Eliminated in urine. Unknown if removed by hemodialysis. ***Half-life:*** 6 hr.

INDICATIONS AND DOSAGES

Parkinson's disease

PO

Adults, Elderly. Initially, 0.25 mg 3 times a day. May increase dosage every 7 days.

Restless leg syndrome

PO

Adults, Elderly. 0.25 mg for days 1 and 2; 0.5 mg for days 3-7; 1 mg for week 2; 1.5 mg for week 3; 2 mg for week 4; 2.5 mg for week 5; 3 mg for week 6; 4 mg for week 7. All doses to be given 1-3 hrs before bedtime.

AVAILABLE FORMS

- *Tablets:* 0.25 mg, 0.5 mg, 1 mg, 2 mg, 3 mg, 4 mg, 5 mg.

CONTRAINDICATIONS: None known.

PREGNANCY AND LACTATION: Pregnancy category C; inhibits lactation

SIDE EFFECTS

Frequent (60%-40%)

Nausea, dizziness, somnolence

Occasional (12%-5%)

Syncope, vomiting, fatigue, viral infection, dyspepsia, diaphoresis, asthenia, orthostatic hypotension, abdominal discomfort, pharyngitis, abnormal vision, dry mouth, hypertension, hallucinations, confusion

Rare (less than 4%)

Anorexia, peripheral edema, memory loss, rhinitis, sinusitis, palpitations, impotence

SERIOUS REACTIONS

- Falling asleep without warning while engaged in activities of daily living, including driving motor vehicles, has been reported.

INTERACTIONS

Drugs

3 *Ciprofloxacin, enoxacin, pefloxacin:* Addition increases ropinirole concentrations

3 *CNS depressants:* May increase CNS depressant effects

3 *Dopamine antagonists:* Diminished anti-Parkinson's effect

3 *Estrogens:* Reduced ropinirole clearance, may need to decrease ropinirole if estrogen stopped

3 *Kava kava:* May decrease the effectiveness of ropinirole

SPECIAL CONSIDERATIONS

- Domperidone 20 mg 1 hr prior to ropinirole prevents drug-induced postural effects
- Discontinue slowly over 1 wk

PATIENT/FAMILY EDUCATION

- Take ropinirole with food if nausea is a problem
- Dizziness, drowsiness, and orthostatic hypotension are common initial responses to the drug; change

positions slowly to help prevent orthostatic hypotension

• Avoid tasks that require mental alertness or motor skills until response to the drug has been established

• The drug may cause hallucinations

MONITORING PARAMETERS

• Assess for relief of symptoms, such as improvement of mask-like facial expression, muscular rigidity, shuffling gait, and resting tremors of the hands and head

rosiglitazone maleate

(roz-ih-gli'-ta-zone mal'-ee-ate)

Rx: Avandia

Combinations

Rx: with metformin (Avandamet)

Chemical Class: Thiazolidinedione

Therapeutic Class: Antidiabetic; hypoglycemic; insulin resistance reducer

CLINICAL PHARMACOLOGY

Mechanism of Action: An antidiabetic that improves target-cell response to insulin without increasing pancreatic insulin secretion. Decreases hepatic glucose output and increases insulin-dependent glucose utilization in skeletal muscle. ***Therapeutic Effect:*** Lowers blood glucose concentration.

Pharmacokinetics

Rapidly absorbed. Protein binding: 99%. Metabolized in the liver. Excreted primarily in urine, with a lesser amount in feces. Not removed by hemodialysis. ***Half-life:*** 3-4 hr.

INDICATIONS AND DOSAGES

Diabetes mellitus, combination therapy

PO (with sulfonylureas, metformin)

Adults, Elderly. Initially, 4 mg as a single daily dose or in divided doses twice a day. May increase to 8 mg/day after 12 wk of therapy if fasting glucose level is not adequately controlled.

PO (with insulin)

Adults, Elderly. Initially, 4 mg/day in 1 or 2 doses and reduce insulin dose by 10%-25%. If hypoglycemia occurs or plasma glucose falls to less than 100 mg/dl, doses of rosiglitazone greater than 4 mg are not recommended.

Diabetes mellitus, monotherapy

Adults, Elderly. Initially, 4 mg as single daily dose or in divided doses twice a day. May increase to 8 mg/day after 12 wk of therapy.

AVAILABLE FORMS

• *Tablets:* 2 mg, 4 mg, 8 mg.

CONTRAINDICATIONS: Active hepatic disease, diabetic ketoacidosis, increased serum transaminase levels, including ALT greater than 2.5 times the normal serum level, type 1 diabetes mellitus

PREGNANCY AND LACTATION: Pregnancy category C; no adequate and well controlled studies in pregnant women available; abnormally high glucose levels during pregnancy associated with higher incidence of congenital anomalies, morbidity, and mortality, insulin monotherapy preferred agent; drug detected in lactating rats; no information in humans

SIDE EFFECTS

Frequent (9%)

Upper respiratory tract infection

Occasional (4%-2%)

Headache, edema, back pain, fatigue, sinusitis, diarrhea

SERIOUS REACTIONS

• Hepatotoxicity occurs rarely.

INTERACTIONS

Drugs

3 *Fenugreek, ginseng, glucomannan, bitter melon, eucalyptus, guar gum, St. John's wort:* Additive blood glucose lowering; increased risk of hypoglycemia

3 *Glucosamine, licorice:* May reduce the effectiveness of rosiglitazone

3 *Gemfibrozil:* May increase plasma concentrations of rosiglitazone

Labs

• Elevations of AST, ALT, bilirubin, LDH, LDL cholesterol (15%); HDL cholesterol (15%); decreases in hematocrit, hemoglobin, alkaline phosphatase

SPECIAL CONSIDERATIONS

• *Expected hypoglycemic effects:* Decreases in serum glucose: 50-75 mg/dL; decreases in HbA1c 1.2%-1.5%

PATIENT/FAMILY EDUCATION

• Caloric restriction, weight loss, and exercise essential adjuvant therapy

• Blood draws for LFT monitoring along with routine diabetes mellitus labs; review symptoms of hepatitis (unexplained nausea, vomiting, abdominal pain, fatigue, anorexia, or dark urine)

• Notify clinician of rapid increases in weight or edema or symptoms of heart failure (shortness of breath)

• OK to take with food

• Review hypoglycemia risks and symptoms when added to other hypoglycemic agents

• Follow prescribed diet

• Carry candy, sugar packets, or other sugar supplements for immediate response to hypoglycemia and wear medical alert identification stating he or she has diabetes

• Avoid alcohol

MONITORING PARAMETERS

• "Poly" diabetes mellitus symptoms, periodic serum glucose and HbA1c measurements; LFT (AST, ALT) prior to initiation of therapy and periodically thereafter; hemoglobin/hematocrit, signs and symptoms of heart failure

---

rosuvastatin calcium

(roe-soo'-va-sta-tin kal'-see-um)

Rx: Crestor

Chemical Class: Substituted heptenoic acid derivative

Therapeutic Class: HMG-CoA reductase inhibitor; antilipemic

CLINICAL PHARMACOLOGY

Mechanism of Action: An antihyperlipidemic that interferes with cholesterol biosynthesis by inhibiting the conversion of the enzyme hydroxamethylglutaryl-CoA (HMG-CoA) to mevalonate, a precursor to cholesterol. ***Therapeutic Effect:*** Decreases LDL cholesterol, VLDL, and plasma triglyceride levels, increases HDL concentration.

Pharmacokinetics

Protein binding: 88%. Minimal hepatic metabolism. Primarily eliminated in the feces. ***Half-life:*** 19 hr (increased in patients with severe renal dysfunction).

INDICATIONS AND DOSAGES

Hyperlipidemia, dyslipidemia

PO

Adults, Elderly. 5-40 mg/day. Usual starting dosage is 10 mg/day, with adjustments based on lipid levels; monitor q2-4wk until desired level is achieved. Maximum: 40 mg/day.

Renal impairment (creatinine clearance less than 30 ml/min)

PO

Adults, Elderly. 5 mg/day; do not exceed 10 mg/day.

Concurrent cyclosporine use
PO
Adults, Elderly. 5 mg/day.
Concurrent lipid-lowering therapy
PO
Adults, Elderly. 10 mg/day.

AVAILABLE FORMS

• *Tablets:* 5 mg, 10 mg, 20 mg, 40 mg.

CONTRAINDICATIONS: Active hepatic disease, breast-feeding, pregnancy, unexplained, persistent elevations of serum transaminase levels

PREGNANCY AND LACTATION: Pregnancy category X; not recommended for nursing mothers

SIDE EFFECTS

Rosuvastatin is generally well tolerated. Side effects are usually mild and transient.

Occasional (9%-3%)
Pharyngitis; headache; diarrhea; dyspepsia, including heartburn and epigastric distress; nausea

Rare (less than 3%)
Myalgia, asthenia or unusual fatigue and weakness, back pain

SERIOUS REACTIONS

• Cases of rhabdomyolysis have been reported.
• Lens opacities may occur.
• Hypersensitivity reaction and hepatitis occur rarely.

INTERACTIONS

Drugs

3 *Cyclosporine:* Increase in rosuvastatin mean C_{max} and mean AUC
3 *Erythromycin:* Reduces the plasma concentration of erythromycin
3 *Ethinyl estradiol, norgestrel:* Increases the plasma concentrations of ethinyl estradiol and norgestrel
3 *Gemfibrozil:* Increase in rosuvastatin mean C_{max} and mean AUC
3 *Magnesium- and aluminum-containing antacids:* Decreased absorption; separate by 2 hr
3 *Niacin:* Increases the risk of myopathy
3 *St. John's wort:* May reduce the effectiveness of rosuvastatin
3 *Warfarin:* Coadministration with stable warfarin therapy resulted in clinically significant hypoprothrombinemia (INR>4)

SPECIAL CONSIDERATIONS

• Base statin selection on lipid-lowering prowess, cost, side effects, and availability of mortality reduction studies
• Rosuvastatin is the most potent statin on the market in its ability to decrease LDL with a significant reduction in total cholesterol, triglycerides, and increase in HDL; however, overall mortality rates are lacking
• Notable proteinuria (persistent) accompanies rosuvastatin use; clinical significance yet unknown; would hesitate to use as first-line statin
• NOTE: not dependent on metabolism by cytochrome P4503A4 to a clinically significant extent

PATIENT/FAMILY EDUCATION

• Report symptoms of myalgia, muscle tenderness, or weakness
• May be taken with or without food and regardless of the time of day
• Adjunctive to diet and exercise
• The female patient of childbearing years should use appropriate contraceptive measures during rosuvastatin therapy; rosuvastatin is pregnancy risk category X
• Periodic laboratory tests are an essential part of therapy

MONITORING PARAMETERS

• *Efficacy:* Fasting lipid panel at 3-6 mos

• AST/ALT at baseline, 12 wks, following any elevation of dose, and then periodically (discontinue if elevations persist at >3 times upper limit of normal)
• CPK in patients complaining of unexplained diffuse myalgia, muscle tenderness, or muscle weakness
• Routine urinalysis for proteinuria; may need to reduce dose with persistent proteinuria

salicylic acid

(sal-i-sill'-ik as'-id)

Rx: Compound W, Compound W One Step Wart Remover, DHS Sal, Dr. Scholl's Callus Remover, Dr. Scholl's Clear Away, DuoFilm, DuoPlant, Freezone, Fung-O, Gordofilm, Hydrisalic, Ionil, Ionil Plus, Keralyt, LupiCare, Dandruff, LupiCare II Psoriasis, LupiCare Psoriasis, Mediplast, MG217 Sal-Acid, Mosco Corn and Callus Remover, NeoCeuticals Acne Spot Treatment, Neutrogena Acne Wash, Neutrogena Body Clear, NeutrogenaClear Pore, Neutrogena Clear Pore Shine Control, Neutrogena Healthy Scalp, Neutrogena Maximum Strength T/Sal, Neutrogena On The Spot Acne Patch, Occlusal-HP, Oxy Balance, Oxy Balance Deep Pore, Palmer's Skin Success Acne Cleanser, Pedisilk, Propa pH, SalAc, Sal-Acid, Salactic, Sal-Plant, Stri-dex, Stri-dex Body Focus, Stri-dex Facewipes To Go, Stri-dex Maximum Strength, Tinamed, Tiseb, Trans-Ver-Sal, Wart-Off Maximum Strength, Zapzyt Acne Wash, Zapzyt Pore Treatment, Salac

Combinations

Rx: with sodium thiosulfate (Versiclear)

Chemical Class: Salicylate derivative

Therapeutic Class: Keratolytic

CLINICAL PHARMACOLOGY

Mechanism of Action: A keratolytic agent that produces desquamation of hyperkeratotic epithelium by dissolution of intercellular cement and causes the cornified tissue to swell, soften, macerate, and desquamate. ***Therapeutic Effect:*** Decreases acne, psoriasis, and wart removal.

Pharmacokinetics

Absorption differs between formulations. Protein binding: 50%-80%. Bound to serum albumin. Metabolized to salicylate glucoronides and salicyluric acid. Excreted in urine.

INDICATIONS AND DOSAGES

Acne

Topical

Adults, Elderly, Children. Apply cream, foam, gel, liquid, pads, patch, or soap 1-3 times/day.

Callus, corn, wart removal

Topical

Adults, Elderly, Children. Apply gel, liquid, plaster, or patch to wart 1-2 times/day.

Dandruff, psoriasis, seborrheic dermatitis

Topical

Adults, Elderly, Children. Apply cream, ointment, or shampoo 3-4 times/day.

AVAILABLE FORMS

• *Cream:* 2% (Neutrogena Acne Wash), 2.5% (LupiCare Dandruff, LupiCare Psoriasis, LupiCare II).

• *Gel:* 0.5% (Neutrogena Clean Pore Shine Control), 2% (NeuCeuticals Acne Spot Treatment, Neutrogena Clean Pore, Oxy Balance, Stri-dex Body Focus, Zapzyt Acne Wash, Zapzyt Pore Treatment), 6% (Hydrisalic, Keralyt), 17% (Compound W, DuoPlant, Sal-Plant).

• *Foam:* 2% (Neutrogena Acne Wash, Salac).

• *Liquid:* 2% (NeoCeuticals Acne Spot Treatment, Neutrogena Acne Wash, Neutrogena Body Clear, Propa pH, SalAc), 17% (Compound W, DuoFilm, Freezone, Fung-O, Gordofilm, Mosco Corn and Callus Remover, Occlusal-HP, Pedisilk, Salactic, Tinamed, Wart-Off).

• *Ointment:* 3% (MG217 Sal-Acid).

• *Pads:* 0.5% (Oxy Balance, Oxy Balance Deep Pore, Stri-dex, Stri-dex Facewipes To Go), 2% (Neutrogena Acne Wash, Stri-dex Maximum Strength).

• *Patch:* 2% (Neutrogena On The Spot Acne Patch), 15% (Trans-Ver-Sal), 40% (Compound W, Dr. Scholl's Callus Remover, Dr. Scholl's Clear Away, DuoFilm).

• *Plaster:* 40% (Mediplast, Sal-Acid, Tinamed).

• *Shampoo:* 1.8% (Neutrogena Healthy Scalp), 2% (Ionil, Ionil Plus, LupiCare Dandruff, LupiCare Psoriasis, Tiseb), 3% (Neutrogena Maximum Strength T/Sal).

• *Soap:* 2%.

• *Solution:* 17% (Compound W).

UNLABELED USES: Tinea pedis

CONTRAINDICATIONS: Children less than 2 yrs old, diabetes, impaired circulation, hypersensitivity to salicylic acid or any of its components

PREGNANCY AND LACTATION: Pregnancy category C

SIDE EFFECTS

Occasional

Burning, erythema, irritation, pruritus, stinging

Rare

Dizziness, nausea, vomiting, diarrhea, hypoglycemia

SERIOUS REACTIONS

• Symptoms of salicylate toxicity include lethargy, hyperpnea, diarrhea, and psychic disturbances.

INTERACTIONS

Drugs

3 *Ammonium sulfate:* Increases plasma salicylate level

3 *Corticosteroids:* Decreases plasma salicylate level; tapering doses of steroids may promote salicylism
3 *Heparin:* Salicylate decreases platelet adhesiveness and interferes with hemostasis in heparin-treated patients
3 *Methotrexate:* Decreases tubular reabsorption; clinical toxicity from methotrexate can result
3 *Pyrazinamide:* Inhibits pyrazinamide-induced hyperuricemia
3 *Tolbutamide:* Potentiates hypoglycemia
3 *Uricosuric agents:* Inhibits the effect of these drugs

SPECIAL CONSIDERATIONS

PATIENT/FAMILY EDUCATION

- For external use only; avoid contact with face, eyes, genitals, mucous membranes, and normal skin surrounding warts
- May cause reddening or scaling of skin
- Soaking area in warm water for 5 min prior to application may enhance effect (remove any loose tissue with brush, washcloth, or emery board and dry thoroughly prior to application)

MONITORING PARAMETERS

- Clinical improvement

salmeterol xinafoate

(sal-me'-te-role zin-na'-foe-ate)

Rx: Serevent, Serevent Diskus

Combinations

Rx: with fluticasone (Advair)

Chemical Class: Sympathomimetic amine; β_2-adrenergic agonist

Therapeutic Class: Antiasthmatic; bronchodilator

CLINICAL PHARMACOLOGY

Mechanism of Action: An adrenergic agonist that stimulates beta$_2$-adrenergic receptors in the lungs, resulting in relaxation of bronchial smooth muscle. ***Therapeutic Effect:*** Relieves bronchospasm and reduces airway resistance.

Pharmacokinetics

Route	Onset	Peak	Duration
Inhalation	10-20 mins	3 hrs	12 hrs

Low systemic absorption; acts primarily in the lungs. Protein binding: 95%. Metabolized by hydroxylation. Primarily eliminated in feces. ***Half-life:*** 3-4 hrs.

INDICATIONS AND DOSAGES

Prevention and maintenance treatment of asthma

Inhalation (Diskus)

Adults, Elderly, Children 4 yr and older. 1 inhalation (50 mcg) q12h.

Prevention of exercise-induced bronchospasm

Inhalation (Diskus)

Adults, Elderly, Children 4 yr and older. 1 inhalation at least 30 min before exercise.

Chronic obstructive pulmonary disorder (COPD)

Inhalation (Diskus)

Adults, Elderly. 1 inhalation q12h.

AVAILABLE FORMS

• *Powder for Oral Inhalation:* 50 mcg.

CONTRAINDICATIONS: History of hypersensitivity to sympathomimetics

PREGNANCY AND LACTATION: Pregnancy category C

SIDE EFFECTS

Frequent (28%)

Headache

Occasional (7%-3%)

Cough, tremor, dizziness, vertigo, throat dryness or irritation, pharyngitis

Rare (3%)

Palpitations, tachycardia, nausea, heartburn, GI distress, diarrhea

SERIOUS REACTIONS

• Salmeterol may prolong the QT interval, which may precipitate ventricular arrhythmias.

• Hypokalemia and hyperglycemia may occur.

INTERACTIONS

Drugs

❷ *β-blockers:* Decreased action of salmeterol, cardioselective β-blockers preferable if concurrent use necessary

❸ *Furosemide:* Potential for additive hypokalemia

SPECIAL CONSIDERATIONS

PATIENT/FAMILY EDUCATION

• Patients receiving salmeterol for asthma should normally *also* be receiving regular and adequate doses of an effective asthma controller medication, such as inhaled corticosteroid

• Proper inhalation technique is vital

• Notify clinician if no response to usual doses, or if palpitations, rapid heartbeat, chest pain, muscle tremors, dizziness, headache occur

• **Do not use to treat acute symptoms or on an as-needed basis**

• Keep the drug canister at room temperature because cold decreases the drug's effects

• When the drug is used to prevent exercise-induced bronchospasm, administer the dose at least 30-60 min before exercising

• Wait at least 1 full min before the second inhalation

• Do not abruptly discontinue the drug or exceed the recommended dosage

• Avoid excessive consumption of caffeinated products, such as chocolate, cocoa, cola, coffee, and tea

• Teach the patient how to measure peak flow readings and keep a log of measurements

MONITORING PARAMETERS

• Blood pressure, pulse rate and quality, and respiratory rate, depth, rhythm, and type

• Periodically evaluate the serum potassium level

salsalate

(sal'-sa-late)

Rx: Amigesic, Disalcid, Mono-Gesic, Salflex, Salsitab

Chemical Class: Salicylate derivative

Therapeutic Class: NSAID; nonnarcotic analgesic

S

CLINICAL PHARMACOLOGY

Mechanism of Action: An NSAID that inhibits prostaglandin synthesis, reducing the inflammatory response and the intensity of pain stimuli reaching the sensory nerve endings. ***Therapeutic Effect:*** Produces analgesic and antiinflammatory effects.

Pharmacokinetics

Rapidly and completely absorbed from the GI tract. Food delays absorption of salsalate. Protein binding: high (to albumin). Metabolized in the liver. Excreted in urine. Removed by hemodialysis. ***Half-life:*** 1 hr.

INDICATIONS AND DOSAGES

Rheumatoid arthritis, osteoarthritis pain

PO

Adults, Elderly. Initially, 3 g/day in 2-3 divided doses. Maintenance: 2-4 g/day.

AVAILABLE FORMS

- *Tablets (Amigesic, Disalcid):* 500 mg, 750 mg.
- *Tablets (Mono-Gesic, Slaflex):* 750 mg.

CONTRAINDICATIONS: Bleeding disorders, hypersensitivity to salicylates or NSAIDs

PREGNANCY AND LACTATION: Pregnancy category C; excreted into breast milk; use caution in nursing mothers due to potential adverse effects in nursing infant

SIDE EFFECTS

Occasional

Nausea, dyspepsia (including heartburn, indigestion, and epigastric pain)

SERIOUS REACTIONS

- There is an increased risk of cardiovascular events, including MI and cerebrovascular accident, and serious—potentially life-threatening—GI bleeding.
- Tinnitus may be the first indication that the serum salicylic acid concentration is reaching or exceeding the upper therapeutic range.
- Salsalate use may also produce vertigo, headache, confusion, drowsiness, diaphoresis, hyperventilation, vomiting, and diarrhea.
- Reye's syndrome may occur in children with chickenpox or the flu.
- Severe overdose may result in electrolyte imbalance, hyperthermia, dehydration, and blood pH imbalance.
- GI bleeding, peptic ulcer, and Reye's syndrome rarely occur.

INTERACTIONS

Drugs

3 *Antacids, urinary alkalinizers:* Increase the excretion of salsalate

3 *Anticoagulants, heparin, thrombolytics:* Increase the risk of bleeding

3 *Antidiabetics:* May increase the effects of these drugs (with large doses of salsalate)

3 *Methotrexate, zidovudine:* May increase the toxicity of these drugs

3 *Ototoxic medications, vancomycin:* May increase the risk of ototoxicity

3 *Probenecid, sulfinpyrazone:* May decrease the effects of these drugs

Labs

- *False increase:* Serum bicarbonate, CSF, protein, serum theophylline
- *False decrease:* Urine cocaine, urine estrogen, serum glucose, urine 17-hydroxycorticosteroids, urine opiates
- *False positive:* Urine ferric chloride test

SPECIAL CONSIDERATIONS

- Consider for patients with GI intolerance to aspirin or patients in whom interference with normal platelet function by aspirin or other NSAIDs is undesirable

PATIENT/FAMILY EDUCATION

- Take salsalate with food and use antacids to relieve upset stomach
- Notify the physician if persistent GI pain or ringing in ears occurs
- Avoid alcohol and NSAIDs during salsalate therapy

MONITORING PARAMETERS

- AST, ALT, bilirubin, creatinine, CBC, hematocrit if patient is on long-term therapy

• Therapeutic response, such as improved grip strength, increased joint mobility, reduced joint tenderness, and relief of pain, stiffness, and swelling

saquinavir

(sa-kwin'-a-veer)

Rx: Fortovase, Invirase

Chemical Class: Protease inhibitor, HIV

Therapeutic Class: Antiretroviral

CLINICAL PHARMACOLOGY

Mechanism of Action: Inhibits HIV protease, rendering the enzyme incapable of processing the polyprotein precursors needed to generate functional proteins in HIV-infected cells. ***Therapeutic Effect:*** Interferes with HIV replication, slowing the progression of HIV infection.

Pharmacokinetics

Poorly absorbed after PO administration (absorption increased with high-calorie and high-fat meals). Protein binding: 99%. Metabolized in the liver to inactive metabolite. Primarily eliminated in feces. Unknown if removed by hemodialysis. ***Half-life:*** 13 hr.

INDICATIONS AND DOSAGES

HIV infection in combination with other antiretrovirals

PO (Fortovase)

Adults, Elderly. 1200 mg 3 times a day or 1000 mg twice a day in combination with ritonavir 100 mg twice a day.

PO (Invirase)

Adults, Elderly. 1000 mg (5×200 mg or 2×500 mg) twice a day in combination with ritonavir 100 mg twice a day.

Dosage adjustments when given in combination therapy:

Delavirdine: Fortovase 800 mg 3 times a day.

Lopinavir/ritonavir: Fortovase 800 mg twice a day.

Nelfinavir: Fortovase 800 mg 3 times a day or 1200 mg twice a day.

Ritonavir: Fortovase or Invirase 1000 mg twice a day.

AVAILABLE FORMS

• *Capsules (Invirase):* 200 mg.

• *Capsules, Gelatin (Fortovase):* 200 mg.

• *Tablets (Invirase):* 500 mg.

CONTRAINDICATIONS: Concurrent use with ergot medications, lovastatin, midazolam, simvastatin, or triazolam

PREGNANCY AND LACTATION: Pregnancy category B

SIDE EFFECTS

Occasional

Diarrhea, abdominal discomfort and pain, nausea, photosensitivity, stomatitis

Rare

Confusion, ataxia, asthenia, headache, rash

SERIOUS REACTIONS

• Ketoacidosis occurs rarely.

INTERACTIONS

Drugs

⚠ *Astemizole:* Increased plasma levels of astemizole

③ *Barbiturates:* Increased clearance of saquinavir; reduced clearance of barbiturates

③ *Calcium channel blockers, clindamycin, dapsone, quinidine:* May increase the plasma concentrations of these drugs

② *Carbamazepine:* Increased clearance of saquinavir, reduced clearance of carbamazepine

⚠ *Cisapride:* Increased plasma levels of cisapride

③ *Clarithromycin:* Reduced clearance of saquinavir; saquinavir reduces clearance of clarithromycin

3 *Delavirdine:* Decreased clearance of saquinavir; reduce dose of Fortovase (saquinavir soft gel capsule) to 800 mg tid

3 *Dexamethasone:* Reduced saquinavir level

⚠ *Efavirenz:* Reduced saquinavir level

⚠ *Ergot alkaloids:* Increased plasma levels of ergot alkaloids

3 *Erythromycin:* Reduced clearance of saquinavir; saquinavir reduces clearance of erythromycin

3 *Garlic, St. John's Wort:* May decrease the plasma concentration and effect of saquinavir

3 *Grapefruit juice:* Increased saquinavir level

⚠ *Indinavir:* Decreased clearance of saquinavir

3 *Ketoconazole:* Increases saquinavir plasma concentration

⚠ *Lovastatin:* Saquinavir reduces clearance of lovastatin

⚠ *Midazolam:* Increased plasma levels of midazolam and prolonged effect

3 *Nelfinavir:* Decreased clearance of saquinavir; reduce dose of Fortovase (saquinavir soft gel capsule) to 800 mg tid

3 *Oral contraceptives:* Saquinavir may reduce efficacy

3 *Phenytoin:* Increased clearance of saquinavir; reduced clearance of phenytoin

⚠ *Rifabutin:* Increased clearance of saquinavir

⚠ *Rifampin:* Increased clearance of saquinavir

3 *Ritonavir:* Decreased clearance of saquinavir; decrease saquinavir dose to 400 mg bid, or less, depending on ritonavir dose

3 *Sildenafil:* Increases sildenafil plasma concentrations

⚠ *Simvastatin:* Saquinavir reduces clearance of simvastatin

⚠ *Terfenadine:* Increased plasma levels of terfenadine

⚠ *Triazolam:* Increased plasma levels of triazolam and prolonged effect

SPECIAL CONSIDERATIONS

- Invirase and fortovase not considered bioequivalent; no food effect on Invirase when taken with ritonavir; take Fortovase with large meal
- Fortovase is the recommended formulation
- Invirase should only be considered if it is to be combined with antiretrovirals that significantly inhibit saquinavir's metabolism

PATIENT/FAMILY EDUCATION

- Take saquinavir within 2 hrs after a full meal
- Space drug doses evenly around the clock and continue taking the drug for the full course of treatment
- Notify the physician if nausea or vomiting or persistent abdominal pain occurs
- Avoid grapefruit products while taking saquinavir
- Avoid exposure to artificial light sources and sunlight
- Saquinavir is not a cure for HIV infection, nor does it reduce the risk of transmitting HIV to others

MONITORING PARAMETERS

- Blood chemistry and serum hepatic enzyme levels, CD4+ cell count and blood glucose, HIV RNA, and serum triglyceride levels
- Monitor for signs and symptoms of GI discomfort
- Assess pattern of daily bowel activity and stool consistency
- Inspect the patient's mouth for signs of mucosal ulceration
- If the patient experience severe toxicities, such as ketoacidosis, withhold the drug and notify the physician

scopolamine

(skoe-pol′-a-meen)

Rx: *Transdermal:* Transderm-Scop

Rx: *Ophth:* Isopto Hyoscine

Rx: *Oral:* Scopace

Chemical Class: Belladonna alkaloid

Therapeutic Class: Anticholinergic; antiemetic; antivertigo agent; cycloplegic; mydriatic

CLINICAL PHARMACOLOGY

Mechanism of Action: An anticholinergic that reduces excitability of labyrinthine receptors, depressing conduction in the vestibular cerebellar pathway. ***Therapeutic Effect:*** Prevents motion-induced nausea and vomiting.

Pharmacokinetics

Well absorbed percutaneously. Crosses blood-brain barrier. Metabolized in liver. Excreted in urine. ***Half-life:*** 9.5 hrs (transdermal).

INDICATIONS AND DOSAGES

Prevention of motion sickness

Transdermal

Adults. 1 system q72h.

Postoperative nausea or vomiting

Transdermal

Adults, Elderly. 1 system no sooner than 1 h before surgery and removed 24 hrs after surgery.

AVAILABLE FORMS

• *Transdermal System (Trans-Derm Scop):* 1.5 mg.

CONTRAINDICATIONS: Angle-closure glaucoma, GI or GU obstruction, myasthenia gravis, paralytic ileus, tachycardia, thyrotoxicosis

PREGNANCY AND LACTATION: Pregnancy category C; no reports of adverse effects reported; compatible with breast-feeding

SIDE EFFECTS

Frequent (greater than 15%)

Dry mouth, somnolence, blurred vision

Rare (5%-1%)

Dizziness, restlessness, hallucinations, confusion, difficulty urinating, rash

SERIOUS REACTIONS

• None known.

INTERACTIONS

Drugs

3 *Antihistamines, phenothiazines, tricyclics:* Additive anticholinergic effect

3 *CNS depressants:* May increase CNS depression

SPECIAL CONSIDERATIONS

PATIENT/FAMILY EDUCATION

• Avoid abrupt discontinuation (taper off over 1 wk)

• Wash hands thoroughly after handling transdermal patches before contacting eyes

• Avoid tasks requiring mental alertness or motor skills until response to the drug has been established

MONITORING PARAMETERS

• BUN level; blood chemistry test results; and serum alkaline phosphatase, bilirubin, creatinine, AST (SGOT), and ALT (SGPT) levels to assess hepatic and renal function

secobarbital sodium

(see-koe-bar'-bi-tal soe'-dee-um)

Rx: Seconal

Combinations

Rx: with amobarbital (Tuinal)

Chemical Class: Barbituric acid derivative

Therapeutic Class: Anesthesia adjunct; anticonvulsant; sedative/hypnotic

DEA Class: Schedule II

CLINICAL PHARMACOLOGY

Mechanism of Action: A barbiturate that depresses the central nervous system (CNS) activity by binding to barbiturate site at the GABA-receptor complex enhancing GABA activity and depressing reticular activity system. ***Therapeutic Effect:*** Produces hypnotic effect due to CNS depression.

Pharmacokinetics

Well absorbed from the gastrointestinal (GI) tract. Protein binding: 52%-57%. Crosses blood-brain barrier. Widely distributed. Metabolized in liver by microsomal enzyme system to inactive and active metabolites. Primarily excreted in urine. Not removed by hemodialysis. ***Half-life:*** 15-40 hrs.

INDICATIONS AND DOSAGES

Insomnia

PO

Adults. 100 mg at bedtime.

Preoperative sedation

PO

Adults. 100-300 mg 1-2 hrs. before procedure.

Children. 2-6 mg/kg 1-2 hrs. before procedure. Maximum: 100 mg/dose.

Sedation, daytime

PO

Adults. 30-50 mg 3-4 times/day.

Children. 2 mg/kg 3 times/day.

AVAILABLE FORMS

• *Capsules:* 50 mg (Seconal sodium).

UNLABELED USES: Chemotherapy-induced nausea and vomiting

CONTRAINDICATIONS: History of manifest or latent porphyria, marked liver dysfunction, marked respiratory disease in which dyspnea or obstruction is evident, and hypersensitivity to secobarbital or barbituates

PREGNANCY AND LACTATION: Pregnancy category D; small amounts excreted in breast milk; drowsiness in infant reported; compatible with breast-feeding

Controlled Substance: Schedule II

SIDE EFFECTS

Frequent

Somnolence

Occasional

Agitation, confusion, hyperkinesia, ataxia, CNS depression, nightmares, nervousness, psychiatric disturbance, hallucinations, insomnia, anxiety, dizziness, abnormality in thinking, hypoventilation, apnea, bradycardia, hypotension, syncope, nausea, vomiting, constipation, headache

Rare

Hypersensitivity reactions, fever, liver damage, megaloblastic anemia

SERIOUS REACTIONS

• Agranulocytosis, megaloblastic anemia, apnea, hypoventilation, bradycardia, hypotension, syncope, hepatic damage, and Stevens-Johnson syndrome rarely occur.

• Tolerance and physical dependence may occur with repeated use.

INTERACTIONS

Drugs

3 *Acetaminophen:* Enhanced hepatotoxic potential of acetaminophen overdoses

3 *Antidepressants:* Reduced serum concentration of cyclic antidepressants

3 *β-adrenergic blockers:* Reduced serum concentrations of β-blockers, which are extensively metabolized

3 *Calcium channel blockers:* Reduced serum concentrations of verapamil and dihydropyridines

3 *Chloramphenicol:* Increased barbiturate concentrations; reduced serum chloramphenicol concentrations

3 *Corticosteroids:* Reduced serum concentrations of corticosteroids; may impair therapeutic effect

3 *Cyclosporine:* Reduced serum concentration of cyclosporine

3 *Digitoxin:* Reduced serum concentration of digitoxin

3 *Disopyramide:* Reduced serum concentration of disopyramide

3 *Doxycycline:* Reduced serum doxycycline concentrations

3 *Estrogen:* Reduced serum concentration of estrogen

3 *Ethanol:* Excessive CNS depression

3 *Griseofulvin:* Reduced griseofulvin absorption

3 *MAOIs:* Prolonged effect of barbiturates

3 *Methoxyflurane:* Enhanced nephrotoxic effect

3 *Narcotic analgesics:* Increased toxicity of meperidine; reduced effect of methadone; additive CNS depression

3 *Neuroleptics:* Reduced effect of either drug

2 *Oral anticoagulants:* Decreased hypoprothrombinemic response to oral anticoagulants

3 *Oral contraceptives:* Reduced efficacy of oral contraceptives

3 *Phenytoin:* Unpredictable effect on serum phenytoin levels

3 *Propafenone:* Reduced serum concentration of propafenone

3 *Quinidine:* Reduced quinidine plasma concentration

3 *Tacrolimus:* Reduced serum concentration of tacrolimus

3 *Theophylline:* Reduced serum theophylline concentrations

3 *Valproic acid:* Increased serum concentrations of secobarbital

2 *Warfarin:* See oral anticoagulants

Labs

- *Glucose:* Falsely low with Clinistix, Diastix
- *17-Ketosteroids:* Falsely increased in urine
- *Phenobarbital:* Falsely increased in serum

SPECIAL CONSIDERATIONS

- Compared to the benzodiazepine sedative hypnotics, secobarbital is more lethal in overdosage, has a higher tendency for abuse and addiction, and is more likely to cause drug interactions via induction of hepatic microsomal enzymes; few advantages if any in safety or efficacy over benzodiazepines

PATIENT/FAMILY EDUCATION

- Avoid driving and other dangerous activities
- Withdrawal insomnia may occur after short-term use; do not start using drug again, insomnia will improve in 1-3 nights
- May experience increased dreaming
- Avoid alcohol and limit caffeine intake

MONITORING PARAMETERS

- Blood pressure, pulse, respiratory rate and rhythm

selegiline hydrochloride

(se-le´-ji-leen)

Rx: Eldepryl

Chemical Class: Phenethylamine derivative

Therapeutic Class: Anti-Parkinson's agent

CLINICAL PHARMACOLOGY

Mechanism of Action: An antiparkinson agent that irreversibly inhibits the activity of monoamine oxidase type B, the enzyme that breaks down dopamine, thereby increasing dopaminergic action. ***Therapeutic Effect:*** Relieves signs and symptoms of Parkinson's disease.

Pharmacokinetics

Rapidly absorbed from the GI tract. Crosses the blood-brain barrier. Metabolized in the liver to the active metabolites. Primarily excreted in urine. ***Half-life:*** 17 hr (amphetamine), 20 hr (methamphetamine).

INDICATIONS AND DOSAGES

Adjunctive treatment for parkinsonism

PO

Adults. 10 mg/day in divided doses, such as 5 mg at breakfast and lunch, given concomitantly with each dose of carbidopa and levodopa.

Elderly. Initially, 5 mg in the morning. May increase up to 10 mg/day.

AVAILABLE FORMS

- *Capsules:* 5 mg.
- *Tablets:* 5 mg.

UNLABELED USES: Treatment of Alzheimer's disease, attention deficit hyperactivity disorder, depression, early Parkinson's disease, extrapyramidal symptoms, negative symptoms of schizophrenia

CONTRAINDICATIONS: Concurrent use with meperidine

PREGNANCY AND LACTATION: Pregnancy category C; excretion in breast milk unknown

SIDE EFFECTS

Frequent (10%-4%)

Nausea, dizziness, light-headedness, syncope, abdominal discomfort

Occasional (3%-2%)

Confusion, hallucinations, dry mouth, vivid dreams, dyskinesia

Rare (1%)

Headache, myalgia, anxiety, diarrhea, insomnia

SERIOUS REACTIONS

- Symptoms of overdose may vary from CNS depression, characterized by sedation, apnea, cardiovascular collapse, and death, to severe paradoxical reactions, such as hallucinations, tremor, and seizures.
- Other serious effects may include involuntary movements, impaired motor coordination, loss of balance, blepharospasm, facial grimaces, feeling of heaviness in the lower extremities, depression, nightmares, delusions, overstimulation, sleep disturbance, and anger.

INTERACTIONS

Drugs

❷ *Antidepressants, serotonin reuptake inhibitors (fluoxetine, fluvoxamine, paroxetine, sertraline):* Serious, sometimes fatal, reactions including hyperthermia, autonomic instability, and mental status changes

❷ *Dexfenfluramine, fenfluramine:* Increased risk of serotonin syndrome

❷ *Dextroamphetamine:* Severe hypertension

❷ *Dextromethorphan:* Increased risk of serotonin syndrome

❸ *Guanadrel, guanethidine:* May inhibit the antihypertensive effects of antihypertensive agents

3 *Insulin:* Excessive hypoglycemia may occur when MAOIs are administered to patients with diabetes
3 *Levodopa:* May precipitate hypertensive crisis
⚠ *Methylphenidate:* Increased risk of hypertensive reactions
3 *Moclobemide:* Increased pressor effects of tyramine; increased risk of adverse drug or food interactions
❷ *Narcotic analgesics (meperidine):* Stupor, muscular rigidity, severe agitation, elevated temperature, hallucinations, and death
3 *Narcotic analgesics (morphine):* Stupor, muscular rigidity, severe agitation, elevated temperature, hallucinations, and death
⚠ *Reserpine:* Loss of antihypertensive effects
⚠ *Sibutramine:* Increased risk of serotonin syndrome
3 *Succinylcholine:* Prolonged muscle relaxation caused by succinylcholine
⚠ *Sympathomimetics (metaraminol, phenylpropanolamine, pseudoephedrine):* Additive pressor response to sympathomimetic
3 *Sympathomimetics (norepinephrine, phenylephrine):* Additive pressor response to sympathomimetic
3 *Tyramine:* Increases the pressor effect of food or drink containing tyramine
⚠ *Venlafaxine:* Increased risk of serotonin syndrome

Labs

- *False positive:* Urine ketones, urine glucose
- *False negative:* Urine glucose (glucose oxidase)
- *False increase:* Uric acid, urine protein

SPECIAL CONSIDERATIONS

- At low doses, irreversible type B MAOI; at higher doses is metabolized to amphetamine, inhibiting both A and B subtypes of MAO
- Several placebo-controlled studies have demonstrated a significant delay in the need to initiate levodopa therapy in patients who receive selegiline in the early phase of the disease
- May have significant benefit in slowing the onset of the debilitating consequences of Parkinson's disease

PATIENT/FAMILY EDUCATION

- Dizziness, drowsiness, light-headedness, and dry mouth are common side effects of the drug but will diminish or disappear with continued treatment
- Change positions slowly and let legs dangle momentarily before standing to reduce the drug's hypotensive effect
- Avoid tasks that require mental alertness or motor skills until response to the drug has been established
- Avoid alcoholic beverages during therapy
- Avoid ingesting large amounts of caffeine or tyramine-rich foods, such as wine and aged cheese, to prevent a hypertensive reaction

MONITORING PARAMETERS

- Monitor the patient for dyskinetic effects
- Assess the patient for clinical reversal of symptoms, including improvement of masklike facial expression, muscular rigidity, shuffling gait, and resting tremor of the hands and head
- Be alert for neurologic effects, including agitation, headache, lethargy, and confusion

senna

(sen'-na)

Rx: Ex-Lax, Senexon, Senna-Glen, Sennatural, Senokot, X-Prep

Chemical Class: Anthraquinone derivative

Therapeutic Class: Laxative, stimulant

CLINICAL PHARMACOLOGY

Mechanism of Action: A GI stimulant that has a direct effect on intestinal smooth musculature by stimulating the intramural nerve plexi. ***Therapeutic Effect:*** Increases peristalsis and promotes laxative effect.

Pharmacokinetics

Route	Onset	Peak	Duration
PO	6-12 hrs	N/A	N/A
Rectal	0.5-2 hrs	N/A	N/A

Minimal absorption after oral administration. Hydrolyzed to active form by enzymes of colonic flora. Absorbed drug metabolized in the liver. Eliminated in feces via biliary system.

INDICATIONS AND DOSAGES

Constipation

PO (Tablets)

Adults, Elderly, Children 12 yrs and older. 2 tablets at bedtime. Maximum: 4 tablets twice a day.

Children 6-11 yrs. 1 tablet at bedtime. Maximum: 2 tablets twice a day.

Children 2-5 yrs. ½ tablet at bedtime. Maximum: 1 tablet twice a day.

PO (Syrup)

Adults, Elderly, Children 12 yrs and older. 10-15 ml at bedtime. Maximum: 15 ml twice a day.

Children 6-11 yrs. 5-7.5 ml at bedtime. Maximum: 7.5 ml twice a day.

Children 2-5 yrs. 2.5-3.75 ml at bedtime. Maximum: 3.75 ml twice a day.

PO (Granules)

Adults, Elderly, Children 12 yrs and older. 1 tsp at bedtime. Maximum: 2 tsp twice a day.

Children 6-11 yrs. one half (½) teaspoon at bedtime up to 1 teaspoon 2 times/day.

Children 2-5 yrs. one quarter (¼) teaspoon at bedtime up to one half (½) teaspoon 2 times/day.

Bowel evacuation

PO

Adults, Elderly, Children older than 1 yr. 75 ml between 2 p.m. and 4 p.m. on day prior to procedure.

AVAILABLE FORMS

- *Granules (Senokot):* 15 mg/tsp.
- *Liquid (X-Prep):* 8.8 mg/5 ml.
- *Syrup (Senokot):* 8.8 mg/5 ml.
- *Tablets (Sennatural, Senokot, Senexon, Senna-Gen):* 8.6 mg, 15 mg.
- *Tablets (Ex-Lax).*

CONTRAINDICATIONS: Abdominal pain, appendicitis, intestinal obstruction, nausea, vomiting

PREGNANCY AND LACTATION: Pregnancy category C

SIDE EFFECTS

Frequent

Pink-red, red-violet, red-brown, or yellow-brown discoloration of urine

Occasional

Some degree of abdominal discomfort, nausea, mild cramps, griping, faintness

SERIOUS REACTIONS

- Long-term use may result in laxative dependence, chronic constipation, and loss of normal bowel function.
- Prolonged use or overdose may result in electrolyte and metabolic disturbances (such as hypokalemia, hypocalcemia, and metabolic acidosis or alkalosis), vomiting, muscle weakness, persistent diarrhea, malabsorption, and weight loss.

INTERACTIONS

Drugs

3 *Oral medications:* May decrease transit time of concurrently administered oral medications, decreasing absorption of senna

SPECIAL CONSIDERATIONS

- Proposed laxative of choice for narcotic-induced constipation

PATIENT/FAMILY EDUCATION

- Urine may turn pink-red, red-violet, red-brown, or yellow-brown
- Institute measures to promote defecation, such as increasing fluid intake, exercising, and eating a high-fiber diet
- Take other oral medications within 1 hr of taking senna because these substances may decrease the effectiveness of senna

MONITORING PARAMETERS

- Bowel sounds for peristalsis
- Pattern of daily bowel activity and stool consistency; record time of evacuation
- Electrolytes

sertraline hydrochloride

(ser'-tra-leen hy-droe-klor'-ide)

Rx: Zoloft

Chemical Class: Naphthalenamine derivative

Therapeutic Class: Antidepressant, selective serotonin reuptake inhibitor (SSRI)

CLINICAL PHARMACOLOGY

Mechanism of Action: An antidepressant, anxiolytic, and obsessive-compulsive disorder adjunct that blocks the reuptake of the neurotransmitter serotonin at CNS neuronal presynaptic membranes, increasing its availability at postsynaptic receptor sites. ***Therapeutic Effect:*** Relieves depression, reduces obsessive-compulsive behavior, decreases anxiety.

Pharmacokinetics

Incompletely and slowly absorbed from the GI tract; food increases absorption. Protein binding: 98%. Widely distributed. Undergoes extensive first-pass metabolism in the liver to active compound. Excreted in urine and feces. Not removed by hemodialysis. ***Half-life:*** 26 hr.

INDICATIONS AND DOSAGES

Depression

PO

Adults. Initially, 50 mg/day. May increase by 50 mg/day at 7-day intervals up to 200 mg/day.

Elderly. Initially, 25 mg/day. May increase by 25-50 mg/day at 7-day intervals up to 200 mg/day.

Obsessive-compulsive disorder

PO

Adults, Children 13-17 yr. Initially, 50 mg/day with morning or evening meal. May increase by 50 mg/day at 7-day intervals.

Elderly, Children 6-12 yr. Initially, 25 mg/day. May increase by 25-50 mg/day at 7-day intervals. Maximum: 200 mg/day.

Panic disorder, posttraumatic stress disorder, social anxiety disorder

PO

Adults, Elderly. Initially, 25 mg/day. May increase by 50 mg/day at 7-day intervals. Range: 50-200 mg/day. Maximum: 200 mg/day.

Premenstrual dysphoric disorder

PO

Adults. Initially, 50 mg/day. May increase up to 150 mg/day in 50-mg increments.

AVAILABLE FORMS

- *Oral Concentrate:* 20 mg/ml.
- *Tablets:* 25 mg, 50 mg, 100 mg.

S

UNLABELED USES: Eating disorders, generalized anxiety disorder (GAD), impulse control disorders

CONTRAINDICATIONS: User within 14 days of MAOIs

PREGNANCY AND LACTATION: Pregnancy category C; excretion into breast milk unknown; use caution in nursing mother

SIDE EFFECTS

Frequent (26%-12%)

Headache, nausea, diarrhea, insomnia, somnolence, dizziness, fatigue, rash, dry mouth

Occasional (6%-4%)

Anxiety, nervousness, agitation, tremor, dyspepsia, diaphoresis, vomiting, constipation, abnormal ejaculation, visual disturbances, altered taste

Rare (less than 3%)

Flatulence, urinary frequency, paresthesia, hot flashes, chills

SERIOUS REACTIONS

• None known.

INTERACTIONS

Drugs

3 *Cimetidine:* Increased plasma sertraline concentrations

3 *Cyproheptadine:* Serotonin antagonist may partially reverse antidepressant and other effects

❷ *Dexfenfluramine:* Duplicate effects on inhibition of serotonin reuptake; inhibition of dexfenfluramine metabolism (CYP2D6) exaggerates effect; both mechanisms increase risk of serotonin syndrome

❷ *Fenfluramine:* Duplicate effects on inhibition of serotonin reuptake; inhibition of dexfenfluramine metabolism (CYP2D6) exaggerates effect; both mechanisms increase risk of serotonin syndrome

3 *Lithium:* Neurotoxicity (tremor, confusion, ataxia, dizziness, dysarthria, and absence seizures) reported in patients receiving fluoxetine-lithium combination; mechanism unknown

▲ *MAOIs (isocarboxazid, phenelzine, tranylcypromine):* Increased CNS serotonergic effects has been associated with severe or fatal reactions with this combination

❷ *Selegiline:* Sporadic cases of mania and hypertension

3 *Sumatriptan:* Concomitant use of SSRI and sumatriptan may increase adverse effects

3 *Tricyclic antidepressants (clomipramine, desipramine, doxepin, imipramine, nortriptyline, trazodone):* Marked increases in tricyclic antidepressant levels due to inhibition of metabolism (CYP2D6)

❷ *Tryptophan:* Additive serotonergic effects

3 *Warfarin:* Increased hypoprothrombinemic response to warfarin

SPECIAL CONSIDERATIONS

• SSRI of choice based on intermediate length $t_{1/2}$, linear pharmacokinetics, absence of appreciable age effect on clearance, substantially less effect on P450 enzymes, reducing potential for drug interactions

• Oral concentrate contains 12% alcohol; dropper contains natural rubber, caution if latex allergy

• Splitting 100-mg tablets to yield 50-mg dose cuts costs

PATIENT/FAMILY EDUCATION

• Oral concentrate must be diluted in water, ginger ale, lemon/lime soda, lemonade, or orange juice only, no other liquids should be used; do not mix in advance

• Avoid alcohol

sevelamer hydrochloride

(seh-vel′-ah-mer hye-droe-klor′-ide)

Rx: Renagel

Chemical Class: Allylamine

Therapeutic Class: Phosphate adsorbent

CLINICAL PHARMACOLOGY

Mechanism of Action: An antihyperphosphatemia agent that binds with dietary phosphorus in the GI tract, thus allowing phosphorus to be eliminated through the normal digestive process and decreasing the serum phosphorus level. ***Therapeutic Effect:*** Decreases incidence of hypercalcemic episodes in patients receiving calcium acetate treatment.

Pharmacokinetics

Not absorbed systemically. Unknown if removed by hemodialysis.

INDICATIONS AND DOSAGES

Hyperphosphatemia

PO

Adults, Elderly. 800-1600 mg with each meal, depending on severity of hyperphosphatemia.

AVAILABLE FORMS

- *Capsules:* 403 mg.
- *Tablets:* 400 mg, 800 mg.

CONTRAINDICATIONS: Bowel obstruction, hypophosphatemia

PREGNANCY AND LACTATION: Pregnancy category C; use caution in nursing mothers due to potential for reductions in serum levels of various vitamins

SIDE EFFECTS

Frequent (20%-11%)

Infection, pain, hypotension, diarrhea, dyspepsia, nausea, vomiting

Occasional (10%-1%)

Headache, constipation, hypertension, thrombosis, increased cough

SERIOUS REACTIONS

- Thrombosis occurs rarely.

INTERACTIONS

Drugs

3 *Antiarrhythmics, anticonvulsants:* Potential for decreased bioavailability of these drugs when concomitantly administered with sevelamer, administer >1 hr before or 3 hr after sevelamer

SPECIAL CONSIDERATIONS

- Has not been studied in ESRD patients not on hemodialysis
- Compared to calcium acetate, may reduce the risk of developing hypercalcemia

PATIENT/FAMILY EDUCATION

- A daily multivitamin supplement may prevent reduction in serum levels of vitamins D, E, K, and folic acid
- Do not chew or take caps apart prior to administration
- Space doses of sevelamer ≥1 hr before or 3 hrs after concomitant medications
- Take with food
- Notify the physician if diarrhea, signs of hypotension (such as lightheadedness), nausea or vomiting, or a persistent headache occurs

MONITORING PARAMETERS

- Serum phosphorus, calcium, bicarbonate, and chloride levels

S

sibutramine hydrochloride

(sih-byoo′-tra-meen)

Rx: Meridia

Chemical Class: Cyclobutanemethamine derivative

Therapeutic Class: Anorexiant

CLINICAL PHARMACOLOGY

Mechanism of Action: A central nervous system (CNS) stimulant inhibits reuptake of serotonin (enhancing satiety) and norepinephrine (raises metabolic rate) centrally. ***Therapeutic Effect:*** Induces and maintains weight loss.

Pharmacokinetics

Rapidly absorbed from the gastrointestinal (GI) tract. Protein binding: 95%-97%. Metabolized in liver, undergoes first-pass metabolism. Primarily excreted in urine, minimal elimination in feces. ***Half-life:*** 1.1 hrs.

INDICATIONS AND DOSAGES

Weight loss

PO

Adults 16 yrs and older. Initially, 10 mg/day. May increase up to 15 mg/day. Maximum: 20 mg/day.

AVAILABLE FORMS

• *Capsules:* 5 mg, 10 mg, 15 mg (Meridia).

CONTRAINDICATIONS: Anorexia nervosa, concomitant MAOI use, concomitant use of centrally acting appetite suppressants, hypersensitivity to sibutramine or any component of the formulation

PREGNANCY AND LACTATION: Pregnancy category C; excretion into breast milk unknown; not recommended in nursing mothers

Controlled Substance: Schedule IV

SIDE EFFECTS

Frequent

Headache, dry mouth, anorexia, constipation, insomnia, rhinitis, pharyngitis

Occasional

Back pain, flu syndrome, dizziness, nausea, asthenia (loss of strength, energy), arthralgia, nervousness, dyspepsia, sinusitis, abdominal pain, anxiety, dysmenorrhea

Rare

Depression, rash, cough, sweating, tachycardia, migraine, increased BP, paresthesia, altered taste

SERIOUS REACTIONS

• Seizures, thrombocytopenia, and deaths have been reported.

• Serotonin syndrome can occur with concomitant use of drugs that increase serotonin.

• Large doses may produce extreme nervousness and tachycardia.

INTERACTIONS

Drugs

❷ *MAOIs:* Potential for the development of serotonin syndrome; at least 14 days should elapse between administration of MAO inhibitors and sibutramine

❷ *Sumatriptan, tryptophan:* Increased risk of serotonin syndrome

SPECIAL CONSIDERATIONS

• Primary pulmonary hypertension and cardiac valve disorders have been associated with other centrally acting weight loss agents that cause release of serotonin from nerve terminals; although sibutramine has not been associated with these effects in premarketing clinical studies, patients should be informed of the potential for these side effects and monitored closely for their occurrence

• Substantially increases blood pressure in some patients

• Maintenance of weight loss beyond 18 mos has not been studied

PATIENT/FAMILY EDUCATION

• Avoid alcohol

• May be habit-forming

• Do not take OTC medications with first consulting the physician

MONITORING PARAMETERS

• Regular blood pressure monitoring

• Heart rate, weight

sildenafil citrate

(sill-den'-a-fill sye'-trate)

Rx: Revatio, Viagra

Chemical Class: CGMP-specific phosphodiesterase inhibitor

Therapeutic Class: Antiimpotence agent

CLINICAL PHARMACOLOGY

Mechanism of Action: An erectile dysfunction agent that inhibits phosphodiesterase type 5, the enzyme responsible for degrading cyclic guanosine monophosphate in the corpus cavernosum of the penis, pulmonary vascular smooth muscle, resulting in smooth muscle relaxation and increased blood flow. ***Therapeutic Effects:*** Facilitates an erection, produces pulmonary vasodilation.

Pharmacokinetics

Rapidly absorbed from the GI tract. Protein binding: greater than 96%. Metabolized in liver. Excreted primarily in the feces, urine and semen. ***Half-life:*** 4 hr.

INDICATIONS AND DOSAGES

Erectile dysfunction

PO

Adults. 50 mg (30 min-4 hr before sexual activity). Range: 25-100 mg. Maximum dosing frequency is once daily.

Elderly older than 65 yr. Consider starting dose of 25 mg.

Pulmonary arterial hypertension

PO

Adults, Elderly. 20 mg 3 times a day.

AVAILABLE FORMS

• *Tablets:* 20 mg (Revatio), 25 mg (Viagra), 50 mg (Viagra), 100 mg (Viagra).

UNLABELED USES: Treatment of diabetic gastroparesis, sexual dysfunction associated with the use of selective serotonin reuptake inhibitors

CONTRAINDICATIONS: Concurrent use of sodium nitroprusside or nitrates in any form

PREGNANCY AND LACTATION: Pregnancy category B; use not recommended in women

SIDE EFFECTS

Frequent

Headache (16%), flushing (10%)

Occasional (7%-3%)

Dyspepsia, nasal congestion, UTI, abnormal vision, diarrhea

Rare (2%)

Dizziness, rash

SERIOUS REACTIONS

• Prolonged erections (lasting over 4 hrs) and priapism (painful erections lasting over 6 hrs) occur rarely.

INTERACTIONS

Drugs

3 *Cimetidine, erythromycin, itraconazole, ketoconazole:* Increased sildenafil levels

3 *High-fat meals:* Delay drug's maximum effectiveness by 1 hr

⚠ *Nitrates:* Cardiac arrest, death

3 *Rifampin:* Decreased sildenafil levels

SPECIAL CONSIDERATIONS

• Tablets are priced the same regardless of dose, 100-mg tablets can be broken in half

PATIENT/FAMILY EDUCATION

• Sildenafil is not effective without sexual stimulation

• Seek treatment immediately if an erection lasts longer than 4 hrs

• Avoid using nitrate drugs concurrently with sildenafil

• High-fat meals may affect the drug's absorption rate and effectiveness

MONITORING PARAMETERS

• Blood pressure, heart rate

silver nitrate

Rx: Silver nitrate
Chemical Class: Heavy metal
Therapeutic Class: Antibiotic; cauterizing agent

CLINICAL PHARMACOLOGY

Mechanism of Action: Free silver ions precipitate bacterial proteins by combining with chloride in tissue forming silver chloride; coagulates cellular protein to form an eschar or scab. The germicidal action is credited to precipitation of bacterial proteins by free silver ions. ***Therapeutic Effect:*** Inhibits growth of both gram-positive and gram-negative bacteria.

Pharmacokinetics

Minimal gastrointestinal (GI) tract and cutaneous absorption. Minimal excretion in urine.

INDICATIONS AND DOSAGES

Exuberant granulations

Applicator sticks

Adults, Elderly, Children. Apply to mucous membranes and other moist skin surfaces only on area to be treated 2-3 times/wk for 2-3 wks.

Topical, solution

Adults, Elderly, Children. Apply a cotton applicator dipped in solution on the affected area 2-3 times/wk for 2-3 wks.

Gonococcal ophthalmia neonatorum

Ophthalmic

Neonates. Instill 2 drops in each eye immediately after delivery.

AVAILABLE FORMS

- *Applicator Sticks:* 75% silver nitrate and 25% potassium nitrate.
- *Ophthalmic Solution:* 1%.
- *Topical Solution:* 10%, 25%, 50%.

UNLABELED USES: *Neonates.* Instill 2 drops in each eye immediately after delivery.

CONTRAINDICATIONS: Broken skin, cuts, or wounds, hypersensitivity to silver nitrate or any of its components

PREGNANCY AND LACTATION: Pregnancy category C

SIDE EFFECTS

Occasional

Ophthalmic: Chemical conjunctivitis

Topical: Burning, irritation, staining of the skin

Rare

Hyponatremia, methemoglobinemia

SERIOUS REACTIONS

- Symptoms of overdose include blackening of skin and mucous membranes, pain and burning of the mouth, salivation, vomiting, diarrhea, shock, convulsions, coma, and death.
- Methemoglobinemia is caused by absorbed silver nitrate but occurs rarely.
- Cauterization of the cornea and blindness occur rarely.

SPECIAL CONSIDERATIONS

PATIENT/FAMILY EDUCATION

- Stains skin and utensils (removable with iodine tincture followed by sodium thiosulfate solution)
- Discontinue topical preparation if irritation or redness develops
- Do not use topical preparations near the eyes or abraded areas

MONITORING PARAMETERS

- Skin for irritation, redness, and staining with application
- Methemoglobin levels with prolonged use

silver sulfadiazine

(sul-fa-dye'-a-zeen)

Rx: Silvadene, SSD, SSD AF, Thermazene

Chemical Class: Sulfonamide derivative

Therapeutic Class: Antibiotic, topical

CLINICAL PHARMACOLOGY

Mechanism of Action: An antiinfective that acts upon cell wall and cell membrane. Releases silver slowly in concentrations selectively toxic to bacteria. ***Therapeutic Effect:*** Produces bactericidal effect.

Pharmacokinetics

Variably absorbed. Significant systemic absorption may occur if applied to extensive burns. Absorbed medication excreted and unchanged in urine. ***Half-life:*** 10 hrs (half-life increased with impaired renal function).

INDICATIONS AND DOSAGES

Burns

Topical

Adults, Elderly, Children. Apply 1-2 times daily.

AVAILABLE FORMS

• *Cream:* 1% (Silvadene, SSD, SSD AF).

UNLABELED USES: Treatment of minor bacterial skin infection, dermal ulcer

CONTRAINDICATIONS: Hypersensitivity to silver sulfadiazine or any component of the formulation

PREGNANCY AND LACTATION: Pregnancy category B; contraindicated in neonates (kernicterus)

SIDE EFFECTS

Side effects characteristic of all sulfonamides may occur when systemically absorbed such as extensive burn areas, anorexia, nausea, vomiting, headache, diarrhea, dizziness, photosensitivity, joint pain

Frequent

Burning feeling at treatment site

Occasional

Brown-gray skin discoloration, rash, itching

Rare

Increased sensitivity or skin to sunlight

SERIOUS REACTIONS

• If significant systemic absorption occurs, less often but serious are hemolytic anemia, hypoglycemia, diuresis, peripheral neuropathy, Stevens-Johnson syndrome, agranulocytosis, disseminated lupus erythematosus, anaphylaxis, hepatitis, and toxic nephrosis.

• Fungal superinfections may occur.

• Interstitial nephritis occurs rarely.

INTERACTIONS

Drugs

3 *Proteolytic enzymes:* Silver may inactivate enzymes

SPECIAL CONSIDERATIONS

• Prior to application, burn wounds should be cleansed and debrided (following control of shock and pain)

• Use sterile glove and tongue blade to apply medication; thin layer (1.5 mm) to completely cover wound; dressing as required only

• Continue until no chance of infection

PATIENT/FAMILY EDUCATION

• Continue treatment until satisfactory healing has occurred, or until the burn site is ready for grafting

MONITORING PARAMETERS

• Serum sulfa concentrations

• Renal function

• Urine for sulfa crystals

simethicone

(sye-meth′-i-kone)

OTC: Alka-Seltzer Gas Relief, Gas-X, Genasyme, Infant Mylicon, Mylanta Gas, Phazyme

Combinations

OTC: with calcium carbonate (Titralac Plus); with aluminum hydroxide, magnesium hydroxide (Mylanta Gelisil, Maalox Extra Strength); with calcium carbonate, magnesium hydroxide (Tempo, Rolaids); with Magaldrate, (Riopan Plus); with charcoal (Charcoal Plus, Flatulex)

Chemical Class: Siloxane polymer

Therapeutic Class: Antiflatulent

CLINICAL PHARMACOLOGY

Mechanism of Action: An antiflatulent that changes surface tension of gas bubbles, allowing easier elimination of gas. ***Therapeutic Effect:*** Drug dispersal, prevents formation of gas pockets in the GI tract.

Pharmacokinetics

Does not appear to be absorbed from GI tract. Excreted unchanged in feces.

INDICATIONS AND DOSAGES

Antiflatulent

PO

Adults, Elderly, Children 12 yrs and older. 40-360 mg after meals and at bedtime. Maximum: 500 mg/day.

Children 2-11 yrs. 40 mg 4 times a day.

Children younger than 2 yrs. 20 mg 4 times a day.

AVAILABLE FORMS

- *Oral Drops (Infant Mylicon):* 40 mg/0.6 ml.
- *Softgel:* 125 mg (Alka-Seltzer Gas Relief, Gas-Z, Mylanta Gas), 180 mg (Phazyme).
- *Tablets (Chewable):* 80 mg (Gas-X, Genasyme, Mylanta Gas), 125 mg (Gas-X, Mylanta Gas).

UNLABELED USES: Adjunct to bowel radiography and gastroscopy

CONTRAINDICATIONS: None known.

PREGNANCY AND LACTATION: Pregnancy category C

SIDE EFFECTS

None known.

SERIOUS REACTIONS

- None known.

SPECIAL CONSIDERATIONS

- Commonly prescribed, little evidence for any beneficial effect

PATIENT/FAMILY EDUCATION

- Avoid carbonated beverages during simethicone therapy
- Chew tablets thoroughly before swallowing

MONITORING PARAMETERS

- Therapeutic response (relief of abdominal bloating and flatulence)

simvastatin

(sim′-va-sta-tin)

Rx: Zocor

Combinations

Rx: with ezetimibe (Vytorin)

Chemical Class: Substituted hexahydronaphthalene

Therapeutic Class: HMG-CoA reductase inhibitor; antilipemic

CLINICAL PHARMACOLOGY

Mechanism of Action: A HMG-CoA reductase inhibitor that interferes with cholesterol biosynthesis by inhibiting the conversion of the enzyme HMG-CoA to mevalonate. ***Therapeutic Effect:*** Decreases serum LDL, cholesterol, VLDL, and plasma triglyceride levels; slightly increases serum HDL concentration.

Pharmacokinetics

Route	Onset	Peak	Duration
PO to reduce cholesterol	3 days	14 days	N/A

Well absorbed from the GI tract. Protein binding: 95%. Undergoes extensive first-pass metabolism. Hydrolyzed to active metabolite. Primarily eliminated in feces. Unknown if removed by hemodialysis.

INDICATIONS AND DOSAGES

Prevention of cardiovascular events, hyperlipidemias

PO

Adults, Elderly. 20-40 mg once daily. Range: 5-80 mg/day.

Homozygous familial hypercholesterol

PO

Adults, Elderly. 40 mg once daily in evening or 80 mg/day in divided doses.

Heterozygous familial hypercholesterol

PO

Children 10-17 yr. 10 mg once daily in evening. Range: 10-40 mg/day.

AVAILABLE FORMS

• *Tablets:* 5 mg, 10 mg, 20 mg, 40 mg, 80 mg.

CONTRAINDICATIONS: Active hepatic disease or unexplained, persistent elevations of liver function test results, age younger than 18 yrs, pregnancy

PREGNANCY AND LACTATION: Pregnancy category X; breast milk excretion unknown; other drugs in this class are excreted in small amounts; manufacturer recommends against breast-feeding

SIDE EFFECTS

Simvastatin is generally well tolerated. Side effects are usually mild and transient.

Occasional (3%-2%)

Headache, abdominal pain or cramps, constipation, upper respiratory tract infection

Rare (less than 2%)

Diarrhea, flatulence, asthenia (loss of strength and energy), nausea or vomiting

SERIOUS REACTIONS

• Lens opacities may occur.

• Hypersensitivity reaction and hepatitis occur rarely.

• Myopathy manifested as muscle pain, tenderness or weakness with elevated CK sometimes taking the form of rhabdomyolysis fatalities, have occurred.

INTERACTIONS

Drugs

❷ *Azole antifungals (fluconazole, itraconazole, ketoconazole, miconazole):* Increased simvastatin levels via inhibition of metabolism with increased risk of rhabdomyolysis

❸ *Cholestyramine, colestipol:* Reduced bioavailability of simvastatin

❸ *Cyclosporine:* Concomitant administration increases risk of severe myopathy or rhabdomyolysis

❸ *Danazol:* Inhibition of metabolism (CYP3A4) thought to yield increased simvastatin levels with increased risk of rhabdomyolysis

❷ *Fluoxetine:* Inhibits CYP3A4 hepatic metabolism with risk of rhabdomyolysis

❷ *Gemfibrozil:* Small increased risk of myopathy with combination, especially at high doses of statin

❸ *Isradipine:* Isradipine probably decreases simvastatin (like lovastatin) plasma concentrations minimally

3 *Macrolide antibiotics (clarithromycin, erythromycin, telithromycin, troleandomycin):* Increased simvastatin levels via inhibition of metabolism with increased risk of rhabdomyolysis

3 *Nefazadone:* Inhibit CYP3A4 hepatic metabolism (like lovastatin) with risk of rhabdomyolysis

3 *Niacin:* Concomitant administration increases risk of severe myopathy or rhabdomyolysis

2 *Ritonavir:* Increases the risk of toxicity

3 *St. John's Wort:* Lowers simvastatin plasma concentrations

3 *Tacrolimus:* Increased risk of developing rhabdomyolysis

3 *Warfarin:* Addition of simvastatin may increase hypoprothrombinemic response to warfarin via inhibition of metabolism (CYP2C9)

SPECIAL CONSIDERATIONS

- Superior to fibrates, cholestyramine, and probucol in lowering total and LDL cholesterol levels
- Statin selection based on lipid-lowering prowess, cost, and availability

PATIENT/FAMILY EDUCATION

- Report symptoms of myalgia, muscle tenderness, or weakness
- Take daily doses in the evening for increased effect
- Use appropriate contraceptive measures while taking simvastatin; this drug is pregnancy risk category X
- Periodic laboratory tests are an essential part of therapy

MONITORING PARAMETERS

- Cholesterol (max therapeutic response 4-6 wks)
- LFTs (AST, ALT) at baseline and at 12 wk of therapy; if no change, no further monitoring necessary (discontinue if elevations persist at >3 × upper limit of normal)
- CPK at baseline and in patients complaining of diffuse myalgia, muscle tenderness, or weakness
- Pattern of daily bowel activity

sirolimus

(sir-oh'-li-mus)

Rx: Rapamune

Chemical Class: Macrolide derivative

Therapeutic Class: Immunosuppressant

CLINICAL PHARMACOLOGY

Mechanism of Action: An immunosuppressant that inhibits T-lymphocyte proliferation induced by stimulation of cell surface receptors, mitogens, alloantigens, and lymphokines. Prevents activation of the enzyme target of rapamycin, a key regulatory kinase in cell cycle progression. ***Therapeutic Effect:*** Inhibits proliferation of T and B cells, essential components of the immune response; prevents organ transplant rejection.

Pharmacokinetics

Rapidly absorbed from the GI tract. Protein binding: 92%. Extensively metabolized in liver. Primarily eliminated in feces; minimal excretion in urine. ***Half-life:*** 57-63 hrs.

INDICATIONS AND DOSAGES

Prevention of organ transplant rejection

PO

Adults. Loading dose: 6 mg. Maintenance: 2 mg/day.

Children 13 yrs and older weighing less than 40 kg. Loading dose: 3 mg/m^2. Maintenance: 1 mg/m^2/day.

AVAILABLE FORMS

- *Oral Solution:* 1 mg/ml.
- *Tablets:* 1 mg, 2 mg, 5 mg.

UNLABELED USES: Immunosuppression of other organ transplants

CONTRAINDICATIONS: Malignancy

PREGNANCY AND LACTATION: Pregnancy category C; excretion into breast milk unknown; use caution in nursing mothers

SIDE EFFECTS

Occasional

Hypercholesterolemia, hyperlipidemia, hypertension, rash; with high doses (5 mg/day): anemia, arthralgia, diarrhea, hypokalemia, and thrombocytopenia

Rare

Peripheral edema, hypertension

SERIOUS REACTIONS

- Pancytopenia and hepatotoxicity occur rarely.

INTERACTIONS

Drugs

3 *Azole antifungals, bromocriptine, calcium channel blockers, cimetidine, danazol, ethinyl estradiol, GI prokinetic agents, macrolide antibiotics, protease inhibitors:* Decreased metabolism or increased bioavailability of sirolimus

3 *Carbamazepine, phenobarbital, phenytoin, rifabutin, rifapentine:* Decreased sirolimus concentrations possible

3 *Cyclosporine:* Increased sirolimus concentrations when given concurrently. Sirolimus should be taken 4 hr after cyclosporine

3 *Diltiazem:* Increased sirolimus concentrations

▲ *Grapefruit juice:* Increased sirolimus concentrations, grapefruit juice should not be administered with sirolimus

▲ *Ketoconazole:* Significant increase in rate and extent of absorption of sirolimus, concurrent administration not recommended

▲ *Live vaccines:* Avoid use of live vaccines, vaccinations may be less effective

2 *Rifampin:* Sirolimus clearance significantly increased, decreased sirolimus concentrations; consider alternative therapeutic agents to rifampin

3 *St. John's wort (hypericum perforatum):* Potential for decreased plasma tacrolimus concentrations

SPECIAL CONSIDERATIONS

- Tablets and solution are not bioequivalent (tab has 27% > bioavailability); however, 2-mg tabs clinically equivalent to 2 mg oral sol; not known if higher doses of oral sol are clinically equivalent to higher doses of tabs
- Allows cyclosporine dose reduction
- Experience limited with use as rescue therapy
- Black patients had higher rejection rates (56% vs 13%) than non-blacks given same regimen; no significant differences in trough sirolimus concentrations at equal doses between blacks and non-blacks
- IV formulation is under development

PATIENT/FAMILY EDUCATION

- Take medication the same each day with regard to timing of meals and other medications
- Limit UV/sunlight exposure, wear protective clothing and use sunsreen due to increased risk of skin cancer
- Due to potential risks to fetus, effective contraception should be used before, during and 12 wks after sirolimus therapy in women of childbearing potential
- Avoid grapefruit or grapefruit juice during therapy
- Avoid contact with people with colds or other infections

MONITORING PARAMETERS

- Whole-blood sirolimus levels (drawn 1 hr prior to next dose), 5-7 days after initiation or dose change. Maintain levels at 10-15 ng/ml for

first month, then consider increasing to 15-20 ng/ml, especially in patients receiving little cyclosporine
- CBC, platelets, lipids
- Liver function tests periodically

sodium bicarbonate

(sew'-dee-um bye-car'-bon-ate)

Rx: Neut

Combinations

OTC: with alginic acid, (AlOH, Mg Trisilicate Gastrocote); with sodium citrate (Citrocarbonate)

Chemical Class: Monosodium salt of carbonic acid

Therapeutic Class: Alkalinizing agent, systemic/urinary; antacid; electrolyte supplement

CLINICAL PHARMACOLOGY

Mechanism of Action: An alkalinizing agent that dissociates to provide bicarbonate ion. ***Therapeutic Effect:*** Neutralizes hydrogen ion concentration, raises blood and urinary pH.

Pharmacokinetics

Route	Onset	Peak	Duration
PO	15 min	N/A	1-3 hr
IV	Immediate	N/A	8-10 min

After administration, sodium bicarbonate dissociates to sodium and bicarbonate ions. With increased hydrogen ion concentrations, bicarbonate ions combine with hydrogen ions to form carbonic acid, which then dissociates to CO_2, which is excreted by the lungs.

INDICATIONS AND DOSAGES

Cardiac arrest

IV

Adults, Elderly. Initially, 1 mEq/kg (as 7.5%-8.4% solution). May repeat with 0.5 mEq/kg q10min during continued cardiopulmonary arrest. Use in the postresuscitation phase is based on arterial blood pH, partial pressure of carbon dioxide in arterial blood ($PaCO_2$), and base deficit calculation.

Children, Infants. Initially, 1 mEq/kg.

Metabolic acidosis (not severe)

IV

Adults, Elderly, Children. 2-5 mEq/kg over 4-8 hr. May repeat based on laboratory values.

Metabolic acidosis (associated with chronic renal failure)

PO

Adults, Elderly. Initially, 20-36 mEq/day in divided doses.

Renal tubular acidosis (distal)

PO

Adults, Elderly. 0.5-2 mEq/kg/day in 4-6 divided doses.

Children. 2-3 mEq/kg/day in divided doses.

Renal tubular acidosis (proximal)

PO

Adults, Elderly, Children. 5-10 mEq/kg/day in divided doses.

Urine alkalinization

PO

Adults, Elderly. Initially, 4 g, then 1-2 g q4h. Maximum: 16 g/day.

Children. 84-840 mg/kg/day in divided doses.

Antacid

PO

Adults, Elderly. 300 mg-2 g 1-4 times a day.

Hyperkalemia

IV

Adults, Elderly. 1 mEq/kg over 5 mins.

AVAILABLE FORMS

- *Tablets:* 325 mg, 650 mg.
- *Injection:* 4%, 0.5 mEq/ml (4.2%), 0.6 mEq/ml (5%), 0.9 mEq/ml (7.5%), 1 mEq/ml (8.4%).

CONTRAINDICATIONS: Excessive chloride loss due to diarrhea, diuretics, GI suctioning, or vomiting; hypocalcemia; metabolic or respiratory alkalosis

PREGNANCY AND LACTATION: Pregnancy category C

SIDE EFFECTS

Frequent

Abdominal distention, flatulence, belching

SERIOUS REACTIONS

• Excessive or chronic use may produce metabolic alkalosis (characterized by irritability, twitching, paresthesias, cyanosis, slow or shallow respirations, headache, thirst, and nausea).

• Fluid overload results in headache, weakness, blurred vision, behavioral changes, incoordination, muscle twitching, elevated BP, bradycardia, tachypnea, wheezing, coughing, and distended neck veins.

• Extravasation may occur at the IV site, resulting in tissue necrosis and ulceration.

INTERACTIONS

Drugs

3 *Amphetamines:* Sodium bicarbonate inhibits the elimination and increases the effects of amphetamines

3 *β-blockers:* Reduced absorption

3 *Calcium-containing products:* May result in milk-alkali syndrome

3 *Cefpodoxime:* Reduced absorption

3 *Cefuroxime:* Reduced serum levels with reduced antibiotic efficacy

3 *Corticosteroids:* May cause edema and hypertension

3 *Ephedrine:* Large doses of sodium bicarbonate increase the serum concentrations of ephedrine

3 *Flecainide:* Increased urine pH will increase flecainide serum concentration

3 *Glipizide:* Enhanced rate of glipizide absorption

3 *Glyburide:* Enhanced rate of glyburide absorption

3 *Iron:* Reduced iron absorption

3 *Ketoconazole:* Decreased ketoconazole absorption

3 *Lithium:* Sodium bicarbonate may lower lithium plasma concentrations

3 *Methenamine compound:* Sodium bicarbonate-induced urinary pH changes interfere with antibacterial activity of methenamine compounds

3 *Mexiletine:* Increased urine pH increases mexiletine concentrations

3 *Pseudoephedrine:* Sodium bicarbonate–induced urinary pH changes may markedly inhibit the elimination of pseudoephedrine

3 *Quinidine:* Sodium bicarbonate–induced urinary pH changes may increase quinidine concentrations

3 *Quinolones:* Reduced absorption

3 *Salicylates:* Sodium bicarbonate–induced urinary pH changes can decrease serum salicylate concentrations

3 *Tetracyclines:* Reduced absorption

Labs

• *Protein:* Falsely elevates urine protein

SPECIAL CONSIDERATIONS

PATIENT/FAMILY EDUCATION

• Milk-alkali syndrome (may result from excessive antacid use): confusion, headache, nausea, vomiting, anorexia, urinary stones, hypercalcemia

• To avoid drug interactions due to reduced absorption, separate intake by 2 hr
• The female patient considering breast-feeding should consult with her physician before taking sodium bicarbonate
• Check with the physician before taking OTC drugs because they may contain sodium

MONITORING PARAMETERS
• Electrolytes, blood pH, PO_2, HCO_3, during treatment
• ABGs frequently during emergencies
• Serum calcium, phosphate, and uric acid levels
• Signs and symptoms of fluid overload and metabolic alkalosis
• Pattern of daily bowel activity and stool consistency
• Relief of gastric distress
• Clinical improvement of metabolic acidosis, including relief from disorientation, hyperventilation, and weakness

sodium chloride

(soe'-dee-um klor'-ide)

OTC: Muro 128, Nasal Mist, Nasal Moist, Ocean, SalineX, SeaMist, Slo-Salt

Chemical Class: Monovalent cation

Therapeutic Class: Electrolyte supplement; irrigant; moisturizing agent

CLINICAL PHARMACOLOGY

Mechanism of Action: Sodium is a major cation of extracellular fluid that controls water distribution, fluid and electrolyte balance, and osmotic pressure of body fluids; it also maintains acid-base balance.

Pharmacokinetics
Well absorbed from the GI tract. Widely distributed. Primarily excreted in urine.

INDICATIONS AND DOSAGES

Prevention and treatment of sodium and chloride deficiencies; source of hydration
IV
Adults, Elderly. 1-2 L/day 0.9% or 0.45% or 100 ml 3% or 5% over 1 hr; assess serum electrolyte levels before giving additional fluid.

Prevention of heat prostration and muscle cramps from excessive perspiration
PO
Adults, Elderly. 1-2 g 3 times a day.

Relief of dry and inflamed nasal membranes
Intranasal
Adults, Elderly. Use as needed.

Diagnostic aid in ophthalmoscopic exam, treatment of corneal edema
Ophthalmic solution
Adults, Elderly. Apply 1-2 drops q3-4h.
Ophthalmic ointment
Adults, Elderly. Apply once a day or as directed.

AVAILABLE FORMS
• *Tablets:* 1 g
• *Injection (Concentrate):* 23.4% (4 mEq/ml).
• *Injection:* 0.45%, 0.9%, 3%.
• *Irrigation:* 0.45%, 0.9%.
• *Nasal Gel (Nasal Moist):* 0.65%.
• *Nasal Solution (OTC):* 0.4% (SalineX), 0.65% (Nasal Moist, SeaMist).
• *Ophthalmic Solution (OTC [Muro 128]):* 5%.
• *Ophthalmic Ointment (OTC [Muro 128]):* 5%.

CONTRAINDICATIONS: Fluid retention, hypernatremia

PREGNANCY AND LACTATION: Pregnancy category C

SIDE EFFECTS

Frequent

Facial flushing

Occasional

Fever; irritation, phlebitis, or extravasation at injection site

Ophthalmic: Temporary burning or irritation

SERIOUS REACTIONS

• Too-rapid administration may produce peripheral edema, CHF, and pulmonary edema.

• Excessive dosage may cause hypokalemia, hypervolemia, and hypernatremia.

INTERACTIONS

Drugs

3 *Lithium:* High sodium intake may reduce serum lithium concentrations, while restriction of sodium tends to increase serum lithium

2 *Hypertonic saline solution, oxytocics:* May cause uterine hypertonus, ruptures, or lacerations

SPECIAL CONSIDERATIONS

• One g of sodium chloride provides 17.1 mEq sodium and 17.1 mEq chloride

PATIENT/FAMILY EDUCATION

• Temporary burning or irritation after instillation of the ophthalmic drug may occur

• Discontinue the ophthalmic medication and notify the physician if acute redness of eyes, floating spots, severe eye pain or pain on exposure to light, a rapid change in vision (side and straight ahead), or headache occurs

MONITORING PARAMETERS

• IV site for extravasation

• Fluid balance, acid-base balance, blood pressure, electrolytes

• Signs and symptoms of hypernatremia (edema, hypertension, and weight gain) and hyponatremia (dry mucous membranes, muscle cramps, nausea, and vomiting)

sodium fluoride

(flur'-eyed)

Rx: Control Rx, Denta 5000 Plus, Ethedent, Ethedent Chewable, Fluorabon, Fluor-A-Day, Fluorinse, Fluoritab, Flura-Drops, Flura-Loz, Flura-Tab, Gel-Kam, Gel-Kam Dentinbloc, Gel-Kam Sensitivity Therapy, Karidium, Lozi-Flur, Luride, Nafrinse, Nafrinse Solution, Neutracare Mint Gel, NeutroGard, Omnii Gel, Omni Perio-Med, Pediaflor Drops, Perio Med, Pharmaflur, Pharmaflur 1.1, Phos-Flur, Prevident, Prevident 5000 Plus, Prevident 500 Plus Boost, Prevident Dental Rinse, SF, SF 5000 Plus, Thera-Flur-N

OTC: Fluorigard, Gel-Tin

Chemical Class: Fluoride ion

Therapeutic Class: Anti–dental caries agent; antiosteoporotic

S

CLINICAL PHARMACOLOGY

Mechanism of Action: A trace element that increases tooth resistance to acid dissolution. ***Therapeutic Effect:*** Promotes remineralization of decalcified enamel, inhibits dental plaque bacteria, increases resistance to development of caries, maintains bone strength.

Pharmacokinetics

Not protein bound. Excreted in urine.

INDICATIONS AND DOSAGES

Dietary supplement for prevention of dental caries in children

Fluoride Level in Water	*Age*	*Dosage*
less than 0.3 ppm*	younger than 2 yrs	0.25 mg/day
	2-3 yrs	0.5 mg/day
	4-13 yrs	1 mg/day
0.3-0.7 ppm*	younger than 2 yrs	None
	2-3 yrs	0.25 mg/day
	4-13 yrs	0.5 mg/day
greater than 0.7 ppm*	None	None

AVAILABLE FORMS

- *Lozenge:* 2.2 mg (Fluor-A-Day, Lozi-Flur).
- *Oral Liquid:* 0.125 mg/drop (Fluor-A-Day, Flura-Drops), 0.25 mg/drop (Fluoritab), 0.25 mg/0.6 ml (Fluorabon).
- *Oral Solution (Luride, Pediaflor):* 1.1 mg/ml.
- *Oral Solution Drops:* 1.1 mg/ml.
- *Oral Solution Rinse:* 0.5% (Fluorigard), 0.2% (Fluorinse), 0.44% (Phos-Flur).
- *Tablets (Flura-Tab, Fluoritab, Karidium):* 1 mg.
- *Tablets (Chewable):* 0.25 mg (Ethedent Chewable, Fluor-A-Day, Fluoritab, Luride), 0.5 mg (Ethedent Chewable, Fluor-A-Day, Fluoritab, Luride, Pharmaflur 1.1), 0.58 mg (Ethedent Chewable, Fluorabon, Fluor-A-Day, Fluoritab, Flura-Loz, Luride, Nafrinse, Pharmaflur), 1 mg (Ethedent Chewable, Fluorabon, Fluor-A-Day, Fluoritab, Flura-Loz, Luride, Nafrinse, Pharmaflur), 1.1 mg (Fluor-A-Day, Luride Lozi-Tabs), 2.2 mg (Fluor-A-Day, Luride Lozi-Tabs).
- *Topical Cream (Denta 5000 Plus, Ethedent):* 1.1%.
- *Topical Gel:* 0.4% (Omnii Gel), 1.1% (Ethedent, Neutracare Mint Gel, Prevident, Prevident 500 Plus Boost, SF, Thera-Flur-N).
- *Topical Gel-Drops (Thera-Flur-N):* 1.1%.
- *Topical Kit (Gel-Kam Dentinbloc, Gel-Kam Sensitivity Therapy):* 0.14%-1.09%-0.4%.
- *Topical Paste (Control Rx, Prevident 5000 Plus, SF 5000 Plus):* 1.1%.
- *Topical Solution:* 0.02% (Nafrinse, Phos-Flur), 0.2% (Fluorinse, Omni Perio-Med, Prevident Dental Rinse), 0.63% (Gel-Kam, Perio Med).

CONTRAINDICATIONS: Arthralgia, GI ulceration, severe renal insufficiency, children younger than 3 yr (oral rinse), children younger than 6 mo (drops, tablets)

PREGNANCY AND LACTATION: Administration from third-ninth mo of gestation safe (no information on teratogenicity); small amounts excreted into breast milk, inadequate therapeutically due to small amount of excretion and complexation with calcium

SIDE EFFECTS

Rare

Oral mucous membrane ulceration

SERIOUS REACTIONS

- Hypocalcemia, tetany, bone pain (especially in ankles and feet), electrolyte disturbances, and arrhythmias occur rarely.
- Fluoride use may cause skeletal fluorosis, osteomalacia, and osteosclerosis.

INTERACTIONS

Drugs

3 *Aluminum hydroxide, calcium:* May decrease the absorption of fluoride

SPECIAL CONSIDERATIONS

• Therapy begun prenatally and continued through age 16 is effective in reducing the number of decayed, missing, or filled surfaces and teeth; especially beneficial in areas where fluoride content of drinking water is below 0.7 ppm

• Treatment of osteoporosis, combined with 1 or more of the following—calcium, estrogen, or vitamin D—increases bone density, reduces rate of new vertebral fractures, if correct dose and in slow-release preparation; role in steroid-induced osteoporosis being investigated, reports to date indicate a poor response rate

PATIENT/FAMILY EDUCATION

• Avoid use with dairy products
• Use gels and rinse at bedtime after brushing and flossing; expectorate excess fluoride—do not swallow it
• Do not drink, eat, or rinse the mouth after application
• Do not take fluoride with dairy products, which may decrease fluoride's absorption

MONITORING PARAMETERS

• Perform dental exams once or twice per year

sodium oxybate

(soe'-dee-um ok'-si-bate)

Rx: Xyrem

Chemical Class: Hydroxybutyrate

Therapeutic Class: Anticataplectic; central nervous system depressant

CLINICAL PHARMACOLOGY

Mechanism of Action: A naturally occurring inhibitory neurotransmitter that binds to gamma aminobutyric acid (GABA)-B receptors and sodium oxybate–specific receptors with its highest concentrations in the basal ganglia, which meditates sleep cycles, temperature regulation, cerebral glucose metabolism and blood flow, memory, and emotion control. ***Therapeutic Effect:*** Reduces the number of sleep episodes.

Pharmacokinetics

Rapidly and incompletely absorbed. Absorption is delayed and decreased by a high-fat meal. Protein binding: less than 1%. Widely distributed, including in cerebrospinal fluid (CSF). Metabolized in liver. Excretion is less than 5% in the urine and negligible in feces. Unknown if removed by hemodialysis. ***Half-life:*** 20-53 min.

INDICATIONS AND DOSAGES

Cataplexy of narcolepsy

PO

Adults, Elderly. 4.5 g/day in 2 equal doses of 2.25 g, the first taken at bedtime while in bed and the second 2.5-4 hrs. later. Maximum: 9 g/day in two weekly increments of 1.5 g/day.

AVAILABLE FORMS

• *Oral Solution:* 500 mg/ml (Xyrem).

UNLABELED USES: Alcohol withdrawal

CONTRAINDICATIONS: Metabolic/respiratory alkalosis, current treatment with sedative hypnotics, succinic semialdehyde dehydrogenase deficient, hypersensitivity to sodium oxybate or any component of the formulation

PREGNANCY AND LACTATION: Pregnancy category B; excretion into breast milk unknown; use caution in nursing mothers

Controlled Substance: Schedule III

SIDE EFFECTS

Frequent

Mild bradycardia

Occasional
Headache, vertigo, dizziness, restless legs, abdominal pain, muscle weakness
Rare
Dreamlike state of confusion

SERIOUS REACTIONS

• Agitation, excitation, increased blood pressure (BP), and insomnia may occur upon abrupt discontinuation of sodium oxybate.

INTERACTIONS

Drugs

❷ *Barbiturates:* Additive CNS and respiratory depression
❷ *Benzodiazepines:* Additive CNS and respiratory depression
❷ *Centrally acting muscle relaxants:* Additive CNS and respiratory depression
❷ *Opioid analgesics:* Additive CNS and respiratory depression
❷ *Ethanol:* Additive CNS and respiratory depression

SPECIAL CONSIDERATIONS

• Sodium oxybate is effective and indicated for the treatment of cataplexy in patients with narcolepsy; it could also be effective for general anesthesia, narcolepsy, fibromyalgia syndrome, insomnia, alcoholism, and opiate withdrawal, but its potential for abuse is unacceptable

PATIENT/FAMILY EDUCATION

• Prepare both doses prior to bedtime; each dose must be diluted with 2 oz (60 ml) of water in the child-resistant dosing cups before ingestion
• The first dose is to be taken at bedtime while in bed and the second taken 2.5-4 hr later while sitting in bed; patients will probably need to set an alarm to awaken for the second dose
• The second dose must be prepared before ingesting the first dose, and should be placed in close proximity to the patient's bed
• After ingesting each dose the patient should then lie down and remain in bed
• Avoid tasks that require mental alertness or motor skills until response to the drug is established
• Avoid alcohol
• Avoid high-fat meals because they may delay the absorption of the drug

MONITORING PARAMETERS

• *History/physical exam:* Review signs and symptoms for efficacy, toxicity, and abuse, including tremor and coma
• *Laboratory:* Sodium and potassium plasma levels, hepatic functions, blood gas analysis

sodium polystyrene sulfonate

(soe'-dee-um po-lee-stye'-reen sul'-foe-nate)

Rx: Kayexalate, Kionex, SPS
Chemical Class: Cation exchange resin
Therapeutic Class: Antihyperkalemic

CLINICAL PHARMACOLOGY

Mechanism of Action: An ion exchange resin that releases sodium ions in exchange primarily for potassium ions. ***Therapeutic Effect:*** Moves potassium from the blood into the intestine so it can be expelled from the body.

Pharmacokinetics

Not absorbed from GI tract. Not metabolized. Completely excreted in feces.

INDICATIONS AND DOSAGES

Hyperkalemia

PO

Adults, Elderly. 60 ml (15 g) 1-4 times a day.
Children. 1 g/kg/dose q6h.

Rectal
Adults, Elderly. 30-50 g as needed q6h.
Children. 1 g/kg/dose q2-6h.

AVAILABLE FORMS

- *Suspension (SPS):* 15 g/60 ml.
- *Powder for Suspension (Kayexalate, Kionex):* 454 g.
- *Rectal Enema:* 15 g/60 ml.

CONTRAINDICATIONS: Hypokalemia, hypernatremia, intestinal obstruction or perforation

PREGNANCY AND LACTATION: Pregnancy category C; excretion in breast milk not expected

SIDE EFFECTS

Frequent
High dosage: Anorexia, nausea, vomiting, constipation
High dosage in elderly: Fecal impaction characterized by severe stomach pain with nausea or vomiting
Occasional
Diarrhea, sodium retention marked by decreased urination, peripheral edema, and increased weight

SERIOUS REACTIONS

- Potassium deficiency may occur. Early signs of hypokalemia include confusion, delayed thought processes, extreme weakness, irritability, and EKG changes (including prolonged QT interval; widening, flattening, or inversion of T wave; and prominent U waves).
- Hypocalcemia, manifested by abdominal or muscle cramps, occurs occasionally.
- Arrhythmias and severe muscle weakness may be noted.

INTERACTIONS

Drugs

3 *Antacids:* Combined use of magnesium- or calcium-containing antacids with resin may result in systemic alkalosis

3 *Laxatives (such as magnesium hydroxide):* May decrease effect of sodium polystyrene sulfonate, and cause systemic alkalosis in patients with renal impairment

SPECIAL CONSIDERATIONS

- Exchange efficacy of resin is approx 33%; 1 g of resin (4.1 mEq of sodium) exchanges approximately 1 mEq of potassium
- Rectal route is less effective than oral administration
- Powder formulations very hydrophobic, difficult to mix. Pre-prepared suspensions in sorbitol preferable

PATIENT/FAMILY EDUCATION

- Do not mix with orange juice
- Drink the entire amount of resin for best results
- When used rectally, try to retain the solution for several hours, if possible

MONITORING PARAMETERS

- Serum K, Ca, Mg, Na, acid-base balance, bowel function, possibly ECG

solifenacin

(sol-i-fen′-a-cin)
Rx: VESIcare
Chemical Class: Antimuscarinic substituted amine
Therapeutic Class: Genitourinary muscle relaxant

CLINICAL PHARMACOLOGY

Mechanism of Action: A urinary antispasmodic that acts as a direct antagonist at muscarinic acetylcholine receptors in cholinergically innervated organs. Reduces tonus (elastic tension) of smooth muscle in the bladder and slows parasympathetic contractions. ***Therapeutic Effect:*** Decreases urinary bladder contractions, increases residual urine volume, and decreases detrusor muscle pressure.

Pharmacokinetics

Well absorbed following PO administration. Protein binding: 98%. Metabolized by liver. Excreted in feces and urine. ***Half-life:*** 40-68 hr.

INDICATIONS AND DOSAGES

Overactive bladder

PO

Adults, Elderly. 5 mg/day; if tolerated, may increase to 10 mg/day.

Dosage in renal or hepatic impairment

For patients with severe renal impairment or moderate hepatic impairment, maximum dosage is 5 mg/day.

AVAILABLE FORMS

• *Tablets:* 5 mg, 10 mg.

CONTRAINDICATIONS: Breast-feeding, GI obstruction, uncontrolled angle-closure glaucoma, urine retention

PREGNANCY AND LACTATION: Pregnancy category C; breast milk excretion unknown

SIDE EFFECTS

Frequent (11%-5%)

Dry mouth, constipation, blurred vision

Occasional (5%-3%)

UTI, dyspepsia, nausea

Rare (2%-1%)

Dizziness, dry eyes, fatigue, depression, edema, hypertension, upper abdominal pain, vomiting, urine retention

SERIOUS REACTIONS

• Angioneurotic edema and GI obstruction occur rarely.

• Overdose can result in severe central anticholinergic effects.

INTERACTIONS

Drugs

3 *CYP3A4 inhibitors:* CYP3A4 inhibitors increases levels of solifenacin, reduce dose to 5 mg qday

3 *Ketoconazole:* Ketoconazole increases levels of solifenacin, reduce dose to 5 mg qday

SPECIAL CONSIDERATIONS

• Studies have not shown that solifenacin is better than generically available drugs for the same purpose

PATIENT/FAMILY EDUCATION

• May precipitate urinary retention or narrow angle glaucoma

---

somatropin/somatrem

(soe-mah-troe′-pin/soe′-ma-trem)

Rx: (somatropin) Genotropin, Genotropin Miniquick, Humatrope, Norditropin, Norditropin Cartridge, Nutropin, Nutropin AQ, Nutropin Depot, Saizen, Serostim, Zorbitive

Rx: (somatrem) Protopin

Chemical Class: Growth hormone; recombinant human peptide

Therapeutic Class: Anti-cachexic; growth hormone

CLINICAL PHARMACOLOGY

Mechanism of Action: A polypeptide hormone that stimulates cartilaginous growth areas of long bones, increases the number and size of skeletal muscle cells, influences the size of organs, and increases RBC mass by stimulating erythropoietin. Influences the metabolism of carbohydrates (decreases insulin sensitivity), fats (mobilizes fatty acids), minerals (retains phosphorus, sodium, potassium by promotion of cell growth), and proteins (increases protein synthesis). ***Therapeutic Effect:*** Stimulates growth.

Pharmacokinetics
Well absorbed after subcutaneous or IM administration. Localized primarily in the kidneys and liver. ***Half-life:*** IV, 20-30 min; subcutaneous, IM, 3-5 hr.

INDICATIONS AND DOSAGES
Growth hormone deficiency
Subcutaneous (Humatrope)
Adults. 0.006 mg/kg once daily.
Children. 0.18-0.3 mg/kg weekly divided into alternate-day doses or 6 doses/wk.
Subcutaneous (Nutropin)
Adults. 0.006 mg/kg once daily.
Children. 0.3-0.7 mg/kg weekly divided into daily doses.
Subcutaneous (Nutropin AQ)
Adults. 0.006 mg/kg once daily.
Subcutaneous (Genotropin)
Adults. 0.04-0.08 mg/kg weekly divided into 6-7 equal doses/wk.
Children. 0.16-0.24 mg/kg weekly divided into daily doses.
Subcutaneous (Protopin)
Children. 0.3 mg/kg weekly divided into daily doses.
Subcutaneous (Norditropin)
Children. 0.024-0.036 mg/kg/dose 6-7 times a week.
Subcutaneous (Saizen)
Children. 0.06 mg/kg 3 times a week.
Subcutaneous only (Nutropin Depot)
Children. 0.75 mg/kg twice monthly or 1.5 mg/kg once monthly.
Chronic renal insufficiency
Subcutaneous (Nutropin, Nutropin AQ)
Children. 0.35 mg/kg weekly divided into daily doses.
Turner syndrome
Subcutaneous (Humatrope, Nutropin, Nutropin AQ)
Children. 0.375 mg/kg weekly divided into equal doses 3-7 times a week.
AIDS-related wasting
Subcutaneous
Adults weighing more than 55 kg. 6 mg once a day at bedtime.
Adults weighing 45-55 kg. 5 mg once a day at bedtime.
Adults weighing 35-44 kg. 4 mg once a day at bedtime.
Adults weighing less than 35 kg. 0.1 mg/kg once a day at bedtime.
Short bowel syndrome
Subcutaneous (Zorbitive)
Adults. 0.1 mg/kg/day. Maximum: 8 mg/day.

AVAILABLE FORMS
- *Injection Powder for Reconstitution (somatrem [Protopin]):* 5 mg.
- *Injection Powder for Reconstitution (somatropin):* 0.4 mg (Genotropin Miniquick), 0.6 mg (Genotropin Miniquick), 0.8 mg (Genotropin Miniquick), 1 mg (Genotropin Miniquick), 1.2 mg (Genotropin Miniquick), 1.4 mg (Genotropin Miniquick), 1.5 mg (Genotropin, Genotropin Miniquick), 1.6 mg (Genotropin Miniquick), 1.8 mg (Genotropin Miniquick), 2 mg (Genotropin Miniquick), 4 mg (Norditropin, Serostim, Zorbitive), 5 mg (Humatrope, Nutropin, Saizen, Serostim, Zorbitive), 5.8 mg (Genotropin), 6 mg (Humatrope, Serostim, Zorbitive), 8 mg (Norditropin), 8.8 mg (Saizen, Zorbitive), 10 mg (Nutropin), 12 mg (Humatrope), 13.5 mg (Nutropin Depot), 18 mg (Nutropin Depot), 22.5 mg (Nutropin Depot), 24 mg (Humatrope).
- *Solution for Injection (somatropin [Norditropin Cartridge]):* 15 mg/1.5 ml.
- *Injection Solution (somatropin [Nutropin AQ]):* 5 mg/ml.

CONTRAINDICATIONS: Active neoplasia (either newly diagnosed or recurrent), critical illness, hypersensitivity to growth hormone

PREGNANCY AND LACTATION: Pregnancy category B (for Genotropin, Genotropin Miniquick, Saizen, Serostim, Zorbitive); C (for Humatrope, Norditropin, Norditropin Cartridge, Nutropin, Nutropin AQ, Nutropin Depot, Protopin); excretion into breast milk unknown

SIDE EFFECTS

Frequent

Otitis media, other ear disorders (with Turner's syndrome)

Occasional

Carpal tunnel syndrome; gynecomastia; myalgia; swelling of hands, feet, or legs; fatigue; asthenia

Rare

Rash, pruritus, altered vision, headache, nausea, vomiting, injection site pain and swelling, abdominal pain, hip or knee pain

SERIOUS REACTIONS

• Glucose intolerance can occur with overdosage. Long-term overdosage with growth hormone could result in signs and symptoms of acromegaly.

INTERACTIONS

Drugs

3 *Corticosteroids:* May inhibit growth response

SPECIAL CONSIDERATIONS

MONITORING PARAMETERS

• Individualize doses for growth hormone inadequacy
• Check for hypothyroidism, malnutrition, antibodies or opportunistic infections (AIDs patients) if no response to initial dose
• TSH
• Evaluate if child limps
• Follow with fundoscopy (papilledema)
• Bone density, blood glucose level, serum calcium and phosphorus levels

---

sorbitol

(sor'-bi-tole)

Rx: Sorbitol

Chemical Class: Polyalcoholic sugar

Therapeutic Class: Diuretic, osmotic; laxative, osmotic

CLINICAL PHARMACOLOGY

Mechanism of Action: An polyalcoholic sugar with osmotic cathartic actions. Specific mechanism unknown. ***Therapeutic Effect:*** Catharsis, urinary irrigation.

Pharmacokinetics

Onset of action within 15-60 mins. Poorly absorbed by both oral and rectal route. Metabolized in live to primary metabolite, fructose.

INDICATIONS AND DOSAGES

Hyperosmotic laxative

PO

Adults, Elderly, Children 12 yrs and older: 30-150 mL as a 70% solution.

Children 2-11 yrs: 2 mL/kg as a 70% solution.

Rectal

Adults, Elderly, Children 12 yrs and older: 120 mL as a 25%-30% solution.

Children 2-11 yrs: 30-60 mL as a 25%-30% solution.

Transurethral surgical procedure

Topical

Adults, Elderly: 3-3.3% as transurethral surgical procedure irrigation.

AVAILABLE FORMS

• *Solution:* 3%.

CONTRAINDICATIONS: Anuria

PREGNANCY AND LACTATION: Pregnancy category C

SIDE EFFECTS

Acidosis, electrolyte loss, marked diuresis, urinary retention, edema, dryness of mouth and thirst, dehydration, pulmonary congestion, hypotension, tachycardia, angina-like pains, blurred vision, convulsions, nausea, vomiting, diarrhea, rhinitis, chills, vertigo, backache, urticaria

SERIOUS REACTIONS

• Life-threatening adverse reactions with IV sorbitol infusions have been reported in patients with fructose intolerance.

SPECIAL CONSIDERATIONS

• Just as effective as lactulose as a laxative at reduced expense

PATIENT/FAMILY EDUCATION

• Notify the physician if dry mouth, nausea, vomiting, diarrhea, chills, dizziness, or backache occurs

MONITORING PARAMETERS

• Fluid and electrolytes
• Blood glucose

sotalol hydrochloride

(soe′-ta-lole hye-droe-klor′-ide)

Rx: Betapace, Betapace AF, Sorine

Chemical Class: β-adrenergic blocker, nonselective

Therapeutic Class: Antiarrhythmic, class III

CLINICAL PHARMACOLOGY

Mechanism of Action: A beta-adrenergic blocking agent that prolongs action potential, effective refractory period, and QT interval. Decreases heart rate and AV node conduction; increases AV node refractoriness. ***Therapeutic Effect:*** Produces antiarrhythmic activity.

Pharmacokinetics

Well absorbed from the GI tract. Protein binding: none. Widely distributed. Primarily excreted unchanged in urine. Removed by hemodialysis. ***Half-life:*** 12 hr (increased in the elderly and patients with impaired renal function).

INDICATIONS AND DOSAGES

Documented, life-threatening arrhythmias

PO (Betapace, Sorine)

Adults, Elderly. Initially, 80 mg twice a day. May increase gradually at 2-3-day intervals. Range: 240-320 mg/day.

Atrial fibrillation, atrial flutter

PO (Betapace AF)

Adults, Elderly. 80 mg twice a day.

Dosage in renal impairment

Betapace, Sorine

Dosage interval is modified based on creatinine clearance.

Creatinine Clearance	*Dosage Interval*
31-60 ml/min	24 hr
10-30 ml/min	36-48 hr
less than 10 ml/min	Individualized

Betapace AF

Creatinine Clearance	*Dosage Interval*
greater than 60 ml/min	12 hr
40-60 ml/min	24 hr
less than 40 ml/min	Contraindicated

AVAILABLE FORMS

• *Tablets:* 80 mg (Betapace, Betapace AF Sorine), 120 mg (Betapace, Betapace AF, Sorine), 160 mg (Betapace, Betapace AF, Sorine), 240 mg (Betapace, Sorine).

UNLABELED USES: Maintenance of normal heart rhythm in chronic or recurring atrial fibrillation or flutter; treatment of anxiety, chronic angina pectoris, hypertension, hypertrophic cardiomyopathy, MI, mitral valve prolapse syndrome, pheo-

S

chromocytoma, thyrotoxicosis, tremors

CONTRAINDICATIONS: Bronchial asthma, cardiogenic shock, prolonged QT syndrome (unless functioning pacemaker is present), second- and third-degree heart block, sinus bradycardia, uncontrolled cardiac failure

PREGNANCY AND LACTATION: Pregnancy category B (D if used in second or third trimester); similar drug, atenolol, frequently used in the third trimester for treatment of hypertension (many studies of efficacy and safety of atenolol in pregnancy-induced hypertension); long-term use has been associated with intrauterine growth retardation; concentrated in breast milk (levels 3-5 times those of plasma); symptoms of β-blockade possible in infant, but considered compatible with breastfeeding

SIDE EFFECTS

Frequent

Diminished sexual function, drowsiness, insomnia, unusual fatigue or weakness

Occasional

Depression, cold hands or feet, diarrhea, constipation, anxiety, nasal congestion, nausea, vomiting

Rare

Altered taste, dry eyes, itching, numbness of fingers, toes, or scalp

SERIOUS REACTIONS

• Bradycardia, CHF, hypotension, bronchospasm, hypoglycemia, prolonged QT interval, torsades de pointes, ventricular tachycardia, and premature ventricular complexes may occur.

INTERACTIONS

Drugs

3 *Adenosine:* Bradycardia aggravated

3 *α_1-adrenergic blockers:* Potential enhanced first-dose response (marked initial drop in blood pressure), particularly on standing (especially prazocin)

3 *Antacids:* Reduced sotalol absorption with aluminum- and magnesium-containing antacids, separate dose by 2 hrs

▲ *Antiarrhythmics, Class Ia (disopyramide, moricizine, quinidine, procainamide) and Class III (amiodarone, bretylium, dofetilide, ibutilide):* Concomitant therapy not recommended due to potential to prolong refractoriness, hold antiarrhythmics for at least 3 half-lives prior to doing with sotalol

❷ *β_2-receptor agonists (albuterol, isoproterenol, terbutaline):* β-agonists may have to be administered in increased dosages when used concomitantly with sotalol

3 *Calcium channel blockers:* Possible additive effects on AV conduction or ventricular function, possible additive effects on BP

3 *Catecholamine-depleting agents (guanethidine, reserpine):* Hypotension and marked bradycardia possible due to excessive reduction of resting sympathetic nervous tone with concomitant use

3 *Cholinesterase inhibitors (neostigmine, physostigmine, tacrine):* Bradycardia aggravated

3 *Cimetidine:* Renal clearance reduced; AUC increased with cimetidine coadministration

3 *Cisapride:* Dual prolongation of QT interval; increased risk of ventricular tachyarrhythmias

3 *Clonidine, guanabenz, guanfacine:* Exacerbation of rebound hypertension upon discontinuation of clonidine

3 *Cocaine:* Cocaine-induced vasoconstriction potentiated; reduced coronary blood flow

3 *Contrast media:* Increased risk of anaphylaxis

3 *Digitalis:* Enhances bradycardia

3 *Dipyridamole:* Bradycardia aggravated

3 *Epinephrine, phenylephrine:* Potentiates pressor response; resultant hypertension and bradycardia

3 *Flecainide:* Additive negative inotropic effects; case report of bradycardia, AV block, and cardiac arrest following switch from flecainide to sotalol

3 *Fluoxetine:* Increased β-blockade activity

3 *Hypoglycemic agents (insulin, oral antidiabetics):* Masked hypoglycemia, hyperglycemia may occur requiring dosage adjustment of insulin or antidiabetic agents

3 *Lidocaine:* Increased serum lidocaine concentrations possible

⚠ *Macrolide antibiotics (clarithromycin, erythromycin):* Increased risk of QT prolongation and life-threatening arrhythmias

3 *Neuroleptics:* Both drugs inhibit each other's metabolism; additive hypotension

3 *NSAIDs:* Reduced hemodynamic effects of sotalol

⚠ *Phenothiazines:* Increased risk of QT prolongation and life-threatening arrhythmias

⚠ *Quinolone antibiotics (gatifloxacin, levofloxacin, moxifloxacin, sparfloxacin):* Increased risk of QT prolongation and life-threatening arrhythmias

❷ *Theophylline:* Antagonistic pharmacodynamic effects

⚠ *Tricyclic antidepressants:* Increased risk of QT prolongation and life-threatening arrhythmias

⚠ *Ziprasidone:* Increased risk of QT prolongation and life-threatening arrhythmias

Labs

• *Metanephrines total:* Falsely increases urine levels (may be double)

SPECIAL CONSIDERATIONS

PATIENT/FAMILY EDUCATION

• Do not discontinue abruptly; may require taper; rapid withdrawal may produce rebound hypertension or angina

• Avoid tasks that require mental alertness or motor skills until response to the drug has been established

• Periodic laboratory tests and EKGs are a necessary part of therapy

MONITORING PARAMETERS

• *Angina:* Reduction in nitroglycerin usage; frequency, severity, onset, and duration of angina pain; heart rate

• *Arrhythmias:* Heart rate and rhythm; monitor QT intervals (discontinue or reduce dose if QT >520 msec)

• *Congestive heart failure:* Functional status, cough, dyspnea on exertion, paroxysmal nocturnal dyspnea, exercise tolerance, and ventricular function

• *Hypertension:* Blood pressure

• *Toxicity:* Blood glucose, bronchospasm, hypotension, bradycardia, depression, confusion, hallucination, sexual dysfunction

• Because of prodysrhythmic risk, begin and increase drug in setting with cardiac rhythm monitoring

sparfloxacin

(spar-floks'-a-sin)

Rx: Zagam

Chemical Class: Fluoroquinolone derivative

Therapeutic Class: Antibiotic

CLINICAL PHARMACOLOGY

Mechanism of Action: A fluoroquinolone that interferes with DNA-gyrase in susceptible microorganisms. ***Therapeutic Effect:*** Inhibits DNA replication and repair. Bactericidal.

Pharmacokinetics

Well absorbed from the gastrointestinal (GI) tract after PO administration. Widely distributed. Metabolized in liver. Primarily excreted in urine with a lesser amount eliminated in the feces. ***Half-life:*** 16-30 hrs.

INDICATIONS AND DOSAGES

Bronchitis, pneumonia

PO

Adults 18 yrs and older, Elderly. Initially, two 200-mg tablets as a loading dose on first day. Then one 200-mg tablet q24h for a total of 10 days.

Dosage in renal impairment (creatinine clearance <50 ml/min)

PO

Adults 18 yrs and older, Elderly. Initially, two 200-mg tablets as a loading dose on first day. Then one 200-mg tablet q48h for a total of 9 days.

AVAILABLE FORMS

• *Tablets:* 200 mg (Zagam).

CONTRAINDICATIONS: Hypersensitivity to fluoroquinolones, cinoxacin, nalidixic acid

PREGNANCY AND LACTATION: Pregnancy category C; excretion into breast milk unknown; due to the potential for arthropathy and osteochondrosis, use extreme caution in nursing mothers

SIDE EFFECTS

Occasional

Photosensitivity, diarrhea, nausea, headache

Rare

Dyspepsia, dizziness, insomnia, abdominal pain, change in taste

SERIOUS REACTIONS

• Superinfection (particularly enterococcal or fungal overgrowth of nonsusceptible organisms) due to altered bacterial balance may occur (genital/anal pruritus, ulceration or changes in oral mucosa, moderate to severe diarrhea, new or increased fever).

• Hypersensitivity reactions have occurred in those receiving fluoroquinolone therapy.

INTERACTIONS

Drugs

3 *Aluminum:* Reduced absorption of sparfloxacin; do not take within 4 hr of dose

3 *Antacids:* Reduced absorption of sparfloxacin; do not take within 4 hr of dose

3 *Antipyrine:* Inhibits metabolism of antipyrine; increased plasma antipyrine level

3 *Calcium:* Reduced absorption of sparfloxacin; do not take within 4 hr of dose

3 *Diazepam:* Inhibits metabolism of diazepam; increased plasma diazepam level

3 *Didanosine:* Markedly reduced absorption of sparfloxacin; take sparfloxacin 2 hr before didanosine

3 *Foscarnet:* Coadministration increases seizure risk

3 *Iron:* Reduced absorption of sparfloxacin; do not take within 4 hr of dose

3 *Magnesium:* Reduced absorption of sparfloxacin; do not take within 4 hr of dose

3 *Metoprolol:* Inhibits metabolism of metoprolol; increased plasma metoprolol level

3 *Phenytoin:* Inhibits metabolism of phenytoin; increased plasma phenytoin level

3 *Propranolol:* Inhibits metabolism of propranolol; increased plasma propranolol level

3 *Ropinirole:* Inhibits metabolism of ropinirole; increased plasma ropinirole level

3 *Sodium bicarbonate:* Reduced absorption of sparfloxacin; do not take within 4 hr of dose

3 *Sucralfate:* Reduced absorption of sparfloxacin; do not take within 4 hr of dose

3 *Warfarin:* Inhibits metabolism of warfarin; increases hypoprothrombinemic response to warfarin

3 *Zinc:* Reduced absorption of sparfloxacin; do not take within 4 hr of dose

3 *Ziprasidone:* Prolongs the QTc interval

SPECIAL CONSIDERATIONS

PATIENT/FAMILY EDUCATION

- Avoid direct or indirect sunlight during treatment and for 5 days after completion of therapy; drink fluids liberally
- Take antacids 2 hrs before or after taking the medication
- Continue the medication for the full length of treatment

MONITORING PARAMETERS

- Be alert for superinfection such as genital/anal pruritus, ulceration or changes in oral mucosa, moderate to severe diarrhea, new or increased fever

---

spectinomycin

(spek-ti-noe-mye'-sin)

Rx: Trobicin

Chemical Class: Aminoglycoside derivative

Therapeutic Class: Antibiotic

CLINICAL PHARMACOLOGY

Mechanism of Action: An antiinfective that inhibits protein synthesis of bacterial cells. ***Therapeutic Effect:*** Produces bacterial cell death.

Pharmacokinetics

Rapid, complete absorption after intramuscular (IM) administration. Protein binding: unknown. Widely distributed. Excreted unchanged in urine. Partially removed by hemodialysis. ***Half-life:*** 1.7 hrs.

INDICATIONS AND DOSAGES

Treatment of acute gonococcal urethritis and proctitis in males, acute gonococcal cervicitis and proctitis in females

IM

Adults, Elderly. 2 g once. In areas where antibiotic resistance is known to be prevalent, 4 g (10 ml) divided between 2 injection sites is preferred.

AVAILABLE FORMS

- *Powder for Reconstitution:* 2 g (Trobicin).

UNLABELED USES: Treatment of disseminated gonorrhea

CONTRAINDICATIONS: Hypersensitivity to spectinomycin or any component of the formulation

PREGNANCY AND LACTATION: Pregnancy category B; excretion into breast milk unknown

SIDE EFFECTS

Frequent

Pain at IM injection site

Occasional

Dizziness, insomnia

Rare

Decreased urine output

SERIOUS REACTIONS

- Hypersensitivity reaction characterized as chills, fever, nausea, vomiting, urticaria, and anaphylaxis.

SPECIAL CONSIDERATIONS

- Follow with doxycycline 100 mg bid for 7 days (erythromycin if pregnant or allergic)
- Ineffective against syphilis and may mask symptoms
- Give in gluteal muscle; dose >2 g must be divided in 2 gluteal injections

PATIENT/FAMILY EDUCATION
• IM injection may cause discomfort

MONITORING PARAMETERS
• Observe patient 1 hr after injection due to potential for anaphylaxis

spironolactone

(speer-on-oh-lak'-tone)

Rx: Aldactone

Combinations

Rx: with hydrochlorothiazide (Aldactazide)

Chemical Class: Aldosterone antagonist

Therapeutic Class: Antihypertensive; diuretic, potassium-sparing

CLINICAL PHARMACOLOGY

Mechanism of Action: A potassium-sparing diuretic that interferes with sodium reabsorption by competitively inhibiting the action of aldosterone in the distal tubule, thus promoting sodium and water excretion and increasing potassium retention. ***Therapeutic Effect:*** Produces diuresis; lowers BP; diagnostic aid for primary aldosteronism.

Pharmacokinetics

Route	*Onset*	*Peak*	*Duration*
PO	24-48 hrs	48-72 hrs	48-72 hrs

Well absorbed from the GI tract (absorption increased with food). Protein binding: 91%-98%. Metabolized in the liver to active metabolite. Primarily excreted in urine. Unknown if removed by hemodialysis. ***Half-life:*** 0-24 hrs (metabolite, 13-24 hrs).

INDICATIONS AND DOSAGES

Edema

PO

Adults, Elderly. 25-200 mg/day as a single dose or in 2 divided doses.

Children. 1.5-3.3 mg/kg/day in divided doses.

Neonates. 1-3 mg/kg/day in 1-2 divided doses.

Hypertension

PO

Adults, Elderly. 25-50 mg/day in 1-2 doses/day.

Children. 1.5-3.3 mg/kg/day in divided doses.

Hypokalemia

PO

Adults, Elderly. 25-200 mg/day as a single dose or in 2 divided doses.

Male hirsutism

PO

Adults, Elderly. 50-200 mg/day as a single dose or in 2 divided doses.

Primary aldosteronism

PO

Adults, Elderly. 100-400 mg/day as a single dose or in 2 divided doses.

Children. 100-400 mg/m^2/day as a single dose or in 2 divided doses.

CHF

PO

Adults, Elderly. 25 mg/day adjusted based on patient response and evidence of hyperkalemia.

Dosage in renal impairment

Dosage interval is modified based on creatinine clearance.

Creatinine Clearance	*Interval*
10-50 ml/min	Usual dose q12-24h
less than 10 ml/min	Avoid use

AVAILABLE FORMS
• *Tablets:* 25 mg, 50 mg, 100 mg.

UNLABELED USES: Treatment of edema and hypertension in children; female acne, hirsutism, polycystic ovary disease

CONTRAINDICATIONS: Acute renal insufficiency, anuria, BUN and serum creatinine levels more than twice normal values, hyperkalemia

PREGNANCY AND LACTATION: Pregnancy category D; feminization occurs in male rat fetuses; active metabolite excreted in breast milk; compatible with breast-feeding but alternate options preferred; therapy for existing hypertension can be continued throughout pregnancy with minimal risk; initiating for simple edema not recommended; few unequivocal indications for diuretic therapy in pregnancy except for pulmonary edema or congestive heart failure

SIDE EFFECTS

Frequent

Hyperkalemia (in patients with renal insufficiency and those taking potassium supplements), dehydration, hyponatremia, lethargy

Occasional

Nausea, vomiting, anorexia, abdominal cramps, diarrhea, headache, ataxia, somnolence, confusion, fever

Male: Gynecomastia, impotence, decreased libido

Female: Menstrual irregularities (including amenorrhea and postmenopausal bleeding), breast tenderness

Rare

Rash, urticaria, hirsutism

SERIOUS REACTIONS

• Severe hyperkalemia may produce arrhythmias, bradycardia, and EKG changes (tented T waves, widening QRS complex, and ST segment depression). These may proceed to cardiac standstill or ventricular fibrillation.

• Cirrhosis patients are at risk for hepatic decompensation if dehydration or hyponatremia occurs.

• Patients with primary aldosteronism may experience rapid weight loss and severe fatigue during high-dose therapy.

INTERACTIONS

Drugs

3 *Ammonium chloride:* Combination may produce systemic acidosis

3 *Angiotensin-converting enzyme inhibitors:* Concurrent mechanisms to decrease potassium excretion; increased risk of hyperkalemia

3 *Angiotensin II receptor antagonists:* Concurrent mechanisms to decrease potassium excretion; increased risk of hyperkalemia

3 *Anticoagulants, heparin:* May decrease the effects of these drugs

3 *Digitalis glycosides:* False or true increase in digoxin concentrations

3 *Disopyramide:* Increased potassium concentrations may enhance disopyramide effects on myocardial conduction

3 *Lithium:* May decrease the clearance and increase the risk of toxicity of lithium

▲ *Mitotane:* Spironolactone antagonizes the activity of mitotane

3 *NSAIDs:* May decrease the antihypertensive effect of spironolactone

❷ *Potassium:* Increased risk of hyperkalemia

3 *Salicylates:* Decreased diuretic (not antihypertensive effect) due to decreased tubular secretion of active metabolite

Labs

• *Corticosteroids:* Marked false increase in plasma corticosteroids

• *Cortisol:* Falsely increased fluorometric methods of measurement

• *Digoxin:* False increases in digoxin concentrations

• *17-Hydroxycorticosteroids:* False increases in urine measurements

• *17-Ketogenic steroids:* Falsely increases urine concentrations

SPECIAL CONSIDERATIONS

PATIENT/FAMILY EDUCATION

- Expect an increase in the frequency and volume of urination
- The drug's therapeutic effect takes several days to begin and can last for several days once the drug is discontinued (unless he or she is taking a potassium-losing drug concomitantly)
- Avoid consuming potassium supplements and foods high in potassium, including apricots, bananas, raisins, orange juice, potatoes, legumes, meat, and whole grains (such as cereals)
- Notify the physician if irregular heartbeat, diarrhea, muscle twitching, cold and clammy skin, confusion, drowsiness, dry mouth, or excessive thirst occurs
- Avoid performing tasks that require mental alertness or motor skills until response to the drug has been established

MONITORING PARAMETERS

- When used for diagnosis of primary hyperaldosteronism, positive results are: (long test) correction of hyperkalemia and hypertension; (short test) serum potassium increases during administration, but falls upon discontinuation
- Blood pressure, edema, urine output, ECG (if hyperkalemia exists), urine electrolytes, BUN, creatinine, gynecomastia, impotence

stanozolol

(stan-oh'-zoe-lole)

Rx: Winstrol

Chemical Class: Anabolic steroid; testosterone derivative

Therapeutic Class: Androgen; antiangioedema agent

DEA Class: Schedule III

CLINICAL PHARMACOLOGY

Mechanism of Action: A synthetic testosterone derivative that increases circulating levels of C1 INH and C4 through an increase in general protein anabolism, and, more specifically, through an increase in the synthesis of messenger RNA. ***Therapeutic Effect:*** Decreases swelling of the face, extremities, genitalia, bowel wall, and upper respiratory tract

Pharmacokinetics

Metabolized in liver. Primarily excreted in urine. Unknown if removed by hemodialysis.

INDICATIONS AND DOSAGES

Hereditary angioedema prophylaxis

PO

Adults. Initially, 2 mg 2 times/day. Decrease at 1-3-mos intervals. Maintenance: 2 mg/day.

AVAILABLE FORMS

- *Tablets:* 2 mg (Winstrol).

UNLABELED USES: Antithrombin III deficiency, arterial occlusions, hemophilia A, lichen sclerosus et atrophicus, liposclerosis, necrobiosis lipoidica, osteoporosis, protein C deficiency, rheumatoid arthritis, thrombosis, urticaria

CONTRAINDICATIONS: Cardiac impairment, hypercalcemia, pregnancy, prostatic or breast cancer in males, severe liver or renal disease, hypersensitivity to stanozolol or its components

PREGNANCY AND LACTATION: Pregnancy category X (masculinization); excretion into breast milk unknown; use extreme caution in nursing mothers

SIDE EFFECTS

Frequent

Gynecomastia, acne

Females: Amenorrhea or other menstrual irregularities, hirsutism, deepening of voice, clitoral enlargement that may not be reversible when drug is discontinued

Occasional

Edema, nausea, insomnia, oligospermia, male pattern baldness, bladder irritability, hypercalcemia in immobilized patients or those with breast cancer, hypercholesterolemia

SERIOUS REACTIONS

• Peliosis hepatitis or liver, spleen replaced with blood-filled cysts, hepatic neoplasms, and hepatocellular carcinoma have been associated with prolonged high dosage.

INTERACTIONS

Drugs

❷ *Oral anticoagulants:* Enhanced hypoprothrombinemic response

3 *Antidiabetic agents:* Enhanced hypoglycemic response

❷ *Cyclosporine:* Increased cyclosporine concentrations

3 *HMG-CoA reductase inhibitors (lovastatin, pravastatin):* Myositis risk increased

SPECIAL CONSIDERATIONS

• Anabolic steroids have potential for abuse, especially in the athlete

PATIENT/FAMILY EDUCATION

• Do not take more of the medicine than prescribed due to an increase risk of severe side effects

• Do not take any other medications, including OTC drugs, without first consulting the physician

• Notify the physician if acne, nausea, pedal edema, or vomiting occurs

• The female patient should promptly report deepening of voice, hoarseness, and menstrual irregularities

• The male patient should report difficulty urinating, frequent erections, and gynecomastia

MONITORING PARAMETERS

• LFTs, lipids

• Growth rate in children (X-rays for bone age q6mo)

• Signs of virilization

• Blood Hgb and Hct periodically

• Electrolytes

stavudine

(stav'-yoo-deen)

Rx: Zerit, Zerit XR

Chemical Class: Nucleoside analog

Therapeutic Class: Antiretroviral

CLINICAL PHARMACOLOGY

Mechanism of Action: Inhibits HIV reverse transcriptase by terminating the viral DNA chain. Also inhibits RNA- and DNA-dependent DNA polymerase, an enzyme necessary for HIV replication. ***Therapeutic Effect:*** Impedes HIV replication, slowing the progression of HIV infection.

Pharmacokinetics

Rapidly and completely absorbed after PO administration. Undergoes minimal metabolism. Excreted in urine. ***Half-life:*** 1.5 hr (increased in renal impairment).

INDICATIONS AND DOSAGES

HIV infection

PO

Adults, Elderly, Children weighing 60 kg and more. 40 mg q12h.

Children weighing 30-59 kg. 30 mg q12h.
Neonates 14 days and older, Infants, Children weighing less than 30 kg. 1 mg/kg/dose q12h. Maximum: 30 mg q12h.
Neonates 0-13 days. 0.5 mg/kg/dose q12h.

Dosage in renal impairment

Dosage and frequency are modified based on creatinine clearance and patient weight.

Creatinine Clearance	*Weight 60 kg or More*	*Weight Less than 60 kg*
greater than 50 ml/min	40 mg q12h	30 mg q12h
26-50 ml/min	20 mg q12h	15 mg q12h
10-25 ml/min	20 mg q24h	15 mg q24h

AVAILABLE FORMS

- *Capsules:* 15 mg, 20 mg, 30 mg, 40 mg.
- *Oral Solution:* 1 mg/ml.

CONTRAINDICATIONS: None known.

PREGNANCY AND LACTATION: Pregnancy category C; excreted in breast milk

SIDE EFFECTS

Frequent

Headache (55%), diarrhea (50%), chills and fever (38%), nausea and vomiting, myalgia (35%), rash (33%), asthenia (28%), insomnia, abdominal pain (26%), anxiety (22%), arthralgia (18%), back pain (20%), diaphoresis (19%), malaise (17%), depression (14%)

Occasional

Anorexia, weight loss, nervousness, dizziness, conjunctivitis, dyspepsia, dyspnea

Rare

Constipation, vasodilation, confusion, migraine, urticaria, abnormal vision

SERIOUS REACTIONS

- Peripheral neuropathy, (numbness, tingling, or pain in the hands and feet) occurs in 15%-21% of patients.
- Ulcerative stomatitis (erythema or ulcers of oral mucosa, glossitis, gingivitis), pneumonia, and benign skin neoplasms occur occasionally.
- Pancreatitis, hepatomegaly, and lactic acidosis have been reported.

INTERACTIONS

Drugs

3 *Didanosine, ethambutol, isoniazid, lithium, phenytoin, zalcitabine:* May increase the risk of peripheral neuropathy development

3 *Didanosine, hydroxyurea:* May increase the risk of hepatotoxicity

▲ *Zidovudine:* Competitive inhibition of the intracellular phosphorylation of stavudine, concomitant use not recommended

SPECIAL CONSIDERATIONS

PATIENT/FAMILY EDUCATION

- Report neuropathic symptoms (numbness, tingling, or pain in the feet or hands)
- Space doses evenly around the clock and continue taking the drug for the full course of treatment
- Do not take any other medications, OTC drugs, without first notifying the physician
- Stavudine is not a cure for HIV infection, nor does it reduce the risk of transmitting HIV to others

MONITORING PARAMETERS

- CBC, SGOT, SGPT
- Weight
- Skin for rash
- Pattern of daily bowel activity and stool consistency
- Eyes for signs of conjunctivitis
- Monitor for signs and symptoms of peripheral neuropathy, such as numbness, pain, or tingling in the

feet or hands. Be aware that these symptoms usually resolve promptly if stavudine therapy is discontinued, but they may worsen temporarily after the drug is withdrawn. If symptoms resolve completely, expect to resume drug therapy at a reduced dosage

streptokinase

(strep-toe-kin'-ace)

Rx: Kabikinase, Streptase

Chemical Class: Betahemolytic steptococcus filtrate, purified

Therapeutic Class: Thrombolytic

CLINICAL PHARMACOLOGY

Mechanism of Action: An enzyme that activates the fibrinolytic system by converting plasminogen to plasmin, an enzyme that degrades fibrin clots. Acts indirectly by forming a complex with plasminogen, which converts plasminogen to plasmin. Action occurs within the thrombus, on its surface, and in circulating blood. ***Therapeutic Effect:*** Destroys thrombi.

Pharmacokinetics

Rapidly cleared from plasma by antibodies and the reticuloendothelial system. Route of elimination unknown. Duration of action continues for several hours after drug has been discontinued. ***Half-life:*** 23 min.

INDICATIONS AND DOSAGES

Acute evolving transmural MI (given as soon as possible after symptoms occur)

IV Infusion

Adults, Elderly. (1.5 million units diluted to 45 ml). 1.5 million units infused over 60 min.

Intracoronary Infusion

Adults, Elderly. (250,000 units diluted to 125 ml). Initially, 20,000-units (10-ml) bolus; then, 2000 units/min for 60 min. Total dose: 140,000 units.

Pulmonary embolism, deep vein thrombosis (DVT), arterial thrombosis and embolism (given within 7 days of onset)

IV Infusion

Adults, Elderly. (1.5 million units diluted to 90 ml). Initially, 250,000 units infused over 30 min; then, 100,000 units/hr for 24-72 hrs for arterial thrombosis or embolism, and pulmonary embolism, 72 hrs for DVT.

Intraarterial infusion

Adults, Elderly. (1.5 million units diluted to 45 ml). Initially, 250,000 units infused over 30 min; then 100,000 units/hr for maintenance.

AVAILABLE FORMS

- *Powder for Injection (Kabikinase, Streptase):* 250,000 units, 750,000 units, 1.5 million units.

CONTRAINDICATIONS: Carcinoma of the brain, cerebrovascular accident, internal bleeding, intracranial surgery, recent streptococcal infection, severe hypertension

PREGNANCY AND LACTATION: Pregnancy category C; no data available for breast-feeding

SIDE EFFECTS

Frequent

Fever, superficial bleeding at puncture sites, decreased BP

Occasional

Allergic reaction, including rash and wheezing; ecchymosis

SERIOUS REACTIONS

- Severe internal hemorrhage may occur.
- Lysis of coronary thrombi may produce life-threatening arrhythmias.

INTERACTIONS

Drugs

3 *Heparin, oral anticoagulants, drugs that alter platelet function (i.e., aspirin, dipyridamole, abciximab, eptifibitide, tirofiben):* May increase the risk of bleeding

Labs

- *Fibrinogen:* False increase with certain methods
- *Lactate dehydrogenase isoenzymes:* False positive

SPECIAL CONSIDERATIONS

PATIENT/FAMILY EDUCATION

- Use an electric razor and soft toothbrush to prevent bleeding during drug therapy
- Report black or red stool, coffee-ground vomitus, dark or red urine, red-speckled mucus from cough, or other signs of bleeding
- Immediately report chest pain, headache, palpitations, or shortness of breath

MONITORING PARAMETERS

- Clinical response and vital signs
- Hgb and Hct, blood pressure, and platelet count; do not obtain blood pressure in lower extremities because a deep vein thrombus may be present
- aPTT, fibrinogen level, PT, and thrombin every 4 hrs after therapy begins
- Stool for occult blood

streptomycin sulfate

(strep-toe-mye'-sin sul'-fate)

Chemical Class: Aminoglycoside

Therapeutic Class: Antibiotic; antituberculosis agent

CLINICAL PHARMACOLOGY

Mechanism of Action: An aminoglycoside that binds directly to the 30S ribosomal subunits, causing a faulty peptide sequence to form in the protein chain. ***Therapeutic Effect:*** Inhibits bacterial protein synthesis.

Pharmacokinetics

Protein binding: 34%-35%. Excreted in urine. ***Half-life:*** 2.5 hr.

INDICATIONS AND DOSAGES

Tuberculosis

IM

Adults. 15 mg/kg/day. Maximum: 1 g/day.

Elderly. 10 mg/kg/day. Maximum: 750 mg/day.

Children. 20-40 mg/kg/day. Maximum: 1 g/day.

Dosage in renal impairment

Creatinine Clearance	*Dosage Interval*
10-50 ml/min	q24-72h
less than 10 ml/min	q72-96h

AVAILABLE FORMS

- *Injection:* 1 g.

CONTRAINDICATIONS: Hypersensitivity to aminoglycosides, pregnancy

PREGNANCY AND LACTATION: Pregnancy category D; small amounts excreted into breast milk; compatible with breast-feeding (oral absorption poor)

SIDE EFFECTS

Occasional

Hypotension, drowsiness, headache, drug fever, paresthesia, rash, nausea, vomiting, anemia, arthralgia, weakness, tremor

SERIOUS REACTIONS

- Nephrotoxicity (as evidenced by increased BUN and serum creatinine levels and decreased creatinine clearance) may be reversible if the drug is stopped at the first sign of nephrotoxic symptoms.
- Irreversible ototoxicity (manifested as tinnitus, dizziness, ringing or roaring in the ears, and impaired hearing) and neurotoxicity (as evi-

denced by headache, dizziness, lethargy, tremor, and visual disturbances) occur occasionally. Symptoms of ototoxicity, nephrotoxicity, and neuromuscular toxicity may occur.

INTERACTIONS

Drugs

3 *Amphotericin B, cephalosporins, cyclosporine, NSAIDs, loop diuretics:* Additive nephrotoxicity

3 *Carboplatin:* Additive ototoxicity

2 *Ethacrynic acid:* Additive ototoxicity

3 *Methoxyflurane:* Additive nephrotoxicity

2 *Neuromuscular blocking agents:* Respiratory depression

3 *Oral anticoagulants:* Enhanced hypoprothrombinemic response

3 *Penicillins, extended-spectrum:* Inactivation of aminoglycoside

Labs

- *Protein:* Falsely increases CSF-protein
- *Sugar:* Falsely increased urine levels via copper reduction methods
- *Urea nitrogen:* Decreases serum levels

SPECIAL CONSIDERATIONS

- Not usually used for long-term therapy secondary to nephrotoxicity and ototoxicity

PATIENT/FAMILY EDUCATION

- Notify the physician if such symptoms as hearing loss, dizziness, or fullness or roaring in the ears occur

MONITORING PARAMETERS

- Serum drug levels; therapeutic peak levels 20-30 mcg/ml, toxic peak levels (1 hr after IM administration) >50 mcg/ml
- Keep patient well hydrated
- Hearing
- Renal function

succimer

(suks'-si-mer)

Rx: Chemet

Chemical Class: Dimercaprol derivative

Therapeutic Class: Antidote, heavy metal

CLINICAL PHARMACOLOGY

Mechanism of Action: An analog of dimercaprol that forms water soluble chelates with heavy metals, which are excreted renally. ***Therapeutic Effect:*** Treats lead intoxication in children.

Pharmacokinetics

Rapidly absorbed from the gastrointestinal (GI) tract. Extensively metabolized. Excreted in feces (39%), urine (9%-25%), and lungs (1%). Removed by hemodialysis. ***Half-life:*** 2 hrs-2 days.

INDICATIONS AND DOSAGES

Lead poisoning, in pediatric patients with blood lead levels about 45 mcg/L

PO

Children 12 mos and older. 10 mg/kg q8h for 5 days, then 10 mg/kg q12h for 14 days.

AVAILABLE FORMS

- *Capsules:* 100 mg (Chemet).

UNLABELED USES: Lead poisoning in adults, arsenic intoxication, mercury intoxication

CONTRAINDICATIONS: Hypersensitivity to succimer or any component of its formulation

PREGNANCY AND LACTATION: Pregnancy category C; excretion in breast milk unknown; discourage mothers from breast-feeding during therapy

SIDE EFFECTS

Occasional

Anorexia, diarrhea, nausea, vomiting, rash, odor to breath and urine, increased liver function tests

Rare

Neutropenia

SERIOUS REACTIONS

• Elevated blood lead levels and symptoms of intoxication may occur after succimer therapy due to redistribution of lead from bone to soft tissues and blood.

• Elevated liver function tests have been reported.

INTERACTIONS

Drugs

❷ *Other chelators (e.g., EDTA):* Coadministration not recommended

SPECIAL CONSIDERATIONS

PATIENT/FAMILY EDUCATION

• In children unable to swallow capsule, separate capsule and sprinkle beads on food or on spoon followed by fruit drink

• Notify the physician if rash occurs

• A harmless side effect of offensive sulfurous odor to breath and urine may occur; it will subside when succimer is discontinued

MONITORING PARAMETERS

• Serum transaminases at start of therapy, then qwk during therapy

• After therapy, monitor for rebound (because of redistribution of lead from bound stores to soft tissues, blood) qwk until stable

• CBC, WBC, platelet count

sucralfate

(soo'-kral-fate)

Rx: Carafate

Chemical Class: Aluminum complex of sulfated sucrose

Therapeutic Class: Antiulcer agent

CLINICAL PHARMACOLOGY

Mechanism of Action: An antiulcer agent that forms an ulcer-adherent complex with proteinaceous exudate, such as albumin, at ulcer site. Also forms a viscous, adhesive barrier on the surface of intact mucosa of the stomach or duodenum. ***Therapeutic Effect:*** Protects damaged mucosa from further destruction by absorbing gastric acid, pepsin, and bile salts.

Pharmacokinetics

Minimally absorbed from the GI tract. Eliminated in feces, with small amount excreted in urine. Not removed by hemodialysis.

INDICATIONS AND DOSAGES

Active duodenal ulcers

PO

Adults, Elderly. 1 g 4 times a day (before meals and at bedtime) for up to 8 wk.

Maintenance therapy after healing of acute duodenal ulcers

PO

Adults, Elderly. 1 g twice a day.

AVAILABLE FORMS

• *Oral Suspension:* 1 g/10 ml.

• *Tablets:* 1 g.

UNLABELED USES: Prevention and treatment of stress-related mucosal damage, especially in acutely or critically ill patients; treatment of gastric ulcer and rheumatoid arthritis; relief of GI symptoms associated with NSAIDs; treatment of gastroesophageal reflux disease

CONTRAINDICATIONS: None known.

PREGNANCY AND LACTATION: Pregnancy category B; little systemic absorption, so minimal, if any, excretion into milk expected

SIDE EFFECTS

Frequent (2%)

Constipation

Occasional (less than 2%)

Dry mouth, backache, diarrhea, dizziness, somnolence, nausea, indigestion, rash, hives, itching, abdominal discomfort

SERIOUS REACTIONS

• Bezoars (ingested compaction that does not pass into intestine) have been reported in patients treated with sucralfate.

INTERACTIONS

Drugs

3 *Antacids:* May interfere with binding of sucralfate

3 *Digoxin:* May decrease the absorption of digoxin

3 *Ketoconazole:* Reduces plasma levels of antifungal

3 *Phenytoin:* Modest reduction in GI absorption of phenytoin

3 *Quinolones:* Reduced antibiotic levels

3 *Trovafloxacin:* Reduces the bioavailability of trovafloxacin; a loss of therapeutic efficacy may occur

3 *Warfarin:* Isolated cases of reduced hypoprothrombinemic response to warfarin

SPECIAL CONSIDERATIONS

PATIENT/FAMILY EDUCATION

• Take antacids prn for pain relief, but not within ½ hr before or after sucralfate

• Take on an empty stomach

• Take sips of tepid water and suck a hard candy to relieve dry mouth

MONITORING PARAMETERS

• Pattern of daily bowel activity and stool consistency

sulfabenzamide/ sulfacetamide/ sulfathiazole

(sul-fa-ben'-za-mide/sul-fa-see'-ta-mide/sul-fa-thye'-a-zole)

Rx: V.V.S.

Chemical Class: Sulfonamide derivative

Therapeutic Class: Antibiotic

CLINICAL PHARMACOLOGY

Mechanism of Action: Interferes with synthesis of folic acid that bacteria require for growth by inhibition of para-aminobenzoic acid metabolism. ***Therapeutic Effect:*** Prevents further bacterial growth.

Pharmacokinetics

Absorption from vagina is variable and unreliable. Primarily metabolized by acetylation. Excreted in urine. ***Half-life:*** Unknown.

INDICATIONS AND DOSAGES

Treatment of Haemophilus vaginalis vaginitis

Vaginal

Adults, Elderly. Insert one applicatorful into vagina twice daily for 4-6 days. Dosage may then be decreased to ½-¼ of an applicatorful twice daily.

AVAILABLE FORMS

• *Vaginal Cream:* 3.7% sulfabenzamide, 2.86% sulfacetamide, 3.42% sulfathiazole (V.V.S).

CONTRAINDICATIONS: Renal dysfunction, pregnancy (or near term), hypersensitivity to sulfabenzamide, sulfacetamide, sulfathiazole, or any component of preparation

PREGNANCY AND LACTATION: Pregnancy category C (category D if used near term; may cause jaundice, hemolytic anemia, and kernicterus in newborns); excreted into breast milk in low concentrations; compatible with breast-feeding in healthy, full-term infants

SIDE EFFECTS

Occasional

Local irritation

Rare

Pruritus urticaria, allergic reactions

SERIOUS REACTIONS

- Superinfection and Stevens-Johnson syndrome occur rarely.

SPECIAL CONSIDERATIONS

PATIENT/FAMILY EDUCATION

- Insert high into vagina
- Do not engage in vaginal intercourse during treatment
- Complete the full course of therapy

MONITORING PARAMETERS

- Monitor the patient for skin rash or evidence of systemic toxicity; if these develop, discontinue medication

sulfacetamide sodium

(sul-fa-see′-ta-mide soe′-dee-um)

Rx: AK-Sulf, Bleph-10, Isopto Cetamide, Ophthacet, Sodium Sulamyd, Sulfair

Combinations

Rx: with prednisolone (Blephamide, Dioptimyd, Metamyd, Vasocidin, Isopto Cetapred); with sulfer (Sulfacet-R); with sulfabenzamide (Sulfathiazole, Sulfa-Gyn, Sulnac, Trysul); with phenylepherine (Vasosulf); with fluorometholone (FML-S)

Chemical Class: Sulfonamide derivative

Therapeutic Class: Antibiotic

CLINICAL PHARMACOLOGY

Mechanism of Action: Interferes with synthesis of folic acid that bacteria require for growth. ***Therapeutic Effect:*** Prevents further bacterial growth. Bacteriostatic.

Pharmacokinetics

Small amounts may be absorbed into the cornea. Excreted rapidly in urine. ***Half-life:*** 7-13 hrs.

INDICATIONS AND DOSAGES

Treatment of corneal ulcers, conjunctivitis and other superficial infections of the eye, prophylaxis after injuries to the eye/removal of foreign bodies, adjunctive therapy for trachoma and inclusion conjunctivitis

Ophthalmic

Adults, Elderly. Ointment: Apply small amount in lower conjunctival sac 1-4 times/day and at bedtime. Solution: 1-3 drops to lower conjunctival sac q2-3h. Seborrheic dermatitis, seborrheic sicca (dandruff), secondary bacterial skin infections

Topical

Adults, Elderly. Apply 1-4 times/day.

AVAILABLE FORMS

• *Lotion:* 10% (Carmol, Klaron, Ovace).

• *Ophthalmic Ointment:* 10% (AK-Sulf).

• *Ophthalmic Solution:* 10% (Bleph-10, Ocusulf, Sulf-10).

UNLABELED USES: Treatment of bacterial blepharitis, blepharoconjunctivitis, bacterial keratitis, keratoconjunctivitis

CONTRAINDICATIONS: Hypersensitivity to sulfonamides or any component of preparation (some products contain sulfite), use in combination with silver-containing products

PREGNANCY AND LACTATION: Pregnancy category C (category D if used near term); compatible with breast-feeding in healthy, full-term infants

SIDE EFFECTS

Frequent

Transient ophthalmic burning, stinging

Occasional

Headache

Rare

Hypersensitivity (erythema, rash, itching, swelling, photosensitivity)

SERIOUS REACTIONS

• Superinfection, drug-induced lupus erythematosus, Stevens-Johnson syndrome occur rarely; nephrotoxicity w/high dermatologic concentrations.

INTERACTIONS

Drugs

❷ *Silver preparations:* Incompatible with sulfacetamide

SPECIAL CONSIDERATIONS

PATIENT/FAMILY EDUCATION

• May cause sensitivity to bright light

• Do not touch tip of container to any surface

• May cause transient burning and stinging

• Notify the physician if swelling, itching, or rash occurs

MONITORING PARAMETERS

• Monitor for signs of hypersensitivity reaction

---

sulfasalazine

(sul-fa-sal'-a-zeen)

Rx: Azulfidine, Azulfidine EN-Tabs

Chemical Class: Salicylate derivative; sulfonamide derivative

Therapeutic Class: Disease-modifying antirheumatic drug (DMARD); gastrointestinal antiinflammatory

CLINICAL PHARMACOLOGY

Mechanism of Action: A sulfonamide that inhibits prostaglandin synthesis, acting locally in the colon. ***Therapeutic Effect:*** Decreases inflammatory response, interferes with GI secretion.

Pharmacokinetics

Poorly absorbed from the GI tract. Cleaved in colon by intestinal bacteria, forming sulfapyridine and mesalamine (5-ASA). Absorbed in colon. Widely distributed. Metabolized in the liver. Primarily excreted in urine. ***Half-life:*** sulfapyridine, 6-14 hrs; 5-ASA, 0.6-1.4 hrs.

INDICATIONS AND DOSAGES

Ulcerative colitis

PO

Adults, Elderly. 1 g 3-4 times a day in divided doses q4-6h. Maintenance: 2 g/day in divided doses q6-12h. Maximum: 6 g/day.

Children. 40-75 mg/kg/day in divided doses q4-6h. Maintenance: 30-50 mg/kg/day in divided doses q4-8h. Maximum: 2 g/day. Maximum: 6 g/day.

Rheumatoid arthritis

PO

Adults, Elderly. Initially, 0.5-1 g/day for 1 wk. Increase by 0.5 g/wk, up to 3 g/day.

Juvenile rheumatoid arthritis

PO

Children. Initially, 10 mg/kg/day. May increase by 10 mg/kg/day at weekly intervals. Range: 30-50 mg/kg/day. Maximum: 2 g/day.

AVAILABLE FORMS

- *Tablets (Azulfidine):* 500 mg.
- *Tablets (Delayed-Release [Azulfidine EN-Tabs]):* 500 mg.

UNLABELED USES: Treatment of ankylosing spondylitis, collagenous colitis, Crohn's disease, juvenile chronic arthritis, psoriasis, psoriatic arthritis

CONTRAINDICATIONS: Children younger than 2 yrs; hypersensitivity to carbonic anhydrase inhibitors, local anesthetics, salicylates, sulfonamides, sulfonylureas, sunscreens containing PABA, or thiazide or loop diuretics; intestinal or urinary tract obstruction; porphyria; pregnancy at term; severe hepatic or renal dysfunction

PREGNANCY AND LACTATION: Pregnancy category B; excreted into breast milk; should be given to nursing mothers with caution because significant adverse effects (bloody diarrhea) may occur in some nursing infants

SIDE EFFECTS

Frequent (33%)

Anorexia, nausea, vomiting, headache, oligospermia (generally reversed by withdrawal of drug)

Occasional (3%)

Hypersensitivity reaction (rash, urticaria, pruritus, fever, anemia)

Rare (less than 1%)

Tinnitus, hypoglycemia, diuresis, photosensitivity

SERIOUS REACTIONS

- Anaphylaxis, Stevens-Johnson syndrome, hematologic toxicity (leukopenia, agranulocytosis), hepatotoxicity, and nephrotoxicity occur rarely.

INTERACTIONS

Drugs

3 *Digoxin:* Sulfasalazine reduces digoxin serum concentrations

3 *Folic acid:* Reduced absorption of folic acid

3 *Methenamine:* Combination of sulfadiazine and methenamine can result in crystalluria

3 *Phenytoin:* Some sulfonamides (sulfaphenazole, sulmethoxazole) increase phenytoin concentrations, requiring dosage adjustment

3 *Talinolol:* Reduces serum concentrations of talinolol; reduced clinical efficacy is likely to occur

3 *Tolbutamide:* Several sulfonamides (sulfamethizole, sulfaphenazole, sulfisoxasole) can increase plasma sulfonylurea levels and enhance their hypoglycemic effects

3 *Warfarin:* Several sulfonamides (trimethoprim-sulfamethoxazole, sulfamethoxazole, sulfamethizole, sulfaphenazole) increase the hypoprothrombinemic response to warfarin via inhibition of metabolism

Labs

- *Bilirubin, conjugated:* Falsely increased in serum
- *Bilirubin, unconjugated:* Falsely decreased in serum
- *Creatinine:* Falsely increased in serum
- *Potassium:* Falsely decreased in serum

• *False positive:* Urinary glucose tests (Benedict's method)

SPECIAL CONSIDERATIONS

PATIENT/FAMILY EDUCATION

• Adequate hydration and urinary output are essential to prevent crystalluria and stone formation
• Avoid prolonged exposure to sunlight
• Space drug doses around the clock and continue sulfasalazine therapy for the full course of treatment
• It is important to comply with follow-up and laboratory tests
• Inform the dentist or surgeon of sulfasalazine therapy if he or she will have dental or other surgical procedures

MONITORING PARAMETERS

• *Inflammatory bowel disease:* Decrease in rectal bleeding or diarrhea in conjunction with mucosal healing
• *Rheumatoid arthritis:* Tender, swollen joints, visual analog scale for pain; acute phase reactants (ESR, C-reactive protein), duration of early morning stiffness, preservation of function
• Baseline CBC with differential and liver function tests then every second week during the first 3 mos of therapy, monthly during the second 3 mos of therapy, then every 3 mos thereafter; urinalysis and renal function tests periodically
• Skin for rash

sulfinpyrazone

(sul-fin-pie'-ra-zone)

Rx: Anturane

Chemical Class: Pyrazolidine derivative

Therapeutic Class: Antigout agent

CLINICAL PHARMACOLOGY

Mechanism of Action: A uricosuric that increases urinary excretion of uric acid, thereby decreasing blood urate levels. ***Therapeutic Effect:*** Promotes uric acid excretion and reduces serum uric acid levels.

Pharmacokinetics

Rapidly and completely absorbed from gastrointestinal (GI) tract. Widely distributed. Metabolized in liver to two active metabolites, P-hydroxy-sulfinpyrazone and a sulfide analog. Excreted primarily in urine. Not removed by hemodialysis. ***Half-life:*** 2.7-6 hrs.

INDICATIONS AND DOSAGES

Gout

PO

Adults, Elderly. 100-200 mg 2 times/day. Maximum: 800 mg/day.

AVAILABLE FORMS

• *Tablets:* 100 mg (Anturane).

UNLABELED USES: Mitral valve replacement, myocardial infarction

CONTRAINDICATIONS: Active peptic ulcer, blood dyscrasias, GI inflammation, pregnancy (near term), hypersensitivity to sulfinpyrazone, phenylbutazone, other pyrazoles, or any of its components

PREGNANCY AND LACTATION: Pregnancy category C, D

SIDE EFFECTS

Frequent

Nausea, vomiting, stomach pain

Occasional

Flushed face, headache, dizziness, frequent urge to urinate, rash

Rare
Increased bleeding time, hepatic necrosis, nephrotic syndrome, uric acid stones

SERIOUS REACTIONS

- Hematologic toxicity including anemia, leucopenia, agranulocytosis, thrombocytopenia, and aplastic anemia occur rarely.
- Overdose causes a drowsiness, dizziness, anorexia, abdominal pain, hemolytic anemia, acidosis, jaundice, fever, and agranulocytosis.

INTERACTIONS

Drugs

3 *Acetaminophen:* Increased metabolism of acetaminophen by about 20%; increased risk of acetaminophen toxicity

3 *β-blockers:* Reduced hypotensive effects of β-blockers

• *Heparinoids:* Risk of augmented bleeding and epidural or spinal hematomas is increased when used concurrently with another agent that affects hemostasis

❷ *Methotrexate:* Increased methotrexate levels with subsequent increased effect and potential toxicity

❷ *Oral anticoagulants:* Inhibit warfarin metabolism and possibly other oral anticoagulants, increasing prothrombin time response; concomitant antiplatelet effects further complicate combined therapy

3 *Salicylates:* Inhibited uricosuric effect of each other

3 *Tolbutamide:* May increase the hypoglycemic effect of tolbutamide

Labs

• *Cyclosporine:* Falsely decreased serum levels

SPECIAL CONSIDERATIONS

PATIENT/FAMILY EDUCATION

- Take with food, milk, or antacids to decrease stomach upset
- Avoid aspirin and other salicylate-containing products
- Drink plenty of fluids
- Report any unusual side effects

MONITORING PARAMETERS

- Serum uric acid concentrations, renal function, CBC
- Therapeutic response such as reduced joint tenderness, limitation of motion, redness and swelling

sulfisoxazole

(sul-fi-sox'-a-zole)

Rx: Gantrisin, Truxazole

Combinations

Rx: with erythromycin (Pediazole, Sulfimycin)

Chemical Class: Sulfonamide derivative

Therapeutic Class: Antibiotic

CLINICAL PHARMACOLOGY

Mechanism of Action: An antibacterial sulphonamide that inhibits bacterial synthesis of dihydrofolic acid by preventing condensation of pteridine with aminobenzoic acid through competitive inhibition of the enzyme dihydropteroate synthetase. ***Therapeutic Effect:*** Bacteriostatic.

Pharmacokinetics

Rapidly and completely absorbed. Small intestine is major site of absorption, but some absorption occurs in the stomach. Exists in the blood as unbound, protein-bound and conjugated forms. Sulfisoxazole is metabolized primarily by acetylation and oxidation in the liver. The free form is considered to be the therapeutically active form. Protein binding: 85%. ***Half-life:*** 5-8 hrs.

INDICATIONS AND DOSAGES

Acute, recurrent, or chronic urinary tract infections; meningococcal meningitis; acute otitis media due to Haemophilus influenzae

PO

Infants over 2 mos of age, Children. One-half of the 24-hr dose initially, then 150 mg/kg daily or 4 g/m_2 daily for maintanence divided q4-6h. Maximum dose: 6 g daily.

Adults. 2-4 g initially, then 4-8 g daily divided q4-6h.

AVAILABLE FORMS

- *Tablet.* 500 mg.
- Powder. 100%.
- Oral Suspension. 500 mg/5 mL (Gantrisin).

CONTRAINDICATIONS: Patients with a known hypersensitivity to sulfonamides, children younger than 2 mos (except in the treatment of congenital toxoplasmosis as adjunctive therapy with pyrimethamine), pregnant women at term, and mothers nursing infants less than 2 mos of age.

PREGNANCY AND LACTATION: Pregnancy category B, D (if used near term; may cause jaundice, hemolytic anemia, and kernicterus in newborns); excreted into breast milk in low concentrations; compatible with breast-feeding in healthy, full-term infants

SIDE EFFECTS

Anaphylaxis, erythema multiforme (Stevens-Johnson syndrome), toxic epidermal necrolysis, exfoliative dermatitis, angioedema, arteritis and vasculitis, allergic myocarditis, serum sickness, rash, urticaria, pruritus, photosensitivity, conjunctival and scleral injection, generalized allergic reactions, generalized skin eruptions, tachycardia, palpitations, syncope, cyanosis, goiter, diuresis, hypoglycaemia, arthralgia, myalgia, headache, dizziness, peripheral neuritis, paresthesia, convulsions, tinnitus, vertigo, ataxia, intracranial hypertension, cough, shortness of breath, pulmonary infiltrates

SERIOUS REACTIONS

- Fatalities associated with the administration of sulfonamides, including Stevens-Johnson syndrome, toxic epidermal necrolysis, fulminant hepatic necrosis, agranulocytosis, aplastic anemia, and other blood dyscrasias, occur rarely.
- Clinical signs such as rash, sore throat, fever, arthralgia, pallor, purpura, or jaundice may be early indications of serious reactions.

INTERACTIONS

Drugs

❷ *Methotrexate:* May increase free methotrexate concentrations

❷ *Para-aminobenzoic acid (PABA):* PABA may interfere with the antibacterial activity of sulfamethoxazole

❸ *Phenytoin:* Sulfamethoxazole increases phenytoin concentrations, requiring dosage adjustment

❸ *Thiopental:* May reduce the amount of thiopental required for anesthesia and shorten awaken time

❸ *Tolbutamide:* Sulfisoxazole can increase plasma sulfonylurea levels and enhance their hypoglycemic effects

❸ *Warfarin:* Trimethoprim-sulfamethoxazole, sulfamethoxazole increase the hypoprothrombinemic response to warfarin via inhibition of metabolism

Labs

- *Folate:* Falsely decreased serum levels
- *Protein:* Falsely increased in CSF
- *Urobilinogen:* Decreased falsely in feces

SPECIAL CONSIDERATIONS

PATIENT/FAMILY EDUCATION

- Avoid prolonged exposure to sunlight
- Administer with glass of water
- Avoid alcohol

MONITORING PARAMETERS

• CBC, renal function tests, urinalysis

sulindac

(sul-in'-dak)

Rx: Clinoril

Chemical Class: Acetic acid derivative

Therapeutic Class: NSAID; antipyretic; nonnarcotic analgesic

CLINICAL PHARMACOLOGY

Mechanism of Action: An NSAID that produces analgesic and antiinflammatory effects by inhibiting prostaglandin synthesis. ***Therapeutic Effect:*** Reduces inflammatory response and intensity of pain.

Pharmacokinetics

Route	*Onset*	*Peak*	*Duration*
PO (Antirheumatic)	7 days	2-3 wks	N/A

Well absorbed from the GI tract. Metabolized in liver to active metabolite. Primarily excreted in urine. Not removed by hemodialysis. ***Half-life:*** 7.8 hr; metabolite: 16.4 hr.

INDICATIONS AND DOSAGES

Rheumatoid arthritis, osteoarthritis, ankylosing spondylitis

PO

Adults, Elderly. Initially, 150 mg twice a day; may increase up to 400 mg/day.

Acute shoulder pain, gouty arthritis, bursitis, tendinitis

PO

Adults, Elderly. 200 mg twice a day.

AVAILABLE FORMS

• *Tablets:* 150 mg, 200 mg.

CONTRAINDICATIONS: Active peptic ulcer disease, chronic inflammation of GI tract, GI bleeding or ulceration, history of hypersensitivity to aspirin or NSAIDs

PREGNANCY AND LACTATION: Pregnancy category B (category D if used in third trimester); could cause constriction of the ductus arteriosus *in utero,* persistent pulmonary hypertension of the newborn, or prolonged labor

SIDE EFFECTS

Frequent (9%-4%)

Diarrhea or constipation, indigestion, nausea, maculopapular rash, dermatitis, dizziness, headache

Occasional (3%-1%)

Anorexia, abdominal cramps, flatulence

SERIOUS REACTIONS

• Rare reactions with long-term use include peptic ulcer disease, GI bleeding, gastritis, nephrotoxicity (glomerular nephritis, interstitial nephritis, nephrotic syndrome), severe hepatic reactions (cholestasis, jaundice), and severe hypersensitivity reactions (fever, chills, and joint pain).

INTERACTIONS

Drugs

3 *Aminoglycosides:* Reduced clearance with elevated aminoglycoside levels and potential for toxicity (especially indomethacin in premature infants; other NSAIDs probably)

3 *Antacids:* May decrease sulindac blood concentration

3 *Anticoagulants:* Excessive hypoprothrombinemia, decreased platelet aggregation with increased risk of GI bleeding

3 *Antihypertensives (α-blockers, angiotensin-converting enzyme inhibitors, angiotensin II receptor blockers, β-blockers, diuretics):* In-

hibition of antihypertensive and other favorable hemodynamic effects

3 *Bone marrow depressants:* May increase the risk of hematologic reactions

3 *Corticosteroids:* Increased risk of GI ulceration

3 *Cyclosporine:* Increased nephrotoxicity risk

3 *Feverfew:* May decrease the effects of feverfew

3 *Ginkgo biloba:* May increase the risk of bleeding

3 *Lithium:* Decreased clearance of lithium (mediated via prostaglandins), resulting in elevated serum lithium levels and risk of toxicity

3 *Methotrexate:* Decreased renal secretion of methotrexate, resulting in elevated methotrexate levels and risk of toxicity

3 *Phenylpropanolamine:* Possible acute hypertensive reaction

3 *Potassium-sparing diuretics:* Additive hyperkalemia potential

3 *Probenecid:* May increase sulindac blood concentration

3 *Triamterene:* Acute renal failure reported with addition of indomethacin; caution with other NSAIDs

SPECIAL CONSIDERATIONS

- No significant advantage over other NSAIDs; cost should govern use

PATIENT/FAMILY EDUCATION

- Avoid aspirin and alcoholic beverages
- Take with food, milk, or antacids to decrease GI upset
- Antirheumatic action may not be apparent for several weeks
- The female patient should inform the physician if she is or plans to become pregnant
- Avoid performing tasks that require mental alertness or motor skills until response to the drug has been established

MONITORING PARAMETERS

- Initial hemogram and fecal occult blood test within 3 mos of starting regular chronic therapy; repeat every 6-12 mos (more frequently in high-risk patients [>65 years, peptic ulcer disease, concurrent steroids or anticoagulants]); electrolytes, creatinine, and BUN within 3 mo of starting regular chronic therapy; repeat every 6-12 mos

sumatriptan succinate

(soo-ma-trip′-tan suk′-si-nate)

Rx: Imitrex, Imitrex, Imitrex Nasal, Imitrex Statdose, Imitrex Statdose Refill

Chemical Class: Serotonin derivative

Therapeutic Class: Antimigraine agent

CLINICAL PHARMACOLOGY

Mechanism of Action: A serotonin receptor agonist that binds selectively to vascular receptors, producing a vasoconstrictive effect on cranial blood vessels. ***Therapeutic Effect:*** Relieves migraine headache.

Pharmacokinetics

Route	Onset	Peak	Duration
Nasal	15 mins	N/A	24-48 hrs
PO	30 mins	2 hrs	24-48 hrs
Subcutaneous	10 mins	1 hr	24-48 hrs

Rapidly absorbed after subcutaneous administration. Absorption after PO administration is incomplete, with significant amounts undergoing hepatic metabolism, resulting in low bioavailability (about 14%). Protein binding: 10%-21%. Widely distributed. Undergoes first-pass metabolism in the liver. Excreted in urine. ***Half-life:*** 2 hr.

INDICATIONS AND DOSAGES

Acute migraine attack

PO

Adults, Elderly. 25-50 mg. Dose may be repeated after at least 2 hr. Maximum: 100 mg/single dose; 200 mg/24 hr.

Subcutaneous

Adults, Elderly. 6 mg. Maximum: Two 6-mg injections/24 hr (separated by at least 1 hr).

Intranasal

Adults, Elderly. 5-20 mg; may repeat in 2 hr. Maximum: 40 mg/24 hr.

AVAILABLE FORMS

- *Tablets (Imitrex):* 25 mg, 50 mg, 100 mg.
- *Injection (Imitrex, Imitrex Statdose):* 6 mg/0.5 ml.
- *Nasal Spray (Imitrex Nasal):* 5 mg, 20 mg.

CONTRAINDICATIONS: Cerebrovascular accident (CVA), ischemic heart disease (including angina pectoris, history of MI, silent ischemia, and Prinzmetal's angina), severe hepatic impairment, transient ischemic attack, uncontrolled hypertension, use within 14 days of MAOIs, use within 24 hr of ergotamine preparations

PREGNANCY AND LACTATION: Pregnancy category C; excreted in breast milk in animals, no data in humans

SIDE EFFECTS

Frequent

Oral (10%-5%): Tingling, nasal discomfort

Subcutaneous (greater than 10%): Injection site reactions, tingling, warm or hot sensation, dizziness, vertigo

Nasal (greater than 10%): Bad or unusual taste, nausea, vomiting

Occasional

Oral (5%-1%): Flushing, asthenia, visual disturbances

Subcutaneous (10%-2%): Burning sensation, numbness, chest discomfort, drowsiness, asthenia

Nasal (5%-1%): Nasopharyngeal discomfort, dizziness

Rare

Oral (less than 1%): Agitation, eye irritation, dysuria

Subcutaneous (less than 2%): Anxiety, fatigue, diaphoresis, muscle cramps, myalgia

Nasal (less than 1%): Burning sensation

SERIOUS REACTIONS

- Excessive dosage may produce tremor, red extremities, reduced respirations, cyanosis, seizures, and paralysis.
- Serious arrhythmias occur rarely, especially in patients with hypertension, diabetes, or a strong family history of coronary artery disease; obese patients; and smokers.

INTERACTIONS

Drugs

3 *Ergot-containing drugs:* Potential for prolonged vasospastic reactions and additive vasoconstriction, theoretical precaution

3 *MAOIs:* May increase sumatriptan blood concentration and half-life

❷ *Sibutramine:* Increased risk of serotonin syndrome

SPECIAL CONSIDERATIONS

- First inj should be administered under medical supervision

PATIENT/FAMILY EDUCATION

- Use only to treat migraine headache; not for prevention
- Inject the medication and discard the syringe
- Inject the drug into an area with adequate subcutaneous tissue because the needle will penetrate the skin and adipose tissue as deeply as 6 mm
- Do not administer more than two subcutaneous injections during any 24-hr period and allow at least 1 hr between injections

• Notify the physician immediately if palpitations, a rash, wheezing, pain or tightness in the chest or throat, or facial edema occurs
• Lie down in dark, quiet room for additional benefit after taking sumatriptan

MONITORING PARAMETERS

• Evaluate the patient for relief of migraines and associated symptoms, including nausea and vomiting, photophobia, and phonophobia (sound sensitivity)

tacrine hydrochloride

(tak'-reen hye-droe-klor'-ide)

Rx: Cognex

Chemical Class: Cholinesterase inhibitor; monoamine acridine derivative

Therapeutic Class: Antidementia agent

CLINICAL PHARMACOLOGY

Mechanism of Action: A cholinesterase inhibitor that inhibits the enzyme acetylcholinesterase, thus increasing the concentration of acetylcholine at cholinergic synapses and enhancing cholinergic function in the CNS. ***Therapeutic Effect:*** Slows the progression of Alzheimer's disease.

Pharmacokinetics

Rapidly absorbed following PO administration. Protein binding: 55%. Extensively metabolized in liver. Negligible amounts excreted in urine. ***Half-life:*** 2-4 hr.

INDICATIONS AND DOSAGES

Alzheimer's disease

PO

Adults, Elderly. Initially, 10 mg 4 times a day for 6 wk, followed by 20 mg 4 times a day for 6 wk, 30 mg 4 times a day for 12 wk, then 40 mg 4 times a day if needed.

Dosage in hepatic impairment

For patients with ALT greater than 3-5 times normal, decrease the dose by 40 mg/day and resume the normal dose when ALT returns to normal. For patients with ALT greater than 5 times normal, stop treatment and resume it when ALT returns to normal.

AVAILABLE FORMS

• *Capsules:* 10 mg, 20 mg, 30 mg, 40 mg.

CONTRAINDICATIONS: Known hypersensitivity to tacrine, patients previously treated with tacrine who developed jaundice

PREGNANCY AND LACTATION: Pregnancy category C; excretion into breast milk unknown

SIDE EFFECTS

Frequent (28%-11%)

Headache, nausea, vomiting, diarrhea, dizziness

Occasional (9%-4%)

Fatigue, chest pain, dyspepsia, anorexia, abdominal pain, flatulence, constipation, confusion, agitation, rash, depression, ataxia, insomnia, rhinitis, myalgia

Rare (less than 3%)

Weight loss, anxiety, cough, facial flushing, urinary frequency, back pain, tremor

SERIOUS REACTIONS

• Overdose can cause cholinergic crisis, marked by increased salivation, lacrimation, bradycardia, respiratory depression, hypotension, and increased muscle weakness. Treatment usually consists of supportive measures and an anticholinergic such as atropine.

INTERACTIONS

Drugs

3 *Anticholinergics:* Inhibits anticholinergic effect, centrally acting anticholinergics may inhibit effect of tacrine

3 *β-blockers:* Additive bradycardia
3 *Cholinergics:* Increased cholinergic effects
3 *Cimetidine:* Increased tacrine levels
3 *Levodopa:* Decreased levodopa effect
3 *NSAIDs:* May increase the adverse effects of NSAIDs
3 *Quinolones:* Inhibition of tacrine metabolism
3 *Serotonin reuptake inhibitors:* Increased tacrine concentrations
3 *Smoking:* Markedly reduces tacrine levels
3 *Theophylline:* Increased theophylline concentrations
3 *Trihexyphenidyl:* May inhibit the therapeutic effect of trihexyphenidyl

SPECIAL CONSIDERATIONS

- Transaminase elevation is the most common reason for withdrawal of drug (8%); monitor ALT qwk for first 18 wk, then decrease to q3mo; when dose is increased, monitor qwk for 6 wk
- If elevations occur, modify dose as follows: ALT ≤3 times upper limit normal (ULN), continue current dose; ALT >3 to ≤5 times ULN, reduce dose by 40 mg qd and resume dose titration when within normal limits; ALT >5 times ULN, stop treatment; rechallenge may be tried if ALT is <10 times ULN
- Do not rechallenge if clinical jaundice develops
- Improvement in symptoms of dementia statistically, but perhaps not clinically significant; discontinue therapy if improvement not evident to family members and clinician

PATIENT/FAMILY EDUCATION

- Take tacrine at regular intervals, between meals; take the drug with meals if GI upset occurs
- Do not abruptly discontinue tacrine or adjust the drug dosage
- Avoid smoking during tacrine therapy because smoking reduces the drug's blood level
- Tacrine is not a cure for Alzheimer's disease but may slow the progression of its symptoms
- Refer the patient's family to the local chapter of the Alzheimer's Disease Association for a guide to available services

MONITORING PARAMETERS

- AST (SGOT) and ALT (SGPT) levels
- Periodically monitor the EKG and rhythm strips of patients with underlying arrhythmias
- Assess for signs of GI distress
- Monitor behavioral, cognitive, and functional status

tacrolimus

(ta-kroe'-li-mus)
Rx: Prograf, Protopic
Chemical Class: Macrolide derivative
Therapeutic Class: Immunosuppressant

CLINICAL PHARMACOLOGY

Mechanism of Action: An immunologic agent that inhibits T-lymphocyte activation by binding to intracellular proteins, forming a complex, and inhibiting phosphatase activity. ***Therapeutic Effect:*** Suppresses the immunologically mediated inflammatory response; prevents organ transplant rejection.

Pharmacokinetics

Variably absorbed after PO administration (food reduces absorption). Protein binding: 75%-97%. Extensively metabolized in the liver. Excreted in urine. Not removed by hemodialysis. ***Half-life:*** 11.7 hr.

INDICATIONS AND DOSAGES

Prevention of liver transplant rejection

PO

Adults, Elderly. 0.1-0.15 mg/kg/day in 2 divided doses 12 hr apart.

Children. 0.15-0.2 mg/kg/day in 2 divided doses 12 hr apart.

IV

Adults, Elderly, Children. 0.03-0.15 mg/kg/day as a continuous infusion.

Prevention of kidney transplant rejection

PO

Adults, Elderly. 0.2 mg/kg/day in 2 divided doses 12 hrs apart.

IV

Adults, Elderly. 0.03-0.15 mg/kg/day as continuous infusion.

Atopic dermatitis

Topical

Adults, Elderly, Children 2 yrs and older. Apply 0.03% ointment to affected area twice a day. 0.1% ointment may be used in adults and the elderly. Continue until 1 wk after symptoms have cleared.

AVAILABLE FORMS

- *Capsules (Prograf):* 0.5 mg, 1 mg, 5 mg.
- *Injection (Prograf):* 5 mg/ml.
- *Ointment (Protopic):* 0.03%, 0.1%.

UNLABELED USES: Prevention of organ rejection in patients receiving allogeneic bone marrow, heart, pancreas, pancreatic island cell, or small-bowel transplant, treatment of autoimmune disease, severe recalcitrant psoriasis

CONTRAINDICATIONS: Concurrent use with cyclosporine (increases the risk of nephrotoxicity), hypersensitivity to HCO-60 polyoxyl 60 hydrogenated castor oil (used in solution for injection)

PREGNANCY AND LACTATION: Pregnancy category C; excreted in breast milk; avoid nursing

SIDE EFFECTS

Frequent (greater than 30%)

Headache, tremor, insomnia, paresthesia, diarrhea, nausea, constipation, vomiting, abdominal pain, hypertension

Occasional (29%-10%)

Rash, pruritus, anorexia, asthenia, peripheral edema, photosensitivity

SERIOUS REACTIONS

- Nephrotoxicity (characterized by increased serum creatinine level and decreased urine output), neurotoxicity (including tremor, headache, and mental status changes), and pleural effusion are common adverse reactions.
- Thrombocytopenia, leukocytosis, anemia, atelectasis, sepsis, and infection occur occasionally.

INTERACTIONS

Drugs

3 *Azole antifungals, bromocriptine, calcium channel blockers, cimetidine, danazol, ethinyl estradiol, GI prokinetic agents, macrolide antibiotics, nefazodone, omeprazole, protease inhibitors:* Decreased metabolism or increased bioavailability of tacrolimus

3 *Carbamazepine, phenobarbital, phenytoin, rifamycins:* Decreased tacrolimus blood levels

▲ *Cyclosporine:* Additive/synergistic nephrotoxicity, do not coadminister, discontinue tacrolimus or cyclosporine for 24 hr before starting the other

3 *Echinacea:* May decrease the effects of tacrolimus

3 *Grapefruit, grapefruit juice:* May alter the effects of the drug

▲ *Live vaccines:* Avoid use of live vaccines, vaccinations may be less effective

2 *Nephrotoxic agents (aminoglycosides, amphotericin B, cisplatin, ganciclovir):* Potential for additive/synergistic nephrotoxicity

T

❷ *Potassium-sparing diuretics:* Increased risk of hyperkalemia

❸ *St. John's wort (hypericum perforatum):* Potential for decreased plasma tacrolimus concentrations

SPECIAL CONSIDERATIONS

- Black patients may need higher doses in kidney transplant
- Also known as FK 506

PATIENT/FAMILY EDUCATION

- Take the capsules on an empty stomach and do not mix them with grapefruit juice
- Take the drug at the same time each day and notify the physician if a dose is missed
- Avoid crowds and people with infections
- Notify the physician if chest pain, dizziness, headache, decreased urination, rash, respiratory infection, or unusual bleeding or bruising occurs
- Avoid exposure to sunlight and artificial light because this may cause a photosensitivity reaction

MONITORING PARAMETERS

- Regularly assess serum creatinine, potassium, and fasting glucose
- Whole blood tacrolimus concentrations as measured by ELISA may be helpful in assessing rejection and toxicity, median trough concentrations measured after the second week of therapy ranged from 9.8-19.4 mg/ml
- CBC weekly during the first month of therapy, twice monthly during the second and third months of treatment, then monthly for the rest of the first year; liver function test results
- Intake and output

tadalafil

(tah-da'-la-fil)

Rx: Cialis

Chemical Class: CGMP specific phosphodiesterase inhibitor

Therapeutic Class: Antiimpotence agent

CLINICAL PHARMACOLOGY

Mechanism of Action: An erectile dysfunction agent that inhibits phosphodiesterase type 5, the enzyme responsible for degrading cyclic guanosine monophosphate in the corpus cavernosum of the penis, resulting in smooth muscle relaxation and increased blood flow. ***Therapeutic Effect:*** Facilitates an erection.

Pharmacokinetics

Route	*Onset*	*Peak*	*Duration*
PO	16 mins	2 hrs	36 hrs

Rapidly absorbed after PO administration. Drug has no effect on penile blood flow without sexual stimulation. ***Half-life:*** 17.5 hrs.

INDICATIONS AND DOSAGES

Erectile dysfunction

PO

Adults, Elderly. 10 mg 30 min before sexual activity. Dose may be increased to 20 mg or decreased to 5 mg, based on patient tolerance. Maximum dosing frequency is once daily.

Dosage in renal impairment

For patients with a creatinine clearance of 31-50 ml/min, the starting dose is 5 mg before sexual activity once a day and the maximum dose is 10 mg no more frequently than once q48h.

For patients with a creatinine clearance of less than 31 ml/min, the starting dose is 5 mg before sexual activity once a day.

Dosage in mild or moderate hepatic impairment

Patients with Child-Pugh class A or B hepatic impairment should take no more than 10 mg once a day.

AVAILABLE FORMS

• *Tablets:* 5 mg, 10 mg, 20 mg.

CONTRAINDICATIONS: Concurrent use of alpha-adrenergic blockers (other than the minimum dose tamsulosin), concurrent use of sodium nitroprusside or nitrates in any form, severe hepatic impairment

PREGNANCY AND LACTATION: Pregnancy category B; not indicated for use in women

SIDE EFFECTS

Occasional

Headache, dyspepsia, back pain, myalgia, nasal congestion, flushing

SERIOUS REACTIONS

• Prolonged erections (lasting over 4 hrs) and priapism (painful erections lasting over 6 hrs) occur rarely.

• Angina, chest pain, and MI have been reported.

INTERACTIONS

Drugs

3 *Alcohol:* Substantial alcohol consumption can increase risk of blood pressure–lowering effects

⚠ *Alpha-adrenergic blockers:* Concurrent use with tadalafil contraindicated (except tamsulosin at 0.4 mg qd)

3 *CYP3A4 inducers (carbamazepine, phenobarbital, phenytoin, rifampin):* Decreased tadalafil levels likely

2 *CYP3A4 inhibitors (erythromycin, itraconazole, ketoconazole, ritonavir):* Potent inhibitors significantly increase tadalafil levels, max tadalafil dose 10 mg, dosing interval not more frequent than q72hr

⚠ *Nitrates:* Concurrent use with tadalafil contraindicated

SPECIAL CONSIDERATIONS

PATIENT/FAMILY EDUCATION

• Sexual stimulation is required for an erection to occur after taking tadalafil

• Erectile function improved up to 36 hr following dose

• Seek treatment immediately if an erection lasts longer than 4 hrs

• Avoid using nitrate drugs and alpha-adrenergic blockers concurrently with tadalafil

MONITORING PARAMETERS

• Cardiovascular status

• Liver and renal function

tamoxifen citrate

(ta-mox'-i-fen sit'-trate)

Rx: Nolvadex

Chemical Class: Estrogen agonist-antagonist; triphenylethylene derivative

Therapeutic Class: Antineoplastic

CLINICAL PHARMACOLOGY

Mechanism of Action: A nonsteroidal antiestrogen that competes with estradiol for estrogen-receptor binding sites in the breasts, uterus, and vagina. ***Therapeutic Effect:*** Inhibits DNA synthesis and estrogen response.

Pharmacokinetics

Well absorbed from the GI tract. Metabolized in the liver. Primarily eliminated in feces by biliary system. ***Half-life:*** 7 days.

INDICATIONS AND DOSAGES

Adjunctive treatment of breast cancer

PO

Adults, Elderly. 20-40 mg/day. Give doses greater than 20 mg/day in divided doses.

Prevention of breast cancer in high-risk women
PO
Adults, Elderly. 20 mg/day.

AVAILABLE FORMS

• *Tablets (Nolvadex):* 10 mg, 20 mg.

UNLABELED USES: Treatment of mastalgia, gynecomastia, pancreatic carcinoma, ovulation induction, treatment of precocious puberty in females

CONTRAINDICATIONS: Concomitant coumarin-type therapy when used in the treatment of breast cancer in high-risk women, history of deep vein thrombosis or pulmonary embolism in high-risk women, pregnancy

PREGNANCY AND LACTATION: Pregnancy category D; excretion into breast milk unknown

SIDE EFFECTS

Frequent
Women (greater than 10%): Hot flashes, nausea, vomiting
Occasional
Women (9%-1%): Changes in menstruation, genital itching, vaginal discharge, endometrial hyperplasia or polyps
Men: Impotence, decreased libido
Men and women: Headache, nausea, vomiting, rash, bone pain, confusion, weakness, somnolence

SERIOUS REACTIONS

• Retinopathy, corneal opacity, and decreased visual acuity have been noted in patients receiving extremely high dosages (240-320 mg/day) for longer than 17 mos.
• There have been an increased number of incidences of endometrial changes, thromboembolic events, and uterine malignancies while using tamoxifen.

INTERACTIONS

Drugs
❷ *Aminoglutethimide:* Reduces tamoxifen concentrations
❸ *Anticoagulants:* May increase the risk of bleeding
❸ *Estrogens:* May decrease the effects of tamoxifen
❸ *Red Clover, St. John's Wort:* May decrease the effectiveness of tamoxifen

SPECIAL CONSIDERATIONS

• Treatment duration >5 yr may provide no further benefit and increase risk of endometrial cancer for some women; reevaluate the need for continued therapy
• The Gail Model Risk Assessment Tool is available to health care professionals by calling (800) 456-3669 (ext. 3838)
• Premenopausal women should use nonhormonal contraception during treatment

PATIENT/FAMILY EDUCATION

• Notify the physician if leg cramps, weakness, weight gain, or vaginal bleeding, itching, or discharge occurs
• May initially cause an increase in bone and tumor pain, which appears to indicate a good tumor response to tamoxifen
• Notify the physician if nausea and vomiting continue at home
• Intake and output
• Weight
• Be alert for reports of increased bone pain and provide adequate pain relief as ordered
• Assess the patient for signs and symptoms of hypercalcemia, including constipation, deep bone or flank pain, excessive thirst, hypotonicity of muscles, increased urine output, nausea and vomiting, and renal calculi

MONITORING PARAMETERS

• Endometrial biopsy indicated for abnormal vaginal bleeding

tamsulosin hydrochloride

(tam-soo-lo'-sin hye-droe-klor'-ide)

Rx: Flomax

Chemical Class: Quinazoline

Therapeutic Class: α_1-adrenergic blocker

CLINICAL PHARMACOLOGY

Mechanism of Action: An alpha$_1$ antagonist that targets receptors around bladder neck and prostate capsule. ***Therapeutic Effect:*** Relaxes smooth muscle and improves urinary flow and symptoms of prostatic hyperplasia.

Pharmacokinetics

Well absorbed and widely distributed. Protein binding: 94%-99%. Metabolized in the liver. Primarily excreted in urine. Unknown if removed by hemodialysis. ***Half-life:*** 9-13 hr.

INDICATIONS AND DOSAGES

Benign prostatic hyperplasia

PO

Adults. 0.4 mg once a day, approximately 30 min after same meal each day. May increase dosage to 0.8 mg if inadequate response in 2-4 wks.

AVAILABLE FORMS

• *Capsules:* 0.4 mg.

CONTRAINDICATIONS: Concurrent use of sildenafil, tadalafil, or vardenafil

PREGNANCY AND LACTATION: Pregnancy category B; not indicated for use in women

SIDE EFFECTS

Frequent (9%-7%)

Dizziness, somnolence

Occasional (5%-3%)

Headache, anxiety, insomnia, orthostatic hypotension

Rare (less than 2%)

Nasal congestion, pharyngitis, rhinitis, nausea, vertigo, impotence

SERIOUS REACTIONS

• First-dose syncope (hypotension with sudden loss of consciousness) may occur within 30-90 mins after administration of initial dose and may be preceded by tachycardia (pulse rate of 120-160 beats/minute).

INTERACTIONS

Drugs

3 *β-blockers:* Enhanced "first-dose" phenomenon

3 *Other α-adrenergic blocking agents (such as doxazosin, prazosin, terazosin):* May increase the α-blockade effects of both drugs

3 *Warfarin:* May alter the effects of warfarin

SPECIAL CONSIDERATIONS

PATIENT/FAMILY EDUCATION

• Consider administration of first dose at bedtime; caution following first 12 hr after initiation or reinitiation of therapy for "first-dose phenomenon"

• Use caution when getting up from a sitting or lying position

• Avoid tasks that require mental alertness or motor skills until response to the drug has been established

MONITORING PARAMETERS

• Blood pressure and renal function

tazarotene

(ta-zare'-oh-teen)

Rx: Avage, Tazorac

Chemical Class: Retinoid prodrug; vitamin A derivative

Therapeutic Class: Antiacne agent; antipsoriatic

CLINICAL PHARMACOLOGY

Mechanism of Action: Modulates differentiation and proliferation of epithelial tissue, binds selectively to retinoic acid receptors. ***Therapeutic Effect:*** Restores normal differentiation of the epidermis and reduction in epidermal inflammation.

Pharmacokinetics

Minimal systemic absorption occurs through the skin. Binding to plasma proteins is greater than 99%. Metabolism is in the skin and liver. Elimination occurs through the fecal and renal pathways. ***Half-life:*** 18 hrs.

INDICATIONS AND DOSAGES

Psoriasis

Topical

Adults, Adolescents, Children >12 yrs. Thin film applied once daily in the evening; only cover the lesions, and area should be dry before application.

Acne vulgaris

Topical

Adults, Adolescents, Children > 12 yrs. Thin film applied to affected areas once daily in the evening, after face is gently cleansed and dried.

Fine facial wrinkles, facial mottled hyperpigmentation (liver spots), hypopigmentation associated with photoaging

Topical

Adults. Thin film applied to affected areas once daily in the evening, after face is gently cleansed and dried.

AVAILABLE FORMS

- *Gel:* 0.05%, 0.1% (Tazorac).
- *Cream:* 0.05%, 0.1% (Tazorac).

CONTRAINDICATIONS: Should not be used in pregnant women, patients with hypersensitivity to tazarotene, benzyl alcohol, or any one of its components.

PREGNANCY AND LACTATION: Pregnancy category X (some evidence to suggest potential increased safety margin vs other retinoids based on minimal absorption and short half life); excreted into breast milk of rats; no human data

SIDE EFFECTS

Frequent

Desquamation, burning or stinging, dry skin, itching, erythema, worsening of psoriasis, irritation, skin pain, pruritis, xerosis, photosensitivity

Occasional

Irritation, skin pain, fissuring, localized edema, skin discoloration, rash, desquamation, contact dermatitis, skin inflammation, bleeding, dry skin, hypertriglyceridema, peripheral edema, acne vulgaris, cheilitis

SPECIAL CONSIDERATIONS

- Attractive alternative to oral retinoid therapy in psoriasis (e.g., etretinate), primarily due to less toxicity. Structural changes to the basic retinoid structure (e.g., conformational rigidity) are claimed to enhance therapeutic efficacy and reduce the local toxicity associated with topical tretinoin (retinoic acid). However, place in therapy should await direct comparisons vs standard regimens in terms of efficacy, toxicity, and cost

PATIENT/FAMILY EDUCATION

- Burning or stinging after application, dryness, itching, peeling, or redness of the skin may occur during tazarotene therapy
- Avoid direct exposure to sunlight

MONITORING PARAMETERS

• Therapeutic response to medication

tegaserod

(te-gas'-a-rod)

Rx: Zelnorm

Chemical Class: Pentylcarbazimidamide derivative

Therapeutic Class: Gastrointestinal prokinetic agent

CLINICAL PHARMACOLOGY

Mechanism of Action: An antiirritable bowel syndrome (IBS) agent that binds to 5-HT_4 receptors in the GI tract. ***Therapeutic Effect:*** Triggers a peristaltic reflex in the gut, increasing bowel motility.

Pharmacokinetics

Rapidly absorbed. Widely distributed. Protein binding: 98%. Metabolized by hydrolysis in the stomach and by oxidation and conjugation of the primary metabolite. Primarily excreted in feces. ***Half-life:*** 11 hr.

INDICATIONS AND DOSAGES

IBS

PO

Adults, Elderly women. 6 mg twice a day for 4-6 wks.

Chronic constipation

PO

Adults. 6 mg twice a day.

AVAILABLE FORMS

• *Tablets:* 2 mg, 6 mg.

CONTRAINDICATIONS: Abdominal adhesions, diarrhea, history of bowel obstruction, moderate to severe hepatic impairment, severe renal impairment, suspected sphincter of Oddi dysfunction, symptomatic gallbladder disease

PREGNANCY AND LACTATION: Pregnancy category B; excretion in human milk unknown, use caution in nursing mothers (excreted in milk of lactating rats with a high milk to plasma ratio)

SIDE EFFECTS

Frequency (greater than 5%)

Headache, abdominal pain, diarrhea, nausea, flatulence

Occasional (5%-2%)

Dizziness, migraine, back pain, extremity pain

SERIOUS REACTIONS

• Ischemic colitis, mesenteric ischemia, gangrenous bowel, rectal bleeding, syncope, hypotension, hypovolemia, electrolyte disorders, suspected sphincter of Oddi spasm, bile duct stone, cholecystitis with elevated transaminases, and hypersensitivity reaction including rash, urticaria, pruritus and serious allergic Type I reactions have been reported.

SPECIAL CONSIDERATIONS

PATIENT/FAMILY EDUCATION

• Take before a meal

• Consult prescriber if severe diarrhea or diarrhea accompanied by cramping, abdominal pain, or dizziness occurs

MONITORING PARAMETERS

• Therapeutic response (relief from abdominal discomfort, bloating, cramping, and urgency)

telithromycin

(tell-ith'-roe-my-sin)

Rx: Ketek, Ketek Pak

Chemical Class: Macrolide derivative

Therapeutic Class: Antibiotic

CLINICAL PHARMACOLOGY

Mechanism of Action: A ketolide that blocks protein synthesis by binding to ribosomal receptor sites on the bacterial cell wall. ***Therapeutic Effect:*** Bactericidal.

Pharmacokinetics

Protein binding: 60%-70%. More of drug is concentrated in WBCs than in plasma, and drug is eliminated more slowly from WBCs than from plasma. Partially metabolized by the liver. Minimally excreted in feces and urine. ***Half-life:*** 10 hr.

INDICATIONS AND DOSAGES

Chronic bronchitis, sinusitis

PO

Adults, Elderly. 800 mg once a day for 5 days.

Community-acquired pneumonia

PO

Adults, Elderly. 800 mg once a day for 7-10 days.

AVAILABLE FORMS

- *Tablets (Ketek, Ketek Pak):* 400 mg.

UNLABELED USES: Treatment of tonsillitis and pharyngitis due to *S. pyogenes*

CONTRAINDICATIONS: Hypersensitivity to macrolide antibiotics, concurrent use of cisapride or pimozide

PREGNANCY AND LACTATION: Pregnancy category C; excreted in breast milk of rats; unknown if excreted in human milk

SIDE EFFECTS

Occasional (11%-4%)

Diarrhea, nausea, headache, dizziness

Rare (3%-2%)

Vomiting, loose stools, altered taste, dry mouth, flatulence, visual disturbances

SERIOUS REACTIONS

- Hepatic dysfunction, severe hypersensitivity reaction, and atrial arrhythmias occur rarely.
- Antibiotic-associated colitis and other superinfections may result from altered bacterial balance.

INTERACTIONS

Drugs

3 *Carbamazepine, cyclosporine, tacrolimus, phenytoin, sirolimus, hexobarbital (CYP450 substrates):* Increased drug levels

▲ *Cisapride, pimozide:* Increased levels of these drugs, contraindicated per manufacturer

3 *Digoxin, theophylline:* Increased peak and trough levels

❷ *Ergotatime, dihydroergotamine:* Ergot toxicity (vasospasm and dysethesia) reported

3 *Itraconazole, ketoconazole (C3A4 inhibitors):* Increased telithromycin levels

3 *Metoprolol (CYP2D6 substrates):* Increased metoprolol levels but half-life unchanged

❷ *Quinidine, procainamide, dofetilide:* Possible arrhythmia

❷ *Rifampin, phenytoin, carbamazepine, phenobarbital:* Decreased (approx 80% with rifampin) levels of telithromycin

❷ *Simvastatin, lovastatin, atrovastation, midazolam, triazolam (CYP34A substrates):* Increased levels of these drugs and risk of myopathy

3 *Sotalol:* Decreased telithromycin absorption

SPECIAL CONSIDERATIONS

PATIENT/FAMILY EDUCATION

- May take without regard to meals, swallow whole.
- Do not take if you or a close relative has a rare heart condition called prolongation of the QT interval. Notify provider if you faint while on this medication
- Do not take with diuretics or if you have low blood potassium or magnesium levels
- Telithromycin may produce difficulty focusing that may last several hours after the first or second dose

• Avoid tasks that require mental alertness or motor skills until response to the drug has been established

MONITORING PARAMETERS

• Pattern of daily bowel activity and stool consistency
• Hepatic function

telmisartan

(tel-mi-sar'-tan)

Rx: Micardis

Chemical Class: Angiotensin II receptor antagonist

Therapeutic Class: Antihypertensive

CLINICAL PHARMACOLOGY

Mechanism of Action: An angiotensin II receptor, type AT_1, antagonist that blocks vasoconstrictor and aldosterone-secreting effects of angiotensin II, inhibiting the binding of angiotensin II to the AT_1 receptors. ***Therapeutic Effect:*** Causes vasodilation, decreases peripheral resistance, and decreases BP.

Pharmacokinetics

Rapidly and completely absorbed after PO administration. Protein binding: greater than 99%. Undergoes metabolism in the liver to inactive metabolite. Excreted in feces. Unknown if removed by hemodialysis. ***Half-life:*** 24 hr.

INDICATIONS AND DOSAGES

Hypertension

PO

Adults, Elderly. 40 mg once a day. Range: 20-80 mg/day.

AVAILABLE FORMS

• *Tablets:* 20 mg, 40 mg, 80 mg.

UNLABELED USES: Treatment of CHF

CONTRAINDICATIONS: None known.

PREGNANCY AND LACTATION: Pregnancy category C, first trimester—category D, second and third trimesters; drugs acting directly on the renin-angiotensin-aldosterone system are documented to cause fetal harm (hypotension, oligohydramnios, neonatal anemia, hyperkalemia, neonatal skull hypoplasia, anuria, and renal failure); neonatal limb contractures, craniofacial deformities, and hypoplastic lung development

SIDE EFFECTS

Occasional (7%-3%)

Upper respiratory tract infection, sinusitis, back or leg pain, diarrhea

Rare (1%)

Dizziness, headache, fatigue, nausea, heartburn, myalgia, cough, peripheral edema

SERIOUS REACTIONS

• Overdosage may manifest as hypotension and tachycardia. Bradycardia occurs less often.

INTERACTIONS

Drugs

3 *Digoxin:* 49% increase in digoxin peak, 20% increase in trough digoxin concentrations

3 *Warfarin:* Slightly decreases warfarin plasma concentration

SPECIAL CONSIDERATIONS

• Potentially as or more effective than angiotensin-converting enzyme inhibitors, without cough; no evidence for reduction in morbidity and mortality as first-line agents in hypertension, yet; whether they provide the same cardiac and renal protection also still tentative; like ACE inhibitors, less effective in black patients

PATIENT/FAMILY EDUCATION

• Call the clinician immediately if note following side effects: wheezing; lip, throat, or face swelling; hives or rash

• Drink fluids to maintain proper hydration
• Female patients should be aware of the consequences of second- and third-trimester exposure to telmisartan; immediately notify the physician if they become pregnant
• Avoid excessive exertion during hot weather because of the risks of dehydration and hypotension

MONITORING PARAMETERS

• Baseline electrolytes, urinalysis, blood urea nitrogen and creatinine with recheck at 2-4 wk after initiation (sooner in volume-depleted patients); monitor sitting blood pressure; watch for symptomatic hypotension, particularly in volume-depleted patients

temazepam

(te-maz'-e-pam)

Rx: Restoril

Chemical Class: Benzodiazepine

Therapeutic Class: Hypnotic

DEA Class: Schedule IV

CLINICAL PHARMACOLOGY

Mechanism of Action: A benzodiazepine that enhances the action of the inhibitory neurotransmitter gamma-aminobutyric acid, resulting in CNS depression. ***Therapeutic Effect:*** Induces sleep.

Pharmacokinetics

Well absorbed from the GI tract. Protein binding: 96%. Widely distributed. Crosses the blood-brain barrier. Metabolized in the liver. Primarily excreted in urine. Not removed by hemodialysis. ***Half-life:*** 4-18 hr.

INDICATIONS AND DOSAGES

Insomnia

PO

Adults, Children 18 yr and older. 15-30 mg at bedtime.

Elderly, Debilitated. 7.5-15 mg at bedtime.

AVAILABLE FORMS

• *Capsules:* 7.5 mg, 15 mg, 22.5 mg, 30 mg.

UNLABELED USES: Treatment of anxiety, depression, panic attacks

CONTRAINDICATIONS: Angle-closure glaucoma; CNS depression; pregnancy or breast-feeding; severe, uncontrolled pain; sleep apnea

PREGNANCY AND LACTATION: Pregnancy category X; may cause sedation and poor feeding in nursing infant

Controlled Substance: Schedule IV

SIDE EFFECTS

Frequent

Somnolence, sedation, rebound insomnia (may occur for 1-2 nights after drug is discontinued), dizziness, confusion, euphoria

Occasional

Asthenia, anorexia, diarrhea

Rare

Paradoxical CNS excitement or restlessness (particularly in elderly or debilitated patients)

SERIOUS REACTIONS

• Abrupt or too-rapid withdrawal may result in pronounced restlessness, irritability, insomnia, hand tremor, abdominal or muscle cramps, vomiting, diaphoresis, and seizures.
• Overdose results in somnolence, confusion, diminished reflexes, respiratory depression, and coma.

INTERACTIONS

Drugs

3 *Cimetidine, disulfiram:* Increased benzodiazepine levels

3 *Clozapine:* Possible increased risk of cardiorespiratory collapse

3 *Ethanol:* Adverse psychomotor effects

3 *Kava kava, valerian:* May increase CNS depression

3 *Rifampin:* Reduced benzodiazepine levels

SPECIAL CONSIDERATIONS

• Good benzodiazepine choice for elderly and patients with liver disease (phase II metabolism and lack of active metabolites)

PATIENT/FAMILY EDUCATION

• Withdrawal symptoms may occur if administered chronically and discontinued abruptly; symptoms include dysphoria, abdominal and muscle cramps, vomiting, sweating, tremor, and seizure

• May cause impairment the day following administration, exercise caution with hazardous tasks and driving

• Take temazepam about 30 mins before bedtime

• Avoid alcohol and other CNS depressants during therapy

• The female patient should notify the physician if she is or plans to become pregnant during temazepam therapy

MONITORING PARAMETERS

• Cardiovascular, mental, and respiratory status

• Therapeutic response, such as a decrease in the number of nocturnal awakenings and a longer duration of sleep

• Assess elderly or debilitated patients for paradoxical reactions, particularly during early therapy

tenofovir disoproxil fumarate

(te-noe′-fo-veer dye-soe-prox′-il fyoo′-mar-ate)

Rx: Viread

Combinations

Rx: with emtricitabine (Truvada)

Chemical Class: Nucleotide analog

Therapeutic Class: Antiviral

CLINICAL PHARMACOLOGY

Mechanism of Action: A nucleotide analog that inhibits HIV reverse transcriptase by being incorporated into viral DNA, resulting in DNA chain termination. ***Therapeutic Effect:*** Slows HIV replication and reduces HIV RNA levels (viral load).

Pharmacokinetics

Bioavailability in fasted patients is approximately 25%. High-fat meals increase the bioavailability. Protein binding: 0.7%-7.2%. Excreted in urine. Removed by hemodialysis. ***Half-life:*** Unknown.

INDICATIONS AND DOSAGES

HIV infection (in combination with other antiretrovirals)

PO

Adults, Elderly, Children 18 yr and older. 300 mg once a day.

Dosage in renal impairment

Creatinine Clearance	*Dosage*
30-49 ml/min	300 mg q48h
10-29 ml/min	300 mg twice a wk
less than 10 ml/min	Not recommended

AVAILABLE FORMS

• *Tablets:* 300 mg.

CONTRAINDICATIONS: None known.

PREGNANCY AND LACTATION: Pregnancy category B; breast milk excretion unknown; the CDC recommends that HIV-infected mothers not breast-feed their infants to avoid risking postnatal transmission of HIV

SIDE EFFECTS

Occasional

GI disturbances (diarrhea, flatulence, nausea, vomiting)

SERIOUS REACTIONS

• Lactic acidosis and hepatomegaly with steatosis occur rarely, but may be severe.

INTERACTIONS

Drugs

3 *Didanosine (buffered formulation):* Tenofovir decreases didanosine AUC by 44% (When coadministered with didanosine, tenofovir should be administered 2 hrs before or 1 hr after administration of didanosine)

3 *High-fat meals:* Increases tenofovir bioavailability

3 *Lopinavir/ritonavir:* Increases tenofovir AUC by 34%; tenofovir decreases AUC of lopinavir/ritonavir by 24% (when coadministered with lopinavir/ritonavir, tenofovir should be administered 2 hrs before or 1 hr after administration of lopinavir/ritonavir)

SPECIAL CONSIDERATIONS

PATIENT/FAMILY EDUCATION

• When coadministered with didanosine or lopinavir/ritonavir, take tenofovir 2 hrs before or 1 hr after taking them

• Take tenofovir with a meal to increase the drug's absorption

• Continue drug therapy for the full course of treatment

• Notify the physician of nausea, vomiting, or persistent abdominal pain

• Tenofovir is not a cure for HIV infection, nor does it reduce the risk of transmitting HIV to others

MONITORING PARAMETERS

• CBC with platelet count, renal function, liver enzymes

• CD4+ cell count, Hgb and HIV RNA plasma levels, and reticulocyte count

• Pattern of daily bowel activity and stool consistency

terazosin hydrochloride

(ter-a'-zoe-sin hye-droe-klor'-ide)

Rx: Hytrin

Chemical Class: Quinazoline derivative

Therapeutic Class: Antihypertensive; α_1-adrenergic blocker

CLINICAL PHARMACOLOGY

Mechanism of Action: An antihypertensive and benign prostatic hyperplasia agent that blocks alpha-adrenergic receptors. Produces vasodilation, decreases peripheral resistance, and targets receptors around bladder neck and prostate. ***Therapeutic Effect:*** In hypertension, decreases BP. In benign prostatic hyperplasia, relaxes smooth muscle and improves urine flow.

Pharmacokinetics

Route	Onset	Peak	Duration
PO	15 mins	1-2 hrs	12-24 hrs

Rapidly, completely absorbed from the GI tract. Protein binding: 90%-94%. Metabolized in the liver to active metabolite. Primarily eliminated in feces via biliary system; excreted in urine. Not removed by hemodialysis. ***Half-life:*** 12 hr.

INDICATIONS AND DOSAGES

Mild to moderate hypertension

PO

Adults, Elderly. Initially, 1 mg at bedtime. Slowly increase dosage to desired levels. Range: 1-5 mg/day as single or 2 divided doses. Maximum: 20 mg.

Benign prostatic hyperplasia
PO
Adults, Elderly. Initially, 1 mg at bedtime. May increase up to 10 mg/day. Maximum: 20 mg/day.

AVAILABLE FORMS

- *Capsules:* 1 mg, 2 mg, 5 mg, 10 mg.
- *Tablets:* 1 mg, 2 mg, 5 mg, 10 mg.

CONTRAINDICATIONS: None known.

PREGNANCY AND LACTATION: Pregnancy category C; excretion into breast milk unknown

SIDE EFFECTS

Frequent (9%-5%)
Dizziness, headache, unusual tiredness

Rare (less than 2%)
Peripheral edema, orthostatic hypotension, myalgia, arthralgia, blurred vision, nausea, vomiting, nasal congestion, somnolence

SERIOUS REACTIONS

- First-dose syncope (hypotension with sudden loss of consciousness) may occur 30-90 mins after initial dose of 2 mg or more, a too-rapid increase in dosage, or addition of another antihypertensive agent to therapy. First-dose syncope may be preceded by tachycardia (pulse rate of 120-160 beats/min).

INTERACTIONS

Drugs

3 *Angiotensin-converting enzyme inhibitors (enalapril):* Potential for exaggerated first-dose hypotensive episode when α-blockers added

3 *Nonsteroidal antiinflammatory drugs (ibuprofen, indomethacin):* NSAIDs may inhibit antihypertensive effects

3 *β-adrenergic blockers:* Potential for exaggerated first-dose hypotensive episode when α-blockers added

3 *Dong quai, ginseng, garlic, yohimbe:* May decrease the effects of terazosin

3 *Estrogens, other sympathomimetics:* May decrease the effects of terazosin

3 *Hypotension-producing medications:* May increase the effects of terazosin

Labs

- False positive urinary metabolites of norepinephrine and VMA
- No effect on prostate specific antigen (PSA)

SPECIAL CONSIDERATIONS

- The doxazosin arm of the ALLHAT study was stopped early; the doxazosin group had a 25% greater risk of combined cardiovascular disease events, which was primarily accounted for by a doubled risk of CHF vs the chlorthalidone group; doxazosin was also found to be less effective at controlling systolic BP an average of 3 mm Hg; may want to consider primary antihypertensives in addition to α-blockers for BPH symptoms
- Use as a single antihypertensive agent limited by tendency to cause sodium and water retention and increased plasma volume

PATIENT/FAMILY EDUCATION

- Alert patients to the possibility of syncopal and orthostatic symptoms, especially with the first dose ("first dose syncope"); initial dose should be administered at bedtime in the smallest possible dose
- Consume dry toast, noncola carbonated beverages, and unsalted crackers to relieve nausea
- Nasal congestion may occur
- Full therapeutic effect of terazosin may not occur for 3-4 wks
- Use caution when driving, performing tasks requiring mental alertness, and rising from a sitting or lying position

• Notify the physician if dizziness or palpitations occurs

MONITORING PARAMETERS

• Blood pressure, pulse

terbinafine hydrochloride

(ter-bin'-a-feen hye-droe-klor'-ide)

Rx: Lamisil, Lamisil AT

Chemical Class: Allylamine derivative

Therapeutic Class: Antifungal

CLINICAL PHARMACOLOGY

Mechanism of Action: A fungicidal antifungal that inhibits the enzyme squalene epoxidase, thereby interfering with fungal biosynthesis. ***Therapeutic Effect:*** Results in death of fungal cells.

Pharmacokinetics

Well absorbed following PO administration. Protein binding: 99%. Metabolized by liver. Primarily excreted in urine; minimal elimination in feces. ***Half-life:*** (oral): 36 hr, (topical): 22-26 hr.

INDICATIONS AND DOSAGES

Tinea pedis

Topical

Adults, Elderly, Children 12 yrs and older. Apply twice a day until signs and symptoms significantly improve.

Tinea cruris, tinea corporis

Topical

Adults, Elderly, Children 12 yrs and older. Apply 1-2 times a day until signs and symptoms significantly improve.

Onychomycosis

PO

Adults, Elderly, Children 12 yrs and older. 250 mg/day for 6 wk (fingernails) or 12 wk (toenails).

Tinea versicolor

Topical solution

Adults, Elderly. Apply to the affected area twice a day for 7 days.

Systemic mycosis

PO

Adults, Elderly. 250-500 mg/day for up to 16 mo.

AVAILABLE FORMS

• *Tablets (Lamisil):* 250 mg.
• *Cream (Lamisil AT):* 1%.
• *Topical Solution (Lamisil, Lamisil AT):* 1%.
• *Topical Spray (Lamisil AT):* 1%.

CONTRAINDICATIONS: Oral: Children younger than 12 yrs, preexisting hepatic or renal impairment (creatinine clearance of 50 ml/min or less)

PREGNANCY AND LACTATION: Pregnancy category B; it is recommended that treatment of onychomycosis be delayed until after pregnancy; small amounts of terbinafine are excreted into breast milk when administered orally; not recommended in nursing mothers; avoid application to the breast when breast-feeding

SIDE EFFECTS

Frequent (13%)

Oral: Headache

Occasional (6%-3%)

Oral: Diarrhea, rash, dyspepsia, pruritus, taste disturbance, nausea

Oral: Abdominal pain, flatulence, urticaria, visual disturbance

Topical: Irritation, burning, pruritus, dryness

SERIOUS REACTIONS

• Hepatobiliary dysfunction (including cholestatic hepatitis), serious skin reactions, and severe neutropenia occur rarely.
• Ocular lens and retinal changes have been noted.

INTERACTIONS

Drugs

3 *Alcohol, other hepatotoxic medications:* May increase the risk of hepatotoxicity

3 *Hepatic enzyme inducers, including rifampin:* May increase terbinafine clearance

3 *Hepatic enzyme inhibitors, including cimetidine:* May decrease terbinafine clearance

SPECIAL CONSIDERATIONS

PATIENT/FAMILY EDUCATION

- Optimal clinical effect in onychomycosis may not be apparent for several mo following completion of therapy
- Rub topical terbinafine well into the affected and surrounding areas and do not cover the treated area with an occlusive dressing
- Keep the affected area clean and dry and wear light clothing to promote ventilation
- Separate personal items that come in contact with the affected area
- Do not let topical forms come in contact with eyes, mouth, nose, or other mucous membranes
- Notify the physician if diarrhea or skin irritation occurs

MONITORING PARAMETERS

- Topical terbinafine should be used for at least 1 wk but no more than 4 wks
- Assess for signs of a therapeutic response
- Discontinue the drug and notify the physician if a local reaction (such as blistering, burning, irritation, pruritus, oozing, erythema, or edema) occurs

terbutaline sulfate

(ter-byoo′-ta-leen sul′-fate)

Rx: Brethine

Chemical Class: Sympathomimetic amine; β_2-adrenergic agonist

Therapeutic Class: Antiasthmatic; bronchodilator; tocolytic

CLINICAL PHARMACOLOGY

Mechanism of Action: An adrenergic agonist that stimulates beta$_2$-adrenergic receptors, resulting in relaxation of uterine and bronchial smooth muscle. ***Therapeutic Effect:*** Relieves bronchospasm and reduces airway resistance. Also inhibits uterine contractions.

Pharmacokinetics

Partially absorbed in GI tract following oral administration. Protein binding: 14%-25%. Metabolized in liver. Excreted in feces and urine. ***Half-life:*** 3-4 hr.

INDICATIONS AND DOSAGES

Bronchospasm

PO

Adults, Elderly, Children 15 yr and older. Initially, 2.5 mg 3-4 times a day. Maintenance: 2.5-5 mg 3 times a day q6h while awake. Maximum: 15 mg/day.

Children 12-14 yr. 2.5 mg 3 times a day. Maximum: 7.5 mg/day.

Children younger than 12 yr. Initially, 0.05 mg/kg/dose q8h. May increase up to 0.15 mg/kg/dose. Maximum: 5 mg.

Subcutaneous

Adults, Children 12 yr and older. Initially, 0.25 mg. Repeat in 15-30 min if substantial improvement does not occur. Maximum: 0.5 mg/4 hr.

Children younger than 12 yr. 0.005-0.01 mg/kg/dose to a maximum of 0.4 mg/dose q15-20min for 2 doses.

Preterm labor
PO
Adults. 2.5-10 mg q4-6h.
IV
Adults. 2.5-10 mcg/min. May increase gradually q15-20 min up to 17.5-30 mcg/min.

AVAILABLE FORMS
- *Tablets:* 2.5 mg, 5 mg.
- *Injection:* 1 mg/ml.

CONTRAINDICATIONS: History of hypersensitivity to sympathomimetics

PREGNANCY AND LACTATION: Pregnancy category B; compatible with breast-feeding

SIDE EFFECTS
Frequent (23%-18%)
Tremor, anxiety
Occasional (11%-10%)
Somnolence, headache, nausea, heartburn, dizziness
Rare (3%-1%)
Flushing, asthenia, mouth and throat dryness or irritation (with inhalation therapy)

SERIOUS REACTIONS
- Too-frequent or excessive use may lead to decreased drug effectiveness and severe, paradoxical bronchoconstriction.
- Excessive sympathomimetic stimulation may cause palpitations, extrasystoles, tachycardia, chest pain, a slight increase in BP followed by a substantial decrease, chills, diaphoresis, and blanching of skin.

INTERACTIONS
Drugs
❷ *β-blockers:* Decreased action of terbutaline, cardioselective β-blockers preferable if concurrent use necessary; metoprolol inhibits terbutaline metabolism
❸ *Digoxin, sympathomimetics:* May increase the risk of arrhythmias
❸ *Furosemide:* Potential for additive hypokalemia
❸ *MAOIs:* May increase the risk of hypertensive crisis
❸ *Tricyclic antidepressants:* May increase cardiovascular effects

SPECIAL CONSIDERATIONS
PATIENT/FAMILY EDUCATION
- Notify the physician if chest pain, difficulty breathing, dizziness, flushing, headache, muscle tremors, or palpitations occurs
- May cause anxiety, nervousness, and shakiness
- Avoid excessive consumption of caffeinated products, such as chocolate, cocoa, cola, coffee, and tea

MONITORING PARAMETERS
- Pulse rate and quality and respiratory rate, depth, rhythm, and type
- Breath sounds for rhonchi and wheezing
- Serum potassium level
- ABG levels
- Observe the patient's fingernails and lips for a blue or dusky color in light-skinned patients and a gray color in dark-skinned patients, which are signs of hypoxemia
- Clinical improvement, such as cessation of clavicular retractions, quieter and slower respirations, and a relaxed facial expression
- When the drug is used for preterm labor, monitor the duration and frequency of contractions and diligently monitor the fetal heart rate

terconazole

(ter-kon'-a-zole)

Rx: Terazol 3, Terazol 7

Chemical Class: Triazole derivative

Therapeutic Class: Antifungal

CLINICAL PHARMACOLOGY

Mechanism of Action: An antifungal that disrupts fungal cell membrane permeability. ***Therapeutic Effect:*** Produces antifungal activity.

Pharmacokinetics

Extent of systemic absorption after vaginal administration may be dependent on presence of a uterus, 5%-8% in women who had a hysterectomy vs 12%-16% in nonhysterectomy women.

INDICATIONS AND DOSAGES

Vulvovaginal candidiasis

Intravaginal

Adults, Elderly. 1 suppository vaginally at bedtime for 3 days.

Adults, Elderly. 1 applicatorful at bedtime for 7 days (0.4% cream) or for 3 days (0.8% cream).

AVAILABLE FORMS

- *Suppository:* 80 mg (Terazol 3).
- *Cream:* 0.4 % (Terazol 7), 0.8% (Terazol 3).

CONTRAINDICATIONS: Hypersensitivity to terconazole or any component of the formulation

PREGNANCY AND LACTATION: Pregnancy category C; systemic absorption occurs; excretion into breast milk unknown

SIDE EFFECTS

Frequent

Headache, vulvovaginal burning

Occasional

Dysmenorrhea, pain in female genitalia, abdominal pain, fever, itching

Rare

Chills

SERIOUS REACTIONS

- Flu-like syndrome has been reported.

SPECIAL CONSIDERATIONS

- No significant advantage over less expensive OTC products

PATIENT/FAMILY EDUCATION

- Insert the vaginal form high into the vagina
- Complete for the full course of therapy
- Notify the physician if itching or burning occurs

MONITORING PARAMETERS

- Watch for local irritation

teriparatide (rDNA origin)

(ter-i-par'-a-tide)

Rx: Forteo

Chemical Class: Recombinant human parathyroid hormone (rDNA origin)

Therapeutic Class: Parathyroid hormone

CLINICAL PHARMACOLOGY

Mechanism of Action: A synthetic polypeptide hormone that acts on bone to mobilize calcium; also acts on kidney to reduce calcium clearance, increase phosphate excretion. ***Therapeutic Effect:*** Promotes an increased rate of release of calcium from bone into blood, stimulates new bone formation.

INDICATIONS AND DOSAGES

Osteoporosis

SC

Adults, Elderly. 20 mcg once daily into the thigh or abdominal wall.

AVAILABLE FORMS

- *Injection:* 3 ml prefilled pen containing 750 mcg teriparatide (Forteo).

T

CONTRAINDICATIONS: Serum calcium above normal level, those at increased risk for osteosarcoma (Paget's disease, unexplained elevations of alkaline phosphatase, open epiphyses, prior radiation therapy that include the skeleton), hypercalcemic disorder (e.g., hyperparathyroidism), hypersensitivity to teriparatide or any of the components of the formulation

PREGNANCY AND LACTATION: Pregnancy category C; not indicated for use in premenopausal women

SIDE EFFECTS

Occasional

Leg cramps, nausea, dizziness, headache, orthostatic hypotension, increased heart rate

SERIOUS REACTIONS

• None known.

INTERACTIONS

Drugs

3 *Digoxin:* Transient increase in serum calcium may increase risk of digitalis toxicity

SPECIAL CONSIDERATIONS

• Treatment not recommended beyond 2 yr as safety and efficacy not established
• Postural hypotension, if it occurs, happens within 4 hr and with the first several doses; does not preclude continued treatment
• Inform patients teriparatide caused osteosarcoma in rats; clinical relevance in humans unknown
• Maximal serum calcium levels occur 4-6 hr post dose

PATIENT/FAMILY EDUCATION

• Initially administer lying down (postural hypotension)
• Inject into thigh or abdominal wall
• Refrigerate, minimize time out of refrigerator
• Recap pen to protect from light
• Discard if not used within 28 days
• Notify provider of nausea, vomiting, constipation, lethargy, muscle weakness (possible hypercalcemia)

MONITORING PARAMETERS

• Bone mineral density, parathyroid hormone level, and urinary and serum calcium levels
• Blood pressure for hypotension and pulse rate for tachycardia
• Signs and symptoms of hypercalcemia

testosterone

(tes-tos'-ter-one)

Rx: Androderm, AndroGel, Delatestryl, Depandro 100, Depo-Testosterone, FIRST-Testosterone, FIRST-Testosterone MC, Striant, Testim, Testoderm, Testro AQ, Testro-L.A.

Chemical Class: Androgen

Therapeutic Class: Androgen; antineoplastic

DEA Class: Schedule III

CLINICAL PHARMACOLOGY

Mechanism of Action: A primary endogenous androgen that promotes growth and development of male sex organs and maintains secondary sex characteristics in androgen-deficient males. ***Therapeutic Effect:*** Helps relieve androgen deficiency.

Pharmacokinetics

Well absorbed after IM administration. Protein binding: 98%. Undergoes first-pass metabolism in the liver. Primarily excreted in urine. Unknown if removed by hemodialysis. ***Half-life:*** 10-20 min.

INDICATIONS AND DOSAGES

Male hypogonadism

IM

Adults. 50-400 mg q2-4wk.

Adolescents. Initially 40-50 mg/m^2/dose monthly until growth rate falls to prepubertal levels. 100 mg/m^2/dose until growth ceases. Maintenance virilizing dose: 100 mg/m^2/dose twice a month.

Subcutaneous (Pellets)

Adults, Adolescents. 150-450 mg q3-6mo.

Transdermal (Patch [Testoderm])

Adults, Elderly. Start therapy with 6 mg/day patch. Apply patch to scrotal skin.

Transdermal (Patch [Testoderm TTS])

Adults, Elderly. Apply TTS patch to arm, back, or upper buttocks.

Transdermal (Patch [Androderm])

Adults, Elderly. Start therapy with 5 mg/day patch applied at night. Apply patch to abdomen, back, thighs, or upper arms.

Transdermal (Gel [AndroGel])

Adults, Elderly. Initial dose of 5 mg delivers 50 mg testosterone and is applied once daily to the abdomen, shoulders, or upper arms. May increase to 7.5 g, then to 10 g, if necessary.

Transdermal (Gel [Testim])

Adults, Elderly. Initial dose of 5 g delivers 50 mg testosterone and is applied once a day to the shoulders or upper arms. May increase to 10 g.

Buccal system (Striant)

Adults, Elderly. 30 mg q12h.

Delayed puberty

IM

Adults. 50-200 mg q2-4wk.

Adolescents. 40-50 mg/m^2/dose every month for 6 mo.

Subcutaneous (Pellets)

Adults, Adolescents. 150-450 mg q3-6mo.

Breast carcinoma

IM (testosterone aqueous)

Adults. 50-100 mg 3 times a week.

IM (testosterone cypionate or testosterone ethanate)

Adults. 200-400 mg q2-4wk.

IM (testosterone propionate)

Adults. 50-100 mg 3 times a week.

AVAILABLE FORMS

- *Cypionate Injection (Depo-Testosterone):* 100 mg/ml, 200 mg/ml.
- *Ethanate Injection (Andro LA 200, Delatestryl, Testro-L.A.):* 200 mg/ml.
- *Propionate Injection Solution (Depandro 100):* 100 mg/ml.
- *Intramuscular Solution:* 50 mg/ml (Testro), 100 mg/ml (Testro AQ).
- *Subcutaneous Pellets (Testopel):* 75 mg.
- *Topical Gel:* 25 mg/2.5 g (AndroGel) 50 mg/5 g (AndroGel, Testim).
- *Topical Cream (FIRST-Testosterone MC):* 2%.
- *Topical Ointment (FIRST-Testosterone):* 2%.
- *Transdermal Patch:* 2.5 mg/day (Androderm), 4 mg/day (Testoderm), 5 mg/day (Androderm), 6 mg/day (Testoderm).
- *Buccal (Striant):* 30 mg.

CONTRAINDICATIONS: Breastfeeding, cardiac impairment, hypercalcemia, pregnancy, prostate or breast cancer in males, severe hepatic or renal disease

PREGNANCY AND LACTATION: Pregnancy category X; excretion into breast milk unknown; use extreme caution in nursing mothers

SIDE EFFECTS

Frequent

Gynecomastia, acne

Females: Hirsutism, amenorrhea or other menstrual irregularities, deepening of voice, clitoral enlargement that may not be reversible when drug is discontinued

Occasional

Edema, nausea, insomnia, oligospermia, priapism, male-pattern baldness, bladder irritability, hypercalcemia (in immobilized patients

or those with breast cancer), hypercholesterolemia, inflammation and pain at IM injection site
Transdermal: Pruritus, erythema, skin irritation
Rare
Polycythemia (with high dosage), hypersensitivity

SERIOUS REACTIONS

- Peliosis hepatitis (presence of blood-filled cysts in parenchyma of liver), hepatic neoplasms, and hepatocellular carcinoma have been associated with prolonged high-dose therapy.
- Anaphylactic reactions occur rarely.

INTERACTIONS

Drugs

3 *Cyclosporine:* Increased cyclosporine concentrations
3 *Hepatotoxic medications:* May increase the risk of hepatotoxicity
2 *Oral anticoagulants:* Increased hypoprothrombinemic response

SPECIAL CONSIDERATIONS

PATIENT/FAMILY EDUCATION

- Apply the patch to a clean, dry, hairless area of the skin, avoiding bony prominences
- Do not take any other medications, including OTC drugs, without first consulting the physician
- Consume a diet high in calories and protein; food may be better tolerated if he or she eats small, frequent meals
- Weigh oneself every day and report to the physician weight gain of 5 lb or more per week
- Notify the physician if acne, nausea, vomiting, or foot swelling occurs
- The female patient should promptly report deepening of the voice, hoarseness, and menstrual irregularities
- The male patient should report difficulty urinating, frequent erections, and gynecomastia
- Regular monitoring tests and visits to the physician are important

MONITORING PARAMETERS

- LFTs, lipids, Hct and Hgb
- Growth rate in children (X-rays for bone age q6mo)
- Blood pressure
- Weight
- Intake and output
- Electrolytes
- Signs of virilization

tetracaine hydrochloride

(tet'-ra-cane hye-droe-klor'-ide)
Rx: AK-T Caine, Opticaine, Pontocaine
OTC: Cepacol, Viractin
Chemical Class: Benzoic acid derivative
Therapeutic Class: Anesthetic, local

CLINICAL PHARMACOLOGY

Mechanism of Action: Tetracaine causes a reversible blockade of nerve conduction by decreasing nerve membrance permeability to sodium. ***Therapeutic Effect:*** Local anesthetic.

Pharmacokinetics

Systemic absorption of tetracaine is variable. Metabolized by plasma pseudocholinesterasis. Excreted in the urine.

INDICATIONS AND DOSAGES

Anesthetize lower abdomen

Spinal
Adults. 3-4 ml (9-12 mg) of a 0.3% solution.

Anesthetize perineum

Spinal
Adults. 1-2 ml (3-6 mg) of a 0.3% solution.

Anesthetize upper abdomen
Spinal
Adults. 5 ml (15 mg) of a 0.3% solution.

Obstetric anesthesia, low spinal (saddle block) anesthesia
Spinal
Adults. 1-2 ml (2-14 mg) of a 0.2% solution.

Anesthesia of the perineum
Intrathecal
Adults. 0.5 ml (5 mg) as a 1% solution, diluted with equal amount of CSF or 10% dextrose injection.

Anesthesia of the perineum and lower extremeties
Intrathecal
Adults. 1 ml (10 mg) as a 1% solution, diluted with equal amount of CSF or 10% dextrose injection.

Anesthesia up to the costal margin
Intrathecal
Adults. 1.5-2 ml (15-20 mg) as a 1% solution, diluted with equal amount of CSF.

Topical anesthesia
Topical
Adults. Apply to the affected areas as needed. Maximum dosage is 28 g per 24 hrs.
Children. Apply to the affected areas as needed. Maximum dosage is 7 g in a 24-hr period.

Topical anesthesia of nose and throat, abolish laryngeal and esophageal reflexes prior to diagnostic procedure
Topical
Adults. Direct application of a 0.25% or 0.5% topical solution or by oral inhalation of a nebulized 0.5% solution. Total dose should not exceed 20 mg.

Mild pain, burning and/or pruritis associated with herpes labialis (cold sores or fever blisters)
Topical
Adults, Children 2 yrs and older. Apply to the affected area no more than 3-4 times a day.

Ophthalmic anesthesia
Topical
Adults. 1-2 drops of a 0.5% solution.

AVAILABLE FORMS
- *Solution for Injection:* 0.2%, 0.3%, 1%, 2% (Pontocaine).
- *Cream:* 1%.
- *Ointment:* 0.5%.

CONTRAINDICATIONS: Hypersensitivity to esther local anesthetics, sulfites, PABA; infection or inflammation at the injection site; bactermia; platelet abnormalities; thrombocytopenia; increased bleeding time; uncontrolled coagulopathy, or anticoagulant therapy; sulfonamide therapy

PREGNANCY AND LACTATION: Pregnancy category C; excretion into breast milk unknown

SIDE EFFECTS
Frequent
Burning, stinging, or tenderness; skin rash, itching, redness, or inflammation; numbness or tingling of the face or mouth; pain at the injection site; sensitivity to light; swelling of the eye or eyelid; watering of the eyes; acute ocular pain and ocular irritation (burning, stinging, or redness)
Occasional
Paresthesias, weakness and paralysis of lower extremity, hypotension, high or total spinal block, urinary retention or incontinence, fecal incontinence, headache, back pain, septic meningitis, meningismus, arachnoiditis, shivering cranial nerve palsies due to traction on nerves from loss of CSF, and loss of perineal sensation and sexual function

T

Rare

Anxiety, restlessness, difficulty breathing, shortness of breath, dizziness, drowsiness, lightheadedness, nausea, vomiting, seizures (convulsions), slow, irregular heartbeat (palpitations), swelling of the face or mouth, skin rash, itching (hives), tremors, visual impairment

SERIOUS REACTIONS

• Tetracaine-induced CNS toxicity usually presents with symptoms of a CNS stimulation such as anxiety, apprehension, restlessness, nervousness, disorientation, confusion, dizziness, tinnitus, blurred vision, tremor, and/or seizures. Subsequently, depressive symptoms may occur, including drowsiness, respiratory arrest, or coma.

• Depression or cardiac excitability and contractility may cause AV block, ventricular arrhythmias, or cardiac arrest. Symptoms of local anesthetic CNS toxicity, such as dizziness, tongue numbness, visual impairment or disturbances, and muscular twitching appear to occur before cardiotoxic effects. Cardiotoxic effects include angina, QT prolongation, PR prolongation, atrial fibrillation, sinus bradycardia, hypotension, palpitations, and cardiovascular collapse. Maternal seizures and cardiovascular collapse may occur following paracervical block in early pregnancy due to rapid systemic absorption.

Alert: Tetracaine is more likely than any other topical anesthetic to cause contact reactions, including skin rash (unspecified), mucous membrane irritation, erythema, pruritis, urticaria, burning, stinging, edema, or tenderness.

Alert: During labor and obstetric delivery, local anesthetics can cause varying degrees of maternal, fetal, and neonatal toxicities. Fetal heart rate should be monitored continuously because fetal bradycardia may occur in patients receiving tetracaine anesthesia and may be associated with fetal acidosis. Maternal hypotension can result from regional anesthesia; patient position can alleviate this problem. Spinal tetracaine may cause decreased uterine contractility or maternal expulsion efforts and alter the forces of parturition.

INTERACTIONS

Drugs

3 *Propranolol:* Enhanced sympathomimetic side effects resulting in hypertensive reactions; acute discontinuation of β-blockers prior to local anesthesia may increase side effects of tetracaine

3 *Sulfonamides:* Inhibits the action of sulfonamides

Labs

• *Interference:* CSF protein

SPECIAL CONSIDERATIONS

• Previously used as component of "Magic Numbing Solution" or TAC Sol (epinephrine 1:2000, tetracaine 0.5%, cocaine 11.8%) and LET Sol (lidocaine 4%, epinephrine 0.1%, tetracaine 0.5%), which are used as topical anesthesia for repair of minor lacerations, especially in pediatric patients. Topical tetracaine solutions no longer available

PATIENT/FAMILY EDUCATION

• Notify the physician of any trouble breathing

MONITORING PARAMETERS

• Assess the effectiveness of anesthesia

tetracycline hydrochloride

(tet-ra-sye'-kleen)

Rx: Panmycin, Sumycin, Tetracon

Chemical Class: Tetracycline

Therapeutic Class: Antibiotic

CLINICAL PHARMACOLOGY

Mechanism of Action: A tetracycline antibiotic that inhibits bacterial protein synthesis by binding to ribosomes. ***Therapeutic Effect:*** Bacteriostatic.

Pharmacokinetics

Readily absorbed from the GI tract. Protein binding: 30%-60%. Widely distributed. Excreted in urine; eliminated in feces through biliary system. Not removed by hemodialysis. ***Half-life:*** 6-11 hr (increased in impaired renal function).

INDICATIONS AND DOSAGES

Inflammatory acne vulgaris, Lyme disease, mycoplasmal disease, Legionella infections, Rocky Mountain spotted fever, chlamydial infections in patients with gonorrhea

PO

Adults, Elderly. 250-500 mg q6-12h.

Children 8 yrs and older. 25-50 mg/kg/day in 4 divided doses. Maximum: 3 g/day.

H. pylori infections

PO

Adults, Elderly. 500 mg 2-4 times a day (in combination).

Topical

Adults, Elderly. Apply twice a day (once in the morning, once in the evening).

Dosage in renal impairment

Dosage interval is modified based on creatinine clearance.

Creatinine Clearance	*Dosage Interval*
50-80 ml/min	Usual dose q8-12h
10-50 ml/min	Usual dose q12-24h
less than 10 ml/min	Usual dose q24h

AVAILABLE FORMS

- *Capsules:* 250 mg (Ala-Tet, Panmycin, Sumycin, Tetracon), 500 mg (Sumycin, Tetracon).
- *Oral Suspension (Sumycin):* 125 mg/5 ml.
- *Tablets (Sumycin):* 250 mg, 500 mg.
- *Topical Solution.* 2.2 mg/ml.
- *Topical Ointment:* 3%.

CONTRAINDICATIONS: Children 8 yrs and younger, hypersensitivity to sulfites

PREGNANCY AND LACTATION: Pregnancy category D (systemic), category B (topical); systemic tetracycline excreted into breast milk in low concentrations; theoretically, dental staining could occur, but serum levels in infants undetectable, so considered compatible with breast-feeding

SIDE EFFECTS

Frequent

Dizziness, light-headedness, diarrhea, nausea, vomiting, abdominal cramps, possibly severe photosensitivity

Topical: Dry, scaly skin; stinging or burning sensation

Occasional

Pigmentation of skin or mucous membranes, rectal or genital pruritus, stomatitis

Topical: Pain, redness, swelling, or other skin irritation

SERIOUS REACTIONS

- Superinfection (especially fungal), anaphylaxis, and benign intracranial hypertension may occur.
- Bulging fontanelles occur rarely in infants.

T

INTERACTIONS

Drugs

3 *Antacids:* Reduced tetracycline concentrations
3 *Anticoagulants:* May depress plasma prothrombin activity; may require downward adjustment of anticoagulant dosage
2 *Bismuth subsalicylate:* Reduced tetracycline concentrations
3 *Calcium:* Reduced tetracycline concentrations
3 *Carbamazepine, phenytoin:* May decrease tetracycline blood concentration
3 *Cholestyramine colestipol:* Reduced tetracycline concentrations
3 *Dairy products:* Inhibits tetracycline absorption
3 *Digoxin:* Decreased digoxin concentrations due to reduced GI flora
3 *Food:* Reduced tetracycline concentrations
3 *Iron:* Reduced tetracycline concentrations
3 *Magnesium:* Reduced tetracycline concentrations
2 *Methoxyflurane:* Increased renal toxicity
3 *Oral contraceptives:* Possible decreased contraceptive effect
3 *Penicillin:* Impaired efficacy of penicillin
3 *Sodium bicarbonate:* Reduced tetracycline concentrations
3 *St. John's Wort:* May increase the risk of photosensitivity
3 *Zinc:* Reduced tetracycline concentrations

Labs

- *False negative:* Urine glucose with Clinistix or TesTape
- *False increase:* Serum glucose
- *False decrease:* Serum acetaminophen concentration, serum folate
- *Interference:* Plasma catecholamines, urinary porphyrins, CSF protein

SPECIAL CONSIDERATIONS

PATIENT/FAMILY EDUCATION

- Avoid milk products, antacids, or separate by 2 hr; take with a full glass of water
- Use in children ≤8 yr causes permanent discoloration of teeth, enamel hypoplasia, and retardation of skeletal development; risk greatest for children <4 yr and receiving high doses
- Side effects noted for systemic administration not observed with topical formulations
- Take oral tetracycline on an empty stomach
- Space drug doses evenly around the clock and continue taking tetracycline for the full course of treatment
- Notify the physician if diarrhea, rash, or any other new symptoms occur
- Avoid overexposure to the sun or ultraviolet light to prevent photosensitivity reactions
- Do not take any other medications, including OTC drugs, without consulting the physician
- Topical tetracycline may turn skin yellow but washing removes the solution; fabrics may be stained by heavy topical application
- Do not apply topical tetracycline to deep or open wounds
- Avoid performing tasks that require mental alertness or motor skills until response to the drug has been established

MONITORING PARAMETERS

- Pattern of daily bowel activity and stool consistency
- Skin for rash
- Blood pressure
- Be alert for signs and symptoms of superinfection, such as anal or genital pruritus, diarrhea, and stomatitis

tetrahydrozoline hydrochloride

(tet-ra-hye-droz′-a-leen hye-droe-klor′-ide)

Rx: Tyzine

OTC: Visine

Chemical Class: Sympathomimetic amine

Therapeutic Class: Decongestant

CLINICAL PHARMACOLOGY

Mechanism of Action: A vasoconstrictor that stimulates alpha-adrenergic receptors in sympathetic nervous system. Constricts arterioles. ***Therapeutic Effect:*** Reduces redness, irritation, and congestion.

Pharmacokinetics

May be systemically absorbed. Metabolic, elimination rates unknown.

INDICATIONS AND DOSAGES

Relief of itching, minor irritation and to control hyperemia with superficial corneal vascularity

Ophthalmic

Adults, Elderly, Children. 1-2 drops 2-4 times/day.

Relief of nasal congestion of rhinitis, the common cold, sinusitis, hay fever, or other allergies; reduces swelling and improves visualization for surgery or diagnostic procedures; opens obstructed eustachian ostia with ear inflammation

Intranasal

Adults, Elderly, Children older than 6 yrs. 2-4 drops (0.1% solution) to each nostril q4-6h (no sooner than q3h).

Children 2-6 yrs. 2-3 drops (0.05% solution) to each nostril q4-6h (no sooner than q3h).

AVAILABLE FORMS

- *Nasal Solution:* 0.05%, 0.1% (Tyzine).
- *Ophthalmic Solution:* 0.05% (Visine).

CONTRAINDICATIONS: Children less than 2 yrs of age, the 0.1% nasal solution is contraindicated in children less than 6 yrs of age, angle-closure glaucoma or other serious eye diseases, hypersensitivity to tetrahydrozyline or any component of the formulation

PREGNANCY AND LACTATION: Pregnancy category C; excretion into breast milk unknown

SIDE EFFECTS

Occasional

Intranasal: Transient burning, stinging, sneezing, dryness of mucosa

Ophthalmic: Irritation, blurred vision, mydriasis

Systemic sympathomimetic effects may occur with either route: headache, hypertension, weakness, sweating, palpitations, tremors. Prolonged use may result in rebound congestion

SERIOUS REACTIONS

- Overdosage may result in CNS depression with drowsiness, decreased body temperature, bradycardia, hypotension, coma, and apnea.

INTERACTIONS

Drugs

3 *MAOIs:* May cause hypertension

SPECIAL CONSIDERATIONS

- Manage rebound congestion by stopping tetrahydrozoline: one nostril at a time, substitute systemic decongestant, substitute inhaled steroid

PATIENT/FAMILY EDUCATION

- Do not use for >3-5 days or rebound congestion may occur
- Discontinue and consult physician immediately if ocular pain or visual changes occur or if condition worsens or continues for more than 72 hrs

thalidomide

(tha li' doe mide)

Rx: Thalomid

Chemical Class: Glutamic acid derivative

Therapeutic Class: Leprostatic

CLINICAL PHARMACOLOGY

Mechanism of Action: An immunomodulator whose exact mechanism is unknown. Has sedative, antiinflammatory, and immunosuppressive activity, which may be due to selective inhibition of the production of tumor necrosis factor-alpha.

Therapeutic Effect: Improves muscle wasting in HIV patients; reduces local and systemic effects of leprosy.

Pharmacokinetics

Protein binding: 55%. Metabolism and elimination are not known. ***Half-life:*** 5-7 hr.

INDICATIONS AND DOSAGES

AIDS-related muscle wasting

PO

Adults. 100-300 mg a day.

Leprosy

PO

Adults, Elderly. Initially, 100-300 mg/day as single bedtime dose, at least 1 hr after the evening meal. Continue until active reaction subsides, then reduce dose q2-4wk in 50-mg increments.

AVAILABLE FORMS

- *Capsules:* 50 mg, 100 mg, 200 mg.

UNLABELED USES: Prevention and treatment of discoid lupus erythematosus, erythema fultiforme, graft vs host reactions following bone marrow transplantation, rheumatoid arthritis; treatment of Behcet's syndrome, Crohn's disease, GI bleeding, multiple myeloma, pruritus, recurrent aphthous ulcers in HIV patients, wasting syndrome associated with HIV or cancer

CONTRAINDICATIONS: Neutropenia, peripheral neuropathy; pregnancy

PREGNANCY AND LACTATION: Pregnancy category X; breast milk excretion unknown

SIDE EFFECTS

Frequent

Somnolence, dizziness, mood changes, constipation, dry mouth, peripheral neuropathy

Occasional

Increased appetite, weight gain, headache, loss of libido, edema of face and limbs, nausea, alopecia, dry skin, rash, hypothyroidism

SERIOUS REACTIONS

- Neutropenia, peripheral neuropathy, and thromboembolism occur rarely.

INTERACTIONS

Drugs

3 *Barbiturates:* Additive sedative effects

3 *Chlorpromazine:* Additive sedative effects

3 *Ethanol:* Additive sedative effects

3 *Medications associated with peripheral neuropathy (such as isoniazid, lithium, metronidazole, phenytoin):* May increase peripheral neuropathy

3 *Reserpine:* Additive sedative effects

SPECIAL CONSIDERATIONS

PATIENT/FAMILY EDUCATION

- Teratogenic in human whether taken by male or female
- Sedation common; usually taken at bedtime
- Avoid consuming alcohol or using other drugs that cause drowsiness during thalidomide therapy
- Female patients of childbearing age should perform a pregnancy test within 24 hrs before beginning thalidomide therapy, and then every 2-4 wks

• Avoid performing tasks that require mental alertness or motor skills until response to the drug has been established

MONITORING PARAMETERS

• Pregnancy test (weekly during first mo of use, then monthly)
• ALT, AST
• CBC
• Signs and symptoms of peripheral neuropathy

theophylline

(thee-off'-i-lin)

Rx: Elixophyllin, Slo-Bid Gyrocaps, Quibron-T, Theochron, Theo-Dur, Theolair, Theolair SR, T-Phyl, Truxophyllin, Uniphyl

Combinations

Rx: with guaifenesin (Elixophyllin-GG, Quibron); with potassium iodide (Elixophylline KI)

Chemical Class: Xanthine derivative

Therapeutic Class: COPD agent; antiasthmatic; bronchodilator

CLINICAL PHARMACOLOGY

Mechanism of Action: An antiasthmatic medication with two distinct actions in the airways of patients with reversible obstruction: smooth muscle relaxation and suppression of the response of airways to stimuli. Mechanisms of action are not known with certainty. It is known theophylline increases force of contraction of diaphragmatic muscles by enhancing calcium uptake through adenosine-mediated channels. ***Therapeutic Effect:*** Causes bronchodilation and decreased airway reactivity.

Pharmacokinetics

The pharmacokinetics of theophylline vary widely among similar patients and cannot be predicted by age, sex, body weight, or other demographic characteristics. Rapidly and completely absorbed after oral administration in solution or immediate-release solid oral dosage form. Distributed freely into fat-free tissues. Extensively metabolized in liver. ***Half-life:*** 4-8 hrs.

INDICATIONS AND DOSAGES

Chronic asthma/lung diseases

PO

Adults. Acute symptoms: 5 mg/kg as a loading dose, maintenance 3 mg/kg every 8 hrs (nonsmokers), 3 mg/kg every 6 hrs (smokers), 2 mg/kg every 8 hrs (older patients), 1-2 mg/kg every 12 hrs (CHF); IV 5 mg/kg load over 20 mins, maintenance 0.2 mg/kg/hr (CHF, elderly), 0.43 mg/kg/hr (nonsmokers), 0.7 mg/kg/hr (young adult smokers).

Slow titration: Initial dose 16 mg/kg/day or 400 mg daily, whichever is less, doses divided every 6-8 hrs

Dosage adjustment after serum theophylline measurement. Serum level 5-10 mcg/ml, maintain dose by 25%, recheck level in 3 days. Serum level 10-20 mcg/ml, maintain dosage if tolerated, recheck level every 6-12 mos. Serum level 20-25 mcg/ml, decrease dose by 10%, recheck level in 3 days. Serum level 25-30 mcg/ml, skip next dose, decrease dose by 25%, recheck level in 3 days. Serum level > 30 mcg/ml, skip next 2 doses, decrease dose by 50%, recheck level in 3 days.

Children 9-16 yrs. 5 mg/kg as a loading dose, maintenance 3 mg/kg every 6 hrs; IV 5 mg/kg load over 20 minutes, maintenance 0.7 mg/kg/hr.

Children 1-9 yrs. 5 mg/kg as a loading dose, maintenance 4 mg/kg every 6 hrs; IV 5 mg/kg load over 20 mins, maintenance 0.8 mg/kg/hr.
Infants. [(0.2 × age in weeks) +5] × kg = 24-hr dose in mg; divide into every 8 hr dosing (6 wks-6 mos), every 6 hr dosing (6-12 mos); IV 5 mg/kg load over 20 mins, maintenance dose in mg/kg/hr [(0.0008 × age in weeks) + 0.21].

AVAILABLE FORMS

- *Capsule, extended release:* 100 mg (Slo-Bid Gyrocaps); 125 mg; 200 mg (Slo-Bid Gyrocaps); 300 mg (Slo-Bid Gyrocaps).
- *Elixir:* 80 mg/15 ml (Elixophyllin).
- *Solution, intravenous:* 40 mg/100 ml, 80 mg/100 ml, 160 mg/100 ml, 200 mg/100 ml, 200 mg/50 ml, 320 mg/100 ml, 400 mg/100 ml.
- *Solution, oral:* 80 mg/15 ml (Truxophyllin).
- *Tablet:* 100 mg.
- *Tablet, extended release:* 100 mg (Theo-Dur, Theochron, Theo-Time), 200 mg (Theo-Dur, Theochron, Theo-Time), 300 mg (Theo-Dur, Theochron, Theo-Time), 400 mg (Uni-Dur), 450 mg (Theochron).

UNLABELED USES: Apnea, bradycardia of prematurity

CONTRAINDICATIONS: Hypersensitivity to theophylline or any component of the formulation, active peptic ulcer disease, underlying seizure disorders unless receiving appropriate anticonvulsant medication

PREGNANCY AND LACTATION: Pregnancy category C; no reports of malformations; compatible with breast-feeding with precaution that rapidly absorbed preparations may cause irritability in the infant

SIDE EFFECTS

Anxiety, dizziness, headache, insomnia, lightheadedness, muscle twitching, restlessness, seizures, dysrhythmias, fluid retention with tachycardia, hypotension, palpitations, pounding heartbeat, sinus tachycardia, anorexia, bitter taste, diarrhea, dyspepsia, gastroesophageal reflux, nausea, vomiting, urinary frequency, increased respiratory rate, flushing, urticaria

SERIOUS REACTIONS

- Severe toxicity from theophylline overdose is a relatively rare event.

INTERACTIONS

Drugs

3 *Adenosine:* Inhibited hemodynamic effects of adenosine

3 *Allopurinol, amiodarone, cimetidine, ciprofloxacin, disulfiram, erythromycin, interferon alfa, isoniazid, methimazole, metoprolol, norfloxacin, pefloxacin, pentoxyfylline, propafenone, propylthiouracil, radioactive iodine, tacrine, thiabendazole, ticlopidine, verapamil:* Increased theophylline concentrations

3 *Aminoglutethamide, barbiturates, carbamazepine, moricizine, phenytoin, rifampin, ritonavir, thyroid hormone:* Reduced theophylline levels; decreased serum phenytoin concentrations

3 *β-blockers:* Reduced bronchodilating response to theophylline

2 *Enoxacin, fluvoxamine, mexiletine, propranolol, troleandomycin:* Markedly increased theophylline concentrations

3 *Imipenem:* Some patients on theophylline have developed seizures following the addition of imipenem

3 *Lithium:* Reduced lithium concentrations

3 *Smoking:* Increased theophylline dosing requirements

Labs

- *False increase:* Serum barbiturate concentrations, urinary uric acid
- *False decrease:* Serum bilirubin
- *Interference:* Plasma somatostatin

SPECIAL CONSIDERATIONS

PATIENT/FAMILY EDUCATION

- Contents of beaded capsules may be sprinkled over food for children
- Avoid excessive amounts of caffeine, as well as extremes in dietary protein and carbohydrates
- Charbroiled foods may increase elimination and reduce the half-life
- Nervousness, restlessness, and increased heart rate may occur during theophylline therapy

MONITORING PARAMETERS

- Blood levels; therapeutic level is 10-20 mcg/ml (6-14 mcg/ml for apnea, bradycardia of prematurity); toxicity may occur with small increase above 20 mcg/ml and occasionally at levels below this; obtain serum levels 1-2 hr after administration for immediate-release products and 5-9 hr after the a.m. dose for sustained-release formulations
- Recent evidence indicates that blood levels of 8-12 mcg/ml may provide adequate therapeutic effect with a lower risk of adverse events
- Signs of toxicity include nausea, vomiting, anxiety, insomnia, seizures, ventricular dysrhythmias

thiabendazole

(thye-a-ben′-da-zole)

Rx: Mintezol

Chemical Class: Benzimidazole derivative

Therapeutic Class: Antihelmintic

CLINICAL PHARMACOLOGY

Mechanism of Action: An antihelmintic agent that inhibits helminth-specific mitochondrial fumarate reductase. ***Therapeutic Effect:*** Suppresses parasite production.

Pharmacokinetics

Rapidly and well absorbed from the gastrointestinal (GI) tract. Rapidly metabolized in liver. Primarily excreted in urine; partially eliminated in feces. ***Half-life:*** 1.2 hrs.

INDICATIONS AND DOSAGES:

Dose is based on patient's body weight.

Cutaneous lava migrans (creeping eruption)

PO

Adults, Elderly, Children. 50 mg/kg/day q12h for 2 days. Maximum: 3 g/day.

Intestinal roundworms

PO

Adults, Elderly, Children. 50 mg/kg/day q12h for 2 days. Maximum: 3 g/day.

Strongloidiasis (threadworms)

PO

Adults, Elderly, Children. 50 mg/kg/day q12h for 2 days. Maximum: 3 g/day.

Trichinosis

PO

Adults, Elderly, Children. 50 mg/kg/day q12h for 2-4 days. Maximum: 3 g/day.

T

Visceral larva migrans

PO

Adults, Elderly, Children. 50 mg/kg/day q12h for 7 days. Maximum: 3 g/day.

AVAILABLE FORMS

- *Suspension:* 500 mg/5 ml (Mintezol).
- *Tablets:* 500 mg (Mintezol).

UNLABELED USES: Angiostrongyliasis, capillaria infestations, dracunculus infestations, pediculosis capitis, tinea infections

CONTRAINDICATIONS: Prophylactic treatment of pinworm infestation, hypersensitivity to thiabendazole or its components

PREGNANCY AND LACTATION: Pregnancy category C

SIDE EFFECTS

Occasional

Dizziness, drowsiness, nausea, vomiting, diarrhea

Rare

Erythema multiform, liver damage

SERIOUS REACTIONS

- Overdose includes symptoms of altered mental status and visual problems.
- Erythema multiform, liver damage, and Stevens-Johnsons syndrome occur rarely.

INTERACTIONS

Drugs

3 *Carbamazepine:* Decreased thiabendazole concentrations, therapeutic failure possible

3 *Theophylline:* May inhibit metabolism of xanthines, potentially elevating serum concentrations

SPECIAL CONSIDERATIONS

PATIENT/FAMILY EDUCATION

- Take after meals; chew before swallowing
- Proper hygiene after bowel movement, including handwashing technique; change bed linen
- Urine may turn red-brown or dark brown during drug therapy
- Avoid tasks that require mental alertness or motor skills until response to the drug is established

MONITORING PARAMETERS

- Renal and hepatic function

thiamine hydrochloride (vitamin B_1)

(thy'-a-min)

Rx: (Beta-Sol [AUS], Betaxin[CAN], Thiamilate)

CLINICAL PHARMACOLOGY

Mechanism of Action: A water-soluble vitamin that combines with adenosine triphosphate in the liver, kidneys, and leukocytes to form thiamine diphosphate, a coenzyme that is necessary for carbohydrate metabolism. ***Therapeutic Effect:*** Prevents and reverses thiamine deficiency.

Pharmacokinetics

Readily absorbed from the GI tract, primarily in duodenum, after IM administration. Widely distributed. Metabolized in the liver. Primarily excreted in urine.

INDICATIONS AND DOSAGES

Dietary supplement

PO

Adults, Elderly. 1–2 mg/day.

Children. 0.5–1 mg/day.

Infants. 0.3–0.5 mg/day.

Thiamine deficiency

PO

Adults, Elderly. 5–30 mg/day, as a single dose or in 3 divided doses, for 1 mo.

Children. 10–50 mg/day in 3 divided doses.

Thiamine deficiency in patients who are critically ill or have malabsorption syndrome

IV, IM

Adults, Elderly. 5–100 mg, 3 times a day.

Children. 10–25 mg/day.

Metabolic disorders

PO

Adults, Elderly, Children. 10–20 mg/day; increased up to 4 g/day in divided doses.

AVAILABLE FORMS

- *Tablets:* 50 mg, 100 mg, 250 mg, 500 mg.
- *Injection:* 100 mg/ml.

CONTRAINDICATIONS: None known.

SIDE EFFECTS

Frequent

Pain, induration, and tenderness at IM injection site

SERIOUS REACTIONS

- IV administration may result in a rare, severe hypersensitivity reaction marked by a feeling of warmth, pruritus, urticaria, weakness, diaphoresis, nausea, restlessness, tightness in throat, angioedema, cyanosis, pulmonary edema, GI tract bleeding, and cardiovascular collapse.

thiethylperazine maleate

(thye-eth-il-per'-azeen mal'-ee-ate)

Rx: Torecan

Chemical Class: Piperazine phenothiazine derivative

Therapeutic Class: Antiemetic

CLINICAL PHARMACOLOGY

Mechanism of Action: A piperazine phenothiazine that acts centrally to block dopamine receptors in chemoreceptor trigger zone (CTZ) in central nervous system (CNS). ***Therapeutic Effect:*** Relieves nausea and vomiting.

INDICATIONS AND DOSAGES

Nausea or vomiting

PO/Rectal/IM

Adults, Elderly. 10 mg 1-3 times/day.

AVAILABLE FORMS

- *Injection:* 5 mg/ml (Torecan).
- *Tablets:* 10 mg (Torecan).

CONTRAINDICATIONS: Comatose states, severe CNS depression, pregnancy, hypersensitivity to phenothiazines

PREGNANCY AND LACTATION: Pregnancy category X; excretion into breast milk unknown; use caution in nursing mothers

SIDE EFFECTS

Frequent

Drowsiness, dizziness

Occasional

Blurred vision, decreased color/night vision, fever, headache, orthostatic hypotension, rash, ringing in ears, constipation, dry mouth, decreased sweating

SERIOUS REACTIONS

- Extrapyramidal symptoms manifested as torticollis (neck muscle spasm), oculogyric crisis (rolling back of eyes), and akathisia (motor restlessness, anxiety) occur rarely.

INTERACTIONS

Drugs

3 *Anticholinergics, antiparkinson drugs, antidepressants:* Increased anticholinergic action

3 *Barbiturates:* Induction, decreased effect of thiethylperazine

3 *β-blockers:* Augmented pharmacologic action of both drugs

3 *Bromocriptine:* Neuroleptic drugs inhibit bromocriptine's ability to lower prolactin concentration

3 *Epinephrine:* Reversed pressor response to epinephrine

3 *Levodopa:* Inhibited antiparkinsonian effect of levodopa

3 *Lithium:* Lowered serum concentration of both drugs in combination

3 *Narcotic analgesics:* Hypotension with meperidine, caution with other narcotic analgesics

3 *Orphenadrine:* Lower thiethylperazine concentration and excessive anticholinergic effects

SPECIAL CONSIDERATIONS

- Effective antiemetic agent for the treatment of postoperative nausea and vomiting, nausea and vomiting secondary to mildly emetic chemotherapeutic agents, and vomiting secondary to radiation therapy and toxins
- No comparisons with prochlorperazine
- More extrapyramidal reactions than chlorpromazine and promazine; thiethylperazine would be less desirable than these agents in patients where the occurrence of a dystonic reaction would be hazardous (i.e., head and neck surgery patients, patients with severe pulmonary disease, patients with a history of dyskinetic reactions)

PATIENT/FAMILY EDUCATION
- Avoid hazardous activities, activities requiring alertness
- Notify the physician of any visual disturbances

MONITORING PARAMETERS
- Respiratory status initially
- Blood pressure
- Intake and output

---

thioridazine hydrochloride

(thye-or-rid'-a-zeen)

Rx: Mellaril, Thioridazine Intensol

Chemical Class: Piperazine phenothiazine derivative

Therapeutic Class: Antipsychotic

CLINICAL PHARMACOLOGY

Mechanism of Action: A phenothiazine that blocks dopamine at postsynaptic receptor sites. Possesses strong anticholinergic and sedative effects. ***Therapeutic Effect:*** Suppresses behavioral response in psychosis; reduces locomotor activity and aggressiveness.

INDICATIONS AND DOSAGES

Psychosis

PO

Adults, Elderly, Children 12 yr and older. Initially, 25-100 mg 3 times a day; dosage increased gradually. Maximum: 800 mg/day.

Children 2-11 yr. Initially, 0.5 mg/kg/day in 2-3 divided doses. Maximum: 3 mg/kg/day.

AVAILABLE FORMS
- *Oral Solution (Concentrate [Thioridazine Intensol]):* 30 mg/ml.
- *Tablets (Mellaril):* 10 mg, 15 mg, 25 mg, 50 mg, 100 mg, 150 mg, 200 mg.

UNLABELED USES: Treatment of behavioral problems in children, dementia, depressive neurosis

CONTRAINDICATIONS: Angle-closure glaucoma, blood dyscrasias, cardiac arrhythmias, cardiac or hepatic impairment, concurrent use of drugs that prolong QT interval, severe CNS depression

PREGNANCY AND LACTATION: Pregnancy category C

SIDE EFFECTS

Occasional

Drowsiness during early therapy, dry mouth, blurred vision, lethargy, constipation or diarrhea, nasal congestion, peripheral edema, urine retention

Rare

Ocular changes, altered skin pigmentation (in those taking high doses for prolonged periods), photosensitivity, darkening of urine

SERIOUS REACTIONS
- Prolonged QT interval may produce torsades de pointes, a form of ventricular tachycardia, and sudden death.

INTERACTIONS

Drugs

3 *Alcohol, CNS depressants:* May increase respiratory depression and the hypotensive effects of thioridazine

3 *Anticholinergics, antiparkinson drugs, antidepressants:* Increased anticholinergic action

3 *Antithyroid agents:* May increase the risk of agranulocytosis

3 *Barbiturates:* Induction, decreased effect of thioridazine

3 *β-blockers:* Augmented pharmacologic action of both drugs

3 *Bromocriptine:* Neuroleptic drugs inhibit bromocriptine's ability to lower prolactin concentration; reverse not common

3 *Epinephrine:* Reversed pressor response
3 *Levodopa:* Inhibited antiparkinsonian effect
3 *Lithium:* Lowered serum concentration of both drugs in combination
3 *MAOIs, tricyclic antidepressants:* May increase the anticholinergic and sedative effects of thioridazine
3 *Narcotic analgesics:* Hypotension with meperidine, caution with other narcotic analgesics
3 *Orphenadrine:* Lower thioridazine concentration and excessive anticholinergic effects
3 *Phenylpropanolamine:* Patient on thioridazine died after single dose of phenylpropanolamine; a causal relationship was not established
2 *Ziprasidone:* May prolong the QTc interval and ECG; may increase the risk of ventricular arrhythmias

Labs

- *False positive:* Pregnancy tests, serum tricyclic antidepressants screen

SPECIAL CONSIDERATIONS

- Phenothiazine with weak potency, low incidence of EPS, but high incidence of sedation, anticholinergic effects, and cardiovascular effects

PATIENT/FAMILY EDUCATION

- Arise slowly from reclining position
- Avoid abrupt withdrawal
- Use a sunscreen during sun exposure
- Caution with activities requiring complete mental alertness (e.g., driving), may cause sedation
- Provide full information on risks of tardive dyskinesia
- Full therapeutic effect may take up to 6 wks to appear
- Notify the physician of any visual disturbances
- Avoid alcohol and exposure to artificial light and sunlight during thioridazine therapy

MONITORING PARAMETERS

- Blood pressure, CBC, EKG, serum potassium level, and liver function test results, including serum alkaline phosphatase, bilirubin, AST (SGOT), and ALT (SGPT) levels
- Therapeutic response, such as improvement in self-care and ability to concentrate, increased interest in surroundings, and relaxed facial expression
- Therapeutic serum level for thioridazine is 0.2-2.6 mcg/ml, and the toxic serum level is not established

---

thiothixene

(thye-oh-thix′-een)

Rx: Navane

Chemical Class: Thioxanthene derivative

Therapeutic Class: Antipsychotic

CLINICAL PHARMACOLOGY

Mechanism of Action: An antipsychotic that blocks postsynaptic dopamine receptor sites in brain. Has alpha-adrenergic blocking effects, and depresses the release of hypothalamic and hypophyseal hormones. ***Therapeutic Effect:*** Suppresses psychotic behavior.

Pharmacokinetics

Well absorbed from the GI tract after IM administration. Widely distributed. Metabolized in the liver. Primarily excreted in urine. Unknown if removed by hemodialysis. ***Half-life:*** 34 hr.

INDICATIONS AND DOSAGES
Mild to moderate psychosis
PO
Adults, Elderly, Children 12 yr and older. 2 mg 3 times a day up to 20-30 mg/day.
Severe psychosis
PO
Adults, Elderly, Children 12 yr and older. Initially, 5 mg twice a day. May increase gradually up to 60 mg/day.
Rapid tranquilization of agitated patient
PO
Adults, Elderly. 5-10 mg q15-30min. Total dose: 15-30 mg.
AVAILABLE FORMS
• *Capsules:* 1 mg, 2 mg, 5 mg, 10 mg, 20 mg.
• *Oral Concentrate:* 5 mg/ml.
• *Injection:* 5 mg of thiothixene and 59.6 mg of mannitol per ml when reconstituted with 2.2 ml of sterile water for injection.
CONTRAINDICATIONS: Blood dyscrasias, circulatory collapse, CNS depression, coma, history of seizures
PREGNANCY AND LACTATION: Pregnancy category C
SIDE EFFECTS
Expected
Hypotension, dizziness, syncope (occur frequently after first injection, occasionally after subsequent injections, and rarely with oral form)
Frequent
Transient drowsiness, dry mouth, constipation, blurred vision, nasal congestion
Occasional
Diarrhea, peripheral edema, urine retention, nausea
Rare
Ocular changes, altered skin pigmentation (in those taking high doses for prolonged periods), photosensitivity
SERIOUS REACTIONS
• The most common extrapyramidal reaction is akathisia, characterized by motor restlessness and anxiety. Akinesia, marked by rigidity, tremor, increased salivation, mask-like facial expression, and reduced voluntary movements, occurs less frequently. Dystonias, including torticollis, opisthotonos, and oculogyric crisis, occur rarely.
• Tardive dyskinesia, characterized by tongue protrusion, puffing of the cheeks, and chewing or puckering of the mouth, occurs rarely but may be irreversible. Elderly female patients have a greater risk of developing this reaction.
• Grand mal seizures may occur in epileptic patients, especially those receiving the drug by IM administration.
• Neuroleptic malignant syndrome occurs rarely.
INTERACTIONS
Drugs
3 *Alcohol, other CNS depressants:* May increase CNS and respiratory depression and the hypotensive effects of thiothixene
3 *Anticholinergics, antiparkinson drugs, antidepressants:* Increased anticholinergic action
3 *Barbiturates:* Induction, decreased effect of thiothixene
3 *β-blockers:* Augmented pharmacologic action of both drugs
3 *Bromocriptine:* Thiothixene inhibits bromocriptine's ability to lower prolactin concentration, reverse not common
3 *Epinephrine:* Reversed pressor response
3 *Guanethidine:* Inhibited antihypertensive response to guanethidine

3 *Kava kava, St. John's wort, valerian:* May increase CNS depression
3 *Levodopa:* Inhibited antiparkinsonian effect
3 *Lithium:* Lowered serum concentration of both drugs in combination
3 *Narcotic analgesics:* Hypotension with meperidine, caution with other narcotic analgesics
3 *Orphenadrine:* Lower thiothixene concentration and excessive anticholinergic effects
3 *Quinidine:* May increase cardiac effects

SPECIAL CONSIDERATIONS

- High-potency antipsychotic with a relatively high incidence of EPS, but a low incidence of sedation, anticholinergic effects, and cardiovascular effects

PATIENT/FAMILY EDUCATION

- Informed consent regarding risks of tardive dyskinesia; orthostatic hypotension
- Full therapeutic effect may take up to 6 wks to appear
- Avoid tasks that require mental alertness or motor skills until response to the drug has been established; drowsiness generally subsides during continued therapy
- Avoid alcohol and artificial light or direct sunlight
- Take sips of tepid water and chew sugarless gum to relieve dry mouth

MONITORING PARAMETERS

- Blood pressure hypotension
- Pattern of daily bowel activity and stool consistency
- Monitor the patient for extrapyramidal reactions and early signs of tardive dyskinesia and potentially fatal neuroleptic malignant syndrome (such as altered mental status, fever, irregular pulse or blood pressure, and muscle rigidity)
- Therapeutic response, such as improvement in self-care and ability to concentrate, increased interest in surroundings, and relaxed facial expression

---

thyroid

(thye'-roid)

Rx: Armour Thyroid, Nature-Throid NT, Westhroid

Chemical Class: Thyroid hormone in natural state

Therapeutic Class: Thyroid hormone

CLINICAL PHARMACOLOGY

Mechanism of Action: A natural hormone derived from animal sources, usually beef or pork, that is involved in normal metabolism, growth, and development, especially the central nervous system (CNS) of infants. Possesses catabolic and anabolic effects. Provides both levothyroxine and liothyronine hormones. ***Therapeutic Effect:*** Increases basal metabolic rate, enhances gluconeogenesis, stimulates protein synthesis.

Pharmacokinetics

Partially absorbed from the gastrointestinal (GI) tract. Protein binding: 99%. Widely distributed. Metabolized in liver to active, liothyronine (T_3), and inactive, reverse triiodothyronine (rT_3), metabolites. Eliminated by biliary excretion. ***Half-life:*** 2-7 days.

INDICATIONS AND DOSAGES

Hypothyroidism

PO

Adults, Elderly. Initially, 15-30 mg. May increase by 15-mg increments q2-4wks. Maintenance: 60-120 mcg/day. Use 15 mg in patients with cardiovascular disease or myxedema.

Children 12 yrs and older. 90 mg/day.
Children 6-12 yrs. 60-90 mg/day.
Children older than 1-5 yrs. 45-60 mg/day.
Children older than 6-12 mos. 30-45 mg/day.
Children 3 mos and younger. 15-30 mg/day.

AVAILABLE FORMS

- *Capsules:* 15 mg, 30 mg, 60 mg, 90 mg, 120 mg, 180 mg, 240 mg.
- *Tablets:* 30 mg, 32.5 mg, 60 mg, 65 mg, 120 mg, 130 mg, 180 mg.
- 15 mg, 30 mg, 60 mg, 90 mg, 120 mg, 180 mg, 240 mg, 300 mg (Armour Thyroid).
- 32.4 mg, 64.8 mg, 129.6 mg, 194.4 mg (Nature-Throid NT, Westhroid).

CONTRAINDICATIONS: Uncontrolled adrenal cortical insufficiency, untreated thyrotoxicosis, treatment of obesity, uncontrolled angina, uncontrolled hypertension, uncontrolled myocardial infarction, and hypersensitivity to any component of the formulations

PREGNANCY AND LACTATION: Pregnancy category A; little or no transplacental passage at physiologic serum concentrations; excreted into breast milk in low concentrations (inadequate to protect a hypothyroid infant; too low to interfere with neonatal thyroid screening programs)

SIDE EFFECTS

Rare

Dry skin, GI intolerance, skin rash, hives, severe headache

SERIOUS REACTIONS

- Excessive dosage produces signs and symptoms of hyperthyroidism including weight loss, palpitations, increased appetite, tremors, nervousness, tachycardia, hypertension, headache, insomnia, and menstrual irregularities.
- Cardiac arrhythmias occur rarely.

INTERACTIONS

Drugs

3 *Antidiabetics:* May decrease the effects of insulin and oral hypoglycemics

3 *Bile acid sequestrants:* Reduced serum thyroid hormone concentrations

3 *Carbamazepine, phenytoin, rifampin:* Increases elimination of thyroid hormones; may increase dosage requirements

3 *Estrogens, oral contraceptives:* May decrease the effects of thyroid hormones

3 *Oral anticoagulants:* Thyroid hormones increase catabolism of vitamin K–dependent clotting factors; an increase or decrease in clinical thyroid status will increase or decrease the hypoprothrombinemic response to oral anticoagulants

3 *Theophylline:* Reduced serum theophylline concentrations with initiation of thyroid therapy

SPECIAL CONSIDERATIONS

- Although used traditionally, natural hormones less clinically desirable due to varying potencies, inconsistent clinical effects, and more adverse stimulatory effects; synthetic derivatives (i.e., levothyroxine) preferred

PATIENT/FAMILY EDUCATION

- Do not discontinue the drug
- Follow-up office visits and thyroid function tests are essential
- Take drug at the same time each day, preferably in the morning
- Notify the physician if chest pain, insomnia, nervousness, tremors, or weight loss occurs

MONITORING PARAMETERS

- TSH yearly

tiagabine hydrochloride

(tye-ah'-gah-been hye-droe-klor'-ide)

Rx: Gabitril

Chemical Class: Nipecotic acid derivative

Therapeutic Class: Anticonvulsant

CLINICAL PHARMACOLOGY

Mechanism of Action: An anticonvulsant that enhances the activity of gamma-aminobutyric acid, the major inhibitory neurotransmitter in the CNS. ***Therapeutic Effect:*** Inhibits seizures.

Pharmacokinetics

Rapidly and nearly completely absorbed after PO administration. Protein binding: 96%. Metabolized in liver. Eliminated in urine and feces. Not removed by hemodialysis. ***Half-life:*** 7-9 hr.

INDICATIONS AND DOSAGES

Adjunctive treatment of partial seizures

PO

Adults, Elderly. Initially, 4 mg once a day. May increase by 4-8 mg/day at weekly intervals. Maximum: 56 mg/day.

Children 12-18 yr. Initially, 4 mg once a day. May increase by 4 mg at week 2 and by 4-8 mg at weekly intervals thereafter. Maximum: 32 mg/day.

AVAILABLE FORMS

• *Tablets:* 2 mg, 4 mg, 12 mg, 16 mg.

UNLABELED USES: Bipolar disorder

CONTRAINDICATIONS: None known.

PREGNANCY AND LACTATION: Pregnancy category C

SIDE EFFECTS

Frequent (34%-20%)

Dizziness, asthenia, somnolence, nervousness, confusion, headache, infection, tremor

Occasional

Nausea, diarrhea, abdominal pain, impaired concentration

SERIOUS REACTIONS

• Overdose is characterized by agitation, confusion, hostility, and weakness. Full recovery occurs within 24 hrs.

INTERACTIONS

Drugs

3 *Anticonvulsants (hepatic enzyme inducers—i.e., barbiturates, carbamazepine, phenytoin, primidone):* Decreased tiagabine levels and effect

3 *Ginkgo biloba:* May increase anticonvulsant effectiveness

3 *Rifampin:* Decreased tiagabine levels and effect via hepatic enzyme induction

3 *Valproate:* Increased tiagabine free blood levels

SPECIAL CONSIDERATIONS

• Patients should exercise caution with initiation and dosage titration when driving, operating hazardous machinery, or other activities requiring mental concentration; patients should be advised to take the medication with food, to delay peak effects to avoid many CNS adverse effects

PATIENT/FAMILY EDUCATION

• Change positions slowly from recumbent to sitting position before standing if patient experiences dizziness

• Avoid tasks that require mental alertness or motor skills until response to the drug is established

• Avoid alcohol while taking tiagabine

MONITORING PARAMETERS

- Perform periodic CBCs and blood chemistry tests to assess hepatic and renal function
- Signs of clinical improvement, such as a decrease in the frequency or intensity of seizures

ticarcillin disodium/clavulanate potassium

(tye-car-sill'-in/klav'-yoo-lan-ate)

Rx: Timentin

Chemical Class: Penicillin derivative, extended-spectrum

Therapeutic Class: Antibiotic

CLINICAL PHARMACOLOGY

Mechanism of Action: Ticarcillin binds to bacterial cell walls, inhibiting cell wall synthesis. Clavulanate inhibits the action of bacterial beta-lactamase. ***Therapeutic Effect:*** Ticarcillin is bactericidal in susceptible organisms. Clavulanate protects ticarcillin from enzymatic degradation.

Pharmacokinetics

Widely distributed. Protein binding: ticarcillin 45%-60%, clavulanate 9%-30%. Minimally metabolized in the liver. Primarily excreted unchanged in urine. Removed by hemodialysis. ***Half-life:*** 1-1.2 hr (increased in impaired renal function).

INDICATIONS AND DOSAGES

Skin and skin-structure, bone, joint, and lower respiratory tract infections; septicemia; endometriosis

IV

Adults, Elderly. 3.1 g (3 g ticarcillin) q4-6h. Maximum: 18-24 g/day.

Children 3 mos and older. 200-300 mg (as ticarcillin) q4-6h.

UTIs

IV

Adults, Elderly. 3.1 g q6-8h.

Dosage in renal impairment

Dosage interval is modified based on creatinine clearance.

Creatinine Clearance	*Dosage Interval*
10-30 ml/min	Usual dose q8h
less than 10 ml/min	Usual dose q12h

AVAILABLE FORMS

- *ADD-Vantage Vial:* 3.1 g.
- *Powder for Injection:* 3.1 g.
- *Premixed Solution for Infusion:* 3.1 g/100 ml.

CONTRAINDICATIONS: Hypersensitivity to any penicillin or clavulanic acid

PREGNANCY AND LACTATION: Pregnancy category B; excreted into breast milk in low concentrations; compatible with breast-feeding

SIDE EFFECTS

Frequent

Phlebitis or thrombophlebitis (with IV dose), rash, urticaria, pruritus, altered smell or taste

Occasional

Nausea, diarrhea, vomiting

Rare

Headache, fatigue, hallucinations, bleeding or ecchymosis

SERIOUS REACTIONS

- Overdosage may produce seizures and other neurologic reactions.
- Antibiotic-associated colitis and other superinfections may result from bacterial imbalance.
- Severe hypersensitivity reactions, including anaphylaxis, occur rarely.

INTERACTIONS

Drugs

3 *Aminoglycosides:* Inactivation of aminoglycosides *in vitro* and *in vivo,* reducing the aminoglycoside effect

3 *Anticoagulants, heparin, NSAIDs, thrombolytics:* Increased risk of bleeding

3 *Probenecid:* May increase ticarcillin blood concentration and risk of toxicity

Labs

• *False increase:* Urine glucose

SPECIAL CONSIDERATIONS

• Synergistic with aminoglycosides
• Sodium content, 5.2 mEq/g ticarcillin
• For reliable activity against *Pseudomonas,* must be dosed q4h

PATIENT/FAMILY EDUCATION

• Notify the physician of pain, redness, or swelling at infusion site

MONITORING PARAMETERS

• Signs and symptoms of superinfection, including anal or genital pruritus, diarrhea, increased fever, sore throat, vomiting, and pain or stomatitis
• Electrolytes

ticlopidine hydrochloride

(tye-kloe′-pi-deen hye-droe-klor′-ide)

Rx: Ticlid

Chemical Class: Thienopyridine derivative

Therapeutic Class: Antiplatelet agent

CLINICAL PHARMACOLOGY

Mechanism of Action: An aggregation inhibitor that inhibits the release of adenosine diphosphate from activated platelets, which prevents fibrinogen from binding to glycoprotein IIb/IIIa receptors on the surface of activated platelets. ***Therapeutic Effect:*** Inhibits platelet aggregation and thrombus formation.

Pharmacokinetics

Rapidly absorbed following PO administration. Protein binding: 98%. Extensively metabolized in liver. Primarily excreted in urine; partially eliminated in feces. ***Half-life:*** 12.6 hr.

INDICATIONS AND DOSAGES

Prevention of stroke

PO

Adults, Elderly. 250 mg twice a day.

AVAILABLE FORMS

• *Tablets:* 250 mg.

UNLABELED USES: Prevention of postoperative deep vein thrombosis (DVT), protection of aortocoronary bypass grafts, reduction of graft loss after renal transplant, treatment of intermittent claudication, sickle cell disease, subarachnoid hemorrhage, diabetic microangiopathy, ischemic heart disease

CONTRAINDICATIONS: Active pathologic bleeding, such as bleeding peptic ulcer and intracranial bleeding; hematopoietic disorders, including neutropenia and thrombocytopenia; presence of hemostatic disorder; severe hepatic impairment

PREGNANCY AND LACTATION: Pregnancy category B; use caution in nursing mothers

SIDE EFFECTS

Frequent (13%-5%)

Diarrhea, nausea, dyspepsia, including heartburn, indigestion, GI discomfort, and bloating

Rare (2%-1%)

Vomiting, flatulence, pruritus, dizziness

SERIOUS REACTIONS

• Neutropenia occurs in approximately 2% of patients.
• Thrombotic thrombocytopenia purpura, agranulocytosis, hepatitis, cholestatic jaundice, and tinnitus occur rarely.

INTERACTIONS

Drugs

3 *Aspirin, heparin, oral anticoagulants, thrombolytics:* May increase the risk of bleeding with these drugs

3 *Cyclosporine:* Potential for reduction in blood cyclosporine concentrations

3 *Phenytoin:* Inhibition of hepatic metabolism (CYP2C9) of phenytoin; potential for development of phenytoin toxicity, reduction in phenytoin dose may be necessary

3 *Theophylline:* Increased theophylline level via inhibition of metabolism, increased risk of toxicity

SPECIAL CONSIDERATIONS

• Due to the risk of life-threatening neutropenia or agranulocytosis and cost, ticlopidine should be reserved for patients intolerant to aspirin or who fail aspirin

MONITORING PARAMETERS

• CBC q2wk for first 3 mo of therapy, then periodically thereafter
• Pattern of daily bowel activity and stool consistency
• Heart sounds
• Blood pressure for hypotension
• Skin for erythema and rash
• Hepatic enzyme levels
• Observe for signs of bleeding

tiludronate disodium

(tye-loo-droe'-nate dye-soe'-dee-um)

Rx: Skelid

Chemical Class: Pyrophosphate analog

Therapeutic Class: Bisphosphonate; bone resorption inhibitor

CLINICAL PHARMACOLOGY

Mechanism of Action: A calcium regulator that inhibits functioning osteoclasts through disruption of cytoskeletal ring structure and inhibition of osteoclastic proton pump. ***Therapeutic Effect:*** Inhibits bone resorption.

Pharmacokinetics

Well absorbed following PO administration. Protein binding: 90%. Not metabolized in liver. ***Half-life:*** 150 hr.

INDICATIONS AND DOSAGES

Paget's disease

PO

Adults, Elderly. 400 mg once a day for 3 mo. Must take with 6-8 oz plain water. Do not give within 2 hr of food intake. Avoid giving aspirin, calcium supplements, mineral supplements, or antacids within 2 hr of tiludronate administration.

AVAILABLE FORMS

• *Tablets:* 200 mg.

CONTRAINDICATIONS: GI disease, such as dysphagia and gastric ulcer, impaired renal function

PREGNANCY AND LACTATION: Pregnancy category C; dose-related scoliosis; avoid exposure in children

SIDE EFFECTS

Frequent (9%-6%)

Nausea, diarrhea, generalized body pain, back pain, headache

Occasional
Rash, dyspepsia, vomiting, rhinitis, sinusitis, dizziness

SERIOUS REACTIONS

• Dysphagia, esophagitis, esophageal ulcer, and gastric ulcer occur rarely.

INTERACTIONS

Drugs

❷ *Food:* Reduces bioavailability 90%

❷ *Antacids/calcium:* Reduces bioavailability 60%-80%

❸ *Aspirin:* Decreases bioavailability of tiludronate by 50%

❸ *Indomethacin:* Bioavailability of NSAID increased 2-4-fold

SPECIAL CONSIDERATIONS

• Studies needed to assess place in therapy with other bisphosphonates
• Inhibition of bone loss in osteoporosis may persist up to 2 yr after 6 mo of treatment and discontinuation of drug

PATIENT/FAMILY EDUCATION

• Take with 6-8 oz plain water; do not take within 2 hr of food or other medications
• Consult the physician to determine if patient needs calcium and vitamin D supplements

MONITORING PARAMETERS

• Adjusted serum calcium, serum alkaline phosphatase, osteocalcin, and urinary hydroxyproline levels to assess the effectiveness of tiludronate

timolol maleate

(tim'-oh-lol)

Rx: Betimol, Blocadren, Istadol Timolol Ophthalmic, Timoptic, Timoptic OccuDose, Timoptic Ocumeter, Timoptic Ocumeter Plus, Timoptic XE

Combinations

Rx: Ophthalmic with dorzolamide (Cosopt)

Chemical Class: β-adrenergic blocker, nonselective

Therapeutic Class: Antianginal; antiglaucoma agent; antihypertensive

CLINICAL PHARMACOLOGY

Mechanism of Action: An antihypertensive, antimigraine, and antiglaucoma agent that blocks $beta_1$- and $beta_2$-adrenergic receptors. ***Therapeutic Effect:*** Reduces intraocular pressure (IOP) by reducing aqueous humor production, lowers BP, slows the heart rate, and decreases myocardial contractility.

Pharmacokinetics

Route	Onset	Peak	Duration
PO	15-45 mins	0.5-2.5 hrs	4 hrs
Ophthalmic	30 mins	1-2 hrs	12-24 hrs

Well absorbed from the GI tract. Protein binding: 60%. Minimal absorption after ophthalmic administration. Metabolized in the liver. Primarily excreted in urine. Not removed by hemodialysis. ***Half-life:*** 4 hr. Systemic absorption may occur with ophthalmic administration.

INDICATIONS AND DOSAGES

Mild to moderate hypertension

PO

Adults, Elderly. Initially, 10 mg twice a day, alone or in combination with other therapy. Gradually increase at intervals of not less than 1 wk. Maintenance: 20-60 mg/day in 2 divided doses.

Reduction of cardiovascular mortality in definite or suspected acute MI

PO

Adults, Elderly. 10 mg twice a day, beginning 1-4 wks after infarction.

Migraine prevention

PO

Adults, Elderly. Initially, 10 mg twice a day. Range: 10-30 mg/day.

Reduction of IOP in open-angle glaucoma, aphakic glaucoma, ocular hypertension, and secondary glaucoma

Ophthalmic

Adults, Elderly, Children. 1 drop of 0.25% solution in affected eye(s) twice a day. May be increased to 1 drop of 0.5% solution in affected eye(s) twice a day. When IOP is controlled, dosage may be reduced to 1 drop once a day. If patient is switched to timolol from another antiglaucoma agent, administer concurrently for 1 day. Discontinue other agent on following day.

Ophthalmic (Timoptic XE)

Adults, Elderly. 1 drop/day.

Ophthalmic (Istalol)

Adults, Elderly. Apply once daily.

AVAILABLE FORMS

• *Tablets (Blocadren):* 5 mg, 10 mg, 20 mg.

• *Ophthalmic Gel (Timoptic-XE):* 0.25%, 0.5%.

• *Ophthalmic Solution (Betimol, Timoptic, Timoptic OccuDose, Timoptic Ocumeter, Timoptic Ocumeter Plus):* 0.25%, 0.5%.

UNLABELED USES: *Systemic:* Treatment of anxiety, cardiac arrhythmias, chronic angina pectoris, hypertrophic cardiomyopathy, migraine, pheochromocytoma, thyrotoxicosis, tremors

Ophthalmic: To decrease IOP in acute or chronic angle-closure glaucoma, treatment of angle-closure glaucoma during and after iridectomy, malignant glaucoma, secondary glaucoma

CONTRAINDICATIONS: Bronchial asthma, cardiogenic shock, CHF unless secondary to tachyarrhythmias, chronic obstructive pulmonary disorder (COPD), patients receiving MAOI therapy, second- or third-degree heart block, sinus bradycardia, uncontrolled cardiac failure

PREGNANCY AND LACTATION: Pregnancy category C (D if used in second or third trimester); similar drug, atenolol, frequently used in the third trimester for treatment of hypertension (many studies of efficacy and safety of atenolol in pregnancy-induced hypertension; long-term use has been associated with intrauterine growth retardation; mean milk:plasma ratio, 0.80 in one study; quantity of drug ingested by breast-feeding infant unlikely to be therapeutically significant

SIDE EFFECTS

Frequent

Diminished sexual function, drowsiness, difficulty sleeping, unusual tiredness or weakness

Ophthalmic: Eye irritation, visual disturbances

Occasional

Depression, cold hands or feet, diarrhea, constipation, anxiety, nasal congestion, nausea, vomiting

Rare

Altered taste, dry eyes, itching, numbness of fingers, toes, or scalp

SERIOUS REACTIONS

• Overdose may produce profound bradycardia, hypotension, and bronchospasm.

• Abrupt withdrawal may result in diaphoresis, palpitations, headache, and tremors.

• Timolol administration may precipitate CHF and MI in patients with cardiac disease; thyroid storm in those with thyrotoxicosis; and peripheral ischemia in those with existing peripheral vascular disease.

• Hypoglycemia may occur in patients with previously controlled diabetes.

• Ophthalmic overdose may produce bradycardia, hypotension, bronchospasm, and acute cardiac failure.

INTERACTIONS

Drugs

3 *α_1-adrenergic blockers:* Potential enhanced first-dose response (marked initial drop in blood pressure, particularly on standing [especially prazocin])

3 *Amiodarone:* Combined therapy may lead to bradycardia, cardiac arrest, or ventricular dysrhythmia

3 *Antidiabetics:* β-blockers increase blood glucose and impair peripheral circulation; altered response to hypoglycemia by prolonging the recovery of normoglycemia, causing hypertension, and blocking tachycardia

3 *Clonidine:* Hypertension occurring upon withdrawal of clonidine may be exacerbated by timolol

3 *Digoxin:* Additive prolongation of atrioventricular (AV) conduction time

3 *Dihydropyridine calcium channel blockers:* Additive hypotension (kinetic and dynamic)

3 *Diltiazam:* Potentiates β-adrenergic effects; hypotension, left ventricular failure, and AV conduction disturbances problematic in elderly, patients with left ventricular dysfunction, aortic stenosis, or with large doses of either drug

3 *Disopyramide:* Additive negative inotropic cardiac effects

3 *Epinephrine:* Enhanced pressor response (hypertension and bradycardia)

3 *Hypoglycemic agents:* Masked hypoglycemia, hyperglycemia

3 *Isoproterenol:* Reduced isoproterenol efficacy in asthma

3 *Methyldopa:* Potential for development of hypertension in the presence of increased catecholamines

3 *Nonsteroidal antiinflammatory drugs:* Reduced antihypertensive effects of timolol

3 *Phenylephrine:* Potential for hypertensive episodes when administered together

3 *Prazosin:* First-dose response to prazosin may be enhanced by β-blockade

3 *Quinidine:* Increased timolol concentrations

3 *Sympathomimetics, xanthines:* May mutually inhibit effects

3 *Tacrine:* Additive bradycardia

3 *Theophylline:* Antagonistic pharmacodynamic effects

3 *Verapamil:* Potentiates β-adrenergic effects; hypotension, left ventricular failure, and AV conduction disturbances problematic in elderly, patients with left ventricular dysfunction, aortic stenosis, or with large doses of either drug

SPECIAL CONSIDERATIONS

• Currently available β-blockers appear to be equally effective; cardioselective or combined α- and β-adrenergic blockade are less likely to cause undesirable effects and may be preferred

PATIENT/FAMILY EDUCATION

• Do not discontinue abruptly; may require taper; rapid withdrawal may produce rebound hypertension or angina

• Avoid tasks that require mental alertness or motor skills until response to the drug has been established

• Notify the physician if excessive fatigue, prolonged dizziness or headache, or shortness of breath occurs
• Do not use nasal decongestants and OTC cold preparations, especially those containing stimulants, without physician approval
• Limit alcohol and salt intake

MONITORING PARAMETERS
• *Angina:* Reduction in nitroglycerin usage; frequency, severity, onset, and duration of angina pain; heart rate
• *Arrhythmias:* Heart rate
• *Congestive heart failure:* Functional status, cough, dyspnea on exertion, paroxysmal nocturnal dyspnea, exercise tolerance, and ventricular function
• *Hypertension:* Blood pressure
• *Migraine headache:* Reduction in the frequency, severity, and duration of attacks
• *Post myocardial infarction:* Left ventricular function, lower resting heart rate
• *Toxicity:* Blood glucose, bronchospasm, hypotension, bradycardia, depression, confusion, hallucination, sexual dysfunction

tinidazole

(tin-nid'-ah-zole)

Rx: Tindamax

Chemical Class: Nitroimidazole derivative

Therapeutic Class: Antibiotic; antiprotozoal

CLINICAL PHARMACOLOGY

Mechanism of Action: A nitroimidazole derivative that is converted to the active metabolite by reduction of cell extracts of *Trichomonas*. The active metabolite causes DNA damage in pathogens. ***Therapeutic Effect:*** Produces antiprotozoal effect.

Pharmacokinetics

Rapidly and completely absorbed. Protein binding: 12%. Distributed in all body tissues and fluids; crosses blood-brain barrier. Significantly metabolized. Primarily excreted in urine; partially eliminated in feces. ***Half-life:*** 12-14 hr.

INDICATIONS AND DOSAGES

Intestinal amebiasis

PO

Adults, Elderly. 2 g/day for 3 days.

Children 3 yrs and older. 50 mg/kg/day (up to 2 g) for 3 days.

Amebic hepatic abscess

PO

Adults, Elderly. 2 g/day for 3-5 days.

Children 3 yrs and older. 50 mg/kg/day (up to 2 g) for 3-5 days.

Giardiasis

PO

Adults, Elderly. 2 g as a single dose.

Children 3 yrs and older. 50 mg/kg (up to 2 g) as a single dose.

Trichomoniasis

PO

Adults, Elderly. 2 g as a single dose.

AVAILABLE FORMS
• *Tablets:* 250 mg, 500 mg.

CONTRAINDICATIONS: First trimester of pregnancy, hypersensitivity to nitroimidazole derivatives

PREGNANCY AND LACTATION: Pregnancy category C

SIDE EFFECTS

Occasional (4%-2%)

Metallic or bitter taste, nausea, weakness, fatigue or malaise

Rare (less than 2%)

Epigastric distress, anorexia, vomiting, headache, dizziness, red-brown or darkened urine

SERIOUS REACTIONS

- Peripheral neuropathy, characterized by paresthesia, is usually reversible if tinidazole treatment is stopped as soon as neurologic symptoms appear.
- Superinfection, hypersensitivity reaction, and seizures occur rarely.

INTERACTIONS

Drugs

3 *Alcohol:* May cause a disulfiram-type reaction

3 *Cholestyramine, oxytetracycline:* May decrease the effectiveness of tinidazole; separate dosage times

3 *Cimetidine, fosphenytoin, ketoconazole, phenobarbital, rifampin:* Decreases the metabolism of tinidazole

3 *Cyclosporine, fluorouracil, lithium, phenytoin (IV), tacrolimus:* May increase blood levels of these drugs

3 *Disulfiram:* May increase the risk of psychotic reactions (separate dose by 2 wks)

3 *Oral anticoagulants:* Increases the risk of bleeding

SPECIAL CONSIDERATIONS

- Also effective for bacterial vaginosis, but not FDA approved

PATIENT/FAMILY EDUCATION

- For trichomoniasis, treat sexual partner; tinidazole may induce candidiasis
- Take with food
- May turn urine red-brown or darken it
- Avoid alcoholic beverages and alcohol-containing preparations (such as cough syrups) during therapy and for 3 days afterward
- Avoid performing tasks that require mental alertness or motor skills if dizziness occurs as a side effect of tinidazole use

MONITORING PARAMETERS

- CBC with WBC differential if retreatment is necessary
- Be alert for neurologic symptoms, including dizziness and paresthesia of the extremities
- Assess for nausea and vomiting and initiate appropriate measures
- Observe for evidence of superinfection, such as anal or genital pruritus, furry tongue, stomatitis, and vaginal discharge

tinzaparin sodium

(tin-za'-pa-rin soe'-dee-um)

Rx: Innohep

Chemical Class: Heparin derivative, depolymerized; low-molecular-weight heparin

Therapeutic Class: Anticoagulant

CLINICAL PHARMACOLOGY

Mechanism of Action: A low-molecular-weight heparin that inhibits factor Xa. Causes less inactivation of thrombin, inhibition of platelets, and bleeding than standard heparin. Does not significantly influence bleeding time, PT, aPTT. ***Therapeutic Effect:*** Produces anticoagulation.

Pharmacokinetics

Well absorbed after subcutaneous administration. Primarily eliminated in urine. ***Half-life:*** 3-4 hr.

INDICATIONS AND DOSAGES

Deep vein thrombosis (DVT)

Subcutaneous

Adults, Elderly. 175 anti-Xa international units/kg once a day. Continue for at least 6 days and until patient is sufficiently anticoagulated with warfarin (INR of 2 or more for 2 consecutive days).

AVAILABLE FORMS

• *Injection:* 20,000 anti-Xa international units/ml.

CONTRAINDICATIONS: Active major bleeding, concurrent heparin therapy, hypersensitivity to heparin, sulfites, benzyl alcohol, or pork products, thrombocytopenia associated with positive *in vitro* test for antiplatelet antibody

PREGNANCY AND LACTATION: Pregnancy category B; low-molecular-weight heparins have been used to prevent and treat thromboembolic disease during pregnancy in lieu of warfarin, which is a known teratogen; excretion into breast milk unknown but thought to be minimal based on pharmacokinetic parameters; use caution in nursing mothers

SIDE EFFECTS

Frequent (16%)

Injection site reaction, such as inflammation, oozing, nodules, and skin necrosis

Rare (less than 2%)

Nausea, asthenia, constipation, epistaxis

SERIOUS REACTIONS

• Overdose may lead to bleeding complications ranging from local ecchymoses to major hemorrhage. Antidote: Dose of protamine sulfate (1% solution) should be equal to dose of tinzaparin injected. One mg protamine sulfate neutralizes 100 units of tinzaparin. A second dose of 0.5 mg tinzaparin per 1 mg protamine sulfate may be given if aPTT tested 2-4 hrs after the initial infusion remains prolonged.

INTERACTIONS

Drugs

3 *Antiplatelet agents (aspirin, ticlopidine, clopidogrel, dipyridamole, NSAIDs), thrombolytics:* Increased risk of hemorrhage

3 *Ginkgo biloba:* Increased risk of bleeding

3 *Oral anticoagulants:* Additive anticoagulant effects

Labs

• *Increase:* AST, ALT

SPECIAL CONSIDERATIONS

• Cannot be used interchangeably with unfractionated heparin or other low-molecular-weight heparin products

PATIENT/FAMILY EDUCATION

• Administer by deep SC inj into abdominal wall; alternate inj sites

• Do not rub inj site after completion of the inj

• Report any unusual bruising or bleeding to clinician

MONITORING PARAMETERS

• Periodic CBC with platelets

• Monitoring aPTT is not required

• Consider anti-factor Xa monitoring in patients with impaired renal function, during pregnancy, and in very small or obese patients

• Assess signs of bleeding, including bleeding at injection or surgical sites or from gums, blood in stool, bruising, hematuria, and petechiae

tioconazole

(tye-oh-kon′-a-zole)

OTC: Vagistat-1, Monistat-1

Chemical Class: Imidazole derivative

CLINICAL PHARMACOLOGY

Mechanism of Action: An imidazole derivative that inhibits synthesis of ergosterol (vital component of fungal cell formation). ***Therapeutic Effect:*** Damaging fungal cell membrane. Fungistatic.

Pharmacokinetics

Negligible absorption from vaginal application.

T

INDICATIONS AND DOSAGES

Vulvovaginal candidiasis

Intravaginal

Adults, Elderly. 1 applicatorful just before bedtime as a single dose.

AVAILABLE FORMS

• *Vaginal Ointment:* 6.5% (Monistat-1, Vagistat-1).

CONTRAINDICATIONS: Hypersensitivity to tioconazole or other imidazole antifungal agents

PREGNANCY AND LACTATION: Pregnancy category C; excretion into breast milk unknown

SIDE EFFECTS

Frequent (25%)

Headache

Occasional (6%-1%)

Burning, itching

Rare (less than 1%)

Irritation, vaginal pain, dysuria, dryness of vaginal secretions, vulvar edema/swelling

SERIOUS REACTIONS

• None reported.

SPECIAL CONSIDERATIONS

• Similar in efficacy to miconazole, econazole, and clotrimazole for the topical management of fungal skin infections; choice determined by cost and availability; additional efficacy vs trichomoniasis with longer course of therapy

PATIENT/FAMILY EDUCATION

• Avoid contact with eyes

• Separate personal items that come in contact with affected areas

• Avoid using condoms or diaphragms within 72 hrs of administration of tioconazole

MONITORING PARAMETERS

• Assess the patient for vaginal irritation

tiopronin

(tye-o-pro′-nin)

Rx: Thiola

Chemical Class: Thiol derivative

Therapeutic Class: Anti-kidney stone agent

CLINICAL PHARMACOLOGY

Mechanism of Action: A sulfhydryl compound with similar properties to those of penicillamine and glutathione that undergoes thiol-disulfide exchange with cysteine to form tiopronin-cysteine, a mixed disulfide. This disulfide is water soluble, unlike cysteine, and does not crystallize in the kidneys. May break disulfide bonds present in bronchial secretions and break the mucus complexes. ***Therapeutic Effect:*** Decreases cysteine excretion.

Pharmacokinetics

Moderately absorbed from the gastrointestinal (GI) tract. Primarily excreted in urine. Following oral administration, up to 48% of dose appears in urine during the first 4 hrs and up to 78% by 72 hrs. ***Half-life:*** 53 hrs.

INDICATIONS AND DOSAGES

Crystinuria

PO

Adults, Elderly. Initially, 800 mg in 3 divided doses. Adjust and maintain crystine concentration below its solubility limit (usually less than 250 mg/L).

Children 9 yrs and older. 15 mg/kg/day in 3 divided doses. Adjust and maintain crystine concentration below its solubility limit (usually less than 250 mg/L).

AVAILABLE FORMS

• *Tablets:* 100 mg (Thiola).

UNLABELED USES: Cataracts, epilepsy, hepatitis, rheumatoid arthritis
CONTRAINDICATIONS: History of agranulocytosis, aplastic anemia, or thrombocytopenia while on tiopronin, pregnancy and lactation, hypersensitivity to tiopronin or its components
PREGNANCY AND LACTATION: Pregnancy category C; excreted in breast milk and may cause adverse effects in nursing infant; mothers taking tiopronin should avoid nursing
SIDE EFFECTS
Frequent
Pain, swelling, tenderness of skin, rash, hives, itching, oral ulcers
Occasional
GI upset, taste or smell impairment, bloody or cloudy urine, chills, difficulty in breathing, high blood pressure, hoarseness, joint pain, swelling of feet or lower legs, tenderness of glands
Rare
Chest pain, cough, difficulty in chewing, talking, swallowing, double vision, general feeling of discomfort, illness, weakness, muscle weakness, spitting up blood, swelling of lymph glands
SERIOUS REACTIONS
- Hematologic abnormalities, including myelosuppression, unusual bleeding, drug fever, renal complications, and lupus erythematous-like reaction including fever, arthralgia, and lymphadenopathy rarely occur.

SPECIAL CONSIDERATIONS
- May be associated with fever and less severe adverse reactions than *d*-penicillamine

PATIENT/FAMILY EDUCATION
- Take on an empty stomach
- Increase fluid intake to at least 3 L of fluid

MONITORING PARAMETERS
- CBC
- Liver function
- Urinary cystine

tiotropium bromide
(tee-oh-tro′-pee-um bro′-mide)
Rx: Spiriva
Chemical Class: Quaternary ammonium compound
Therapeutic Class: COPD agent; bronchodilator

CLINICAL PHARMACOLOGY
Mechanism of Action: An anticholinergic that binds to recombinant human muscarinic receptors at the smooth muscle, resulting in long-acting bronchial smooth-muscle relaxation. ***Therapeutic Effect:*** Relieves bronchospasm.
Pharmacokinetics

Route	*Onset*	*Peak*	*Duration*
Inhalation	N/A	N/A	24-36 hrs

Binds extensively to tissue. Protein binding: 72%. Metabolized by oxidation. Excreted in urine. ***Half-life:*** 5-6 days.
INDICATIONS AND DOSAGES
Chronic obstructive pulmonary disease (COPD)
Inhalation
Adults, Elderly. 18 mcg (1 capsule)/day via HandiHaler inhalation device.
AVAILABLE FORMS
- *Powder for Inhalation:* 18 mcg/capsule (in blister packs containing 6 capsules with inhaler).

CONTRAINDICATIONS: History of hypersensitivity to atropine or its derivatives, including ipratropium
PREGNANCY AND LACTATION: Pregnancy category C; based on rodent studies, tiotropium is excreted into breast milk; the excretion in hu-

man milk is unknown but due to quaternary chemical structure, low degree of systemic absorption following INH, and minimal systemic absorption following oral ingestion, the expected exposure in a nursing infant would not be high; carefully assess risks and benefits in nursing mothers

SIDE EFFECTS

Frequent (16%-6%)

Dry mouth, sinusitis, pharyngitis, dyspepsia, UTI, rhinitis

Occasional (5%-4%)

Abdominal pain, peripheral edema, constipation, epistaxis, vomiting, myalgia, rash, oral candidiasis

SERIOUS REACTIONS

• Angina pectoris, depression, and flu-like symptoms occur rarely.

INTERACTIONS

Drugs

3 *Iptratropium:* Potential for additive anticholinergic effects

SPECIAL CONSIDERATIONS

• Compared to ipratropium is more expensive, but once-daily administration will likely improve adherence with therapy

PATIENT/FAMILY EDUCATION

• Capsules should NOT be swallowed; use only 1 capsule for inhalation at a time

• Refer to product information for instructions on how to administer tiotropium via the HandiHaler device

• Should NOT be used for immediate relief of breathing problems, i.e., as a rescue medication

• Do NOT store capsules in the HandiHaler

• Rinse the mouth with water immediately after inhalation to prevent mouth and throat dryness and oral candidiasis

• Drink plenty of fluids to decrease the thickness of lung secretions

• Avoid excessive consumption of caffeine products, such as chocolate, cocoa, cola, coffee, and tea

MONITORING PARAMETERS

• Improvement in symptoms, such as cessation of clavicular retractions, quieter and slower respirations, and a relaxed facial expression, reduction in the need for rescue short-acting $beta_2$-agonists

• Pulse rate and quality and respiratory rate, depth, rhythm, and type

• ABG levels

• Examine lips and fingernails for signs of cyanosis, such as a blue or gray color in light-skinned patients and a gray color in dark-skinned patients

---

tirofiban hydrochloride

(tye-roe-fye′-ban hye-droe-klor′-ide)

Rx: Aggrastat

Chemical Class: Glycoprotein (GP) IIb/IIIa inhibitor

Therapeutic Class: Antiplatelet agent

CLINICAL PHARMACOLOGY

Mechanism of Action: An antiplatelet and antithrombotic agent that binds to platelet receptor glycoprotein IIb/IIIa, preventing binding of fibrinogen. ***Therapeutic Effect:*** Inhibits platelet aggregation and thrombus formation.

Pharmacokinetics

Poorly bound to plasma proteins; unbound fraction in plasma: 35%. Limited metabolism. Primarily eliminated in the urine (65%) and, to a lesser amount, in the feces. Removed by hemodialysis. ***Half-life:*** 2 hrs. Clearance is significantly decreased in severe renal impairment (creatinine clearance less than 30 ml/min).

INDICATIONS AND DOSAGES

Inhibition of platelet aggregation

IV

Adults, Elderly. Initially, 0.4 mcg/kg/min for 30 min; then continue at 0.1 mcg/kg/min through procedure and for 12-24 hrs after procedure.

Severe renal insufficiency (creatinine clearance less than 30 ml/min)

Adults, Elderly. Half the usual rate of infusion.

AVAILABLE FORMS

• *Injection Premix:* 12.5 mg/250 ml, 25 mg/500 ml (50 mcg/ml).

• *Vial:* 250 mcg/ml.

CONTRAINDICATIONS: Active internal bleeding or a history of bleeding diathesis within previous 30 days, arteriovenous malformation or aneurysm, history of intracranial hemorrhage, history of thrombocytopenia after prior exposure to tirofiban, intracranial neoplasm, major surgical procedure within previous 30 days, severe hypertension, stroke

PREGNANCY AND LACTATION: Pregnancy category B; excretion into breast milk unknown; use caution in nursing mothers

SIDE EFFECTS

Occasional (6%-3%)

Pelvis pain, bradycardia, dizziness, leg pain

Rare (2%-1%)

Edema and swelling, vasovagal reaction, diaphoresis, nausea, fever, headache

SERIOUS REACTIONS

• Signs and symptoms of overdose include generally minor mucocutaneous bleeding and bleeding at the femoral artery access site.

• Thrombocytopenia occurs rarely.

INTERACTIONS

Drugs

3 *Antithrombotics (aspirin, heparin, warfarin, ticlopidine, clopidogrel):* Increased risk of bleeding

SPECIAL CONSIDERATIONS

• When bleeding cannot be controlled with pressure discontinue INF

• Most major bleeding occurs at arterial access site for cardiac catheterization; prior to pulling femoral artery sheath, discontinue heparin for 3-4 hrs and document activated clotting time (ACT) <180 sec or aPTT <45 sec; achieve sheath hemostasis ≥ 4 hr before discharge

• In clinical studies, patients received ASA unless it was contraindicated

• Tirofiban, eptifibitide, and abciximab can all decrease the incidence of cardiac events associated with acute coronary syndromes; direct comparisons are needed to establish which, if any, is superior; for angioplasty, until more data become available, abciximab appears to be the drug of choice

PATIENT/FAMILY EDUCATION

• It may take longer to stop bleeding during tirofiban therapy

• Report unusual bleeding

• The patient should notify his or her dentist and other physicians of tirofiban therapy before surgery is scheduled or new drugs are prescribed

MONITORING PARAMETERS

• Platelet count, hemoglobin, hematocrit, PT/aPTT (baseline, within 6 hr following bolus dose, then daily thereafter)

• Closely monitor the patient for bleeding, particularly at other arterial and venous puncture sites and IM injection sites

tizanidine hydrochloride

(tye-zan'-i-deen hye-droe-klor'-ide)

Rx: Zanaflex

Chemical Class: Imidazoline derivative

Therapeutic Class: Skeletal muscle relaxant

CLINICAL PHARMACOLOGY

Mechanism of Action: A skeletal muscle relaxant that increases presynaptic inhibition of spinal motor neurons mediated by alpha$_2$-adrenergic agonists, reducing facilitation to postsynaptic motor neurons. ***Therapeutic Effect:*** Reduces muscle spasticity.

Pharmacokinetics

Route	*Onset*	*Peak*	*Duration*
PO	N/A	1-2 hrs	3-6 hrs

Well absorbed following PO administration. Protein binding: 30%. Extensive first-pass metabolism. Metabolized in the liver. Partially excreted in urine; minimal elimination in feces. ***Half-life:*** 4-8 hr.

INDICATIONS AND DOSAGES

Muscle spasticity

PO

Adults, Elderly. Initially, 2-4 mg, gradually increased in 2- to 4-mg increments and repeated q6-8h. Maximum: 3 doses/day or 36 mg/24 hr.

AVAILABLE FORMS

- *Tablets:* 2 mg, 4 mg.

UNLABELED USES: Low back pain, spasticity associated with multiple sclerosis or spinal cord injury, tension headaches, trigeminal neuralgia

CONTRAINDICATIONS: None known.

PREGNANCY AND LACTATION: Pregnancy category C; lipid soluble, may pass into breast milk

SIDE EFFECTS

Frequent (49%-41%)

Dry mouth, somnolence, asthenia

Occasional (16%-4%)

Dizziness, UTI, constipation

Rare (3%)

Nervousness, amblyopia, pharyngitis, rhinitis, vomiting, urinary frequency

SERIOUS REACTIONS

- Hypotension (a reduction in either diastolic or systolic BP) may be associated with bradycardia, orthostatic hypotension and, rarely, syncope. The risk of hypotension increases as dosage increases; BP may decrease within 1 hr after administration.

INTERACTIONS

Drugs

3 *Alcohol, other CNS depressants:* May increase CNS depressant effects

3 *Antihypertensives:* May increase tizanidine's hypotensive potential

2 *Clonidine, guanabenz, guanadrel, guanethidine, guanfacine:* Potential for hypotension, avoid concurrent use

3 *Oral contraceptives:* Decreased clearance of tizanidine

3 *Phenytoin:* May increase serum levels and risk of toxicity of phenytoin

SPECIAL CONSIDERATIONS

PATIENT/FAMILY EDUCATION

- Arise slowly from a reclining position
- Tizanidine may cause low blood pressure, impaired coordination, and sedation
- Avoid tasks that require mental alertness or motor skills until response to the drug has been established
- Change positions slowly to help prevent dizziness

MONITORING PARAMETERS

- Perform periodic liver and renal function tests
- Evaluate the patient for a therapeutic response, such as decreased stiffness, tenderness, and intensity of skeletal muscle pain and improved mobility

---

tobramycin sulfate

(toe-bra-mye'-sin sul'-fate)

Rx: AK-Tob, Nebcin, Nebcin Pediatric, PMS-Tobramycin, TOBI, Tobrex

Combinations

Rx: Ophthalmic: with dexamethasone (Tobradex)

Chemical Class: Aminoglycoside

Therapeutic Class: Antibiotic

CLINICAL PHARMACOLOGY

Mechanism of Action: An aminoglycoside antibiotic that irreversibly binds to protein on bacterial ribosomes. ***Therapeutic Effect:*** Interferes with protein synthesis of susceptible microorganisms.

Pharmacokinetics

Rapid, complete absorption after IM administration. Protein binding: less than 30%. Widely distributed (does not cross the blood-brain barrier; low concentrations in cerebrospinal fluid (CSF). Excreted unchanged in urine. Removed by hemodialysis. ***Half-life:*** 2-4 hr (increased in impaired renal function and neonates; decreased in cystic fibrosis and febrile or burn patients).

INDICATIONS AND DOSAGES

Usual parenteral dosage

IV

Adults, Elderly. 3-6 mg/kg/day in 3 divided doses. Once-daily dosing: 4-7 mg/kg every 24 hr.

Children 7 days and older. 6-7.5 mg/kg/day in 3-4 divided doses.

Children younger than 7 days. 2.5-4 mg/kg/day in 2 divided doses.

Superficial eye infections, including blepharitis, conjunctivitis, keratitis, and corneal ulcers

Ophthalmic ointment

Adults, Elderly. Usual dosage, apply a thin strip to conjunctiva q8-12h (q3-4h for severe infections).

Ophthalmic solution

Adults, Elderly. Usual dosage, 1-2 drops in affected eye q4h (2 drops/hr for severe infections).

Bronchopulmonary infections in patients with cystic fibrosis

Inhalation solution

Adults. Usual dosage, 60-80 mg twice a day for 28 days, then off for 28 days.

Children. 40-80 mg 2-3 times a day.

Dosage in renal impairment

Dosage and frequency are modified based on the degree of renal impairment and the serum drug concentration. After a loading dose of 1-2 mg/kg, the maintenance dose and frequency are based on serum creatinine levels and creatinine clearance.

AVAILABLE FORMS

- *Injection Solution:* 10 mg/ml (Nebcin Pediatric), 40 mg/ml (Nebcin).
- *Injection Powder for Reconstitution (Nebcin):* 1.2 g.
- *Ophthalmic Ointment (Tobrex):* 0.3%.
- *Ophthalmic Solution (AKTob, Tobrex):* 0.3%.
- *Nebulization Solution (TOBI):* 60 mg/ml.

CONTRAINDICATIONS: Hypersensitivity to other aminoglycosides (cross-sensitivity) and their components

PREGNANCY AND LACTATION: Pregnancy category C (B, opthalmic form); excreted into breast milk; given poor oral absorption, toxicity minimal; limited to modification of bowel flora and interference with interpretation of culture results if fever workup required

SIDE EFFECTS

Occasional

IM: Pain, induration

IV: Phlebitis, thrombophlebitis

Topical: Hypersensitivity reaction (fever, pruritus, rash, urticaria)

Ophthalmic: Tearing, itching, redness, eyelid swelling

Rare

Hypotension, nausea, vomiting

SERIOUS REACTIONS

- Nephrotoxicity (as evidenced by increased BUN and serum creatinine levels and decreased creatinine clearance) may be reversible if the drug is stopped at the first sign of nephrotoxic symptoms.
- Irreversible ototoxicity (manifested as tinnitus, dizziness, ringing or roaring in ears, and hearing loss) and neurotoxicity (manifested as headache, dizziness, lethargy, tremor, and visual disturbances) occur occasionally. The risk of these reactions increases with higher dosages or prolonged therapy and when the solution is applied directly to the mucosa.
- Superinfections, particularly fungal infections, may result from bacterial imbalance with any administration route.
- Anaphylaxis may occur.

INTERACTIONS

Drugs

3 *Amphotericin B:* Synergistic nephrotoxicity

2 *Atracurium:* Tobramycin potentiates respiratory depression by atracurium

3 *Carbenicillin:* Potential for inactivation of tobramycin in patients with renal failure

3 *Carboplatin:* Additive nephrotoxicity or ototoxicity

3 *Cephalosporins:* Increased potential for nephrotoxicity in patients with preexisting renal disease

3 *Cisplatin:* Additive nephrotoxicity or ototoxicity

3 *Cyclosporine:* Additive nephrotoxicity

2 *Ethacrynic acid:* Additive ototoxicity

3 *Indomethacin:* Reduced renal clearance of tobramycin in premature infants

3 *Methoxyflurane:* Additve nephrotoxicity

2 *Neuromuscular blocking agents:* Tobramycin potentiates respiratory depression by neuromuscular blocking agents

3 *NSAIDs:* May reduce renal clearance of tobramycin

3 *Penicillins (extended spectrum):* Potential for inactivation of tobramycin in patients with renal failure

3 *Piperacillin:* Potential for inactivation of tobramycin in patients with renal failure

2 *Succinylcholine:* Tobramycin potentiates respiratory depression by succinylcholine

3 *Ticarcillin:* Potential for inactivation of tobramycin in patients with renal failure

3 *Vancomycin:* Additive nephrotoxicity or ototoxicity

2 *Vecuronium:* Tobramycin potentiates respiratory depression by vecuronium

SPECIAL CONSIDERATIONS

- Gentamicin is first-line aminoglycoside of choice; differences in toxicity between gentamicin and tobramycin not likely to be clinically important in most patients with normal renal function given short courses of

treatment; consider tobramycin in patients who are more likely to develop toxicity (prolonged and/or recurrent aminoglycoside therapy, those with renal failure) and in patients infected with *Pseudomonas aeruginosa* because of increased antibacterial activity
• Has been administered via nebulizer to treat resistant pneumonia in patients with cystic fibrosis

PATIENT/FAMILY EDUCATION
• Notify the physician if any balance, hearing, urinary, or vision problems develop, even after therapy is completed
• The patient using ophthalmic tobramycin should know that irritation, redness, blurred vision, or tearing may occur briefly after application
• Notify the physician if these symptoms persist

MONITORING PARAMETERS
• Serum Ca, Mg, Na; serum concentrations, peak (30 min following IV INF or 1 hr after IM inj) and trough (just prior to next dose); prolonged concentrations above 12 mcg/ml or trough levels above 2 mcg/ml may indicate tissue accumulation; such accumulation, advanced age, and cumulative dosage may contribute to ototoxicity and nephrotoxicity; perform serum concentration assays after 2 or 3 doses, so that the dosage can be adjusted if necessary, and at 3- to 4-day intervals during therapy; in the event of changing renal function, more frequent serum concentrations should be obtained and the dosage or dosage interval adjusted according to more detailed guidelines

tocainide hydrochloride

(toe-kay'-nide)

Rx: Tonocard

Chemical Class: Lidocaine derivative

Therapeutic Class: Antiarrhythmic, class IB

CLINICAL PHARMACOLOGY

Mechanism of Action: An amide-type local anesthetic that shortens the action potential duration and decreases the effective refractory period and automaticity in the His-Purkinje system of the myocardium by blocking sodium transport across myocardial cell membranes. ***Therapeutic Effect:*** Suppresses ventricular arrhythmias.

Pharmacokinetics

Very rapidly and completely absorbed following PO administration. Protein binding: 10%. Metabolized in liver. Excreted in urine. ***Half-life:*** 15 hr.

INDICATIONS AND DOSAGES

Suppression and prevention of ventricular arrhythmias

PO

Adults, Elderly. Initially, 400 mg q8h. Maintenance: 1.2-1.8 g/day in divided doses q8h. Maximum: 2400 mg/day.

AVAILABLE FORMS
• *Tablets:* 400 mg, 600 mg.

UNLABELED USES: Trigeminal neuralgia

CONTRAINDICATIONS: Hypersensitivity to local anesthetics, second- or third-degree AV block

PREGNANCY AND LACTATION: Pregnancy category C; excreted into breast milk; not recommended in nursing mothers

SIDE EFFECTS

Tocainide is generally well tolerated.

Frequent (10%-3%)

Minor, transient light-headedness, dizziness, nausea, paresthesia, rash, tremor

Occasional (3%-1%)

Clammy skin, night sweats, myalgia

Rare (less than 1%)

Restlessness, nervousness, disorientation, mood changes, ataxia (muscular incoordination), visual disturbances

SERIOUS REACTIONS

- High dosage may produce bradycardia or tachycardia, hypotension, palpitations, increased ventricular arrhythmias, premature ventricular contractions (PVCs), chest pain, and exacerbation of CHF.

INTERACTIONS

Drugs

3 *Antacids:* Antacids that increase urinary pH may increase tocainide serum concentrations

3 *β-blockers:* May increase pulmonary wedge pressure and decrease cardiac index

3 *Other antiarrhythmics:* May increase risk of adverse cardiac effects

3 *Rifampin:* Reduction of serum tocainide concentrations

SPECIAL CONSIDERATIONS

- Can be considered oral lidocaine; antidysrhythmic drugs have not been shown to improve survival in patients with ventricular dysrhythmias; class I antidysrhythmic drugs (e.g., tocainide) have increased the risk of death when used in patients with non–life-threatening dysrhythmias
- Initiate therapy in facilities capable of providing continuous ECG monitoring and managing life-threatening dysrhythmias

PATIENT/FAMILY EDUCATION

- Avoid tasks that require mental alertness or motor skills until response to the drug has been established
- Notify the physician of any breathing difficulties, palpitations, or tremor
- May be taken with food

MONITORING PARAMETERS

- Blood concentrations (therapeutic concentrations 4-10 mcg/ml)
- Monitor the patient's EKG for changes, particularly shortening of the QT interval; notify the physician of significant interval changes
- Fluid status and serum electrolyte levels
- Intake and output
- Weight
- Assess the patient's hand movements for tremor, which is usually the first sign that the maximum dose is being reached
- Monitor the patient for numbness or tingling in the feet or hands
- Assess the patient's skin for clamminess and rash
- Observe the patient for CNS disturbances, including disorientation, incoordination, mood changes, and restlessness
- Assess the patient for signs and symptoms of CHF, including distended neck veins, dyspnea (particularly on exertion or lying down), night cough, and peripheral edema

tolazamide

(tole-az'-a-mide)

Rx: Tolinase

Chemical Class: Sulfonylurea (1st generation)

Therapeutic Class: Antidiabetic; hypoglycemic

CLINICAL PHARMACOLOGY

Mechanism of Action: A first-generation sulfonylurea that promotes release of insulin from beta cells of pancreas. ***Therapeutic Effect:*** Lowers blood glucose concentration.

Pharmacokinetics

Well absorbed from the gastrointestinal (GI) tract. Extensively metabolized in liver to 5 metabolites, 3 which are active. Primarily excreted in urine. Unknown if removed by hemodialysis. ***Half-life:*** 7 hrs.

INDICATIONS AND DOSAGES

Diabetes mellitus

PO

Adults, Elderly. Initially, 100-250 mg once a day, with breakfast or first main meal. Maintenance: 100-1000 mg once a day. May increase by increments of 100-250 mg at weekly intervals, based on blood glucose response. May increase by 100-250 mg/day at weekly intervals. Maximum: 1000 mg/day. Doses more than 500 mg/day should be given in 2 divided doses with meals.

AVAILABLE FORMS

• *Tablets:* 100 mg, 250 mg, 500 mg; 100 mg, 250 mg (Tolinase).

UNLABELED USES: None known.

CONTRAINDICATIONS: Diabetic complications, such as ketosis, acidosis, and diabetic coma; sole therapy for type 1 diabetes mellitus; hypersensitivity to tolazamide or its components

PREGNANCY AND LACTATION: Pregnancy category D; inappropriate for use during pregnancy due to inadequacy for blood glucose control, potential for prolonged neonatal hypoglycemia, and risk for congenital abnormalities; insulin is the drug of choice for control of blood sugars during pregnancy; breast milk excretion data is not available—again, the potential for neonatal hypoglycemia dictates caution in nursing mothers

SIDE EFFECTS

Frequent

Altered taste sensation, dizziness, drowsiness, weight gain, constipation, diarrhea, heartburn, nausea, vomiting, stomach fullness, headache

Occasional

Increased sensitivity of skin to sunlight, peeling of skin, itching, rash

SERIOUS REACTIONS

• Severe hypoglycemia may occur due to overdosage and insufficient food intake, especially with increased glucose demands.

• GI hemorrhage, cholestatic hepatic jaundice, leukopenia, thrombocytopenia, pancytopenia, agranulocytosis, and aplastic or hemolytic anemia occurs rarely.

INTERACTIONS

Drugs

3 *Anabolic steroids, chloramphenicol, clofibrate, cyclic antidepressants, MAOIs, sulfonamides:* Enhanced hypoglycemic effects

3 *β-blockers:* Alter response to hypoglycemia, increase blood glucose concentrations

3 *Clonidine:* Diminished symptoms of hypoglycemia

3 *Ethanol:* Altered glycemic control, usually hypoglycemia

3 *Oral anticoagulants:* Dicoumarol, not warfarin, enhances hypoglycemic response

3 *Oral contraceptives:* Impaired glucose tolerance

3 *Rifampin:* Reduced serum levels, reduced hypoglycemic activity

SPECIAL CONSIDERATIONS

• Similar clinical effect as second generations (e.g., glyburide, glipizide); usually less expensive

PATIENT/FAMILY EDUCATION

• Home blood glucose monitoring
• Multiple drug interactions, including alcohol and salicylates
• Symptoms of hypoglycemia: tingling lips/tongue, nausea, confusion, fatigue, sweating, hunger, visual changes (spots)
• Carry candy, sugar packets, or other sugar supplements for immediate reponse to hypoglycemia
• Notify the physician when glucose demands are altered, such as with fever, heavy physical activity, infection, stress, or trauma

MONITORING PARAMETERS

• Self-monitored blood glucoses; glycosolated hemoglobin q3-6 mos

tolbutamide

(tole-byoo'-ta-mide)

Rx: Orinase, Orinase Diagnostic

Chemical Class: Sulfonylurea (1st generation)

Therapeutic Class: Antidiabetic; hypoglycemic

CLINICAL PHARMACOLOGY

Mechanism of Action: A first-generation sulfonylurea that promotes the release of insulin from beta cells of pancreas. ***Therapeutic Effect:*** Lowers blood glucose concentration.

Pharmacokinetics

Route	Onset	Peak	Duration
PO	1 hr	5-8 hrs	12-24 hrs
IV	N/A	30-45 min	90-181 min

Well absorbed from the gastrointestinal (GI) tract. Protein binding: 80%-99%. Extensively metabolized in liver to 2 inactive metabolites, primarily via oxidation. Excreted in urine. Removed by hemodialysis. ***Half-life:*** 4.5-6.5 hrs.

INDICATIONS AND DOSAGES

Diabetes mellitus

PO

Adults. Initially, 1 g daily, with breakfast or first main meal, or in divided doses. Maintenance: 0.25-3 g once a day. After dose of 2 g is reached, dosage should be increased in increments of up to 2 mg q1-2wks, based on blood glucose response. Maximum: 3 g/day.

Endocrine tumor diagnosis

IV

Adults. 1 g infused over 2-3 mins.

AVAILABLE FORMS

• *Tablets:* 500 mg (Orinase, Tol-Tab).
• *Injection, powder for reconstitution:* 1 g (Orinase Diagnostic).

CONTRAINDICATIONS: Diabetic ketoacidosis with or without coma, sole therapy for type 1 diabetes mellitus, use in children, hypersensitivity to tolbutamide or any component of its formulation

PREGNANCY AND LACTATION: Pregnancy category C; inappropriate for use during pregnancy due to inadequacy for blood glucose control, potential for prolonged neonatal hypoglycemia, and risk of congenital abnormalities; insulin is the drug of choice for control of blood sugars during pregnancy; milk-to-plasma ratio of 0.25 reported; the potential for neonatal hypoglycemia dictates caution in nursing mothers

SIDE EFFECTS

Frequent

Increased sensitivity of skin to sunlight, peeling of skin, itching, rash, dizziness, drowsiness, weight gain, constipation, diarrhea, heartburn, nausea, headache, pain at injection site

Occasional

Altered taste sensation, constipation, vomiting, stomach fullness

SERIOUS REACTIONS

- Severe hypoglycemia may occur because of overdosage or insufficient food intake, especially with increased glucose demands.
- Cardiovascular mortality has been reported as higher in patients treated with tolbutamide.
- GI hemorrhage, cholestatic hepatic jaundice, leukopenia, thrombocytopenia, pancytopenia, agranulocytosis, and aplastic or hemolytic anemia occurs rarely.

INTERACTIONS

Drugs

3 *Anabolic steroids, aspirin, chloramphenicol, MAOIs, sulfonamides:* Enhanced hypoglycemic effects

3 *β-blockers:* Alter response to hypoglycemia

⚠ *Ethanol:* Altered glycemic control, usually hypoglycemia; "Antabuse"-like reaction

3 *Fluconazole, halofenate, itraconazole, ketoconazole, miconazole:* Increased serum concentrations of tolbutamide and other sulfonylureas

3 *Oral anticoagulants:* Dicoumarol, not warfarin, enhances hypoglycemic response to tolbutamide

❷ *Phenylbutazone:* Increased hypoglycemic action

3 *Rifabutin, rifampin:* Reduced serum levels, reduced hypoglycemic activity

3 *Trimethoprim-sulfamethoxazole:* Increases plasma concentration of tolbutamide; may enhance hypoglycemic effects

Labs

- *False increase:* Serum AST, CSF protein
- *Interference:* Urinary albumin

SPECIAL CONSIDERATIONS

- Possible differences exist for tolbutamide (short duration of action, hepatic clearance), potential preferred choice in older patients with poor general physical status and renal impairment

PATIENT/FAMILY EDUCATION

- Multiple drug interactions, including alcohol and salicylates
- Symptoms of hypoglycemia: tingling lips/tongue, nausea, confusion, fatigue, sweating, hunger, visual changes (spots)
- Carry candy, sugar packets, or other sugar supplements for immediate response to hypoglycemia
- Notify the physician when glucose demands are altered, such as with fever, heavy physical activity, infection, stress, or trauma

MONITORING PARAMETERS

- Self-monitored blood glucoses; glycosolated hemoglobin q3-6 mo

---

tolcapone

(tole′-ka-pone)

Rx: Tasmar

Chemical Class: Catechol-*O*-methyl-tranferase (COMT) inhibitor; nitrocatechol

Therapeutic Class: Anti-Parkinson's agent

CLINICAL PHARMACOLOGY

Mechanism of Action: An antiparkinson agent that inhibits the enzyme catechol-*O*-methyltransferase (COMT), potentiating dopamine activity and increasing the duration of action of levodopa. ***Therapeutic Effect:*** Relieves signs and symptoms of Parkinson's disease.

Pharmacokinetics

Rapidly absorbed after PO administration. Protein binding: 99%. Metabolized in the liver. Eliminated primarily in urine (60%) and, to a lesser extent, in feces (40%). Unknown if removed by hemodialysis. ***Half-life:*** 2-3 hr.

INDICATIONS AND DOSAGES

Adjunctive treatment of Parkinson's disease

PO

Adults, Elderly. Initially, 100-200 mg 3 times a day concomitantly with each dose of carbidopa and levodopa. Maximum: 600 mg/day.

Dosage in hepatic impairment

Patients with moderate to severe cirrhosis should not receive more than 200 mg tolcapone 3 times a day.

AVAILABLE FORMS

- *Tablets:* 100 mg, 200 mg.

CONTRAINDICATIONS: None known.

PREGNANCY AND LACTATION: Pregnancy category C; use caution in nursing mothers

SIDE EFFECTS

Alert: Frequency of side effects increases with dosage. The following effects are based on a 200-mg dose.

Frequent (35%-16%)

Nausea, insomnia, somnolence, anorexia, diarrhea, muscle cramps, orthostatic hypotension, excessive dreaming

Occasional (11%-4%)

Headache, vomiting, confusion, hallucinations, constipation, diaphoresis, bright yellow urine, dry eyes, abdominal pain, dizziness, flatulence

Rare (3%-2%)

Dyspepsia, neck pain, hypotension, fatigue, chest discomfort

SERIOUS REACTIONS

- Upper respiratory tract infection and UTI occur in 7%-5% of patients.
- Too-rapid withdrawal from therapy may produce withdrawal-emergent hyperpyrexia, characterized by fever, muscular rigidity, and altered level of consciousness (LOC).
- Dyskinesia and dystonia occur frequently.

INTERACTIONS

Drugs

3 *Food:* Decrease tolcapone bioavailability by 10%-20% if given within 1 hr before or 2 hrs after drug administration

❷ *Nonselective MAO inhibitors (phenelzine, tranycypromine):* Inhibition of the majority of the pathways responsible for normal catecholamine metabolism

3 *Warfarin:* Possible increased hypoprothrombinemic effect of warfarin

SPECIAL CONSIDERATIONS

- Because of the risk of liver failure, use only in patients who are experiencing symptom fluctuations and are not responding to, or are not candidates for, other adjunctive therapies
- Withdraw drug from patients who fail to show substantial clinical benefit within 3 wk of initiation
- Consider having patients sign informed consent alerting them to potential risks and benefits of this drug

PATIENT/FAMILY EDUCATION

- Monitor for signs of liver disease (clay-colored stools, jaundice, dark urine, right upper quadrant tenderness, pruritus, fatigue, appetite loss, lethargy)
- Take tolcapone with food if nausea occurs

• Dizziness, drowsiness, and nausea may occur initially but will diminish or disappear with continued treatment
• Orthostatic hypotension commonly occurs during initial therapy but changing positions slowly can help prevent or minimize this effect
• Avoid tasks that require mental alertness or motor skills until response to the drug has been established
• Hallucinations occur more often in elderly patients, typically within the first 2 wks of therapy
• Urine may turn bright yellow
• The female patient should notify the physician if she is or plans to become pregnant
• Report to the physician if frequent falls occur

MONITORING PARAMETERS

• ALT/AST at baseline then q2wk for first yr of therapy, q4wk for next 6 mo, then q8wk thereafter; repeat this cycle if dose increased to 200 mg tid; **discontinue tolcapone if ALT or AST exceeds upper limit of normal or if clinical signs and symptoms suggest onset of hepatic failure**
• Plan to reduce the levodopa dosage if the patient experiences hallucinations. Keep in mind that hallucinations are usually accompanied by confusion and, to a lesser extent, insomnia
• Assess for relief of symptoms, such as improvement of mask-like facial expression, muscular rigidity, shuffling gait, and resting tremors of the hands and head

tolmetin sodium

(tole'-met-in soe'-dee-um)
Rx: Tolectin, Tolectin DS
Chemical Class: Acetic acid derivative
Therapeutic Class: NSAID; antipyretic; nonnarcotic analgesic

CLINICAL PHARMACOLOGY

Mechanism of Action: A nonsteroidal antiinflammatory that produces analgesic and antiinflammatory effect by inhibiting prostaglandin synthesis. ***Therapeutic Effect:*** Reduces inflammatory response and intensity of pain stimulus reaching sensory nerve endings.

Pharmacokinetics
Rapdily absorbed from the gastrointestinal (GI) tract. Metabolized in liver. Excreted in urine. Minimally removed by hemodialysis. ***Half-life:*** 5 hrs.

INDICATIONS AND DOSAGES

Rheumatoid arthritis, osteoarthritis
PO
Adults, Elderly. Initially, 400 mg 3 times/day (including 1 dose upon arising, 1 dose at bedtime). Adjust dose at 1-2-wk intervals. Maintenance: 600-1800 mg/day in 3-4 divided doses.

Juvenile rheumatoid arthritis
PO
Children more than 2 yrs. Initially, 20 mg/kg/day in 3-4 divided doses. Maintenance: 15-30 mg/kg/day in 3-4 divided doses.

AVAILABLE FORMS

• *Tablets:* 200 mg, 600 mg (Tolectin).
• *Capsules:* 400 mg (Tolectin DS).

UNLABELED USES: Treatment of ankylosing spondylitis, psoriatic arthritis

CONTRAINDICATIONS: Severely incapacitated, bedridden, wheelchair bound, hypersensitivity to aspirin or other NSAIDs

PREGNANCY AND LACTATION: Pregnancy category B (category D near term); small amounts excreted into breast milk; compatible with breast-feeding

SIDE EFFECTS

Occasional

Nausea, vomiting, diarrhea, abdominal cramping, dyspepsia (heartburn, indigestion, epigastric pain), flatulence, dizziness, headache, weight decrease or increase

Rare

Constipation, anorexia, rash, pruritus

SERIOUS REACTIONS

- Peptic ulcer, GI bleeding, gastritis, and severe hepatic reaction (cholestasis, jaundice) occur rarely.
- Nephrotoxicity (dysuria, hematuria, proteinuria, nephrotic syndrome) and severe hypersensitivity reaction (fever, chills, bronchospasm) occur rarely.

INTERACTIONS

Drugs

3 *Aminoglycosides:* Reduced clearance with elevated aminoglycoside levels and potential for toxicity (especially indomethacin in premature infants; other NSAIDs probably)

3 *Anticoagulants:* Excessive hypoprothrombinemia, decreased platelet aggregation with increased risk of GI bleeding

3 *Antihypertensives (α-blockers, angiotensin-converting enzyme inhibitors, angiotensin II receptor blockers, β-blockers, diuretics):* Inhibition of antihypertensive and other favorable hemodynamic effects

3 *Corticosteroids:* Increased risk of GI ulceration

3 *Cyclosporine:* Increased nephrotoxicity risk

3 *Lithium:* Decreased clearance of lithium (mediated via prostaglandins), resulting in elevated serum lithium levels and risk of toxicity

3 *Methotrexate:* Decreased renal secretion of methotrexate, resulting in elevated methotrexate levels and risk of toxicity

3 *Phenylpropanolamine:* Possible acute hypertensive reaction

3 *Potassium-sparing diuretics:* Additive hyperkalemia potential

3 *Triamterene:* Acute renal failure reported with addition of indomethacin; caution with other NSAIDs

Labs

- *False positive:* Proteinuria (use dye-impregnated reagent strips), urinary drugs of abuse screen

SPECIAL CONSIDERATIONS

PATIENT/FAMILY EDUCATION

- Therapeutic effect is usually noted in 1-3 wks
- Avoid alcohol and aspirin during therapy
- Take with food or milk if GI upset occurs
- Notify the physician if headache or GI distress occurs

MONITORING PARAMETERS

- Initial hemogram and fecal occult blood test within 3 mo of starting regular chronic therapy; repeat every 6-12 mo (more frequently in high-risk patients [>65 years, peptic ulcer disease, concurrent steroids or anticoagulants]); electrolytes, creatinine, and BUN within 3 mo of starting regular chronic therapy; repeat every 6-12 mo

tolnaftate

(tole-naf'-tate)

Rx: Absorbine Jr. Antifungal, Aftate Antifungal, Fungi-Guard, Tinactin Antifungal, Tunactin Antifungal Jock Itch, Tinaderm, Ting

Chemical Class: Carbamothioic acid derivative

Therapeutic Class: Antifungal

CLINICAL PHARMACOLOGY

Mechanism of Action: An antifungal that distorts hyphae and stunts mycelial growth in susceptible fungi. ***Therapeutic Effect:*** Results in fungal cell death.

INDICATIONS AND DOSAGES

Tinea pedis, tinea cruris, tinea corporis

Topical

Adults, Elderly, Children 2 yrs and older. Spray aerosol or apply 1-3 drops of solution or a small amount of cream, gel, or powder 2 times daily for 2-4 wks.

AVAILABLE FORMS

- *Aerosol, liquid, topical:* 1% (Aftate, Tinactin Antifungal, Ting).
- *Aerosol, powder, topical:* 1% (Aftate, Tinactin Antifungal, Tinactin Antifungal Jock Itch, Ting).
- *Cream:* 1% (Fungi-Guard, Tinactin Antifungal, Tinactin Antifungal Jock Itch).
- *Gel:* 1% (Absorbine Jr. Antifungal).
- *Powder:* 1% (Tinactin Antifungal).
- *Solution, topical:* 1% (Absorbine Jr. Antifungal, Tinaderm).

UNLABELED USES: Onchomycosis

CONTRAINDICATIONS: Nail and scalp infections, hypersensitivity to tolnaftate or any component of its formulation

PREGNANCY AND LACTATION: Pregnancy category C

SIDE EFFECTS

Rare

Irritation, burning, pruritus, contact dermatitis

SERIOUS REACTIONS

- None known.

SPECIAL CONSIDERATIONS

- Nonprescription topical antifungal agent not effective in the treatment of deeper fungal infections of the skin, nor is it reliable in the treatment of fungal infections involving the scalp or nail beds; *Candida* is resistant; useful for patients desiring self-medication of mild tinea infections; patients must be advised of limitations
- Powders generally used as adjunctive therapy, but may be acceptable as primary therapy in very mild cases

PATIENT/FAMILY EDUCATION

- Keep affected areas clean and dry and wear light clothing to promote ventilation
- Separate personal items that come in contact with affected areas
- Avoid topical cream contact with eyes, mouth, nose, or other mucous membranes
- Rub topical form well into affected and surrounding area

MONITORING PARAMETERS

- Therapeutic response

tolterodine tartrate

(tol-tare'-oh-deen tar'-trate)
Rx: Detrol, Detrol LA
Chemical Class: Tertiary amine
Therapeutic Class: Genitourinary muscle relaxant

CLINICAL PHARMACOLOGY

Mechanism of Action: An antispasmodic that exhibits potent antimuscarinic activity by interceding via cholinergic muscarinic receptors, thereby inhibiting urinary bladder contraction. ***Therapeutic Effect:*** Decreases urinary frequency, urgency.

Pharmacokinetics

Rapidly and well absorbed after PO administration. Protein binding: 96%. Extensively metabolized in the liver to active metabolite. Primarily excreted in urine. Unknown if removed by hemodialysis. ***Half-life:*** 1.9-3.7 hrs.

INDICATIONS AND DOSAGES

Overactive bladder

PO

Adults, Elderly. 1-2 mg twice a day.

Dosage in severe renal or hepatic impairment

PO

Adults, Elderly. 1 mg twice a day.

PO (extended-release)

Adults, Elderly. 2-4 mg once a day.

AVAILABLE FORMS

- *Tablets (Detrol):* 1 mg, 2 mg.
- *Capsules (Extended-Release [Detrol LA]):* 2 mg, 4 mg.

CONTRAINDICATIONS: Gastric retention, uncontrolled angle-closure glaucoma, urine retention

PREGNANCY AND LACTATION: Pregnancy category C; probably excreted in breast milk; not recommended during lactation

SIDE EFFECTS

Frequent (40%)

Dry mouth

Occasional (11%-4%)

Headache, dizziness, fatigue, constipation, dyspepsia (heartburn, indigestion, epigastric discomfort), upper respiratory tract infection, UTI, dry eyes, abnormal vision (accommodation problems), nausea, diarrhea

Rare (3%)

Somnolence, chest or back pain, arthralgia, rash, weight gain, dry skin

SERIOUS REACTIONS

- Overdose can result in severe anticholinergic effects, including abdominal cramps, facial warmth, excessive salivation or lacrimation, diaphoresis, pallor, urinary urgency, blurred vision, and prolonged QT interval.

INTERACTIONS

Drugs

3 *Clarithromycin:* Increased blood tolterodine concentration

3 *Cyclosporine:* Increased blood tolterodine concentration

3 *Erythromycin:* Increased blood tolterodine concentration

3 *Fluoxetine:* May inhibit tolterodine metabolism

3 *Itraconazole:* Increased blood tolterodine concentration

3 *Ketoconazole:* Increased blood tolterodine concentration

3 *Vinblastine:* Increased blood tolterodine concentration

SPECIAL CONSIDERATIONS

PATIENT/FAMILY EDUCATION

- Dry mouth occurs in 40% of treated patients at a dose of 2 mg bid; incidence is dose-dependent
- May cause blurred vision, GI upset or constipation, and dry eyes

MONITORING PARAMETERS

- Monitor the patient for incontinence and residual urine in the bladder

• Determine if the patient experiences a change in vision

topiramate

(toe-pyre'-a-mate)

Rx: Topamax

Chemical Class: Sulfamate-substituted monosaccharide derivative

Therapeutic Class: Anticonvulsant

CLINICAL PHARMACOLOGY

Mechanism of Action: An anticonvulsant that blocks repetitive, sustained firing of neurons by enhancing the ability of gamma-aminobutyric acid to induce an influx of chloride ions into the neurons; may also block sodium channels. ***Therapeutic Effect:*** Decreases seizure activity.

Pharmacokinetics

Rapidly absorbed after PO administration. Protein binding: 13%-17%. Not extensively metabolized. Primarily excreted unchanged in urine. Removed by hemodialysis. ***Half-life:*** 21 hrs.

INDICATIONS AND DOSAGES

Adjunctive treatment of partial seizures, Lennox-Gastant syndrome, tonic-clonic seizures

PO

Adults, Elderly, Children older than 17 yrs. Initially, 25-50 mg for 1 wk. May increase by 25-50 mg/day at weekly intervals. Maximum: 1600 mg/day.

Children 2-16 yrs. Initially, 1-3 mg/kg/day to maximum of 25 mg. May increase by 1-3 mg/kg/day at weekly intervals. Maintenance: 5-9 mg/kg/day in 2 divided doses.

Monotherapy with partial, tonic-clonic seizures

PO

Adults, Elderly, Children 10 yr and older. Initially, 25 mg twice a day. Increase at weekly intervals up to 400 mg/day according to the following schedule:

- Week 1, 25 mg twice a day
- Week 2, 50 mg twice a day
- Week 3, 75 mg twice a day
- Week 4, 100 mg twice a day
- Week 5, 150 mg twice a day
- Week 6, 200 mg twice a day

Migraine prevention

PO

Adults, Elderly. Initially, 25 mg/day. May increase by 25 mg/day at 7-day intervals up to a total daily dose of 100 mg/day in 2 divided doses.

Dosage in renal impairment

Expect to reduce drug dosage by 50% in patients with tonic-clonic seizures who have a creatinine clearance of less than 70 ml/min.

AVAILABLE FORMS

• *Capsules (Sprinkle):* 15 mg, 25 mg.

• *Tablets:* 25 mg, 50 mg, 100 mg, 200 mg.

UNLABELED USES: Treatment of alcohol dependence

CONTRAINDICATIONS: Bipolar disorder

PREGNANCY AND LACTATION: Pregnancy category C

SIDE EFFECTS

Frequent (30%-10%)

Somnolence, dizziness, ataxia, nervousness, nystagmus, diplopia, paresthesia, nausea, tremor

Occasional (9%-3%)

Confusion, breast pain, dysmenorrhea, dyspepsia, depression, asthenia, pharyngitis, weight loss, anorexia, rash, musculoskeletal pain, abdominal pain, difficulty with coordination, sinusitis, agitation, flu-like symptoms

Rare (3%-2%)
Mood disturbances, such as irritability and depression; dry mouth; aggressive behavior

SERIOUS REACTIONS

• Psychomotor slowing, impaired concentration, language problems (such as word-finding difficulties), and memory disturbances occur occasionally. These reactions are generally mild to moderate but may be severe enough to require discontinuation of drug therapy.

INTERACTIONS

Drugs

3 *Alcohol, other CNS depressants:* May increase CNS depression

3 *Phenytoin, carbamazepine, valproic acid:* Lowers topiramate concentrations

3 *Carbonic anhydrase inhibitors:* May increase the risk of renal calculi

3 *Ethinyl estradiol:* Increased clearance of estrogen

3 *Oral contraceptives:* May decrease the effectiveness of oral contraceptives

SPECIAL CONSIDERATIONS

PATIENT/FAMILY EDUCATION

• Drink plenty of fluids to prevent kidney stone formation

• Avoid breaking tablets to avoid their bitter taste

• Do not abruptly discontinue topiramate because this may precipitate seizures; strict maintenance of drug therapy is essential for seizure control

• May cause dizziness, drowsiness, or impaired thinking; avoid tasks that require mental alertness or motor skills until response to the drug is established; drowsiness usually diminishes with continued therapy

• Avoid alcohol and other CNS depressants while on topiramate therapy

• Notify the physician if blurred vision or other visual changes occurs

• The female patient should use additional or alternative means of contraception if she takes oral contraceptives because topiramate decreases contraceptive effectiveness

• The patient should always carry an identification card or wear an identification bracelet that displays seizure disorder and anticonvulsant therapy

MONITORING PARAMETERS

• Assess for clinical improvement, such as a decrease in the frequency and intensity of seizures

• Renal function test results, including BUN and serum creatinine levels

torsemide

(tore'-se-mide)

Rx: Demadex, Demadex I.V.

Chemical Class: Pyridine-sulfonamide derivative

Therapeutic Class: Antihypertensive; diuretic, loop

CLINICAL PHARMACOLOGY

Mechanism of Action: A loop diuretic that enhances excretion of sodium, chloride, potassium, and water at the ascending limb of the loop of Henle; also reduces plasma and extracellular fluid volume. ***Therapeutic Effect:*** Produces diuresis; lowers BP.

Pharmacokinetics

Route	Onset	Peak	Duration
PO	1 hr	1-2 hrs	6-8 hrs
IV	10 mins	1 hr	6-8 hrs

Rapidly and well absorbed from the GI tract. Protein binding: 97%-99%. Metabolized in the liver. Primarily excreted in urine. Not removed by hemodialysis. ***Half-life:*** 3.3 hrs.

INDICATIONS AND DOSAGES

Hypertension

PO

Adults, Elderly. Initially, 2.5-5 mg/day. May increase to 10 mg/day if no response in 4-6 wks. If no response, additional antihypertensive added.

CHF

PO, IV

Adults, Elderly. Initially, 10-20 mg/day. May increase by approximately doubling dose until desired therapeutic effect is attained. Doses greater than 200 mg have not been adequately studied.

Chronic renal failure

PO, IV

Adults, Elderly. Initially, 20 mg/day. May increase by approximately doubling dose until desired therapeutic effect is attained. Doses greater than 200 mg have not been adequately studied.

Hepatic cirrhosis

PO, IV

Adults, Elderly. Initially, 5 mg/day given with aldosterone antagonist or potassium-sparing diuretic. May increase by approximately doubling dose until desired therapeutic effect is attained. Doses greater than 40 mg have not been adequately studied.

AVAILABLE FORMS

- *Tablets (Demadex):* 5 mg, 10 mg, 20 mg, 100 mg.
- *Injection (Demadex I.V.):* 10 mg/ml.

CONTRAINDICATIONS: Anuria, hepatic coma, severe electrolyte depletion

PREGNANCY AND LACTATION: Pregnancy category B; cardiovascular disorders such as pulmonary edema, severe hypertension, or CHF are probably the only valid indications for loop diuretics during pregnancy

SIDE EFFECTS

Frequent (10%-4%)

Headache, dizziness, rhinitis

Occasional (3%-1%)

Asthenia, insomnia, nervousness, diarrhea, constipation, nausea, dyspepsia, edema, EKG changes, pharyngitis, cough, arthralgia, myalgia

Rare (less than 1%)

Syncope, hypotension, arrhythmias

SERIOUS REACTIONS

- Ototoxicity may occur with high doses or a too-rapid IV administration.
- Overdose produces acute, profound water loss; volume and electrolyte depletion; dehydration; decreased blood volume; and circulatory collapse.

INTERACTIONS

Drugs

❷ *Aminoglycosides (gentamicin, kanamycin, neomycin, streptomycin):* Additive ototoxicity (ethacrynic acid > furosemide, torsemide, bumetanide)

❸ *Amphotericin B, nephrotoxic medications, ototoxic medications:* May increase the risk of nephrotoxicity and ototoxicity

❸ *Angiotensin-converting enzyme inhibitors:* Initiation of ACEI with intensive diuretic therapy may result in precipitous fall in blood pressure; ACEIs may induce renal insufficiency in the presence of diuretic-induced sodium depletion

❸ *Anticoagulants, heparin, thrombolytics:* May decrease the effects of these drugs

❸ *Barbiturates (phenobarbital):* Reduced diuretic response

❸ *Bile acid-binding resins (cholestyramine, colestipol):* Resins markedly reduce the bioavailability and diuretic response of furosemide

❸ *Carbenoxolone:* Severe hypokalemia from coadministration

3 *Cephalosporins (cephaloridine, cephalothin):* Enhanced nephrotoxicity with coadministration
2 *Cisplatin:* Additive ototoxicity (ethacrynic acid > furosemide, torsemide, bumetanide)
3 *Clofibrate:* Enhanced effects of both drugs, especially in hypoalbuminemic patients
3 *Corticosteroids:* Concomitant loop diuretic and corticosteroid therapy can result in excessive potassium loss
3 *Digitalis glycosides (digoxin, digitoxin):* Diuretic-induced hypokalemia may increase risk of digitalis toxicity
3 *Lithium:* May increase the risk of lithium toxicity
3 *Other hypokalemia-causing medications:* May increase the risk of hypokalemia
3 *Nonsteroidal antiinflammatory drugs (flurbiprofen, ibuprofen, indomethacin, naproxen, piroxicam, aspirin, sulindac):* Reduced diuretic and antihypertensive effects
3 *Phenytoin:* Reduced diuretic response
3 *Serotonin-reuptake inhibitors (fluoxetine, paroxetine, sertraline):* Case reports of sudden death; enhanced hyponatremia proposed; causal relationships not established
3 *Terbutaline:* Additive hypokalemia
3 *Tubocurarine:* Prolonged neuromuscular blockade

SPECIAL CONSIDERATIONS

• Offers potential advantages over other loop diuretics, including a longer duration of action and fewer adverse electrolyte and metabolic effects; available data not extensive or convincing enough at present to recommend replacement of standard loop diuretic (furosemide); considered alternative in refractory patients

PATIENT/FAMILY EDUCATION

• Take torsemide in the morning to prevent nocturia
• Expect an increase in the frequency and volume of urination
• Notify the physician if cramps, dizziness, an irregular heartbeat, muscle weakness, nausea, or hearing abnormalities occur
• Do not take other medications, including OTC drugs, without first consulting the physician
• Eat foods high in potassium, including apricots, bananas, raisins, orange juice, potatoes, legumes, meat, and whole grains (such as cereals)

MONITORING PARAMETERS

• Urine volume, creatinine clearance, BUN, electrolytes, reduction in edema, increased diuresis, decrease in body weight, reduction in blood pressure, glucose, uric acid, serum calcium (tetany), tinnitus, vertigo, hearing loss (especially in those at risk for ototoxicity—IV doses >120 mg; concomitant ototoxic drugs; renal disease)

tramadol hydrochloride

(traah'-ma-doll hye-droe-klor'-ide)

Rx: Ultram
Combinations
Rx: with acetaminophen (Ultracet)

Chemical Class: Cyclohexanol derivative
Therapeutic Class: Centrally acting synthetic analgesic

CLINICAL PHARMACOLOGY

Mechanism of Action: An analgesic that binds to mu-opioid receptors and inhibits reuptake of norepinephrine and serotonin. Reduces the intensity of pain stimuli reaching sensory nerve endings. ***Therapeutic Effect:*** Alters the perception of and emotional response to pain.

Pharmacokinetics

Route	*Onset*	*Peak*	*Duration*
PO	less than 1 hr	2-3 hrs	4-6 hrs

Rapidly and almost completely absorbed after PO administration. Protein binding: 20%. Extensively metabolized in the liver to active metabolite (reduced in patients with advanced cirrhosis). Primarily excreted in urine. Minimally removed by hemodialysis. ***Half-life:*** 6-7 hr.

INDICATIONS AND DOSAGES

Moderate to moderately severe pain

PO (Immediate-Release, Orally Disintegrating)

Adults, Elderly. 50-100 mg q4-6h. Maximum: 400 mg/day for patients 75 yr and younger; 300 mg/day for patients older than 75 yr.

PO (Extended-Release)

Adults, Elderly. 100-300 mg once daily.

Dosage in renal impairment

For patients with creatinine clearance of less than 30 ml/min, increase dosing interval to q12h. Maximum: 200 mg/day.

Dosage in hepatic impairment

Dosage is decreased to 50 mg q12h.

AVAILABLE FORMS

- *Tablets:* 50 mg.
- *Orally Disintegrating Tablets:* 50 mg.
- *Extended-Release Tablets:* 100 mg, 200 mg, 300 mg.

CONTRAINDICATIONS: Acute alcohol intoxication; concurrent use of centrally acting analgesics, hypnotics, opioids, or psychotropic drugs; hypersensitivity to opioids

PREGNANCY AND LACTATION: Pregnancy category C; small amounts excreted into breast milk

SIDE EFFECTS

Frequent (25%-15%)

Dizziness or vertigo, nausea, constipation, headache, somnolence

Occasional (10%-5%)

Vomiting, pruritus, CNS stimulation (such as nervousness, anxiety, agitation, tremor, euphoria, mood swings, and hallucinations), asthenia, diaphoresis, dyspepsia, dry mouth, diarrhea

Rare (less than 5%)

Malaise, vasodilation, anorexia, flatulence, rash, blurred vision, urine retention or urinary frequency, menopausal symptoms

SERIOUS REACTIONS

- Seizures have been reported in patients receiving tramadol within the recommended dosage range.
- Overdose results in respiratory depression and seizures.
- Tramadol may have a prolonged duration of action and cumulative effect in patients with hepatic or renal impairment.

INTERACTIONS

3 *Carbamazepine:* CNS depression; increased tramadol metabolism, may require significantly increased tramadol dosing for equianalgesic effects

3 *Ethanol, opioids, anesthetic agents, phenothiazines, tranquilizers, sedative-hypnotics:* CNS depression

3 *MAOIs:* Potential exaggerated norepinephrine and serotonin effects, as tramadol inhibits reuptake

3 *Mirtazapine:* Increased risk of developing serotonin syndrome

3 *SSRIs:* Increased risk of seizures

3 *Venlafaxine:* Increased risk of developing serotonin syndrome

T

SPECIAL CONSIDERATIONS

- Expensive, nonnarcotic, "narcotic"-tricyclic antidepressant combination analgesic; potential use in chronic pain; demonstrated efficacy in a variety of pain syndromes; minimal cardiovascular and respiratory side effects
- Does not completely bind to opioid receptors; caution in addicted patients
- Has more potential for abuse than previously thought
- Tolerance and withdrawal symptoms milder than with opiates
- Not chemically related to opiates

PATIENT/FAMILY EDUCATION

- Tramadol use may cause dependence
- Avoid alcohol and OTC drugs such as analgesics and sedatives during tramadol therapy
- Tramadol may cause blurred vision, dizziness, and drowsiness; avoid tasks requiring mental alertness or motor skills until reaction to the drug has been established
- Notify the physician about chest pain, difficulty breathing, excessive sedation, muscle weakness, palpitations, seizures, severe constipation, or tremors

MONITORING PARAMETERS

- Blood pressure, pulse rate
- Pattern of daily bowel activity
- Clinical improvement, and record the onset of pain relief

trandolapril

(tran-dole'-a-pril)

Rx: Mavik

Combinations

Rx: with verapamil (Tarka)

Chemical Class: Angiotensin-converting enzyme (ACE) inhibitor, nonsulfhydryl

Therapeutic Class: Antihypertensive

CLINICAL PHARMACOLOGY

Mechanism of Action: An angiotensin-converting enzyme (ACE) inhibitor that suppresses the renin-angiotensin-aldosterone system and prevents the conversion of angiotensin I to angiotensin II, a potent vasoconstrictor; may also inhibit angiotensin II at local vascular and renal sites. Decreases plasma angiotensin II, increases plasma renin activity, and decreases aldosterone secretion. ***Therapeutic Effect:*** Reduces peripheral arterial resistance and pulmonary capillary wedge pressure; improves cardiac output and exercise tolerance.

Pharmacokinetics

Slowly absorbed from the GI tract. Protein binding: 80%. Metabolized in the liver and GI mucosa to active metabolite. Primarily excreted in urine. Removed by hemodialysis. ***Half-life:*** 24 hr.

INDICATIONS AND DOSAGES

Hypertension (without diuretic)

PO

Adults, Elderly. Initially, 1 mg once a day in non-black patients, 2 mg once a day in black patients. Adjust dosage at least at 7-day intervals. Maintenance: 2-4 mg/day. Maximum: 8 mg/day.

Heart failure or left ventricular dysfunction post-MI

PO

Adults, Elderly. Initially, 0.5-1 mg, titrated to target dose of 4 mg/day.

AVAILABLE FORMS

• *Tablets:* 1 mg, 2 mg, 4 mg.

UNLABELED USES: Treatment of systolic CHF

CONTRAINDICATIONS: History of angioedema from previous treatment with ACE inhibitors, pregnancy

PREGNANCY AND LACTATION: Pregnancy category C (first trimester), category D (second and third trimesters); ACE inhibitors can cause fetal and neonatal morbidity and death when administered to pregnant women; when pregnancy is detected, discontinue ACE inhibitors as soon as possible

SIDE EFFECTS

Frequent (35%-23%)

Dizziness, cough

Occasional (11%-3%)

Hypotension, dyspepsia (heartburn, epigastric pain, indigestion), syncope, asthenia (loss of strength), tinnitus

Rare (less than 1%)

Palpitations, insomnia, drowsiness, nausea, vomiting, constipation, flushed skin

SERIOUS REACTIONS

• Excessive hypotension ("first-dose syncope") may occur in patients with CHF and in those who are severely salt or volume depleted.

• Angioedema and hyperkalemia occur rarely.

• Agranulocytosis and neutropenia may be noted in those with collagen vascular disease, including scleroderma and systemic lupus erythematosus, and impaired renal function.

• Nephrotic syndrome may be noted in those with history of renal disease.

INTERACTIONS

Drugs

3 *Alcohol:* May increase the effects of trandolapril

3 *Azathioprine:* Increased myelosuppression

3 *Lithium:* Increased risk of serious lithium toxicity

3 *Loop diuretics:* Initiation of ACE inhibitor therapy in the presence of intensive diuretic therapy results in a precipitous fall in blood pressure in some patients; ACE inhibitors may induce renal insufficiency in the presence of diuretic-induced sodium depletion

3 *NSAIDs:* Inhibition of the antihypertensive response to ACE inhibitors

3 *Potassium-sparing diuretics:* Increased risk for hyperkalemia

3 *Trimethoprim:* Additive risk of hyperkalemia, especially in patient predisposed to renal insufficiency

Labs

• ACE inhibition can account for approximately 0.5 mEq/L rise in serum potassium

SPECIAL CONSIDERATIONS

PATIENT/FAMILY EDUCATION

• Caution with salt substitutes containing potassium chloride

• Rise slowly to sitting/standing position to minimize orthostatic hypotension

• Dizziness, fainting, lightheadedness may occur during first few days of therapy

• May cause altered taste perception or cough; persistent dry cough usually does not subside unless medication is stopped; notify clinician if these symptoms persist

• Do not abruptly discontinue the drug

• Notify the physician if chest pain, cough, diarrhea, difficulty swallowing, fever, palpitations, sore throat, swelling of the face, or vomiting occurs

MONITORING PARAMETERS

- BUN, creatinine, potassium within 2 wk after initiation of therapy (increased levels may indicate acute renal failure)
- Intake and output and urinary frequency
- Urinalysis for proteinuria
- Pattern of daily bowel activity and stool consistency

tranylcypromine sulfate

(tran-ill-sip'-roe-meen sul'-fate)

Rx: Parnate

Chemical Class: Cyclopropylamine, substituted; nonhydrazine derivative

Therapeutic Class: Antidepressant, monoamine oxidase inhibitor (MAOI)

CLINICAL PHARMACOLOGY

Mechanism of Action: An MAOI that inhibits the activity of the enzyme monoamine oxidase at CNS storage sites, leading to increased levels of the neurotransmitters epinephrine, norepinephrine, serotonin, and dopamine at neuronal receptor sites. ***Therapeutic Effect:*** Relieves depression.

Pharmacokinetics

Well absorbed from GI tract. Metabolized in the liver. Primarily excreted in urine. Removed by hemodialysis. ***Half-life:*** 1.5-3.5 hr.

INDICATIONS AND DOSAGES

Depression refractory to or intolerant of other therapy

PO

Adults, Elderly. Initially, 10 mg twice a day. May increase by 10 mg/day at 1- to 3-wk intervals up to 60 mg/day in divided doses.

AVAILABLE FORMS

- *Tablets:* 10 mg.

UNLABELED USES: Post-traumatic stress disorder

CONTRAINDICATIONS: CHF, children younger than 16 years, pheochromocytoma, severe hepatic or renal impairment, uncontrolled hypertension

PREGNANCY AND LACTATION: Pregnancy category C; excreted into breast milk

SIDE EFFECTS

Frequent

Orthostatic hypotension, restlessness, GI upset, insomnia, dizziness, lethargy, weakness, dry mouth, peripheral edema

Occasional

Flushing, diaphoresis, rash, urinary frequency, increased appetite, transient impotence

Rare

Visual disturbances

SERIOUS REACTIONS

- Hypertensive crisis occurs rarely and is marked by severe hypertension, occipital headache radiating frontally, neck stiffness or soreness, nausea, vomiting, diaphoresis, fever or chills, clammy skin, dilated pupils, palpitations, tachycardia or bradycardia, and constricting chest pain.
- Intracranial bleeding has been reported in association with severe hypertension.

INTERACTIONS

Drugs

▲ *Amphetamines, sympathomimetics, tyramine containing foods:* Severe hypertensive reactions

3 *Antidiabetics:* Prolonged hypoglycemia

3 *Barbiturates:* Prolonged effect of barbiturates

3 *Buproprion:* Enhanced toxicity of buproprion, concomitant use contraindicated

3 *Buspirone:* Hypertension, concomitant use not recommended
3 *Caffeine:* May increase the risk of cardiac arrhythmias and hypertension
⚠ *Clomipramine, fluoxetine, fluvoxamine, paroxetine, sertraline:* Severe or fatal reactions, serotonin related
❷ *Dextromethorphan:* Psychosis or bizarre behavior reported
❷ *Dopamine, guanethidine, methyldopa, reserpine:* Hypertension, headache, and related symptoms
⚠ *Entacapone, tolcapone:* Inhibition of catecholamine metabolism, concomitant use contraindicated
⚠ *Ethanol:* Hypertensive response with alcoholic beverages containing tyramine
⚠ *Furazolidone, procarbazine:* Additive MAO inhibition
3 *Levodopa:* Hypertensive response; carbidopa minimizes the reaction
❷ *Lithium:* Hyperpyrexia with phenelzine
⚠ *Meperidine:* Serotonin accumulation—agitation, blood pressure elevations, hyperpyrexia, ***seizures***
3 *Norepinephrine:* Increased pressor response to norepinephrine
⚠ *Selective serotonin reuptake inhibitors (SSRIs):* Severe or fatal reactions (serotonin syndrome)
⚠ *Sumatriptan:* Increased sumatriptan concentrations, possible toxicity
⚠ *Tricyclic antidepressants:* Increased risk of hypertensive crisis, tricyclics should never be added to an existing MAOI regimen
⚠ *Tryptophan:* Severe or fatal reactions (serotonin syndrome)
⚠ *Venlafaxine:* Increased risk of serotonin syndrome

SPECIAL CONSIDERATIONS

- Irreversible nonselective MAOI effective for typical and atypical depression; equal efficacy to other MAOIs with quicker onset of action, and an amphetamine-like activity with a higher potential for abuse; no anticholinergic or cardiac effects

PATIENT/FAMILY EDUCATION

- Therapeutic effects may take 1-4 wk
- Avoid alcohol ingestion, CNS depressants, OTC medications (cold, weight loss, hay fever, cough syrup)
- Prodromal signs of hypertensive crisis are increased headache, palpitations; discontinue drug immediately
- Do not discontinue medication abruptly after long-term use
- Avoid high-tyramine foods (aged cheese, sour cream, beer, wine, pickled products, liver, raisins, bananas, figs, avocados, meat tenderizers, chocolate, yogurt)

MONITORING PARAMETERS

- Blood pressure, temperature, weight
- Behavior, level of interest, mood, sleep pattern
- Evaluate the patient for an occipital headache radiating frontally and neck stiffness or soreness, which may be the first symptoms of an impending hypertensive crisis. If hypertensive crisis occurs, administer phentolamine 5 to 10 mg IV, as prescribed

trazodone hydrochloride

(tray'-zoe-done)

Rx: Desyrel, Desyrel Dividose

Chemical Class: Triazolopyridine derivative

Therapeutic Class: Antidepressant

CLINICAL PHARMACOLOGY

Mechanism of Action: An antidepressant that blocks the reuptake of serotonin at neuronal presynaptic membranes, increasing its availability at postsynaptic receptor sites. ***Therapeutic Effect:*** Relieves depression.

Pharmacokinetics

Well absorbed from the GI tract. Protein binding: 85%-95%. Metabolized in the liver. Primarily excreted in urine. Unknown if removed by hemodialysis. ***Half-life:*** 5-9 hr.

INDICATIONS AND DOSAGES

Depression

PO

Adults. Initially, 150 mg/day in equally divided doses. Increase by 50 mg/day at 3- to 4-day intervals until therapeutic response is achieved. Maximum: 600 mg/day.

Elderly. Initially, 25-50 mg at bedtime. May increase by 25-50 mg every 3-7 days. Range: 75-150 mg/day.

Children 6-18 yrs. Initially, 1.5-2 mg/kg/day in divided doses. May increase gradually to 6 mg/kg/day in 3 divided doses.

AVAILABLE FORMS

- *Tablets:* 50 mg (Desyrel), 100 mg (Desyrel), 150 mg (Desyrel Dividose), 300 mg (Desyrel Dividose).

UNLABELED USES: Treatment of neurogenic pain

CONTRAINDICATIONS: None known.

PREGNANCY AND LACTATION: Pregnancy category C; excreted into human breast milk; effects on nursing infant unknown, but of possible concern

SIDE EFFECTS

Frequent (9%-3%)

Somnolence, dry mouth, lightheadedness, dizziness, headache, blurred vision, nausea, vomiting

Occasional (3%-1%)

Nervousness, fatigue, constipation, generalized aches and pains, mild hypotension

Rare

Photosensitivity reaction

SERIOUS REACTIONS

- Priapism, diminished or improved libido, retrograde ejaculation, and impotence occur rarely.
- Trazodone appears to be less cardiotoxic than other antidepressants, although arrhythmias may occur in patients with preexisting cardiac disease.

INTERACTIONS

Drugs

3 *Antihypertensives:* May increase the effects of antihypertensives

3 *Clonidine:* Inhibited antihypertensive response to clonidine

3 *Digoxin, phenytoin:* May increase the blood concentration of these drugs

3 *Ethanol:* Additive impairment of motor skills; abstinent alcoholics may eliminate cyclic antidepressants more rapidly than non-alcoholics

3 *Fluoxetine:* Increased plasma trazodone concentrations

3 *Indinavir, ketoconazole, ritonavir:* May increase the blood concentration and toxicity of trazodone

▲ *MAOIs:* Potential for fatal serotonin syndrome

3 *Neuroleptics:* Additive hypotension

3 *St. John's Wort:* May increase the adverse effects of trazodone

SPECIAL CONSIDERATIONS

- Very sedating antidepressant with minimal anticholinergic effects; good choice for elderly patients in whom sedating properties would be desirable

PATIENT/FAMILY EDUCATION

- Take with food
- Use caution driving or performing other tasks requiring alertness
- Take trazodone at bedtime if drowsiness occurs while taking the drug

• Change positions slowly to avoid the drug's hypotensive effect
• The male patient should notify the physician immediately if a painful, prolonged penile erection occurs
• Photosensitivity to sunlight may occur during trazodone therapy
• Notify the physician if visual disturbances occur
• Avoid alcohol while taking trazodone
• Take sips of tepid water or chew sugarless gum to relieve dry mouth

MONITORING PARAMETERS
• Behavior, level of interest, mood, and sleep pattern
• Serum neutrophil and WBC counts
• ECG for arrhythmias

---

treprostinil sodium
(treh-prost'-tin-il)
Rx: Remodulin
Chemical Class: Prostacyclin analog
Therapeutic Class: Vasodilator

CLINICAL PHARMACOLOGY
Mechanism of Action: An antiplatelet that directly dilates pulmonary and systemic arterial vascular beds, inhibiting platelet aggregation. ***Therapeutic Effect:*** Reduces symptoms of pulmonary arterial hypertension associated with exercise.
Pharmacokinetics
Rapidly, completely absorbed after subcutaneous infusion; 91% bound to plasma protein. Metabolized by the liver. Excreted mainly in the urine with a lesser amount eliminated in the feces. ***Half-life:*** 2-4 hr.

INDICATIONS AND DOSAGES
Pulmonary arterial hypertension
Continuous subcutaneous infusion, IV Infusion
Adults, Elderly. Initially, 1.25 ng/kg/min. Reduce infusion rate to 0.625 ng/kg/min if initial dose cannot be tolerated. Increase infusion rate in increments of no more than 1.25 ng/kg/min per wk for the first 4 wk and then no more than 2.5 ng/kg/min per wk for the duration of infusion.
Hepatic impairment (mild to moderate)
Adults, Elderly. Decrease the initial dose to 0.625 ng/kg/min based on ideal body weight and increase cautiously.

AVAILABLE FORMS
• *Injection:* 1 mg/ml, 2.5 mg/ml, 5 mg/ml, 10 mg/ml.

CONTRAINDICATIONS: None known.

PREGNANCY AND LACTATION: Pregnancy category B; excretion into human breast milk unknown; use caution in nursing mothers

SIDE EFFECTS
Frequent
Infusion site pain, erythema, induration, rash
Occasional
Headache, diarrhea, jaw pain, vasodilation, nausea
Rare
Dizziness, hypotension, pruritus, edema

SERIOUS REACTIONS
• Abrupt withdrawal or sudden large reductions in dosage may result in worsening of pulmonary arterial hypertension symptoms.

INTERACTIONS
Drugs
3 *Diuretics, antihypertensives, vasodilators:* Exacerbated reductions in blood pressure, increased potential for hypotension
3 *Anticoagulants, antiplatelet agents:* Increased risk for bleeding

SPECIAL CONSIDERATIONS

PATIENT/FAMILY EDUCATION

- Patient must be able to administer drug via continuous sc INF and care for the infusion system
- Therapy may be required for prolonged periods of time
- Solutions should be administered without additional dilution
- Report signs of increased pulmonary artery pressure, such as dyspnea, cough, or chest pain

MONITORING PARAMETERS

- Blood pressure, clinical symptoms
- BUN, hepatic enzyme, and serum creatinine levels

---

tretinoin

(tret'-i-noyn)

Rx: Altinac, Avita, Renova, Retin-A, Retin-A Micro, Vesanoid

Combinations

Rx: with fluocinolone/hydroquinone (Tri-Luma)

Chemical Class: Retinoid; vitamin A derivative

Therapeutic Class: Antiacne agent

CLINICAL PHARMACOLOGY

Mechanism of Action: A retinoid that decreases cohesiveness of follicular epithelial cells. Increases turnover of follicular epithelial cells. Bacterial skincounts are not altered. Transdermal: Exerts its effects on growth and differentiation of epithelial cells. Antineoplastic: Induces maturation, decreases proliferation of acute promyelocytic leukemia (APL) cells. ***Therapeutic Effect:*** Causes expulsion of blackheads; alleviates fine wrinkles, hyperpigmentation; causes repopulation of bone marrow and blood by normal hematopoietic cells.

Pharmacokinetics

Topical: Minimally absorbed. Oral: Well absorbed following oral administration. Protein binding: 95%. Metabolized in liver. Primarily excreted in urine, minimal excretion in feces. ***Half-life:*** 0.5-2 hrs.

INDICATIONS AND DOSAGES

Acne

Topical

Adults. Apply once daily at bedtime.

Transdermal

Transdermal

Adults. Apply to face once daily at bedtime.

Acute promyelocytic leukemia

PO

Adults. 45 mg/m^2/day given as 2 evenly divided doses until complete remission is documented. Discontinue therapy 30 days after complete remission or after 90 days of treatment, whichever comes first.

AVAILABLE FORMS

- *Capsules:* 10 mg (Vesanoid).
- *Cream:* 0.025% (Altinac, Avita, Retin-A), 0.02% (Renova), 0.05% (Altinac, Renova, Retin-A), 0.1 % (Altinac, Retin-A).
- *Gel:* 0.01% (Retin-A), 0.025% (Avita, Retin-A), 0.04% (Retin-A Micro), 0.1% (Retin-A Micro).
- *Topical Liquid:* 0.05% (Retin-A).

UNLABELED USES: Treatment of disorders of keratinization, including photo-aged skin, liver spots

CONTRAINDICATIONS: Sensitivity to parabens (used as preservative in gelatin capsule)

PREGNANCY AND LACTATION: Pregnancy category D (oral), C (topical)

SIDE EFFECTS

Expected

Topical: Temporary change in pigmentation, photosensitivity, Local inflammatory reactions (peeling, dry skin, stinging, erythema, pruritus) are to be expected and are reversible with discontinuation of tretinoin

Frequent

PO: Headache, fever, dry skin/oral mucosa, bone pain, nausea, vomiting, rash

Occasional

PO: Mucositis, earache or feeling of fullness in ears, flushing, pruritus, increased sweating, visual disturbances, hypo/hypertension, dizziness, anxiety, insomnia, alopecia, skin changes

Rare

PO: Change in visual acuity, temporary hearing loss

SERIOUS REACTIONS

PO:

- Retinoic acid syndrome (fever, dyspnea, weight gain, abnormal chest auscultatory findings, episodic hypotension) occurs commonly, as does leukocytosis.
- Syndrome generally occurs during first month of therapy (sometimes occurs following first dose).
- Pseudo tumor cerebri may be noted, especially in children (headache, nausea, vomiting, visual disturbances).
- Possible tumorigenic potential when combined with ultraviolet radiation.

Topical:

- Possible tumorigenic potential when combined with ultraviolet radiation.

INTERACTIONS

Drugs

3 *Cimetidine, cyclosporine, diltiazem, erythromycin, ketoconazole, verapamil:* May inhibit tretinoin metabolism; increases risk of tretinoin toxicity

3 *Glucocorticoids, pentobarbital, phenobarbital, rifampicin:* May decrease the efficacy of tretinoin

3 *Sulfur, resorcinol, benzoyl peroxide, salicylic acid:* Concomitant topical acne products may cause significant skin irritation

SPECIAL CONSIDERATIONS

- Oral therapy should be prescribed only by those knowledgeable in the treatment of APL

PATIENT/FAMILY EDUCATION

- Keep away from eyes, mouth, angles of nose, and mucous membranes
- Avoid exposure to ultraviolet light
- Acne may worsen transiently
- Normal use of cosmetics is permissible
- Take oral tretinoin with food

MONITORING PARAMETERS

- *Oral:* Liver function, coagulation profile, cholesterol, triglycerides

T

triamcinolone/ triamcinolone acetonide/ triamcinolone diacetate/ triamcinolone hexacetonide

(trye-am-sin'-oh-lone)

Rx: (triamcinolone) Aristocort

Rx: (itriamcinolone acetonide) Acetocot, Aristocort, Aristocort Forte, Aristospan Injection, Clinacort, Clinalog, Kenalog, Kenalog-10, Kenalog-40, Ken-Jec 40, Triam-A, Triamcot, Triam-Forte, Triamonide 40, Triderm, Tri-nasal, U-Tri-Lone

Rx: (triamcinolone diacetate) Amcort, Aristocort Intralesional

Rx: (triamcinolone hexacetonide) Aristospan

Chemical Class: Glucocorticoid, synthetic

Therapeutic Class: Corticosteroid, inhaled; corticosteroid, systemic; corticosteroid, topical

CLINICAL PHARMACOLOGY

Mechanism of Action: An adrenocortical steroid that inhibits accumulation of inflammatory cells at inflammation sites, phagocytosis, lysosomal enzyme release and synthesis, and release of mediators of inflammation. ***Therapeutic Effect:*** Prevents or suppresses cell-mediated immune reactions. Decreases or prevents tissue response to inflammatory process.

Pharmacokinetics

Minimal absorption following nasal and topical administration. Moderate absorption from the lungs and GI tract following administration of inhaled form. Rapidly and almost completely absorbed following PO administration. Metabolized in liver. Excreted in urine. ***Half-life:*** Unknown.

INDICATIONS AND DOSAGES

Immunosuppression, relief of acute inflammation

PO

Adults, Elderly. 4-60 mg/day.

IM (triamcinolone acetonide)

Adults, Elderly. Initially, 2.5-60 mg/day.

IM (triamcinolone diacetate)

Adults, Elderly. 40 mg/wk.

IM (triamcinolone hexacetonide)

Adults, Elderly. Initially, 2.5-40 mg up to 100 mg; 2-20 mg.

Intraarticular, Intralesional

Adults, Elderly. 5-40 mg.

Control of bronchial asthma

Inhalation

Adults, Elderly. 2 inhalations 3-4 times a day.

Children 6-12 yr. 1-2 inhalations 3-4 times a day. Maximum: 12 inhalations/day.

Rhinitis

Intranasal

Adults, Elderly, Children 6 yr and older. Initially, 2 sprays (55 mcg/spray) in each nostril once daily. Maintenance: 1 spray in each nostril once daily.

Relief of inflammation or pruritus associated with corticoid-responsive dermatoses

Topical

Adults, Elderly. 2-4 times a day. May give 1-2 times a day or as intermittent therapy.

AVAILABLE FORMS

• *Oral (Topical Paste [Kenalog in Orabase]):* 0.1% or 5 g.

• *Tablets (Aristocort):* 4 mg, 8 mg.

• *Inhalation (Oral [Azmacort]):* 100 mcg/actuation.

• *Nasal Spray:* 50 mcg/inhalation (Tri-Nasal), 55 mcg/inhalation (Nasacort AQ).

• *Cream:* 0.025% (Aristocort A), 0.05% (Aristocort A), 0.1% (Aristocort A, Kenalog, Triderm).

• *Ointment (Aristocort A, Kenalog):* 0.025%, 0.1%.

• *Injection (acetonide):* 10 mg/ml (Kenalog-10), 40 mg/ml (Acetocot, Clinalog, Kenalog-40, Ken-Jec 40, Triam-A, Triamcot, Triamonide 40, U-Tri-Lone).

• *Injection (diacetate):* 25 mg/ml (Aristocort), 40 mg/ml (Aristocort Forte, Clinacort, Triam-Forte).

• *Injection (hexacetonide [Aristospan Injection]):* 5 mg/ml, 20 mg/ml.

CONTRAINDICATIONS: Administration of live-virus vaccines, especially smallpox vaccine; hypersensitivity to corticosteroids or tartrazine; IM injection or oral inhalation in children younger than 6 yrs; peptic ulcer disease (except life-threatening situations); systemic fungal infection

Topical: Marked circulation impairment

PREGNANCY AND LACTATION: Pregnancy category C (D if used in first trimester); excreted in breast milk and could interfere with infant's growth and endogenous corticosteroid production

SIDE EFFECTS

Frequent

Insomnia, dry mouth, heartburn, nervousness, abdominal distention, diaphoresis, acne, mood swings, increased appetite, facial flushing, delayed wound healing, increased susceptibility to infection, diarrhea or constipation

Occasional

Headache, edema, change in skin color, frequent urination

Rare

Tachycardia, allergic reaction (including rash and hives), mental changes, hallucinations, depression

Topical: Allergic contact dermatitis

SERIOUS REACTIONS

• Long-term therapy may cause muscle wasting in the arms or legs, osteoporosis, spontaneous fractures, amenorrhea, cataracts, glaucoma, peptic ulcer disease, and CHF.

• Abruptly withdrawing the drug following long-term therapy may cause anorexia, nausea, fever, headache, arthralgia, rebound inflammation, fatigue, weakness, lethargy, dizziness, and orthostatic hypotension.

• Anaphylaxis occurs rarely with parenteral administration.

• Suddenly discontinuing triamcinolone may be fatal.

• Blindness has occurred rarely after intralesional injection around face and head.

INTERACTIONS

Drugs

3 *Aminoglutethamide:* Increased clearance of steroid; doubling of dose may be necessary

3 *Amphotericin:* May increase hypokalemia

3 *Antidiabetics:* Increased blood glucose

3 *Barbiturates, carbamazepine:* Reduced serum concentrations of corticosteroids

3 *Cholestyramine, colestipol:* Possible reduced absorption of corticosteroids

3 *Cyclosporine:* Possible increased concentration of both drugs, seizures

3 *Digoxin:* May increase the risk of digoxin toxicity caused by hypokalemia

3 *Diuretics:* May decrease the effects of these drugs

3 *Erythromycin, troleandomycin, clarithromycin, ketoconazole:* Possible enhanced steroid effect

3 *Estrogens, oral contraceptives:* Enhanced effects of corticosteroids

3 *Isoniazid:* Reduced plasma concentrations of isoniazid

3 *IUDs:* Inhibition of inflammation may decrease contraceptive effect

3 *Live-virus vaccines:* May decrease the patient's antibody response to vaccine, increase vaccine side effects, and potentiate virus replication

3 *NSAIDs:* Increased risk of GI ulceration

3 *Rifampin:* Reduced therapeutic effect of corticosteroids

3 *Salicylates:* Increased elimination of salicylates

Labs

- *False increase:* Urinary amino acids

SPECIAL CONSIDERATIONS

PATIENT/FAMILY EDUCATION

- May cause GI upset, take with meals or snacks (systemic)
- Do not give live-virus vaccines to patients on prolonged systemic therapy
- Take PO as single daily dose in a.m.
- Signs of adrenal insufficiency include fatigue, anorexia, nausea, vomiting, diarrhea, weight loss, weakness, dizziness, and low blood sugar
- Avoid abrupt withdrawal of therapy following high-dose or long-term therapy
- Increased dose of rapidly acting corticosteroids may be necessary in patients subjected to unusual stress
- To be used on a regular basis, not for acute symptoms (nasal and inhalation)
- Use bronchodilators before oral inhaler (for patients using both)
- Rinse mouth to prevent oral candidiasis
- Nasal sol may cause drying and irritation of nasal mucosa, clear nasal passages prior to use

MONITORING PARAMETERS

- Serum K and glucose
- Growth of children on prolonged therapy
- Blood pressure, intake and output, weight
- Be alert to signs and symptoms of infection such as fever, pharyngitis, and vague symptoms
- Evaluate the patient for signs and symptoms of hypocalcemia (such as cramps, muscle twitching, and positive Chvostek's or Trousseau's signs), or hypokalemia (such as EKG changes, irritability, muscle cramps and weakness, nausea and vomiting, and numbness and tingling in the lower extremities)

---

triamterene

(try-am'-ter-een)

Rx: Dyrenium

Combinations

Rx: with hydrochlorothiazide (Dyazide, Maxzide)

Chemical Class: Pteridine derivative

Therapeutic Class: Antihypertensive; diuretic, potassium-sparing

---

CLINICAL PHARMACOLOGY

Mechanism of Action: A potassium-sparing diuretic that inhibits sodium, potassium, ATPase. Interferes with sodium and potassium exchange in distal tubule, cortical collecting tubule, and collecting duct. Increases sodium and decreases potassium excretion. Also increases magnesium, decreases calcium loss. ***Therapeutic Effect:*** Produces diuresis and lowers BP.

Pharmacokinetics

Route	Onset	Peak	Duration
PO	2-4 hrs	N/A	7-9 hrs

Incompletely absorbed from the GI tract. Widely distributed. Metabolized in the liver. Primarily eliminated in feces via biliary route. ***Half-life:*** 1.5-2.5 hrs (increased in renal impairment).

INDICATIONS AND DOSAGES

Edema, hypertension

PO

Adults, Elderly. 25-100 mg/day as a single dose or in 2 divided doses. Maximum: 300 mg/day.

Children. 2-4 mg/kg/day as a single dose or in 2 divided doses. Maximum: 6 mg/kg/day or 300 mg/day.

AVAILABLE FORMS

- *Capsules:* 50 mg, 100 mg.

UNLABELED USES: Treatment adjunct for hypertension, prevention and treatment of hypokalemia

CONTRAINDICATIONS: Anuria, drug-induced or preexisting hyperkalemia, progressive or severe renal disease, severe hepatic disease

PREGNANCY AND LACTATION: Pregnancy category B; therapy for preexisting hypertension can be continued throughout pregnancy with minimal risk; initiating for simple edema not recommended; few unequivocal indications for diuretic therapy in pregnancy except for pulmonary edema or congestive heart failure; may decrease placental perfusion; excreted in cow's milk, no human data

SIDE EFFECTS

Occasional

Fatigue, nausea, diarrhea, abdominal pain, leg cramps, headache

Rare

Anorexia, asthenia, rash, dizziness

SERIOUS REACTIONS

- Triamterene use may result in hyponatremia (somnolence, dry mouth, increased thirst, lack of energy) or severe hyperkalemia (irritability, anxiety, heaviness of legs, paresthesia, hypotension, bradycardia, EKG changes [tented T waves, widening QRS complex, ST segment depression]), particularly in those with renal impairment or diabetes, the elderly, or severely ill patients.
- Agranulocytosis, nephrolithiasis, and thrombocytopenia occur rarely.

INTERACTIONS

Drugs

3 *ACE inhibitors:* Hyperkalemia in predisposed patients

3 *Amantadine:* Increased toxicity of amantadine

3 *Angiotensin II receptor antagonists:* Concurrent mechanisms to decrease potassium excretion; increased risk of hyperkalemia

3 *Anticoagulants, heparin:* May decrease the effects of these drugs

3 *Cimetidine:* Increased triamterene bioavailability and decreased renal clearance

3 *Lithium:* May decrease the clearance and increase the risk of toxicity of lithium

3 *NSAIDs:* Acute renal failure with indomethacin and possibly other NSAIDs

2 *Potassium preparation:* Concurrent use increases the risk of hyperkalemia

Labs

- *False increase:* Serum digoxin concentrations
- *Interference:* Urinary catecholamines

SPECIAL CONSIDERATIONS

PATIENT/FAMILY EDUCATION

- Take with meals
- Avoid prolonged exposure to sunlight

- Take single daily doses in a.m.
- The drug's therapeutic effect takes several days to begin and can last for several days after the drug is discontinued
- Expect an increase in the frequency and volume of urination
- Notify the physician if dry mouth, fever, headache, nausea and vomiting, persistent or severe weakness, sore throat, or unusual bleeding or bruising occurs
- Avoid consuming salt substitutes and foods high in potassium

MONITORING PARAMETERS

- Blood pressure, edema, urine output, urine electrolytes, BUN, creatinine, ECG (if hyperkalemic), gynecomastia, impotence, weight

triazolam

(trye-ay'-zoe-lam)

Rx: Halcion

Chemical Class: Benzodiazepine

Therapeutic Class: Hypnotic

DEA Class: Schedule IV

CLINICAL PHARMACOLOGY

Mechanism of Action: A benzodiazepine that enhances the action of the inhibitory neurotransmitter gamma-aminobutyric acid, resulting in CNS depression. ***Therapeutic Effect:*** Induces sleep.

Pharmacokinetics

Rapidly and completely absorbed from GI tract. Protein binding: 89%-94%. Metabolized in the liver. Primarily excreted in urine. ***Half-life:*** 1.5-5.5 hr.

INDICATIONS AND DOSAGES

Insomnia

PO

Adults, Children 18 yr and older. 0.125-0.5 mg at bedtime.

Elderly. 0.0625-0.125 mg at bedtime.

AVAILABLE FORMS

- *Tablets:* 0.125 mg, 0.25 mg.

CONTRAINDICATIONS: Angle-closure glaucoma; CNS depression; hypersensitivity to other benzodiazepines; pregnancy or breast-feeding; severe, uncontrolled pain; sleep apnea

PREGNANCY AND LACTATION: Pregnancy category X (according to manufacturer); no congenital anomalies have been attributed to use during human pregnancies; other benzodiazepines have been suspected of producing fetal malformations after first-trimester exposure

Controlled Substance: Schedule IV

SIDE EFFECTS

Frequent

Somnolence, sedation, dry mouth, headache, dizziness, nervousness, lightheadedness, incoordination, nausea, rebound insomnia (may occur for 1-2 nights after drug is discontinued)

Occasional

Euphoria, tachycardia, abdominal cramps, visual disturbances

Rare

Paradoxical CNS excitement or restlessness (particularly in elderly or debilitated patients)

SERIOUS REACTIONS

- Abrupt or too-rapid withdrawal may result in pronounced restlessness, irritability, insomnia, hand tremors, abdominal or muscle cramps, vomiting, diaphoresis, and seizures.
- Overdose results in somnolence, confusion, diminished reflexes, respiratory depression, and coma.

INTERACTIONS

Drugs

3 *Carbamazepine, phenytoin:* Reduced effect of triazolam

3 *Cimetidine, clarithromycin, disulfiram, erythromycin, fluvoxamine, grapefruit juice, isoniazid, troleandomycin:* Increased plasma triazolam concentrations

2 *Ethanol:* Enhanced adverse psychomotor effects of benzodiazepines

2 *Fluconazole, itraconazole, ketoconazole:* Increased plasma triazolam concentrations

3 *Grapefruit, grapefruit juice:* May alter the absorption of triazolam

3 *Kava kava, valerian:* May increase CNS depression

3 *Smoking:* Reduces the drug's effectiveness

SPECIAL CONSIDERATIONS

- Prescriptions should be written for short-term use (7-10 days); drug should not be prescribed in quantities exceeding a 1-mo supply

PATIENT/FAMILY EDUCATION

- Avoid alcohol and other CNS depressants
- Do not discontinue abruptly after prolonged therapy
- May cause drowsiness or dizziness, use caution while driving or performing other tasks requiring alertness
- May be habit-forming
- Avoid consuming grapefruit or grapefruit juice during triazolam therapy because grapefruit decreases the drug's absorption
- Smoking reduces the drug's effectiveness

MONITORING PARAMETERS

- Sleep pattern
- Cardiovascular, mental, and respiratory status
- Hepatic function of patients on long-term therapy
- Assess elderly or debilitated patients for a paradoxical reaction, particularly during early therapy
- Therapeutic response, such as a decrease in the number of nocturnal awakenings and a longer duration of sleep

trientine hydrochloride

(trye-en'-teen hye-droe-klor'-ide)

Rx: Syprine

Chemical Class: Thiol derivative

Therapeutic Class: Antidote, copper

CLINICAL PHARMACOLOGY

Mechanism of Action: An oral chelating agent that foms complexes by binding metal ions, particularly copper. ***Therapeutic Effect:*** Binds to copper and induces cupruresis.

Pharmacokinetics

None reported.

INDICATIONS AND DOSAGES

Wilson's disease

PO

Adults, Elderly. 750-1250 mg/day in 2-4 divided doses. Maximum: 2 g/day.

Children 12 yrs and older. 500-750 mg/day in 2-4 divided doses. Maximum: 1500 mg/day.

AVAILABLE FORMS

- *Capsules:* 250 mg (Syprine).

CONTRAINDICATIONS: Hypersensitivity to trientine or its components

PREGNANCY AND LACTATION: Pregnancy category C

SIDE EFFECTS

Occasional

Contact dermatitis, dystonia, muscular spasm, myasthenia gravis

SERIOUS REACTIONS

- Iron deficiency anemia and systemic lupus erythematosus rarely occur.

INTERACTIONS

Drugs

3 *Iron preparations:* May decrease absorption of both drugs

SPECIAL CONSIDERATIONS

PATIENT/FAMILY EDUCATION

- Take on empty stomach
- Swallow capsules whole
- Notify the physician if pale skin, swelling of lymph glands, skin rash, fever, joint pain, or general feeling of weakness occurs
- Maintain adequate fluid intake

MONITORING PARAMETERS

- Free serum copper (goal is <10 mcg/dl); increase daily dose only when clinical response is not adequate or concentration of free serum copper is persistently above 20 mcg/dL (determine optimal long-term maintenance dosage at 6-12-mos intervals)
- 24-hr urinary copper analysis at 6-12-mos intervals (adequately treated patients will have 0.5-1 mg copper/24 hr collection of urine)
- Temperature

trifluoperazine hydrochloride

(trye-floo-oh-per'-a-zeen)

Rx: Stelazine

Chemical Class: Piperidine phenothiazine derivative

Therapeutic Class: Antipsychotic

CLINICAL PHARMACOLOGY

Mechanism of Action: A phenothiazine derivative that blocks dopamine at postsynaptic receptor sites. Possesses strong extrapyramidal and antiemetic effects and weak anticholinergic and sedative effects. ***Therapeutic Effect:*** Suppresses behavioral response in psychosis; reduces locomotor activity and aggressiveness.

Pharmacokinetics

Readily absorbed following PO administration. Protein binding: 90%-99%. Metabolized in liver. Excreted in urine. ***Half-life:*** 24 hr.

INDICATIONS AND DOSAGES

Psychotic disorders

PO

Adults, Elderly, Children 12 yr and older. Initially, 2-5 mg once or twice a day. Range: 15-20 mg/day. Maximum: 40 mg/day.

Children 6-11 yr. Initially, 1 mg once or twice a day. Maintenance: Up to 15 mg/day.

IM

Adults. 1-2 mg q4-6h. Maximum: 10 mg/24 h.

Elderly. 1 mg q4-6h. Maximum: 6 mg/24 h.

Children. 1 mg 2 times/day.

AVAILABLE FORMS

- *Tablets:* 1 mg, 2 mg, 5 mg, 10 mg.
- *Injection:* 2 mg/ml.

CONTRAINDICATIONS: Angle-closure glaucoma, circulatory collapse, myelosuppression, severe cardiac or hepatic disease, severe hypertension or hypotension

PREGNANCY AND LACTATION: Pregnancy category C; has been used as an antiemetic during normal labor without producing any observable effect on newborn; bulk of evidence indicates safety for mother and fetus

SIDE EFFECTS

Frequent

Hypotension, dizziness, and syncope (occur frequently after first injection, occasionally after subsequent injections, and rarely with oral form)

Occasional
Drowsiness during early therapy, dry mouth, blurred vision, lethargy, constipation or diarrhea, nasal congestion, peripheral edema, urine retention
Rare
Ocular changes, altered skin pigmentation (in those taking high doses for prolonged periods), photosensitivity

SERIOUS REACTIONS

• Extrapyramidal symptoms appear to be dose related (particularly high doses) and are divided into 3 categories: akathisia (inability to sit still, tapping of feet), parkinsonian symptoms (such as mask-like face, tremors, shuffling gait, and hypersalivation), and acute dystonias (such as torticollis, opisthotonos, and oculogyric crisis). Dystonic reactions may also produce diaphoresis and pallor.

• Tardive dyskinesia, marked by tongue protrusion, puffing of the cheeks, and chewing or puckering of the mouth, occurs rarely but may be irreversible.

• Abrupt withdrawal after long-term therapy may precipitate nausea, vomiting, gastritis, dizziness, and tremors.

• Blood dyscrasias, particularly agranulocytosis, and mild leukopenia may occur.

• Trifluoperazine may lower the seizure threshold.

INTERACTIONS

Drugs

3 *Alcohol, other CNS depressants:* May increase CNS and respiratory depression and the hypotensive effects of trifluoperazine

3 *Antacids:* May inhibit absorption of trifluoperazine if given within 1 hr of drug

3 *Anticholinergics:* Inhibited therapeutic response to antipsychotic; enhanced anticholinergic side effects

3 *Antidepressants:* Increased serum concentrations of some cyclic antidepressants

3 *Antithyroid agents:* May increase the risk of agranulocytosis

3 *Barbiturates:* Reduced effect of antipsychotic

3 *Bromocriptine, lithium:* Reduced effects of both drugs

3 *Extrapyramidal symptom–producing medications:* May increase extrapyramidal symptoms

3 *Guanethidine:* Inhibited antihypertensive response to guanethidine

3 *Hypotension-producing agents:* May increase hypotension

2 *Levodopa:* Inhibited effect of levodopa on Parkinson's disease

3 *Narcotic analgesics:* Excessive CNS depression, hypotension, respiratory depression

3 *Orphenadrine:* Reduced serum neuroleptic concentrations; excessive anticholinergic effects

Labs

• *False increase:* Urinary protein

SPECIAL CONSIDERATIONS

PATIENT/FAMILY EDUCATION

• Arise slowly from reclining position
• Do not discontinue abruptly
• Use a sunscreen during sun exposure; take special precautions to stay cool in hot weather
• Avoid tasks requiring mental alertness or motor skills until response to the drug has been established
• Do not take antacids within 1 hr of trifluoperazine
• Avoid alcohol

MONITORING PARAMETERS

• Observe closely for signs of tardive dyskinesia
• Periodic CBC with platelets during prolonged therapy

• WBC count for blood dyscrasias, such as anemia, neutropenia, pancytopenia, and thrombocytopenia
• Blood pressure for hypotension
• Therapeutic response, such as improvement in self-care and ability to concentrate, increased interest in surroundings, and relaxed facial expression

trifluridine

(trye-flure'-i-deen)

Rx: Viroptic

Chemical Class: Nucleoside analog

Therapeutic Class: Ophthalmic antiviral

CLINICAL PHARMACOLOGY

Mechanism of Action: An antiviral agent that incorporates into DNS, causing increased rate of mutation and errors in protein formation. ***Therapeutic Effect:*** Prevents viral replication.

Pharmacokinetics

Intraocular solution is undetectable in serum. ***Half-life:*** 12 min.

INDICATIONS AND DOSAGES

Herpes simplex virus ocular infections

Ophthalmic

Adults, Elderly, Children older than 6 yrs. 1 drop onto cornea q2h while awake. Maximum: 9 drops/day. Continue until corneal ulcer has completely reepithelialized; then, 1 drop q4h while awake (minimum: 5 drops/day) for an additional 7 days.

AVAILABLE FORMS

• *Ophthalmic Solution:* 1% (Viroptic).

CONTRAINDICATIONS: Hypersensitivity to trifluridine or any component of the formulation

PREGNANCY AND LACTATION: Pregnancy category C

SIDE EFFECTS

Frequent

Transient stinging or burning with instillation

Occasional

Edema of eyelid

Rare

Hypersensitivity reaction

SERIOUS REACTIONS

• Ocular toxicity may occur if used longer than 21 days.

SPECIAL CONSIDERATIONS

PATIENT/FAMILY EDUCATION

• Notify clinician if no improvement after 7 days
• Report any itching, swelling, redness, or increased irritation
• Avoid contact with eyes

MONITORING PARAMETERS

• Therapeutic response

trihexyphenidyl hydrochloride

(trye-hex-ee-fen'-i-dill hye-droe-klor'-ide)

Rx: Artane

Chemical Class: Tertiary amine

Therapeutic Class: Anti-Parkinson's agent; anticholinergic

CLINICAL PHARMACOLOGY

Mechanism of Action: An anticholinergic agent that blocks central cholinergic receptors (aids in balancing cholinergic and dopaminergic activity). ***Therapeutic Effect:*** Decreases salivation, relaxes smooth muscle.

Pharmacokinetics

Well absorbed from gastrointestinal (GI) tract. Primarily excreted in urine. ***Half-life:*** 3.3-4.1 hrs.

INDICATIONS AND DOSAGES

Parkinsonism

PO

Adults, Elderly. Initially, 1 mg on first day. May increase by 2 mg/day at 3-5-day intervals up to 6-10 mg/day (12-15 mg/day in patients with postencephalitic parkinsonism).

Drug-induced extrapyramidal symptoms

PO

Adults, Elderly. Initially, 1 mg/day. Range: 5-15 mg/day.

AVAILABLE FORMS

- *Elixir:* 2 mg/5 ml (Artane).
- *Tablets:* 2 mg, 5 mg (Artane).

CONTRAINDICATIONS: Angle-closure glaucoma, GI obstruction, paralytic ileus, intestinal atony, severe ulcerative colitis, prostatic hypertrophy, myasthenia gravis, megacolon, hypersensitivity to trihexyphenidyl or any component of the formulation

PREGNANCY AND LACTATION: Pregnancy category C; nursing infants may be particularly sensitive to anticholinergic effects

SIDE EFFECTS

Elderly (more than 60 yrs) tend to develop mental confusion, disorientation, agitation, psychotic-like symptoms

Frequent

Drowsiness, dry mouth

Occasional

Blurred vision, urinary retention, constipation, dizziness, headache, muscle cramps

Rare

Seizures, depression, rash

SERIOUS REACTIONS

- Hypersensitivity reaction (eczema, pruritus, rash, cardiac disturbances, photosensitivity) may occur.
- Overdosage may vary from CNS depression (sedation, apnea, cardiovascular collapse, death) to severe paradoxical reaction (hallucinations, tremor, seizures).

INTERACTIONS

Drugs

3 *Alcohol, CNS depressants:* May increase sedative effect

3 *Amantadine:* Potentiates the side effects of amantadine

3 *Antacids, antidiarrheals:* May decrease absorption and effects of trihexyphenidyl

3 *Anticholinergics:* Increased anticholinergic side effects

3 *MAOIs:* Increased anticholinergic side effects

3 *Neuroleptics:* Inhibition of therapeutic response to neuroleptics; excessive anticholinergic effects

3 *Tacrine:* Reduced therapeutic effects of both drugs

Labs

- *False increase:* Serum T_3 and T_4

SPECIAL CONSIDERATIONS

PATIENT/FAMILY EDUCATION

- Do not discontinue abruptly
- Use caution in hot weather; drug may increase susceptibility to heat stroke
- Avoid alcohol
- Chew sugarless gum or take sips of tepid water to relieve dry mouth
- Avoid tasks requiring mental alertness or motor skills until response to the drug has been established

MONITORING PARAMETERS

- Clinical reversal of symptoms

trimethobenzamide hydrochloride

(trye-meth-oh-ben'-za-mide)

Rx: Benzacot, Benzocaine-Trimethobenzamide Adult, Benzocaine-Trimethobenzamide Pediatric, Navogan, Tebamide, Tebamide Pediatric, Tigan, Tigan Adult, Tigan Pediatric

Chemical Class: Ethanolamine derivative

Therapeutic Class: Antiemetic

CLINICAL PHARMACOLOGY

Mechanism of Action: An anticholinergic that acts at the chemoreceptor trigger zone in the medulla oblongata. ***Therapeutic Effect:*** Relieves nausea and vomiting.

Pharmacokinetics

Route	Onset	Peak	Duration
PO	10-40 min	N/A	3-4 hr
IM	15-30 min	N/A	2-3 hr

Partially absorbed from the GI tract. Distributed primarily to the liver. Metabolic fate unknown. Excreted in urine. ***Half-life:*** 7-9 hr.

INDICATIONS AND DOSAGES

Nausea and vomiting

PO

Adults, Elderly. 300 mg 3-4 times a day.

Children weighing 30-100 lb. 100-200 mg 3-4 times a day.

IM

Adults, Elderly. 200 mg 3-4 times a day.

Rectal

Adults, Elderly. 200 mg 3-4 times a day.

Children weighing 30-100 lb. 100-200 mg 3-4 times a day.

Children weighing less than 30 lb. 100 mg 3-4 times a day.

AVAILABLE FORMS

- *Capsules (Tigan):* 250 mg, 300 mg.
- *Injection (Benzacot, Tigan):* 100 mg/ml.
- *Suppositories:* 100 mg (Benzocaine-Trimethobenzamide Pediatric, Navogan, Tebamide, Tebamide Pediatric, Tigan Pediatric), 200 mg (Benzocaine-Trimethobenzamide Adult, Tebamide, Tigan Adult, Tigan Pediatric).

CONTRAINDICATIONS: Hypersensitivity to benzocaine or similar local anesthetics; use of parenteral form in children or suppositories in premature infants or neonates

PREGNANCY AND LACTATION: Pregnancy category C; has been used to treat nausea and vomiting during pregnancy

SIDE EFFECTS

Frequent

Somnolence

Occasional

Blurred vision, diarrhea, dizziness, headache, muscle cramps

Rare

Rash, seizures, depression, opisthotonos, parkinsonian syndrome, Reye's syndrome (marked by vomiting, seizures)

SERIOUS REACTIONS

- A hypersensitivity reaction, manifested as extrapyramidal symptoms (EPS) such as muscle rigidity and allergic skin reactions, occurs rarely.
- Children may experience paradoxical reactions, marked by restlessness, insomnia, euphoria, nervousness, and tremor.
- Overdose may produce CNS depression (manifested as sedation, apnea, cardiovascular collapse, and death) or severe paradoxical reactions (such as hallucinations, tremor, and seizures).

INTERACTIONS

Drugs

3 *Alcohol:* Increased adverse reactions

3 *CNS depressants:* May increase CNS depression

Labs

- *False positive:* Urinary amphetamine

SPECIAL CONSIDERATIONS

- Less effective than phenothiazines

PATIENT/FAMILY EDUCATION

- Relief from nausea or vomiting generally occurs within 30 mins of drug administration
- Trimethobenzamide causes drowsiness—avoid tasks that require mental alertness or motor skills until response to the drug has been established

MONITORING PARAMETERS

- Blood pressure, especially in elderly patients, who are at an increased risk for hypotension
- Electrolytes
- Intake and output
- Hydration status

trimethoprim

(trye-meth'-oh-prim)

Rx: Primsol, Proloprim, Trimpex

Combinations

Rx: with sulfamethoxazole (see co-trimoxazole monograph); with polymixin B sulfate (Polytrim Ophthalmic)

Chemical Class: Folate-antagonist, synthetic

Therapeutic Class: Antibiotic

CLINICAL PHARMACOLOGY

Mechanism of Action: A folate antagonist that blocks bacterial biosynthesis of nucleic acids and proteins by interfering with the metabolism of folinic acid. ***Therapeutic Effect:*** Bacteriostatic.

Pharmacokinetics

Rapidly and completely absorbed from the GI tract. Protein binding: 42%-46%. Widely distributed, including to CSF. Metabolized in the liver. Primarily excreted in urine. Moderately removed by hemodialysis. ***Half-life:*** 8-10 hrs (increased in impaired renal function and newborns; decreased in children).

INDICATIONS AND DOSAGES

Acute, uncomplicated UTI

PO

Adults, Elderly, Children 12 yrs and older. 100 mg q12h or 200 mg once a day for 10 days.

Children younger than 12 yrs. 4-6 mg/kg/day in 2 divided doses for 10 days.

Dosage in renal impairment

Dosage and frequency are modified based on creatinine clearance.

Creatinine Clearance	*Dosage Interval*
greater than 30 ml/min	No change
15-29 ml/min	50 mg q12h

AVAILABLE FORMS

- *Oral Solution (Primsol):* 50 mg/5 ml.
- *Tablets (Trimpex, Proloprim):* 100 mg, 200 mg.

UNLABELED USES: Prevention of bacterial UTIs, treatment of pneumonia caused by *Pneumocystis carinii*

CONTRAINDICATIONS: Infants younger than 2 mos, megaloblastic anemia due to folic acid deficiency

PREGNANCY AND LACTATION: Pregnancy category C; because trimethoprim is a folate antagonist, caution should be used during the first trimester; excreted into breast milk in low concentrations; compatible with breast-feeding

SIDE EFFECTS

Occasional

Nausea, vomiting, diarrhea, decreased appetite, abdominal cramps, headache

Rare

Hypersensitivity reaction (pruritus, rash), methemoglobinemia (bluish fingernails, lips, or skin; fever; pale skin; sore throat; unusual tiredness), photosensitivity

SERIOUS REACTIONS

- Stevens-Johnson syndrome, erythema multiforme, exfoliative dermatitis, and anaphylaxis occur rarely.
- Hematologic toxicity (thrombocytopenia, neutropenia, leukopenia, megaloblastic anemia) is more likely to occur in elderly, debilitated, or alcoholic patients; in patients with impaired renal function; and in those receiving prolonged high dosage.

INTERACTIONS

Drugs

3 *Dapsone:* Increased serum concentrations of both drugs

3 *Folate antagonists (including methotrexate):* May increase the risk of megaloblastic anemia

3 *Phenytoin:* Increased serum phenytoin concentrations, potential for toxicity

3 *Procainamide:* Increased serum concentrations of procainamide and N-acetylprocainamide

SPECIAL CONSIDERATIONS

- Good alternative to co-trimoxazole in patients taking warfarin

PATIENT/FAMILY EDUCATION

- Space drug doses evenly around the clock and complete the full course of trimethoprim therapy, which usually lasts 10-14 days
- Take trimethoprim with food if stomach upset occurs
- Avoid sun and ultraviolet light and use sunscreen and wear protective clothing when outdoors
- Immediately report bleeding, bruising, skin discoloration, fever, pallor, rash, sore throat, and tiredness

MONITORING PARAMETERS

- Skin for rash
- Serum hematology reports
- Liver and renal function
- Signs and symptoms of hematologic toxicity, such as bleeding, ecchymosis, fever, malaise, pallor, and sore throat

trimetrexate

(tri-me-trex'-ate)

Rx: Neutrexin

Chemical Class: Dihydrofolate reductase inhibitor; substituted quinazoline

Therapeutic Class: Antiprotozoal

CLINICAL PHARMACOLOGY

Mechanism of Action: A folate antagonist that inhibits the enzyme dihydrofolate reductase (DHFR). ***Therapeutic Effect:*** Disrupts purine, DNA, RNA, protein synthesis, with consequent cell death.

Pharmacokinetics

Following IV administration, distributed readily into ascitic fluid. Metabolized in liver. Eliminated in urine. ***Half-life:*** 11-20 hrs.

INDICATIONS AND DOSAGES

Pneumocystis carinii pneumonia (PCP)

IV Infusion

Adults. Trimetrexate: 45 mg/m^2 once daily over 60-90 min. Leucovorin: 20 mg/m^2 over 5-10 min q6h for total daily dose of 80 mg/m^2, or orally as 4 doses of 20 mg/m^2 spaced equally throughout the day. Round up the oral dose to the next higher 25-mg increment. Recommended course of therapy: 21 days trimetrexate, 24 days leucovorin.

AVAILABLE FORMS

• *Powder for Injection:* 25 mg (Neutrexin).

UNLABELED USES: Treatment of non-small cell lung, prostate, and colorectal cancer

CONTRAINDICATIONS: Clinically significant hypersensitivity to trimetrexate, leucovorin, or methotrexate

PREGNANCY AND LACTATION: Pregnancy category D; breast milk excretion unknown, but women should not breastfeed while taking trimetrexate

SIDE EFFECTS

Occasional

Fever, rash, pruritus, nausea, vomiting, confusion

Rare

Fatigue

SERIOUS REACTIONS

• Trimetrexate given without concurrent leucovorin may result in serious or fatal hematologic, hepatic, and/or renal complications, including bone marrow suppression, oral and GI mucosal ulceration, and renal and hepatic dysfunction.

• In event of overdose, stop trimetrexate and give leucovorin 40 mg/m^2 q6h for 3 days.

• Anaphylaxis occurs rarely.

INTERACTIONS

Drugs

❷ *Cimetidine:* Reduced trimetrexate metabolism

❷ *Erythromycin:* Reduced trimetrexate metabolism

❷ *Ketoconazole:* Reduced trimetrexate metabolism

❷ *Rifabutin:* Increased trimetrexate metabolism

❷ *Rifampin:* Increased trimetrexate metabolism

SPECIAL CONSIDERATIONS

• Reserve for patients intolerant of or refractory to trimethoprim-sulfamethoxazole

• Randomized trials show trimetrexate is less effective than trimethoprim-sulfamethoxazole (failure rates 40% and 24%, respectively)

PATIENT/FAMILY EDUCATION

• Use two forms of contraception during therapy

• Avoid persons with bacterial infections

• Notify the physician if fever, chills, cough or hoarseness, lower back or side pain, or painful urination occurs

• Report any unusual bleeding or bruising

MONITORING PARAMETERS

• Check at least twice per week: CBC with platelets, hepatic and renal function

trimipramine maleate

(trye-mi′-pra-meen)

Rx: Surmontil

Chemical Class: Dibenzazepine derivative; tertiary amine

Therapeutic Class: Antidepressant, tricyclic

CLINICAL PHARMACOLOGY

Mechanism of Action: A tricyclic antibulimic, anticataplectic, antidepressant, antinarcoleptic, antineuralgic, antineuritic, and antipanic agent that blocks the reuptake of neurotransmitters, such as norepinephrine and serotonin, at presynaptic membranes, increasing their concentration at postsynaptic receptor sites. May demonstrate less autonomic toxicity than other tricyclic antidepressants. ***Therapeutic Effect:*** Results in antidepressant effect. Anticholinergic effect controls nocturnal enuresis.

Pharmacokinetics

Rapidly, completely absorbed after PO administration, and not affected by food. Protein binding: 95%. Metabolized in liver (significant first-pass effect). Primarily excreted in urine. Not removed by hemodialysis. ***Half-life:*** 16-40 hrs.

INDICATIONS AND DOSAGES

Depression

PO

Adults. 50-150 mg/day at bedtime. Maximum: 200 mg/day for outpatients, 300 mg/day for inpatients.

Elderly. Initially, 25 mg/day at bedtime. May increase by 25 mg q3-7days. Maximum: 100 mg/day.

AVAILABLE FORMS

- *Capsules:* 25 mg, 50 mg, 100 mg (Surmontil).

CONTRAINDICATIONS: Acute recovery period after myocardial infarction (MI), within 14 days of MAOI ingestion, hypersensitivity to trimipramine or any component of the formulation

PREGNANCY AND LACTATION: Pregnancy category C; excreted into breast milk; effect on nursing infant unknown, but may be of concern

SIDE EFFECTS

Frequent

Drowsiness, fatigue, dry mouth, blurred vision, constipation, delayed micturition, postural hypotension, diaphoresis, disturbed concentration, increased appetite, urinary retention, photosensitivity.

Occasional

Gastrointestinal (GI) disturbances, such as nausea, and a metallic taste sensation.

Rare

Paradoxical reaction, marked by agitation, restlessness, nightmares, insomnia, extrapyramidal symptoms, particularly fine hand tremors.

SERIOUS REACTIONS

- High dosage may produce cardiovascular effects, such as severe postural hypotension, dizziness, tachycardia, palpitations, arrhythmias and seizures. High dosage may also result in altered temperature regulation, including hyperpyrexia or hypothermia.
- Abrupt withdrawal from prolonged therapy may produce headache, malaise, nausea, vomiting, and vivid dreams.

INTERACTIONS

Drugs

3 *Anticholinergics, propantheline:* Excessive anticholinergic effects

3 *Barbiturates, carbamazepine:* Reduced serum concentrations of cyclic antidepressants

3 *Cimetidine:* Increases trimipramine level

2 *Clonidine:* Reduced antihypertensive response to clonidine; enhanced hypertensive response with abrupt clonidine withdrawal

2 *Epinephrine, norepinephrine:* Markedly enhanced pressor response to IV epinephrine

3 *Ethanol:* Additive impairment of motor skills; abstinent alcoholics may eliminate cyclic antidepressants more rapidly than non-alcoholics

3 *Fluoxetine:* Marked increases in cyclic antidepressant plasma concentrations

2 *Guanadrel, guanethidine:* Inhibited antihypertensive response to guanethidine

▲ *MAOIs:* Excessive sympathetic response; mania or hyperpyrexia possible

❷ *Moclobemide:* Potential association with fatal or non-fatal serotonin syndrome

❸ *Phenylephrine:* Markedly enhanced pressor response to IV epinephrine

❸ *Propoxyphene:* Enhanced effect of cyclic antidepressants

❸ *Quinidine:* Increased cyclic antidepressant serum concentrations

SPECIAL CONSIDERATIONS

PATIENT/FAMILY EDUCATION

- Therapeutic effects may take 2-3 wk
- Avoid rising quickly from sitting to standing, especially in elderly
- Do not discontinue abruptly after long-term use
- Take sips of tepid water and chew sugarless gum to relieve dry mouth

MONITORING PARAMETERS

- CBC, ECG
- Blood pressure, pulse

trioxsalen

(trye-ox'-sa-len)

Rx: Trisoralen

Chemical Class: Psoralen derivative

Therapeutic Class: Pigmenting agent

CLINICAL PHARMACOLOGY

Mechanism of Action: A member of the family of psoralens that induces the process of melanogenesis by a mechanism that is not known. ***Therapeutic Effect:*** Enhances pigmentation.

Pharmacokinetics

Rapidly absorbed from the gastrointestinal (GI) tract. ***Half-life:*** 2 hrs. (skin sensitivity to light remains for 8-12 hrs).

INDICATIONS AND DOSAGES

Pigmentation

PO

Adults, Elderly, Children 12 yrs and older. 10 mg/day 2 hrs before exposure to UVA light or sun exposure.

Vitiligo

PO

Adults, Elderly, Children 12 yrs and older. 10 mg/day 2-4 hrs before exposure to UVA light.

AVAILABLE FORMS

- *Tablets:* 5 mg (Trisoralen).

UNLABELED USES: Polymorphous light eruption, psoriasis, sunlight sensitivity

CONTRAINDICATIONS: Concomitant disease states associated with photosensitivity (acute lupus erythematosus, porphyria, leukoderma of infectious origin), concomitant use of preparations with any internal or external photosensitizing capacity, children under 12 yrs old, hypersensitivity to trioxsalen or any component of the formulation

PREGNANCY AND LACTATION: Pregnancy category C; excretion into breast milk unknown; use caution in nursing mothers

SIDE EFFECTS

Occasional

Gastric discomfort, photosensitivity, pruritus

SERIOUS REACTIONS

- Overdose or overexposure may result in serious blistering and burning.

INTERACTIONS

Drugs

❸ *Anthralin, coal tar, griseofulvin, phenothiazines, nalidixic acid, halogenated salicylanilides, sulfonamides, tetracyclines, thiazides:* Increased photosensitivity to these agents

T

SPECIAL CONSIDERATIONS

PATIENT/FAMILY EDUCATION

- Do not sunbathe during 24 hr prior to ingestion and UVA exposure
- Wear UVA-absorbing sunglasses for 24 hr following treatment to prevent cataract
- Avoid sun exposure for at least 8 hr after ingestion
- Avoid furocoumarin-containing foods (e.g., limes, figs, parsley, parsnips, mustard, carrots, celery)
- Repigmentation may begin after 2-3 wk but full effect may require 6-9 mo

MONITORING PARAMETERS

- Skin for therapeutic response

trospium chloride

(trose′-pee-um klor′-ide)

Rx: Sanctura

Chemical Class: Antimuscarinic substituted amine

Therapeutic Class: Genitourinary muscle relaxant

CLINICAL PHARMACOLOGY

Mechanism of Action: An anticholinergic that antagonizes the effect of acetylcholine on muscarinic receptors, producing parasympatholytic action. ***Therapeutic Effect:*** Reduces smooth muscle tone in the bladder.

Pharmacokinetics

Minimally absorbed after PO administration. Protein binding: 50%-85%. Distributed in plasma. Excreted mainly in feces and, to a lesser extent, in urine. ***Half life:*** 20 hr.

INDICATIONS AND DOSAGES

Overactive bladder

PO

Adults. 20 mg twice a day.

Elderly (75 yr and older). Titrate dosage down to 20 mg once a day, based on tolerance.

Dosage in renal impairment

For patients with creatinine clearance less than 30 ml/min, dosage reduced to 20 mg once a day at bedtime.

AVAILABLE FORMS

- *Tablets:* 20 mg.

CONTRAINDICATIONS: Decreased GI motility, gastric retention, uncontrolled angle-closure glaucoma, urine retention

PREGNANCY AND LACTATION: Pregnancy category C; breast milk excretion unknown

SIDE EFFECTS

Frequent (20%)

Dry mouth

Occasional (10%-4%)

Constipation, headache

Rare (less than 2%)

Fatigue, upper abdominal pain, dyspepsia, flatulence, dry eyes, urine retention

SERIOUS REACTIONS

- Overdose may result in severe anticholinergic effects, such as abdominal pain, nausea and vomiting, confusion, depression, diaphoresis, facial flushing, hypertension, hypotension, respiratory depression, irritability, lacrimation, nervousness, and restlessness.
- Supraventricular tachycardia and hallucinations occur rarely.

INTERACTIONS

Drugs

3 *Digoxin, metformin, morphine, pancuronium, tenofovir, vancomycin:* May increase trospium blood concentration

3 *Other anticholinergic agents:* Increases the severity and frequency of side effects and may alter the absorption of other drugs because of anticholinergic effects on GI motility

3 *Procainamide:* Additive antivagal effects at atrioventricular node

SPECIAL CONSIDERATIONS

- Studies have not shown that trospium is better than generically available drugs for the same purpose

PATIENT/FAMILY EDUCATION

- May precipitate urinary retention or narrow angle glaucoma
- Do not take trospium with high-fat meals because they may reduce drug absorption
- Notify the health care provider if increased salivation or sweating, an irregular heartbeat, nausea and vomiting, or severe abdominal pain occurs

MONITORING PARAMETERS

- Intake and output
- Pattern of daily bowel activity and stool consistency
- Symptomatic relief

trovafloxacin/ alatrofloxacin

(troe′-va-flox-a-sin/a-lat-roe-flox′-a-sin)

Rx: Trovan

Combinations

Rx: with azithromycin (Trovan/Zithromax compliance pak)

Chemical Class: Fluoroquinolone derivative

Therapeutic Class: Antibiotic

CLINICAL PHARMACOLOGY

Mechanism of Action: A fluoroquinolone that inhibits the DNA enzyme gyrase in susceptible microorganisms, interfering with bacterial DNA replication and repair. ***Therapeutic Effect:*** Produces bactericidal activity.

Pharmacokinetics

Well absorbed from the gastrointestinal (GI) tract. Protein binding: 76%. Widely distributed, including to cerebrospinal fluid (CSF). Metabolized in liver by conjugation. Excreted in feces. Not removed by hemodialysis. ***Half-life:*** 9-13 hrs.

INDICATIONS AND DOSAGES

Pneumonia

PO/IV

Adults, Elderly. 200 mg q24h for 7-14 days.

Skin and skin-structure infections

PO/IV

Adults, Elderly. 200 mg q24h for 10-14 days.

Gynecologic infections

IV

Adults, Elderly. 300 mg q24h for 7-14 days.

PO

Adults, Elderly. 100 mg q24h for 7-14 days.

Abdominal infection

Adults, Elderly. 300 mg q24h for 7-14 days.

Bronchitis

PO

Adults, Elderly. 100 q24h for 7-10 days.

AVAILABLE FORMS

- *Tablets:* 100 mg, 200 mg (Trovan).
- *Injection:* 200 mg/40 ml, 300 mg/60 ml (Trovan).

CONTRAINDICATIONS: History of hypersensitivity to other fluoroquinolones

PREGNANCY AND LACTATION: Pregnancy category C; excreted in breast milk

SIDE EFFECTS

Occasional

Diarrhea, dizziness, drowsiness, headache, lightheadedness, vaginal pain and discharge

Rare
Confusion, hallucinations, restlessness, seizures, tremors, rapid heartbeat, shortness of breath, abdominal pain, dark urine, fatigue, loss of appetite, nausea, vomiting, jaundice, pain at injection site, stomach cramps, diarrhea, tendon rupture, increased sensitivity of skin to sunlight

SERIOUS REACTIONS

- Pseudomembranous colitis, as evidenced by severe abdominal pain and cramps, severe watery diarrhea, and fever, may occur.
- Superinfection manifested as genital or anal pruritus, ulceration or changes in oral mucosa, and moderate to severe diarrhea, may occur.
- Hypersensitivity reactions, including photosensitivity as evidenced by rash, pruritus, blistering, swelling, and the sensation of the skin burning, have occurred in patients receiving fluoroquinolone therapy.

INTERACTIONS

Drugs

3 *Aluminum:* Reduced absorption of trovafloxacin; do not take within 4 hr of dose

3 *Antacids:* Reduced absorption of trovafloxacin; do not take within 4 hr of dose

3 *Antidaibetics:* May increase changes in blood glucose and increase risk of hypo/hyperglycemia

3 *Antipyrine:* Inhibits metabolism of antipyrine; increased plasma antipyrine level

3 *Calcium:* Reduced absorption of trovafloxacin; do not take within 4 hr of dose

3 *Diazepam:* Inhibits metabolism of diazepam; increased plasma diazepam level

3 *Didanosine:* Markedly reduced absorption of trovafloxacin; take trovafloxacin 2 hr before didanosine

3 *Foscarnet:* Coadministration increases seizure risk

3 *Iron:* Reduced absorption of trovafloxacin; do not take within 4 hr of dose

3 *Magnesium:* Reduced absorption of trovafloxacin; do not take within 4 hr of dose

3 *Metoprolol:* Inhibits metabolism of metoprolol; increased plasma metoprolol level

3 *Morphine:* Reduced absorption of trovafloxacin; do not take within 2 hr of dose

3 *Pentoxifylline:* Inhibits metabolism of pentoxifylline; increased plasma pentoxifylline level

3 *Phenytoin:* Inhibits metabolism of phenytoin; increased plasma phenytoin level

3 *Propranolol:* Inhibits metabolism of propranolol; increased plasma propranolol level

3 *Ropinirole:* Inhibits metabolism of ropinirole; increased plasma ropinirole level

3 *Sodium bicarbonate:* Reduced absorption of trovafloxacin; do not take within 4 hr of dose

3 *Sucralfate:* Reduced absorption of trovafloxacin; do not take within 4 hr of dose

3 *Warfarin:* Inhibits metabolism of warfarin; increases hypoprothrombinemic response to warfarin

3 *Zinc:* Reduced absorption of trovafloxacin; do not take within 4 hr of dose

SPECIAL CONSIDERATIONS

PATIENT/FAMILY EDUCATION

- Do not take antacids (aluminum-, calcium-, or magnesium-containing) or iron within 2 hr of taking trovafloxacin. Take at bedtime or with food to minimize dizziness associ-

ated with trovafloxacin. Avoid excessive sunlight during treatment
• Drink 6-8 glasses of fluid a day
• Avoid tasks that require mental alertness or motor skills until response to the drug is established
• Notify the physician if chest pain, difficulty breathing, palpitations, persistent diarrhea, swelling, or tendon pain occurs

MONITORING PARAMETERS
• Transaminases if given for more than 7 days
• Signs of hypersensitivity reactions
• Be alert for signs and symptoms of superinfection, manifested as anal or genital pruritus, moderate to severe diarrhea, new or increased fever, and ulceration or changes in oral mucosa

undecylenic acid

(un-de-sill-enn'-ik)

OTC: Caldesene Medicated Powder, Cruex Antifgungal Cream, Cruex Antifungal Powder, Cruex Antifungal Spray Powder, Decylenes Powder, Desenex Antifungal Cream, Desenex Antifungal Liquid, Desenex Antifungal Ointment, Desenex Antifungal Penetrating Foam, Desenex Antifungal Powder, Desenex Antifungal Spray Powder, Godochom Solution

Chemical Class: Hendecenoic acid derivative

Therapeutic Class: Antifungal

CLINICAL PHARMACOLOGY

Mechanism of Action: An antifungal whose mechanism of action is not well understood. ***Therapeutic Effect:*** Fungistatic.

INDICATIONS AND DOSAGES

Tinea pedis, tinea corporis

Topical

Adults, Children 2 yrs and older. Apply 2 times/day to affected area for 4 wks.

AVAILABLE FORMS
• *Aerosol Powder:* 10% (Cruex Antifungal Spray Powder, Desenex Antifungal Spray Powder).
• *Aerosol Foam:* 10% (Desenex Antifungal Penetrating Foam).
• *Cream:* 20% (Cruex Antifungal Cream, Desenex Antifungal Cream).
• *Solution, topical:* 10% (Desenex Antifungal Liquid), 25% (Gordochom Solution).
• *Ointment:* 20% (Desenex Antifungal Ointment).
• *Powder:* 10% (Caldesene Medicated Powder, Cruex Antifungal Powder, Decylenes Powder), 19% (Desenex Antifungal Powder).

CONTRAINDICATIONS: Hypersensitivity to undecylenic acid or any component of its formulation

PREGNANCY AND LACTATION: Problems not documented in breast-feeding

SIDE EFFECTS

Occasional

Skin irritation, rash

SERIOUS REACTIONS
• Hypersensitivity reactions, characterized by rash, facial swelling, pruritus, and a sensation of warmth, may occur.

SPECIAL CONSIDERATIONS
• Newer topical antifungals more effective
• Powders are generally used as adjunctive therapy, but may be useful for primary therapy in very mild cases

PATIENT/FAMILY EDUCATION
• Avoid contact with the eyes
• Separate personal items that come in direct contact with affected area

• Rub the topical form well into the affected area

MONITORING PARAMETERS

• Skin for itching, rash, and urticaria

---

urea

(yoor-ee'-a)

Rx: Carmol-40, Epimide 50, Gordons Urea, Vanamide

OTC: *Topical:* Aqua Care, Carmol, Gormel, Lanaphilic, UltraMide, Ureacin

Chemical Class: Carbonic acid diamide salt

Therapeutic Class: Antiglaucoma agent; osmotic agent

CLINICAL PHARMACOLOGY

Mechanism of Action: A diuretic that rapidly increases blood tonicity, causing a greater urea concentration gradient in the blood than in the extravascular fluid, resulting in movement of fluid from the tissues, including the brain and cerebrospinal fluid, into the blood. A keratolytic that dissolves the intercellular matrix and thereby softens hyperkeratotic areas by enhancing the shedding of scales. ***Therapeutic Effect:*** Decreases ocular hypertension and cerebral edema.

Pharmacokinetics

None known.

INDICATIONS AND DOSAGES

Reduction in intracranial/intraocular pressure

Adults, Elderly. 1-1.5 g/kg. Maximum 120 g daily.

Children 2 yrs and older. 0.5-1.5 g/kg

Children 2 yrs and younger. 0.1 g/kg may be adequate.

Skin/nail debridement

Topical

Adults, Elderly, Children. Apply urea cream, 40% to affected areas. If desired, cover with occlusive dressing. Keep dry and occlusive for 3-7 days.

AVAILABLE FORMS

• *Cream:* 22% (Gordons Urea), 40% (Gordons Urea, Carmol-40, Vanamide).
• *Gel:* 40% (Carmol-40).
• *Lotion:* 40% (Carmol-40).
• *Paste:* 50% (Epimide 50).
• *Powder:* 100% (Urea Rea).

UNLABELED USES: None known.

CONTRAINDICATIONS: Severely impaired renal function, active intracranial bleeding, marked dehydration, frank liver failure,

PREGNANCY AND LACTATION: Pregnancy category C; no data on breast-feeding available

SIDE EFFECTS

Common

Transient stinging, burning, itching, irritation, headaches, nausea, vomiting, infection at site of injection, venous thrombosis or phlebitis extending from site of injection, extravasation, hypervolemia

Occasional

Syncope, disorientation

Rare

Transient agitated confusional state, chemical phlebitis and thrombosis near site of injection

SERIOUS REACTIONS

• No serious reactions have been noted when solutions have been infused slowly, provided renal function is not seriously impaired or there is no evidence of active intracranial bleeding.

• Signs of overdosage include unusually elevated blood urea nitrogen (BUN) levels.

SPECIAL CONSIDERATIONS

• Do not infuse into lower extremity veins

• Monitor for extravasation, tissue necrosis may occur

PATIENT/FAMILY EDUCATION

• Headaches, nausea and vomiting, occasionally syncope and disorientation may occur following intravenous administration

• If redness or irritation occurs with topical use, discontinue use

• Wash excess cream from unaffected skin areas thoroughly after contact

MONITORING PARAMETERS

• BUN

• Serum and urine sodium concentrations

• Electrolytes

---

urokinase

(yoor-oh-kin′-ace)

Rx: Abbokinase, Abbokinase Open-Cath (not for systemic administration)

Chemical Class: Renal enzyme

Therapeutic Class: Thrombolytic

CLINICAL PHARMACOLOGY

Mechanism of Action: A thrombolytic agent that activates fibrinolytic system by converting plasminogen to plasmin (enzyme that degrades fibrin clots). Acts indirectly by forming complex with plasminogen, which converts plasminogen to plasmin. Action occurs within thrombus, on its surface, and in circulating blood. ***Therapeutic Effect:*** Destroys thrombi.

Pharmacokinetics

Rapidly cleared from circulation by liver. Small amounts eliminated in urine and via bile. ***Half-life:*** 20 min.

INDICATIONS AND DOSAGES

Pulmonary embolism

IV

Adults, Elderly. Initially, 4400 IU/kg at rate of 90 ml/hr over 10 min; then, 4400 IU/kg at rate of 15 ml/hr for 12 hrs. Flush tubing. Follow with anticoagulant therapy.

Coronary artery thrombi

Intracoronary

Adults, Elderly. 6000 IU/min for up to 2 hrs.

Occluded IV catheter

Adults, Elderly. Disconnect IV tubing from catheter; attach a 1-ml TB syringe with 5000 U urokinase to catheter; inject urokinase slowly (equal to volume of catheter). Connect empty 5-ml syringe; aspirate residual clot. When patency is restored, irrigate with 0.9% NaCl; reconnect IV tubing to catheter.

AVAILABLE FORMS

• *Powder for Injection:* 250,000 IU/vial, 5000 IU/ml (Abbokinase).

CONTRAINDICATIONS: Active internal bleeding, atrioventricular (AV) malformation or aneurysm, bleeding diathesis, intracranial neoplasm, intracranial or intraspinal surgery or trauma, recent (within the past 2 mos) cerebrovascular accident

PREGNANCY AND LACTATION: Pregnancy category B; no data available on breast-feeding

SIDE EFFECTS

Frequent

Superficial or surface bleeding at puncture sites (venous cutdowns, arterial punctures, surgical sites, IM sites, retroperitoneal/intracerebral sites); internal bleeding (GI/GU tract, vaginal).

Rare

Mild allergic reaction such as rash or wheezing

SERIOUS REACTIONS

• Severe internal hemorrhage may occur. Lysis of coronary thrombi may produce atrial/ventricular arrhythmias

INTERACTIONS

Drugs

3 *Heparin, oral anticoagulants, drugs that alter platelet function (i.e., aspirin, dipyridamole, abciximab, eptifibitide, tirofiban):* May increase the risk of bleeding

SPECIAL CONSIDERATIONS

PATIENT/FAMILY EDUCATION

- Follow measures to reduce the risk of bleeding, such as using an electric razor and a soft toothbrush
- Immediately report signs of bleeding, such as oozing from cuts or gums

MONITORING PARAMETERS

- Before beginning therapy, obtain a hematocrit, platelet count, and a thrombin time (TT), activated partial thromboplastin time (APTT), or prothrombin time (PT)
- Following the intravenous infusion before (re) instituting heparin, the TT or APTT should be less than twice the upper limits of normal
- Blood pressure, pulse rate

---

ursodiol

(er'-soe-dye-ol)

Rx: Actigall, Urso

Chemical Class: Ursodeoxycholic acid

Therapeutic Class: Cholelitholytic

CLINICAL PHARMACOLOGY

Mechanism of Action: A gallstone solubilizing agent that suppresses hepatic synthesis and secretion of cholesterol; inhibits intestinal absorption of cholesterol. ***Therapeutic Effect:*** Changes the bile of patients with gallstones from precipitating (capable of forming crystals) to cholesterol solubilizing (capable of being dissolved).

Pharmacokinetics

Absorbed from the small bowel following PO administration. Protein binding: 70%. Metabolized in colon. Primarily excreted in feces; small amount eliminated in urine. ***Half-life:*** 3.5-5.8 days.

INDICATIONS AND DOSAGES

Dissolution of radiolucent, noncalcified gallstones when cholecystectomy is not recommended; treatment of biliary cirrhosis

PO

Adults, Elderly. 8-10 mg/kg/day in 2-3 divided doses. Treatment may require months. Obtain ultrasound image of gallbladder at 6-mo intervals for first year. If gallstones have dissolved, continue therapy and repeat ultrasound within 1-3 mo.

Prevention of gallstones

PO

Adults, Elderly. 300 mg twice a day.

AVAILABLE FORMS

- *Capsules (Actigall):* 300 mg.
- *Tablets (Urso):* 250 mg.

UNLABELED USES: Prophylaxis of liver transplant rejection, treatment of alcoholic cirrhosis, biliary atresia, chronic hepatitis, gallstone formation, sclerosing cholangitis

CONTRAINDICATIONS: Allergy to bile acids, calcified cholesterol stones, chronic hepatic disease, radiolucent bile pigment stones, radiopaque stones

PREGNANCY AND LACTATION: Pregnancy category B; excretion into breast milk unknown

SIDE EFFECTS

Occasional

Diarrhea

SERIOUS REACTIONS

- None significant.

INTERACTIONS

Drugs

3 *Aluminum-containing antacids, cholestyramine:* May decrease the absorption and effects of ursodiol

3 *Estrogens, oral contraceptives:* May decrease the effects of ursodiol

SPECIAL CONSIDERATIONS

- Complete dissolution may not occur; likelihood of success is low if partial stone dissolution not seen by 12 mo
- Stones recur within 5 yr in 50% of patients

PATIENT/FAMILY EDUCATION

- Administer with food to facilitate dissolution in the intestine
- Therapy requires months
- Avoid taking antacids within hours of taking ursodiol

MONITORING PARAMETERS

- Liver function

valacyclovir hydrochloride

(val-a-sye'-kloh-vir hye-droe-klor'-ide)

Rx: Valtrex

Chemical Class: Acyclic purine nucleoside analog; acyclovir derivative

Therapeutic Class: Antiviral

CLINICAL PHARMACOLOGY

Mechanism of Action: A virustatic antiviral that is converted to acyclovir triphosphate, becoming part of the viral DNA chain. ***Therapeutic Effect:*** Interferes with DNA synthesis and replication of herpes simplex virus and varicella-zoster virus.

Pharmacokinetics

Rapidly absorbed after PO administration. Protein binding: 13%-18%. Rapidly converted by hydrolysis to the active compound acyclovir. Widely distributed to tissues and body fluids (including cerebrospinal fluid [CSF]). Primarily eliminated in urine. Removed by hemodialysis. ***Half-life:*** 2.5-3.3 hr (increased in impaired renal function).

INDICATIONS AND DOSAGES

Herpes zoster (shingles)

PO

Adults, Elderly. 1 g 3 times a day for 7 days.

Herpes simplex (cold sores)

PO

Adults, Elderly. 2 g twice a day for 1 day.

Initial episode of genital herpes

PO

Adults, Elderly. 1 g twice a day for 10 days.

Recurrent episodes of genital herpes

PO

Adults, Elderly. 500 mg twice a day for 3 days.

Prevention of genital herpes

PO

Adults, Elderly. 500-1000 mg/day.

Dosage in renal impairment

Dosage and frequency are modified based on creatinine clearance.

Creatinine Clearance	*Herpes Zoster*	*Genital Herpes*
50 ml/min or higher	1 g q8h	500 mg q12h
30-49 ml/min	1 g q12h	500 mg q12h
10-29 ml/min	1 g q24h	500 mg q24h
less than 10 ml/min	500 mg q24h	500 mg q24h

AVAILABLE FORMS

- *Caplets:* 500 mg, 1000 mg.

UNLABELED USES: To reduce the risk of heterosexual transmission of genital herpes

CONTRAINDICATIONS: Hypersensitivity to or intolerance of acyclovir, valacyclovir, or their components

PREGNANCY AND LACTATION: Pregnancy category B; acyclovir excreted into breast milk; safety not established but should be compatible with breast-feeding

SIDE EFFECTS

Frequent

Herpes zoster (17%-10%): Nausea, headache

Genital herpes (17%): Headache

Occasional

Herpes zoster (7%-3%): Vomiting, diarrhea, constipation (50 yr or older), asthenia, dizziness (50 yr and older)

Genital herpes (8%-3%): Nausea, diarrhea, dizziness

Rare

Herpes zoster (3%-1%): Abdominal pain, anorexia

Genital herpes (3%-1%): Asthenia, abdominal pain

SERIOUS REACTIONS

• Thrombotic thrombocytopenic purpura/hemolytic uremic syndrome (TTP/HUS) has occurred in patients with advanced HIV disease and also in allogenic bone marrow transplant and renal transplant recipients taking valacyclovir at doses of 8 g/day.

INTERACTIONS

Drugs

3 *Cimetidine, probenecid:* May increase acyclovir blood concentration

SPECIAL CONSIDERATIONS

• Acyclovir 400 mg PO bid less expensive for chronic suppression of genital herpes

PATIENT/FAMILY EDUCATION

• Drink adequate fluids

• Start valacyclovir treatment at the first sign of a recurrent episode of genital herpes or herpes zoster; treatment is most effective when started within 48 hrs after symptoms first appear

• Do not touch lesions to avoid spreading the infection to new sites

• Space doses evenly around the clock and continue taking the drug for the full course of treatment

• Avoid sexual intercourse while lesions are present to prevent infecting his or her partner

• Notify the physician if lesions do not improve or if they recur

• The female patient with genital herpes should have a Pap test at least annually because of the increased risk of cervical cancer associated with genital herpes

MONITORING PARAMETERS

• CBC, liver and renal function test results, and urinalysis results

• Evaluate for cutaneous lesions

valganciclovir hydrochloride

(val-gan-sye'-kloh-veer hye-droe-klor'-ide)

Rx: Valcyte

Chemical Class: Acyclic purine nucleoside analog; ganciclovir derivative

Therapeutic Class: Antiviral

CLINICAL PHARMACOLOGY

Mechanism of Action: A synthetic nucleoside that competes with viral DNA esterases and is incorporated directly into growing viral DNA chains. ***Therapeutic Effect:*** Interferes with DNA synthesis and viral replication.

Pharmacokinetics

Well absorbed and rapidly converted to ganciclovir by intestinal and hepatic enzymes. Widely distributed. Slowly metabolized intracellularly. Primarily excreted unchanged in urine. Removed by hemodialysis. ***Half-life:*** 18 hr (increased in impaired renal function).

INDICATIONS AND DOSAGES

Cytomegalovirus (CMV) retinitis in patients with normal renal function

PO

Adults. Initially, 900 mg (two 450-mg tablets) twice a day for 21 days. Maintenance: 900 mg once a day.

Prevention of CMV after transplant

PO

Adults, Elderly. 900 mg once a day beginning within 10 days of transplant and continuing until 100 days post-transplant.

Dosage in renal impairment

Dosage and frequency are modified based on creatinine clearance.

Creatinine Clearance	*Induction Dosage*	*Maintenance Dosage*
60 ml/min or higher	900 mg twice a day	900 mg once a day
40-59 ml/min	450 mg twice a day	450 mg once a day
25-39 ml/min	450 mg once a day	450 mg every 2 days
10-24 ml/min	450 mg every 2 days	450 mg twice a wk

AVAILABLE FORMS

• *Tablets:* 450 mg.

CONTRAINDICATIONS: Hypersensitivity to acyclovir or ganciclovir

PREGNANCY AND LACTATION: Pregnancy category C (teratogenic in animals); breast milk excretion unknown but breast-feeding not recommended if taking valganciclovir; do not resume nursing for at least 72 hr after last dose of valganciclovir

SIDE EFFECTS

Frequent (16%-9%)

Diarrhea, neutropenia, headache

Occasional (8%-3%)

Nausea, anemia, thrombocytopenia

Rare (less than 3%)

Insomnia, paresthesia, vomiting, abdominal pain, fever

SERIOUS REACTIONS

• Hematologic toxicity, including severe neutropenia (most common), anemia, and thrombocytopenia, may occur.

• Retinal detachment occurs rarely.

• An overdose may result in renal toxicity.

• Valganciclovir may decrease sperm production and fertility.

INTERACTIONS

Drugs

3 *Didanosine:* Didanosine may increase valganciclovir level; increased hematologic toxicity possible

❷ *Mycophenolate:* Mycophenolate may increase valganciclovir level; valganciclovir may increase mycophenolate level; increased hematologic toxicity possible

❷ *Probenecid:* Probenecid reduces ganciclovir clearance; increased hematologic toxicity possible

⚠ *Zidovudine:* Additive hematologic toxicity

SPECIAL CONSIDERATIONS

PATIENT/FAMILY EDUCATION

• Take with food

• Do not take during pregnancy or lactation

• Men should use a condom during sex while using this medicine for at least 3 mos after treatment ends because valganciclovir interferes with normal sperm formation

MONITORING PARAMETERS

• CBC, platelet count, creatinine

valproic acid/ valproate sodium/ divalproex sodium

(val-proe'-ik)

Rx: (valproic acid) Depakene

Rx: (valproate sodium) Depakene syrup

Rx: (divalproex sodium) Depacon, Depakote, Depakote ER, Depakote Sprinkle

Chemical Class: Carboxylic acid derivative

Therapeutic Class: Anticonvulsant

CLINICAL PHARMACOLOGY

Mechanism of Action: An anticonvulsant, antimanic, and antimigraine agent that directly increases concentration of the inhibitory neurotransmitter gamma-aminobutyric acid. ***Therapeutic Effect:*** Reduces seizure activity.

Pharmacokinetics

Well absorbed from the GI tract. Protein binding: 80%-90%. Metabolized in the liver. Primarily excreted in urine. Not removed by hemodialysis. ***Half-life:*** 6-16 hrs (may be increased in hepatic impairment, the elderly, and children younger than 18 mos).

INDICATIONS AND DOSAGES

Seizures

PO

Adults, Elderly, Children 10 yrs and older. Initially, 10-15 mg/kg/day in 1-3 divided doses. May increase by 5-10 mg/kg/day at weekly intervals up to 30-60 mg/kg/day. Usual adult dosage: 1000-2500 mg/day.

IV

Adults, Elderly, Children. Same as oral dose but given q6h.

Manic episodes

PO

Adults, Elderly. Initially, 750 mg/day in divided doses. Maximum: 60 mg/kg/day.

Prevention of migraine headaches

PO (Extended-Release)

Adults, Elderly. Initially, 500 mg/day for 7 days. May increase up to 1000 mg/day.

PO (Delayed-Release)

Adults, Elderly. Initially, 250 mg twice a day. May increase up to 1000 mg/day.

AVAILABLE FORMS

- *Capsules (Depakene):* 250 mg.
- *Syrup (Depakene):* 250 mg/5 ml.
- *Tablets (Delayed-Release [Depakote]):* 125 mg, 250 mg, 500 mg.
- *Tablets (Extended-Release [Depakote ER]):* 250 mg, 500 mg.
- *Capsules Sprinkles (Depakote Sprinkle):* 125 mg.
- *Injection (Depacon):* 100 mg/ml.

UNLABELED USES: Prevention of migraine; treatment of behavior disorders in Alzheimer's disease; bipolar disorder; chorea, myoclonic, simple partial, and tonic-clonic seizures; organic brain syndrome; schizophrenia; status epilepticus; tardive dyskinesia

CONTRAINDICATIONS: Active hepatic disease, urea cycle disorders

PREGNANCY AND LACTATION: Pregnancy category D; teratogenic; increased risk of neural tube defects (1%-2% when used between day 17-30 after fertilization); compatible with breast-feeding

SIDE EFFECTS

Frequent

Epilepsy: Abdominal pain, irregular menses, diarrhea, transient alopecia, indigestion, nausea, vomiting, tremors, weight gain or loss

Mania (22%-19%): Nausea, somnolence

Occasional
Epilepsy: Constipation, dizziness, drowsiness, headache, skin rash, unusual excitement, restlessness
Mania (12%-6%): Asthenia, abdominal pain, dyspepsia (heartburn, indigestion, epigastric distress), rash
Rare
Epilepsy: Mood changes, diplopia, nystagmus, spots before eyes, unusual bleeding or ecchymosis

SERIOUS REACTIONS

Alert: Hepatotoxicity may occur, particularly in the first 6 mos of valproic acid therapy. It may be preceded by loss of seizure control, malaise, weakness, lethargy, anorexia, and vomiting rather than abnormal serum liver function test results.

• Blood dyscrasias may occur.

INTERACTIONS

Drugs

3 *Carbamazepine, phenytoin:* Increase, decrease, or no effect on carbamazepine and phenytoin concentrations
3 *Cholestyramine, colestipol:* Reduced absorption of valproic acid
3 *Clarithromycin, erythromycin, troleandomycin:* Increased valproic acid concentrations
3 *Clonazepam:* Absence seizure reported with concurrent use
3 *Clozapine:* Reduced serum clozapine concentrations
3 *Felbamate:* Increased valproic acid concentrations
3 *Isoniazid:* Increased valproic acid concentrations
3 *Lamotrigine:* Increased plasma lamotrigine concentrations; decreased valproic acid concentrations
3 *Nimodipine:* Increased nimodipine area under the plasma concentration-time curve
3 *Phenobarbital, primidone:* Increased phenobarbital levels
3 *Salicylates:* Increased valproate levels
3 *Zidovudine:* Increased zidovudine levels

Labs

• *False increase:* Serum free fatty acids
• *False positive:* Urinary ketones

SPECIAL CONSIDERATIONS

PATIENT/FAMILY EDUCATION

• Administer with food to decrease GI side effects
• Do not administer with carbonated beverages or milk

MONITORING PARAMETERS

• Therapeutic levels (draw just before next dose) 50-100 mcg/ml
• ALT, AST, coagulation studies, and platelet count prior to and during therapy, especially first 6 mo
• Minor elevations in ALT, AST are frequent and dose related

valsartan

(val-sar'-tan)
Rx: Diovan
Combinations
Rx: with hydrochlorothiazide (Diovan HCT)
Chemical Class: Angiotensin II receptor antagonist
Therapeutic Class: Antihypertensive

CLINICAL PHARMACOLOGY

Mechanism of Action: An angiotensin II receptor, type AT_1, antagonist that blocks vasoconstrictor and aldosterone-secreting effects of angiotensin II, inhibiting the binding of angiotensin II to the AT_1 receptors. ***Therapeutic Effect:*** Causes vasodilation, decreases peripheral resistance, and decreases BP.

Pharmacokinetics

Poorly absorbed after PO administration. Food decreases peak plasma concentration. Protein binding: 95%. Metabolized in the liver. Recovered primarily in feces and, to a lesser extent, in urine. Unknown if removed by hemodialysis. ***Half-life:*** 6 hr.

INDICATIONS AND DOSAGES

Hypertension

PO

Adults, Elderly. Initially, 80-160 mg/day in patients who are not volume depleted. May increase up to a maximum: 320 mg/day.

CHF

PO

Adults, Elderly. Initially, 40 mg twice a day. May increase up to 160 mg twice a day. Maximum: 320 mg/day.

Post heart attack

PO

Adults, Elderly. Initially, 20 mg twice a day. May increase within 7 days to 40 mg twice a day. May further increase up to target dose of 160 mg twice a day.

AVAILABLE FORMS

• *Tablets:* 40 mg, 80 mg, 160 mg, 320 mg.

UNLABELED USES: Diabetic nephropathy

CONTRAINDICATIONS: Bilateral renal artery stenosis, biliary cirrhosis or obstruction, hypoaldosteronism, severe hepatic impairment

PREGNANCY AND LACTATION: Pregnancy category C, first trimester—category D, second and third trimesters; drugs acting directly on the renin-angiotensin-aldosterone system are documented to cause fetal harm (hypotension, oligohydramnios, neonatal anemia, hyperkalemia, neonatal skull hypoplasia, anuria, and renal failure); neonatal limb contractures, craniofacial deformities, and hypoplastic lung development

SIDE EFFECTS

Rare (2%-1%)

Insomnia, fatigue, heartburn, abdominal pain, dizziness, headache, diarrhea, nausea, vomiting, arthralgia, edema

SERIOUS REACTIONS

• Overdosage may manifest as hypotension and tachycardia. Bradycardia occurs less often.

• Viral infection and upper respiratory tract infection (cough, pharyngitis, sinusitis, rhinitis) occur rarely.

INTERACTIONS

3 *Diuretics:* Produces additive hypotensive effects

3 *Food:* Decreases peak plasma concentration of valsartan

SPECIAL CONSIDERATIONS

• Potentially as or more effective than angiotensin-converting enzyme inhibitors, without cough; no evidence for reduction in morbidity and mortality as first-line agents in hypertension, yet; whether they provide the same cardiac and renal protection also still tentative; like ACE inhibitors, less effective in black patients

PATIENT/FAMILY EDUCATION

• Call the clinician immediately if note following side effects: wheezing; lip, throat, or face swelling; hives or rash

• Female patients should be aware of the consequences of second- and third-trimester exposure to valsartan

• The female patient should immediately notify the physician if she becomes pregnant

• Valsartan must be taken for the rest of patient's life to control hypertension

• Do not exercise outside during hot weather because of the risks of dehydration and hypotension

MONITORING PARAMETERS

• Baseline electrolytes, urinalysis, BUN and creatinine with recheck at 2-4 wk after initiation (sooner in volume-depleted patients); monitor sitting blood pressure; watch for symptomatic hypotension, particularly in volume-depleted patients

• Assess for signs and symptoms of an upper respiratory tract infection

vancomycin hydrochloride

(van-koe-mye'-sin)

Rx: Vancocin, Vancocin HCl Pulvules

Chemical Class: Tricyclic glycopeptide derivative

Therapeutic Class: Antibiotic

CLINICAL PHARMACOLOGY

Mechanism of Action: A tricyclic glycopeptide antibiotic that binds to bacterial cell walls, altering cell membrane permeability and inhibiting RNA synthesis. ***Therapeutic Effect:*** Bactericidal.

Pharmacokinetics

PO: Poorly absorbed from the GI tract. Primarily eliminated in feces. Parenteral: Widely distributed. Protein binding: 55%. Primarily excreted unchanged in urine. Not removed by hemodialysis. ***Half-life:*** 4-11 hr (increased in impaired renal function).

INDICATIONS AND DOSAGES

Treatment of bone, respiratory tract, skin and soft-tissue infections, endocarditis, peritonitis, and septicemia; prevention of bacterial endocarditis in those at risk (if penicillin is contraindicated) when undergoing biliary, dental, GI, GU, or respiratory surgery or invasive procedures

IV

Adults, Elderly. 500 mg q6h or 1 g q12h.

Children older than 1 mo. 40 mg/kg/day in divided doses q6-8h. Maximum: 3-4 g/day.

Neonates. Initially, 15 mg/kg, then 10 mg/kg q8-12h.

Staphylococcal enterocolitis, antibiotic-associated pseudomembranous colitis caused by Clostridium difficile

PO

Adults, Elderly. 0.5-2 g/day in 3-4 divided doses for 7-10 days.

Children. 40 mg/kg/day in 3-4 divided doses for 7-10 days. Maximum: 2 g/day.

Dosage in renal impairment

After a loading dose, subsequent dosages and frequency are modified based on creatinine clearance, the severity of the infection, and the serum concentration of the drug.

AVAILABLE FORMS

• *Capsules (Vancocin HCl Pulvules):* 125 mg, 250 mg.

• *Powder for Oral Suspension (Vancocin):* 1 g (provides 250 mg/5 ml after mixing).

• *Powder for Injection (Lyphocin, Vancocin HCl):* 500 mg, 1 g, 5 g, 10 g.

• *Infusion (Premix [Vancocin HCl]):* 500 mg/100 ml, 1 g/200 ml.

UNLABELED USES: Treatment of brain abscess, perioperative infections, staphylococcal or streptococcal meningitis

CONTRAINDICATIONS: None known.

PREGNANCY AND LACTATION: Pregnancy category C (oral), B (IV); excreted into breast milk, milk level 4 hr after steady-state dose, 12.7 mcg/ml (similar to mother's trough level); poorly absorbed orally, systemic absorption not expected; problems limited to modification of bowel flora, allergic sensitization, and interference with interpretation of culture results during fever workup

SIDE EFFECTS

Frequent

PO: Bitter or unpleasant taste, nausea, vomiting, mouth irritation (with oral solution)

Rare

Parenteral: Phlebitis, thrombophlebitis, or pain at peripheral IV site; dizziness; vertigo; tinnitus; chills; fever; rash; necrosis with extravasation

PO: Rash

SERIOUS REACTIONS

- Nephrotoxicity and ototoxicity may occur.
- "Red-neck" syndrome (redness on face, neck, arms, and back; chills; fever; tachycardia; nausea or vomiting; pruritus; rash; unpleasant taste) may result from too-rapid injection.

INTERACTIONS

Drugs

3 *Aminoglycosides:* Enhanced nephrotoxicity

3 *Amphotericin B, aspirin, bumetanide, carmustine, cisplatin, cyclosporine, ethacrynic acid, furosemide, streptozocin:* Enhanced ototoxicity and nephrotoxicity of parenteral vancomycin

3 *Cholestyramine, colestipol:* May decrease the effects of oral vancomycin

3 *Indomethacin:* Increased vancomycin in neonates, possible vancomycin toxicity

3 *Methotrexate:* Reduced methotrexate concentrations with oral vancomycin

Labs

- *False increase:* CSF protein

SPECIAL CONSIDERATIONS

PATIENT/FAMILY EDUCATION

- Space drug doses evenly around the clock and continue vancomycin therapy for the full course of treatment
- Notify the physician if a rash, tinnitus, or signs and symptoms of nephrotoxicity occur
- Laboratory tests are an important part of the therapy regimen

MONITORING PARAMETERS

- Audiograms, BUN, creatinine, serum vancomycin concentrations
- Renal function
- Intake and output
- Vancomycin therapeutic peak serum level is 20-40 mcg/ml, and the trough level is 5-15 mcg/ml. The toxic peak serum level is greater than 40 mcg/ml, and the trough level is greater than 15 mcg/ml

vardenafil hydrochloride

(var-den'-a-fil hye-droe-klor'-ide)

Rx: Levitra

Chemical Class: CGMP specific phosphodiesterase inhibitor

Therapeutic Class: Antiimpotence agent

CLINICAL PHARMACOLOGY

Mechanism of Action: An erectile dysfunction agent that inhibits phosphodiesterase type 5, the enzyme responsible for degrading cyclic guanosine monophosphate in the corpus cavernosum of the penis, resulting in smooth muscle relaxation and increased blood flow. ***Therapeutic Effect:*** Facilitates an erection.

Pharmacokinetics

Rapidly absorbed after PO administration. Extensive tissue distribution. Protein binding: 95%. Metabolized in the liver. Excreted primarily in feces; a lesser amount eliminated in urine. Drug has no effect on penile blood flow without sexual stimulation. ***Half-life:*** 4-5 hr.

INDICATIONS AND DOSAGES

Erectile dysfunction

PO

Adults. 10 mg approximately 1 hr before sexual activity. Dose may be increased to 20 mg or decreased to 5 mg, based on patient tolerance. Maximum dosing frequency is once daily.

Elderly, older than 65 yr. 5 mg.

Dosage in moderate hepatic impairment

PO

For patients with Child-Pugh class B hepatic impairment, dosage is 5 mg 60 min before sexual activity.

Dosage with concurrent ritonavir

PO

Adults. 2.5 mg in a 72-hr period.

Dosage with concurrent ketoconazole or itraconazole (at 400 mg/day), or indinavir

PO

Adults. 2.5 mg in a 24-hr period.

Dosage with concurrent ketoconazole or itraconazole (at 200 mg/day), or erythromycin

PO

Adults. 5 mg in a 24-hr period.

AVAILABLE FORMS

• *Tablets:* 2.5 mg, 5 mg, 10 mg, 20 mg.

CONTRAINDICATIONS: Concurrent use of alpha-adrenergic blockers, sodium nitroprusside, or nitrates in any form

PREGNANCY AND LACTATION: Pregnancy category B; not indicated for use in women

SIDE EFFECTS

Occasional

Headache, flushing, rhinitis, indigestion

Rare (less than 2%)

Dizziness, changes in color vision, blurred vision

SERIOUS REACTIONS

• Prolonged erections (lasting over 4 hrs) and priapism (painful erections lasting over 6 hrs) occur rarely.

INTERACTIONS

Drugs

▲ *Alpha-adrenergic blockers:* Concurrent use with vardenafil contraindicated

❷ *Erythromycin:* Erythromycin increases vardenafil C_{max} by factor of 4

❸ *High-fat meals:* Delays drug's maximum effectiveness

❷ *Indinavir:* Indinavir increases vardenafil C_{max} by factor of 7, vardenafil reduces indinavir C_{max} by 40%

❷ *Itraconazole:* Itraconazole increases vardenafil C_{max} by factor of 4

❷ *Ketoconazole:* Ketoconazole increases vardenafil C_{max} by factor of 4

▲ *Nitrates:* Concurrent use with vardenafil contraindicated

❷ *Ritonavir:* Ritonavir increases vardenafil C_{max} by factor of 13, vardenafil reduces ritonavir C_{max} by 20%

SPECIAL CONSIDERATIONS

PATIENT/FAMILY EDUCATION

• Sexual stimulation is required for an erection to occur after taking vardenafil

• Take vardenafil approximately 60 mins before sexual activity, fatty meal may reduce effect

• Rates of erection sufficient for penetration were 65%, 75%, and 80% with 5 mg, 10 mg, and 20 mg doses, respectively

- For diabetics, rates of erection sufficient for penetration were 61% and 64% with 10 mg and 20 mg doses, respectively
- For men after radical prostatectomy, rates of erection sufficient for penetration were 47% and 48% with 10 mg and 20 mg doses, respectively
- Seek treatment immediately if an erection lasts longer than 4 hrs
- Avoid using nitrate drugs and alpha-adrenergic blockers concurrently with vardenafil

MONITORING PARAMETERS

- Cardiovascular status

vasopressin

(vay-soe-press'-in)

Rx: Pitressin

Chemical Class: Arginine vasopressin

Therapeutic Class: Antidiuretic; hemostatic

CLINICAL PHARMACOLOGY

Mechanism of Action: A posterior pituitary hormone that increases reabsorption of water by the renal tubules. Increases water permeability at the distal tubule and collecting duct. Directly stimulates smooth muscle in the GI tract. ***Therapeutic Effect:*** Causes peristalsis and vasoconstriction.

Pharmacokinetics

Route	*Onset*	*Peak*	*Duration*
IV	N/A	N/A	0.5-1 hrs
IM, Subcutaneous	1-2 hrs	N/A	2-8 hrs

Distributed throughout extracellular fluid. Metabolized in the liver and kidney. Primarily excreted in urine. ***Half-life:*** 10-20 mins.

INDICATIONS AND DOSAGES

Cardiac arrest

IV

Adults, Elderly. 40 units as a one-time bolus.

Diabetes insipidus

IV Infusion

Adults, Children. 0.5 mUnits/kg/hr. May double dose q30min. Maximum: 10 mUnits/kg/hr.

IM, Subcutaneous

Adults, Elderly. 5-10 units 2-4 times a day. Range: 5-60 unit/day.

Children. 2.5-10 units, 2-4 times a day.

Abdominal distention, intestinal paresis

IM

Adults, Elderly. Initially, 5 units. Subsequent doses, 10 units q3-4h.

GI hemorrhage

IV Infusion

Adults, Elderly. Initially, 0.2-0.4 unit/min progressively increased to 0.9 unit/min.

Children. 0.002-0.005 unit/kg/min. Titrate as needed. Maximum: 0.01 unit/kg/min.

Vasodilatory shock

IV

Adults, Elderly. Initially, 0.04-0.1 unit/min. Titrate to desired effect.

AVAILABLE FORMS

- *Injection:* 20 units/ml.

UNLABELED USES: Adjunct in treatment of acute, massive hemorrhage

CONTRAINDICATIONS: None known.

PREGNANCY AND LACTATION: Pregnancy category B; breast-feeding reported without complications

SIDE EFFECTS

Frequent

Pain at injection site (with vasopressin tannate)

Occasional
Abdominal cramps, nausea, vomiting, diarrhea, dizziness, diaphoresis, pale skin, circumoral pallor, tremors, headache, eructation, flatulence
Rare
Chest pain; confusion; allergic reaction, including rash or hives, pruritus, wheezing or difficulty breathing, facial and peripheral edema; sterile abscess (with vasopressin tannate)

SERIOUS REACTIONS

- Anaphylaxis, MI, and water intoxication have occurred.
- The elderly and very young are at higher risk for water intoxication.

INTERACTIONS

Drugs

3 *Alcohol, demeclocycline, lithium, norepinephrine:* May decrease the effects of vasopressin
3 *Carbamazepine, chlorpropamide, clofibrate:* May increase the effects of vasopressin

SPECIAL CONSIDERATIONS

- For diabetes insipidus, vasopressin sol for injection may be administered intranasally on cotton pledgets, by nasal spray or by dropper; dose must be individualized

PATIENT/FAMILY EDUCATION

- Common adverse effects (skin blanching, abdominal cramps, and nausea) may be reduced by taking 1-2 glasses of water with the dose of vasopressin; self-limited in minutes
- Report chest pain, headache, shortness of breath, or other symptoms
- Avoid alcohol
- Monitor fluid intake and output

MONITORING PARAMETERS

- ECG, fluid and electrolyte status, urine-specific gravities
- Extravasation may cause tissue necrosis
- Blood pressure, pulse rate
- Intake and output

venlafaxine hydrochloride

(ven'-la-fax-een hye-droe-klor'-ide)
Rx: Effexor, Effexor XR
Chemical Class: Phenethylamine derivative
Therapeutic Class: Antidepressant

CLINICAL PHARMACOLOGY

Mechanism of Action: A phenethylamine derivative that potentiates CNS neurotransmitter activity by inhibiting the reuptake of serotonin, norepinephrine and, to a lesser degree, dopamine. ***Therapeutic Effect:*** Relieves depression.

Pharmacokinetics

Well absorbed from the GI tract. Protein binding: 25%-30%. Metabolized in the liver to active metabolite. Primarily excreted in urine. Not removed by hemodialysis. ***Half-life:*** 3-7 hrs; metabolite, 9-13 hrs (increased in hepatic or renal impairment).

INDICATIONS AND DOSAGES

Depression

PO
Adults, Elderly. Initially, 75 mg/day in 2-3 divided doses with food. May increase by 75 mg/day at intervals of 4 days or longer. Maximum: 375 mg/day in 3 divided doses.
PO (Extended-Release)
Adults, Elderly. 75 mg/day as a single dose with food. May increase by 75 mg/day at intervals of 4 days or longer. Maximum: 225 mg/day.

Social anxiety disorder, generalized anxiety disorder
PO (Extended-Release)
Adults, Elderly. Initially, 37.5-75 mg/day. May increase by 75 mg/day at 4-day intervals up to 225 mg/day.
Dosage in renal and hepatic impairment
Expect to decrease venlafaxine dosage by 50% in patients with moderate hepatic impairment, 25% in patients with mild to moderate renal impairment, and 50% in patients on dialysis (withhold dose until completion of dialysis).

AVAILABLE FORMS
- *Capsules (Extended-Release [Effexor XL]):* 37.5 mg, 75 mg, 150 mg.
- *Tablets (Effexor):* 25 mg, 37.5 mg, 50 mg, 75 mg, 100 mg.

UNLABELED USES: Prevention of relapses of depression; treatment of attention-deficit hyperactivity disorder, autism, chronic fatigue syndrome, obsessive-compulsive disorder

CONTRAINDICATIONS: Use within 14 days of MAOIs

SIDE EFFECTS
Frequent (greater than 20%)
Nausea, somnolence, headache, dry mouth
Occasional (20%-10%)
Dizziness, insomnia, constipation, diaphoresis, nervousness, asthenia, ejaculatory disturbance, anorexia
Rare (less than 10%)
Anxiety, blurred vision, diarrhea, vomiting, tremor, abnormal dreams, impotence

SERIOUS REACTIONS
- A sustained increase in diastolic BP of 10-15 mm Hg occurs occasionally.

INTERACTIONS
Drugs
3 *MAOIs:* May cause neuroleptic malignant syndrome, autonomic instability (including rapid fluctuations of vital signs), extreme agitation, hyperthermia, mental status changes, myoclonus, rigidity, and coma
3 *St. John's Wort:* May increase the sedative-hypnotic effect of venlafaxine

SPECIAL CONSIDERATIONS

PATIENT/FAMILY EDUCATION
- Take venlafaxine with food to minimize GI distress
- Do not abruptly discontinue the drug or decrease or increase the dosage
- Avoid tasks that require mental alertness or motor skills until response to the drug has been established
- The female patient should notify the physician if she is breast-feeding, pregnant, or planning to become pregnant
- Avoid alcohol while taking venlafaxine

MONITORING PARAMETERS
- Blood pressure, weight
- Closely supervise the suicidal patient during early therapy; as depression lessens, the patient's energy level improves, increasing the suicide potential
- Assess appearance, behavior, level of interest, mood, and sleep patterns for evidence of a therapeutic response

verapamil hydrochloride

(ver-ap'-a-mill hye-droe-klor'-ide)

Rx: Calan, Calan SR, Covera-HS, Isoptin, Isoptin I.V., Isoptin SR, Verelan, Verelan PM

Combinations

Rx: with trandolapril (Tarka)

Chemical Class: Phenylalkylamine

Therapeutic Class: Antianginal; antiarrhythmic, class IV; antihypertensive; calcium channel blocker

CLINICAL PHARMACOLOGY

Mechanism of Action: A calcium channel blocker and antianginal, antiarrhythmic, and antihypertensive agent that inhibits calcium ion entry across cardiac and vascular smooth-muscle cell membranes. This action causes the dilation of coronary arteries, peripheral arteries, and arterioles. ***Therapeutic Effect:*** Decreases heart rate and myocardial contractility and slows SA and AV conduction. Decreases total peripheral vascular resistance by vasodilation.

Pharmacokinetics

Route	Onset	Peak	Duration
PO	30 mins	1-2 hrs	6-8 hrs
PO (Extended-Release)	30 mins	N/A	N/A
IV	1-2 mins	3-5 mins	10-60 mins

Well absorbed from the GI tract. Protein binding: 90% (60% in neonates.) Undergoes first-pass metabolism in the liver to active metabolite. Primarily excreted in urine. Not removed by hemodialysis. ***Half-life:*** 2-8 hr.

INDICATIONS AND DOSAGES

Supraventricular tachyarrhythmias (SVT)

IV

Adults, Elderly. Initially, 2.5-5 mg over 2 min. May give 5-10 mg 30 min after initial dose. Maximum initial dose: 20 mg.

Children 1-15 yrs. 0.1-0.3 mg/kg over 2 min. Maximum initial dose: 5 mg. May repeat in 15 min. Maximum second dose: 10 mg.

Children younger than 1 yr. 0.1-0.2 mg/kg over 2 min. May repeat 30 min after initial dose.

Arrhythmias, including prevention of recurrent paroxysmal supraventricular tachycardia and control of ventricular resting rate in chronic atrial fibrillation or flutter (with digoxin)

PO

Adults, Elderly. 240-480 mg/day in 3-4 divided doses.

Vasospastic angina (Prinzmetal's variant), unstable (crescendo or preinfarction) angina, chronic stable (effort-associated) angina

PO

Adults. Initially, 80-120 mg 3 times a day. For elderly patients and those with hepatic dysfunction, 40 mg 3 times a day. Titrate to optimal dose. Maintenance: 240-480 mg/day in 3-4 divided doses.

Hypertension

PO (Immediate-Release)

Adults, Elderly. 80 mg 3 times a day. Range: 80-320 mg/day in 2 divided doses.

PO (Sustained-Release)

Adults, Elderly. 120-240 mg/day. Range: 120-360 mg/day as single dose or in 2 divided doses.

PO (Extended-Release [Covera-HS])

Adults, Elderly. 120-360 mg once daily at bedtime.

PO (Extended-Release [Verelan PM])

Adults, Elderly. 200-400 mg once daily at bedtime.

AVAILABLE FORMS

- *Caplet (Calan SR):* 120 mg, 180 mg, 240 mg.
- *Capsules (Extended-Release [Verelan PM]):* 100 mg, 200 mg, 300 mg.
- *Capsules (Sustained-Release [Verelan]):* 120 mg, 180 mg, 240 mg, 360 mg.
- *Tablets (Calan):* 40 mg, 80 mg, 120 mg.
- *Tablets (Extended-Release [Covera-HS]):* 180 mg, 240 mg.
- *Tablets (Sustained-Release [Isoptin SR]):* 120 mg, 180 mg, 240 mg.
- *Injection:* 2.5 mg/ml.

UNLABELED USES: Treatment of bipolar disorder, hypertrophic cardiomyopathy, vascular headaches

CONTRAINDICATIONS: Atrial fibrillation or flutter and an accessory bypass tract, cardiogenic shock, heart block, hypotension, sinus bradycardia, ventricular tachycardia

PREGNANCY AND LACTATION: Pregnancy category C; excreted in breast milk (approx 25% of maternal serum); compatible with breast-feeding

SIDE EFFECTS

Frequent (7%)

Constipation

Occasional (4%-2%)

Dizziness, lightheadedness, headache, asthenia (loss of strength, energy), nausea, peripheral edema, hypotension

Rare (less than 1%)

Bradycardia, dermatitis or rash

SERIOUS REACTIONS

- Rapid ventricular rate in atrial flutter or fibrillation, marked hypotension, extreme bradycardia, CHF, asystole, and second- and third-degree AV block occur rarely.

INTERACTIONS

Drugs

3 *Amiodarone:* Cardiotoxicity with bradycardia and decreased cardiac output

3 *Barbiturates:* Reduced plasma concentrations of verapamil

3 *Benzodiazepines:* Marked increase in midazolam concentrations, increased sedation likely to result

3 *β-blockers:* β-blocker serum concentrations increased *(atenolol, metoprolol, propranolol)*; increased risk of bradycardia, hypotension, AV conduction, and myocardial contractility

2 *Carbamazepine:* Increased carbamazepine toxicity when verapamil added to chronic anticonvulsant regimens; reduced metabolism

3 *Cimetidine:* Increased verapamil concentrations and effect by cimetidine

3 *Cyclosporine, tacrolimus:* Increased concentrations of these drugs, nephrotoxicity possible

3 *Dantrolene:* Hyperkalemia and myocardial depression may occur; consider a dihydropyridine calcium blocker

3 *Diclofenac:* Reduced verapamil concentrations

3 *Digitalis glycosides:* Increased digoxin concentrations by approximately 70%

3 *Disopyramide:* May increase negative inotropic effect

3 *Doxazosin, prazosin, terazosin:* Enhanced hypotensive effects

3 *Doxorubicin:* Increased doxorubicin concentrations

3 *Encainide:* Increased encainide concentrations

3 *Ethanol:* Increased ethanol concentrations, prolonged and increased levels of intoxication

3 *Fentanyl:* Severe hypotension or increased fluid volume requirements

3 *Grapefruit, grapefruit juice:* May increase verapamil blood concentration

3 *Histamine H_2-antagonists:* Increased blood levels of verapamil with cimetidine

3 *Hydantoins:* Serum verapamil levels may fall if used concurrently

3 *Imipramine:* Increased imipramine concentrations

3 *Lithium:* Potential for neurotoxicity

3 *Neuromuscular blocking agents:* Prolonged neuromuscular blockade

3 *Procainamide:* May increase risk of QT-interval prolongation

3 *Quinidine:* Quinidine toxicity via inhibition of metabolism

3 *Rifampin, rifabutin:* Induced metabolism; reduced verapamil concentrations

3 *Sulfinpyrazone:* Increased clearance of verapamil

3 *Theophylline:* Verapamil inhibits its metabolism, increases theophylline levels

3 *Vitamin D:* Therapeutic efficacy of verapamil may be reduced

SPECIAL CONSIDERATIONS

- Dihydropyridine calcium channel blockers preferred over verapamil and diltiazem in patients with sinus bradycardia, conduction disturbances, and for combination with a β-blocker
- Differentiate PSVT from narrow complex ventricular tachycardia prior to IV administration; failure to do so has resulted in fatalities

PATIENT/FAMILY EDUCATION

- Do not abruptly discontinuing verapamil; compliance with the treatment regimen is essential to control anginal pain
- To avoid the orthostatic effects of verapamil, rise slowly from a lying to a sitting position and to wait momentarily before standing
- Avoid tasks that require mental alertness or motor skills until response to the drug has been established
- Avoid consuming grapefruit or grapefruit juice and limit caffeine intake while taking verapamil
- Notify the physician if anginal pain not reduced by the drug, constipation, dizziness, irregular heartbeat, nausea, shortness of breath, or swelling of the hands and feet occurs

MONITORING PARAMETERS

- Pulse for rate, rhythm, and quality
- EKG for changes, particularly PR-interval prolongation
- Assess stool consistency and frequency
- Therapeutic serum level for verapamil is 0.08-0.3 mcg/ml

vitamin A

(vye'-tah-min A)

Rx: Aquasol A, Palmitate A

Chemical Class: Vitamin, fat soluble

Therapeutic Class: Vitamin

CLINICAL PHARMACOLOGY

Mechanism of Action: A fat-soluble vitamin that may act as a cofactor in biochemical reactions. ***Therapeutic Effect:*** Is essential for normal function of retina, visual adaptation to darkness, bone growth, testicular and ovarian function, and embryonic development; preserves integrity of epithelial cells.

Pharmacokinetics
Rapidly absorbed from the GI tract if bile salts, pancreatic lipase, protein, and dietary fat are present. Transported in blood to the liver, where it is metabolized; stored in parenchymal hepatic cells, then transported in plasma as retinol, as needed. Excreted primarily in bile and, to a lesser extent, in urine.

INDICATIONS AND DOSAGES

Severe vitamin A deficiency
PO
Adults, Elderly, Children 8 yrs and older. 500,000 units/day for 3 days; then 50,000 units/day for 14 days, then 10,000-20,000 units/day for 2 mo.
Children 1-7 yrs. 5000 units/kg/day for 5 days, then 5000-10,000 units/day for 2 mo.
Children younger than 1 yr. 5000-10,000 units/day for 2 mo.
IM
Adults, Elderly, Children 8 yrs and older. 100,000 units/day for 3 days; then 50,000 units/day for 14 days.
Children 1-7 yrs. 17,500-35,000 units/day for 10 days.
Children younger than 1 yr. 7500-15,000 units/day.

Malabsorption syndrome
PO
Adults, Elderly, Children 8 yr and older. 10,000-50,000 units/day.

Dietary supplement
PO
Adults, Elderly. 4000-5000 units/day.
Children 7-10 yrs. 3300-3500 units/day.
Children 4-6 yr. 2500 units/day.
Children 6 mo-3 yrs. 1500-2000 units/day.
Neonates younger than 5 mos. 1500 units/day.

AVAILABLE FORMS
- *Capsules:* 10,000 units, 25,000 units.
- *Injection (Aquasol A):* 50,000 units/ml.
- *Tablets (Palmitate A):* 5000 units, 15,000 units.

CONTRAINDICATIONS: Hypervitaminosis A, oral use in malabsorption syndrome

PREGNANCY AND LACTATION: Pregnancy category X

SIDE EFFECTS
None known.

SERIOUS REACTIONS
- Chronic overdose produces malaise, nausea, vomiting, drying or cracking of skin or lips, inflammation of tongue or gums, irritability, alopecia, and night sweats.
- Bulging fontanelles have occurred in infants.

INTERACTIONS

Drugs
3 *Acitretin, etretinate:* Large doses of vitamin A should be avoided with these retinoids
3 *Cholestyramine, colestipol, mineral oil:* May decrease the absorption of vitamin A
3 *Isotretinoin:* May increase the risk of toxicity

SPECIAL CONSIDERATIONS

PATIENT/FAMILY EDUCATION
- Administer with food for better PO absorption
- Foods high in vitamin A: yellow and dark green vegetables, yellow and orange fruits, A-fortified foods, liver, egg yolks

vitamin D

(vye'-ta-min D)

Rx: Calciferol, Drisdol

Chemical Class: Vitamin, fat soluble

Therapeutic Class: Vitamin

CLINICAL PHARMACOLOGY

Mechanism of Action: A fat-soluble vitamin that stimulates calcium and phosphate absorption from small intestine, promotes secretion of calcium from bone to blood, and promotes resorption of phosphate in renal tubules; also acts on bone cells to stimulate skeletal growth and on parathyroid gland to suppress hormone synthesis and secretion. ***Therapeutic Effect:*** Essential for absorption and utilization of calcium and phosphate and normal bone calcification. Reduces parathyroid hormone level. Improves phosphorus and calcium homeostasis in chronic renal failure.

Pharmacokinetics

Readily absorbed from small intestine. Concentrated primarily in liver and fat deposits. Activated in the liver and kidneys. Eliminated by biliary system; excreted in urine. ***Half-life:*** 19-48 hr for ergocalciferol.

INDICATIONS AND DOSAGES:

Alert: Oral dosing is preferred. Administer the drug IM only in patients with GI, hepatic, or biliary disease associated with malabsorption of vitamin D.

Dietary supplement

PO

Adults, Elderly, Children. 10 mcg (400 units)/day.

Neonates. 10-20 mcg (400-800 units)/day.

Renal failure

PO

Adults, Elderly. 0.5 mg/day.

Children. 0.1-1 mg/day.

Hypoparathyroidism

PO

Adults, Elderly. 625 mcg-5 mg/day (with calcium supplements).

Children. 1.25-5 mg/day (with calcium supplements).

Nutritional rickets, osteomalacia

PO

Adults, Elderly, Children. 25-125 mcg/day for 8-12 wk.

Adults, Elderly (with malabsorption syndrome). 250-7500 mcg/day.

Children (with malabsorption syndrome). 250-625 mcg/day.

Vitamin D-dependent rickets

PO

Adults, Elderly. 250 mcg-1.5 mg/day.

Children. 75-125 mcg/day. Maximum: 1500 mcg/day.

Vitamin D-resistant rickets

PO

Adults, Elderly. 250-1500 mcg/day (with phosphate supplements).

Children. Initially 1000-2000 mcg/day (with phosphate supplements). May increase in 250- to 600-mcg increments q3-4mo.

Osteoporosis prevention

PO

Adults, Elderly. 400-600 units/day. Maximum: 2000 units/day.

AVAILABLE FORMS

- *Capsules (Drisdol):* 50,000 units (1.25 mg).
- *Injection (Calciferol):* 500,000 units/ml (12.5 mg).
- *Oral Liquid Drops (Calciferol, Drisdol):* 8000 units/ml.

CONTRAINDICATIONS: Abnormal sensitivity to toxic effects of hypervitaminosis D, hypercalcemia, malabsorption syndrome

PREGNANCY AND LACTATION: Pregnancy category A (400 IU/d); category D (doses above recommended daily allowance) associated with supravalvular aortic stenosis, elfin facies, and mental retardation; caution should be exercised when ergocalciferol is administered to nursing women; vitamin D and metabolites appear in breast milk; compatible with breast-feeding, but infant should be monitored for hypercalcemia if doses exceed recommended daily allowance

SIDE EFFECTS

Frequency not defined

Nausea, constipation, stiffness, weakness, weight loss

SERIOUS REACTIONS

- Early signs and symptoms of overdose are weakness, headache, somnolence, nausea, vomiting, dry mouth, constipation, muscle and bone pain, and metallic taste.
- Later signs and symptoms of overdose include polyuria, polydipsia, anorexia, weight loss, nocturia, photophobia, rhinorrhea, pruritus, disorientation, hallucinations, hyperthermia, hypertension, and cardiac arrhythmias.

INTERACTIONS

Drugs

3 *Aluminum-containing antacids (long-term use):* May increase aluminum blood concentration and risk of aluminum bone toxicity

3 *Calcium-containing preparations, thiazide diuretics:* May increase the risk of hypercalcemia

3 *Magnesium-containing antacids:* May increase magnesium blood concentration

3 *Mineral oil:* Excessive use of mineral oil decreases vitamin D absorption

Labs

- *Interference:* Serum cholesterol

SPECIAL CONSIDERATIONS

- IM therapy should be reserved for patients with GI, liver, or biliary disease associated with vitamin D malabsorption
- Ensure adequate calcium intake; maintain serum calcium levels between 9-10 mg/dL

PATIENT/FAMILY EDUCATION

- Encourage the patient to consume foods rich in vitamin D, including milk, eggs, leafy vegetables, margarine, meats, and vegetable oils and shortening
- Do not take mineral oil during vitamin D therapy
- The patient receiving chronic renal dialysis should not take magnesium-containing antacids during vitamin D therapy
- Drink plenty of fluids

MONITORING PARAMETERS

- Serum calcium and phosphorus levels (vitamin D levels also helpful, although less frequently)
- Height and weight in children
- X-ray bones monthly until condition is corrected and stabilized
- Periodically determine magnesium and alk phosphatase
- Serum calcium times phosphorous should not exceed 70 mg/dL to avoid ectopic calcification

vitamin E

(vye'-tah-min E)

Rx: Aqua Gem E, Aquasol E, E-Gems, Key-E, Key-E Kaps

Chemical Class: Vitamin, fat soluble

Therapeutic Class: Vitamin

CLINICAL PHARMACOLOGY

Mechanism of Action: An antioxidant that prevents oxidation of vitamins A and C, protects fatty acids from attack by free radicals, and protects RBCs from hemolysis by oxidizing agents. ***Therapeutic Effect:*** Prevents and treats vitamin E deficiency.

Pharmacokinetics

Variably absorbed from the GI tract (requires bile salts, dietary fat, and normal pancreatic function). Primarily concentrated in adipose tissue. Metabolized in the liver. Primarily eliminated by biliary system.

INDICATIONS AND DOSAGES

Vitamin E deficiency

PO

Adults, Elderly. 60-75 units/day.

Children. 1 unit/kg/day.

AVAILABLE FORMS

- *Capsules (E-Gems):* 100 units, 600 units, 800 units, 1000 units, 1200 units.
- *Capsules (Aqua-Gem E, Key-E Kaps):* 200 units, 400 units.
- *Tablets (Key-E):* 100 units, 200 units, 400 units, 800 units.

UNLABELED USES: To decrease severity of tardive dyskinesia

CONTRAINDICATIONS: None known.

PREGNANCY AND LACTATION: Pregnancy category A (C if used in doses above recommended daily allowance)

SIDE EFFECTS

None known.

SERIOUS REACTIONS

- Chronic overdose may produce fatigue, weakness, nausea, headache, blurred vision, flatulence, and diarrhea.

INTERACTIONS

Drugs

3 *Cholestyramine, colestipol, mineral oil:* May decrease the absorption of vitamin E

3 *Iron:* Impaired hematologic response to iron in children with iron-deficiency anemia

3 *Oral anticoagulants:* Vitamin E increases hypoprothombinemic response to oral anticoagulants, especially in doses >400 IU/day

SPECIAL CONSIDERATIONS

- Recommended daily allowance adult male 15 IU, adult female 12 IU

PATIENT/FAMILY EDUCATION

- Swallow tablets and capsules whole; do not chew, open, or crush them
- Notify the physician if signs and symptoms of toxicity, including blurred vision, diarrhea, nausea, dizziness, flu-like symptoms, or headache, occur
- Consume foods rich in vitamin E, including eggs, meats, milk, leafy vegetables, margarine, and vegetable oils and shortening

MONITORING PARAMETERS

- Signs and symptoms of hypervitaminosis E, including headache, fatigue, nausea, weakness, and diarrhea

voriconazole

(vohr-ih-kon′-uh-zohl)

Rx: Vfend

Chemical Class: Triazole derivative

Therapeutic Class: Antifungal

CLINICAL PHARMACOLOGY

Mechanism of Action: A triazole derivative that inhibits the synthesis of ergosterol, a vital component of fungal cell wall formation. ***Therapeutic Effect:*** Damages fungal cell wall membrane.

Pharmacokinetics

Rapidly and completely absorbed after PO administration. Widely distributed. Protein binding: 98%. Metabolized in the liver. Primarily excreted as a metabolite in urine. ***Half-life:*** 6 hr.

INDICATIONS AND DOSAGES

Invasive aspergillosis, other serious fungal infections caused by

Scedosporium apiospermum and Fusarium species

PO

Adults, Elderly weighing 40 kg and more. Initially, 400 mg q12h for 2 doses on day 1. Maintenance: 200 mg q12h (may increase to 200 mg q12h).

Adults, Elderly weighing less than 40 kg. Initially, 200 mg q12h for 2 doses on day 1. Maintenance: 100 mg q12h (may increase to 150 mg q12h).

Usual parenteral dosage

IV

Adults, Elderly, Children. Initially, 6 mg/kg/dose q12h for 2 doses, then 4 mg/kg/dose q12h (may decrease to 3 mg/kg/dose if patient is unable to tolerate 4 mg/kg/dose).

Candidemia in non-neutropenic patients

PO

Adults, Elderly. 200 mg q12h.

IV

Adults, Elderly. Initially, 6 mg/kg/dose q12h for 2 doses, then 3-4 mg/kg/dose q12h.

Esophageal candidiasis

PO

Adults, Elderly weighing 40 kg and more. 200 mg q12h for minimum of 14 days, then at least 7 days following resolution of symptoms.

Adults, Elderly weighing less than 40 kg. 100 mg q12h for minimum of 14 days, then at least 7 days following resolution of symptoms.

AVAILABLE FORMS

- *Tablets:* 50 mg, 200 mg.
- *Injection Powder for Reconstitution:* 200 mg.
- *Powder for Oral Suspension:* 200 mg/5 ml.

CONTRAINDICATIONS: Concurrent administration of carbamazepine; ergot alkaloids; pimozide or quinidine (may cause prolonged QT interval or torsades de pointes); rifabutin; rifampin; or sirolimus

PREGNANCY AND LACTATION: Pregnancy category D; breast milk excretion unknown

SIDE EFFECTS

Frequent (20%-5%)

Abnormal vision, fever, nausea, rash, vomiting

Occasional (5%-2%)

Headache, chills, hallucinations, photophobia, tachycardia, hypertension

SERIOUS REACTIONS

- Hepatotoxicity (e.g., jaundice, hepatitis, hepatic failure, acute renal failure) has been observed in severely ill patients.

INTERACTIONS

Drugs

3 *Alprazolam:* Increased alprazolam effect

⚠ *Astemizole:* Increased astemizole level

⚠ *Barbiturates:* Significantly increased voriconazole metabolism

⚠ *Carbamazepine:* Significantly increased voriconazole metabolism

⚠ *Cisapride:* Increased cisapride level

❷ *Cyclosporine:* Increased cyclosporine level (reduce cyclosporine dose to one-half)

❷ *Delavirdine:* Decreased or increased voriconazole metabolism

3 *Dihydropyridine calcium channel blockers:* Increased dihydropyridine level

❷ *Efavirenz:* Decreased or increased voriconazole metabolism

⚠ *Ergot alkaloids:* Increased ergot alkaloid level

3 *HMG-CoA reductase inhibitors (statins):* Increased statin level

3 *Midazolam:* Increased midazolam effect

❷ *Omeprazole:* Increased omeprazole level (reduce omeprazole dose by one-half if taking 40 mg qd or more)
❷ *Phenytoin:* Increased voriconazole metabolism (adjust dose, see dosage); increased phenytoin level
⚠ *Pimozide:* Increased pimozide level
⚠ *Quinidine:* Increased quinidine level
⚠ *Rifabutin:* Significantly increased voriconazole metabolism
⚠ *Rifampin:* Significantly increased voriconazole metabolism
❸ *Ritonavir:* Decreased voriconazole metabolism
⚠ *Sirolimus:* Increased sirolimus level
❸ *Sulfonylureas:* Increased sulfonylurea level
⚠ *Terfenadine:* Increased terfenadine level
❷ *Tacrolimus:* Increased tacrolimus level (reduce tacrolimus dose to one-third)
❸ *Triazolam:* Increased triazolam effect
❸ *Vinca alkaloids:* Increased vinca alkaloid level
❷ *Warfarin:* Increased hypoprothrombinemic effect

SPECIAL CONSIDERATIONS

- Do not take PO within 1 hr of meals
- Do not drive at night while taking voriconazole
- Avoid direct sunlight
- Voriconazole may have detrimental effects on a fetus; it is important to use effective contraception to avoid becoming pregnant while taking this drug

MONITORING PARAMETERS

- Visual acuity, field, and color perception if taken more than 28 days
- ALT, AST, alkaline phosphatase, bilirubin, electrolytes, renal function

warfarin sodium

(war′-far-in soe′-dee-um)

Rx: Coumadin, Jantoven

Chemical Class: Coumarin derivative

Therapeutic Class: Anticoagulant

CLINICAL PHARMACOLOGY

Mechanism of Action: A coumarin derivative that interferes with hepatic synthesis of vitamin K-dependent clotting factors, resulting in depletion of coagulation factors II, VII, IX, and X. ***Therapeutic Effect:*** Prevents further extension of formed existing clot; prevents new clot formation or secondary thromboembolic complications.

Pharmacokinetics

Route	*Onset*	*Peak*	*Duration*
PO	1.5-3 days	5-7 days	N/A

Well absorbed from the GI tract. Metabolized in the liver. Primarily excreted in urine. Not removed by hemodialysis. ***Half-life:*** 1.5-2.5 days.

INDICATIONS AND DOSAGES

Anticoagulant

PO

Adults, Elderly. Initially, 5-15 mg/day for 2-5 days; then adjust based on INR. Maintenance: 2-10 mg/day.

Children. Initially, 0.1-0.2 mg/kg (maximum 10 mg). Maintenance: 0.05-0.34 mg/kg/day.

Usual elderly dosage (maintenance)

PO, IV

Elderly. 2-5 mg/day.

AVAILABLE FORMS

- *Tablets (Coumadin, Jantoven):* 1 mg, 2 mg, 2.5 mg, 3 mg, 4 mg, 5 mg, 6 mg, 7.5 mg, 10 mg.

UNLABELED USES: Prevention of myocardial infarction, recurrent cerebral embolism; treatment adjunct in transient ischemic attacks

CONTRAINDICATIONS: Neurosurgical procedures, open wounds, pregnancy, severe hypertension, severe hepatic or renal damage, spinal puncture, uncontrolled bleeding, ulcers

PREGNANCY AND LACTATION: Pregnancy category X; use in first trimester carries significant risk to the fetus; exposure in the sixth-ninth wk of gestation may produce a pattern of defects termed the fetal warfarin syndrome with an incidence up to 25% in some series; compatible with breast-feeding for normal, full-term infants

SIDE EFFECTS

Occasional

GI distress, such as nausea, anorexia, abdominal cramps, diarrhea

Rare

Hypersensitivity reaction, including dermatitis and urticaria, especially in those sensitive to aspirin

SERIOUS REACTIONS

- Bleeding complications ranging from local ecchymoses to major hemorrhage may occur. Drug should be discontinued immediately and vitamin K or phytonadione administered. Mild hemorrhage: 2.5-10 mg PO, IM, or IV. Severe hemorrhage: 10-15 mg IV and repeated q4h, as necessary.
- Hepatotoxicity, blood dyscrasias, necrosis, vasculitis, and local thrombosis occur rarely.

INTERACTIONS

Drugs

3 *Acetaminophen:* Repeated doses of acetaminophen may increase the hypoprothrombinemic response to warfarin

3 *Allopurinol, amiodarone, ciprofloxacin, clarithromycin, erythromycin, fluconazole, fluorouracil, fluvastatin, fluvoxamine, glucagon, isoniazid, itraconazole, ketoconazole, lovastatin, miconazole, nalidixic acid, neomycin (oral), norfloxacin, ofloxacin, propafenone, propoxyphene, quinidine, sertraline, sulfonamides, sulfonylureas, thyroid hormones, triclofos, troleandomycin, vitamin E, zafirlukast:* Enhanced hypoprothrombinemic response to warfarin

3 *American ginseng, St. John's wort:* May decrease the effectiveness of warfarin

3 *Aminoglutethimide, carbamazepine, cyclophosphamide, ethchlorvynol, griseofulvin, mercaptopurine, methimazole, mitotane, nafcillin, propylthiouracil, vitamin K:* Reduced hypoprothrombinemic response to warfarin

❷ *Aspirin:* Increased risk of bleeding complications

❷ *Azathioprine, chloramphenicol, cimetidine, clofibrate, co-trimoxazole, danazole, dextrothyroxine, disulfiram, gemfibrozil, metronidazole, sulfinpyrazone, testosterone derivatives:* Enhanced hypoprothrombinemic response to warfarin

❷ *Barbiturates, glutethimide, rifampin:* Reduced hypoprothrombinemic response to warfarin

3 *Bile acid-binding resins:* Variable effect on hypoprothrombinemic effect of warfarin

❷ *Cephalosporins:* Enhanced hypoprothrombinemic response to warfarin with moxalactam, cefoperazone, cefamandole, cefotetan, and cefmetazole

3 *Chloral hydrate:* Transient increase in hypoprothrombinemic response to warfarin

3 *Ethanol:* Enhanced hypoprothrombinemic response to warfarin with acute ethanol intoxication

3 *Feverfew, garlic, ginkgo biloba, ginseng, glucosamine-chondroitin:* May increase the risk of bleeding

3 *Heparin:* Prolonged activated partial thromboplastin time in patients receiving heparin; prolonged prothrombin times in patients receiving warfarin

3 *Mesalamine:* Warfarin effect inhibited in one case report

2 *NSAIDs:* Increased risk of bleeding in anticoagulated patients

2 *Oral contraceptives:* Increase or decrease in anticoagulant response; increased risk of thromboembolic disorders

3 *Phenytoin:* Transient increase in hypoprothrombinemic response to warfarin with initiation of phenytoin therapy, followed within 1-2 wk by inhibition of hypoprothrombinemic response to warfarin

3 *Salicylates:* Increased risk of bleeding in anticoagulated patients; enhanced hypoprothrombinemic response to warfarin with large salicylate doses

Labs

- *Interference:* May cause orange-red discoloration of urine, which may interfere with some lab tests

SPECIAL CONSIDERATIONS

- Avoid use of initial doses >5 mg
- INR during first 5 days of therapy does not correlate with degree of anticoagulation
- Anticoagulant effect of warfarin may be reversed by administration of vitamin K or fresh frozen plasma; should only use in situations where INR is severely elevated >10, or when patient is actively bleeding

PATIENT/FAMILY EDUCATION

- Strict adherence to prescribed dosage schedule is necessary
- Avoid alcohol, salicylates, and drastic changes in dietary habits
- Do not change from one brand to another without consulting clinician
- Consult the physician before having dental work
- May turn urine red-orange
- Use an electric razor and soft toothbrush to prevent bleeding during warfarin therapy
- Do not take other medications, including OTC drugs, without physician approval
- Report black stool, bleeding; brown, dark, or red urine; coffee-ground vomitus; or red-speckled mucus from cough

MONITORING PARAMETERS

- Dosage of anticoagulants must be individualized and adjusted according to INR determinations; it is recommended that INR determinations be performed prior to initiation of therapy, at 24-hr intervals while maintenance dosage is being established, then once or twice weekly for the following 3-4 wk, then at 1-4 wk intervals for the duration of treatment
- Maintain INR at 2-3 (2.5-3.5 for mechanical valves, recurrent systemic thromboembolism)
- Hct, platelet count, AST (SGOT) and ALT (SGPT) levels, and stool and urine cultures for occult blood, regardless of administration route
- Blood pressure, pulse rate
- Determine the amount of female patient's menstrual discharge and monitor for any increase
- Assess the patient's gums for erythema and gingival bleeding, skin for ecchymosis and petechiae, and urine for hematuria
- Examine the patient for excessive bleeding from minor cuts or scratches

xylometazoline

(zye-loe-met-az′-oh-leen)

OTC: Otrivin Measured-Dose Pump with Moisturizers, Otrivin Nasal Drops, Otrivin Nasal Spray, Otrivin Nasal Spray with Eucalyptol, Otrivin Nasal Spray with Moisturizers, Otrivin Pediatric Nasal Drops, Otrivin Pediatric Nasal Spray, Otrivin With Measured-Dose Pump

Chemical Class: Imidazoline derivative

Therapeutic Class: Decongestant

CLINICAL PHARMACOLOGY

Mechanism of Action: A sympathomimetic that directly acts on alpha-adrenergic receptors in arterioles of the nasal mucosa to produce vasoconstriction resulting in decreased blood flow. ***Therapeutic Effect:*** Decreased nasal congestion.

Pharmacokinetics

Onset of action occurs within 5-10 mins for a duration of action of 5-6 hrs. Well absorbed through nasal mucosa. May also be systemically absorbed from both nasal mucosa and gastrointestinal (GI) tract. ***Half-life:*** Unknown.

INDICATIONS AND DOSAGES

Rhinitis

Intranasal

Adults, Elderly, Children 12 yrs and older. 1-3 drops (0.1%) in each nostril q8-10h or 1-2 sprays (0.1%) in each nostril q8-10h. Maximum: 3 doses/day.

Children 2-12 yrs. 2 or 3 drops (0.05%) in each nostril q8-10h.

AVAILABLE FORMS

- *Nasal Drops:* 0.05% (Otrivin Pediatric Nasal Drops), 0.1% (Otrivin Nasal Drops).
- *Nasal Spray:* 0.1% (Otrivin Nasal Spray).

CONTRAINDICATIONS: Narrow-angle glaucoma, rhinitis sicca, children under 6 yrs, hypersensitivity to xylometazoline or other adrenergic agents

PREGNANCY AND LACTATION: Pregnancy category C

SIDE EFFECTS

Occasional

Nasal: Burning, stinging, drying nasal mucosa, sneezing, rebound congestion

SERIOUS REACTIONS

- Large doses may produce tachycardia, palpitations, lightheadedness, nausea, and vomiting.
- Overdosage in patients older than 60 yrs of age may produce hallucinations, CNS depression, and seizures.

SPECIAL CONSIDERATIONS

- Manage rebound congestion by stopping xylometazoline: one nostril at a time, substitute systemic decongestant, substitute inhaled steroid

PATIENT/FAMILY EDUCATION

- Do not use for >3-5 days or rebound congestion may occur
- Use caution when performing tasks that require visual acuity during therapy

MONITORING PARAMETERS

- Therapeutic response

yohimbine hydrochloride

(yo-him'-been hye'-droe-klor'-ide)

Rx: Actibine, Aphrodyne, Dayto-Himbin, Yocon, Yohimbe, Yohimex, Yovital

Chemical Class: Indolalkylamine derivative

Therapeutic Class: Antiimpotence agent

CLINICAL PHARMACOLOGY

Mechanism of Action: An herb that produces genital blood vessel dilation, improves nerve impulse transmission to genital area. Increases penile blood flow, central sympathetic excitation impulses to genital tissues. ***Therapeutic Effect:*** Improves sexual vigor, affects impotence.

Pharmacokinetics

Rapidly absorbed. Extensive metabolism in liver and kidneys. Minimal excretion in urine as unchanged drug. ***Half-life:*** 36 min.

INDICATIONS AND DOSAGES

Impotence

PO

Adults, Elderly. 5.4 mg 3 times/day.

Orthostatic hypotension

PO

Adults, Elderly. 12.5 mg/day.

AVAILABLE FORMS

• *Tablets:* 5 mg (Actibine), 5.4 mg (Aphrodyne, Dayto-Himbin, Yocon, Yovital, Yohimex).

UNLABELED USES: Treatment of SSRI-induced sexual dysfunction, weight loss, sympathicolytic and mydriatic, aphrodisiac

CONTRAINDICATIONS: Renal disease, hypersensitivity to yohimbine or any component of the formulation

PREGNANCY AND LACTATION: Do not use during pregnancy

SIDE EFFECTS

Excitement, tremors, insomnia, anxiety, hypertension, tachycardia, dizziness, headache, irritability, salivation, dilated pupils, nausea, vomiting, hypersensitivity reaction

SERIOUS REACTIONS

• Paralysis, severe hypotension, irregular heartbeats, and cardiac failure may occur. Overdose can be fatal.

INTERACTIONS

Drugs

3 *Antidiabetics, antihypertensives:* May interfere with the effects of these drugs

3 *Clonidine:* May antagonize the effects of clonidine

3 *MAOIs, linezolid, sympathomimetics, tricyclic antidepressants:* Additive effects with these drugs

SPECIAL CONSIDERATIONS

PATIENT/FAMILY EDUCATION

• Do not use other medications, including OTC drugs, without first notifying the physician

MONITORING PARAMETERS

• Blood pressure

• Liver and renal function

zafirlukast

(za-feer'-loo-kast)

Rx: Accolate

Chemical Class: Tolylsulfonyl benzamide derivative

Therapeutic Class: Antiasthmatic; leukotriene receptor antagonist

CLINICAL PHARMACOLOGY

Mechanism of Action: An antiasthmatic that binds to leukotriene receptors, inhibiting bronchoconstriction due to sulfur dioxide, cold air, and specific antigens, such as grass, cat dander, and ragweed. ***Therapeutic Effect:*** Reduces airway edema and smooth muscle constriction; alters cellular activity associated with the inflammatory process.

Pharmacokinetics

Rapidly absorbed after PO administration (food reduces absorption). Protein binding: 99%. Extensively metabolized in the liver. Primarily excreted in feces. Unknown if removed by hemodialysis. ***Half-life:*** 10 hr.

INDICATIONS AND DOSAGES

Bronchial asthma

PO

Adults, Elderly, Children 12 yrs and older. 20 mg twice a day.

Children 5-11 yrs. 10 mg twice a day.

AVAILABLE FORMS

- *Tablets:* 10 mg, 20 mg.

UNLABELED USES: Exercise-induced bronchospasm

CONTRAINDICATIONS: None known.

PREGNANCY AND LACTATION: Pregnancy category C; breast milk excretion unknown

SIDE EFFECTS

Frequent (13%)

Headache

Occasional (3%)

Nausea, diarrhea

Rare (less than 3%)

Generalized pain, asthenia, myalgia, fever, dyspepsia, vomiting, dizziness

SERIOUS REACTIONS

- Concurrent administration of inhaled corticosteroids increases the risk of upper respiratory tract infection.

INTERACTIONS

Drugs

3 *Aspirin:* Increases zafirlukast blood concentration

3 *Astemizole, terfenadine:* Zafirlukast inhibits drug metabolism with potential for cardiac dysrhythmias

3 *Erythromycin, theophylline:* Decreases zafirlukast blood concentration

3 *Warfarin:* Zafirlukast increases hypoprothrombinemic effect

SPECIAL CONSIDERATIONS

PATIENT/FAMILY EDUCATION

- Take regularly, even during symptom-free periods
- Do not alter the dosage or abruptly discontinue other asthma medications
- Zafirlukast is not intended to treat acute asthma episodes
- Drink plenty of fluids to decrease the thickness of lung secretions
- Notify the physician if abdominal pain, nausea, flu-like symptoms, jaundice, or worsening of asthma occurs
- Women should not breast-feed during zafirlukast therapy

MONITORING PARAMETERS

- ALT, AST, CBC
- Pulse rate and quality and respiratory rate, depth, rhythm, and type
- Observe the patient's fingernails and lips for cyanosis, manifested as a blue or dusky color in light-skinned patients and a gray color in dark-skinned patients

zalcitabine

(zal-site'-a-been)

Rx: Hivid

Chemical Class: Nucleoside analog

Therapeutic Class: Antiretroviral

CLINICAL PHARMACOLOGY

Mechanism of Action: A nucleoside reverse transcriptase inhibitor that inhibits viral DNA synthesis. ***Therapeutic Effect:*** Prevents replication of HIV-1.

Pharmacokinetics

Readily absorbed from the GI tract (absorption decreased by food). Protein binding: less than 4%. Undergoes phosphorylation intracellularly to the active metabolite. Primarily excreted in urine. Removed by hemodialysis. ***Half-life:*** 1-3 hr; metabolite, 2.6-10 hr (increased in impaired renal function).

INDICATIONS AND DOSAGES

HIV infection (in combination with other antiretrovirals)

PO

Adults, Children 13 yr and older. 0.75 mg q8h.

Children younger than 13 yr. 0.01 mg/kg q8h. Range: 0.005-0.01 mg/kg q8h.

Dosage in renal impairment

Dosage and frequency are modified based on creatinine clearance.

Creatinine Clearance	Dosage
10-40 ml/min	0.75 mg q12h
less than 10 ml/min	0.75 mg q24h

AVAILABLE FORMS

- *Tablets:* 0.375 mg, 0.75 mg.

CONTRAINDICATIONS: Moderate or severe peripheral neuropathy

PREGNANCY AND LACTATION: Pregnancy category C

SIDE EFFECTS

Frequent (28%-11%)

Peripheral neuropathy, fever, fatigue, headache, rash

Occasional (10%-5%)

Diarrhea, abdominal pain, oral ulcers, cough, pruritus, myalgia, weight loss, nausea, vomiting

Rare (4%-1%)

Nasal discharge, dysphagia, depression, night sweats, confusion

SERIOUS REACTIONS

- Peripheral neuropathy (characterized by numbness, tingling, burning, and pain in the lower extremities) occurs in 17%-31% of patients. These symptoms may be followed by sharp, shooting pain and progress to a severe, continuous, burning pain that may be irreversible if the drug is not discontinued in time.
- Pancreatitis, leukopenia, neutropenia, eosinophilia, and thrombocytopenia occur rarely.

INTERACTIONS

Drugs

3 *Medications associated with peripheral neuropathy (including cisplatin, disulfiram, phenytoin, vincristine):* May increase the risk of neuropathy

3 *Medications causing pancreatitis (including IV pentamidine):* May increase the risk of pancreatitis

SPECIAL CONSIDERATIONS

- Consult the most recent guidelines for HIV antiviral therapy prior to prescribing

PATIENT/FAMILY EDUCATION

- Notify the physician of any signs or symptoms of pancreatitis or peripheral neuropathy
- The female patient of childbearing age should avoid pregnancy during therapy
- Zalcitabine is not a cure for HIV, nor does it reduce the risk of transmitting HIV to others

MONITORING PARAMETERS

- Periodic CBC, serum chemistry tests, transaminase levels
- Serum amylase and triglyceride concentrations in patients with history of elevated amylase, pancreatitis, ethanol abuse, or receiving parenteral nutrition
- Assess the patient for evidence of potentially fatal pancreatitis, including abdominal pain, nausea and vomiting, and increasing serum amylase and triglyceride levels. If the patient develops any of these

signs or symptoms, particularly abdominal pain, withhold the drug and notify the physician immediately

zaleplon

(zal'-e-plon)

Rx: Sonata

Chemical Class: Pyrazolopyrimidine derivative

Therapeutic Class: Sedative/ hypnotic

CLINICAL PHARMACOLOGY

Mechanism of Action: A nonbenzodiazepine that enhances the action of the inhibitory neurotransmitter gamma-aminobutyric acid. ***Therapeutic Effect:*** Induces sleep.

Pharmacokinetics

Rapidly and almost completely absorbed following PO administration. Protein binding: 60%. Metabolized in liver. Primarily excreted in urine. Partially eliminated in feces. ***Half-life:*** 1 hr.

INDICATIONS AND DOSAGES

Insomnia

PO

Adults 10 mg at bedtime. Range: 5-20 mg.

Elderly. 5 mg at bedtime.

AVAILABLE FORMS

• *Capsules:* 5 mg, 10 mg.

CONTRAINDICATIONS: Severe hepatic impairment

PREGNANCY AND LACTATION: Pregnancy category C; small amount excreted in breast milk, with highest excreted amount during a feeding 1 hr after zaleplon administration

SIDE EFFECTS

Expected

Somnolence, sedation, mild rebound insomnia (on first night after drug is discontinued)

Frequent (28%-7%)

Nausea, headache, myalgia, dizziness

Occasional (5%-3%)

Abdominal pain, asthenia, dyspepsia, eye pain, paresthesia

Rare (2%)

Tremors, amnesia, hyperacusis (acute sense of hearing), fever, dysmenorrhea

SERIOUS REACTIONS

• Zaleplon may produce altered concentration, behavior changes, and impaired memory.

• Taking the drug while up and about may result in adverse CNS effects, such as hallucinations, impaired coordination, dizziness, and lightheadedness.

• Overdose results in somnolence, confusion, diminished reflexes, and coma.

INTERACTIONS

Drugs

❷ *Alcohol, other CNS depressants:* Additive CNS depression

❸ *Carbamazepine:* CYP3A4 inducer; may reduce efficacy of zaleplon by lowering AUC, C_{max}

❷ *Cimetidine:* Inhibits both CYP3A4 and aldehyde oxidase; concomitant administration increases zaleplon AUC and C_{max} 85%

❸ *Diphenhydramine:* Weak inhibitor of aldehyde oxidase; might reduce hepatic clearance of zaleplon; additive CNS depressant effects

❸ *Imipramine:* Additive effects on decreased alertness and psychomotor performance

❸ *Phenytoin:* CYP3A4 inducer; may reduce efficacy of zaleplon by lowering AUC, C_{max}

❸ *Phenobarbital:* CYP3A4 inducer; may reduce efficacy of zaleplon by lowering AUC, C_{max}

3 *Rifampin:* Inducer of CYP3A4; reduced AUC, C_{max} of zaleplon 80%—may compromise efficacy

3 *Thioridazine:* Additive effects on decreased alertness and psychomotor performance

Labs

- *Liver function tests:* Transaminases (ALT, AST), bilirubin increased
- *Cholesterol:* Increased
- *Uric acid:* Increased
- *Glucose:* Increased or decreased

SPECIAL CONSIDERATIONS

- Because of the short $t_{1/2}$, agent best for problems with sleep latency, rather than duration of sleep or number of awakenings (e.g., shift workers)
- Abuse potential similar to benzodiazepines
- Advantage over triazolam, given big cost difference, difficult to justify, if used correctly

PATIENT/FAMILY EDUCATION

- *Timing of administration:* Immediately before bedtime or after the patient has gone to bed and has experienced difficulty falling asleep
- Do not take with alcohol or OTC cimetidine
- Avoid activities requiring mental alertness or motor skills until response to the drug has been established

MONITORING PARAMETERS

- Sleep latency, number of awakenings, daytime function (hangover effect), dizziness, confusion

zanamivir

(za-na'-mi-veer)

Rx: Relenza

Chemical Class: Carboxylic acid ethyl ester

Therapeutic Class: Antiviral

CLINICAL PHARMACOLOGY

Mechanism of Action: An antiviral that appears to inhibit the influenza virus enzyme neuraminidase, which is essential for viral replication. ***Therapeutic Effect:*** Prevents viral release from infected cells.

Pharmacokinetics

Systemically absorbed, approximately 4%-17%. Protein binding: low. Not metabolized. Partially excreted unchanged in urine. ***Half-life:*** 1.6-5.1 hr.

INDICATIONS AND DOSAGES

Influenza virus

Inhalation

Adults, Elderly, Children 7 yr and older. 2 inhalations (one 5-mg blister per inhalation for a total dose of 10 mg) twice a day (approximately 12 hr apart) for 5 days.

Prevention of influenza virus

Inhalation

Adults, Elderly. 2 inhalations once a day for the duration of the exposure period.

AVAILABLE FORMS

- *Powder for Inhalation:* 5 mg/blister.

UNLABELED USES: Influenza prophylaxis

CONTRAINDICATIONS: None known.

PREGNANCY AND LACTATION: Pregnancy category C; breast milk excretion unknown

SIDE EFFECTS

Occasional (3%-2%)

Diarrhea, sinusitis, nausea, bronchitis, cough, dizziness, headache

Rare (less than 1.5%)
Malaise, fatigue, fever, abdominal pain, myalgia, arthralgia, urticaria

SERIOUS REACTIONS

- Neutropenia may occur.
- Bronchospasm may occur in those with a history of chronic obstructive pulmonary disease (COPD) or bronchial asthma.

SPECIAL CONSIDERATIONS

- Off-label use to prevent influenza in family members of influenza patients (N Engl J Med 2000 Nov 2;343(18):1282-9): Attack rate reduced from 19% to 4%

PATIENT/FAMILY EDUCATION

- Expected benefit of zanamivir is 1 day of shortening of overall symptoms
- Patients with less severe symptoms get less benefit from therapy
- Influenza vaccine remains the best way to prevent influenza and use of zanamivir should not affect the evaluation of individuals for annual influenza vaccination
- Patients scheduled to use an inhaled bronchodilator at the same time as zanamivir should use their bronchodilator before taking zanamivir
- Two doses should be taken on the first day of treatment whenever possible provided there is at least 2 hrs between doses

MONITORING PARAMETERS

- Pattern of daily bowel activity and stool consistency

zidovudine

(zye-doe′-vyoo-deen)

Rx: Retrovir

Combinations

Rx: with lamivudine (Combivir)

Chemical Class: Nucleoside analog

Therapeutic Class: Antiretroviral

CLINICAL PHARMACOLOGY

Mechanism of Action: A nucleoside reverse transcriptase inhibitor that interferes with viral RNA-dependent DNA polymerase, an enzyme necessary for viral HIV replication. ***Therapeutic Effect:*** Interferes with HIV replication, slowing the progression of HIV infection.

Pharmacokinetics

Rapidly and completely absorbed from the GI tract. Protein binding: 25%-38%. Undergoes first-pass metabolism in the liver. Crosses the blood-brain barrier and is widely distributed, including to cerebrospinal fluid (CSF). Primarily excreted in urine. Minimal removal by hemodialysis. ***Half-life:*** 0.8-1.2 hr (increased in impaired renal function).

INDICATIONS AND DOSAGES

HIV infection

PO

Adults, Elderly, Children older than 12 yr. 200 mg q8h or 300 mg q12h.

Children 12 yr and younger. 160 mg/m^2/dose q8h. Range: 90-180 mg/m^2/dose q6-8h.

Neonates. 2 mg/kg/dose q6h.

IV

Adults, Elderly, Children older than 12 yr. 1-2 mg/kg/dose q4h.

Children 12 yr and younger. 120 mg/m^2/dose q6h.

Neonates. 1.5 mg/kg/dose q6h.

AVAILABLE FORMS

- *Capsules (Retrovir):* 100 mg.
- *Syrup (Retrovir):* 50 mg/5 ml.
- *Tablets (Retrovir):* 300 mg.
- *Injection (Retrovir):* 10 mg/ml.

UNLABELED USES: Prophylaxis in health care workers at risk of acquiring HIV after occupational exposure

CONTRAINDICATIONS: Life-threatening allergic reactions to zidovudine or its components

PREGNANCY AND LACTATION: Pregnancy category C; indicated for pregnant women >14 wk gestation for prevention of maternal-fetus HIV transmission; excreted in breast milk; breast-feeding by HIV+ mothers not recommended

SIDE EFFECTS

Expected (46%-42%)

Nausea, headache

Frequent (20%-16%)

Abdominal pain, asthenia, rash, fever, acne

Occasional (12%-8%)

Diarrhea, anorexia, malaise, myalgia, somnolence

Rare (6%-5%)

Dizziness, paresthesia, vomiting, insomnia, dyspnea, altered taste

SERIOUS REACTIONS

- Serious reactions include anemia, which occurs most commonly after 4-6 wks of therapy, and granulocytopenia; both effects are more likely to occur in patients who have a low Hgb level or granulocyte count before beginning therapy.
- Neurotoxicity (as evidenced by ataxia, fatigue, lethargy, nystagmus, and seizures) may occur.

INTERACTIONS

Drugs

3 *Bone marrow depressants:* May increase myelosuppression

3 *Clarithromycin:* May decrease zidovudine blood concentration

⚠ *Doxorubicin:* Antagonism of therapeutic effect; concomitant use should be avoided

3 *Fluconazole:* Increased plasma concentrations of zidovudine

⚠ *Ganciclovir:* Increased hematologic toxicity

⚠ *Interferon-α:* Increased hematologic toxicity

3 *Probenecid:* Increased plasma concentration of zidovudine

⚠ *Ribavirin:* Antagonism of therapeutic effect; concomitant use should be avoided

3 *Rifampin:* Reduced plasma concentrations of zidovudine

⚠ *Stavudine:* Antagonism of therapeutic effect; concomitant use should be avoided

3 *Valproic acid:* Increased plasma concentrations of zidovudine

SPECIAL CONSIDERATIONS

- Consult the most recent guidelines for HIV antiviral therapy prior to prescribing

PATIENT/FAMILY EDUCATION

- Close monitoring of blood counts is extremely important; does not reduce risk of transmitting HIV to others through sexual contact or blood contamination
- Space zidovudine doses evenly around the clock
- Report bleeding from the gums, nose, or rectum to the physician immediately
- Have dental work done before therapy or postpone it until blood counts return to normal, which may be weeks after therapy has stopped
- Do not take any other medications without the physician's prior approval
- Notify physician if difficulty breathing, headache, inability to sleep, muscle weakness, a rash, signs of infection, or unusual bleeding occurs

MONITORING PARAMETERS

- CBC with differential and platelets q2wk initially for 2 mo, then q4-8 wk
- CD4+ cell count, Hgb and HIV RNA plasma levels, mean corpuscular volume, and reticulocyte count
- Pattern of daily bowel activity and stool consistency
- Skin for acne or a rash
- Assess the patient for signs and symptoms of opportunistic infections, such as chills, cough, fever, and myalgia
- Intake and output
- Serum renal and liver function test results

zileuton

(zi-loo′-ton)

Rx: Zyflo

Chemical Class: Urea derivative

Therapeutic Class: Antiasthmatic; lipoxygenase inhibitor

CLINICAL PHARMACOLOGY

Mechanism of Action: A leukotriene inhibitor that inhibits the enzyme responsible for producing inflammatory response. Prevents formation of leukotrienes (leukotrienes induce bronchoconstricton response, enhance vascular permeability, stimulate mucus secretion). ***Therapeutic Effect:*** Prevents airway edema, smooth muscle contraction, and the inflammatory process, relieving signs and symptoms of bronchial asthma.

Pharmacokinetics

Rapidly absorbed from gastrointestinal (GI) tract. Potein binding: 93%. Metabolized in liver. Primarily excreted in urine. Unknown if removed by hemodialysis. ***Half-life:*** 2.1-2.5 hrs.

INDICATIONS AND DOSAGES

Bronchial asthma

PO

Adults, Elderly, Children 12 yrs and older. 600 mg 4 times/day. Total daily dosage: 2400 mg.

AVAILABLE FORMS

- *Tablets:* 600 mg (Zyflo).

CONTRAINDICATIONS: Active liver disease, impaired liver function, hypersensitivity to zileuton or any component of the formulation

PREGNANCY AND LACTATION: Pregnancy category C; breast milk excretion unknown

SIDE EFFECTS

Frequent

Headache

Occasional

Dyspepsia, nausea, abdominal pain, asthenia (loss of strength), myalgia

Rare

Conjunctivitis, constipation, dizziness, flatulence, insomnia

SERIOUS REACTIONS

- Liver dysfunction occurs rarely and may be manifested as right upper quadrant pain, nausea, fatigue, lethargy, pruritus, jaundice or flu-like symptoms.

SPECIAL CONSIDERATIONS

PATIENT/FAMILY EDUCATION

- Must be taken regularly, even during symptom-free periods
- Not a bronchodilator, do not use to treat acute episodes of asthma
- Increase fluid intake

MONITORING PARAMETERS

- CBC, renal function, and transaminase levels periodically during first year of prolonged therapy
- Rate, depth, and rhythm of respirations, pulse rate

zinc oxide/zinc sulfate

(zink'- ox'-eyed/zink'- sul'-fate)

Rx: (zinc oxide) Balmex, Desitin

Rx: (zinc sulfate) Orazinc

Chemical Class: Divalent cation

Therapeutic Class: Chelating agent; ophthalmic astringent; trace element

CLINICAL PHARMACOLOGY

Mechanism of Action: A mineral that acts as a co-factor for enzymes that are important for protein and carbohydrate metabolism. ***Therapeutic Effect:*** Zinc oxide acts as a mild astringent and skin protectant. Zinc sulfate helps maintain normal growth and tissue repair as well as skin hydration.

INDICATIONS AND DOSAGES

Mild skin irritations and abrasions (such as chapped skin, diaper rash)

Topical (zinc oxide)

Adults, Elderly, Children. Apply as needed.

Treatment and prevention of zinc deficiency, wound healing

PO (zinc sulfate)

Adults, Elderly. 220 mg 3 times a day.

AVAILABLE FORMS

Zinc oxide

- *Ointment:* 10%, 20%, 40%.

Zinc sulfate

- *Capsules:* 110 mg, 220 mg.
- *Tablets:* 110 mg.
- *Injection:* 1 mg/ml.

UNLABELED USES: *Zinc sulfate:* Wilson's disease

CONTRAINDICATIONS: None known.

PREGNANCY AND LACTATION: Pregnancy category C (in doses not exceeding recommended daily allowance); for zinc acetate, zinc has appeared in breast milk and zinc-induced copper deficiency may occur; nursing not recommended

SIDE EFFECTS

Frequency not defined

Nausea, vomiting, epigastric discomfort

SERIOUS REACTIONS

- Hypotension, arrhythmias, anemia, and thrombocytopenia occur rarely.

INTERACTIONS

Drugs

3 *H_2-blockers:* May decrease zinc absorption

3 *Ciprofloxacin, enoxacin, norfloxacin:* Reduced serum concentrations of these drugs

3 *Coffee, dairy products:* May decrease zinc absorption

3 *Tetracycline:* Reduced serum tetracycline concentrations

SPECIAL CONSIDERATIONS

- Acetate not recommended for initial therapy of symptomatic Wilson's disease (should be treated initially with chelating agents)

PATIENT/FAMILY EDUCATION

- Take acetate on an empty stomach
- Coffee and dairy products may decrease the absorption of oral zinc sulfate capsules and tablets
- Notify the physician if the skin condition does not improve after 7 days of treatment

MONITORING PARAMETERS

- 24 hr urine copper, LFTs (acetate)

ziprasidone

(zi-pray'-si-done)

Rx: Geodon

Chemical Class: Benzisothiazole derivative

Therapeutic Class: Antipsychotic

CLINICAL PHARMACOLOGY

Mechanism of Action: A piperazine derivative that antagonizes alpha-adrenergic, dopamine, histamine, and serotonin receptors; also inhibits reuptake of serotonin and norepinephrine. ***Therapeutic Effect:*** Diminishes symptoms of schizophrenia and depression.

Pharmacokinetics

Well absorbed after PO administration. Food increases bioavailability. Protein binding: 99%. Extensively metabolized in the liver. Not removed by hemodialysis. ***Half-life:*** 7 hr.

INDICATIONS AND DOSAGES

Schizophrenia

PO

Adults, Elderly. Initially, 20 mg twice a day with food. Titrate at intervals of no less than 2 days. Maximum: 80 mg twice a day.

IM

Adults, Elderly. 10 mg q2h or 20 mg q4h. Maximum: 40 mg/day.

Mania in bipolar disorder

PO

Adults, Elderly. Initially, 40 mg twice a day. May increase to 60-80 mg twice a day on second day of treatment. Range: 40-80 mg twice a day.

AVAILABLE FORMS

• *Capsules:* 20 mg, 40 mg, 60 mg, 80 mg.

• *Injection:* 20 mg/ml.

UNLABELED USES: Tourette's syndrome

CONTRAINDICATIONS: Conditions that prolong the QT interval, such as congenital long QT syndrome

PREGNANCY AND LACTATION: Pregnancy category C; animal, not human studies demonstrated developmental toxicity, including possible teratogenic effects at doses similar to human therapeutic doses; breast milk excretion—unknown

SIDE EFFECTS

Frequent (30%-16%)

Headache, somnolence, dizziness

Occasional

Rash, orthostatic hypotension, weight gain, restlessness, constipation, dyspepsia

Rare

Hyperglycemia, priapism

SERIOUS REACTIONS

• Prolongation of QT interval may produce torsades de pointes, a form of ventricular tachycardia. Patients with bradycardia, hypokalemia, or hypomagnesemia are at increased risk.

INTERACTIONS

Drugs

3 *Alcohol, other CNS depressants:* May increase CNS depression

▲ *Antiarrhythmics (amiodarone, bretylium, disopyramide, dofetilide, encainide, flecainide, ibutilide, moricizine, procainamide, propafenone, quinidine, sotalol, tocainide):* Increased risk of QT prolongation and life-threatening arrhythmias

3 *Carbamazepine:* Added carbamazepine (induces CYP3A4) decreased AUC 35%; other inducers predicted to produce similar effects: barbiturates, oxcarbazepine, phenytoin, rifampin

3 *Ketoconazole:* Added ketoconazole (inhibits CYP3A4) results in increased AUC and C_{max} (35%-40%); other inhibitors predicted to produce similar effects: cisapride, clarithro-

mycin, erythromycin, fluconazole, itraconazole (all azole antifungals), quinine

3 *Levodopa, dopamine agonists:* Ziprasidone may antagonize the therapeutic effects of these drugs

⚠ *Macrolide antibiotics (erythromycin, clarithromycin):* Increased risk of QT prolongation and life-threatening arrhythmias

⚠ *Phenothiazines:* Increased risk of QT prolongation and life-threatening arrhythmias

⚠ *Quinolone antibiotics (gatifloxacin, levofloxacin, moxifloxacin, sparfloxacin):* Increased risk of QT prolongation and life-threatening arrhythmias

⚠ *Tricyclic antidepressants:* Increased risk of QT prolongation and life-threatening arrhythmias

SPECIAL CONSIDERATIONS

• Atypical agents with less risk of movement disorders best for: Patients resistant to standard antipsychotic agents; patients with therapy-limiting extrapyramidal symptoms, other adverse effects; comparisons with other atypical agents, shorter half-life and bid dosing requirement potential disadvantage, but perhaps less weight gain

PATIENT/FAMILY EDUCATION

• Review presentation of cardiac (prolonged QT - torsades de pointes) and movement disorders; avoid electrolyte disturbance and drug interactions

• Take with food

• Avoid tasks requiring mental alertness or motor skills until response to the drug has been established

MONITORING PARAMETERS

• Improvement of symptomatology (both positive and negative symptoms), complete blood counts, liver function tests, serum prolactin, routine chemistry (especially K^+, Mg^{++} during prolonged therapy); signs/symptoms of akathisia, abnormal movements, persistent constipation

• Weight

zoledronic acid

(zole-eh-drone'-ick as'-id)

Rx: Zometa

Chemical Class: Bisphosphonic acid

Therapeutic Class: Bisphosphonate; bone resorption inhibitor

CLINICAL PHARMACOLOGY

Mechanism of Action: A bisphosphonate that inhibits the resorption of mineralized bone and cartilage; inhibits increased osteoclastic activity and skeletal calcium release induced by stimulatory factors produced by tumors. ***Therapeutic Effect:*** Increases urinary calcium and phosphorus excretion; decreases serum calcium and phosphorus levels.

Pharmacokinetics

Protein binding: 22%. Not metabolized. More than 95% excreted in urine. ***Half-life:*** 167 hr.

INDICATIONS AND DOSAGES

Hypercalcemia

IV Infusion

Adults, Elderly. 4 mg IV infusion given over no less than 15 min. Retreatment may be considered, but at least 7 days should elapse to allow for full response to initial dose.

Multiple myeloma, bone metastases of solid tumors

IV

Adults, Elderly. 4 mg q3-4wk.

AVAILABLE FORMS

• *Injection Powder for Reconstitution:* 4 mg.

• *Injection Solution:* 4 mg/5 ml.

UNLABELED USES: Prevention of bone metastases from breast, prostate cancer, treatment of bone diseases

CONTRAINDICATIONS: Hypersensitivity to other bisphosphonates, including alendronate, etidronate, pamidronate, risedronate, and tiludronate

PREGNANCY AND LACTATION: Pregnancy category C (developmental and embryocidal effects noted in animals, no adequate and well-controlled studies in pregnant women); information on excretion into human breast milk is not available

SIDE EFFECTS

Frequent (44%-26%)

Fever, nausea, vomiting, constipation

Occasional (15%-10%)

Hypotension, anxiety, insomnia, flu-like symptoms (fever, chills, bone pain, myalgia, and arthralgia)

Rare

Conjunctivitis

SERIOUS REACTIONS

• Renal toxicity may occur if IV infusion is administered in less than 15 mins.

INTERACTIONS

Drugs

3 *Aminoglycosides:* Additive nephrotoxicity

3 *Calcium-containing medications, vitamin D:* May antagonize the effects of zoledronic acid in treatment of hypercalcemia

3 *Diuretics (loop):* Additive hypocalcemia

SPECIAL CONSIDERATIONS

• Reconstitute with 5 ml sterile water, then further diluted in 100 ml 0.9% sodium chloride or 5% dextrose; do not mix with calcium-containing infusion solutions (i.e., lactated Ringer's)

• Most potent bisphosphonate available

PATIENT/FAMILY EDUCATION

• Avoid drugs containing calcium and vitamin D, such as antacids, because they might antagonize the effects of zoledronic acid

MONITORING PARAMETERS

• Serum creatinine, electrolytes, phosphate, magnesium, CBC

• Assess for fever

• Monitor fluid intake and output, especially in patients with impaired renal function

zolmitriptan

(zohl-mi-trip'-tan)

Rx: Zomig, Zomig ZMT

Chemical Class: Serotonin derivative

Therapeutic Class: Antimigraine agent

CLINICAL PHARMACOLOGY

Mechanism of Action: A serotonin receptor agonist that binds selectively to vascular receptors, producing a vasoconstrictive effect on cranial blood vessels. ***Therapeutic Effect:*** Relieves migraine headache.

Pharmacokinetics

Rapidly but incompletely absorbed after PO administration. Protein binding: 15%. Undergoes first-pass metabolism in the liver to active metabolite. Eliminated primarily in urine (60%) and, to a lesser extent, in feces (30%). ***Half-life:*** 3 hr.

INDICATIONS AND DOSAGES

Acute migraine attack

PO

Adults, Elderly, Children older than 18 yr. Initially, 2.5 mg or less. If headache returns, may repeat dose in 2 hr. Maximum: 10 mg/24 hr.

Intranasal

Adults, Elderly. 5 mg. May repeat in 2 hr. Maximum: 10 mg/24 hr.

AVAILABLE FORMS

- *Tablets (Zomig):* 2.5 mg, 5 mg.
- *Tablets (Orally Disintegrating [Zomig-ZMT]):* 2.5 mg, 5 mg.
- *Nasal Spray (Zomig):* 5 mg/0.1 ml.

CONTRAINDICATIONS: Arrhythmias associated with conduction disorders, basilar or hemiplegic migraine, coronary artery disease, ischemic heart disease (including angina pectoris, history of MI, silent ischemia, and Prinzmetal's angina), uncontrolled hypertension, use within 24 hr of ergotamine-containing preparations or another serotonin receptor agonist, use within 14 days of MAOIs, Wolff-Parkinson-White syndrome

PREGNANCY AND LACTATION: Pregnancy category C; excretion into breast milk unknown, use caution in nursing mothers

SIDE EFFECTS

Frequent (8%-6%)

Oral: Dizziness; tingling; neck, throat, or jaw pressure; somnolence

Nasal: Altered taste, paresthesia

Occasional (5%-3%)

Oral: Warm or hot sensation, asthenia, chest pressure

Nasal: Nausea, somnolence, nasal discomfort, dizziness, asthenia, dry mouth

Rare (2%-1%)

Diaphoresis, myalgia, paresthesia

SERIOUS REACTIONS

- Cardiac reactions (including ischemia, coronary artery vasospasm, and MI) and noncardiac vasospasm-related reactions (such as hemorrhage and cerebrovascular accident [CVA]) occur rarely, particularly in patients with hypertension, diabetes, or a strong family history of coronary artery disease; obese patients; smokers; males older than 40 yrs; and postmenopausal women.

INTERACTIONS

Drugs

3 *Cimetidine:* Increased zolmitriptan concentration

3 *Ergot-containing drugs:* Potential for prolonged vasospastic reactions and additive vasoconstrictions, theoretic precaution

3 *Fluoxetine, fluvoxamine, paroxetine, sertraline:* May produce hyperreflexia, incoordination, and weakness

2 *MAO inhibitors:* Increased zolmitriptan concentrations, increased potential for serotonin-related toxicity

3 *Oral contraceptives:* Decrease zolmitriptan clearance and volume of distribution

2 *Sibutramine:* Increased risk for serotonin syndrome

SPECIAL CONSIDERATIONS

- Alternative to sumatriptan for the treatment of migraine headache; has not been compared head-to-head with sumatriptan; choice should be based on cost and availability
- First dose should be administered in medical office in case cardiac symptoms occur; take great care to exclude the possibility of silent cardiovascular disease prior to prescribing
- Doses >2.5 mg were not associated with more headache relief, but were associated with increased side effects; if no relief is obtained after first dose, a second dose is unlikely to provide any benefit

PATIENT/FAMILY EDUCATION

- Take a single dose of zolmitriptan as soon as migraine symptoms appear
- Zolmitriptan is intended to relieve migraines, not to prevent them or reduce the number of attacks

- Avoid tasks that require mental alertness or motor skills until response to the drug has been established
- Notify the physician if blood in urine or stool, chest pain, palpitations, easy bruising, numbness or pain in the arms or legs, throat tightness, or swelling of the eyelids, face, or lips occurs
- Lie down in dark, quiet room for additional benefit after taking zolmitriptan

MONITORING PARAMETERS

- Blood pressure, especially in patients with hepatic impairment
- Assess the patient for relief of migraines and associated symptoms, including nausea and vomiting, photophobia, and phonophobia (sound sensitivity)

---

zolpidem tartrate

(zole-pi'-dem tar'-trate)

Rx: Ambien, Ambien CR

Chemical Class: Imidazopyridine derivative

Therapeutic Class: Hypnotic

DEA Class: Schedule IV

CLINICAL PHARMACOLOGY

Mechanism of Action: A nonbenzodiazepine that enhances the action of the inhibitory neurotransmitter gamma-aminobutyric acid. ***Therapeutic Effect:*** Induces sleep and improves sleep quality.

Pharmacokinetics

Route	*Onset*	*Peak*	*Duration*
PO	30 mins	N/A	6-8 hrs

Rapidly absorbed from the GI tract. Protein binding: 92%. Metabolized in the liver; excreted in urine. Not removed by hemodialysis. ***Half-life:*** 1.4-4.5 hr (increased in hepatic impairment).

INDICATIONS AND DOSAGES

Insomnia

PO

Adults. 10 mg at bedtime.

Elderly, Debilitated. 5 mg at bedtime.

PO (Extended-Release)

Adults. 12.5 mg.

Elderly, Debilitated. 6.25 mg.

AVAILABLE FORMS

- *Tablets (Ambien):* 5 mg, 10 mg.
- *Tablets (Extended-Release [Ambien CR]):* 6.25 mg, 12.5 mg.

CONTRAINDICATIONS: None known.

PREGNANCY AND LACTATION: Pregnancy category B; excreted into breast milk in small amounts

Controlled Substance: Schedule IV

SIDE EFFECTS

Occasional (7%)

Headache

Rare (less than 2%)

Dizziness, nausea, diarrhea, muscle pain

SERIOUS REACTIONS

- Overdose may produce severe ataxia, bradycardia, altered vision (such as diplopia), severe drowsiness, nausea and vomiting, difficulty breathing, and unconsciousness.
- Abrupt withdrawal of the drug after long-term use may produce asthenia, facial flushing, diaphoresis, vomiting, and tremor.
- Drug tolerance or dependence may occur with prolonged, high-dose therapy.

INTERACTIONS

Drugs

3 *Alcohol, other CNS depressants:* May increase CNS depression

SPECIAL CONSIDERATIONS

PATIENT/FAMILY EDUCATION

- Take immediately prior to retiring
- Avoid alcohol
- Use caution driving or performing other tasks requiring alertness

• Do not abruptly stop zolpidem after long-term use
• Drug dependence or tolerance may occur with prolonged use of high doses

MONITORING PARAMETERS

• Assess sleep pattern, including time needed to fall asleep and number of nocturnal awakenings
• Evaluate for therapeutic response, such as a decrease in the number of nocturnal awakenings and an increased duration of sleep

zonisamide

(zoh-nis'-a-mide)

Rx: Zonegran

Chemical Class: Sulfonamide derivative

Therapeutic Class: Anticonvulsant

CLINICAL PHARMACOLOGY

Mechanism of Action: A succinimide that may stabilize neuronal membranes and suppress neuronal hypersynchronization by blocking sodium and calcium channels. ***Therapeutic Effect:*** Reduces seizure activity.

Pharmacokinetics

Well absorbed after PO administration. Extensively bound to RBCs. Protein binding: 40%. Primarily excreted in urine. ***Half-life:*** 63 hr (plasma), 105 hr (RBCs).

INDICATIONS AND DOSAGES

Partial seizures

PO

Adults, Elderly, Children older than 16 yr. Initially, 100 mg/day for 2 wk. May increase by 100 mg/day at intervals of 2 wk or longer. Range: 100-600 mg/day.

AVAILABLE FORMS

• *Capsules:* 25 mg, 50 mg, 100 mg.

UNLABELED USES: Treatment of binge eating disorder, bipolar disorder, obesity

CONTRAINDICATIONS: Allergy to sulfonamides

PREGNANCY AND LACTATION: Pregnancy category C (teratogenic, embryolethal in animals; no adequate and well-controlled studies in pregnant women); breast milk excretion in women unknown

SIDE EFFECTS

Frequent (17%-9%)

Somnolence, dizziness, anorexia, headache, agitation, irritability, nausea

Occasional (8%-5%)

Fatigue, ataxia, confusion, depression, impaired memory or concentration, insomnia, abdominal pain, diplopia, diarrhea, speech difficulty

Rare (4%-3%)

Paresthesia, nystagmus, anxiety, rash, dyspepsia, weight loss

SERIOUS REACTIONS

• Overdose is characterized by bradycardia, hypotension, respiratory depression, and coma.
• Leukopenia, anemia, and thrombocytopenia occur rarely.

INTERACTIONS

Drugs

3 *Alcohol, other CNS depressants:* May increase zonisamide's sedative effect

3 *Carbamazepine:* Increased clearance of zonisamide via CYP3A4 induction ($t_{1/2}$ decreased to 38 hr); no appreciable effect on carbamazepine kinetics

3 *Phenytoin:* Increased clearance of zonisamide via CYP3A4 induction ($t_{1/2}$ decreased to 27 hr); no appreciable effect on phenytoin kinetics

3 *Phenobarbital:* Increased clearance of zonisamide via CYP3A4 induction ($t_{1/2}$ decreased to 38 hr)

3 *Valproic acid:* Increased clearance of zonisamide via CYP3A4 induction ($t_{1/2}$ decreased to 46 hr); no appreciable effect on valproate kinetics

Labs

- *Liver function tests (ALT/AST/LDH):* Increased
- *Glucose:* Decreased
- *Sodium:* Decreased

SPECIAL CONSIDERATIONS

- Due to long $t_{1/2}$, steady-state achievable with stable dosing for 2 wks
- Adjunctive therapy for wide variety of seizure disorders, especially those refractory to other drugs

PATIENT/FAMILY EDUCATION

- Low threshold for discussing signs and symptoms related to skin rash, liver problems, or blood problems with clinician
- Do not abruptly discontinue the drug after long-term use because this may precipitate seizures
- Avoid tasks that require mental alertness or motor skills until response to the drug is established
- Avoid alcohol and CNS depressants while taking zonisamide

MONITORING PARAMETERS

- Frequency and severity of seizures, neurotoxicity, hypersensitivity reactions, serum creatinine, BUN

Therapeutic Index

The therapeutic index is arranged by condition/disorder. *Italics* indicate category of drug.

THERAPEUTIC INDEX

Index

Entries can be identified as follows: generic name, Trade Name.

Entries can be identified as follows: generic name, Trade Name.

B

Entries can be identified as follows: generic name, Trade Name.

Entries can be identified as follows: generic name, Trade Name.

Entries can be identified as follows: generic name, Trade Name.

E

Entries can be identified as follows: generic name, Trade Name.

Entries can be identified as follows: generic name, Trade Name.

Entries can be identified as follows: generic name, Trade Name.

Entries can be identified as follows: generic name, Trade Name.

G

H

I

Entries can be identified as follows: generic name, Trade Name.

Entries can be identified as follows: generic name, Trade Name.

Entries can be identified as follows: generic name, Trade Name.

Entries can be identified as follows: generic name, Trade Name.

P

Entries can be identified as follows: generic name, Trade Name.

Q

R

Entries can be identified as follows: generic name, Trade Name.

S

T

Entries can be identified as follows: generic name, Trade Name.

Entries can be identified as follows: generic name, Trade Name.

Entries can be identified as follows: generic name, Trade Name.

Entries can be identified as follows: generic name, Trade Name.

IDEAL BODY WEIGHT (IBW)

ADULTS (>18 YRS):

Male IBW (kg) = 50 + 2.3 for each inch over 60 inches

Female IBW (kg) = 45.5 + 2.3 for each inch over 60 inches

CHILDREN:

Age 1 to 18 yrs, height <60 inches: IBW (kg) = $[1.65 \times \text{height}^2 \text{ (cm)}]/1000$

BODY MASS INDEX (BMI)

$$\text{BMI} = \frac{\text{weight (kg)}}{\text{height}^2 \text{ (m)}}$$

Normal range:

Male: 21.9-22.4

Female: 21.3-22.1

CREATININE CLEARANCE CALCULATION

ADULTS (AGE >18; SERUM CREAT <5 MG/DL AND NOT CHANGING RAPIDLY):

$$\text{CrCl (ml/min)} = \frac{(140 - \text{age})\ (\text{weight in kg})}{(\text{serum creat [mg/dl]})\ (72)}$$

NOTES:

1. Multiply by 0.85 for females
2. Use the following value for weight:
   a. If actual weight <IBW, use actual weight
   b. If actual weight is 100%-130% of IBW, use IBW
   c. If actual weight >130% of IBW, easiest approximation is by using IBW + (actual weight − IBW)/3
3. Accuracy reduced in muscle wasting diseases (e.g., neuromuscular disease) and amputees

CHILDREN:

CrCl (ml/min/1.73m^2) = $[0.48 \times \text{height (cm)}]$/serum creat (mg/dl)

Conversion Information

WEIGHTS AND MEASURES

PREFIXES FOR FRACTIONS

deci = 10^{-1}
centi = 10^{-2}
milli = 10^{-3}
micro = 10^{-6}
nano = 10^{-9}
pico = 10^{-12}

TEMPERATURE MEASURES

$°C = 5/9 \times (°F - 32)$
$°F = 9/5 \times (°C) + 32$

PERCENTAGE EQUIVALENTS

0.1% solution contains: 1 mg per ml
1% solution contains: 10 mg per ml
10% solution contains: 100 mg per ml

MILLIEQUIVALENT CONVERSIONS

1 mEq Na = 23 mg Na = 58.5 mg NaCl
1 g Na = 2.54 g NaCl = 43 mEq Na
1 g NaCl = 0.39 g Na = 17 mEq Na

1 mEq K = 39 mg K = 74.5 mg KCl
1 g K = 1.91 g KCl = 26 mEq K
1 g KCl = 0.52 g K = 13 mEq K

1 mEq Ca = 20 mg Ca
1 g Ca = 50 mEq Ca

1 mEq Mg = 0.12 g $MgSO_4 \cdot 7H_2O$
1 g Mg = 10.2 g $MgSO_4 \cdot 7H_2O$ = 82 mEq Mg

10 mmol P_i = 0.31 g P_i = 0.95 g PO_4
1 g P_i = 3.06 g PO_4 = 32 mmol P_i

METRIC CONVERSIONS

VOLUME MEASUREMENTS

Teaspoonful = 5 ml
Tablespoonful = 15 ml
Fluid ounce = 30 ml
Pint = 473 ml
Quart = 946 ml